Diagnostic Imaging of the Head and Neck

MRI with CT & PET Correlations

EDITOR

Anton N. Hasso, MD, FACR

Professor, Department of Radiological Sciences
Director of Neuroimaging Research
University of California, Irvine
Irvine, CA

Wolters Kluwer | Lippincott Williams & Wilkins
Health

Philadelphia • Baltimore • New York • London
Buenos Aires • Hong Kong • Sydney • Tokyo

Executive Editor: Charles W. Mitchell
Product Manager: Ryan Shaw
Vendor Manager: Bridgett Dougherty
Senior Manufacturing Manager: Benjamin Rivera
Senior Marketing Manager: Angela Panetta
Creative Director: Doug Smock
Production Service: Aptara, Inc.

© 2012 by LIPPINCOTT WILLIAMS & WILKINS, a WOLTERS KLUWER business
Two Commerce Square
2001 Market Street
Philadelphia, PA 19103 USA
LWW.com

All rights reserved. This book is protected by copyright. No part of this book may be reproduced in any form by any means, including photocopying, or utilized by any information storage and retrieval system without written permission from the copyright owner, except for brief quotations embodied in critical articles and reviews. Materials appearing in this book prepared by individuals as part of their official duties as U.S. government employees are not covered by the above-mentioned copyright.

Printed in China

Library of Congress Cataloging-in-Publication Data
Diagnostic imaging of the head and neck : MRI with CT & PET correlations /
editor, Anton N. Hasso.
   p. ; cm.
   Includes bibliographical references and index.
   Summary: "This book explores concepts and methods of mastering the nuances and unique diagnostic information offered by MR imaging, when applied to the head and neck. Benign or malignant processes may cause lymphadenopathy; an infected or hemorrhagic congenital mass may be detected in adulthood; serous fluid or pus may appear similar on imaging studies, are typical examples of why this region of the human body appears mysterious to many radiologists and other imaging experts. Solving these mysteries can often be accomplished by corroborative data obtained from CT or CT/PET studies, as highlighted in this product"—Provided by publisher.
   ISBN 978-0-397-51537-0 (hardback : alk. paper)
   I. Hasso, Anton N.
   [DNLM: 1. Head–pathology.   2. Neck–pathology.   3. Head–radiography.   4. Magnetic Resonance Imaging–methods.   5. Neck–radiography.   6. Tomography, Emission-Computed–methods. WE 705]
   LC-classification not assigned
   617.5′10754—dc23

                                                                                                2011030171

Care has been taken to confirm the accuracy of the information presented and to describe generally accepted practices. However, the authors, editors, and publisher are not responsible for errors or omissions or for any consequences from application of the information in this book and make no warranty, expressed or implied, with respect to the currency, completeness, or accuracy of the contents of the publication. Application of the information in a particular situation remains the professional responsibility of the practitioner.

   The authors, editors, and publisher have exerted every effort to ensure that drug selection and dosage set forth in this text are in accordance with current recommendations and practice at the time of publication. However, in view of ongoing research, changes in government regulations, and the constant flow of information relating to drug therapy and drug reactions, the reader is urged to check the package insert for each drug for any change in indications and dosage and for added warnings and precautions. This is particularly important when the recommended agent is a new or infrequently employed drug.

   Some drugs and medical devices presented in the publication have Food and Drug Administration (FDA) clearance for limited use in restricted research settings. It is the responsibility of the health care provider to ascertain the FDA status of each drug or device planned for use in their clinical practice.

To purchase additional copies of this book, call our customer service department at (800) 638-3030 or fax orders to (301) 223-2320. International customers should call (301) 223-2300.

Visit Lippincott Williams & Wilkins on the Internet: at LWW.com. Lippincott Williams & Wilkins customer service representatives are available from 8:30 am to 6 pm, EST.

                                                                  10 9 8 7 6 5 4 3 2 1

Contents

Preface v
Acknowledgments vii
Contributors ix

1 Basic Physics and Applications of MR Imaging in the Head and Neck 1
Anton N. Hasso, MD, FACR
Michael Lee, MD

2 The Orbit and Globe 13
Anton N. Hasso, MD, FACR
Mindy J. Kim-Miller, MD, PhD
Michelle M. Chandler, MD

3 Sinonasal, Facial, and Mandibular Embryology, Anatomy, and Anomalies 87
Mindy J. Kim-Miller, MD, PhD
Anton N. Hasso, MD, FACR

4 Sinonasal Endoscopic Surgery, Infections and Neoplasms 131
Michael Kim, MD
Mindy J. Kim-Miller, MD, PhD
Christopher R. Trimble, MD, MBA
Anton N. Hasso, MD, FACR

5 The Larynx 193
David Floriolli, MD
Anton N. Hasso, MD, FACR

6 The Pharynx and Oral Cavity 225
Stephanie Channual, MD
Christopher R. Trimble, MD, MBA
Anton N. Hasso, MD, FACR

7 The Neck and Brachial Plexus 267
Wende N. Gibbs, MS, MD
Vincent Whelan, BS
Anton N. Hasso, MD, FACR

8 Vascular Anomalies and Vascular Tumors of the Head and Neck 339
Jose A. Ospina, MD, PhD
Wende N. Gibbs, MS, MD
Anton N. Hasso, MD, FACR

9 The Cranial Nerves 356
Christopher R. Trimble, MD, MBA
Anton N. Hasso, MD, FACR

10 The Craniocervical Junction 419
Anton N. Hasso, MD, FACR
Ramana V. Yedavalli, MD
Danh T. Nguyen, MD
Henry W. Pribram, MD

11 The Temporal Bone 454
Anton N. Hasso, MD, FACR
Wende N. Gibbs, MS, MD
Max Cho, MD
Sahar Farzin, MD
Christopher R. Trimble, MD, MBA

Index 537

Preface

This book explores concepts and methods of mastering the nuances and unique diagnostic information offered by MR imaging, when applied to the head and neck. Benign or malignant processes may cause lymphadenopathy; an infected or hemorrhagic congenital mass may be detected in adulthood; serous fluid or pus may appear similar on imaging studies, are typical examples of why this region of the human body appears mysterious to many radiologists and other imaging experts. Solving these mysteries can often be accomplished by corroborative data obtained from CT or CT/PET studies, as highlighted in this product.

There are several unique features in this textbook that can aid learners in their quest to understand and apply the principles of MRI to the head and neck regions. The manuscript is completely managed by a single senior author with contributions by many students, residents, fellows and colleagues, all of who are associated in some way with the senior author in the same department. Syntax and writing styles are consistent and uniform. There is selective emphasis of specific topics, without boring or tedious repetition of textual materials.

Equally important are an overall consistency of image quality, diagrammatic enhancements and the inclusion of tables, charts and "call outs" throughout the chapters. These teaching aids can improve the readers' understanding and the application of the most appropriate differential diagnosis.

Finally, the prime purpose of the senior author is to generate a ready reference, available for daily use by all trainees during routine readouts of imaging studies. More comprehensive textbooks on the same subject are available to the reader for research or in-depth study of specific disease entities. This text is designed to generate successful learning by daily application and repetition of basic useful principles of MRI to the head and neck regions.

Anton N. Hasso, MD, FACR

Acknowledgments

My warmest thanks go to my early mentors during the 1970s. Professor William Hanafee at the University of California Los Angeles and Dr. Jacqueline Vignaud at the Foundation Adolph de Rothschild, Paris who were instrumental in guiding me to the newly emerging subspecialty of head and neck radiology. During the last three decades, with the advent of CT and later MRI, my colleagues and fellow faculty at Loma Linda University (LLU) and at the University of California Irvine (UCI) gave me helpful advice, for which I'm grateful. Their support allowed me to develop teaching files of cases and other materials that resulted in the early outlines for this text.

I would also like to thank my special friends in Otolaryngology, Head and Neck Surgery and Neuro-otology for valuable assistance over many years. During my sojourn at LLU, I want to thank Drs. George Chonkich, George Petti, and Charles Stewart. More recently at UCI, I want to thank Drs. Roger Crumley, William Armstrong, Terry Shibuya, Jason Kim, Brian Wong and Hamid Djallilian. These clinical colleagues offered me many patient referrals and much useful clinical insights and follow-up for which I'm grateful. The residents and fellows in the departments that worked with me also deserve special thanks for supporting this project through effective management of imaging studies for the best care of their patients.

I want to thank David Metzger for his skill and talent as a medical illustrator. His original work is evident in all of the line drawings and diagrams utilized throughout the chapters in this book. Over the past 2 to 3 years, Dr. Chris Trimble has doggedly and tirelessly produced an electronic version of the manuscript. His unique skills in both text and image management insured efficient production of the final product. His dedication and hard work will be long remembered and highly appreciated.

Over the last decade and a half, my publisher Lippincott, Williams and Wilkins has consistently supported the project. I want to thank my editor Lisa McAllister for her initial enthusiastic encouragement. She later handed the project to Ryan Shaw as the project manager and Charley Mitchell as the editor who have been equally effective in getting the book into final production and print. Finally, I would like to express my heartfelt gratitude to all of my co-authors collectively and individually.

Anton N. Hasso, MD, FACR

Acknowledgements

Contributors

Michelle M. Chandler, MD
Staff Radiologist
Children's Hospital & Research at Oakland
Oakland, California

Stephanie Channual, MD
Intern
Kaiser Permanente
Los Angeles, California

Max Cho, MD
Intern
Alameda Country Medicine Center
Oakland, California

Sahar Farzin, MD
Neuroradiologist
Department of Radiology
Sutter Medical Group/Sutter Health Sacramento Sierra Region
Sacramento, California

David Floriolli, MD
Resident
Department of Radiological Sciences
University of California Irvine
Irvine, California

Wende N. Gibbs, MS, MD
Resident
Department of Radiology
Baylor University Medicine Center
Dallas, Texas

Anton N. Hasso, MD, FACR
Professor
Department of Radiological Sciences
Director of Neuroimaging Research
University of California Irvine
Irvine, California

Michael Jevin Kim, MD
Neuroradiology Fellow
Division of Neuroradiology
Department of Radiology
Keck School of Medicine
University of Southern California
Los Angeles, California

Mindy J. Kim-Miller, MD, PhD
Scan Reader
Department of Nuclear Imaging
Amen Clinics
Newport Beach, California

Michael Byron Lee, MD
Neurophysiology Fellow
Department of Neurology
University of California Los Angeles
Los Angeles, California

Danh T. Nguyen, MD
Staff Radiologist
Department of Radiology
St. Jude Medical Center
Fullerton, California

Jose Ospina, MD, PhD
Neuroradiology Fellow
Department of Radiological Sciences
University of California Irvine
Irvine, California

Henry W. Pribram, MD
Professor Emeritus
Department of Radiological Sciences
University of California Irvine
Irvine, California

Christopher R. Trimble, MD, MBA
Resident Physician
Department of Diagnostic Radiology and Nuclear Medicine
University of Maryland Medical Center
Baltimore, Maryland

Vincent P. Whelan, BS
Medical Student
School of Medicine
University of California Irvine
Irvine, California

Ramana V. Yedavalli, MD, MS
Interventional Radiologist
Associated Radiologists of Joliet, SC
Joliet, Illinois

Basic Physics and Applications of MR Imaging in the Head and Neck

Anton N. Hasso, MD, FACR
Michael Lee, MD

GENERATING AN IMAGE

Unlike X-ray or CT, where image reconstruction is based on the attenuation of X-rays as they pass through tissue and strike a detector, there is no inherent signal localization in MRI. That is, if a tissue sample is excited by a radiofrequency (RF) pulse during a scan and in turn emits a detectable signal, the signal itself does not tell you where it is coming from. Localizing signal from a scan is based on the Larmor equation, which states that the frequency of a precessing nucleus is directly proportional to the magnetic field strength at that point. By systematically altering the Larmor frequency of an area of interest with imaging gradients at different times and along three orthogonal axes, three-dimensional (3D) voxels can be resolved.

Receiver Coils

Because of inherently poor signal to noise ratio (SNR) in the head and neck area, dedicated surface or phased array coils are often needed to boost signal to acceptable levels.[1] In general, the smallest possible coil that fits the anatomical region is recommended. In a phased array coil, receiver coils contribute data that are combined to form a composite image. Although expensive in terms of signal processing and hardware, phased array coils increase SNR without compromising uniform coverage.

Arrays of detection coils have recently been used to encode spatial information as well as to receive the MR signal. Simultaneous acquisition of spatial harmonics (SMASH), and simultaneous detection of spatial harmonics (SENSE) are parallel imaging techniques that take advantage of the geometry of a coil array to encode multiple lines of MR image data simultaneously.[2] In this way, scan time can be reduced by an integer factor up to 6 in both basic and advanced sequences such as contrast-enhanced magnetic resonance angiography (MRA)[3] and echo planar imaging (EPI).[4,5]

Section (Slice) Selection

When a RF pulse is delivered during a sequence, not all protons within the imaging volume are affected. Only those spins precessing at a certain frequency – the same frequency of the RF pulse itself – will resonate. A gradient that alters the resonant frequency of protons during the RF pulse is known as the section-select gradient. Imaging in the axial, coronal, or sagittal plane simply involves turning on gradients of the appropriate orientation. Similarly, oblique sections can be obtained by combining gradients along various axes.

Frequency Encoding

The "read out" or frequency-encoding gradient also takes advantage of the Larmor equation to encode location along an axis. The only difference between section (slice) selection and frequency-encoding gradients is the timing of their application. A frequency-encoding gradient is generated during the measurement of the MR signal and causes a linear variation in the precessional frequency of the spins (i.e., protons) based on their position within the gradient. This allows the localization of MR signal along one dimension within a previously excited slice.

Phase Encoding

Following the determination of the spatial location of a slice and one of its in-plane axes, another gradient is applied that takes advantage of the Larmor equation to determine the second in-plane axes. Again, the only difference between frequency encoding lies in the timing of the phase-encoding gradient to induce a phase change in selected protons.

After the initial 90 degrees pulse of an imaging sequence, a transient gradient is applied perpendicular to the section-select and frequency-encoding axes. This brief magnetic field causes a change in the precessional frequency of protons and then is switched off to allow spins to return to their previous frequency. However, a systematic phase change has been introduced that can be determined during signal measurement. In order to resolve each voxel along the phase axis, the phase-encoding gradient must be repeated at different strengths a number of times that corresponds to the number of phase-encoding steps in the image. This is costly in terms of imaging time. For a spin echo sequence, the time required by an examination is given by the repletion time (TR) multiplied by the number of excitations (Nex) multiplied by the phase-encoding steps.

3D Imaging

The phase-encoding gradient can be used to encode two axes within a region to generate a high-resolution 3D acquisition without gaps. In this technique, the excitation pulse targets the entire volume and each echo contains signal from that entire volume. Thus, SNR is excellent and the image can be reformatted in thin sections in an arbitrary plane. The primary drawback is imaging time since this is given by TR multiplied by Nex multiplied by phase-encoding step one multiplied by phase-encoding step two.

K Space

Although "K space" may sound like a term best left to theoretical physicists, understanding K space and its properties is helpful for the use and optimization of common MR pulse sequences. Consider a digitized drawing of a house. Each pixel within the image is assigned an X coordinate, a Y coordinate, and a certain signal intensity. It so happens that another, mathematically equivalent way of depicting that same house is based on frequency, phase, and signal intensity of a sine function. The Fourier transform serves as a kind of mathematical toggle switch from "real space" (X, Y, intensity) to "K space" (frequency, phase, amplitude) and is based on the fact that any given function can be approximated by an appropriate infinite series of sines and cosines. In reality, the Fourier transform is applied sequentially across different dimensions, hence the terms 2 DFT and 3 DFT, but the basic idea is the same.

K space also has some interesting properties that directly relate to the image and the production of image contrast. The number of rows of K space correspond to the number of frequency encoding steps in an image, and the number of columns in K space correspond to the number of phase-encoding steps. K space possesses "conjugate symmetry" across both the phase and frequency axes that can be used to decrease TE or acquisition time in exchange for a modest reduction in SNR.[6] Half Fourier (half Nex) techniques acquire slightly more than half the data along the phase axis and synthesize the other half to decrease acquisition time.

The collection of slightly more than half the data in the frequency axis is known as a fractional echo and reduces TE for fast scanning or increased T1 weighting (T1-W). The central region of K space provides most of the MR image signal intensity and determines overall tissue contrast. Edge detail and high resolution are filled out by more peripheral K space. This difference is exploited in keyhole image techniques that use the outer portions of K space from previous excitations to reduce acquisition time. The central K space that determines most tissue contrast is still acquired for each section. This can be used to improve imaging resolution with fat suppression techniques,[7] perfusion,[8] or to produce further reduction in scan times for other rapid imaging sequences.[9]

MR CONTRAST AGENTS

MR imaging has high spatial resolution and proven capacity for differentiating soft tissues. However, poor contrast between healthy and diseased tissues can occur if they lack variation in relaxation times, and thus, demonstrate similar signal intensities. In these situations, contrast enhancement is required to increase lesion detection and improve lesion characterization.

MR contrast agents are not visualized directly, but act indirectly by affecting the relaxation times of nearby water protons. These contrast agents are categorized as T1 or T2 agents, based upon which relaxation time is primarily affected. The most common T1 relaxation agents are paramagnetic contrast agents based on chelates of gadolinium. These agents are administered intravenously, and are available in ionic (Magnevist, MultiHance) and nonionic (ProHance, Omniscan, Optimark, and Gadovist) formulations. While these agents do not show statistically significant differences in the incidence of adverse reactions at normal doses, the creation of nonionic agents was important for the development of contrast-enhanced MR angiography, which uses larger doses administered by power injection.[10] The gadolinium-based agents diffuse rapidly from the vascular space into the tissue interstitial space, and are eliminated through glomerular filtration and renal excretion. Their half-life is approximately 90 minutes, with total elimination from the body occurring within 24 hours. The doses required are small, and they produce fewer adverse reactions than iodinated CT contrast agents.

The T2 agents are typically macromolecules with a superparamagnetic iron core. The magnetic susceptibility of these molecules distorts the local magnetic field, causing rapid dephasing of the nearby water protons. This results in significant signal loss in T2-weighted images. In the last decade, tissue-specific contrast agents composed of superparamagnetic iron oxide particles (SPIO) and ultrasmall superparamagnetic iron oxide particles (USPIO) have been developed for use in visualizing the reticuloendothelial system, and have shown great utility in imaging the liver, spleen, gastrointestinal tract, and lymph nodes. Imaging with SPIO and USPIO allows for physiologic characterization of tissues, rather than the purely morphological enhancement provided by gadolinium.

Gadolinium Contrast Agents

Gadolinium, a heavy earth metal, is the primary atom used in contrast media for MRI. Gadolinium contrast agents have pharmacokinetics, volume of distribution, and contrast features similar to iodinated contrast agents.[11] In its free form, gadolinium is toxic, but chelation with diethylene triamine penta-acetic acid (DTPA) allows for rapid renal excretion. Other examples of gadolinium chelates are gadopentetate dimeglumine, HP-DO3A, DTPA-BMA, and DOTA. Unlike iodinated contrast media, however, MR contrast agents rarely cause side effects, nephrotoxicity, or anaphylactoid reactions.[12] They are therefore safer and may be used in patients with impaired renal function or a prior history of drug allergy to iodinated contrast agents. Intravenous (IV) injection of 0.1 mmol/kg into an ante-cubital vein is most commonly used.

Unlike iodine, gadolinium chelates do not produce a signal directly. Rather, they shorten both T1 and T2 relaxation times of nearby mobile protons. Since T2 is much shorter than T1, a much higher concentration of gadolinium is needed to produce appreciable T2 shortening, so gadolinium is known as a T1 enhancement agent that increases signal on a T1-W sequence.

After IV infusion, a variety of pulse sequences and timing windows can be used to visualize gadolinium as it sequentially distributes intravascularly, within the blood pool, and extracellularly. Dynamic images and tissue perfusion can be visualized after the first 30 seconds of a power-injection with fast T1-W gradient echo techniques and may be useful in distinguishing normal tissue from hypervascularized, more rapidly perfused malignancy such as an osteoid osteoma,[13] metastatic cervical lymphadenopathy,[14] or salivary gland tumors.[15] Exact timing is established empirically by means of a small timing bolus with navigator echoes.

Within a minute post-injection, distribution approximates the blood pool. Several minutes after IV injection, interstitial space enhancement is more prominent and blood pool enhancement is less conspicuous. At this interval, edema, inflammation, fibrous tissue, necrosis, and metastates enhance due to their larger interstitial space. Within the CNS, gadolinium plays an important role in the identification of breakdowns of the blood–brain barrier such as tumor, infection, infarction, and inflammation (**Table 1-1**).

Table 1-1 Gadolinium Contrast in Head and Neck Imaging

Tumor Masses
- Allows for tumor delineation and definition of tumor extent
- Enables differentiation of residual tumor from scar and edema
- Increases detection of metastases and small tumors

Infectious or Inflammatory Processes
- Permits visualization of abscesses and necrosis
- Allows characterization of inflammation surrounding infectious foci

Vascular Lesions
- Facilitates identification and characterization of vasoformative malformations
- Differentiates vascular and lymphatic components

Superparamagnetic Iron Oxide Particles

Iron oxide-based contrast agents are a relatively new advance in MR imaging. The superparamagnetic iron oxide particles consist of iron oxide crystals coated with dextran or carboxydextran, or less commonly, with other biocompatible composites of starch, albumin, and arabinogalactose.[16] These agents are administered intravenously, and are phagocytosed by cells of the reticuloendothelial system (RES), primarily in the liver and spleen. Iron particles accumulate within the cells, producing dramatically reduced signal intensity due to their magnetic susceptibility and T2 relaxation shortening effects. Functioning RES cells will appear dark on T2- and T2*-weighted images, while lesions with dysfunctional or absent RES cells do not take up the agent, and therefore contribute relatively high signal.

The properties of different formulations of these agents depend on their size, coating, and charge. The larger SPIO agents, such as ferumoxides (Feridex) and SHU-555 (Resovist) are typically 60 to 100 nm in diameter.[17] These large particles are engulfed by the RES and liver Kupffer cells within minutes, and are used to image bowel, liver, and spleen. Ultrasmall superparamagnetic iron oxide particles, created by size fractionation of ferumoxides, are typically between 10 and 20 nm. These smaller particles are not as readily engulfed by Kupffer cells, and stay in the vascular compartment for a much longer period of time (24 to 36 hours), allowing them entry into less accessible tissues, such as lymph nodes and brain.[18] The promising USPIO, ferumoxtran-10, is in phase III clinical trials for use in lymph node imaging. Ferumoxtran-10 has demonstrated a significant advantage over traditional lymphography by allowing for visualization of all lymph nodes with one injection of contrast, as opposed to the previous method, in which only lymph nodes in the drainage path of the interstitial injection are enhanced.[19] Ferumoxtran-10 is also being investigated for use as a blood pool agent for MR angiography, where the USPIO permits a longer acquisition time window and demonstrates less interstitial background enhancement than current techniques. In this case, the T1 brightening effects of the contrast are exploited. In tissue perfusion imaging, the dose limit ceiling of gadolinium-based agents is overcome by the low toxicity of USPIO agents, allowing for serial measurements. Macrophages in atherosclerotic plaques have been shown to take up the iron oxide particles of USPIO, which may permit MR imaging of these lesions.[20] Monocrystalline iron oxide nanoparticles (MION) are a still smaller formulation of iron oxide-based contrast agent, which are being investigated for receptor-directed MR imaging and magnetically labeled cell probe MR imaging to assess tissue function at the cell and molecular levels.[21]

In the field of head and neck imaging, USPIO contrast agents have shown great promise in imaging lymph nodes, a historically problematic area. There is a significant overlap of the T1 and T2 relaxivities of normal, inflammatory, and metastatic lymph nodes, and for this reason, unenhanced MR imaging, and imaging with nonspecific contrast agents, such as gadolinium, cannot distinguish between them. Imaging with ferumoxtran-10 allows for the differentiation of benign from metastatic nodes based upon the signal intensity change between pre- and post-contrast scans. The small iron oxide particles are able to pass through the vascular endothelium into the interstitium, and are drained through lymphatic vessels to the lymph nodes. Within healthy nodes, the macrophages phagocytose and accumulate the iron oxide particles, leading to decreased signal intensity and the appearance of "darkening" of the node on postcontrast T2-weighted MR images. Metastatic nodes retain high signal intensity on postcontrast images because cancerous cells have replaced macrophages and there is little or no particle phagocytosis. The initial studies with ferumoxtran-10 have shown great promise, demonstrating increased sensitivity and specificity over gadolinium-enhanced imaging in classifying cervical lymph nodes.[22–24]

USPIO agents may also improve delineation of primary tumor margins, due to the T1 enhancement effects of the smaller SPIO and USPIO formulations. Recent studies utilizing ferumoxtran-10 to visualize brain and nasopharyngeal tumors demonstrated a rim of decreased signal surrounding the tumor, creating a sharp margin which could be visualized for several days.[25,26] This is in contrast to gadolinium, which diffuses into normal surrounding brain tissue with a half-life of hours, causing progressive blurring of the tumor margins. It is believed that this accumulation of iron oxide at the intersection between normal and cancerous tissue results from iron uptake by inflammatory cells surrounding the tumor. The ability of the USPIO contrast agents to enhance visualization of the tumor boundaries, as well as their long half-life, may make them a useful tool for preoperative planning and postoperative evaluation of tumor resection.

Iron oxide-based contrast agents have the added advantage being very well tolerated. The biodegradable SPIO is even less toxic than other MR contrast agents.[27] As SPIO agents degrade, the iron enters the plasma iron pool and is subsequently incorporated into other natural uses of iron in the body. Eventually, it is secreted with the normal turnover of body iron stores.

MR PREPULSE SEQUENCES

Magnetization Transfer Contrast

The magnetization transfer (MT) prepulse can precede almost any sequence and is commonly used to diminish signal from background tissue by delivering multiple off-resonant RF pulses. This is often used in angiography to enhance the conspicuity of vessels. To understand magnetization transfer, it will be helpful to distinguish between bound protons and mobile protons. Mobile protons such as those found in free water have a long T2 and a narrow resonant frequency. Protons bound in macromolecules such as protein have a broad resonance peak and very short T2 that makes them invisible on most pulse sequences. However, signal from the bound pool transfers to the mobile pool via dipole–dipole interactions in conventional spin echo sequences. The upshot of this is that macromolecules appear brighter than they would if the magnetization transfer phenomenon did not occur. The broad, off-resonance MT prepulses saturate and hence eliminate signal contribution from bound protons without affecting the narrow resonance of mobile protons. This suppresses signal from background tissue. Applications include greater contrast in GRE sequences otherwise prone toward overestimating foraminal stenosis, increasing the conspicuity of disease processes such as hemorrhage,[28] and to improve vessel contrast in TOF-MRA images by suppressing background tissue.[29]

Other emerging applications include the characterization of parotid masses,[30] head and neck neoplasms,[31] optic nerves,[32] and cervical spine abnormalities in multiple sclerosis.[33] However, the spinal cord region poses additional challenges due to CSF or vascular pulsations and susceptibility artifacts.[34]

Spatially Selective Saturation

Spatially selective saturation applies an RF pulse that is applied to a region that is subsequently spoiled with a dephasing gradient. This is frequently used to eliminate pulsatile flow artifacts in spin echo acquisitions.[35]

Gradient Moment Nulling

Motion that occurs between the 90 degrees RF pulse and data collection (within-view) causes dephasing errors that can be corrected with gradient moment nulling.[36] Vendor-specific acronyms are motion artifact suppression technique (MAST), gradient moment rephasing (GMR), flow compensation (FC), and flow-adjustable gradients (FLAG). In these techniques, more complicated gradient waveforms can be delivered to reduce dephasing from changes in velocity, acceleration, or higher order motion. As gradient moment nulling increases TE, and hence the time available for motion to occur, high bandwidth to reduce TE may be equally effective in reducing within-view artifacts. A common application of this technique is to reduce flow artifacts in gradient echo imaging of the cervical spine.[37]

Chemically Selective Saturation

One of the most commonly used and technically important prepulses in the head and neck region is the chemically selective saturation RF pulse or fat saturation (fat-sat), as it is commonly known. This is because fatty tissue, contrast enhancement, and fat suppression failure, all appear bright on T1-W images and may be confused for one another. Because protons in lipid resonate approximately 220 Hz slower than the protons in water, they can be selectively excited by a RF pulse of the appropriate frequency range and subsequently spoiled by a dephasing gradient to null their transverse magnetization. Hence, only protons from water contribute signal to the resulting image.

The fat-sat technique is commonly employed in contrast studies of the orbits[38] or other regions where lipid could potentially mask enhancement such as perineural extension of tumor.[39] There may be an emerging role for fat suppression in the characterization of normal thymus and the hyperplastic thymus of early adulthood.[40]

In general, fat-sat is recommended for suppression of signal from large amounts of fat and reliable acquisition of contrast material-enhanced images.[41] In this setting, the STIR sequence would be self-defeating since T1-shortening from gadolinium may cause tumor to have the same zero point as fat. Any alteration in local magnetic fields also affects resonance and may cause a fat-sat pulse to produce artifactual changes in signal intensity. An example of this is the bulk susceptibility artifact that occurs between large changes of imaging volume such as the craniocervical junction. Local field heterogeneities from air–tissue interfaces can inadvertently suppress water during a fat-sat pulse as well. This is commonly observed as a loss of signal intensity in the mucosa of the pharynx or paranasal sinus. Fat suppression failure in the lower retrobulbar region and upper pharynx is also a result of air–tissue susceptibility artifact.[42] Comparison of pre- and postcontrast images helps to avoid mistaking fat suppression failure for contrast enhancement.

MR PULSE SEQUENCES

See **Tables 1-2** and **1-3**.

T1-weighted Imaging

The head and neck is known to be an area where identifying the anatomical compartment of a lesion is of key importance. This is because localization provides insight to potential etiology and differential diagnosis. T1-weighted images are useful for visualizing distortion of normal anatomic boundaries and disruption of fascial planes. Loss of bright signal from fat or fatty bone marrow can be helpful for the detection of osteomyelitis[43] or osseous tumor extension.[44]

Spin Echo

Conventional spin echo (CSE or SE), the traditional workhorse of MR imaging, uses a 90 degrees RF pulse followed by a 180 degrees rephasing pulse to produce a spin echo. Although more than one spin echo can be generated per TR (typically 1 to 4), each echo has the same phase-encoding gradient within a pulse cycle but may be used to form an image with a different contrast weighting. The first echo does not require additional time to acquire and in that sense is "free," hence the popularity of SE to produce proton density and T2-weighted images in a single acquisition. However, since both echoes have the same TR, neither image has optimal contrast weighting. In a SE sequence, the number of slices that can be acquired depends on the TE of the last echo.

The advantages of SE include decreased susceptibility to artifacts relative to other sequences and many years of experience in using SE to produce T1-weighted images. *Scan time for a two-dimensional technique is given by the equation:*

$$\text{Scan Time} = TR \times (\textit{No. of phase-encoding steps}) \times (\textit{No. of signal averages}).$$

Fast Spin Echo or Turbo Spin Echo

Due to its greater SNR, speed, and conspicuity of disease processes, fast spin echo (FSE) has often replaced SE for T2-weighted imaging[45–48] in many settings. In a FSE sequence, a 90 degrees RF pulse is followed by multiple 180 degrees rephasing pulses to produce multiple spin echoes within a given TR. This can improve efficiency by a factor of 2X to 32X or more, in direct proportion to echo train length (ETL), the number of spin echoes within a TR. Other new terminology for FSE such as echo spacing (ES), that is the time between echoes, and echo duration, that is the times required for the ETL also affect image quality. Efficiency gains from a FSE sequence can be bartered into a combination of higher resolution (increased phase encoding steps), better SNR (increased Nex), increased coverage, stronger T2-weighting (longer TR), or faster imaging. This is especially useful for the head and neck region where lack of coverage, low resolution, and long imaging times were of particular concern.

FSE Image Optimization

Because FSE image formation depends on combining data from a number of spin echoes with a range of TEs, image contrast, and resolution are slightly different from SE. This is less of an issue than one might expect because assigning effective TE (Tef) to the central, contrast-determining portion of K-space preserves similar image weighting. However, because T2 decay continues throughout the echo train, later echoes have decreased magnitude and spatial resolution degrades slightly for a given matrix size. Edge blurriness can be avoided by using gains in imaging efficiency to increase matrix size. More generally, edge detail improves with larger matrices, short echo train length, short echo train duration, and long Tef.

Echo spacing should be minimized to allow a longer ETL for a given echo train duration. High bandwidth is useful for fast echo sampling and hence short echo spacing. Because increasing bandwidth reduces SNR, longer ES may be necessary to image regions with poor inherent signal (e.g., the sinus regions).

Differences from SE

One of the most obvious differences from SE is that fat remains bright on T2-weighted images. This is due to diffusion and J-coupling from multiple 180 degrees pulses.[49] These pulses also cause a magnetization transfer effect that diminishes signal from macromolecules and may make disc desiccation and dehydration less noticeable. Therefore, when imaging the vertebral bodies for metastatic disease or bone marrow abnormalities, a STIR sequence is recommended.[50] Another consequence of the echo train is that FSE resists chemical shift artifact and magnetic field susceptibility from local paramagnetic effects even better than SE. This is helpful in the imaging of air/tissue; bone/tissue interfaces and makes the presence of calcium and hemosiderin less obvious.

One limitation of FSE to bear in mind is that there is no "free lunch" in using a FSE sequence to produce both T2 and proton density weighted images within a given TR. Each acquisition must be separate, but superior contrast weighting can be achieved by optimizing parameters for each image series. Compared to SE, FSE is more vulnerable to ghost artifact from motion, e.g., in the cervical spine, where CSF flows relatively quickly. Swapping the phase and frequency axis may project artifact in a less obtrusive direction.[51]

FSE can also be applied to 3D and single-shot acquisitions. Single-shot FSE (SS-FSE), also known as HASTE (half-acquisition single-shot turbo echo), fills half of K-space with a long echo train and recreates the other half using conjugate synthesis. This technique enables dynamic imaging studies[52] while 3D-FSE allows 1-mm isotropic resolution, oblique reformations, less CSF motion artifact, and may be especially useful in neuroimaging[53] and for the visualization of the inner ear.[54]

Table 1-2 MR Pulse Sequences Image Optimization Parameters and Tradeoffs

Parameter	Advantages	Disadvantages
TR increased	Increased SNR Increased number of slices per acquisition	Increased scan time Decreased T1 weighting
TR decreased	Decreased scan time Increased T1 weighting	Decreased SNR Decreased number of slices per acquisition
TE increased	Increased T2 weighting	Decreased SNR
TE decreased	Increased SNR	Decreased T2 weighting
Nex increased	Increased SNR in all tissues	Direct proportional increase in scan time
Nex decreased	Direct proportional decrease in scan time	Decreased SNR in all tissues Increased flow artifact from less signal averaging
Slice thickness increased	Increased SNR in all tissues Increased coverage of anatomy	Decreased spatial resolution and partial voluming in slice select direction
Slice thickness decreased	Increases spatial resolution and reduced partial voluming in slice select direction	Decreased SNR in all tissues Decreased coverage of anatomy
FOV increased	Increased SNR Increased coverage of anatomy Decreased likelihood of aliasing	Decreased spatial resolution
FOV decreased	Decreased SNR in all tissues Decreased coverage of anatomy Increased likelihood of aliasing	Increases spatial resolution
Matrix increased	Increased spatial resolution	Decreased SNR if pixel size decreases. If pixel size remains same, SNR will increase because more phase encoding steps are performed Increased scan time
Matrix decreased	Increased SNR in all tissues if pixel size increases. If pixel remains the same, SNR decreases as fewer phase encoding steps are performed Decreased scan time	Decreased resolution
Receive bandwidth increased	Decreased SNR	Decrease of minimum TE Decrease in chemical shift
Receive bandwidth decreased	Increased SNR	Increase of minimum TE Increase in chemical shift

TR = repletion time; TE = acquisition time; Nex = number of excitations; FOV = field of view; SNR = signal to noise ratio.

Table 1-3 Pulse Sequence Acronyms

Family	Generic Name	General Electric	Marconi	Philips	Siemens	Toshiba
Spin echo	Fast spin echo (FSE)	FSE	FSE	TSE	TSE	FSE
	IR-FSE	IR-FSE	Fast IR	IR-TSE	Turbo-IR	Fast IR
	Single-shot FSE	SS-FSE	Express	UFSE	SS-TSE, HASTE	FASE, DIET
	GRASE (gradient and spin echo)	–	–	GRASE	TGSE	–
Gradient echo	Spoiled GE	SPGR, MP-SPGR	RF-FAST	T1-FFE	FLASH	RF-spoiled FE
	Unspoiled GE	MPGR, GRE	FAST	FFE	FISP	FE
	SSFP (steady-state free precession)	SSFP	CE-FAST	T2 FFE	PSIF	–

Inversion Recovery

A 180 degrees inversion recovery (IR) pulse can delivered before a spin echo sequence in order to obtain special contrast features. After a 180 degrees pulse, the patient's net magnetization vector begins to re-align itself with the main magnetic field, B_0. After a specified inversion time (TI), a 90 degrees pulse rotates that net magnetization vector into the horizontal plane where it can be measured as per a standard spin echo sequence. This allows for heavy T1 weighting because the magnetization vector recovers through a larger distance. Alternately, judicious choice of the TI can "null" the signal from a tissue based on its T1 relaxation properties. A short TI (STIR) sequence that catches the net magnetization when the fat signal has recovered to zero (no longitudinal component) selectively removes signal from lipid while an IR sequence with a long TI (fluid attenuated inversion recovery or FLAIR) attuned to the zero point for water nulls CSF. FLAIR sequences are often used in conjunction with T2-weighted FSE to detect periventricular lesions.[53] STIR imaging allows homogeneous and global fat suppression and can be used with low field strength magnets. However, this technique is not specific for fat, and the signal intensity of tissue with a long T1 and tissue with a short T1 may be ambiguous.[41] For the cervical region, STIR is often recommended rather than fat-sat.[54]

Gradient Echo Sequences

Gradients can also be used to generate an echo and are the foundation of a family of related techniques. Rather than using a 180 degrees pulse, the echo is formed by dephasing and then rephasing the magnetization vector by using gradients of reversed polarity. This lack of a 180 degrees pulse causes sensitivity to magnetic heterogeneities in the main magnetic field as well as local susceptibility differences. Thus, the MR signal decays rapidly according to T2*, and shorter values of TE (<30 ms) are required for heavily T2*-weighted sequences. This may be desirable to detect the so-called "blooming" of signal dropout from hemosiderin but also causes general image degradation. Gradient echo techniques are speedy, with a short TR that necessitates small flip angles that avoid saturating the signal to zero between excitations. Their speed and short TR are especially helpful in achieving reasonable scan times for 3D imaging. After a few RF pulses, the recovery of the magnetization vector exactly matches the effect of the RF pulse and the magnetization vector is in the steady state. When TR is less than T2, some transverse magnetization will remain during the next RF pulse. The fate of this transverse magnetization determines contrast. Spoiled gradient techniques will diphase residual transverse magnetization and are T1 or PD weighted. Unspoiled techniques make use of this added signal and give mixed T2/T1 contrast. Steady-state free precession (SSFP) uses only the transverse magnetization for T2 weighting. Also, because fat and water resonate at slightly different speeds, the choice of TE determines whether their signal is additive or cancels. This opposed-phase effect can demonstrate lesions that contain small amounts of fat but are not reliable for detection of small tumors embedded in fatty tissues.[41]

Coherent (Unspoiled) Gradient Echo

In this technique, also known as gradient recalled acquisition in the steady state (GRASS), gradient recalled echo (GRE), fast imaging with steady-state precession (FISP), Fourier acquired steady-state technique (FAST), and fast field echo (FFE), the steady state is used. Thus, the transverse component of magnetization accumulates and the resulting images have mixed contrast that emphasizes tissues with both short T1 relaxation and long T2 relaxation. Blood, CSF, and joint fluid appear bright and demonstrate an angiographic,[55] myelographic,[56] or arthrographic effect. Longer TRs are frequently used for multi-slice acquisitions in spinal and joint imaging.

Incoherent (Spoiled) Gradient Echo

Also known as fast low-angle shot (FLASH),[57] spoiled gradient recalled echo (SPGR), T1 fast field echo (T1-FFE), RF-spoiled Fourier acquired steady-state technique (FAST), this technique spoils steady-state magnetization with RF or crusher gradients to achieve T1/PD contrast weighting. They are therefore very effective in demonstrating anatomy and can be used with or without contrast.

Steady-state Free Precession (T2)

Steady-state free precession (SSFP) and its vendor-specific acronyms, contrast-enhanced Fourier acquired steady-state technique (CE-FAST), T2 fast field echo (T2 FFE), PSIF (FISP backwards) is a gradient echo technique where each excitation pulse also refocuses transverse magnetization. Only the transverse magnetization portion is used, so the sequence is T2 weighted. This can be used for T2-weighted 3D imaging of the cervical spines,[58] allowing a second opportunity to study contrast-enhanced arterial or venous anatomy with high image SNR and high spatial resolutions.[59]

EPI

Echo planar imaging (EPI) uses multiple gradient echoes per excitation to reduce acquisition time[60] and is the gradient echo equivalent of FSE. In "single-shot" EPI techniques, all of K-space is filled by rapidly oscillating gradients within a single TR. This places great demands on gradient hardware but is becoming increasingly available as the demand for diffusion-weighted imaging, perfusion, and cardiac applications increases. Thus, EPI images are sensitive to magnetic susceptibility effects and are highly T2* weighted. EPI may be useful to depict lesions with paramagnetic susceptibility characteristics,[61] but suffer from image blurring from T2* decay within the long echo train. Multishot techniques allow for increased SNR and resolution at a cost of acquisition time and increased sensitivity to patient motion. If greater T2-weighted contrast is desired, a single 180 degrees refocusing pulse timed to the acquisition of the central lines of K-space can reduce T2* susceptibility.

GRASE

Gradient recalled and spin echo (GRASE) techniques use a hybrid of spin echoes and gradient echoes to form an image. As such, GRASE may offer great flexibility in balancing the time savings from gradient echo with the resistance to magnetic susceptibility offered by spin echo techniques. Similarly, GRASE tends to have less of an MT effect than pure FSE. The GRASE factor refers to the number of gradient echoes to spin echoes. This can be used to generate tissue contrast similar to FSE, but with enhanced visualization of pathology involving susceptibility artifacts. Other trials have proved less successful.[62]

Diffusion-weighted Imaging

The image contrast is determined by the random microscopic motion of water protons in diffusion-weighted imaging (DWI).[63] The addition of bipolar gradients sensitizes the image to diffusion effects and can be used in conjunction with rapid imaging techniques such as EPI or HASTE. The magnitude of this sensitivity in a given axis is determined by a b-value (expressed as s/mm^2) of the bipolar gradients. When diffusion gradients are applied along all three axes they are referred to as isotropic. Often a number of B_0's are used (0, 500, 1,000, 1,500) and an apparent diffusion coefficient (ADC) used for quantification and visualization. DWI signal is high when diffusion is restricted, as occurs in cytotoxic damage from ischemia, inflammation, trauma, or tumors. Although somewhat overlapping, differences in ADC coefficients may be useful in distinguishing various processes from each other. For example, ADCs for lymphoma < carcinoma < solid benign tumor < benign cystic lesion.[61,64,65]

Recent studies suggest a potential role in the evaluation spinal cord lesions,[66–68] myelomalacia,[69] and distinction of benign fracture edema and tumor infiltration of the vertebral bodies.[70]

SUPPLEMENTARY TECHNIQUES: MR SPECTROSCOPY AND MR ANGIOGRAPHY

MR Spectroscopy

The same phenomenon underlying chemical shift between water and lipid can be used to study the chemical composition of tissue. Electrons in a complex chemical environment produce small alterations in the local magnetic field that alter the resonant frequency of adjacent protons. This is known as chemical shift and is visualized as a spectrum of peaks displayed in units of parts per million (ppm) of B_0. Although possible with any nuclei that possess an odd number of protons or neutrons, magnetic resonance spectroscopy (MRS) usually images hydrogen because of its abundance and greater SNR. In the most commonly used technique, spatial localization is determined by the intersection of three orthogonal slice-select gradients, yielding a spectrum of a single $2 \times 2 \times 2$ cm voxel. Because MRS depends on small changes in magnetic resonance caused by chemical shifts, magnetic field homogeneity is of utmost importance. Partially or fully automated shimming of local coils aids in this regard, but care must still be taken to avoid targeting regions of differing magnetic susceptibility. Another technical consideration is the suppression of water and lipid peaks to avoid swamping the relatively small signal from metabolites of interest. Short echo times of 30 ms allow identification of a greater range of metabolites, including Myo-inositol, a product of myelin breakdown (3.6 ppm), Choline (at 3.2 ppm), a marker of cell membrane lipids, creatine compounds (3.0 ppm), glutamine/glutamate (2.1 to 2.5 ppm). The neuronal marker NAA (2.0 ppm), and lactate, a marker for cell death and tissue necrosis. Lactate produces a doublet that characteristically inverts at a TE of 135 ms, which is useful for positive identification and separation from the broader peak from lipids. Although technically easier for intracranial applications,[71] spectroscopy may play an emerging role in the differentiation of metastatic cancer from normal muscular tissue, recurrent tumor vs. post-treatment change, as well as the detection of abscess[72] and monitoring of cancer response in the head and neck region.

Magnetic Resonance Angiography

The general principle of magnetic resonance angiography (MRA) is to acquire images where the signal returned from flowing nuclei is high, and the signal from stationary tissue is low. This allows visualization of vascular anatomy and can be applied in 2D or volumetric sequences. Frequently, more than one technique is necessary to delineate the vascular tree in its entirety. Maximum intensity projection (MIP) algorithms are often used to display the resulting images in contiguous sections for later viewing.

Time of Flight

Time of flight (TOF) MR angiographic techniques employ a spoiled GRE sequence to acquire thin slices from a selected volume. As the images are acquired, multiple RF pulses saturate stationary tissues but blood flowing into the region yields high signal. The specific visualization of the arterial or venous circulation is achieved by spatially selective pulses applied outside the volume of interest. In a 2D-TOF sequence, thin slices grant sensitivity to slow flow, but the associated long TEs reduce signal from turbulence or complex flow patterns. Generally, the shortest possible opposed-phase TE is chosen to reduce undesirable signal intensity from fat.[73]

For 3D-TOF acquisitions, slow moving blood becomes saturated due to longer scan times unless incrementally ramped flip angles or thin slabs are used. This maintains vessel signal by delaying saturation of flowing blood. MOTSA (multiple overlapping thin slab acquisition) acquires a number of thinner overlapping 3D sections, discarding redundant coverage for MIP reconstruction. This may lead to a "Venetian blind" appearance of the composite image. 3D-TOF techniques offer increased SNR and spatial resolution, but with diminished sensitivity to slow flow. 3D-TOF benefits from gadolinium contrast.

Common applications are to demonstrate relatively fast-moving venous and arterial flow in the head, neck, and peripheral vessels,[74] often with contrast[75] and in conjunction with magnetization transfer[76] for background suppression.

Phase Contrast

Phase-contrast angiography (PC-MRA) offers excellent background suppression and does not have difficulty in imaging slow flow, but takes considerably longer to acquire than an equivalent TOF study. In essence, an unspoiled gradient echo subtraction method, in this technique a bipolar gradient is applied between the initial excitation RF pulse and readout gradient to introduce phase shift, and a similar acquisition with a reversed bipolar gradient is then subtracted from the first acquisition. Stationary protons yield zero signal while moving protons in blood have additive phase shift appear bright. The user must specify velocity encoding or VENC in order to visualize flow of the desired velocity, which can be applied in single or multiple planes. Common applications include the demonstration of arterial flow in the head and major veins.

3D PC-MRA has the advantage of thinner slices and superior depiction of slow flow, but at the cost of lengthy imaging time relative to TOF. In addition, the presence of flow-encoding gradients increases TE, causes loss of signal in regions of fluid turbulence, and makes flow compensation impossible. However, this may be useful for the depiction of carotid artery stenosis.[77]

Contrast-enhanced MRA

Although the terminology can be misleading, contrast-enhanced MRA specifically refers to angiography based on T1 shortening of a gadolinium bolus. The in-flow phenomenon is not involved. Saturation is therefore much less of a concern and larger field of view acquisitions can be acquired using 3D gradient echo sequences with short TR and TE. A timing bolus is usually given to capture the first-pass of a contrast agent through the region of interest, and strategic K-space reordering schemes such as elliptic centric phase encoding determine image contrast.[78,79] Magnetization transfer and fat-sat are often used to reduce background signal. Recent reports demonstrate neurovascular compression in trigeminal neuralgia[80] and the characterization of AVMs and their post-treatment follow-up.[81]

ARTIFACTS AND REMIDIES

Artifacts represent any alterations of signal intensity that do not correspond to anatomical structures or pathologic entities. For example, ghosting is a common artifact produced by motion between successive applications of the phase-encoding gradient or motion along the direction of the phase-encoding gradient during data collection. This causes phantom images of bright structures to appear throughout the phase encode direction, regardless of whether the motion occurs within the phase encode axis. In the head and neck region, pulsation from vessels may degrade image clarity. Potential remedies include switching the frequency/phase axes to shift ghosting to a less troublesome axis, spatial presaturations between the origin of the artifact and the FOC, and gradient moment nulling (**Table 1-4**). See a complete list of common artifacts and their remedies in Table IV of Ref. 82.

Table 1-4 Artifacts and Remedies

Artifact	Remedy	Penalty of Remedy
Truncation	Increase phase encoding	Increases scan time
	Increase Nex	Increases scan time
Phase mismapping (ghosting)	Swap phase and frequency	May need over sampling
	Pre-saturation	May lose slices
	Gradient moment nulling	Increases minimum TE
Chemical shift	Reduce bandwidth	Increases TE
	Reduce FOV	Reduces SNR
	Use chemical saturation	Reduces SNR
Aliasing	Over sampling (frequency)	None
	Digital filtering (frequency)	None
	Enlarge FOV	Reduces resolution
Zipper	Call engineer	None
Magnetic susceptibility	Use spin echo sequences	Not flow sensitive
	Remove metal where possible	
Motion	Counseling	None
	All remedies for mismapping	See above
	Fast imaging (EPI, etc.)	Limited to T2 contrast
	Fast imaging (HASTE)	Edge blurring
Cross-talk	Interleaved image slices	Doubles scan time
	Square RF pulses	Reduces SNR (small)

Nex = number of excitations; FOV = field of view; EPI = echo planar imaging; HASTE = half acquisition single-shot turbo echo; RF = radiofrequency; SNR = signal to noise ratio; TE = acquisition time.

REFERENCES

1. Lufkin RB and Hanafee W: Application of surface coils to NMR anatomy of the larynx. Am J Neuroradiol 1985;6:492–497.
2. Hyde JS, Jesmanowicz A, Froncisz, W, et al.: Parallel image acquisition from noninteracting local coils. J Magn Reson 1987;70:512–517.
3. Van den Brink JS, Watanabe Y, and Kohl CK: Implications of SENSE MR in routine clinical practice. Eur J Radiol 2003;46(1):3–27.
4. Bydder M, Atkinson D, and Larkman DJ: SMASH navigators. Magn Reson Med 2003;49(3):493–500.
5. Sodickson DK, Griswold MA, and Jakob PM: SMASH imaging. Magn Reson Imaging Clin N Am 1999;7(2):237–254.
6. Feinberg DA, Hale JD, Watts JC, et al.: Halving MR imaging time by conjugation: demonstration at 3.5 kG. Radiology 1986;161(2):527–531.
7. Flask CA, Salem KA, Moriguchi H, et al.: Keyhole Dixon method for faster, perceptually equivalent fat suppression. J Magn Reson Imaging 2003;18(1):103–112.
8. Heiland S, Margosian P, Benner T, et al.: Does the "keyhole" technique improve spatial resolution in MRI ferfusion measurements? A study in volunteers. Neuroradiology 2001;43(7):518–524.
9. Zaitsev M, Zilles K, and Shah NJ: Shared K-space echo planar imaging with keyhole. Magn Reson Med 2001;45(1):109–117.
10. Runge VM: Safety of magnetic resonance contrast media. Top Magn Reson Imaging 2001;12:309–314.
11. Weinman H-J, Brasch RC, Press WR, et al.: Characteristics of gadolinium-DTPA complex: a potential NMR contrast agent. Am J Roentgenol 1984;142: 619–624.
12. Niendorf HP, Haustein J, and Cornelius I: Safety of gadolinium-DTPA: extended clinical experience. Magn Reson Med 1991;22(2):222–228; discussion 229–232.
13. Liu PT, Chivers FS, Roberts CC, et al.: Imaging of osteoid osteoma with dynamic gadolinium-enhanced MR imaging. Radiology 227(3):691–700, 2003.
14. Fischbein NJ, Noworolski SM, Henry RG, et al.: Assessment of metastatic cervical adenopathy using dynamic contrast-enhanced MR imaging. Am J Neuroradiol 2003;24(3):297.
15. Yabuuchi H, Fukuya T, Tajirna T, et al.: Salivary gland tumors: diagnostic value of gadolinium-enhanced dynamic MR imaging with histopathologic correlation. Radiology 2003;226(2):345–354.
16. Wang YJ, Hussain SM, and Krestin GP: Superparamagnetic iron oxide contrast agents: physiochemical characteristics and applications in MR imaging. Eur Radiol 2001;11:2319–2331.
17. Kirchin MA and Runge VM: Contrast agents for magnetic resonance imaging: safety update. Top Magn Reson Imaging 2003;14:426–435.
18. Raynal I, Prigent P, Peyramaure S, et al.: Macrophage endocytosis of superparamagnetic iron oxide nanoparticles. Invest Radiol 2004;39:56–63.
19. Anzai Y: Superparamagnetic iron oxide nanoparticles: nodal metastases and beyond. Top Magn Reson Imaging 2004;15:103–111.
20. Ruehm SG, Corot C, and Debatin JF: MR imaging of atherosclerotic plaque with ultrasmall paramagnetic iron oxide in hyperlipidemic rabbits. Radiology 2003; 213[Suppl]:267.
21. Artemov D: Molecular magnetic resonance imaging with targeted contrast agents. J Cell Biochem 2003;90:518–524.
22. Mack MG, Balzer JO, Eichler K, et al.: Superparamagnetic iron oxide enhanced MR imaging of head and neck lymph nodes. Radiology 2002;222:239–244.

23. Anzai Y, Piccoli CW, Outwater EK, et al.: Evaluation of neck and body metastases to nodes with furomoxtran 10-enhanced MR imaging: Phase III Safety and efficacy study. Radiology 2003;228:777–788.
24. Anzai Y, Blackwell KE, Hisrshowitz SL, et al.: Initial clinical experience with dextran-coated superparamagnetic iron oxide for etection of lymph node metastases in patients with head and neck cancer. Radiology 1994;192: 709–715.
25. Varallyay P, Nesbit G, Muldoon LL, et al.: Comparison of two superparamagnetic viral-sized iron oxide particles ferumoxides and ferumoxtran-10 with a gadolinium chelate in imaging intracranial tumors. Am J Neuroradiol 2002;223:510–519.
26. Enochs WS, Harsh G, Hochberg F, et al.: Improved delineation of human brain tumors on MR images using a long-circulating, superparamagnetic iron oxide agent. J Magn Reson Imaging 1999;9:228–232.
27. Simonsen CZ, Ostergaard L, Vestrgaard-Poulsen P, et al.: CBF and CBV measurements by USPIO bolus tracking: reproducibility and comparison with Gd-based values. J Magn Reson Imaging 1999;9:342–347.
28. Grossman RI, Gomori JM, Goldberg HI, et al.: MR imaging of hemorrhagic conditions of the head and neck. Radiographics 1988;8(3):441–454.
29. Atkinson D, Brant-Zawadzki M, Gillan G, et al.: Improved MR angiography: magnetization transfer suppression with variable flip angle excitation and increased resolution. Radiology 1994;190(3):890–894.
30. Takashima S, Wang J, Takayama F, et al.: Parotid masses: prediction of malignancy using magnetization transfer and MR imaging findings. Am J Roentgenol 2001;176(6):1577–1584.
31. Yousem DM, Montone KT, Sheppard LM, et al.: Head and neck neoplasms: magnetization transfer analysis. Radiology 1994;192(3):703–707.
32. Inglese M, Ghezzi A, Bianchi S, et al.: Irreversible disability and tissue loss in multiple sclerosis: a conventional and magnetization transfer magnetic resonance imaging study of the optic nerves. Arch Neurol 2002;59(2):250–255.
33. Rovaris M, Holtrnannspotter M, Rocca MA, et al.: Contribution of cervical cord MRI and brain magnetization transfer imaging to the assessment of individual patients with multiple sclerosis: a preliminary study. Mult Scler 2002;8(1):52–58.
34. Quencer RM: Advances in imaging of spinal cord injury: implications for treatment and patient evaluation. Prog Brain Res 2002;137:3–8.
35. Tkach JA, Ruggieri PM, Ross JS, et al.: Pulse sequence strategies for vascular contrast in time-of-flight carotid MR angiography. J Magn Reson Imaging 1993;3(6):811–820.
36. Pattany PM, Phillips JJ, Chiu LC, et al.: Motion artifact suppression technique (MAST) for MR imaging. J Comput Assist Tomogr 1987;11(3):369–377.
37. Held P, Seitz J, Frund R, et al.: Comparison of two-dimensional gradient echo, turbo spin echo and two-dimensional turbo gradient spin echo sequences in MRI of the cervical spinal cord anatomy. Eur J Radiol 2001;38(1):64–71.
38. Tien RD, Chu PK. Hesselink JR, et al.: Intra- and extra-orbital lesions: value of fat-suppression MR imaging with paramagnetic contrast enhancement. Am J Neuroradiol 1991;12(2):245–253.
39. Simon JH and Szumowski J: Chemical shift imaging with paramagnetic contrast material enhancement for improved lesion depiction. Radiology 1996;171:539–543.
40. Takahashi K, lnaoka T, Murakami N, et al.: Characterization of the normal and hyperplastic thymus on chemical-shift MR imaging. Am J Roentgenol 2003;180(5):1265–1269.
41. Delfaut EM, Beltran J, Johnson G, et al.: Fat suppression in MR imaging: techniques and pitfalls. Radiographics 1999;19(2):373–382.
42. Anzai Y, Lufkin RB, Jabour BA, et al.: Fat-suppression failure artifacts simulating pathology on frequency-selective fat-suppression MR images of the head and neck. Am J Neuroradiol 1992;13(3):879–884.
43. Ledermann HP, Schweitzer ME, Morrison WB, et al.: MR imaging findings in spinal infections: rules or myths? Radiology 2003;228(2):506–514.
44. Dosda R, Marti-Bonmati L, Menor F, et al.: Comparison of plain radiographs and magnetic resonance images in the evaluation of periosteal reaction and osteoid matrix in osteosarcomas. MAGMA 1999;9(1–2):72–80.
45. Fulbright R, Panush D, Sze G, et al.: MR of the head and neck: comparison of fast spin-echo and conventional spin-echo sequences. Am J Neuroradiol 1994;15(4):767–773.
46. Zoarski GH, Mackey JK, Anzai Y, et al.: Head and neck: initial clinical experience with fast spin-echo MR imaging. Radiology 1993;188(2):323–327.
47. Renowden SA and Anslow P: The effective use of magnetic resonance imaging in the diagnosis of acoustic neuromas. Clin Radiol 1993;48(1):25–28.
48. Atlas SW, Hackney DB, and Listerud J: Fast spin-echo imaging of the brain and spine. Magn Reson Q 1993;9(2):61–83.
49. Henkelman RM, Hardy PA, and Bishop JE: Why fat is bright in RARE and fast spin-echo imaging. J Magn Reson Imaging 1992;2(5):533–540.
50. Mehta RC, Marks MP, Hinks RS, et al.: MR evaluation of vertebral metastases: T1-weighted, short-inversion-time inversion recovery, fast spin-echo, and inversion-recovery fast spin-echo sequences. Am J Neuroradiol 1995;16(2): 281–288.
51. Gillams AR, Soto JA, and Carter AP: Fast spin echo vs conventional spin echo in cervical spine imaging. Eur Radiol 1997;7(8):1211–1214.
52. Duerinckx AJ, Yu WD, El-Saden S, et al.: MR imaging of cervical spine motion with HASTE. Magn Reson Imaging 1999;17(3):371–381.
53. Castillo M and Mukherji SK: Clinical applications of FLAIR, HASTE, and magnetization transfer in neuroimaging. Semin Ultrasound CT MR. 2000;21(6):417–427.
54. Naganawa S, Itoh T, and Fukatsu H: Three-dimensional fast spin-echo MR of the inner ear: ultra-long echo train length and half-Fourier technique. Am J Neuroradiol 1998;19(4):739–741.
55. Nakatsu M, Hatabu H, Itoh H, et al.: Comparison of short inversion time inversion recovery (STIR) and fat-saturated (chemsat) techniques for background fat intensity suppression in cervical and thoracic MR imaging. J Magn Reson Imaging 2000;11(1):56–60.
56. Atlas SW, Mark AS, Fram EK, et al.: Vascular intracranial lesions: applications of gradient-echo MR imaging. Radiology 1988;169(2):455–461.
57. Georgy HA and Hesselink JR: MR imaging of the spine: recent advances in pulse sequences and special techniques. Am J Roentgenol 1994;162(4): 923–934.
58. Frahm J, Haase A, and Matthaei D: Rapid NMR imaging of dynamic processes using the FLASH technique. Magn Reson Med 1986;3(2):321–327.
59. Haskaran V, Pereles FS, Russell EJ, et al.: Myelographic MR imaging of the cervical spine with a 3D true fast imaging with steady-state precession technique: initial experience. Radiology 2003;227(2):585 592.
60. Foo TK, Ho VB, Marcos HB, et al.: MR angiography using steady-state free precession. Magn Reson Med 2002;48(4):699–706.
61. Butts RK, Riederer SJ, Ehman RI, et al.: Interleaved echo planar imaging on a standard MRI system. Magn Reson Med 1994;31:67–74.
62. Rockwell DT, Melhem ER, and Bhatia RG: GRASE (gradient- and spin-echo) MR of the brain. Am J Neuroradiol 1997;18(10):1923–1928.
63. Brunereau L, Leveque C, and Bertrand P: Familial form of cerebral cavernous malformations: evaluation of gradient-spin-echo (GRASE) imaging in lesion detection and characterization at 1.5 T. Neuroradiology 2001;43(11):973–979.
64. Bammer R: Basic principles of diffusion-weighted imaging. Eur J Radiol 2003;45(3):169–184.
65. Mukherji SK, Chenevert TL, and Castillo M: Diffusion-weighted magnetic resonance imaging. J Neuroophthalmol 2002;22(2):118–122.
66. Wang J, Takashima S, Takayama F, et al.: Head and neck lesions: characterization with diffusion-weighted echo-planar MR imaging. Radiology 2001;220(3):621–630.
67. Bammer R, Augustin M, Prokesch RW, et al.: Diffusion-weighted imaging of the spinal cord: interleaved echo-planar imaging is superior to fast spinecho. J Magn Reson Imaging 2002;15(4):364–373.
68. Fujikawa A, Tsuchiya K, Koppera P, et al.: Case report: spinal cord infarction demonstrated on diffusion-weighted MR imaging with a single-shot fast spin-echo sequence. J Comput Assist Tomogr 2003;27(3):415–419.
69. Moller-Hartmann W, Krings T, and Coenen VA: Preoperative assessment of motor cortex and pyramidal tracts in central cavernoma employing functional and diffusion-weighted magnetic resonance imaging. Surg Neurol 2002;58(5):302–307.
70. Tsuchiya K, Katase S, Fujikawa A, et al.: Diffusion-weighted MRI of the cervical spinal cord using a single-shot fast spin-echo technique: findings in normal subjects and in myelomalacia. Neuroradioldgy 2003;45(2):90–94.
71. Spuentrup E, Buecker A, Koelker C, et al.: Respiratory motion artifact suppression in diffusion-weighted MR imaging of the spine. Eur Radiol 2003;13(2):330–336.
72. Burtscher IM and Holtas S: Proton MR spectroscopy in clinical routine. J Magn Reson Imaging 2001;13(4):560–567.
73. Kendi T, Arikan OK, and Koc C: MR spectroscopy in a cervical abscess. Neuroradiology 2003;45(9):631–633.
74. Laub GA: Time-of-flight method of MR angiography. Magn Reson Imaging Clin N Am. 1995;3(3):391–398.
75. Graves MJ: Magnetic resonance angiography. Br J Radiol 1997;70:6–28.

76. Meaney JF: Magnetic resonance angiography of the peripheral arteries: current status. Eur Radiol 2003;13(4):836–852.
77. Mathews VP, Ulmer JL, White ML, et al.: Depiction of intracranial vessels with MRA: utility of magnetization transfer saturation and gadolinium. J Comput Assist Tomogr 1999;23(4):597–602.
78. Iseda T, Nakano S, Miyahara D, et al.: Poststenotic signal attenuation on 3D phase-contrast MR angiography: a useful finding in haemodynamically significant carotid artery stenosis. Neuroradiology 2000;42(12):868–873.
79. Amano Y, Amano M, and Matsuda T: Fat-suppressed three-dimensional MR angiography technique with elliptical centric view order and no prolonged breath-holding time. J Magn Reson Imaging 2002;16(6):707–715.
80. De Marco JK, Schonfeld S, and Keller I: Contrast-enhanced carotid MR angiography with commercially available triggering mechanisms and elliptic centric phase encoding. Am J Roentgenol 2001;176(1):221–227.
81. Patel NK, Aquilina K, Clarke Y, et al.: How accurate is magnetic resonance angiography in predicting neurovascular compression in patients with trigeminal neuralgia? A prospective, single-blinded comparative study. Br J Neurosurg 2003;17(1):60–64.
82. Suzuki M, Matsui O, Kobayashi K, et al.: Contrast-enhanced MRA for investigation of cerebral arteriovenous malformations. Neuroradiology 2003;45(4):231–235.
83. Arena L, Morehouse HT, and Safir J: MR imaging artifacts that simulate disease: how to recognize and eliminate them. Radiographics 1995;15(6):1373–1394.

The Orbit and Globe

Anton N. Hasso, MD, FACR
Mindy J. Kim-Miller, MD, PhD
Michelle M. Chandler, MD

INTRODUCTION

Many orbital lesions that lie in the anterior portions of the orbit or within the globe are readily accessible to the ophthalmoscope. In order to assess the extent of such lesions and to examine portions of the orbit not so readily assessed with the ophthalmoscope, imaging plays a vital role. MR is useful for evaluating visual loss or suspected cranial nerve dysfunction. Multiplanar high-resolution MR images can be used to examine most diseases within and around the orbits, and to localize soft-tissue lesions within the globe, intraorbital, conal, and extraconal spaces. Overall, CT is most useful for detecting foreign bodies, masses, intraocular calcification, and bony details. Dacryocystography is used to evaluate disorders of the lacrimal drainage apparatus by injecting a water-soluble contrast material into the canaliculi during fluoroscopy. Imaging should be obtained based on the clinical history and physical examination and should include views of the orbit and adjacent regions of the skull, face, and sinuses.

CLINICAL SIGNS AND SYMPTOMS

As part of the visual system, the eye collects light and converts it into electrical impulses that travel from the retina to the midbrain, thalamus, and finally to the visual cortex. Visual perception is the most complex human sensory system; it involves five cranial nerves (CN II, III, IV, V, VI) with approximately 1.1 million nerve fibers in each optic nerve, compared to 30,000 fibers in an auditory nerve.

Visual disturbances can result from lesions anywhere along the visual pathway. **Table 2-1** lists some causes of vision loss. Disturbances in visual acuity include blindness (legal blindness is defined as best-corrected vision no better than 20/200) and amblyopia, commonly known as "lazy eye," a reduction in vision not correctable with glasses. Monocular blindness is usually caused by a refractive error or lens opacity. The most common causes of amblyopia include constant strabismus (constant deviation of one eye), anisometropia (different prescriptions in each eye), and/or visual deprivation in an eye due to trauma, lid droop, etc. Myopia refers to nearsightedness caused by rays focusing in front of the retina and affects about one-third of the population. Hyperopia, or farsightedness, affects about a fourth of the population and results when light rays focus behind the retina. Nasal, temporal, upper, or lower field deficits may occur with preservation of the remaining visual fields depending on the location of the lesion. Most occipital lobe lesions lead to visual field cuts, symmetrically or asymmetrically. In general, lesions to an eye anterior to the optic chiasm cause monocular visual disturbances, and lesions posterior to the optic chiasm cause binocular disturbances.

Diplopia (double vision) can be monocular or binocular and present in primary gaze and/or with eye movement. In binocular diplopia, the double vision is eliminated when either eye is occluded. Causes of binocular diplopia include thyroid eye disease, cranial nerve palsies, nerve or extraocular muscle entrapments, CNS lesions, intranuclear ophthalmoplegia (multiple sclerosis), vascular/ischemic injuries, and pseudotumor cerebri. With monocular diplopia, the double vision remains when the uninvolved eye is occluded. Causes of monocular diplopia include refractive error, cataract, macular disease, corneal opacity, and retinal detachment. Ophthalmoplegia, paralysis of one or more of the motor nerves of the eye, may cause visual abnormalities including decreased visual acuity, afferent pupillary defect, and visual field deficits in addition to diplopia. Ophthalmoplegia may be associated with pain, which is often exacerbated by attempted movement of the eye. When these symptoms are present together, several different lesions may cause them[1] (**Table 2-2**).

Proptosis and Enophthalmos

Many primary diseases of the orbit will present with proptosis with or without visual disturbances. Proptosis refers to abnormal protrusion of the globe and may be differentiated from exophthalmos, which refers to abnormal prominence of the globe (**Fig. 2-1**).

Table 2-1 Isolated Visual Disturbances

Minimal or Variable Pain with Vision Loss
- Optic neuritis
- Retinal detachment/choroidal detachment
- Ocular tumor
- Vitreous hemorrhage
- Central retinal artery occlusion (amaurosis fugax)
- Ischemic optic neuropathy
- Pseudotumor cerebri (papilledema)
- Ischemic or vascular lesions
  - Aneurysm
  - Vascular dolichoectasia
  - Vascular malformation

Pain Present
- Glaucoma
- Iritis
- Corneal ulcer
- Temporal arteritis (giant cell arteritis)
- Optic nerve meningitis
  - Pyogenic
  - Syphilitic
  - Fungal
- Trauma
- Retro-orbital hemorrhage causing compressive neuropathy

Less Common Etiologies
- Complications of radiation therapy (radiation-induced optic neuropathy)
- Complication of chemotherapy
- Toxic or metabolic insult
- Connective tissue diseases (vasculitis):
  - Systemic lupus erythromatosis
  - Rheumatoid arthritis
  - Sjögren disease
- Fulminant demyelination:
  - Acute disseminated encephalomyelitis (ADEM)
  - Progressive leukoencephalopathy (PML)
  - Herpes encephalitis
  - Lyme disease

Table 2-2 Painful Ophthalmoplegia

Inflammatory Conditions
- Idiopathic orbital pseudotumor (IOP) or Idiopathic orbital inflammation (IOI)
- Tolosa-Hunt syndrome (form of IOP involving orbital apex and/or cavernous sinus)
- Sarcoidosis

Vascular
- Aneurysm
- Carotid dissection
- Carotid-cavernous fistula

Neoplasm
- Primary intacranial tumors
- Metastases

Infections
- Fungal
- Mycobacterial

Systemic Diseases
- Dysthyroid orbitopathy
- Amyloidosis

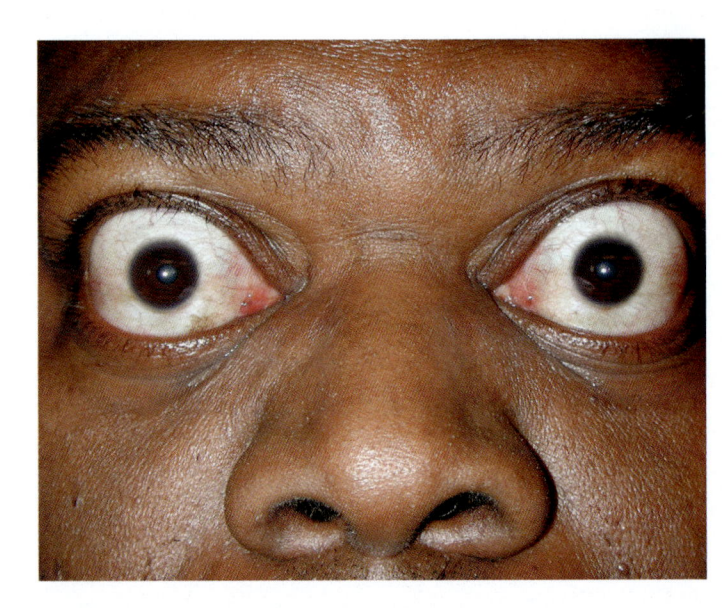

Figure 2-1 Thyroid Ophthalmoplegy
Thyroid ophthalmopathy in a patient with Graves' disease. Note the bilateral proptosis, lid retraction, and scleral show. (Photo courtesy of Jonathan W. Kim, MD, University of California, Irvine.)

Clinically, it may not be possible to diferentiate these two entities without imaging information. Exorbitism refers to a decrease in the total volume of the orbit, resulting in proptosis or exophthalmos.

Clinical proptosis or exophthalmos is measured with an exophthalmometer and is diagnosed whenever there is greater than 21 mm anterior protrusion of the orbital contents beyond the interzygomatic line. Similar guidelines are used for radiologic diagnosis of proptosis, i.e., whenever there is greater than 21 mm anterior protrusion of the orbital contents beyond the interzygomatic line, measured on axial CT or MR images obtained at the level of the ocular lenses.

Proptosis or exophthalmos may be classified into one of three anatomic locations: ocular, retroocular, or extraocular. Ocular or bulbar disorders typically cause exophthalmos, unless there is extraocular spread of an associated mass lesion leading to both exophthalmos and proptosis. Many cases of proptosis are due to primary retrobulbar disorders. Neoplasms of the face, paranasal sinuses, nasal cavities, or frontal cranial fossae can lead to proptosis. Other extraocular causes of proptosis include a variety of infections and inflammations including cellulitis, abscess formation, mucoceles, inflammatory orbital syndrome (IOS), sarcoidosis, or Wegener granulomatosis.

Enophthalmos is a less-than-normal prominence of the globe. The globe may be diffusely small or sunken in as a result of injury or other cause of bone loss in and around the orbit.

Hypertelorism and Hypotelorism

Hypertelorism refers to an increased intraorbital distance. A variety of midline anomalies such as nasal, ethmoidal, or orbital encephaloceles can lead to hypertelorism. Hypotelorism refers to a decreased interorbital distance. Various midface dysplasias or calvarial anomalies such as craniosynostosis can lead to hypotelorism.

Lacrimal Dysfunction

With disturbances of the lacrimal apparatus, there may be excessive tearing referred to as epiphora. Epiphora is a common ophthalmologic problem, and may have a variety of causes. Most commonly, epiphora is due to a blockage of the nasolacrimal sac or duct. Blockage may be secondary to congenital malformation, the presence of stones (dacryolithiasis), or possibly a neoplasm.[2] Epiphora may also be caused by reflex hypersecretion of tears secondary to an infection or by irritation caused by an anatomic lesion, for instance when the patient has an ectropion, entropion, or trichiasis. In some cases, patients may complain of the absence of tears, which is usually secondary to a neurological problem involving cranial nerve VII.[3] This should be distinguished from dry eye syndrome caused by rapid tear evaporation secondary to an imbalance of mucin and oil composition of tears.

Orbital Calcification

The presence of orbital calcification is a sign, not a symptom in a variety of orbital pathologies. Orbital calcification can occur in any structure in the orbit and is often classified into two groups, metastatic or dystrophic. Metastatic calcification refers to the precipitation of calcium phosphate salts attributed to hypercalcemia. The calcium phosphate salts are deposited in normal tissues including the orbit. Dystrophic calcification occurs with cellular injury and may occur after trauma, tissue hypoxia, or tumor growth that exceeds the vascular supply or by vascular stasis. Both types of calcification are easily recognized on CT scans.[4] See **Tables 2-3** and **2-4** for comprehensive lists of differential diagnosis of orbital calcifications.

EMBRYOLOGY

Embryologic development of the orbit and globe is independent of each other. Tissues at the junction of the surface and neural ectoderm give rise to the neural crest cells. These cells will eventually develop into the adnexal structures, bony orbit, fat, and nerve sheaths. The para-axial mesoderm will eventually develop into the vascular endothelium and striated extraocular muscles.

Within the first three weeks after conception, the globe-forming tissues will have been induced by the para-axial mesoderm. The neural ectoderm will have formed the neural plate, which will develop into two neural folds separated by the central neural groove. By the 22nd day of fetal life, the eye-forming tissue on each side of the neural groove is referred to as the optic primordium. The neural folds will eventually meet and form a neural tube.

Evaginations of this neural tube toward the surface ectoderm in the region of the future forebrain are referred to as the optic pits that form by the 24th day. With the closure of the neural tube, later to form the central cavities of the central nervous system, the optic pits have now become optic vesicles. The relationship of the three primordial layers remains intact with the neural ectoderm most central, the neural crest cells in the middle and the surface ectoderm on the outside.

By the 26th day, the optic vesicles are separated from the primitive forebrain by short necks known as the primitive optic stocks. These spherically shaped paired optic vesicles become optic cups as the walls invaginate against each other. The outer layer of these cups will eventually become the retinal pigment epithelium and the inner layer the neurosensory retina. At the same time, cells overlying the optic cup in the surface ectoderm form the lenticular placodes. These placodes will eventually become the ocular lenses on approximately the 33rd day. The "rim" of the optic cup will undergo various changes and develop into the more anterior structures of the eye. Normal formation of the iris is dependent upon the closure of the embryonic fissure, which is completed by the 33rd to 35th day. By the end of the third month, the sclera has surrounded the choroid to form the primitive globe.[5,6]

Vessels

On the inner or ventral surface of the optic cup and extending into the stalk, a fetal embryonic fissure remains. This fissure will allow the hyaloid artery to enter the globe. Under normal circumstances, this fissure is closed between the fifth and seventh

Table 2-3 Dystrophic Orbital Calcification: Differential Diagnosis

Intraocular

- Cataract
- Choroidal osteoma
- Endophthalmitis
- Hyaline plaques
- Idiopathic sclerochoroidal calcification
- Optic nerve drusen
- Phthisis bulbi
- Retinal detachment
- Retinal dysplasia
- Retinoblastoma
- Retinopathy of prematurity
- Retinal astrocytic hamartoma (tuberous sclerosis, neurofibromatosis, linear nevus sebaceous syndrome)
- Retinal angiomatosis (von Hippel-Lindau disease)
- Choroidal hemangioma (Sturge-Weber disease)

Extraocular

Within the Lacrimal Gland Fossa

- Amyloidosis
- Choristoma
- Dermolipoma
- Malignant and benign tumors of the lacrimal gland
- Plasmacytoma
- Pleomorphic adenoma
- Venous varix

Extrinsic to the Lacrimal Gland Fossa

- Amyloid
- Arteriovenous shunt or malformation
- Calcified trochlea
- Cartilaginous tumors
- Cysticercosis
- Epidermoid and dermoid cysts
- Fibro-osseous tumors
- Glioma
- Hemangioma
- Hemangiopericytoma
- Hemorrhage
- Idiopathic orbital pseudotumor
- Lymphangioma
- Lymphoma
- Melanoma
- Meningioma
- Metastatic adenocarcinoma
- Mucocele
- Neuroblastoma
- Neurofibroma
- Orbital bone fragment after trauma
- Teratoma
- Trichinosis
- Venous varix

Modified from Froula PD, Bartley GB, Garrity JA, et al. The differential diagnosis of orbital calcification as detected on computed tomographic scans. Mayo Clin Proc 1993;68:257 and Som PM and Curtin HD. Head and Neck Imaging. 3rd ed. St. Louis, MO: Mosby; 1996:22.

weeks by the development of multipotential cells leaving the hyaloid artery in place. The hyaloid artery is derived from the terminal portion of the ophthalmic artery. This vessel and its branches form the primary vitreous as well as provide nourishment for the eye. By the 33rd day, the primitive vascular system involutes, as does the primary vitreous. The remaining hyaloid branches will eventually become the central retinal vessels.

By the 35th day, endothelial blood spaces give rise to sporadic vessels that are in close proximity to the outer layer of the optic cup. These sporadic vessels coalesce and drain into the supraorbital and infraorbital venous plexuses. Small buds from the ophthalmic artery will eventually form the short and long posterior ciliary arteries. These arterial vessels connect with the coalescence of veins that will eventually develop into the choroid layer of the globe. Vortex veins are formed by the confluence of the collecting venous channels that drain the venous plexuses. These vortex veins will penetrate into the globe at various sites in order to drain the choroid. The choroidal detachments that are seen in patients occur between subjacent vortex veins (**Fig. 2-2**). Development of the vascular system of the entire eye is an ongoing process with the majority of events occurring between the third to sixth months.[5,6]

Optic Nerve and Orbit

By the seventh week, ganglion cells from the retina have migrated into the optic stalk around the hyaloid artery, and glial cells have begun to form. Proliferation of cells into axons and progression toward the forebrain eventually lead to the development of the optic nerve. The optic recess on the floor of the third ventricle is the remnant of the original connection between the eye and the third ventricle.

Table 2-4 Metastatic Orbital Calcification: Differential Diagnosis

Congenital
- Fanconi syndrome
- Milk-alkali syndrome
- Renal tubular acidosis

Endocrine
- Hyperparathyroidism: primary or secondary
- Hypoparathyroidism
- Pseudohypoparathyroidism

Infectious/Inflammatory
- Sarcoidosis
- Cytomegalovirus infection
- Leprosy
- Pyogenic osteomyelitis
- Syphilis
- Toxoplasmosis
- Tuberculosis

Toxic
- Excessive ingestion of calcium phosphate or alkali
- Vitamin D intoxication

Neoplastic
- Bronchogenic carcinoma
- Metastatic involvement of bone
- Multiple myeloma
- Parathyroid adenoma or carcinoma

Modified from Froula PD, Bartley GB, Garrity JA, et al. The differential diagnosis of orbital calcification as detected on computed tomographic scans. Mayo Clin Proc 1993;68:257.

Following development of the orbit cup, the bony orbit is formed and determines the limits of the orbit. The many bones that make up the orbit are mostly derived from cranial neural crest cells. Both the maxillary and frontonasal processes contribute to the walls of the orbit. Partial ossification of the orbit walls is reached by the third month.[5,6]

Adnexal Structures

There are two theories for the development of the extraocular muscles at around the five-week stage. One theory is that the muscles develop from the head somites and grow anteriorly within the orbit. The other theory is that the muscles develop in situ within the orbit and that the individual muscles grow together at the same time.

At approximately the fourth to fifth week of development, mesenchymal condensations develop beneath a proliferating epithelium and give rise to the eyelids. Mesoderm from the second visceral arch give rise to the muscles of the eyelid. The eyelids fuse at approximately 10 weeks.[5,6]

Development of the nasolacrimal drainage apparatus takes place between the fourth and sixth months. The nasolacrimal duct is the result of an irregular cord of ectodermal cells, which via central vacuolization eventually forms the nasolacrimal duct and sac. The persistence of this cord allows for the formation of the nasolacrimal canal. The lacrimal gland is also derived from similar cords of tissue.

ANATOMY

Several anatomic compartments make up the orbit including the bony orbit itself, the globe, the adnexal structures, the optic nerve, and lacrimal apparatus. The orbit can further be divided into extra and intraconal regions and preseptal and postseptal spaces (Fig. 2-3). These distinctions may assist the imaging physician to develop an appropriate differential diagnosis.

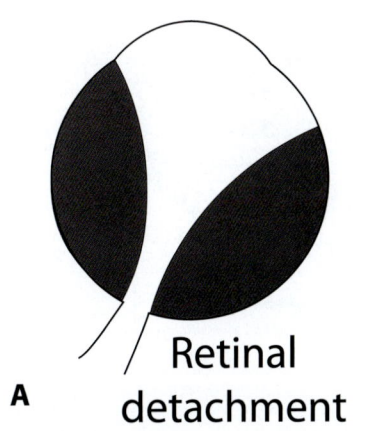

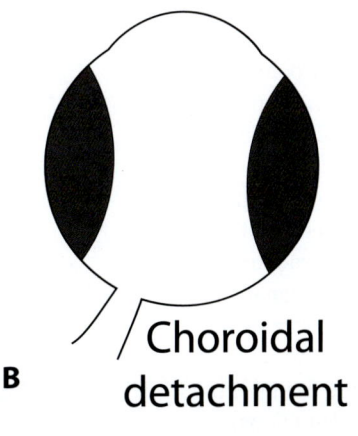

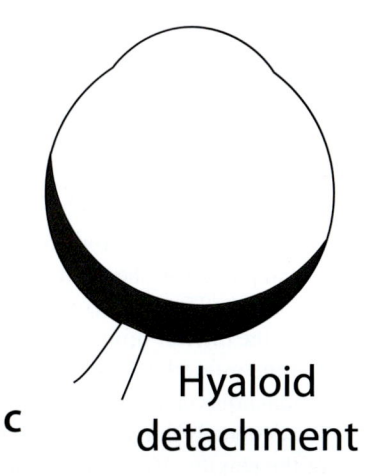

Figure 2-2 Detachments of the Eye
A shows typical choroidal detachment with the margins at the point of venous perforation. B shows the "gull wing" appearance of a classical retinal detachment that spares the optic nerve head. In C the characteristic crescent shape of a hyaloid detachment is illustrated. (Reprinted with permission from Smirniotopoulos JG, Bargallo N, and Mafee MF: Differential diagnosis of leukokoria: radiologic-pathologic correlation. Radiographics 1994;14:1059.)

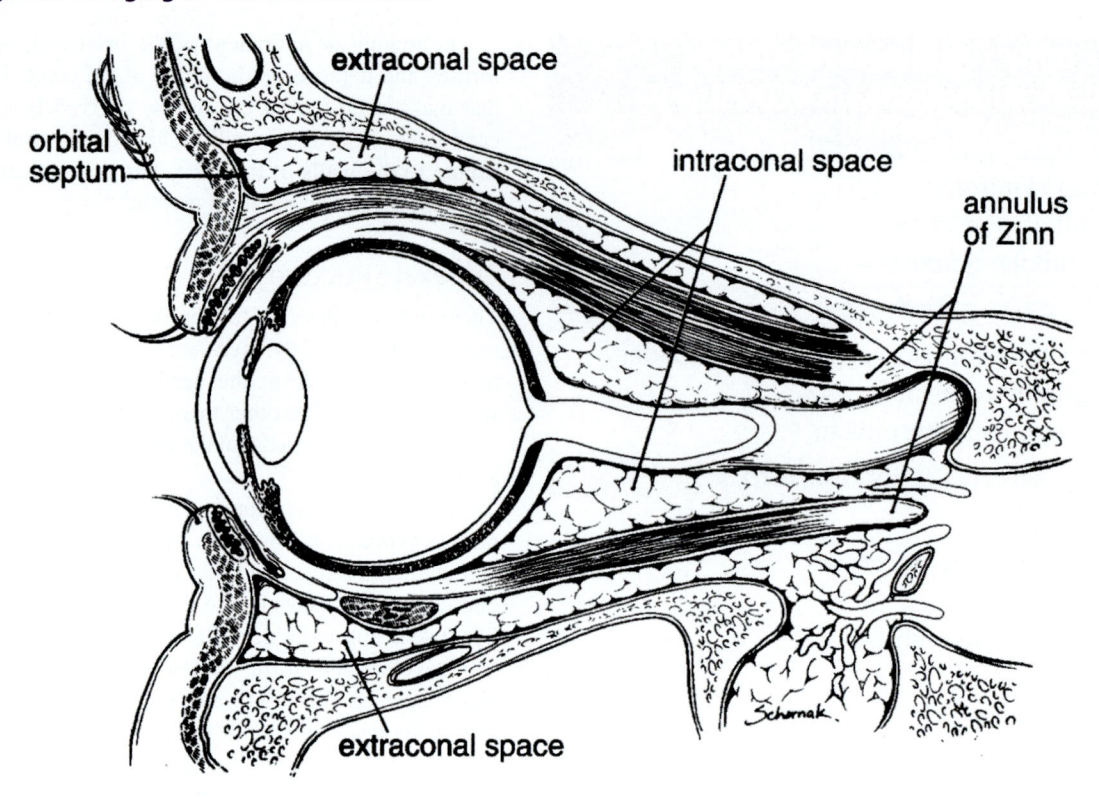

Figure 2-3 Orbital Compartments
(Reprinted with permission and modified from McKenzie JD, Drayer BP: Computed tomography (CT) and magnetic resonance (MR) imaging of the orbits. BNI Q 1993;9:35.)

Bony Orbit and Fibrous Septae

The bony orbit consists of four structures that represent the roof, floor, and medial and lateral walls of the orbit (**Fig. 2-4**). The orbital roof is triangular in shape and formed by the orbital plate of the frontal bone and lesser wing of the sphenoid. It contains the lacrimal fossa, trochlear pit and spine, and optic canal. The structures that pass through the optic canal include the optic nerve, perioptic meninges ophthalmic artery, and sympathetic nerves. The optic canal is separated from the superior orbital fissure by the optic strut. Medially and anteriorly approximately 4 mm from the superior orbital margin is the fovea trochlearis, the site of attachment for the trochlea or pulley of the superior oblique muscle. Composed of hyaline cartilage, the trochlea commonly calcifies with age.[7]

The floor of the orbit formed by the orbital part of the maxilla, orbital process of the zygoma, and the orbital process of the palatine bones. The floor contains the infraorbital groove that runs from the inferior orbital fissure to the infraorbital canal and opens at the infraorbital foramen of the maxilla and carries the infraorbital artery and nerve.

The extremely thin medial wall is formed by the frontal process of the maxilla, lacrimal bone, orbital plate or lamina papyracea of the ethmoid, and body of the sphenoid bone. The medial wall contains the lacrimal groove, which forms a fossa for the lacrimal sac. The groove communicates with the nasolacrimal canal, which is about 1 cm in length and contains the nasolacrimal

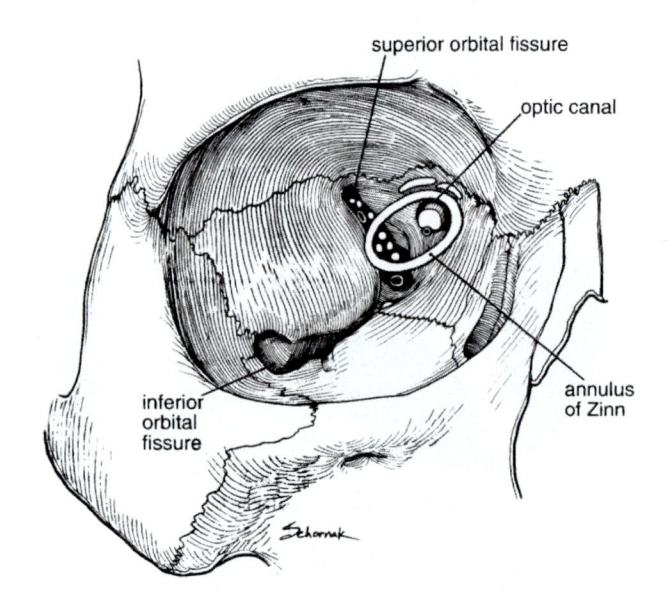

Figure 2-4 Orbital Walls and Apertures
(Reprinted with permission and modified from McKenzie JD, Drayer BP: Computed tomography (CT) and magnetic resonance (MR) imaging of the orbits. BNI Q 1993;9:35.)

duct. Along the frontoethmoidal suture are the anterior and posterior ethmoidal foramina, which carry the anterior and posterior ethmoidal vessels and nerves, respectively. These canals are a way of passage for spread of disease especially infection from the ethmoidal sinuses into the orbit.[6,8,9]

The lateral wall is the thickest and strongest wall of the orbit and is formed by the orbital surfaces of the zygoma in front, and greater wing of the sphenoid bone behind. Both the inferior and superior orbital fissures pass through this wall. The inferior orbital fissure transmits the infraorbital artery and nerve and supplies the venous connection between the inferior ophthalmic vein and pterygoid venous plexus. The superior orbital fissure partially separates the lateral wall from the roof of the orbit and is immediately inferior to the anterior clinoid process that is best seen on coronal scans. The superior orbital fissure communicates with the middle cranial fossa and transmits the third, fourth, sixth, and the ophthalmic portion of the fifth cranial nerves along with superior ophthalmic vein. The apex of the orbit lies at the medial ends of the superior and inferior orbital fissures. Approximately 11 mm below the frontozygomatic suture lies the lateral orbital tubercle of the zygoma. The lateral orbital tubercle is the site of attachment for the check ligament of the lateral rectus muscle, the suspensory ligament of the globe, the lateral palpebral ligament, and the aponeurosis of the levator palpebrae muscle.[7]

The periosteum of the orbit is known as the periorbita and is continuous with the dura and optic nerve sheath posteriorly, and the periosteum of the anterior orbital rim anteriorly. It contributes to the formation of the orbital septum. The orbital septum is a barrier between the lids and the orbit or the preseptal and postseptal compartments. Although the orbital septum is not directly visible on MRI, the preseptal fat lying anteriorly and the orbital fat lying posteriorly define its borders. Clinically, the septum is important, because it limits the spread of infection between the preseptal and postseptal compartments. Other septa in the orbit separate the intra and extraconal fat and contribute to muscular connections. The bulbar fascia, also known as Tenon's capsule, covers the eyeball from the optic nerve to the ciliary muscle.

Extraocular Muscles

The extraocular muscles include the superior, lateral, inferior, and medial recti, the superior and inferior obiques, and the levator palpebrae. A connective tissue spans the recti muscles to form a muscle cone. This fibrous septa separate the retrobulbar space into intra- and extraconal areas (**Fig. 2-5**). The intraconal space lies within the extraocular muscles, while the extraconal space lies outside the extraocular muscles but inside the periorbita of the bony orbit. The four recti muscles orginate from a common tendinous ring, the annulus of Zinn, and extend forward to attach to the sclera at Tenon's capsule. The annulus of Zinn encloses the central superior orbital fissure and optic foramen and transmits the optic nerve, ophthalmic artery, third and sixth cranial nerves. The superior rectus is the longest extraocular muscle and the medial rectus has the largest diameter.

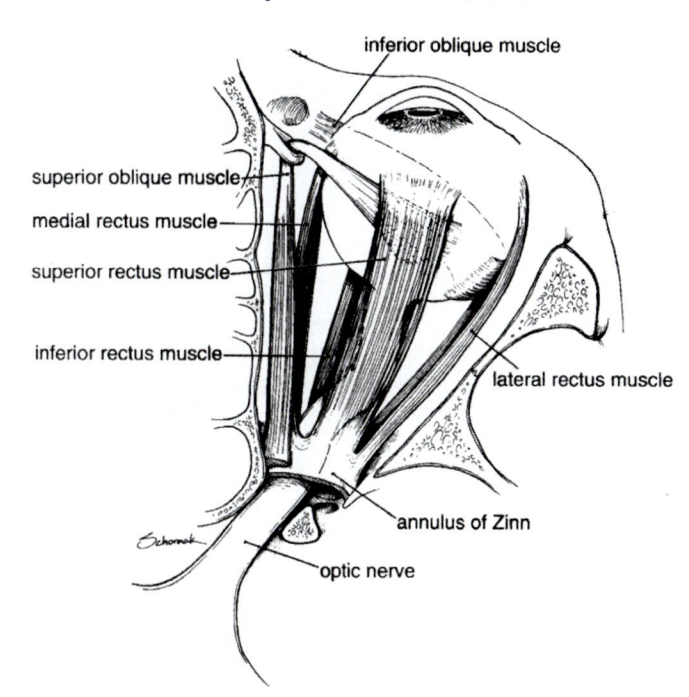

Figure 2-5 Extraocular Muscles
(Reprinted with permission from McKenzie JD, Drayer BP: Computed tomography (CT) and magnetic resonance (MR) imaging of the orbits. BNI Q 1993; 9:35.)

The inferior and superior oblique and levator palpebrae superioris muscles do not originate at the annulus of Zinn. The inferior oblique is the only extraocular muscle to originate anteriorly from the upper surface of the maxilla lateral to the nasolacrimal canal. It lies inferior to the inferior rectus muscle. The superior oblique muscle is the thinnest extraocular muscle and has a tendon that passes through the trochlea at the anteromedial border of the orbit. It lies superior to the medial rectus muscle and arises from the periorbita near the apex of the orbit. The levator palpebra superioris muscle lies above the superior rectus and controls the eyelid.[9] It can be separated from the superior rectus in coronal views, but is typically imaged together with the superior rectus on axial views.[8] Most of the extraocular muscles are innervated by cranial nerve III (oculomotor) except for the superior oblique, which is innervated by cranial nerve IV (trochlear) and the lateral rectus muscle, which is innervated by cranial nerve VI (abducens).

The extraocular muscles are isointense on most MR sequences. These muscles show intense enhancement.[8] The intense enhancement of the extraocular muscles in comparison to other skeletal muscle is probably due to the rich vascularity and increased extracellular space between the muscular bundles when compared to other skeletal muscles in the body.[10,11]

Neurovascular Structures

The optic nerve is a direct extension of the central nervous system (CNS) and therefore the optic nerve sheath complex is enveloped by the meninges (**Fig. 2-6**). There may be cerebrospinal

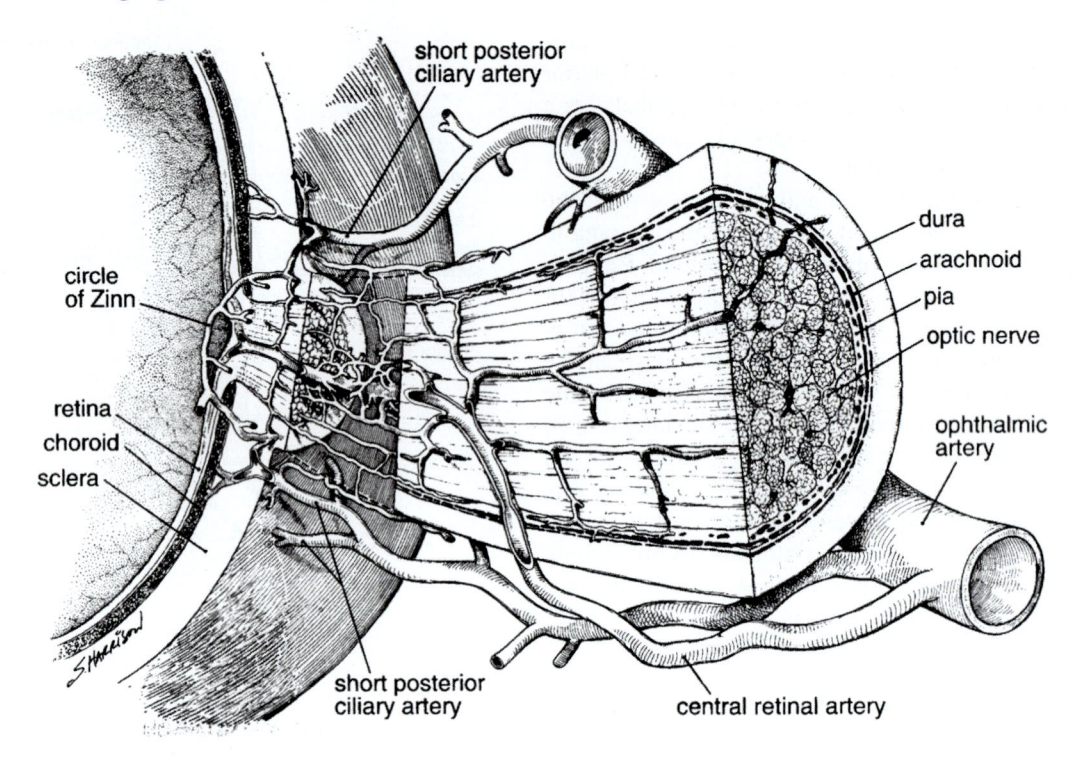

Figure 2-6 Optic Nerve and Blood Supply
(Reprinted with permission from Levy DL, Zabramski JM, and Hodak JA: Current diagnosis and management of traumatic optic neuropathies. BNI Q 1993;9:30.)

fluid (CSF) extending from the CNS to surround the optic nerve, which may be visualized on complex imaging studies. This extension of the CNS may facilitate the extension of intracranial pathology into the orbit.[8]

The optic nerve has three segments: intraorbital, intracanalicular, and intracranial. The nerve connects the third ventricle with the retina (**Fig. 2-7**). It is the narrowest in diameter at the optic foramen measuring approximately 4 to 9 mm, but often is imaged with oblique sections that may cause artificial enlargement due to the course it travels. The general course is ten degrees off the normal anterior-posterior axis and is often sinusoidal as well in order to allow for free movement of the attached eyeball.[6,9] The optic nerve head appears as a slight prominence just nasal to the posterior pole of the globe on axial imaging.

The other cranial nerves enter the orbit through various foramina innervate the various structures of the orbit via both intra and extraconal routes of travel (**Table 2-5** and **Fig. 2-8**). On T1W MR scans the nerves have an isointense or slightly low intense signal.

Vessels are easily visualized within the orbit as flow voids on T1W MR scans contrasted against the intraorbital fat. Most of the blood supply to the orbital structures is derived from the ophthalmic artery, which arises from the internal carotid artery and anastomose with the external carotid artery. It enters the orbit via the optic canal and travels intraconally below the optic nerve (**Fig. 2-6**). The ophthalmic artery gives off several branches and eventually splits into the supratrochlear and dorsal nasal arteries.[9]

The superior ophthalmic vein is the largest vessel in the orbit measuring 2.5 to 3 mm in diameter. It is formed by the supraorbital and angular veins and exits the orbit intraconally via the superior orbital fissure above the optic nerve. The inferior ophthalmic vein is typically not visualized on MR and originates as a plexus on the floor of the orbit to drain either directly into the cavernous sinus or into the superior ophthalmic vein.[9]

Ocular Structures

Most of the components of the globe can be identified using MR imaging techniques. The globe has three layers: the fibrous outer sclera, the middle uvea, and the inner retina (**Fig. 2-9**). The sclera appears as a low-intensity, thin structure surrounding the globe that extends from the corneal margin to the optic nerve. The cornea is also a low-intensity structure, but may have a hyperintense rim due to adherent tears. The uvea is made up of three separate components: iris, ciliary body, and choroid. The iris lies most anteriorly. The ciliary body lies in the middle. The choroid continues from its junction with the ciliary body, known as the ora serrata, to the optic nerve in the posterior globe. The choroid will appear hyperintense on T1W MR scans. The retina is a hyperintense structure on T1W MR scans and is continuous with the optic nerve. It has two layers, which are not discernable under normal circumstances: the internal sensory and external retinal-pigmented epithelium.

The lens divides the globe into anterior and posterior chambers. Its shape varies from spherical to elliptical with increasing age. On MR imaging, the lens appears hypointense. The anterior

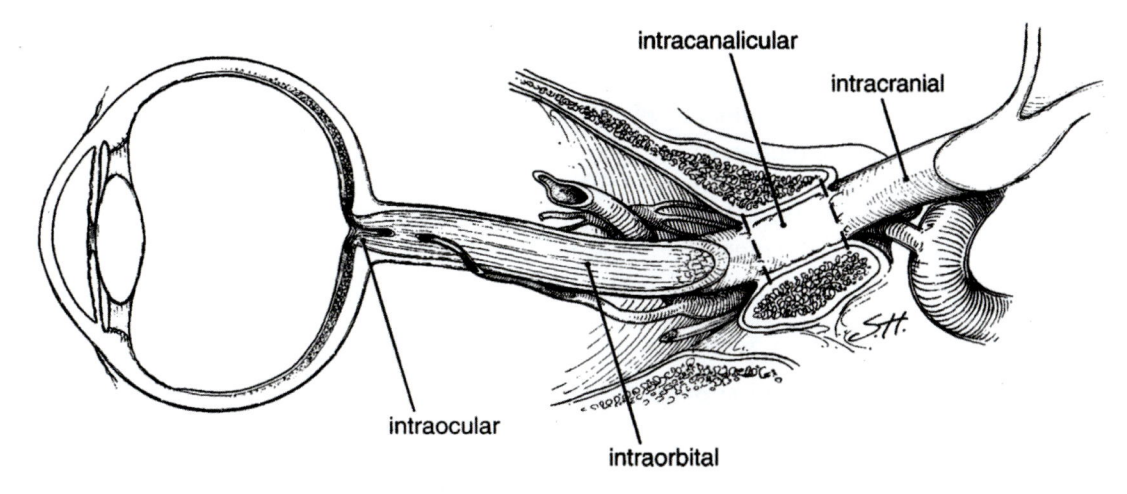

Figure 2-7 Characteristic Portions of the Optic Nerve
(Reprinted with permission from Levy DL, Zabramski JM, and Hodak JA: Current diagnosis and management of traumatic optic neuropathies. BNI Q 1993;9:30.)

chamber contains aqueous humor, whereas the posterior chamber contains vitreous humor. The vitreous humor constitutes two-thirds of the volume of the eye and is made up of almost 99% water. It appears hypointense on T1W MR, and hyperintense on T2W MR scans.

Lacrimal Apparatus and Eyelids

The lacrimal apparatus extends from the anterior portion of the orbit. The lacrimal gland consists of two lobes: the palpebral and the orbital. The anterosuperolateral orbit is home to the orbital lobe that lies in the lacrimal fossa. A smaller structure, the palpebral lobe extends out of the lacrimal fossa into the upper eyelid. At the inferomedial margin of the orbit, the lacrimal sac receives the tears drained via the inferior and superior canaliculi in the lower and upper lid margins, respectively. The nasolacrimal duct leaves the sac to drain into the inferior nasal meatus inferior to the inferior turbinate.

The eyelids consist of the tarsal plates, orbicularis oculi muscles, levator palpebrae superioris muscles, inferior tarsal muscles, canthal tendons, and Whitnall ligaments. The tarsal plates serve to maintain the shape of the eyelids and may appear hyperintense to surrounding tissues on MR imaging. Whitnall ligament, a structure that divides the lacrimal gland into two lobes along with the levator palpebrae aponeurosis may be seen outlined by fat on MR imaging. This ligament extends from the trochlea on the medial orbital rim to the lateral orbital wall.[9]

Table 2-5 Cranial Nerves

Cranial Nerve	Divisions	Structures Innervated
Oculomotor (III)	Superior	Superior rectus muscle, levator palpebrae superioris muscle
	Inferior	Medial rectus muscle, inferior rectus muscle, inferior oblique muscle
		Ciliary branches: sphincter papillae and ciliary muscles
Trochlear (IV)		Superior oblique muscle
Trigeminal (V)	Ophthalmic (V1)	*Nasociliary branch*: sensory for the globe, ciliary ganglion, ethmoidal sinus, nasal cavity, medial upper eyelid, lacrimal sac
		Frontal branch: sensory for the upper eyelid and scalp including forehead
		Lacrimal branch: sensory for the lacrimal gland and adjacent conjunctiva, upper eyelid
Abducens (VI)		Lateral rectus muscle

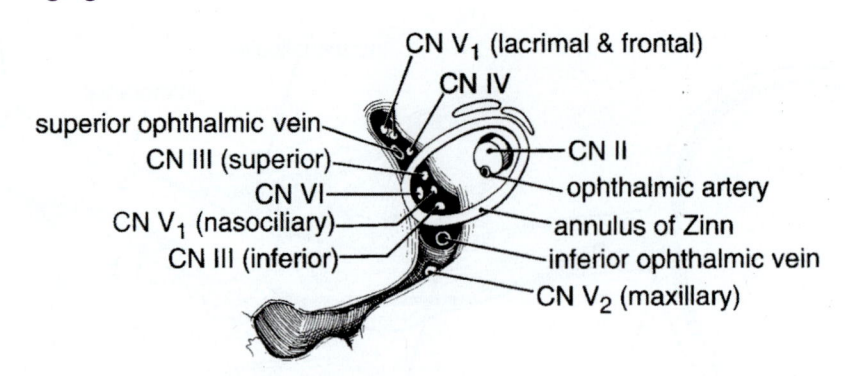

Figure 2-8 Transiting Neurovascular Structures of the Orbit
Diagram of the neurovascular structures as they enter and exit the orbit through the superior orbital fissure, optic canal, and inferior orbital fissure. (Reprinted with permission from McKenzie JD and Drayer BP: Computed tomography (CT) and magnetic resonance (MR) imaging of the orbits. BNI Q 1993;9:35.)

CONGENITAL AND DEVELOPMENTAL DISORDERS

Congenital and developmental lesions of the eye often occur in conjunction with various other developmental abnormalities of the body. Lesions and syndromes affecting the eye as a whole will be discussed in this section. Lesions affecting specific regions of the orbit will be discussed in subsequent sections.

Disorders of the Globe

Anophthalmia is the congenital absence of the eye. This rare occurrence is sporadic, but may be associated with other congenital abnormalities such as trisomies 13 to 15, Klinefelter syndrome, and other complex craniofacial malformations.[12] The abnormality is typically bilateral and occurs when the optic pit fails to form a vesicle. All structures that arise from the neuroectoderm tissue are absent in such cases of primary anophthalmia. However, the extraocular muscles, eyelids, and lacrimal apparatus (structures not derived from the neuroectoderm) are usually present in primary anophthalmia.

If there is gross malformation of the forebrain along with other structures within the orbit, the anomaly is referred to as secondary anophthalmia. If the vesicle forms but then degenerates, the anomaly is referred to as tertiary anophthalmia. The secondary and tertiary forms of this malformation can occur in conjunction with malformation of various adjacent structures arising from the anterior neural tube.[6,9,12]

Cryptophthalmos or "hidden eye" refers to a rare failure of eyelid development. An affected patient has no development of the lid fold and there is absence of the eyelids (ablepharia), eyelashes, meibomian glands, lacrimal glands, lacrimal puncta, and eyebrows. The cornea undergoes metaplastic change to skin. This abnormal skin represents what is clinically observed covering the eyes instead of the eyelids. Imaging is performed to determine the condition and presence of other eye structures. Typically, there is disorganization of structures both anteriorly and posteriorly with lens calcification. This abnormality is commonly associated with other craniofacial, otological, rhinological, urogenital, and extremity malformations.[6,13]

Microphthalmos describes an eye that is smaller than normal. It occurs in many forms and can be divided into three basic types: pure, simple, and complex. Microphthalmos may result from intrauterine toxoplasmosis or rubella, retrolental hyperplasia, radiation therapy, infection, and trauma.

Commonly, microphthalmos is associated with other malformations and syndromes such as Lowe's disease (bilateral microphthalmos and cataracts, abnormalities in the white matter, and renal disease), trisomy 13, Norrie syndrome (see section below), fetal alcohol syndrome, myotonic dystrophy, achrondoplasia, oculodentodigital dysplasia, craniofacial abnormalities, and colobomatous cysts. Imaging typically reveals a small globe and a small, poorly formed orbit.[6,9,12]

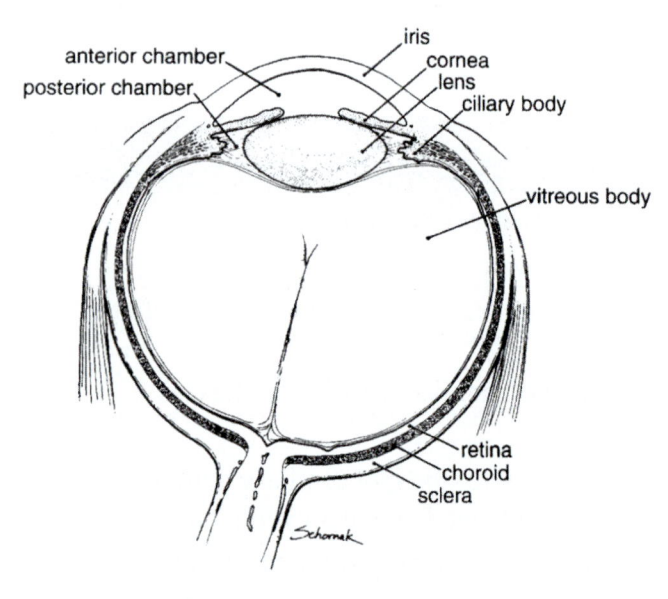

Figure 2-9 Axial View of the Globe
(Reprinted with permission from Levy DL, Zabramski JM, and Hodak JA: Current diagnosis and management of traumatic optic neuropathies. BNI Q 1993;9:30.)

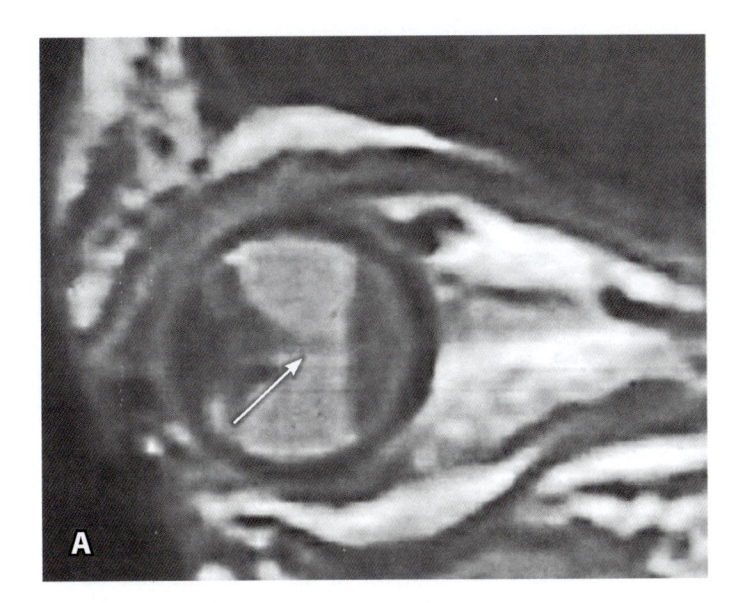

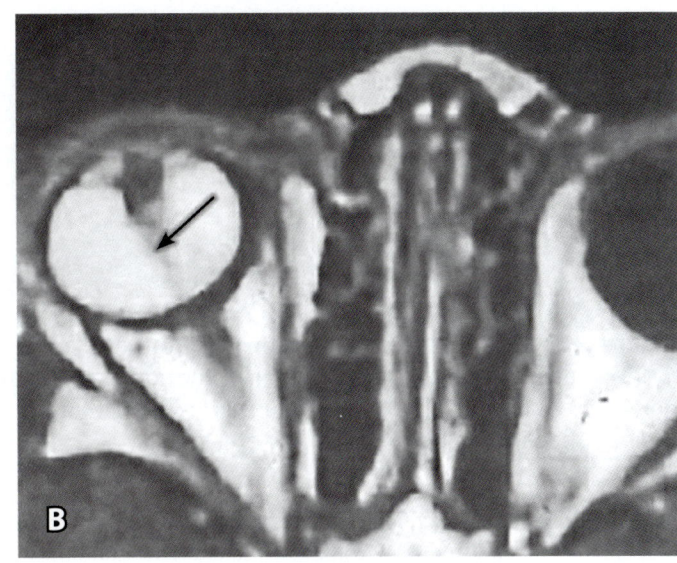

Figure 2-10 Microphthalmos, PHPV

Persistent hypoplastic primary vitreous (PHPV) with microphthalmos of the right eye. There is hemorrhage filling the vitreous, evident by high-signal intensities on both the sagittal T1W (**A**) and axial T2W (**B**) MR images. There is a persistent structure in the center of the vitreous that represents the canal for the hyaloid artery (*arrows,* **A** and **B**), which normally involutes in fetal life but may persist following birth. The connection between the contents of the anterior chamber and the dependent subhyaloid hemorrhage simulates the silhouette of a champagne glass. The eye lacks development, is nonfunctional, and contains both embryonic remnants and blood products.

Pure microphthalmos, or nanophthalmos, refers to a small eye containing a lens of "normal" volume with no gross structural defects. It is thought to result from an arrest in ocular development after the fetal fissure has closed. Because the size of the lens is normal, patients with nanophthalmic eyes display a shallow anterior chamber and are prone to attacks of angle-closure glaucoma. Thickening of the sclera around the exits of the vortex veins may contribute to retinal and choroidal effusion. In addition to hyperopia, vision loss may develop later in life due to secondary complications of this disorder. Nanophthalmos is generally bilateral and these eyes are usually deeply set in shallow orbits.

Simple microphthalmos refers to a small eye that is otherwise normal. Most cases are bilateral and occur sporadically. Approximately 50% of patients with simple microphthalmos have an associated systemic developmental abnormality. Most patients are hyperopic but otherwise have normal vision. The complications that are seen with nanophthalmos do not occur in this disorder. Simple microphthalmos represents a retardation in growth that occurs once the primary optic vesicle has formed and invaginated. It has been caused in animal experiments by radiation, mechanical stimulation, and chemicals.

The term "complex microphthalmos" denotes a small, deformed eye. The malformation(s) may occur as an isolated ocular entity or as part of an associated systemic disorder. Associated ocular deformities can include anterior segment maldevelopment, hyperplastic primary vitreous (**Fig. 2-10**), and other lens, vitreous or retinal abnormalities. Complex microphthalmos may be unilateral or bilateral, and the vision can range from normal to no light perception. Both sporadic and hereditary forms are known.

Microphthalmos with coloboma is one specific type of complex microphthalmos and is caused by an incomplete closure of the embryonic fissure (**Fig. 2-11**). It may also occur as both a sporadic and hereditary form. It may associated with a number of systemic diseases including CHARGE syndrome (Choanal Atresia, Posterior Coloboma, Heart defect, choanal Atresia, Retardation, Genital and Ear anomalies). Recognition of this entity when evaluating a child with microphthalmos is important as the heart defects in the CHARGE association can be lethal. Autosomal dominant colobomatous microphthalmos occurs without an associated systemic abnormality and has variable expressivity and penetrance. Family members of affected patients should receive appropriate genetic counseling.

Macrophthalmos is defined as enlargement of the eye. It is most commonly seen with infantile glaucoma or myopia. When macrophthalmos is present with myopia, there is usually an elongation and enlargement of the globe in the anteroposterior axis. Orbital infection, Grave's disease, or staphyloma may also cause this deformity. It may be unilateral or bilateral and the patient will usually have amblyopia as well. In addition to the oval-shaped eyes demonstrated on imaging, thinning of the sclera is sometimes noted.

If imaging reveals an enlarged globe with a "floppy" contour, a connective tissue disorder such as Marfan syndrome, Ehler-Danlos syndrome, Weill-Marchesani syndrome, or homocystinuria may be the underlying cause. There is usually bilateral

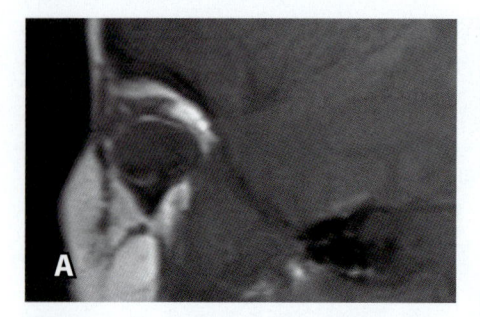

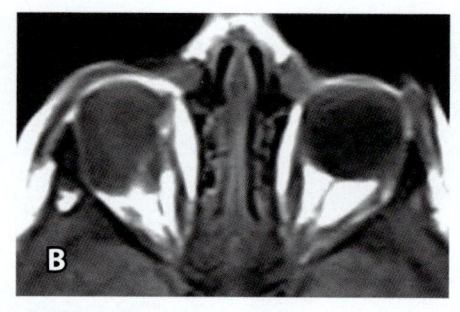

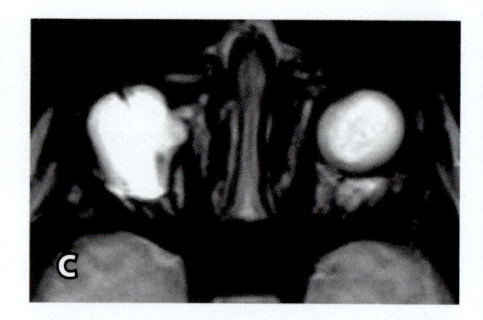

Figure 2-11 Colobomatous Cyst with Microphthalmia
Colobomatous cyst with microphthalmia of the right eye. Sagittal T1W (**A**), axial T1W (**B**), and axial T2W (**C**) MR images demonstrate enlargement of the right orbital contents. However, the colobomatous cyst occupies most of the space, while the native globe is diminished in size.

macrophthalmia and frequently other associated ocular abnormalities.[9,14] In children, the compliant sclera will sometimes also allow intraocular masses to cause macrophthalmos and proptosis.

When there is enlargement of the eye due to increased intraocular pressure, the lesion is referred to as buphthalmos. Elevation of intraocular pressure caused by abnormal outflow or increased production of the aqueous humor can lead to an increase in the size of the globe. Buphthalmos is typically a bilateral condition found in children with glaucoma and may or may not be associated with other abnormalities. There may be a congenitally abnormal trabecular meshwork or secondary blockage of the canal of Schlemm (the canal responsible for aqueous humor resorption). Blockages of this canal may be seen in patients with neurofibromatosis I, and other neurocutaneous syndromes. On imaging studies, the enlargement of the globe may be diffuse and not uniform, and possible responsible pathology may also be identified.[9,14]

Coloboma and Colobomatous Cyst

A coloboma is an absence or defect in the ocular structures due to improper or incomplete closure of the embryonic fissures (**Fig. 2-12**). Colobomas constitute 2% of congenital ocular anomalies, are bilateral in just over one-half of the cases, and inherited in an autosomal dominant pattern. The sclera, uvea, retina, and optic nerve are typically involved. When the anterior segment of the eye is involved, vision may be maintained, but is usually reduced when the posterior segment is involved.

A colobomatous cyst typically arises in a microphthalmic eye due to proliferation of the inner layer of the retina at the border of the unfused embryonic fissure. This proliferation of cells protrudes outward forming a cyst, usually posterior to the globe, that can alter both the size and shape of the disc (**Figs. 2-13** and **2-14**). On imaging studies, this cyst is differentiated from other abnormalities by the inferonasal location of the narrowed neck of the cyst, at the point of attachment to the globe. The cyst may appear hypointense on T1W images and hyperintense on T2W images (**Fig. 2-11**). The orbit is diffusely enlarged on the side of the colobomatous cyst (**Table 2-6**).

A colobomatous cyst must be distinguished from a congenital cystic eye that results from the failure of the optic vesicle to invaginate resulting in a cystic structure instead of a globe. The cyst may be lined by primitive retinal cells and associated with

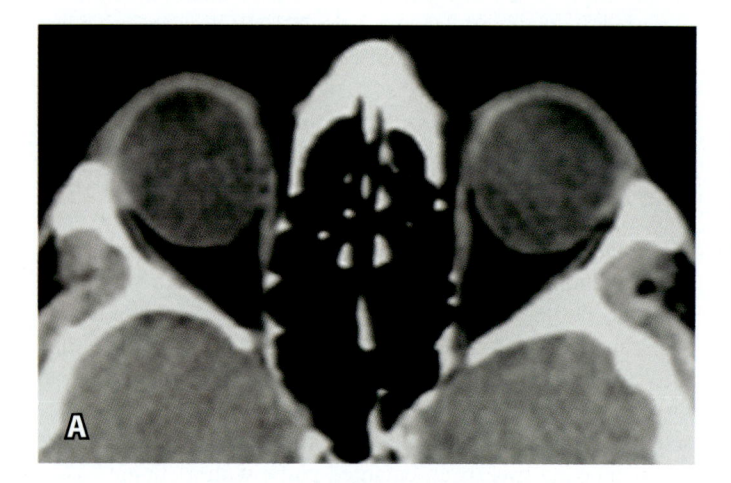

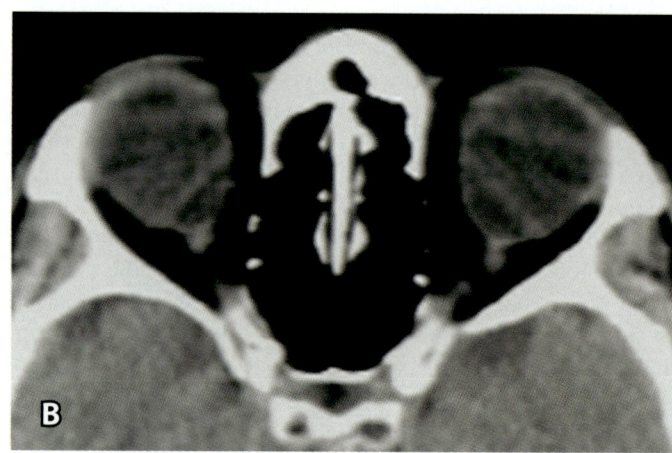

Figure 2-12 Retinal Colobomas: Bilateral
Colobomas of the posterior portions of the globes bilaterally in a middle-aged male. Axial CT scans with contrast (**A–B**) demonstrate a posterior bulge of the globes with absence of the usual hyperdense rim of the globes in this area.

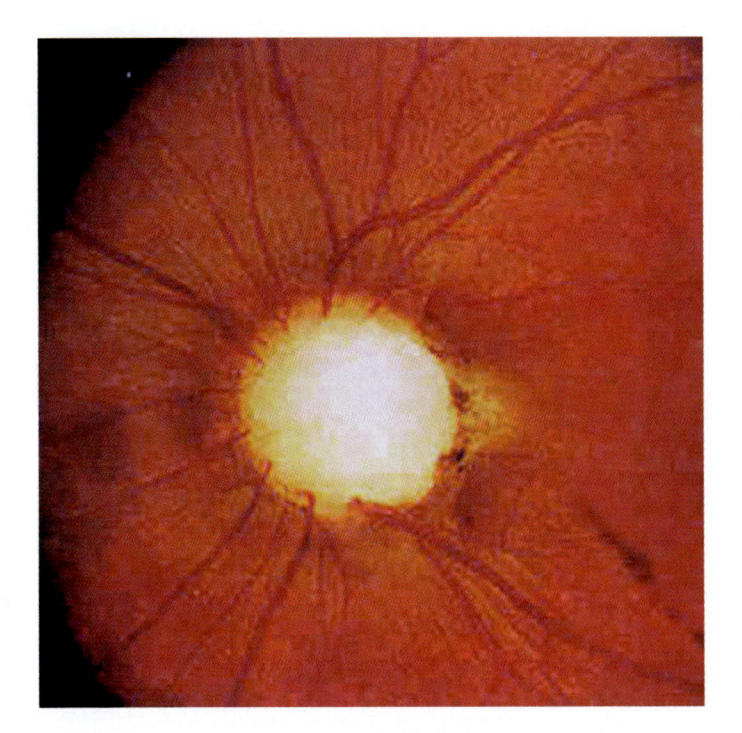

Figure 2-13 Retinal Colobomatous Cyst
Fundus photo of a retinal colobomatous cyst. Note that the blood vessels arise from the periphery of the disc rather than from the center. (Photo courtesy of Jonathan W. Kim, MD, University of California, Irvine.)

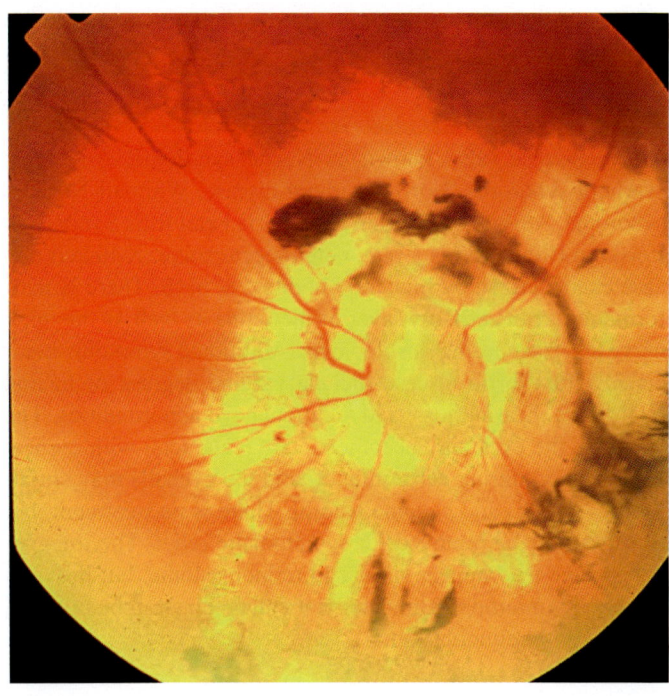

Figure 2-14 Optic Disc Coloboma
Fundus photo of the left eye shows a large, funnel-shaped, excavated disc with central white glial tissue surrounded by areas of elevated pigmentation forming a ring, resembling the appearance of a morning glory flower. (Photo courtesy of Jonathan W. Kim, MD, University of California, Irvine.)

remnants of the optic nerve stalk, lens, and extraocular muscles. Imaging appearance is consistent with a cystic structure with internal septations. The lesion appears isointense to brain on T1W and hyperintense on T2W MR images (**Table 2-6**).

A coloboma involving the optic disc is referred to as the "morning glory" lesion. In such a case, there is an enlarged, posteriorly displaced or excavated optic disc and associated abnormalities of the bordering structures. The characteristic fundoscopic finding of the funnel-shaped, lighter colored area of the optic disc with the surrounding abnormal chorioretinal layer resembles the morning glory flower and assists in the diagnosis (**Fig. 2-14**). Optic nerve colobomas have been associated with encephaloceles, microphthalmos, and agenesis of the corpus callosum that may be observed on imaging. In addition, the

Table 2-6 Distinguishing Colobomatous v. Congenital Cysts	
Colobomatous Cysts	**Congenital Cysts**
• Attached to orbit inferonasally via a narrowed neck • Hypointense on T1W • Hyperintense on T2W • Orbit is diffusely enlarged on the side of cyst • Associated with encephaloceles, microphthalmos, agenesis of the corpus callosum • Outpouching has similar attenuation to vitreous (**Fig. 2-11**)	• Lined by primitive retinal cells • Associated with remnants of optic nerve stalk, lens, and extraocular muscles • Resembles the morning glory flower on ophthalmic examination • Imaging shows cystic structure with internal septations • Isointense to brain on T1W • Hyperintense on T2W
Secondary to proliferation of the inner layer of the retina at the border of the unfused fissure	Secondary to failure of the optic vesicle to invaginate

colobomatous outpouching will appear similar in attenuation to the vitreous.[6,9,15–17]

Norrie Disease

Norrie disease (also known as Norrie syndrome, Andersen-Warburg syndrome, Norrie-Warburg disease, Whitnall-Norman syndrome, Atrophia bulborum hereditaria Fetal Iritis Syndrome, Episkopi Blindness) is a rare, neurodegenerative, X-linked disease characterized by bilateral blindness at birth. There is malformation of the sensory layer of the retina as well as the optic nerve and tract during development. Additional symptoms associated with Norrie disease include varyine degrees of mental retardation, hearing loss, and additional eye abnormalities. The lenses of the eyes may become cloudy (cataracts) with corneal opacification during early infancy, and the eyeballs may shrink (phthisis bulbi) and become painful. There is no treatment, but the eyes may be removed for symptomatic relief. The imaging appearance may appear similar to retinoblastoma, but the eyes are usually microphthalmic and not enlarged as can be noted in patients with retinoblastoma.[6,18]

Cephalocele

A cephalocele of the orbit is usually of the naso-orbital variety. There is an osseous defect in the medial aspect of the orbit that allows the cranial contents to bulge through the defect. Rarely, the defect lies in the pars orbitalis portion of the frontal bone, producing a superior or lateral cephalocele. Although basisphenoidal encephaloceles do not directly involve the orbit, the patient may demonstrate visual symptoms due to a stretching of the optic nerves and optic chiasm.

A cephalocele of the orbit is likely to produce proptosis. The contents of the sac on imaging may show obvious brain tissue or contents with attenuation similar to CSF. There may be a bony defect that is identifiable or the mass may appear attached to the skull. A diagnosis must be made to avoid the potential complications that would be incurred from a biopsy of a lesion of this nature.[9,16,19]

Proteus Syndrome

Proteus syndrome is a rare, sporadic syndrome that occurs with equal distribution between the sexes. Proteus syndrome is due to a lethal somatic mutation that is only expressed in a mosaic pattern allowing for survival of those affected, as the disease never involves a complete organ system or the entire body. Hamartomatous changes are observed throughout the mesoderm and ectoderm of the body. The syndrome has some similarities to both neurofibromatosis and tuberous sclerosis. Noted findings include mental retardation, macrocrania, hemimegaencephaly, periventricular calcifications, subependymal calcified nodules, skull exostoses, asymmetric limbs with gigantism of the hands and feet, skin lesions, venous thrombosis, and increased incidence of neoplasms. The ocular manifestations that have been reported include macro or microphthalmos, myopia, strabismus, cataracts, retinal detachment, chorioretinitis, nystagmus, heterochromia of the irises, and anisocoria. The disease is progressive and without treatment at the current time.[14,20]

EXTRACONAL LESIONS

The extraconal lesions of the orbit include most forms of orbital infections. When and if these infections invade the intraconal space they are seen as combined lesions of both the extraconal and intraconal spaces. Many of the noninfectious inflammatory afflictions of the orbit are primarily seen in the extraconal space with variable involvement of the intraconal space. These noninfectious inflammatory lesions are also discussed in this chapter. The extraorbital osseous and fibro-osseous lesions that secondarily invade the orbits are fully discussed in Chapter 10.[24–26]

Orbital Infections

Orbital infections can be broken down into five clinical stages or groups that form useful categories in determining treatment and prognosis[33] (**Table 2-7**). An orbital infection may first be evident as inflammation and edema of the skin of the anterior orbit that may progress to cellulitis. The orbital septum acts as a barrier to spread of infection from the preseptal to the postseptal area. A subperiosteal abscess or subperiosteal elevation may develop and result in an orbital abscess.

An abscess that has spread behind the muscle cone may cause "orbital apex syndrome." In this syndrome, the nerves and vessels that pass through the optic foramen and superior orbital fissure are affected causing visual loss and ophthalmoplegia. This syndrome may result from direct spread of disease from the sphenoid and ethmoid sinuses and may cause little preseptal inflammation. The final stage of intracranial spread of the infection can then lead to cavernous sinus thrombosis.[30–33]

Cellulitis

Preseptal cellulitis refers to infection and inflammation located anterior to the orbital septum without globe involvement (**Fig. 2-15**). It typically originates from a neighboring skin infection or trauma, whereas 70% to 80% of postseptal infections are secondary to paranasal sinus disease and occurs more commonly in children.[30,31] The second most common cause is from trauma, usually with the introduction of a foreign body into the orbit. Other causes include spread of an odontogenic infection, post surgical infection, septic emboli, and implants.

Orbital cellulitis describes infection posterior to the orbital septum and involves the globe. It usually spreads from a preexisting infection such as paranasal sinusitis, dacryocystitis, dacryoadenitis, but can also be caused by dental or intracranial infections, penetrating trauma, and postorbital surgery.

Several orbital infections develop as complications of sinonasal infections (**Table 2-8**). The ethmoid sinus is the most common source, followed by the maxillary sinus. This is probably due to the thinness of the bones in this region or the presence of congenital dehiscence or anatomical foramina that can facilitate the spread of infection into the orbit. Due to the later pneumatization of the frontal and sphenoidal sinuses, spread of infection from these sources is seen in an older age group. Spread from the frontal sinus is most likely to occur through the valveless

Table 2-7 Classification of Orbital Cellulitis

State	Clinical Findings
Inflammatory edema	Eyelid swelling and erythema
Preseptal cellulitis (Group I)	Eyelid swelling and erythema associated with inflammatory soft-tissue thickening of the orbit anterior to the orbital septum.
	Chemosis may be present. Globe typically remains uninvolved.
Postseptal cellulitis (Group II)	True orbital cellulitis. Diffuse edema of the orbital contents. Proptosis, chemosis, decreased extraocular movement, pain on eye movements, and impaired visual acuity may be noted.
Subperiosteal abscess (Group III)	A collection of inflammatory infiltrates and pus separates the periosteum from the orbital bones. Usually involves the medial orbital wall adjacent to the ethmoid sinuses.
	Globe is often displaced by the abscess and proptotic.
	Ocular motility and vision may also be affected.
Orbital abscess (Group IV)	Abscess formation within the orbital fat or muscles results in more severe proptosis, ophthalmoplegia, and visual loss.
	Displacement of the globe occurs in opposite direction of the abscess.
Cavernous sinus thrombosis (Group V)	Proptosis and ophthalmoplegia with development of similar signs on the contralateral side.
	Associated with cranial nerve palsies (CN III, IV, V, VI) and visual loss.

facial veins, and spread from the sphenoid sinus is probably via the intracanalicular nerve.[30,31]

Clinically, patients may exhibit sinus tenderness, fever, headache, orbital edema, and ocular pain. In children, orbital cellulitis is the most common cause of proptosis.[31] With more extensive involvement of the more posterior eye structures and extension into the cavernous sinus, one may observe venous congestion, cranial nerve palsies, limitation of movement of the extraocular muscles, and papilledema. The lateral rectus is usually the first extraocular muscle to exhibit signs of cavernous sinus thrombosis and cranial nerve involvement. Initial treatment is with oral antibiotics for preseptal infection and intravenous antibiotics for postseptal infection. If medical management fails as evidenced by progressive cranial neuropathy or if intracranial extension is present, surgical drainage is performed to drain any abscesses. Cavernous sinus thrombosis should be treated with anticoagulants as well as antibiotics. Complications of cavernous sinus extension include intracranial extension with cerebritis and brain abscess.[30,31,34]

The etiological agents responsible for orbital infections include bacterial, viral, fungal, and parasitic agents. Staphylococcus aureus and Streptococcus species are the most common bacterial causes, but in children, Haemophiles influenzae should also be considered. Viral causes often originate in the lacrimal apparatus and include mumps, influenza, Epstein-Barr, and herpes simplex. Mycotic orbital infection (Aspergillus, Cryptococcus) are usually seen in patients with diabetes mellitus, metabolic acidosis, malignancy, or immunocompromise (AIDS, steroid, radiation or chemotherapy, septicemia). Cysticercosis and Echinococcus may also cause orbital infection in the appropriate geographical regions.

Although MR is the imaging modality of choice to evaluate the full extent of an orbital infection, CT scans may identify the causative sinusitis with evidence of air–fluid levels and mucosal thickening within the sinus and enlargement of the extraocular muscle adjacent to the affected sinus. There may be ophthalmic vein or optic nerve enlargement, orbital fat infiltration, or a gross abscess that appears as a central low-density collection with an enhancing rim (**Table 2-9**).

Orbital cellulitis appears as a low signal region with diffuse post contrast enhancement on T1W MR images (**Fig. 2-16**) and increased signal in the orbital fat on T2W MR images.

Table 2-8 Orbital Complications of Sinonasal Infections

- Cellulitis (pre- or postseptal)
- Subperiosteal abscess
- Retrobulbar abscess
- Episcleritis

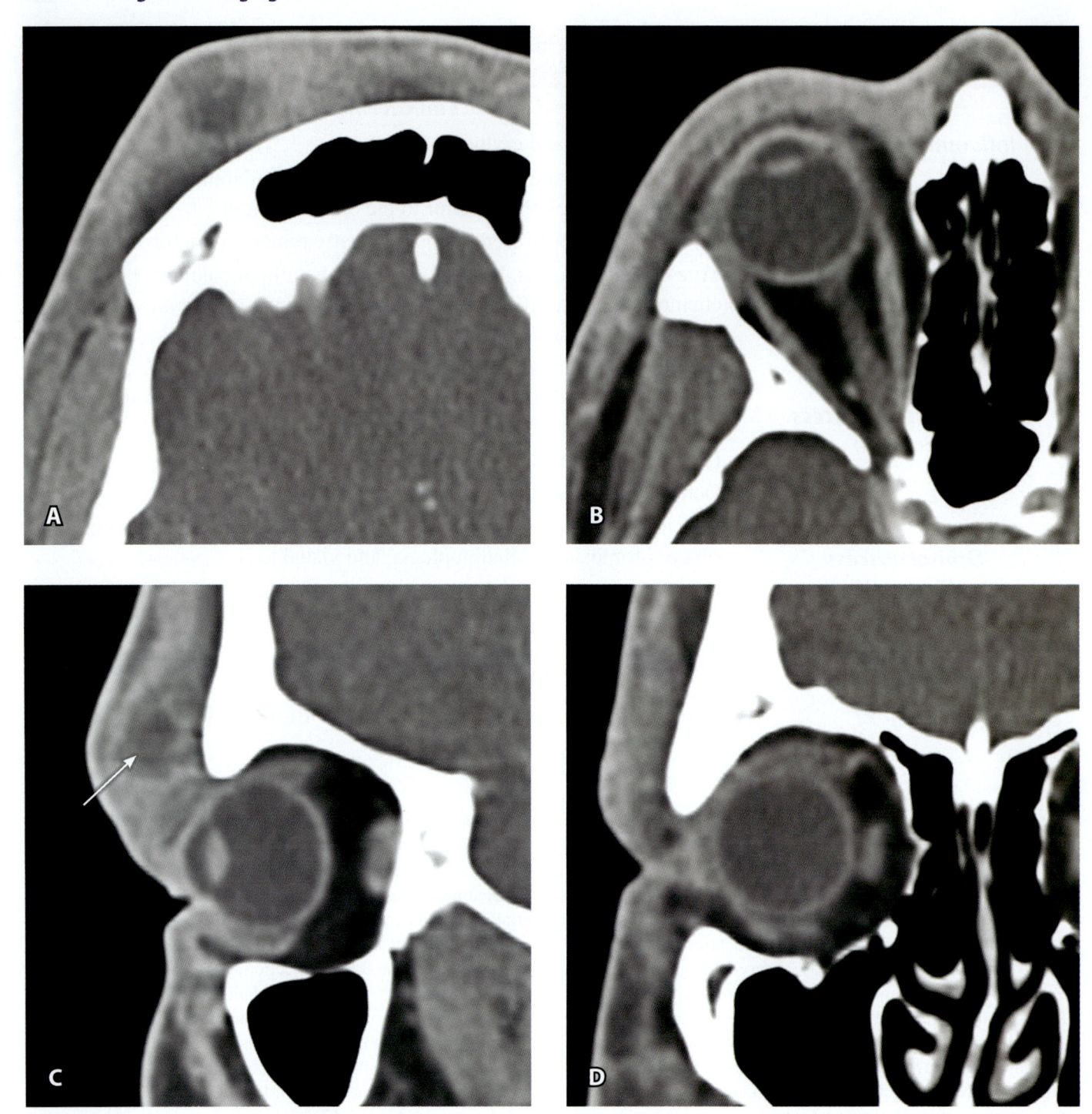

Figure 2-15 Preseptal Cellulitis
Preseptal cellulitis associated with a right forehead abscess. Axial (**A–B**) and sagittal reformatted (**C**) and coronal (**D**) post contrast CT images show marked thickening and enhancement of the preseptal soft tissues of the right face, including the eyelids. There is a focal abscess cavity in the right forehead, located just above the right orbit (*arrow,* **C**).

If a subperiosteal abscess is present there may be a fluid collection with an air–fluid level (**Figs. 2-17** and **2-18**). A subperiosteal abscess will appear as a localized homogeneous elevation of the periorbita typically adjacent to an opacified sinus with or without bone densification. The material within the abscess often cannot be determined, and the abscess may actually enlarge on serial scans during treatment before a decrease in size is observed.[30,33,34]

A bacterial abscess may show rim enhancement with a central low signal on T1W images, but a high signal on T2W images. In contrast, a fungal abscess may be hypointense on both T1 and T2W images and may contain calcifications. Involvement of the extraocular muscles may show intense enhancement and enlargement. If the optic nerve is also involved, it may appear thickened and the sheath may enhance, suggesting meningitis of

Table 2-9 Imaging of Orbital Infections

Lesion	CT May Show	MR May Show
Sinusitis	• Air–fluid level • Mucosal thickening • Extraocular muscle enlargement • Ophthalmic vein enlargement • Optic nerve enlargement • Orbital fat infiltration • Abscess (central low-density collection with an enhancing rim)	
Orbital cellulitis (Fig. 2-15)		• Low signal region • Diffuse post contrast enhancement on T1W
Subperiosteal abscess (Fig. 2-17)	• Localized homogeneous elevation of periorbita adjacent to an opacified sinus +/− bone densification • Fluid collection +/− air–fluid level	
Bacterial abscess		• Rim enhancement with a central low signal on T1W • High signal on T2W
Fungal abscess		• Hypointensity on both T1W and T2W • +/− calcifications
Cavernous sinus thrombosis		• Enlarged cavernous sinus with unenhanced areas representing clots • Ophthalmic veins engorged
Optic nerve involvement		• Nerve thickening • Sheath enhancement (optic sheath meningitis)
Extraocular muscle involvement		• Muscles with intense enhancement, enlargement
Meningitis		• Meninges enhancement
Brain abscess; epidural fluid; subdural fluid		• Low signal on T1W • High signal on T2W • Rim enhancement with contrast in both sequences

the optic sheath. Engorgement of the ophthalmic veins is often noted, especially with thrombosis in the cavernous sinus. Cavernous sinus thrombosis is typically evidenced by enlargement of the cavernous sinus with unenhanced areas representing clots within the sinus.[30]

Infection that has spread intracranially beyond the cavernous sinus may be observed. Meningitis is seen on MR imaging as enhancement of the meninges. Epidural and subdural fluid collections and brain abscesses will typically have a low signal on T1W images and a high signal on T2W images with both sequences showing rim enhancement after contrast administration. If cerebritis is present, there will be areas of ill-defined increased signal on T2W images that have irregular, patchy enhancement after contrast administration.[30]

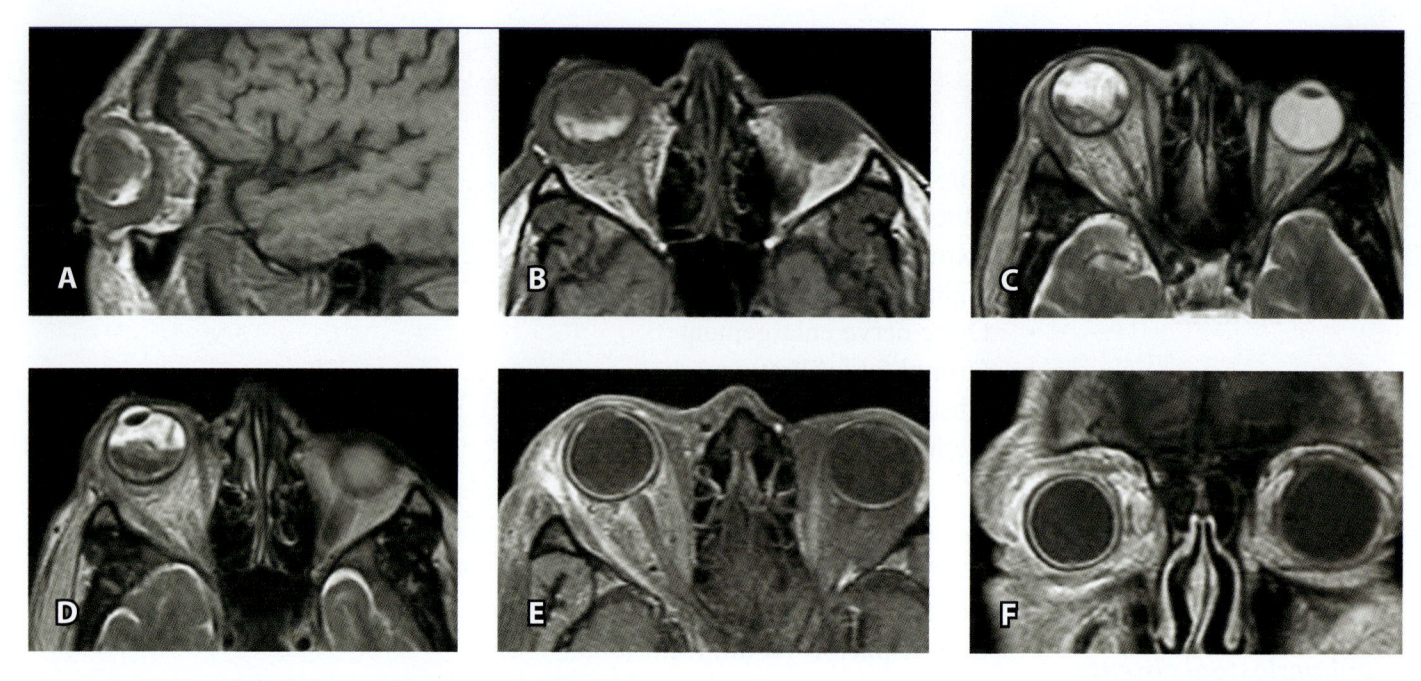

Figure 2-16 Enophthalmitis and Postseptal Cellulitis
Enophthalmitis and celluitis secondary to aspergillosis of the right orbit and globe. Sagittal (**A**) and axial (**B**) T1W MR images show hemorrhage in the right eye, evidenced by high signal intensity. Axial T2W MR images (**C–D**) show the extensive hemorrhage and debris in the vitreous with surrounding soft tissue edema and proptosis. Post contrast axial (**E**) and coronal (**F**) postcontrast T1W MR show enhancement of the layers of the globe and surrounding tissues.

Mycotic Infections

Rhinocerebral mucormycosis is a mycotic infection that is typically seen in a diabetic patient with ketoacidosis or in an immunocompromised individual. This ubiquitous organism enters the body via the nose and may spread systemically as well as locally from the nose to sinuses, orbit, cavernous sinus, skull base, and eventually the brain. The disease is usually of rapid onset although some chronic cases have been reported. The patients clinically present with rapid onset headache, fever, lethargy, mucosal necrosis, proptosis, ptosis, ophthalmoplegia, and visual changes that can lead to coma and death. Spread intracranially may cause thrombosis of the carotid artery or the cavernous sinus.

Imaging of mucormycosis is not specific for a fungal infection (**Table 2-10**). There may be expansion and destruction of the bony walls as the infection spreads from the nose to the anterior cranial fossa. A finding associated with mycotic infection, but not observed in bacterial infection, is the hypointensity of an abscess or of a mycetoma on T2W MR scans. Ideal treatment for this disease is sometimes controversial; however, both surgery and Amphotericin B medical therapy are typically used with variable results.[30,33,35]

Table 2-10 Imaging of Mycotic Infections

Lesion	CT May Show	MR May Show
Mucormycosis	• Expansion, destruction of bony walls as infection spreads	• Hypointensity of abscess or mycetoma on T2 W
Aspergillosis	• Heterogeneous bone destruction and calcifications similar in density to muscle	• Low signal or no signal mass on T1 W and T2 W • Enhancement with contrast • Propensity for vascular invasion → carotid artery thrombosis, hemorrhagic infarction, mycotic aneurysm aspergilloma • Cavernous sinus involvement

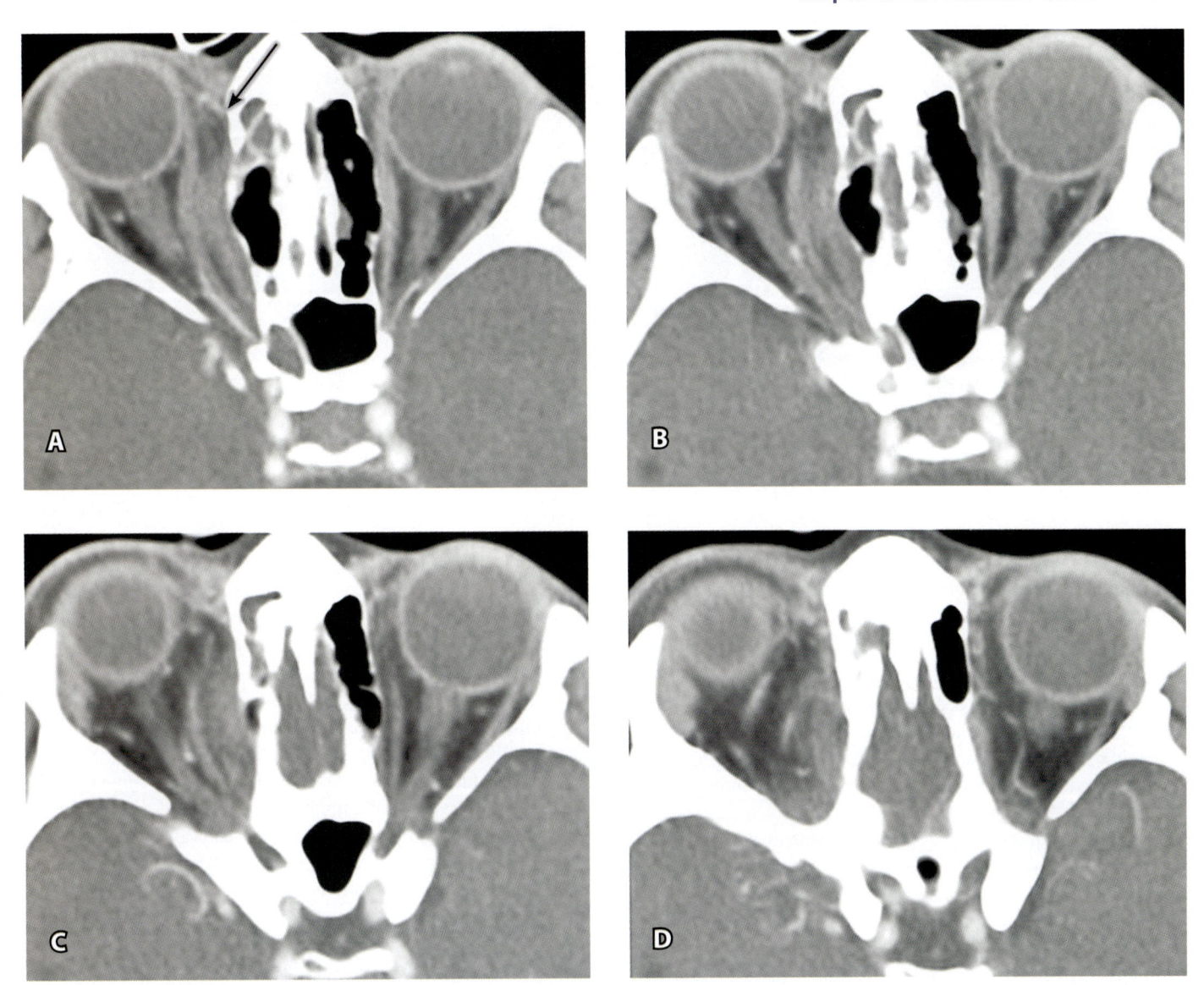

Figure 2-17 Subperiosteal Abscess
Pyogenic right ethmoid sinusitis with subperiosteal abscess. Axial CT scans with contrast (**A–D**) show a low density area with a half moon shape in the medial part of the right orbit, adjacent to the ethmoid air cells (*arrow*, **A**). The low-density area represents pus that has spread along the ophthalmic arteries through the lamina papyracea to involve the subperiosteal space of the orbit. Note the opacification and enhancement of the right ethmoid air cells.

Invasive aspergillosis behaves similarly to mucormycosis once the infection has reached the orbit. Aggressive local spread may cause carotid artery thrombosis, hemorrhagic infarction, or a mycotic aneurysm as Aspergillus has a propensity for vascular invasion. The orbit may also be reached via hematogenous spread of aspergillosis from the lungs. Aspergillosis may also affect the orbit as a more indolent infection forming an aspergilloma (a ball of Aspergillus) or as allergic fungal sinusitis that erodes into the orbit. Surgical removal of such an aspergilloma and local medical treatment of the fungal sinusitis are usually effective.[36,37]

Imaging findings show characteristics of an invasive infection such as bone destruction and calcifications in a heterogeneous mass similar in density to muscle on CT scans and a low signal or no signal mass on MR T1W and T2W images. This mass will enhance after contrast administration. If present, cavernous sinus involvement may be identified as well (**Table 2-10**). Invasive aspergillosis requires emergent aggressive antibiotic and surgical therapy.

Hydatid Infections

Although orbital hydatid disease is rare, it should be identified preoperatively in order to avoid cystic rupture and further dissemination. Echinococcus granulosus is a tapeworm larva that infects dogs and sheep and is passed to humans via fecal–oral contact. The liver and lungs are typically involved, but in 1% of cases, the orbits may be affected. The imaging appearance is that of a unilocular, hypodense cyst with peripheral rim enhancement following contrast administration. The cyst contents have similar

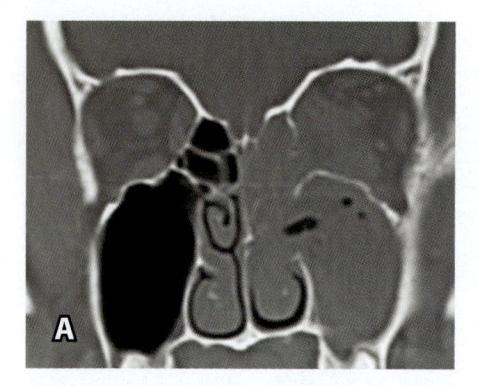

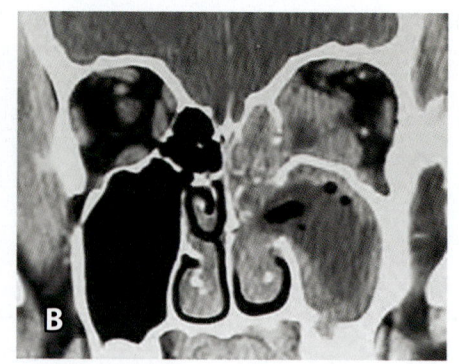

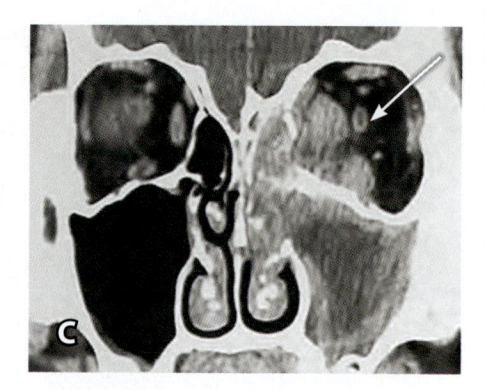

Figure 2-18 Post-traumatic Sino-orbital Abscess

Left orbit medial wall fracture with subperiosteal abscess and traumatic optic atrophy. Coronal CT scans (**A–C**) show a fracture of the left lamina papyracea and disruption of the normal structures of the medial orbital, ethmoid sinus, and nasal structures. An abscess extends from the sinus into the orbit. **C** demonstrates a small optic nerve on the left due to traumatic atrophy (*arrow*, **C**).

attenuation to the vitreous. There may also be bony erosion or displacement of the orbital walls, multilocularity, or hyperdense cyst contents without enhancement. Such an appearance may be confused with orbital soft tissue tumors.[30,38]

Erdheim-Chester Disease

Erdheim-Chester disease is characterized by a lipid-laden histiocytic infiltration of bones and viscera, especially the retroperitoneum, lungs, skin, orbit, and long bones. It is usually found in the Caucasian adult male, who may present with compressive, circumscribed dural granulomas of the brain stem, cerebellum, posterior orbit, and/or optic nerve. Clinically, patients with Erdheim-Chester disease may be asymptomatic or experience bone pain, fever, and weight loss. They may present with diabetes insipidus, ataxia, progressive bilateral exophthalmos, ophthalmoplegia, and/or visual loss due to a compressive optic neuropathy. Intracranial meningiomas have been associated with this disease. Treatment is undetermined and may include anti-inflammatory drugs, chemotherapy, or radiation therapy. The disease may remain localized, or systemic involvement may be quite extensive and fatal.

Imaging in Erdheim-Chester disease depicts subtle homogeneous masses with intense enhancement after contrast administration. Retention of the contrast over 24 hours has been observed but is not always present. There may also be proptosis, extraocular muscle atrophy or enlargement, lacrimal gland enlargement, and/or optic nerve infiltration. Involvement of the long bones shows symmetric sclerosis of the metaphysis, sparing the epiphysis. The differential includes other granulomatous diseases, lymphoma and Hand-Schuller-Christian disease.[28,39,40]

Langerhans Cell Histiocytosis

The term Langerhans cell histiocytosis encompasses what used to be referred to as three separate disease entities: eosinophilic granuloma, Hand-Schuller-Christian disease, and Letterer-Siwe disease or Histiocytosis X. The disease is related to an abnormal immune process or clonal proliferation that causes the sudden onset of a rapidly progressive, painful swelling. The disease most commonly affects children but may occur in any age group.

Although the disease itself is rare, patients with the disease commonly have orbital involvement at some point during their illness. The disease prognosis is worse in younger patients and those with multisystem involvement or evidence of organ system failure. Diabetes insipidus may occur in association with Langerhans cell histiocytosis. Treatment is conservative as spontaneous remission may occur. When treatment is necessary, excisional biopsy, local steroid injection, and radiation therapy or systemic chemotherapy are all options.

The common presenting symptoms in the orbit are unilateral or bilateral proptosis, inflammation of the eyelid and periorbital pain. Bony and soft tissue lesions that usually originate in the sinuses classically involve the superolateral aspects of the orbit and temporal fossa. There may be a single or multiple lesions. CT scans reveal focal bony lysis and irregular, usually intraosseous lesions associated with a soft tissue mass that may be isodense to the extraocular muscles. On MR imaging, there is a solid, well-defined mass that may have a heterogeneous, hypointense signal on T1W images. On T2W images the mass may be hyperintense. After contrast administration the mass enhances markedly and heterogeneously.[21,41–43]

Idiopathic Orbital Pseudotumor

Idiopathic orbital pseudotumor (IOP) also known as idiopathic orbital inflamatory syndrome (IOIS), orbital pseudotumor, or inflammatory fibromyotendinitis is characterized by idiopathic inflammation of the orbital tissues resulting in acute, subacute or chronic proptosis and visual loss. By definition, this is a diagnosis of exclusion and must exclude orbital inflammation due to known causes such as granulomatous diseases, sclerosing hemangioma, sinusitis, or trauma. This disease may appear as a diffuse or focal entity. In the diffuse form, there is inflammatory infiltrate of the orbital fat, extraocular muscles and adnexal structures, particularly in the orbital apex. The more focal forms of IOP involve particular anatomic structures (**Table 2-11**). These commonly involve the tendinous portion of the extraocular muscles (myositic form), the uveal structures (anterior form), the scleral region (posterior form), the outer layer of the dural sheath of the optic nerve,

Table 2-11 Classification of Idiopathic Orbital Pseudotumor based on Anatomic Patterns

- Anterior orbital inflammation (acute and subacute)
- Apical or posterior orbital inflammation (acute and subacute)
- Diffuse orbital inflammation (acute and subacute)
- Lacrimal adenitis or dacryoadenitis
- Myositic orbital inflammation (acute and subacute)
- Perineuritis
- Perisclerotic
- Tolosa-Hunt syndrome (variant of IOP in which inflammation is restricted to the optic canal, superior orbital fissure, or cavernous sinus)

and adjacent fat (perineural form) or the lacrimal gland (lacrimal form). All forms of the disease show extensive histologic infiltration that is composed of polyclonal lymphocytes, plasma cells, neutrophils, and macrophages with various amounts of fibrosis. The disease is nongranulomatous or noncaseating granulomatous and may also be associated with an inflammatory vasculitis. Contrary to previous thought, it is not related to orbital reactive lymphoid hyperplasia (pseudolymphoma) nor is it a lymphoid tumor.

The clinical picture of IOP can vary widely, but is typically characterized by orbital pain, swelling, restricted eye movement, diplopia, proptosis and impaired vision with optic nerve involvement due to mass effect, inflammation, and infiltration. The acute form of IOP is typically unilateral and develops over days to weeks. This form of the disease may relapse after initial response into a subacute variety. The chronic form of the disease develops insidiously over weeks to months and lacks inflammatory symptoms, but there are increasing symptoms of fixation and mass effect. The disease may be seen bilaterally in 10% to 15% of cases. The disease is typically seen in the adult population, and when seen in children, there is a higher incidence of bilateral disease with the additional symptoms of headache, vomiting, and fever.

MR imaging may show intra- or extraconal soft tissue lesions that are diffuse or localized and commonly involve the lacrimal gland and orbital apices (**Table 2-12**). Depending on the degree of fibrosis and dense cellularity, these lesions are usually hypointense on T2 W images and show weak, homogeneous contrast enhancement. Occassionally, there may be a well-defined mass lesion. This lesion is usually of low signal intensity on the T1W images and has variable intensity on the T2W images depending upon the degree of fibrosis. A reticular pattern or "dirty appearance" in the orbital fat is highly suggestive of IOP. Involvement of the extraocular muscles shows asymmetric enlargement, but the enlarged portion is the muscle bundles and tendons in contrast to orbital endocrinopathy in which the muscular bundles only are enlarged. In virtually all cases, there is prominent enhancement on the post contrast MR scans (**Figs. 2-19** and **2-20**).

CT imaging can reveal a broad range of nonspecific pathological changes that may be suggestive of IOP. There may be diffuse thickening of the involved structures, or the lesion may appear as a discrete lesion with well-defined borders resembling a neoplasm or granuloma. If the inflammatory changes remain localized to part of the globe, it may produce an apparent thickening of the scleral border with an effusion under Tenon's capsule. A similar picture is seen in lymphomas and differentiation between the two conditions may be impossible. Although usually confined to the orbital soft tissues, IOP can produce bone destruction or extraorbital extension (**Table 2-12**).

Most cases of acute IOP improve or resolve following systemic steroid therapy. There is a high rate of recurrence and low cure rate. High-intensity lesions may have a better response to therapy with steroids when compared to low-intensity lesions and involvement of the optic nerve may have a better prognosis. In refractory cases, low dose radiation, immunosupressants, and surgery may be helpful. The disease process may progress to a lymphoproliferative disorder or lymphoma in the subacute or chronic forms. The differentiation of IOP from lymphoma is based on histopathological examination with a predominant polyclonal lymphocytic population in the earlier disorder and a monoclonal lymphocytic process in the latter disorder. MR scans may be used to follow the course of the illness until it resolves or recurs in the chronic form of the disease.

Involvement of the optic nerve and ipsilateral cavernous sinus with IOP leads to alterations in visual acuity and ophthalmoplegia. When there is secondary thrombosis of the sphenoidal veins or cavernous sinus, a painful ophthalmoplegia results with the presumptive diagnosis of Tolosa-Hunt syndrome. (See section below on extraocular muscle lesions.)

Subsets of patients with isolated ocular manifestations of IOP also have posterior scleritis. These patients are seen for ocular pain, proptosis, gaze restriction, scleral effusions, disc edema, and intraocular hemorrhages. Posterior scleritis shows inflammatory signs in the sclera with thickening (**Table 2-12**). Such changes may be identified as areas of enhancement. The thickened sclera enhanced by contrast presents as a so-called "ring sign." This phenomenon may be clearly seen on MR images that include fat saturation with the postcontrast images. Without fat saturation, the inherent chemical shift artifact with conventional MR images may preclude the identification of posterior scleritis.[44]

There is another subset of patients with a predominant "sclerosing" variety of IOP. In these cases there is a diffuse increase in density of the orbital fat and obliteration of the optic nerve and extraocular muscles with a histological predominance of sclerosis. The increased fibrosis with less edema of these lesions results in decreased signal intensities on T2 W images (**Table 2-12**). The intraorbital structures become fixated and there is a poor response to steroid therapy. Besides the sclerosing variety, there are several other histologic subclasses of IOP referred to in the literature including granulomatous, vasculitic, and eosinophilic.

The myositic form of IOP extends into the extraocular muscles directly. In this pattern, there is infiltration of the

Table 2-12 Imaging of Idiopathic Orbital Pseudotumor

MR	CT

• Diffuse or localized intra- or extraconal soft tissue lesions
• Commonly involve lacrimal gland and orbital apices
• Hypointense on T2 W
• Weak, homogeneous contrast enhancement
• Reticular pattern or "dirty appearance" in orbital fat
• Asymmetric enlargement of involved extraocular muscles and tendons
• Prominent enhancement post contrast
• "Ring sign" if posterior scleritis is present (scleral thickening that enhances post contrast with fat saturation)
• Occasionally a well-defined mass
  • Usually of low signal intensity on T1 W
  • Variable intensity on T2 W
	• Spectrum:
	  • Diffuse thickening of involved structures, or
	  • Discrete lesion with well-defined borders resembling neoplasm or granuloma
	  • Inflammatory changes may be localized to part of the globe (thickening of scleral border with effusion under Tenon's capsule)
	• Bony involvement is rare but possible

Tolosa-Hunt Syndrome	
Thrombosis of sphenoidal veins or cavernous sinus	
"Sclerosing" Variant of IOP	
• Diffuse increase in density of orbital fat • Obliteration of optic nerve and extraocular muscles • Dense fibrosis results in decreased signal intensities on T2 W	
Myositic Variant of IOP	
• Extraocular muscle enlargement in focal or diffuse pattern	

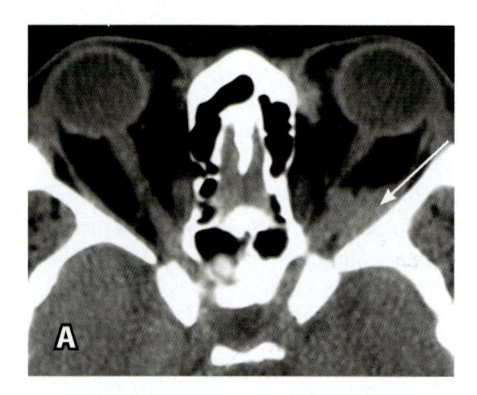

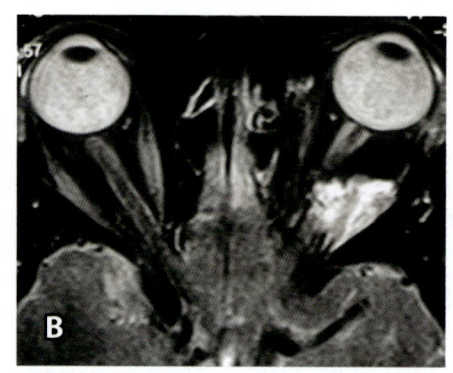

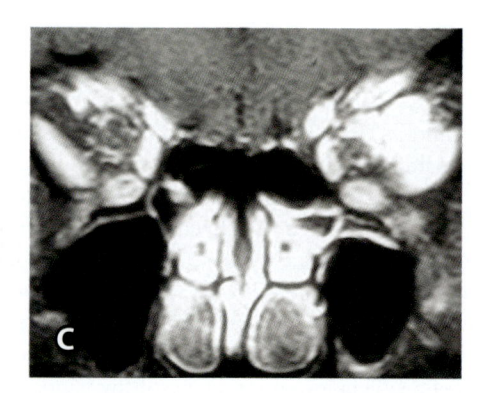

Figure 2-19 Idiopathic Orbital Pseudotumor
Idiopathic orbital pseudotumor (IOP); focal lesion limited to the posterior portion of the left orbit. The axial CT (**A**) shows ill-defined soft tissue in the left orbital apex with extension to the bony margin (*arrow*, **A**). The axial T2W MR image (**B**) shows high signal intensity occupying the left orbital apex involving posterior contents including muscles and posterior portion of the optic nerve. The coronal T1W enhanced MR image (**C**) clearly shows the enhancements of both the extraconal muscles and intraconal optic nerve.

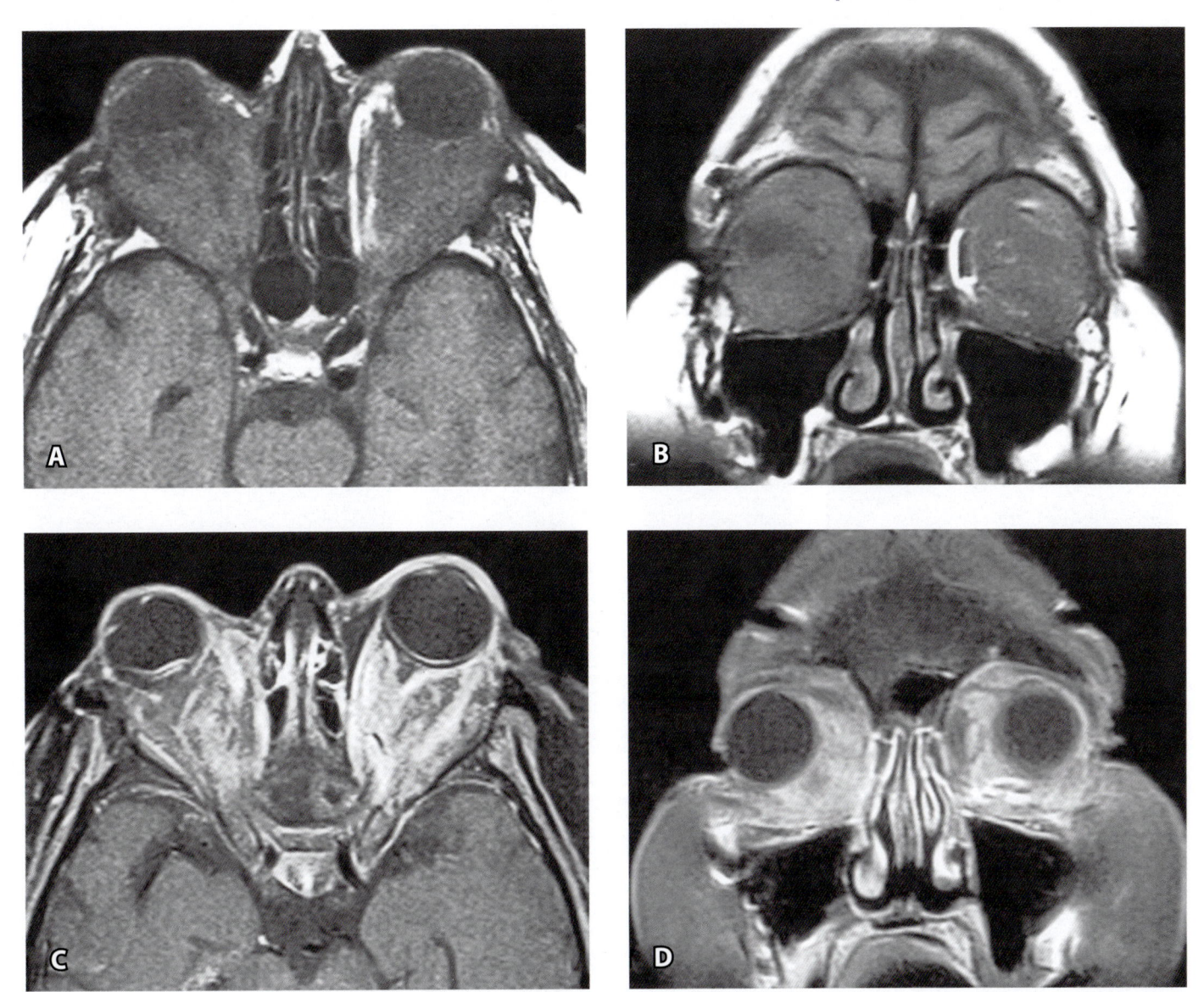

Figure 2-20 Idiopathic Orbital Pseudotumor
Idiopathic orbital pseudotumor (IOP); diffuse lesions involving virtually all of the orbital contents bilaterally. Axial T1W MR images (**A**, **C**) and coronal T1W MR images (**B**, **D**) show the expansion of all the retrobulbar structures leading to profound proptosis. Axial (**C**) and coronal (**D**) fat-saturated enhanced MR images clearly document the combined intraconal and extraconal involvement of both orbits.

muscles with lymphocytes and plasma cells in a focal or diffuse pattern causing swelling of the muscle fibers with intervening edema and fibrosis that has been observed on histologic examination. Fiber degeneration may eventually occur that has also been seen at the microscopic level. The patients may present with diplopia, pain with eye movement, and conjunctival injection and chemosis at the site of the muscle insertions. Enlargement of the muscles may compress the optic nerve or cause perineural inflammation with a resultant optic neuropathy. The symptoms usually resolve with the use of high-dose steroids.

The combination of orbital pain and proptosis can be caused by a variety of infections or inflammations (Table 2-13), all of

Table 2-13 Pain and Proptosis (suspect orbital infection or inflammation)

- Cellulitis or abscess formation
- Idiopathic orbital pseudotumor (IOP)
- Sinus infections or mucoceles
- Wegener's granulomatosis
- Lipogranulomatosis (Erdheim-Chester disease)
- Kimura's disease
- Sarcoidosis

which can simulate IOP. There is no key clinical differentiating feature nor is the response to corticosteroid therapy an indication of the etiology, but may help to support the diagnosis. The definitive diagnosis is made by biopsy that is sometimes omitted, if the diagnosis is suggested by the imaging and clinical findings.[1,22,28,45–47]

Lymphoproliferative Disease

Lymphoproliferative disease is a continuum of entities from benign lymphoid hyperplasia to malignant lymphoma. The orbits are involved in 3% to 4% of cases usually by the non-Hodgkin's variety of lymphoma. It has recently been reported that orbital lymphomas have shown the greatest rise in annual incidence of orbital malignancies and now account for 55% of malignant orbital tumors. There is a slight female predominance, and the disease is typically found in older adults, except for Burkitt's lymphoma and granulocytic sarcoma, which are found more commonly in children. Orbital involvement may be the only manifestation of a lymphoma, and when involved, occurs as an extranodal lesion.

Clinically, patients may present with proptosis, diplopia, mild motility disorders, visual impairment, and/or ptosis. There may be a rubbery, palpable mass in the anterosuperior orbit or anterior tumefactive swelling in the lids, conjunctiva, and lacrimal glands (**Fig. 2-21**). Eyelid disease is most commonly

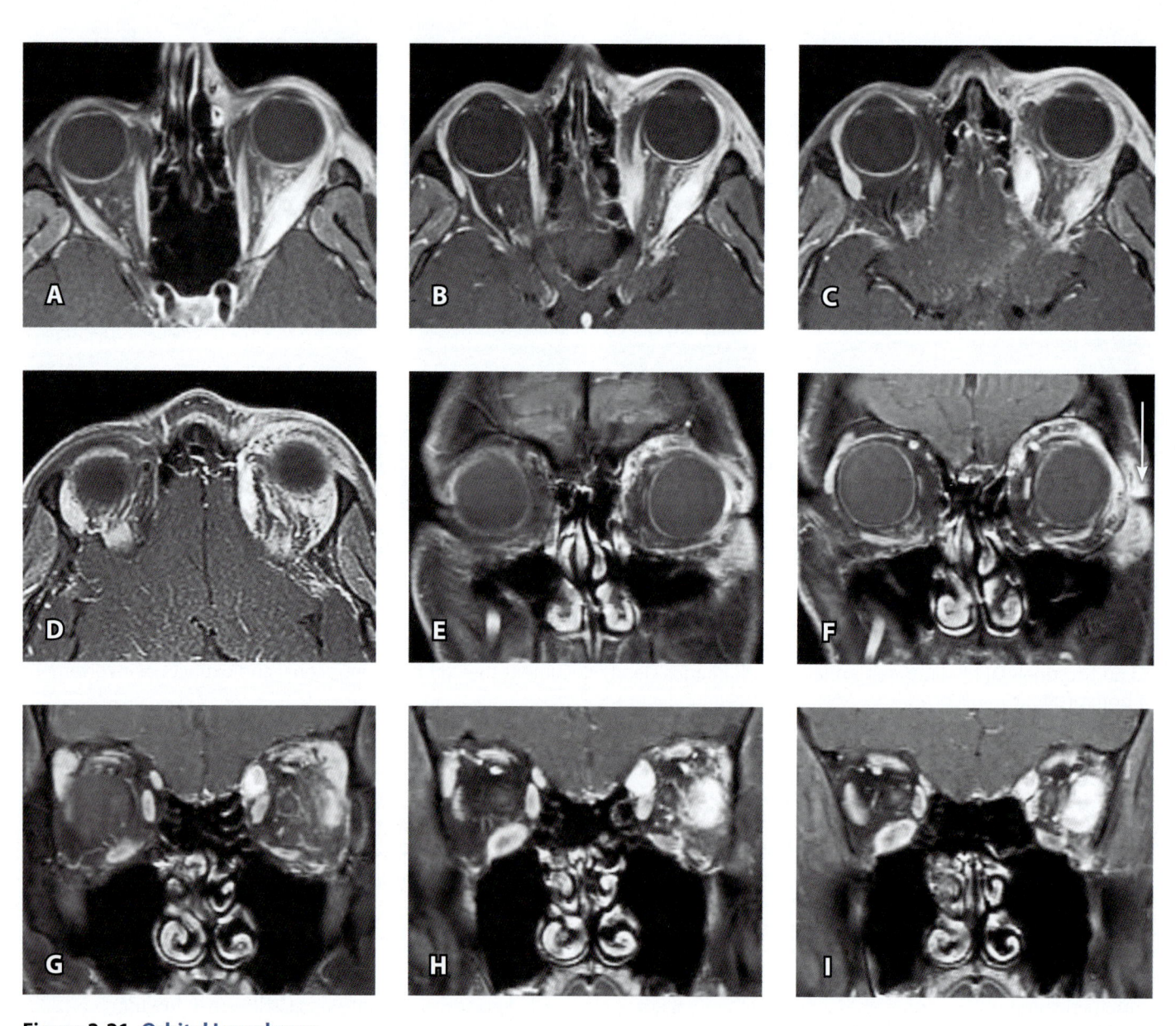

Figure 2-21 Orbital Lymphoma
Orbital lymphoma in a middle-aged female patient. Axial (**A–D**) and coronal (**E–I**) T1W enhanced MR images show diffuse homogenous soft tissue filling the contents of the left orbit with involvement of the extraocular muscles and eyelids. Note the enhancement of the soft tissues of the face and scalp, a characteristic finding in lymphoproliferative diseases (*arrow*, **F**).

associated with systemic disease when lymphoma is found in the orbit.

Lymphoproliferative lesions typically follow the contour of the globe without indentation and are usually oval or round in shape with polypoid projections into the orbital fat. There may be many small masses or a solitary lesion. Bone destruction is not typically observed except in the childhood lymphomas. The benign or malignant nature of a lymphoproliferative lesion cannot be determined with imaging alone.

Direct involvement of the extraocular muscles is rare and is usually secondary to infiltration into the muscle. If the lesion is primarily confined to the muscle, there may be an enlarged, lobulated contour to the muscle. The medial and lateral recti muscles are often obliterated by the tumor due to a close association of the tumor with the muscle margin. Infiltration of Tenon's space will cause thickening of the scleral and uveal coats. There may be enlargement and displacement of the optic nerve sheath complex when involved. The lesions may gain access to adjacent regions via fissures and foramina and are typically obviously enhancing after contrast administration.

MR imaging of lymphomas will demonstrate a low signal lesion on T1W images and typically intermediate signal intensity on T2W images, although the T2W imaging appearance may be variable depending upon the cellular composition of the lesion. Fat suppression techniques should be used, as the fat is usually infiltrated. The lesions will enhance markedly after contrast administration. The combination of fat suppression, contrast administration, and surface coils with MR imaging should be used to allow for the highest possible detection rate (**Table 2-14**).

Differentiation among lymphoproliferative lesions may be difficult. Lymphoproliferative disorders cannot be distinguished from IOP by imaging alone, although the presence of multiple lesions, rounded shape, and molding of orbital structures is supportive of lymphoma and not characteristic of IOP. Plasma cell proliferations may appear similarly, except for the presence of lytic bone destruction with a plasmacytoma.

Biopsy of lymphoproliferative disorders may be performed once an epithelial tumor has been ruled out due to the risk of tumor spillage in squamous cell carcinoma. Total excision is not performed due to the characteristically diffuse and infiltrative nature of lymphoproliferative lesions. If lesions are bilateral, only one side need be sampled because histology is usually the same on both sides. Some small well-circumscribed anterior lesions may be excised, but most orbital lesions will receive radiotherapy. If systemic disease is present, chemotherapy will also be given.[48–50]

Kimura Disease

Kimura disease is a disease characterized by angiolymphoid hyperplasia with eosinophilia. It appears similar to lymphoma radiographically and the diagnosis must be made clinically (**Fig. 2-22**). There is a slight male predominance of this disease in older adults. The clinical presentation may be similar to lymphoma and can include ptosis, proptosis, and sometimes an eyelid mass. There are usually associated systemic abnormalities including eosinophilia, elevated serum IgE, and lymphadenopathy.

Table 2-14 Imaging of Lymphoproliferative Disease

- Follows contour of the globe
- Lesions are usually oval or round with polypoid projections into orbital fat
- Multiple lesions are common, but may have a solitary lesion
- Bone destruction may be found in childhood lymphomas
- Muscle involvement may create an enlarged, lobulated contour
- Medial, lateral recti muscles are often obliterated by tumor
- Scleral thickening if lesion infiltrates into Tenon's space
- Optic nerve sheath involvement causes enlargement and displacement
- Lytic bone destruction with a plasmacytoma
- MR imaging
  - Low signal intensity on T1W
  - Intermediate signal intensity on T2W
  - T2W imaging may be variable depending upon composition of lesion
  - Enhances dramatically post contrast
  - Fat suppression shows fat infiltration

  (**Fig. 2-21**)

Dermoid, Epidermoid, and Teratoma

The dermoid, epidermoid, and teratoma types of lesion are usually the result of a developmental defect. Many cases will present later in life and may be the result of processes unrelated to development. In such cases, they are considered more like neoplasms.

Teratomas are neoplasms that contain tissue from at least one of the germ layers, but more commonly from all three layers and show varying levels of differentiation, from neural tube cells to well-formed teeth. They are thought to arise from ectopic rests of germ cells during development or via the hematogenous spread of ectopic rests of cells. They are most commonly benign and form complex masses of both embryonic and adult tissues. Teratomas are the most common congenital tumor, but are rarely seen in the orbit as compared with dermoids (congenital being defined to include the first 60 days of life).

Teratomas can become quite large causing orbital and facial deformity and remodeling. The majority of lesions are

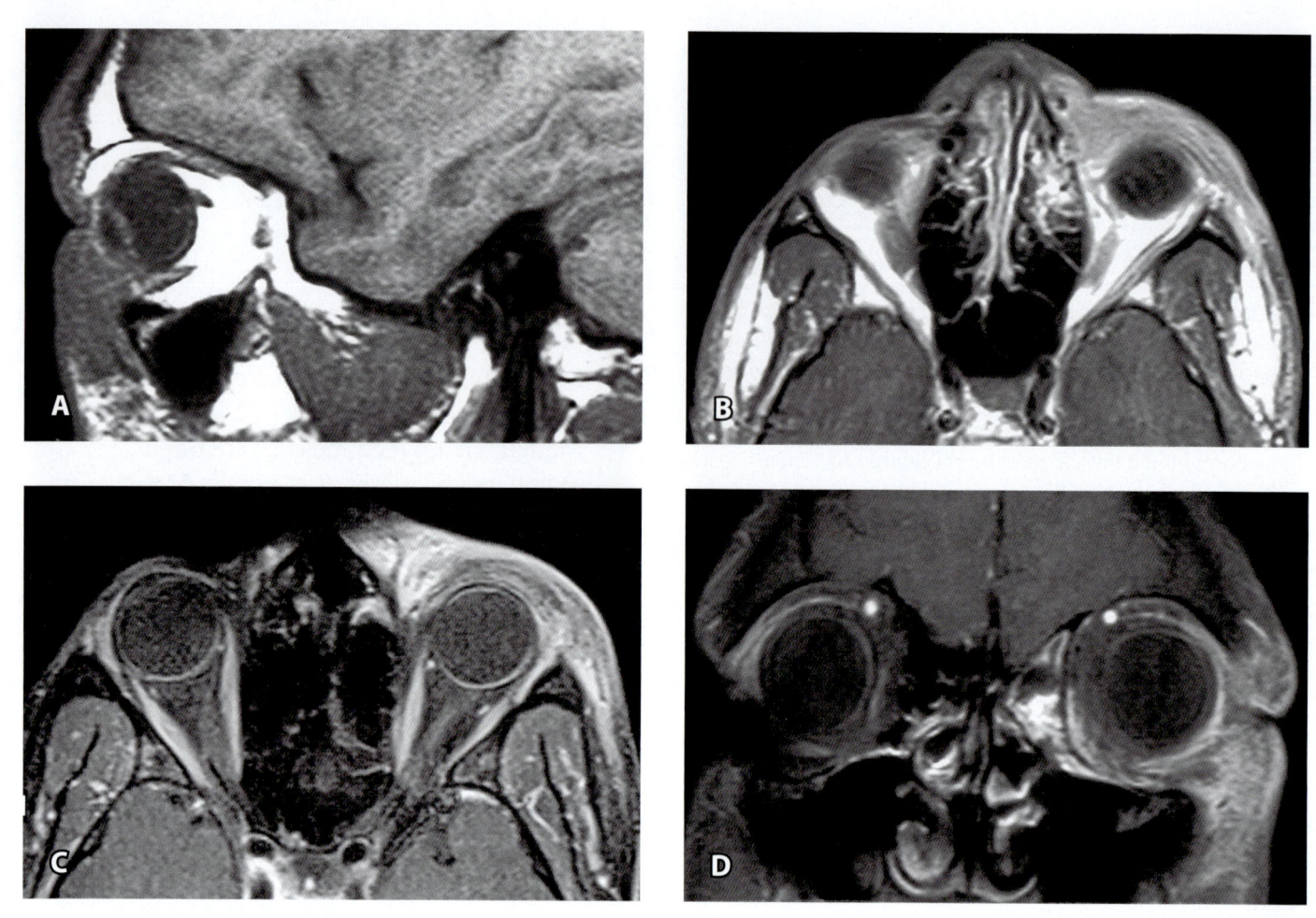

Figure 2-22 Kimura Disease

Kimura disease (a type of lymphoproliferative disorder). Sagittal T1W MR scan (**A**) shows soft tissue mass in both the eyelids and the preseptal space of the left orbit. Axial T1W enhanced MR image without fat saturation (**B**) demonstrates the soft tissue enhancement that encompasses the anterior adnexal structures in the preseptal space. Axial (**C**) and Coronal (**D**) T1W enhanced MR images with fat saturation show enhancement of multiple structures of the left orbit and adjacent scalp and face.

benign and surgical excision is curative with reconstructive surgery performed as needed. Teratomas will grow rapidly after birth and appear as complex solid or multicystic lesions, which may have expanded the bony orbit to 2 to 3 times its normal size. The mass typically shows imaging characteristics consistent with many tissue types and will usually have fatty regions and calcifications. After contrast administration, enhancement may be patchy occurring in the solid regions of the tumor (**Table 2-15**).

Dermoids and epidermoids are ectoderm-lined inclusion cysts. Dermoids contain hair, sebaceous and sweat glands, as well as squamous epithelium; whereas epidermoids only contain squamous epithelium. They are derived from ectopic collections of sequestered ectoderm that develop to form cysts. Dermoid and epidermoid cysts arise when there is failure of separation of the surface ectoderm from the underlying neural tube during development. They may also be the result of abnormal sequestration of ectoderm along embryonic folds and areas of dermal fusion, or may occur when ectoderm is implanted beneath the skin e.g., by a lumbar puncture performed without using a stylet. The dermoid and epidermoid lesions may present as slow-growing masses. Their symptoms are related to compression of nearby structures. Dermoids in general are typically identified during early adulthood, whereas epidermoids present slightly later in the third and fourth decades. Orbital dermoids are the most common pediatric orbital tumor. Dermoids may also have an associated sinus tract or fistula.

Although epidermoids may contain cholesterol or fatty salts, upon imaging they will often appear more homogeneous than dermoids with signal characteristics of water or CSF in the lumen (**Figs. 2-23** and **2-24**). Larger lesions may cause scalloping and expansion of the surrounding orbital walls (**Fig. 2-24**). On MR imaging, the signal intensity of the cyst contents will also be variable. If there is a fat-fluid level in the cyst, the fatty content in the nondependent portion

Table 2-15 Imaging Epidermoids, Dermoids, and Teratomas

Epidermoids and Dermoids	Teratomas
MR	• Contain tissue from all three germ layers • Large size can cause orbital, facial deformity • May have multicystic lesions with many tissue types • Usually see fatty regions and calcifications • Contrast shows patchy enhancement in solid regions of tumor
• Signal intensity of cyst contents may be variable • Larger lesions may cause scalloping and expansion of orbital walls • If there is a fat-fluid level, the fatty content in the nondependent portion of the cyst will have high intensity on T1W and low intensity on T2W • Water and keratin-containing portion of the cyst will have low signal on T1W and high signal on T2W • Calcifications may be evident	
Epidermoids (Figs. 2-23 and 2-24)	
• Contain squamous epithelium • May contain cholesterol or fatty salts • Lumen may appear more homogeneous with signal characteristics of water or CSF • Thin capsule not notable with contrast	
Dermoids (Fig. 2-25)	
• Contain hair, sebaceous glands, sweat glands • May have an associated sinus tract or fistula • Contrast shows enhancing capsule with nonenhancing lumen	

of the cyst will have high intensity on T1W images and low intensity on T2W images. The water and keratin-containing, dependent portion of the cyst will appear the opposite with low signal on T1W and high signal on T2W images. Contrast administration will reveal an enhancing capsule with a non-enhancing lumen in dermoids (**Fig. 2-25**). The thin capsule of epidermoids is typically not demonstrated. Calcifications may be evident in dermoids and epidermoids due to saponification of the fat and subsequent dystrophic calcification[5,51] (**Fig. 2-23** and **Table 2-15**).

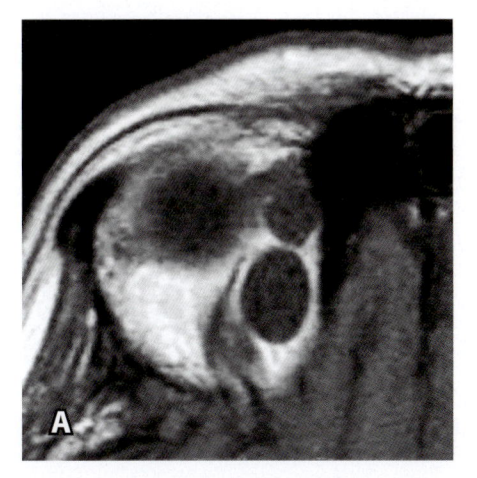

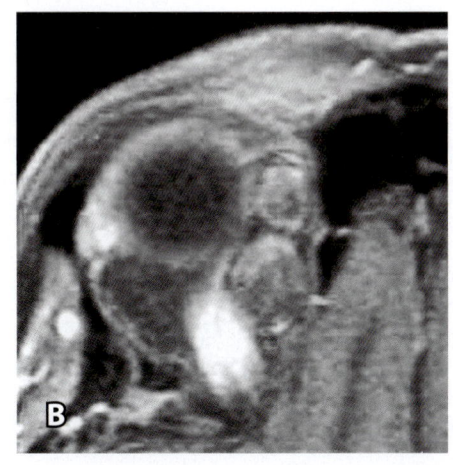

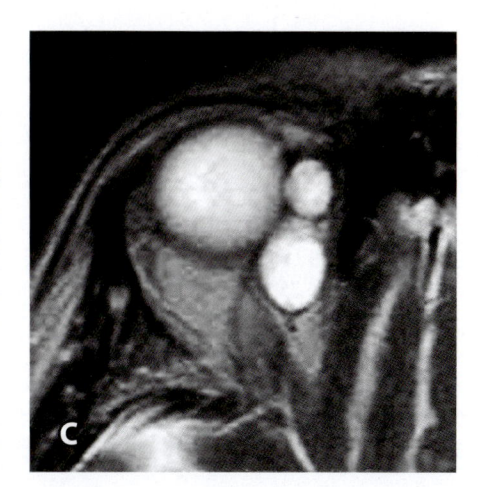

Figure 2-23 Epidermoid Cysts
Epidermoid cyst in the superior medial portion of the right orbit. Axial T1W (**A**) axial T1W enhanced (**B**) and coronal T2W (**C**) images show an encapsulated masses in the right supramedial orbit, which shows distinct enhancement of the capsule following contrast infusion.

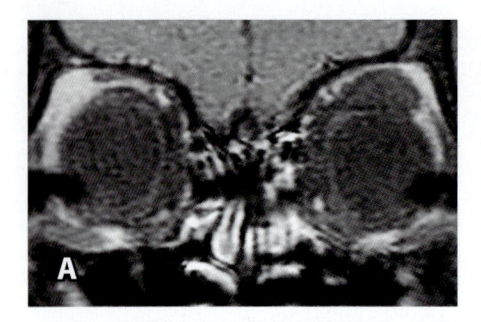

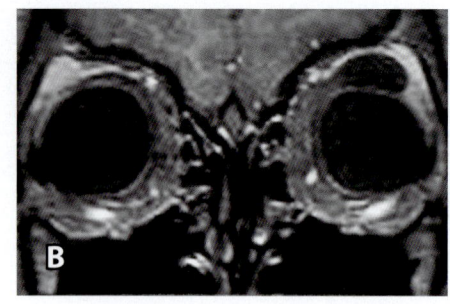

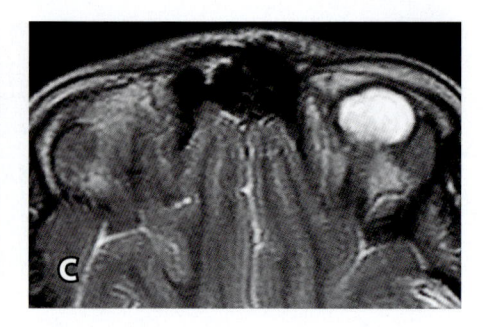

Figure 2-24 Epidermoid Cyst
Epidermoid cyst in the superior orbit. Coronal T1W (**A**) coronal T1W enhanced (**B**) and axial T2W (**C**) axial MR scans show a well-circumscribed cyst above with slight downward compression of the globe. The lesions shows long T1 and long T2 signal intensity, but no enhancement, consistent with an epidermoid cyst.

Metastasis

Metastasis to the orbits is common and typically originates from adjacent structures, although hematogenous spread may occur most commonly from neuroblastoma in children and breast and lung carcinoma in adults. Neuroblastoma will usually spare the globe and may present with the sudden onset of proptosis due to intratumoral hemorrhage.

Imaging of metastatic disease to the orbits is not specific. On ultrasound, solitary or multiple masses may be observed with variable echogenecity and infiltrative borders. MR imaging is often necessary to evaluate the extent of involvement of metastatic tumor. These lesions may appear as poorly defined masses and there may be permeative, lytic bone lesions associated with a soft tissue mass. Metastasis from the prostate gland may show sclerotic bony lesions and have a similar appearance to a meningioma.

MR imaging of metastasis to the extraconal space will typically show soft tissue lesions replacing the normal fat. The lesions will usually have a lower signal than the fat on T1W images and a more variable appearance on T2W images.[22,27,28] Single photon emission computed tomography (SPECT) of bone has been shown to identify lesions of the skull base not recognized by imaging alone and may be a useful adjunct although alone it is less sensitive than either CT or MR imaging.[54]

EXTRAOCULAR MUSCLE LESIONS

The extraocular muscles are most commonly identified as pathologic on imaging studies by their enhancement characteristics and enlargement. Although many diseases may affect the extraocular muscles while involving other parts of the orbit, only those diseases that are characteristic for extraocular muscle involvement will be discussed in this section. Many imaging characteristics of lesions as they affect the extraocular muscles

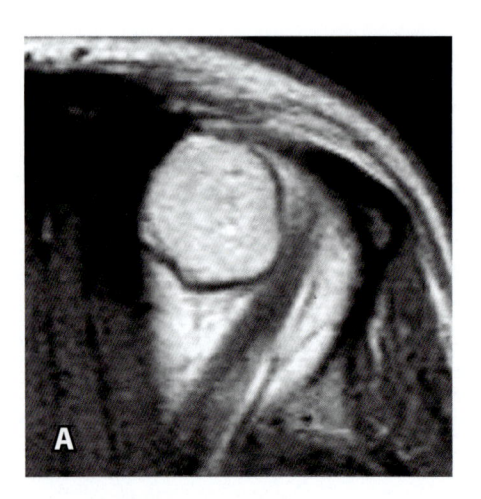

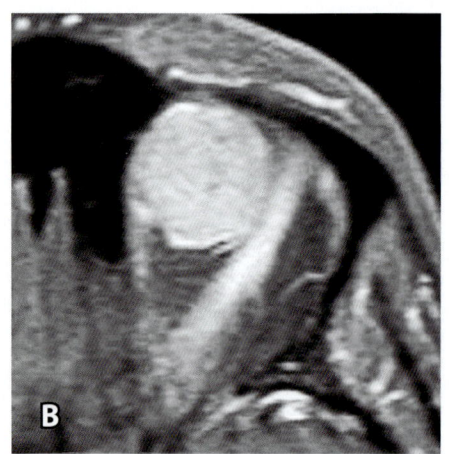

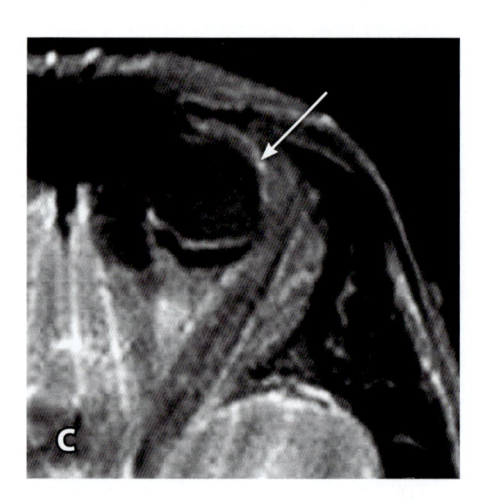

Figure 2-25 Dermoid Cyst
Dermoid cyst of the left superior eyelid of a six-year-old boy. Axial T1W (**A**), T1W enhanced (**B**) and T2W (**C**) MR images show an encapsulated mass in the left supramedial orbit which shows distinct enhancement of the capsule following contrast infusion (*arrow*, **C**). Note that the high signal intensity completely fades on the T2 scan, consistent with fat contents within the dermoid cyst.

are discussed in the anatomical section of the orbit where the lesion is most likely to occur. **Table 2-9** lists some of the many entities that may cause extraocular muscle enlargement.

Endocrine Orbitopathy/Graves' Disease

Endocrine orbitopathy, thyroid ophthalmopathy, thyroid-related orbitopathy, or Graves' disease are all terms used to describe an autoimmune disorder that affects the thyroid gland, orbital soft tissues, and subcutaneous tissues of the extremities. It is the most common diffuse orbital disorder. This disease may be detected in patients who are hyper, hypo, or euthyroid. Most (25–50%) of these cases occur in patients with Graves' hyperthyroidism and occasionally in patients with Hashimoto thyroiditis. The female-to-male ratio is 4 to1 and approximately 15% of patients are under age 15, although the typical patient is 40 to 50 years of age. Disease severity worsens with age and in males. Up to 30% of cases may have a hereditary component. In all age groups, approximately 15% of unilateral orbital proptosis and the majority of bilateral proptosis are secondary to endocrine orbitopathy.

Signs and symptoms of endocrine orbitopathy include proptosis, periobital edema, corneal exposure/ulceration, chemosis, pain, diplopia, upper eyelid lag on downward gaze, upper lid retraction with or without exophthalmos, compressive optic neuropathy (decreased visual acuity, decreased color vision, afferent pupillary defect, visual field defects), extraocular muscle restriction (inferior > medial > superior > lateral rectus), and/or vascular injection at the insertion of the rectus muscles. The clinical features are secondary to overproduction of glycosaminoglycans, which are produced by stimulated fibroblasts. The overstimulation of fibroblasts is centered on the T-cell lymphocytes that recognize the fibroblasts' cross-reactive antigens and release cytokines. The glycosaminoglycans deposit into the bellies of the extraocular muscles in a perivascular location (as well as other tissues of the orbit including the eyelids, sclera, and retrobulbar fat). This deposition results in congestion and hypertrophy and eventual fibrosis and a restrictive myopathy. With the deposition of mucopolysaccharides either in the extraocular muscles causing enlargement with or without venous stasis, or in the retrobulbar fat, patients can develop severe proptosis and optic neuropathy. Lid retraction likely occurs due to fibrosis of the levator or Muller's muscle as well as increased sympathetic tone.

Treatment is usually initiated using corticosteroids and later orbital radiation for the acute inflammatory phase and compressive optic neuropathy. If the proptosis, optic neuropathy, and/or corneal exposure persist, then surgical management should be undertaken. Orbital decompression surgery involves removing the bony walls of the orbit to enlare the orbital volume and allow prolapse of the orbital soft tissues. Typically, the medial wall, orbital floor, anterior lateral wall, and/or posterior lateral wall are removed using either a trans-eyelid, trans-conjunctival, trans-caruncular, trans-antral, or endoscopic approaches. Recent studies have found that the posterior inferomedial orbital decompression using a trans-fornix/transcaruncular approach is an effective procedure with less risk of globe dystopia and/or impairment of the maxillary sinus drainage.[55,56] If diplopia or motility deficits have been stable for six months, then strabismus/extraocular muscle surgery can be performed (typically recession of the inferior and medial rectus muscles). Eyelid surgery can be performed for lid retraction by lowering the upper lid and raising the lower lid, and for periorbital edema by removing excess skin and fat.

On both CT and MR studies, there is enlargement of one or more of the extraocular muscles (**Fig. 2-26**). Recent studies show that multiple muscle involvement is more common than one or two isolated muscle involvement and such involvement is usually diffuse and symmetric. The inferior and medial recti are most commonly involved; therefore, coronal plane imaging should be performed. Although the posterior and middle thirds of the muscle bellies are affected, the tendons near their insertions are usually not thickened. There may be bony remodeling secondary to pressure from the enlarged muscles. The extraocular muscle edges are smooth. Enhancement after contrast administration is characteristic. In patients with eyelid retraction, the levator palpebrae muscles may also be thickened.

The ability to measure the T2W signal intensity offers useful information both in determining which patients will benefit from immunosuppressive or local radiation therapy (those with high T2 values) and which patients are less likely to respond (based on a measurable response on serial MR images). The increased T2W relaxation times in the responsive patients may be due to an increase in edema or water content due to inflammation in those muscles likely to respond. In contrast, chronic endocrine orbitopathy that has already progressed to fibrosis (and shorter T2 relaxation times) usually does not respond to therapy. In addition, the maximal muscle area also predicts a response to therapy. Chronic disease is not responsive to immunosuppressive therapy and surgical decompression of the orbit may need to be performed.

An important role for MRI is to demonstrate the relationship of the extraocular muscles to the optic nerve at the orbital apex. The increase in extraocular muscle size correlates with the degree of optic neuropathy, and as extraocular muscles decrease in size optic neuropathy has been shown to improve. A prolapse of fat intracranially may also be a reliable sign of optic nerve compression. Increasing amounts of orbital fat may also cause stretching and straightening of the optic nerve and anterior bulging of the orbital septum.

There are several other entities that lead to enlargement of the extraocular muscles (**Table 2-16**). Lymphoma and metastatic disease, especially of the breast, may cause muscle enlargement. When idiopathic orbital pseudotumor causes enlargement it is typically diffuse in nature not localized to the muscle bellies as in endocrine orbitopathy. In the presence of a dural arteriovenous fistula dilation of the superior ophthalmic vein may also be noted on imaging. Diffuse enlargement may also be seen in orbital myositis and acromegaly.[57–63]

Tolosa-Hunt Syndrome

Tolosa-Hunt syndrome is a variant of idiopathic orbital pseudotumor (IOP) in which inflammation is restricted to the optic canal, superior orbital fissure, or cavernous sinus (see previous

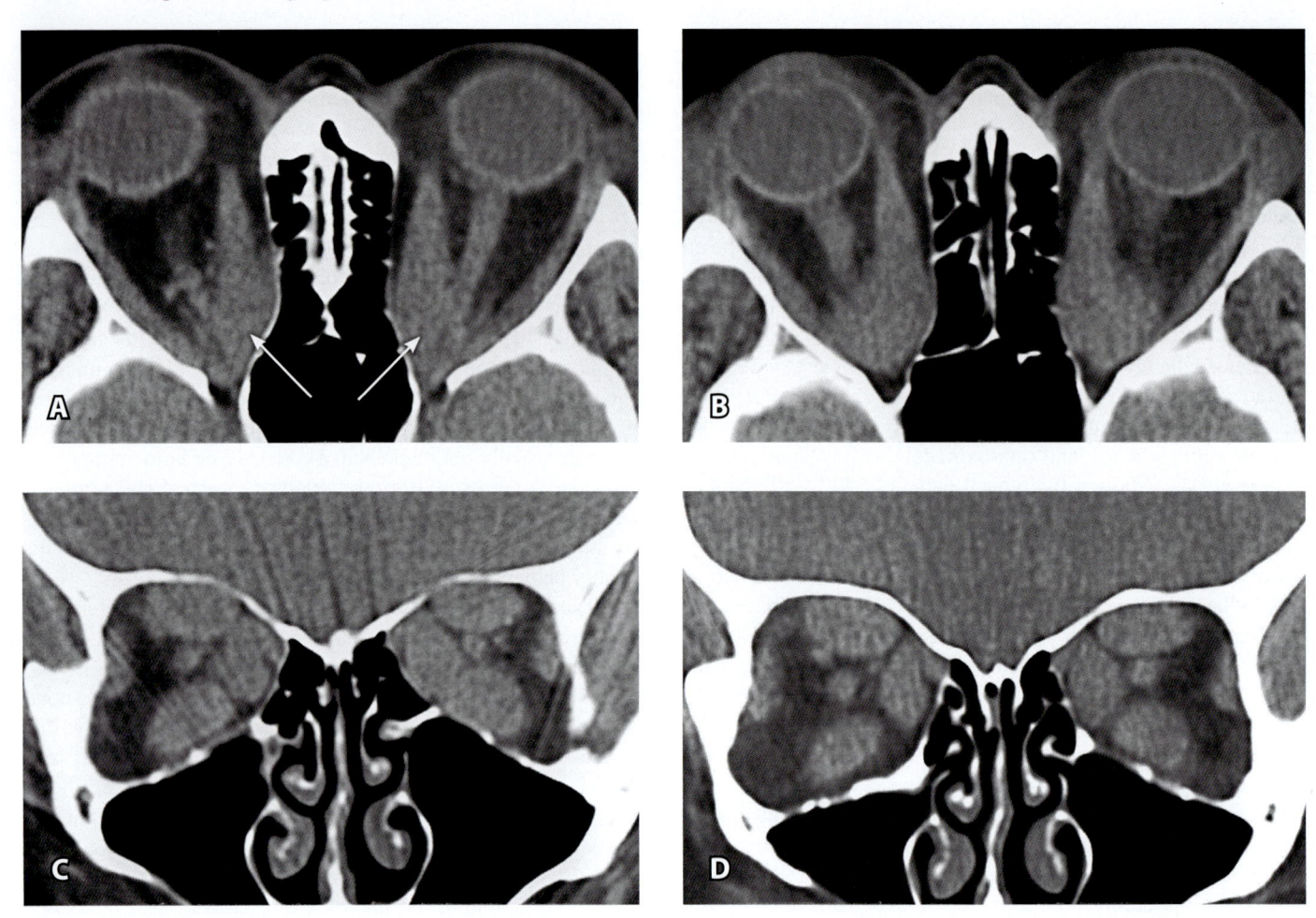

Figure 2-26 Graves Orbitopathy
Endocrine orbitopathy (Graves' disease) in an elderly female with a compressive optic neuropathy. Axial CT scans (**A** and **B**) show markedly enlarged extraocular muscles. The enlargement is predominately in the belly region of the muscle (*arrows,* **A**) and the more anterior areas of tendinous insertion are spared. Coronal CT scans (**C** and **D**) show that all of the extraocular muscles appear to be involved. It is important to evaluate the coronal view because the inferior and medical recti are the most commonly involved muscles. CT is more useful than MR if surgical orbital decompression is planned.

section on IOP). Patients often present with painful ophthalmoplegia and only minimal proptosis. The ophthalmoplegia occurs when the inflammatory process extends from the orbital apex into the cavernous sinus to involve the cranial nerves. In addition to orbital pain, the patients may also have III, IV, and VI cranial nerve palsies and hypesthesia of the periorbital skin due to V1 involvement. Rarely, there may be visual loss and external signs of inflammation. The ophthalmoparesis usually requires weeks to months of treatment with corticosteroids for resolution, but sometimes it may never resolve completely. On imaging studies there may be enlargement of the cavernous sinus on the affected side, or intracavernous carotid artery narrowing with diffuse enhancement around the vessel and marked muscular enhancement.[5,28,47]

Rhabdomyosarcoma and Liposarcoma

Rhabdomyosarcoma and liposarcoma are both primary malignant tumors of children and teenagers. These tumors are thought to arise from undifferentiated mesenchymal elements, not the extraocular muscles themselves. Equal numbers of tumors can arise from the orbits as from invasion directly from adjacent sinuses, or as a result of metastasis.[12] Rhabdomyosarcoma and liposarcoma are both highly malignant tumors that often extend locally into the adjacent bone and soft tissues. There may be single or multiple involvement of the extraocular muscles. The neoplasm usually occurs unilaterally with a rapid onset of unilateral proptosis.

MR imaging should be performed to delineate the extent of the neoplasm. Rhabdomyosarcomas and liposarcomas appear isointense to slightly hyperintense to muscle on T1W images and have variable intensity on proton-density MR images. On T2W images, the lesions usually appear hyperintense. Post contrast administration the tumor shows intense enhancement.

Treatment includes radical excision and local radiation and adjuvant chemotherapy. Triple combination chemotherapy has been shown to improve survival. With little to no residual tumor,

Table 2-16 Extraocular Muscle Enlargement

- Endocrine orbitopathy
- Lymphoproliferative disorders
- Idiopathic orbital pseudotumor (IOP)
- Tolosa-Hunt syndrome (variant of IOP)
- Giant cell polymyositis
- Sarcoidosis
- Vascular lesions (arteriovenous malformation or carotid cavernous fistula)
- Ophthalmic vein or cavernous sinus thrombosis
- Rhabdomyosarcoma
- Metastasis
- Amyloidosis
- Acromegaly
- Trauma
- Trichinosis (typically extraconal)
- Cysticercosis

Table 2-17 Pulsating or Positional (Stress) Proptosis

- Cavernous carotid or dural fistulas
- Arteriovenous malformation
- Venous varix
- Hemangioma

the patency and adequacy of the collateral cerebral blood flow should occlusion of the involved vessels occur during treatment. During the venous phase of the angiogram, it is important to assess the risk of intracerebral venous rupture due to increased collateral cerebral venous drainage or the presence of an underlying venous aneurysm.[53,66]

INTRACONAL LESIONS

Lesions of the intraconal space stem from the optic nerve itself, the soft tissue around the optic nerve, or extend from adjacent regions into the intraconal space. Lesions of the optic nerve typically cause enlargement of the optic nerve, optic nerve sheath or both with or without enhancement. A list of these lesions is presented in **Table 2-18**. First, we will discuss the lesions that directly involve the optic nerve, then the lesions that originate from the surrounding tissues.

Optic Nerve Aplasia and Hypoplasia

The complete absence of the optic nerve or optic nerve aplasia is a rare, usually unilateral, sporadic anomaly. It is typically accompanied by absence of the retinal blood vessels and is frequently associated with anterior colobomas. Aplasia may or may not be associated with other congenital ocular or systemic abnormalities. In optic nerve hypoplasia, the optic nerve starts to develop but then regresses due to a neurological insult early in prenatal development. On inspection, the optic nerve head appears small and is surrounded by a white rim of scleral tissue showing through the underdeveloped nerve. CT images of these patients reveal defects in the septum pelucidum and posterior

survival rates can be 90% after five years. Lesions that should be included in the differential include IOP, aggressive fibromatosis, proliferating hemangiomas, and veno-lymphatic malformations.[23,53,64,65]

Carotid Cavernous Fistula

A carotid cavernous fistula is a connection between the carotid artery and cavernous sinus. The high flow lesions have a direct communication with the carotid artery while the low flow lesions have an intervening collection of dural vessels. These abnormal connections between the arterial and venous systems can lead to increased retrograde drainage into the inferior and superior ophthalmic veins resulting in muscular congestion. These fistulas are typically secondary to trauma (head trauma or iatrogenic trauma) or carotid aneurysm rupture, but may also occur in patients with collagen vascular diseases such as Ehler-Danlos or may develop spontaneously.

Signs and symptoms of pulsating proptosis or proptosis that is aggravated by increases in venous pressure (stress proptosis) are suggestive of an orbital vascular lesion (**Table 2-17**). The additional clinical finding of dilated episcleral vessels is characteristic of a carotid cavernous fistula. These patients may also have increased intraocular pressure, an auscultable bruit over the eye and diplopia. They may complain of tinnitus due to the redirected flow of blood into the petrosal sinuses toward the temporal bones.

The enlargement of the cavernous sinus and the engorgement of the extraocular muscles may be observed on various imaging modalities. Ultrasound will reveal dilation of the superior ophthalmic vein with flow characteristics of arterialization. Angiography remains the imaging method of choice to demonstrate the fistula. Particular attention should be paid to

Table 2-18 Optic Nerve Enlargement

- Optic neuritis
- Optic nerve and sheath tumors
- Metastatic tumors
- Papilledema
- Endocrine orbitopathy
- Idiopathic orbital pseudotumor (IOP)
- Lymphoproliferative disorders
- Central retinal vein occlusion
- Traumatic hematoma of the optic nerve sheath

corpus callosum. Due to the subnormal number of functional nerve axons, visual acuity may be slightly to severely impaired. Optic nerve hypoplasia may result from chronic alcohol and drug abuse by the mother during the prenatal period.[6]

Septo-optic Dysplasia

Septo-optic dysplasia or De Morsier syndrome is a combination of hypoplasia of the optic nerves accompanied by an abnormal or absent septum pellucidum. There are two types of septo-optic dysplasia. The first variant is associated with schizencephaly, which may be a mild form of holoprosencephaly, and seizures. The second type is associated with white matter hypoplasia and hypothalamic-pituitary dysfunction (Fig. 2-27). Type 2 is more common and although many theories have been proposed, a definitive etiology has not been determined for either type. Both types of septo-optic dysplasia may present with normal or decreased vision, blindness and/or nystagmus. Imaging will reveal small optic canals and nerves, small anterior recesses of the third ventricle, and hypotelorism.[67]

Optic Atrophy

Atrophy of the optic nerve may be acquired or congenital. The acquired type may be due to trauma, glaucoma, vascular disturbances (occlusions of the central retinal vein or artery, arteriosclerotic changes within the optic nerve), degenerative retinal disease (papilledema, optic neuritis), metabolic diseases (diabetes), toxicity (alcohol, tobacco, other poisons), or compression of the optic nerve due to space-filling lesions with the orbit. Congenital optic atrophy is usually bilateral and can come in three forms: autosomal dominant, autosomal recessive, and X-linked. The autosomal dominant form is more mild with gradual onset of optic atrophy in childhood. The more severe, autosomal recessive form presents with optic atrophy at birth or within the first two years of life and is associated with nystagmus. Leber's Disease or Leber's Hereditary Optic Neuropathy (LHON) is a mitochodrial, X-linked disease that presents in 20- to 30-year-old males and can progress to total bilateral blindness due to degeneration of the optic nerve. With optic atrophy, the primary symptom is gradual vision loss (over weeks to months), and the disc may appear pale with enlarged disc cupping. Typically, degeneration of the optic nerve fibers is irreversible. However, visual loss due to pressure against the optic nerve may be partially reversed if the pressure is relieved early in the degenerative process.

Pseudotumor Cerebri

Pseudotumor cerebri or benign intracranial hypertension is classically a disease of obese middle-aged women. In this disease there is increased intracranial pressure and papilledema, but no etiology can be identified. The disease is not actually benign in that progressive visual loss may result in some patients and has been shown to correlate with the degree of reversal of the optic nerve head. One explanation for this is that the increased intracranial pressure is transmitted down the optic nerve to the optic nerve head, causing reversed protrusion and a compressive ischemia or disruption of axonal transport.

Imaging findings include reversal of the protrusion of the optic nerve head on CT and fundoscopic examination (Figs. 2-28 and 2-29). Abnormally increased ventricular size has been reported in the past, but a recent controlled and blinded study could only confirm the finding of optic nerve sheath enlargement. Normal ventricular size in patients with pseudotumor cerebri has also been noted in several other recent studies. With current scanning techniques, an empty sella has been noted as a frequent finding in patients with pseudotumor cerebri.[68–70]

Drusen or deposits of hyaline calcified material of the optic nerve head that is buried may mimic the findings of papilledema on fundoscopic exam and hence may require radiological evaluation (Fig. 2-30). In most cases, the calcified deposits may be seen on a CT scan (Fig. 2-31). MR scans do not identify the calcification in drusen deposits, although use of MRI may rule out an intracranial mass lesion at the same time.[71,72]

Optic Neuritis

Optic neuritis is a general term used to describe inflammation or demyelination of the optic nerve resulting in acute visual deficits. Idiopathic optic neuropathy is the most common cause, but of the known etiologies, multiple sclerosis (MS) is most common, followed by infectious and inflammatory diseases (Tables 2-19 and 2-20).

It is usually seen in women between the ages of 15 and 45 years, but may occur in either gender of any age. Of the patients with isolated optic neuritis, approximately 50% will eventually be diagnosed with MS (about 75% of women and 34% of men). Conversely, approximately 70% of MS patients will have an episode of optic neuritis during the course of the disease; it is the presenting diagnosis in 15% to 20% of MS patients.

There are two types of optic neuritis depending on the location of the lesion: papillitis (optic disc swelling is present), and retrobulbar (disc swelling is not present, because the inflammation is behind the globe). Optic disc swelling is found in about 35% of the cases. Clinically, optic neuritis presents with unilateral acute visual deficits (blurred or distorted vision, reduced color vision, or a blind spot), pain on eye movement, and an afferent pupillary defect. Less common symptoms include bilaterality, anterior or posterior segment inflammation, and lack of pain. They symptoms may progress for seven to 10 days, then stabilize for three to eight weeks. Typically, most of the vision will return after six months. Treatment options include observation or IV steroids for three days followed by oral steroid taper over 11 days. The Optic Neuritis Treatment Trial showed that although this regimen had little effect on final visual outcome over the course of three years, the use of IV steroids accelerated the recovery rate by two weeks and reduced the risk of developing MS within two years by half (from 16% to 8%). Interestingly, patients treated with oral steroids alone had an increased rate of recurrent optic neuritis compared to placebo.

MR imaging of the orbits and whole brain is used to assist with diagnosis, look for demyelinating white matter disease, identify the extent of involvement, and measure the effectiveness

Chapter 2: The Orbit and Globe 45

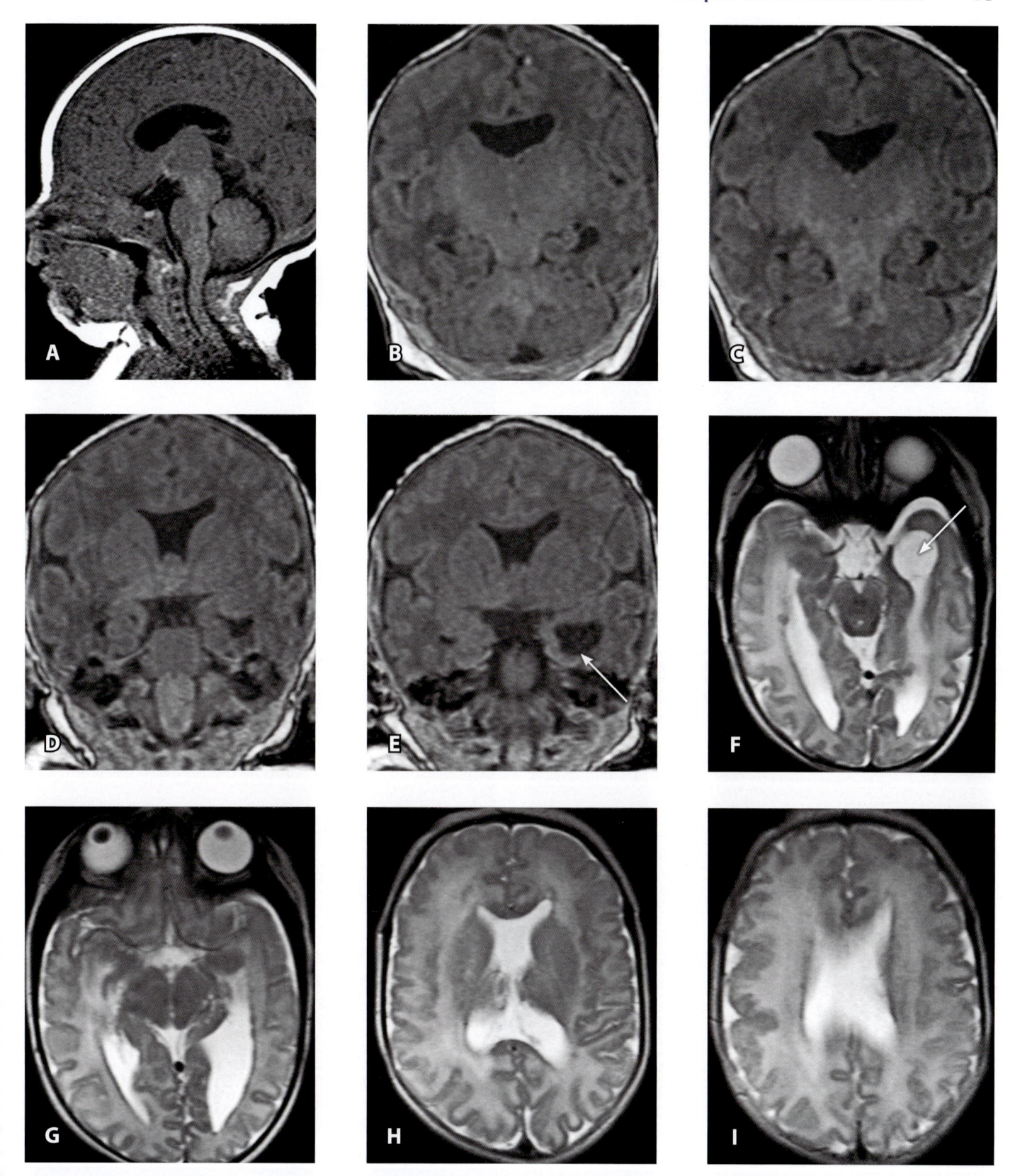

Figure 2-27 Septo-optic Dysplasia with Pachygyria
Septo-optic dysplasia in a two-month-old infant girl. Sagittal T1W MR scan (**A**) demonstrates hypoplasia of the optic chiasm and corpus callosum. Coronal T1W MR scans (**B–E**) shows complete absence of the septum pellucidum from anterior to posterior. There is cystic expansion of the left temporal horn (*arrows*, **E**, **F**). Axial T2W MR scans (**F–I**) demonstrate the absence of the septum pellucidum, as well as abnormal and thickened right posterior temporal and parietal gyria (pachygyria), consistent with a complex CNS malformation.

46 Diagnostic Imaging of the Head and Neck

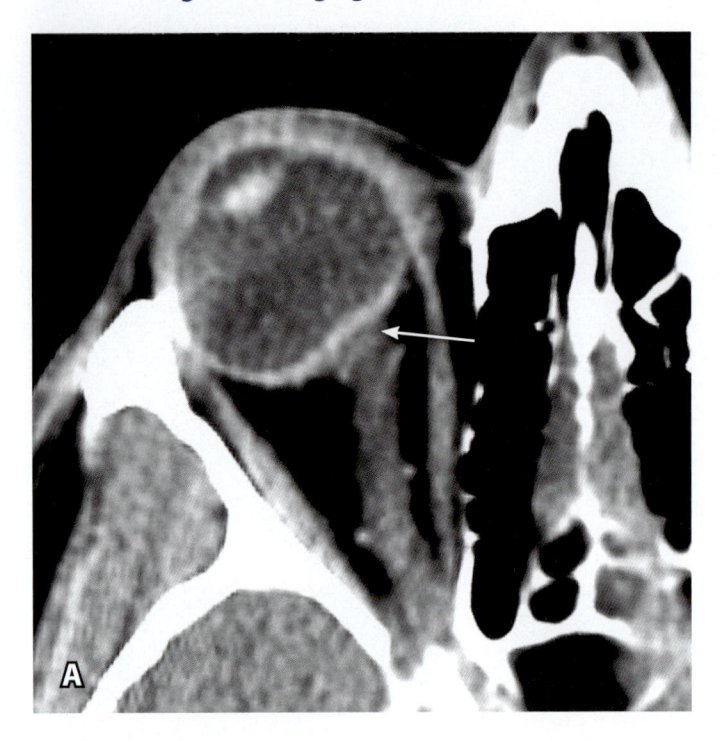

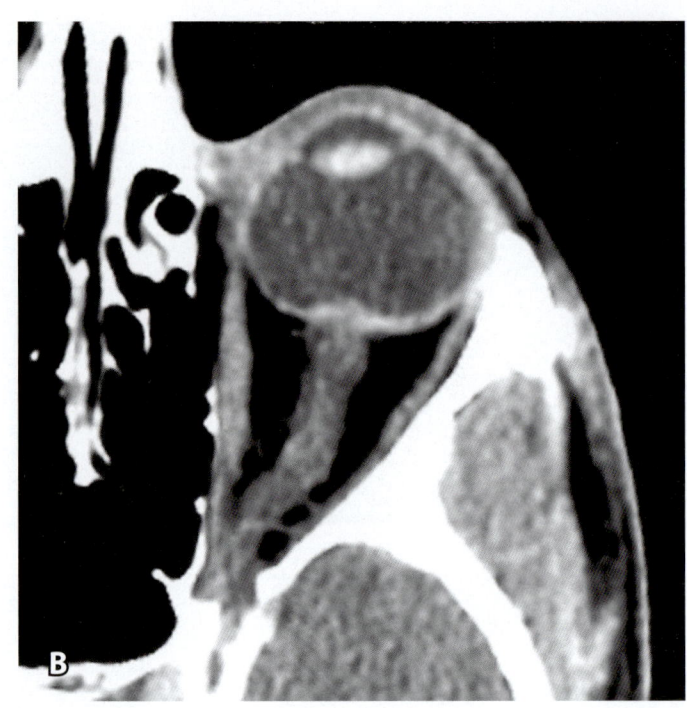

Figure 2-28 Papilledema
Bilateral papilledema due to pseudotumor cerebri. Axial CT scans with contrast. The swollen optic nerve heads obscure the margin between the posterior choroid and optic nerves with flattening of the globe on the right side (*arrow*, **A**) and protrusion into the posterior globe on the left side (**B**).

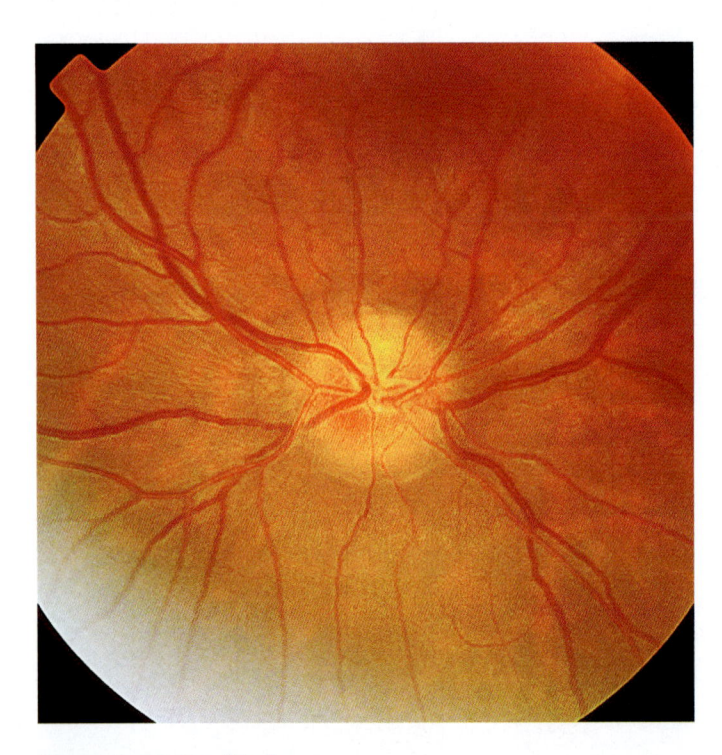

Figure 2-29 Papilledema
Papilledema due to pseudotumor cerebri. Fundus photo shows the swollen optic nerve fiber layer that obscures the disc margins, disc capillaries, and optic cup. There are also some small peripapillary hemorrhages and retinal exudates present. (Photo courtesy of Jonathan W. Kim, MD, University of California, Irvine.)

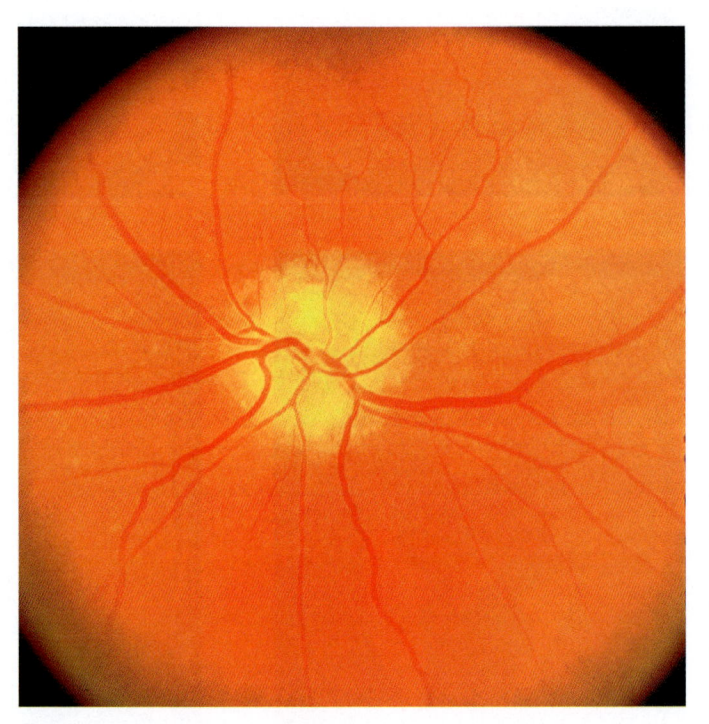

Figure 2-30 Optic Drusen
Fundus photo demonstrates multiple small whitish-yellow lesions that are located deep in the substance of the nerve head just anterior to the lamina cribrosa. The lesions represent mineralization of accumulated axoplasmic material, primarily acid mucopolysaccharide. (Photo courtesy of Jonathan W. Kim, MD, University of California, Irvine.)

Table 2-19 Optic Neuritis: Differential Diagnosis

Idiopathic (most common)

Systemic Diseases	Local Disease Processes
• Multiple sclerosis (most common) • Rheumatic retinitis or choroiditis • Graves' disease • Sarcoidosis • Lymphoma • Leukemia • Blood dyscrasias • Diabetes • Avitaminoses	• Papilledema • Idiopathic orbital pseudotumor (IOP) • Neuromyelitis optica (Devic disease) • Hereditary optic nerve atrophy (Leber disease) • Ischemic arterial occlusion • Congestive venous occlusion • Hematoma of the optic nerve sheath • Direct nerve trauma • Extension of sinus disease/Infection

Systemic Infections	CNS-Related Processes
• Viral • Syphilis • Poliomyelitis • Tuberculosis • Influenza • Cat scratch fever • Mumps • Lyme disease • Measles • Bacterial pneumonia	• Acute disseminated encephalomyelitis (ADEM) • Diffuse periaxial encephalitis (Schilder disease) • Meningioma • Glioma

Orbit Infection	Toxins
• Infectious scleritis • Endophthalmitis • Cytomegalovirus retinitis • Syphilitic chorioretinitis	• Tobacco • Methanol • Quinine • Arsenic • Salicylates

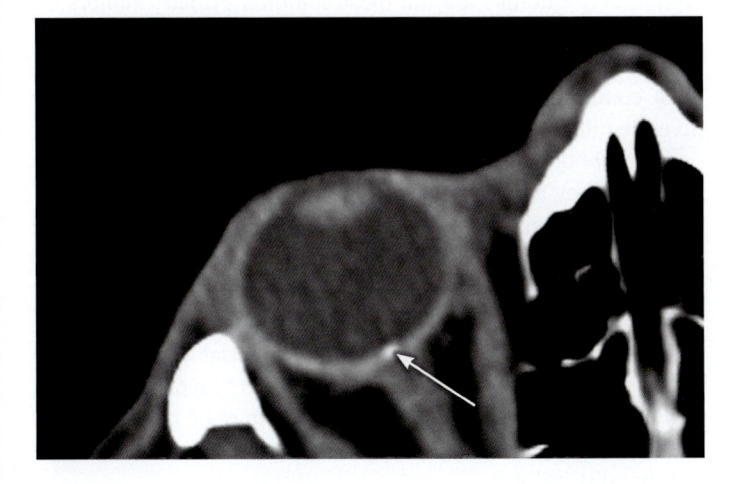

Figure 2-31 Optic Drusen
Axial CT scan without contrast shows focal dense calcifications in the optic nerve head.

Table 2-20 Arthropathies Associated with Optic Neuritis

- Syphilis
- Ulcerative colitis
- Vitamin B deficiency
- Collagen diseases:
    - Progressive systemic sclerosis
    - Systemic lupus erythematosis
    - Reiter's syndrome
    - Rheumatoid arthritis

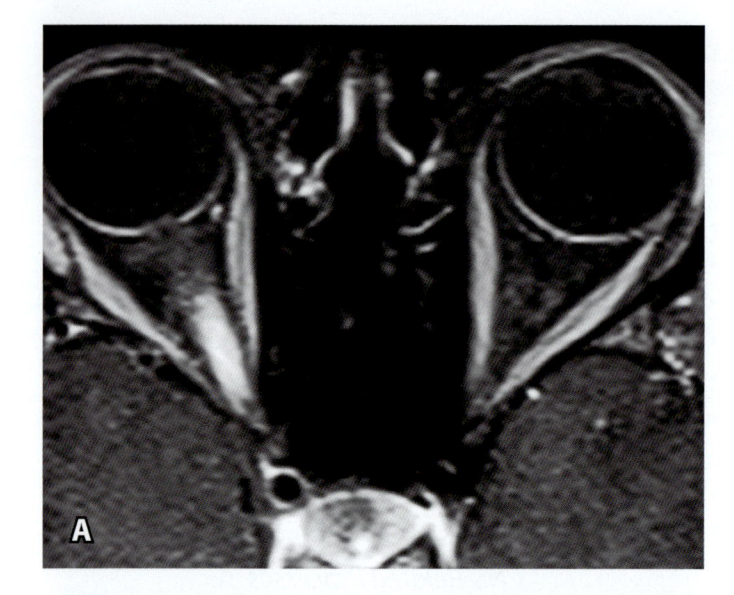

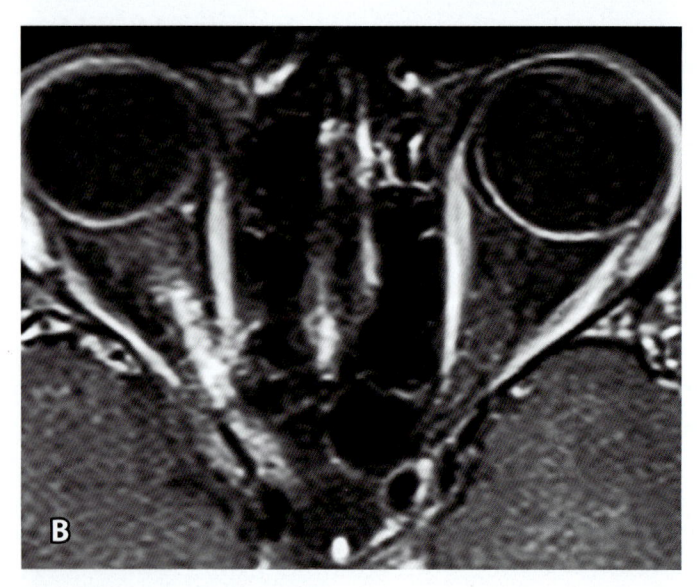

Figure 2-32 Optic Neuritis
Optic Neuritis of the right eye. Axial T1W enhanced MR images show enhancement in both the intraorbital (**A**) and intracanalicular (**B**) portions of the right optic nerve. There is no enlargment of the optic nerve.

of therapy. Although MR imaging is not always necessary for diagnosis in patients with a strong clinical picture of optic neuritis, its ability to rule out other possible causes and to identify the extent of the lesion intracranially is valuable (**Fig. 2-32**). Patients with more lesions are more likely to develop MS sooner, and identification of this subgroup may be useful for treatment decisions and experimental therapy. Of those with a normal MR, only 0% to 5% will develop MS compared to 30% to 50% of patients with three or more periventricular or ovoid white matter lesions. Therefore, high-quality MR imaging with pulse sequences optimized to detect white matter lesions should be performed. Use of fat and water suppression techniques on T2 W images, such as multiecho train T2 W or STIR sequences, allow for the best differentiation of a lesion of increased signal intensity in the optic nerve. In the acute phase, there may be enhancement of optic neuritis lesions, which is best seen on T1 W images with fat suppression[73–78] (**Fig. 2-33**).

Radiation-induced Optic Neuropathy

Radiation-induced optic neuropathy (RION) is a rare condition that has been reported to occur between 3 months to 4 years following treatment by radiation therapy. Affected patients typically receive total doses of greater than 4500cGy or individual, fractionated doses of greater than 200cGy of radiation for a sellar or parasellar tumor. Concomitant treatment with chemotherapy predisposes the patient to RON at lower doses of radiation. The clinical picture is one of a rapid onset of monocular, painless, irreversible visual loss usually resulting in blindness, which may extend to the contra-lateral eye or optic chiasm. The cause of the visual loss may be secondary to microvasculature injury that results in fibrosis, thrombosis and edema. The only known treatment is corticosteroid therapy that delays the onset of ROP and reverses some of the symptoms.

Imaging with MR is the method of choice both to identify the changes in the optic pathway and to rule out a recurrence of tumor as a cause for any visual loss. On T1W images there is enlargement of the optic nerves. There is typically marked enhancement of the affected area after contrast administration, which may or may not persist on follow-up evaluations. Abnormalities on T2W imaging reflect the edema and inflammation of affected structures with intense increased signal of the lesions. Atrophy of the optic nerves during follow-up has also been reported.[79–81]

Optic Nerve Glioma

Optic nerve gliomas are the most common primary tumors of the optic nerve. The peak incidence of these tumors occurs in the first decade of life, and there is a female predominance. The most common subtype to affect the optic nerve is the benign juvenile pilocytic astrocytoma.

Childhood optic nerve gliomas may be unilateral or bilateral, but when they are bilateral they are considered pathognomic of neurofibromatosis-1 (NF-1) (**Table 2-21**). Up to half of patients with optic nerve gliomas also have NF-1. In the tumors associated with NF-1, a para-optic component to the tumor has been observed. This component is due to perineural arachnoidal gliomatosis consisting of a proteinaceous material that seeds and spreads within the optic nerve subarachnoid space and is a portion of the tumor. This process may result in optic nerve elongation and resultant kinking of the nerve just posterior to the dorsal portion of the globe.

There is a much less common subgroup of adult patients with optic nerve gliomas that are highly malignant and not associated with NF-1. In these patients, the clinical presentation and imaging findings are similar to optic neuritis. There is no current curative treatment for these aggressive neoplasms, and in some cases the disease may be fatal one year after diagnosis.

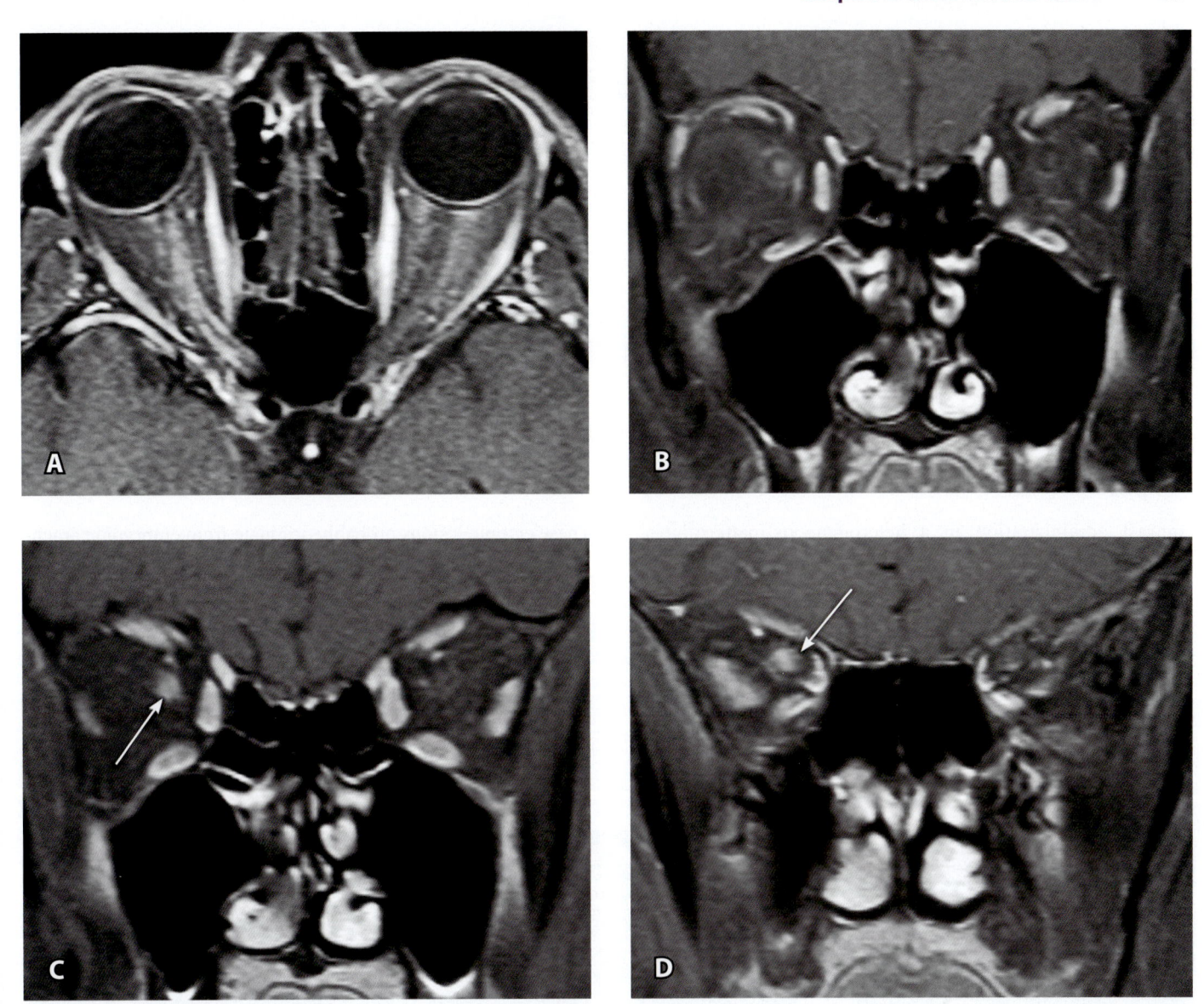

Figure 2-33 Optic Neuritis
Optic neuritis in the right eye of a young woman with relapsing multiple sclerosis. Axial (**A**) and coronal (**B–D**) T1W FS enhanced MR images show enhancement of the right proximal intracranial, intracanalicular, and intraorbital optic nerve. Note that the apparent "tram-like enhancement" suggested on the axial image (**A**) is actually enhancement of the nerve itself as seen on the coronal scans (*arrows*, **C**, **D**). The left optic nerve is normal.

Progressive loss of visual acuity is the classical presentation of optic gliomas. There may be specific field deficits depending upon the location of the tumor (intraocular, intraorbital, or intracranial). Over half of optic nerve gliomas also involve the chiasm or hypothalamus. An afferent pupillary defect and optic nerve atrophy may also be present. Spasmus mutans is a type of nystagmus that has been reported in association with optic nerve gliomas. It is a benign, self-limiting, high frequency, low-amplitude nystagmus in any direction. Proptosis is not typically present until there is extensive involvement of the intraorbital space (**Fig. 2-34**). Treatment is catered to the aggressiveness of the lesion and ranges from watchful waiting to surgical debulking.

The extra and intracranial extent of an optic nerve tumor is best evaluated on MR imaging (**Table 2-22**). The optic nerve may appear fusiform, homogeneous, enlarged, or thickened and tortuous. The normal optic nerve and sheath are isointense to the white matter with an intervening area of hyperintensity represented by the CSF. With tumor obstruction of this space (obstruction may also be caused by other lesions), optic hydrops (also referred to as optic nerve sheath cyst, arachnoid cyst, perioptic hygroma, or dural ectasia) or a dilation of the CSF-filled space may occur. The lesion may appear hyperintense to cerebral cortex on T2 W images, and this signal intensity may appear heterogeneous if there are cystic regions present. The tumors will usually enhance after

Table 2-21 Phakomatoses (Neurocutaneous Syndromes) with Common Orbital Involvement

Neurofibromatosis I	Tuberous Sclerosis and Linear Sebaceous Nevus Syndrome
• Optic nerve and chiasmal tumors • Sphenoid wing dysplasia • Buphthalmos • Plexiform neurofibroma • Retinal astrocytoma	• Retinal astrocytoma
Sturge-Weber Syndrome	**von Hippel-Lindau**
• Buphthalmos • Choroidal hemangioma	• Retinal angiomatosis (capillary angioma)

contrast administration in a heterogeneous pattern[23,53,82,83] (**Fig. 2-34**).

Perioptic (Optic Sheath) Meningioma

Perioptic or optic sheath meningiomas arise from the meningoepithelial cells of the arachnoid. The tumors may develop from intracranial lesions that spread to the orbit, the optic nerve sheath, or in rare instances, from ectopic lesions in the orbit. These ectopic lesions probably originate from embryonic arachnoid cell rests.

Perioptic meningiomas occur most often in women in the third to sixth decades of life. Bilateral involvement is uncommon, and when it does occur may be associated with neurofibromatosis. When the lesion occurs in children, it is much more aggressive and may be associated with neurofibromatosis 2. The most common presenting features are painless, progressive, peripheral, and eventually central loss of vision secondary

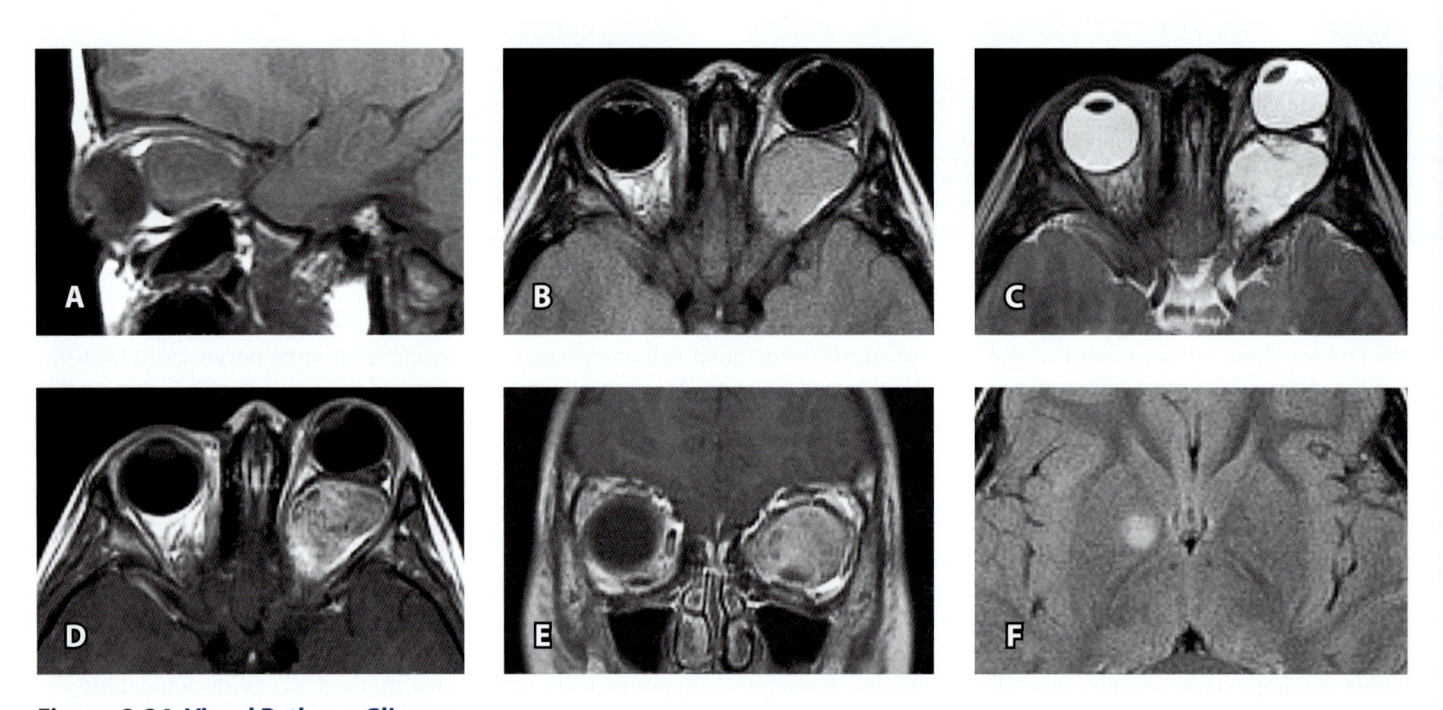

Figure 2-34 Visual Pathway Glioma
Optic glioma in a young child with NF-I and proptosis. Paramedian sagittal T1W MR image (**A**) shows a pear-shaped mass within an expanded muscle cone of the left eye. Axial PDW (**B**) and T2W (**C**) MR images show marked expansion of the silhouette of the optic nerve inside the orbit with proptosis and medial deviation of the globe. Axial (**D**) and coronal (**E**) T1W enhanced MR images show heterogeneous enhancement within the tumor, which surgically proved to be anaplastic astrocytoma. Axial flair image of the brain (**F**) shows abnormal signal in the region of the right optic tract, confirming intracranial extension of a visual pathway glioma.

Table 2-22 Imaging Optic Nerve Gliomas, Perioptic Meningiomas

Optic Nerve Glioma	Perioptic Meningiomas
MR	CT
• Optic nerve may appear fusiform, homogeneous, enlarged, or thickened and tortuous • Optic hydrops or dilation of the CSF-filled space may occur • May appear hyperintense to cerebral cortex on T2 W • May appear heterogeneous if there are cystic regions • Usually enhance post contrast in a heterogeneous pattern (**Fig. 2-34**)	• Tubular or fusiform thickening or area of local, eccentric expansion of optic nerve • Diffuse thickening is more common than segmental thickening • Well-defined lesion • Enhances homogenously post contrast • "Tram-track" sign – lucent area surrounded by enhancement (also seen in IOP, lymphoma, and neuritis) • May see globular or sheet-like (en plaque) calcifications around the optic nerve • May see perioptic cysts or cystic degenerative areas within the tumor
	MR
	• Variable signal intensity • Usually isointense to brain and the optic nerve • Moderate to marked enhancement is post contrast with fat saturation (**Fig. 2-35**)

to compressive optic neuropathy and proptosis. Visual loss may worsen during pregnancy. The degree of proptosis is directly related to the length of symptoms. Some patients report transient visual obscuration (brief periods of dim vision). Fundoscopic findings include optic disc pallor on the side of the lesion, disc swelling, which may cause transient visual obscuration, and optociliary venous shunts.

CT scans of perioptic meningiomas typically show a tubular or fusiform thickening or a local region of eccentric expansion of the optic nerve (**Table 2-22**). Diffuse thickening is seen more commonly than segmental thickening. The lesion is well-defined and enhances homogenously post contrast administration. The appearance of enhancement surrounding a lucent area corresponding to a nerve sheath tumor surrounding the optic nerve itself is referred to as the "tram-track" sign. It is characteristically observed in perioptic meningiomas as well as IOP, lymphoma, and neuritis of the optic nerve. Calcifications seen as a globular lesion or forming a sheet-like tube (en plaque) around the optic nerve are not uncommon (**Fig. 2-35**). Perioptic cysts or cystic degenerative areas within the tumor may also be encountered in the evaluation of perioptic meningiomas.

MRI is the method of choice to evaluate perioptic meningiomas, particularly if there is intracranial involvement. The shapes of the lesions are similar to that seen on CT, but the signal intensity is more variable (**Table 2-22**). Most frequently, the tumors are isointense to brain and the optic nerve. Enhancement is moderate to marked and is best evaluated on postcontrast images with fat saturation.

The long-term clinical course is one of continued worsening of vision. Any proposed treatment is based on preservation of vision. If there is significant deterioration with some vision remaining, radiation therapy has been proposed as an appropriate treatment. If the patient is blind, then surgical intervention and resection is performed. Imaging alone may not be able to distinguish optic nerve meningiomas from a variety of other lesions including sarcoidosis (**Fig. 2-36**), optic neuritis, and optic nerve glioma.[23,53,84,85]

Peripheral Nerve Sheath Tumors

Neurofibromas and schwannomas are peripheral nerve sheath tumors, which constitute 4% of all orbital neoplasms. These tumors are usually benign, but rarely a malignant schwannoma or neurofibrosarcoma may occur in the orbit. Peripheral nerve sheath tumors affect the sensory component of the nerves more frequently than the motor component. This is supported by the fact that patients present with pain and proptosis, but not diplopia until the lesions are large enough to limit muscle movement grossly.

Neurofibromas may occur in one of four patterns: plexiform (**Figs. 2-37** and **2-38**), diffuse, localized, and post amputation. The localized tumors have a tendency to occur in the superior orbit as

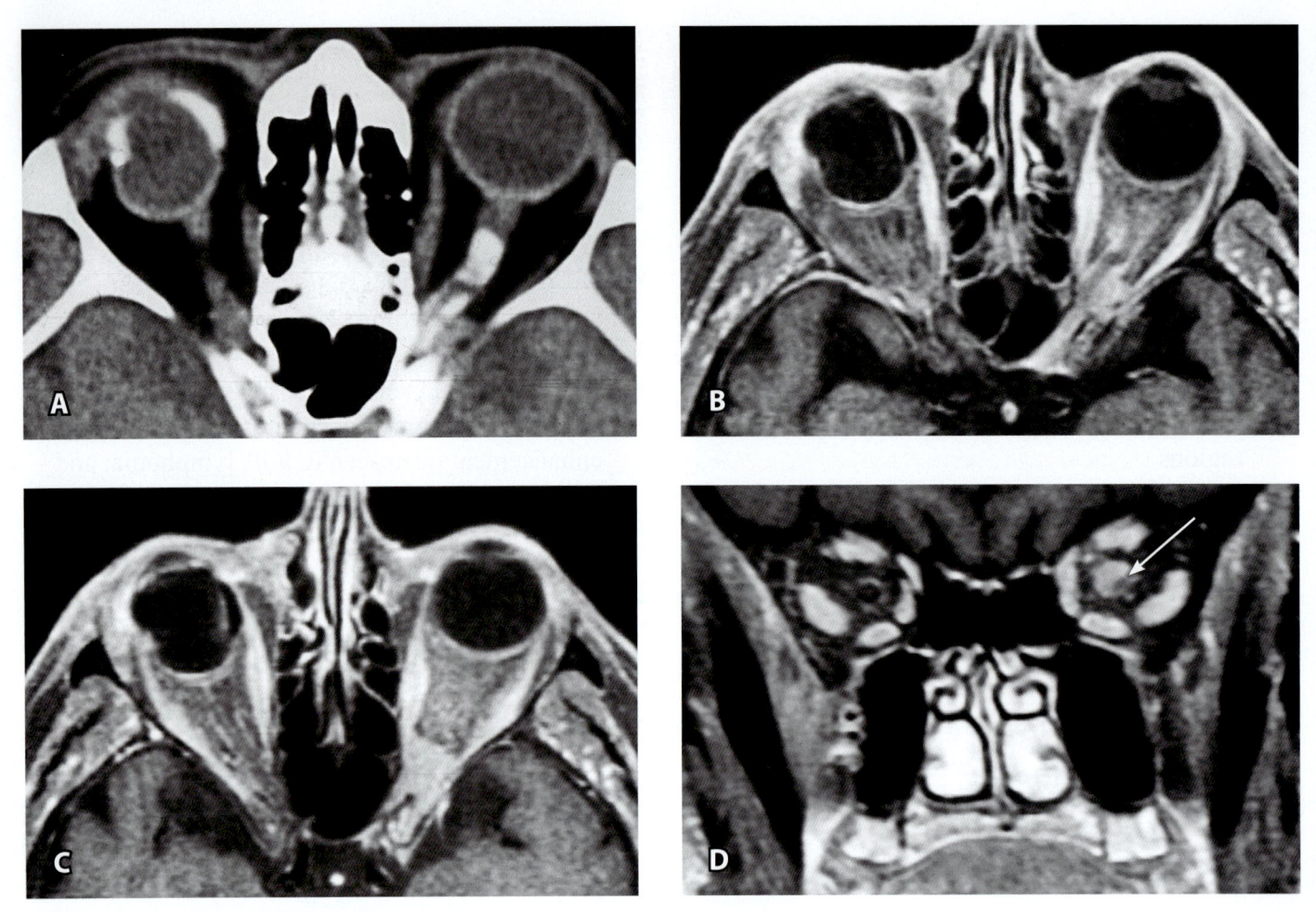

Figure 2-35 Optic Sheath Meningioma
Axial CT scan without contrast (**A**) shows both solid and linear dense calcifications embedded in the left optic nerve. Axial (**B–C**) and coronal (**D**) T1W enhanced MR. **B** and **C** demonstrate enhancement around the optic nerve that extends into the optic canal and spreads along the adjacent intracranial dura, as evidence of meningeal origin. **D** shows that the enhancement extends circumferentially around 80% of the outline of the nerve, with an nonenhancing focus of the intraorbital portion of the optic nerve (*arrow*, **D**). An unrelated banding device is visualized in the right globe.

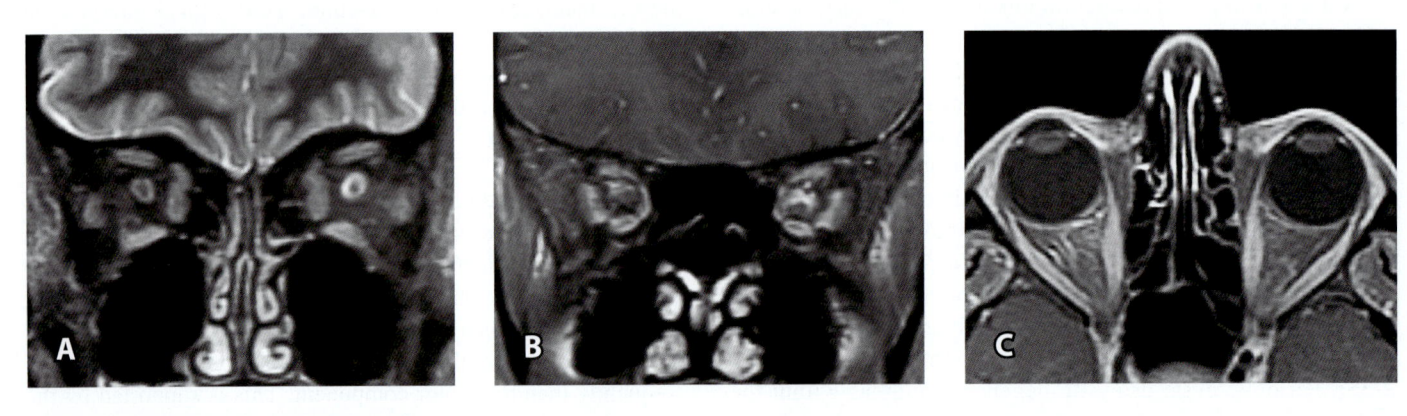

Figure 2-36 Optic Sheath Sarcoid
Optic sheath sarcoid in a young adult woman with left-sided visual blurring. Coronal T2W MR image (**A**) shows high signal within the sheath surrounding the left optic nerve. Coronal T1W enhanced MR image (**B**) shows focal enhancement of the optic nerve sheath. Axial T1W enhanced MR image (**C**) confirms similar changes in the sheath of the left optic nerve.

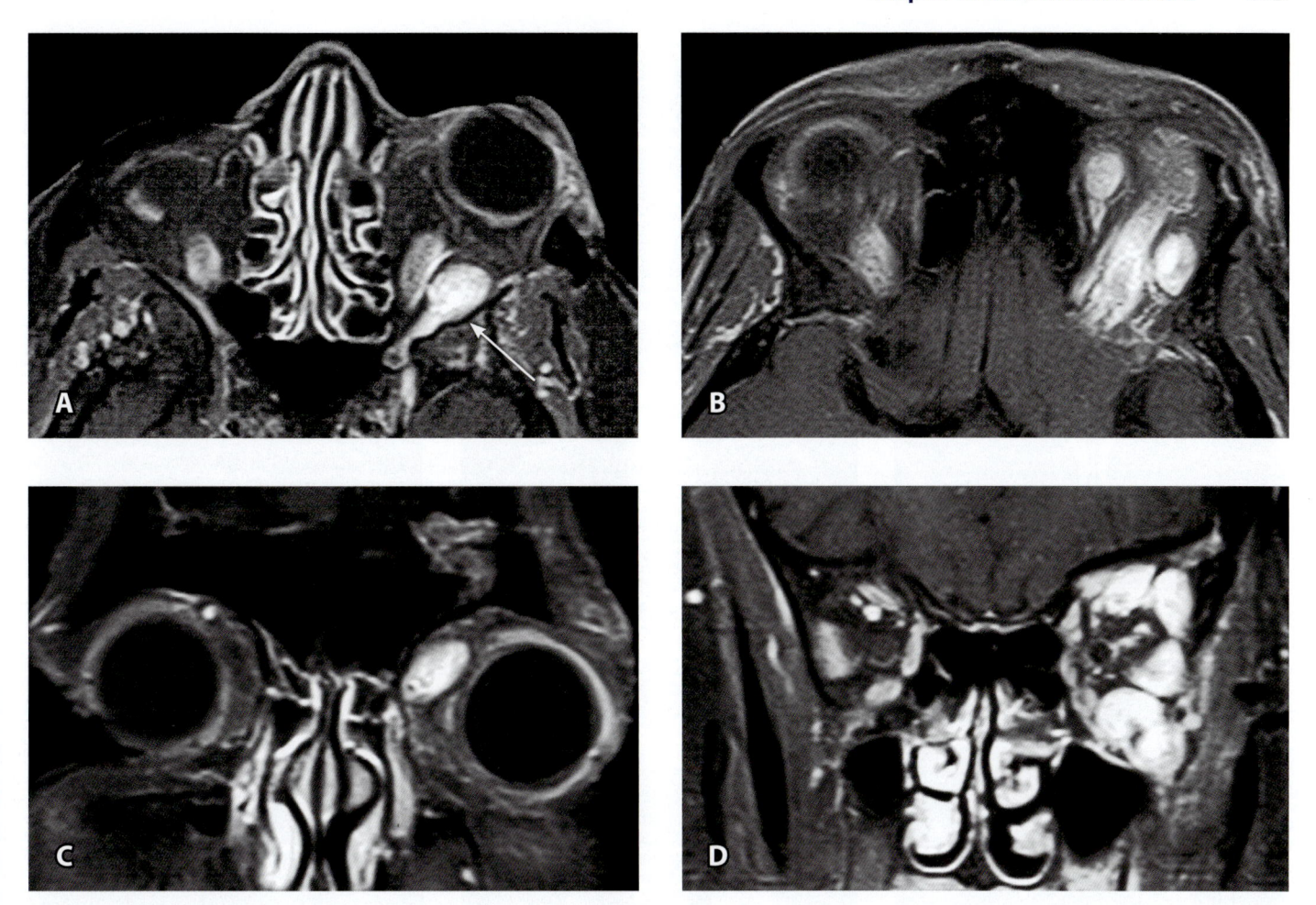

Figure 2-37 Orbital Plexiform Neurofibroma
Orbital plexiform neurofibroma of the oculomotor nerve. T1W enhanced MR scans with fat saturation. Axial images (**A**) and (**B**) show a nodular enhancing tumor insinuating around the conal structures of the orbit. Posteriorly in (**A**) the tumor is seen to extend through the superior orbital fissure towards the left side of the cavernous (*arrow,* **A**), sinus consistent with origin from the V1 division of the trigeminal nerve. Coronal views (**C**) and (**D**) show that the tumor extends along the divisions of V-1 with expansion of the frontal and nasociliary divisions within the orbit which simulates enlargement of the extraocular muscles.

a slow-growing mass in a middle-aged adult. The diffuse form may infiltrate the orbital fat and extraocular muscles, and may or may not be associated with neurofibromatosis. Involvement of the eyelid with a plexiform neurofibroma that most commonly occurs in the extraocular muscles, retrobulbar space, lacrimal gland, skin and eyelid regions is usually indicative of NF-1 (**Table 2-23**).

Patients with the autosomal dominant disease, NF-1, have multiple neurofibromas of the skin, skeleton, and nervous system, and may show a unique and rare facial-orbital disfigurement involving a cluster of several disease processes. These include optic nerve neoplasms, plexiform neurofibromas, orbital osseous dysplasia, and buphthalmos. Plexiform neurofibromas, either isolated or in association with other disease constellations, occur in early childhood or infancy. Most commonly they occur in the eyelid as a characteristic visible or palpable mass referred to as a "bag of worms" secondary to the cords and nodules present within the tumor.

The typical schwannoma is a benign, slow-growing, encapsulated tumor. CT imaging may reveal a well-circumscribed tumor with similar attenuation to brain (**Fig. 2-37**). The tumor may be internally homogeneous or heterogeneous. On T1W MR images, it may have intermediate signal intensity similar to the extraocular muscles and high signal intensity on T2W images. This tumor will enhance markedly after contrast administration (**Fig. 2-38**). The enhancement may be heterogeneous due to areas of cystic degeneration.

Solitary neurofibromas differ from schwannomas in that they are unencapsulated tumors. They will also remodel bone and have a variable appearance on CT examination. MR imaging reveals a heterogeneous lesion with intermediate signal on T1W images and higher signal on T2W images with variable enhancement post contrast administration. The plexiform variety of neurofibroma forms an unencapsulated tumor that shows centripetal growth into the surrounding tissues. The mass will typically appear isodense on CT scan and cause orbital cavity deformity. MR imaging shows a poorly delineated infiltrating mass with hypointense to intermediate heterogeneous intensity

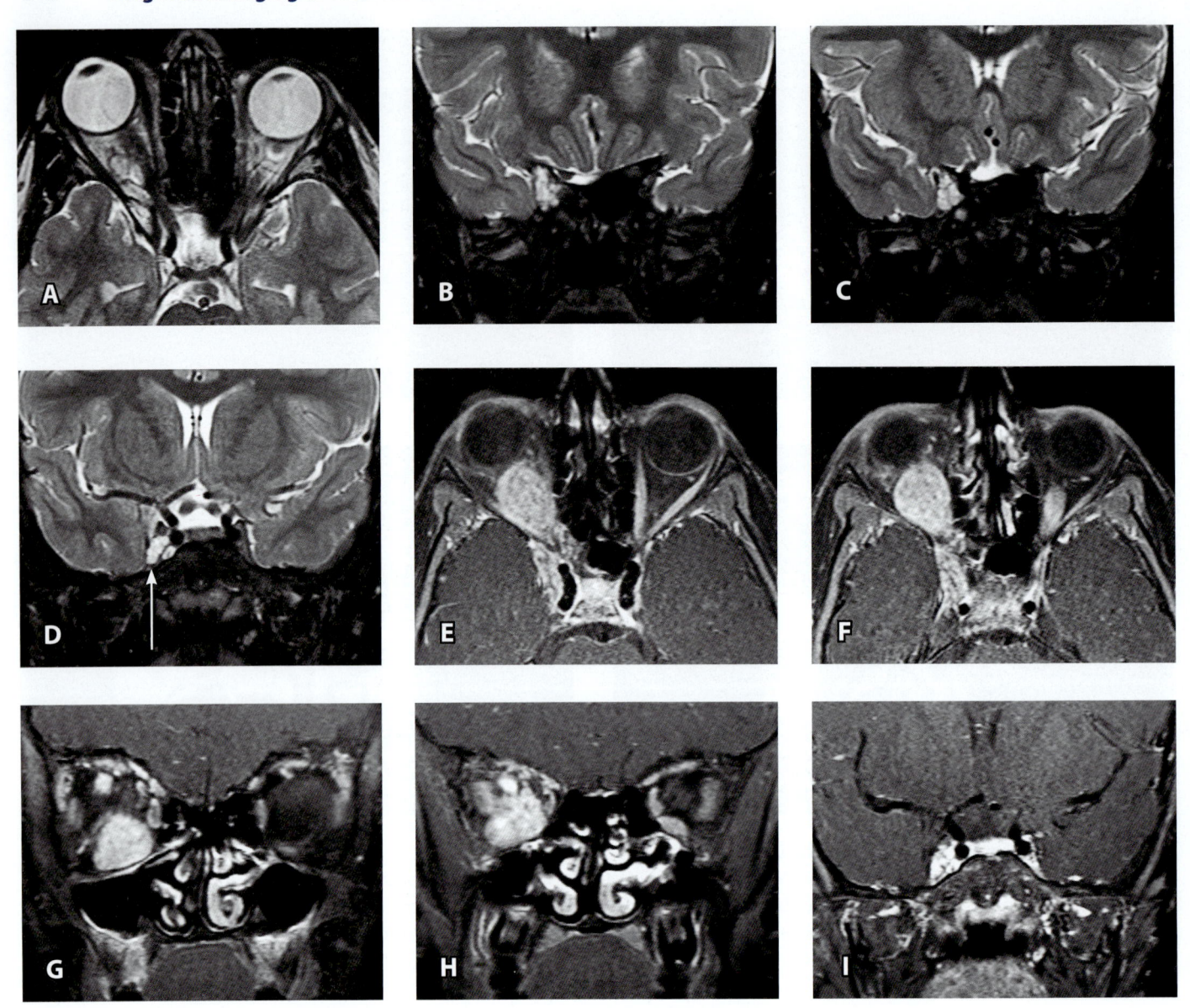

Figure 2-38 Plexiform Neurofibroma
Plexiform neurofibroma in a child with NF-I. Axial T2W (**A**) shows a multilobulated mass in the apex of the orbit, separate from the optic nerve. Coronal T2W MR images (**B–D**) show the extension of the mass beyond the orbit into the right side of the cavernous sinus (*arrow*, **D**). Axial (**E–F**) and coronal (**G–I**) T1W enhanced MR images confirm a discrete, multilobulated mass inferior to the optic nerve with extension into the right cavernous sinus. Extension into the orbital apex and cavernous sinus follows the course of the oculomotor nerve nerve.

on T1W images and hyperintensity on T2W images relative to the orbital fat. Serpentine and cord-like structures are visible within the mass, and involvement of orbital structures causes enlargement and deformity. Enhancement is variable, but the lesion is usually highly vascularized (**Table 2-23**).

Treatment of schwannomas and solitary neurofibromas is local excision due to their benign nature and low rate of malignant transformation. Plexiform neurofibromas are more difficult to treat. They have a small tendency to undergo malignant change and their diffuse infiltrative nature makes complete surgical excision difficult, recurrence rate high, and surgical reconstruction often necessary.[21,23,86–88]

VENOUS VARICES

The orbital varix is a congenital or acquired venous anomaly that is signified by an abnormal enlargement of one or more orbital veins. Such enlargement commonly involves the superior ophthalmic vein and appears similar to other causes of superior ophthalmic vein enlargement (**Table 2-24** and **Figs. 2-39–2-41**). An orbital varix usually dilates with increased systemic venous pressure causing clinically evident positional or stress proptosis (**Table 2-13**). A varix with a small connection to the systemic circulation and presumably slower flow may present acutely with painful proptosis due to hemorrhage or thrombosis. Such

Table 2-23 Imaging Schwannomas and Neurofibromas

Schwannomas	Neurofibromas
CT	**CT**
• Well-circumscribed, encapsulated tumor with similar attenuation to brain • Internally homogeneous or heterogeneous • May have intermediate signal intensity similar to extraocular muscles on T1W • High signal intensity on T2W • Enhances markedly post contrast • Enhancement may be heterogeneous due to cystic degeneration	• Unencapsulated tumors • Bone remodeling/deformities *Solitary Pattern* • Has variable appearance *Plexiform Pattern* • Shows centripetal growth into surrounding tissues • Appears isodense **MR** *Solitary Pattern* • Heterogeneous lesion with intermediate signal on T1W • Higher signal on T2W • Variable enhancement post contrast *Plexiform Pattern* • Poorly delineated infiltrating mass • Hypointense to intermediate heterogeneous intensity on T1W • Hyperintense on T2W • Serpentine and cord-like structures visible within the mass • Involvement of orbital structures causes enlargement and deformity • Enhancement is variable • Lesion is usually highly vascularized

a lesion is less likely to have stress proptosis with increases in venous pressure.

For optimal evaluation of venous varices, CT is the imaging method of choice due to its shorter imaging time (**Fig. 2-39 A** and **B**). In order to view the full extent of varices, there must be an attempt at increasing the systemic venous pressure. This is most commonly accomplished by asking the patient to perform a Valsalva maneuver. Patients can only sustain this artificial elevation of pressure for a limited time; hence the need for rapid scans. Complete imaging should be performed both with and without increased venous pressure to ensure correct diagnosis of an expanding vascular anomaly. CT may also show the presence of phleboliths. Such phleboliths are seen in a variety of vascular abnormalities including varices, thrombosed AVMs, and veno-lymphatic malformations. Phleboliths are identified as concentric calcifications surrounding a lucent center.

Orbital varices most commonly appear as tapering lesions with the larger end located more anteriorly (**Fig. 2-39 C** and **D**). They may also appear as regions of segmental vascular dilations or a mass of venous channels. They are more typically located in the superior orbit and may cause erosion of the orbital roof. Nonthrombosed varices without hemorrhage will appear slightly dense on CT scans, hypointense to intermediate intensity on T1W, and hypointense or hyperintense on T2W MR imaging and will enhance.[12,17,23,52,53,89] MR venography of the orbit with contrast may be necessary to accurately define the nature of the lesion (**Fig. 2-39 E**).

Table 2-24 Superior Ophthalmic Vein Enlargement

- Endocrine orbitopathy
- Idiopathic orbital pseudotumor (IOP)
- Carotid cavernous fistula
- Cavernous sinus thrombosis
- Parasellar or orbital meningioma
- Venous varix

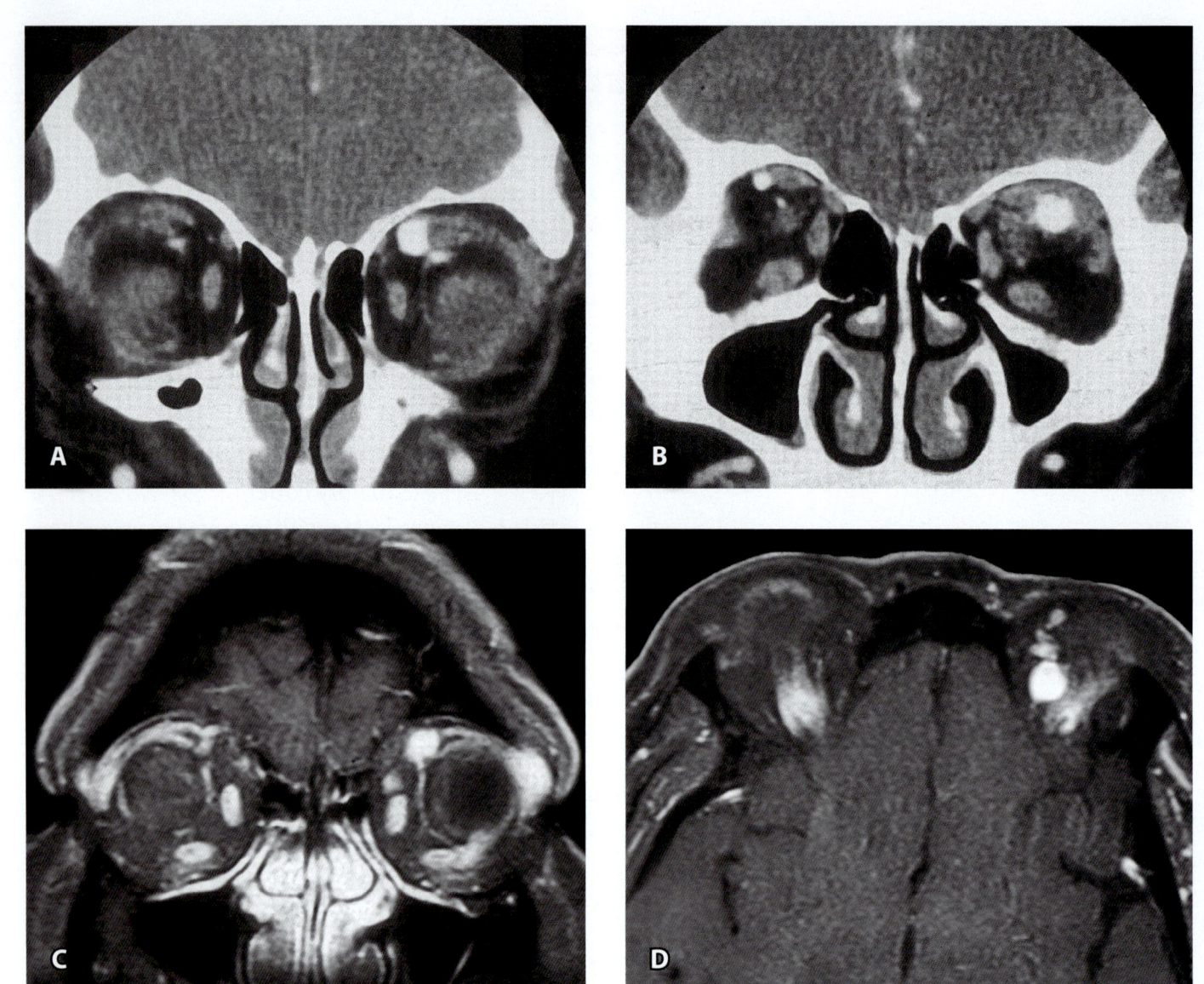

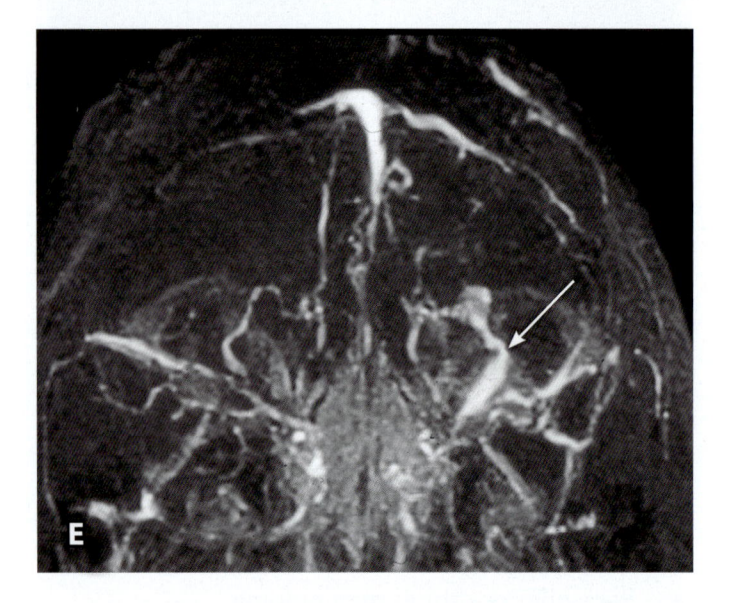

Figure 2-39 Orbital Varix

Orbital varix of the left superior ophthalmic vein. Coronal CT scans with contrast (**A–B**) show intense round enhancement of the anterior portion of a markedly enlarged superior ophthalmic vein. Coronal (**C**) and axial (**D**) T1W enhanced MR scans fat saturation show the enlarged superior ophthalmic vein with a focal dilatation that represents the varix. There is enlargement of the extraocular muscles due to venous congestion. Coronal MR venogram with contrast (**E**) shows a focal varix in the anterior portion of the superior ophthalmic vein and the overall increase in number of prominent veins within the left orbit (*arrow*, **E**).

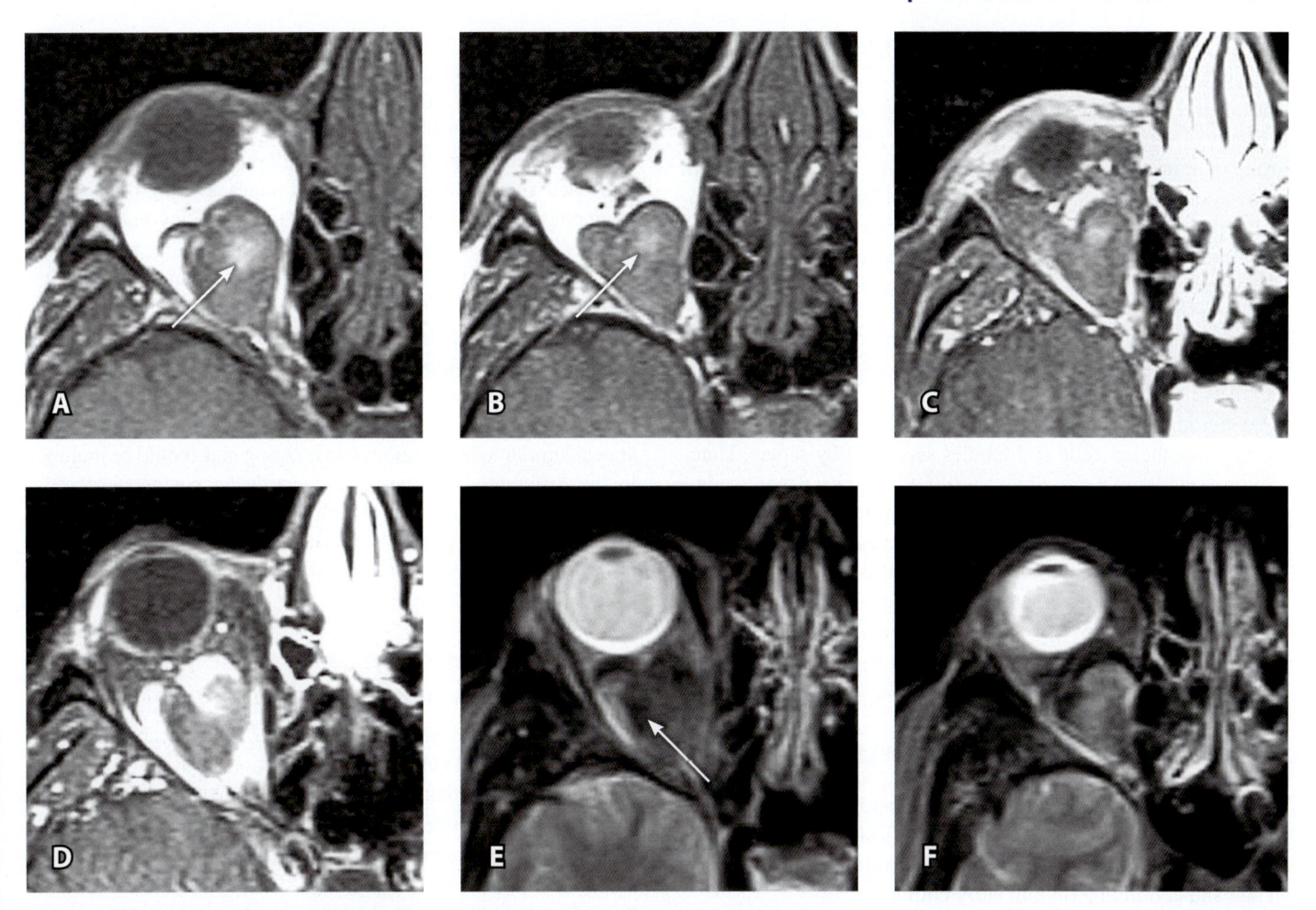

Figure 2-40 Intraconal Varix with Thrombosis
Venous malformation with hemorrhage in a patient with sudden aggravation of positional proptosis. Axial T1W (**A–B**), T1W enhanced (**C–D**), and T2W (**E–F**) MR images show a heart-shaped, intraconal retrobulbar mass with peripheral enhancement which shows intralesional hemorrhage (**A–B**) and decreased T2 signal (**E–F**), consistent with near complete thrombosis of the lesion.

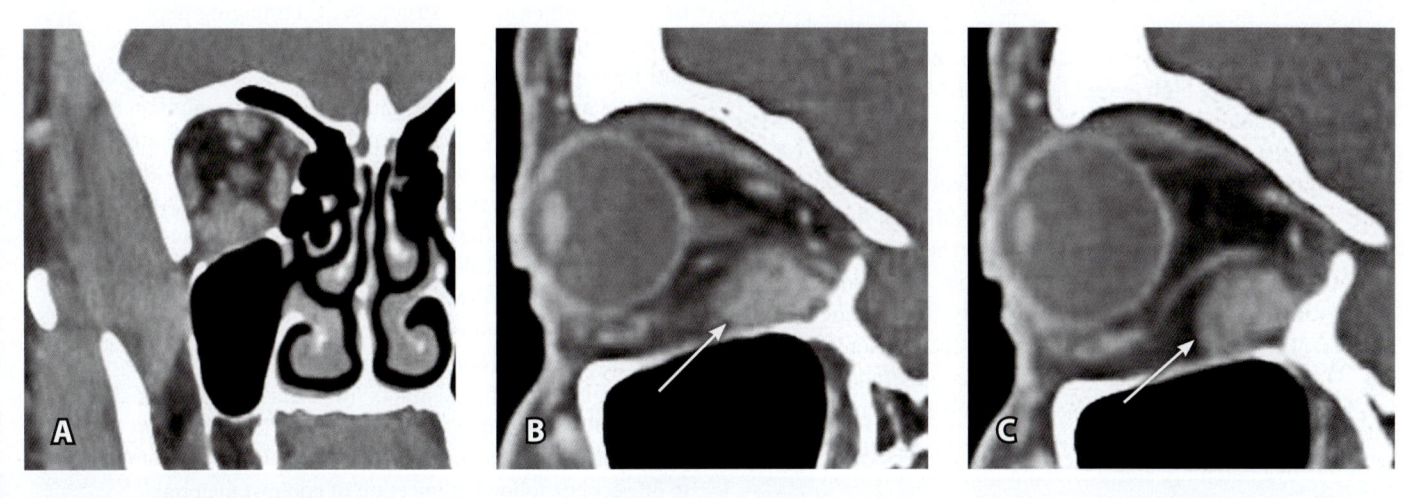

Figure 2-41 Extraconal Varix
Extraconal varix in an adult female complaining of positional or stress proptosis. Coronal (**A**) and reformatted sagittal (**B–C**) enhanced CT scans show a soft tissue mass lying inferiorly in the left orbit that elevates the inferior orbital contents (*arrows,* **B**, **C**), consistent with a varix or venous malformation.

VASOFORMATIVE ANOMALIES

The term vasoformative anomaly is a generic description of a group of congenital tumors (hemangiomas) and a different group of arteriovenous, venous, or lymphatic malformations. An association may be made between some of the intraorbital vasoformative anomalies and intracranial venous anomalies, such as dural arteriovenous fistulas or venous angiomas. If an orbital vasoformative anomaly is identified on imaging, the intracranial structures should be evaluated as well.

Proliferating Hemangioma

Hemangiomas are neoplasms comprising capillaries with proliferating endothelial cells and lobules separated by septae. Hemangiomas undergo a growing or proliferating phase that is completely separate from their subsequent involuting phase. During growth, the histologic appearance is of vascular proliferation with many mast cells. During involution, there are no mast cells and few proliferating vessels. These lesions are both supplied and drained by large vessels in continuation with the systemic circulation. The presence of large vessels signifies a proliferating lesion, while lack of these channels signifies an involuting lesion.

In neonates and infants, hemangiomas are the most common vascular tumors and may be present even in utero. Hemangiomas occur more commonly in girls than boys in a 3:2 ratio. There is usually a growth spurt of these lesions in the first six months of life followed by involution starting at about one year of age and continuing on into early childhood.

An orbital hemangioma is most often seen in the superomedial portion involving the skin of the eyelids. Both "herald spot" and "strawberry nevi" are terms used to describe the cutaneous appearance of a hemangioma. The hemangioma may also appear as a purple "bruise-like" lesion if it is subcutaneous in location. If there is no cutaneous component, proptosis may be the presenting feature in lesions located in the muscle cone or deep orbit. Bleeding disorders due to intratumoral platelet coagulapathies and high output heart failure are rarely seen with orbital hemangiomas, but have been reported with other massive lesions of the head, neck, or trunk.

Orbital hemangiomas may coexist with hemangiomas of other regions within the head and neck. Although these tumors typically involute completely, there may be various sequelae including facial disfigurement, amblyopia, strabismus, optic atrophy, or residual mass effect, especially from larger lesions. Treatment is necessary if a hemangioma affects vision or if there are complications including erosion of the epidermis, high output heart failure, bleeding disorders, or obstruction of the airway. Various treatment modalities have been utilized including selective eye patching, steroids, radiation, and surgery.

MR imaging is the best method to evaluate hemangiomas due to its superior ability to correctly characterize and identify the vascularity and extent of a lesion. Such MR imaging is particularly valuable in tumors that lie deep in the orbit and lack a cutaneous component. Proliferating hemangiomas appear as irregular nonencapsulated masses with visible lobules, septa, and vessels. The lesions may be infiltrative with little distinction between tumors and surrounding normal tissues with finger like extensions into the various compartments of the orbit.

On T1W images, hemangiomas appear of moderate-low to intermediate signal intensity similar to the brain and have increased signal intensity on T2W images. During the proliferating phase, flow voids are notable. During the involuting phase, the lack of flow voids makes the diagnosis more problematic. The uses of fat suppression and contrast enhancement greatly increase the delineation of hemangiomas. These tumors enhance markedly after contrast administration. Such enhancement clearly defines the borders of a lesion and identifies the feeding and draining vessels.

Rhabdomyosarcoma and metastatic neuroblastoma may appear similar to hemangioma on imaging and should be included in the differential diagnosis. If there is no cutaneous component to a hemangioma, other benign lesions that cause a rapidly expanding mass must also be considered such as hemorrhage in a lymphangioma, rupture of a dermoid cyst, or a variety of orbital acute inflammatory conditions.[52,53,90]

Cavernous Hemangioma (Encapsulated Venous Malformation)

The term cavernous hemangioma applies to an encapsulated vascular malformation made of large cavernous spaces lined by flattened endothelium that slowly increases in size over time. Encapsulated venous malformation may be a more correct alternative term to use in reference to cavernous hemangiomas. Cavernous hemangiomas are typically seen in adult patients where they occur more frequently in women than in men. The classical clinical presentation is one of a slowly progressive, painless proptosis. With increasing size, compressive optic nerve symptoms may result.

Imaging of cavernous hemangiomas shows well-defined masses with round or oval shapes (**Fig. 2-42**). These lobulated lesions will usually displace, but not directly involve the optic nerve and other orbital structures. CT imaging depicts a hyperdense homogeneous mass. MR reveals a lesion that is isointense and homogenous to muscle on T1W images and hyperintense on T2W images to muscle and fat. Internal septations may also be visible on T2W images and wide-window scans, if taken soon after contrast administration. Enhancement after contrast administration is variable, but is most evident if images are taken some time after injection. Ultrasound scans may show a homogeneous, well-defined, encapsulated mass that has little or no internal venous flow on Doppler imaging.

A cavernous hemangioma may appear similar to a hemangiopericytoma, schwannoma, neurofibroma, or meningioma on MR imaging. All of these tumors will show early marked vascular stains with angiography, while cavernous hemangiomas are angiographically occult unless delayed filming is carried out for over 20 to 30 seconds following injection of contrast material.[12,13,22,23,52,53]

Lymphangioma

Lymphangiomas are a subtype of the vasoformative anomalies of childhood. Lymphangiomas are not true neoplasms, but consist of a malformation with both venous and lymphatic components

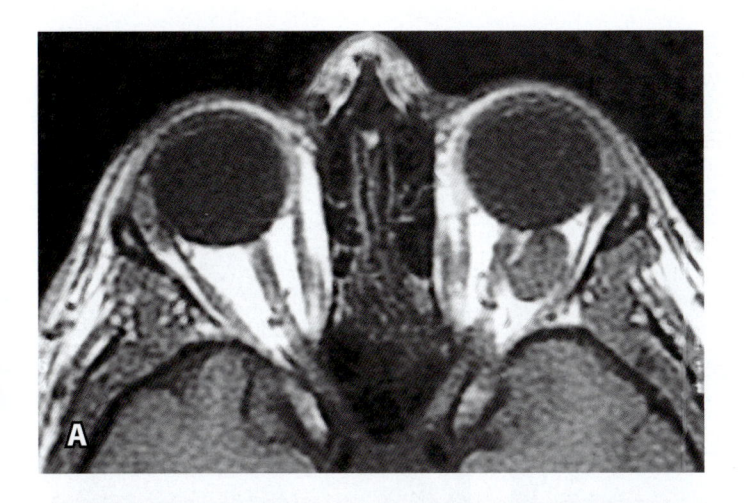

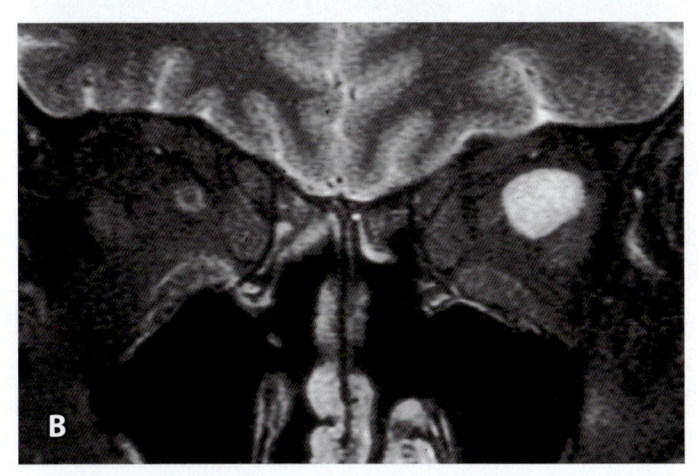

Figure 2-42 Cavernous Hemangioma
Intraconal cavernous hemangioma (encapsulated venous malformation) of the left orbit. T1W axial (**A**) and T2W (**B**) coronal images show a well-circumscribed soft tissue mass within the fat of the muscle cone. Such lesions typically cause gradual onset of progressive proptosis. In this adult female, the mass was relatively asymptomatic, except for mild positional proptosis.

Blood products of various ages may be present. Acute hemorrhage will appear hypointense to fat on both T1W and T2W images due to the presence of deoxyhemoglobin. The presence of subacute blood and blood products will appear hyperintense on T1W and T2W images due to the paramagnetic methemoglobin. In aged hemorrhages, there may be fluid–fluid levels with the lower signal region in the dependent portion containing cellular elements in contrast to the methemoglobin-containing, nondependent regions.

Chronic hemorrhage may appear hypointense due to the presence of hemosiderin and ferretin. The overall appearance of the mass is isointense or hyperintense to brain on T1W images and hyperintense to brain on T2W images and intermediate-weighted MR scans. Postcontrast administration enhancement will occur only in the venous component of these combined lesions.

Veno-lymphatic malformations differ from orbital varices (**Fig. 2-43**) in that they lack a communication with the systemic vascular system. Encapsulated venous malformations, i.e., cavernous hemangiomas (**Fig. 2-42**), are well-defined and unlike lymphangiomas, enhance for long duration. Management of these veno-lymphatic malformations is still controversial ranging from conservative management to surgical debulking.[12,16,17,52,53]

LESIONS OF THE GLOBE

Staphyloma

A staphyloma is defined as a local or generalized corneal or scleral ectasia with a uveal lining. Staphylomas can be divided into four types based on the anatomic location of the bulging or ectatic component: 1) anterior staphylomas occur between the ciliary body and cornea, 2) ciliary staphylomas occur over the ciliary body, 3) equatorial staphyloma at the equator of the globe, 4) and posterior staphylomas occur between the equator and optic nerve.

Posterior staphylomas are commonly the result of axial myopia or glaucoma, whereas the other varieties are due to an increase in intraocular pressure coupled with a local decrease in resistance of the sclera caused by injury or inflammation. These lesions may be unilateral or bilateral and are complicated by chorioretinal degeneration, choroidal hemorrhage, and retinal detachment often causing blindness, cataracts, and secondary glaucoma.

The CT appearance of a posterior staphyloma secondary to axial myopia consists of a defect lying temporal to the optic nerve. This defect appears as a focal bulging with thinning or absence of the scleral-uveal rim (**Figs. 2-44** and **2-45**). Enhancement of the globe is not altered from normal after contrast infusion. Differentiation of a staphyloma from tumor and pseudotumor is based on the presence of scleral-uveal thickening which is typically present in both of these later conditions. In contrast, there is thinning of the scleral-uveal layers in a staphyloma.[14,89,92,93]

Retinoschisis

Retinoschisis is a bulbous lesion found on the temporal side of the retina, usually bilaterally and symmetrically. It is the result of separation of the sensory retinal layers with a cystic collection

and are often seen as combined veno-lymphatic malformations. A veno-lymphatic malformation consists of an unencapsulated mass of dilated endothelial-lined vascular and lymph channels surrounded by lymphoid tissue. These lesions commonly occur in the conjunctiva, eyelid, and retrobulbar regions. Patients may present with proptosis and/or optic nerve compression that may have an acute onset if there is intralesional hemorrhage and formation of a blood-containing cyst. The lesions may also enlarge during infection most probably due to the lymphatic component of the lesion, but will show only minimal if any enlargement with the Valsalva maneuver.

On MR imaging, there may be orbital expansion and exophthalmos (**Fig. 2-43**). The lesion is unencapsulated and diffusely infiltrating, with irregular borders often crossing anatomic boundaries such as the orbital septum. There may be cysts and multiple septations within a veno-lymphatic malformation.

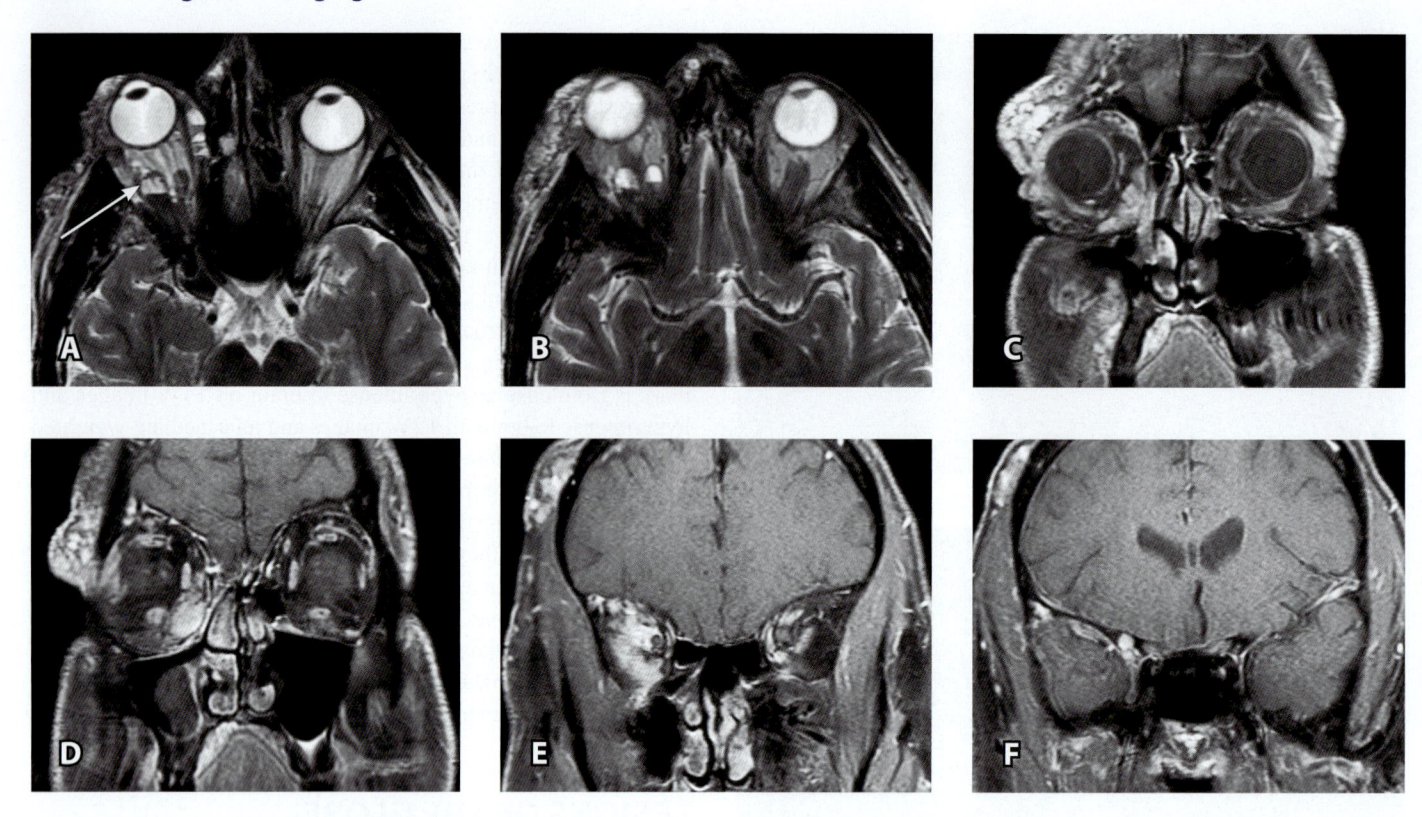

Figure 2-43 Venolymphatic Malformation
Venolymphatic malformation in an adult male presenting with a known deveopmental lesion of the left orbit. Axial T2W MR images (**A–B**) show a heterogeneous cystic mass in the right orbit both in the intraconal and extraconal spaces. The cysts show multiple fluid–fluid levels (*arrow,* **A**) consistent with hemorrhage, accounting for recent aggravation of the proptosis. Coronal T1W enhanced MR images (**D–F**) depict the full extent of the lesion, which involves the forehead, the eyelids, the extrocular muscles, and extends posteriorly into the superior orbital fissure. The venous component shows intense enhancement whereas portions within the muscle cone show less enhancement, consistent with a mixed venous lymphatic origin.

between the layers. Causes include inflammation, trauma, or long-standing retinal detachment. The lesion can also be congenital and heritable in an X-linked recessive pattern usually presenting in children.

Children with retinoschisis are typically symptomatic in school with reading difficulties. Infants with retinoschisis usually present with symptoms of strabismus and nystagmus. There is a bulbous elevation of the retina on fundoscopic examination. The disease is slowly progressive without any known treatment. There is typically a slow decline in vision into the older years, unless the disease is complicated by a retinal detachment or vitreal hemorrhage leading to blindness. On CT scans, the lesion may appear as a fluid–fluid level that layers dependently and contains high attenuation fluid.[53,94]

Retinopathy of Prematurity

Retinopathy of prematurity (ROP), also known as retrolental fibroplasia, is the result of alterations in the oxygenation of the immature retina. These alterations cause a proliferative vascular retinopathy. The lesions of ROP are typically seen in premature infants that receive excess oxygen therapy. The disease affects the globes bilaterally, but not necessarily symmetrically. It is responsible for 3% to 5% of the cases of leukokoria, or "cat's eye reflex".

The different stages of ROP that are visible by the ophthalmoscope include arteriolar vasoconstriction of immature vessels at the border of a hypovascular retina, especially in the temporal region, leading ischemia. The ischemic tissue becomes edematous, and the retinal vessels become elongated, tortuous, and dilated. Neovascularization then develops with ensuing hemorrhage and fibrosis that leads to the development of fiber tracts and eventual retraction of the fibrovascular tissue. Such retraction of the fiber tracts may lead to traction on the retina and contribute to retinal detachment and scarring. There may also be an intraocular temporal mass. This entire process results in microphthalmia with blindness.

CT findings may demonstrate associated microphthalmia, a shallow anterior chamber, hyperattenuation of the entire globe due to neovascularization, and in the late stages of the disease, dystrophic calcifications (**Fig. 2-46**). Microphthalmia may also be documented on MR scans along with hyperintense globes on T1W and T2W images due to chronic subretinal hemorrhages. If there is retinal detachment, the detachment may appear as a hypointense retrolental mass with hyperintense subretinal fluid.[12,53,95]

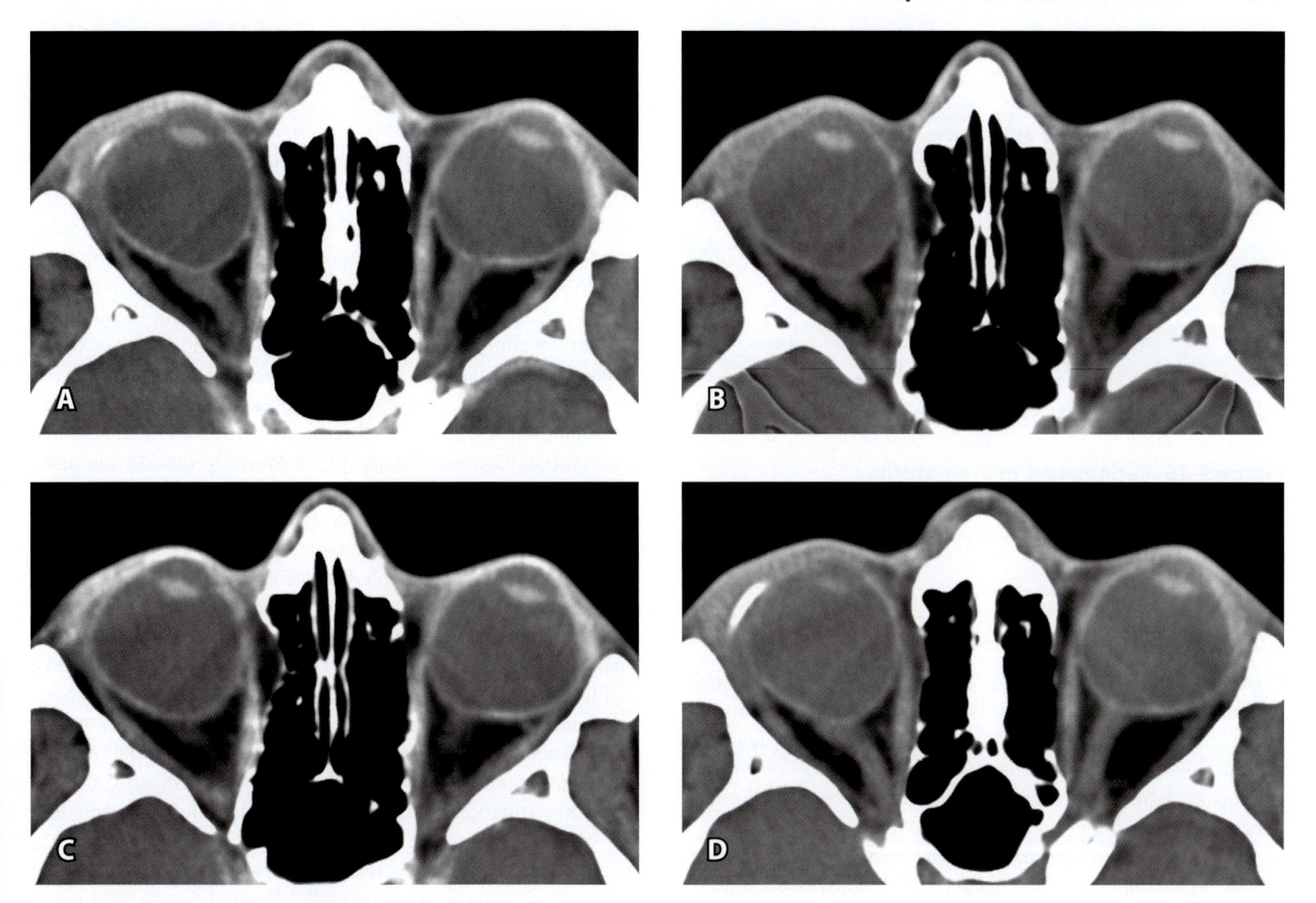

Figure 2-44 Staphyloma: Bilateral
Bilateral staphylomas in a young adult with recent and remote trauma. Axial CT scans without contrast (**A–D**) show an increase in the axial dimensions of both globes with thinning, but persistence, of the hyperdense lines marking the posterior margins. See Fig. 2-12 posterior coloboma: bilateral.

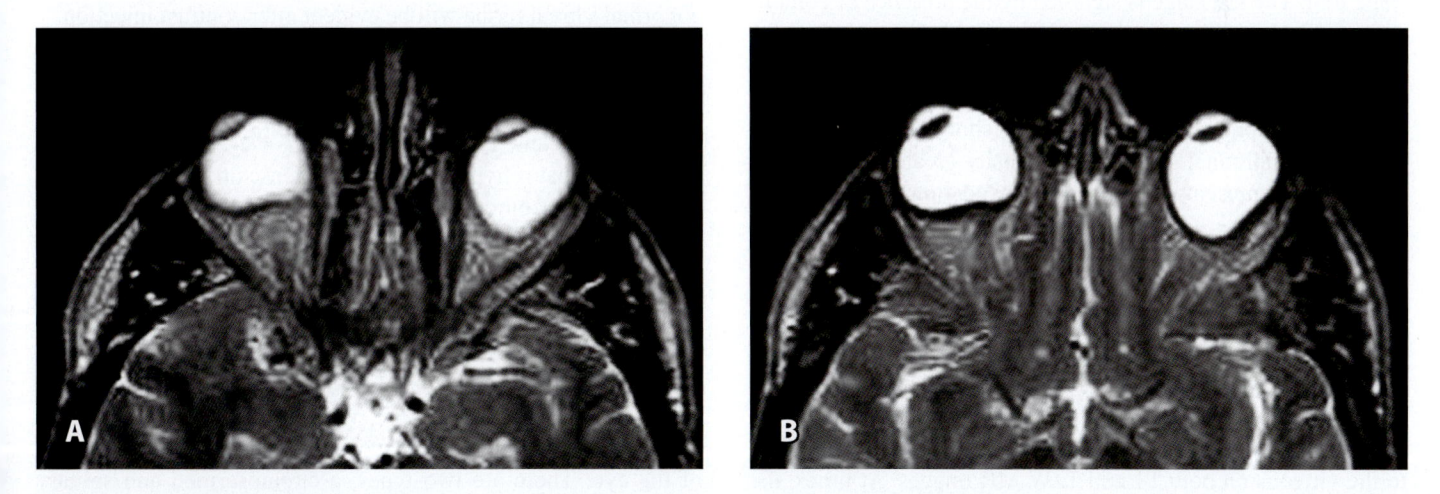

Figure 2-45 Staphyloma: Bilateral
Bilateral staphylomas in an elderly female, presenting with bitemporal hemianopsia. Axial T2W images (**A–B**) show marked deformity and pear-shaped appearance of both globes, consistent with posterior staphylomas.

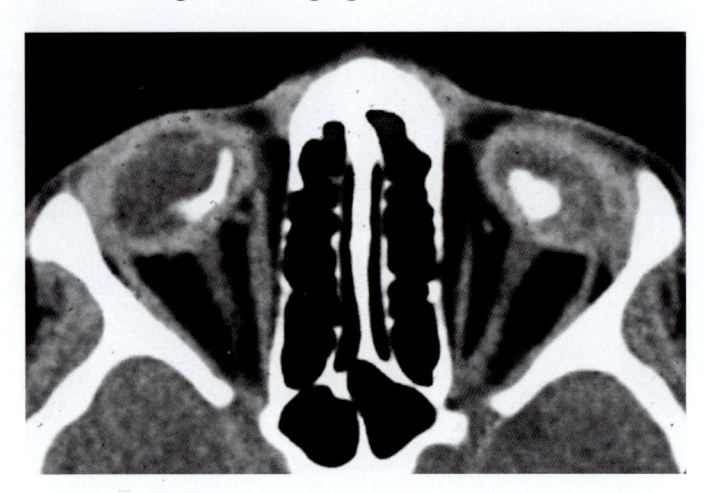

Figure 2-46 Retinopathy of Prematurity
Retinopathy of prematurity in a six-month-old infant. Axial CT scan shows extensive calcification in the globes and bilateral microphthalmos.

Coats' Disease (Primary Retinal Telangiectasia)

Coats' disease is an idiopathic congenital disorder that presents most commonly in young boys. Presenting symptoms and signs include unilateral leukocoria, strabismus, visual loss, and painful angle closure glaucoma. Treatment usually consists of photocoagulation and/or surgery, but has only been moderately successful in this otherwise progressive disease.

Coats' disease or primary retinal telangiectasia is characterized by telangiectatic and aneurysmal blood vessels that are surrounded by intraretinal and subretinal exudates. Compromise of the blood-retinal barrier allows for the leakage of blood products. One classification scheme separates Coats' disease into five stages. First, there are focal exudates, next extensive retinal exudation. The third stage includes partial retinal detachment and progression to complete detachment that classifies the disease as stage four. The last stage is signified by the presence of complications from chronic retinal detachment including rubeosis iridis, neovascular glaucoma, cataracts, uveitis, and phthisis bulbi.

Imaging of Coats' disease shows subretinal fluid with or without microphthalmos. CT imaging shows a homogeneous area in the subretinal space with a density greater than the vitreous. This represents the subretinal exudation. After contrast administration the neovascularized retina will show enhancement but the subretinal space will not. The location of the enhancement will depend upon the degree of retinal detachement and helps to distinguish this lesion from a retinoblastoma that is likely to show enhancement in the subretinal space. Calcifications, although rare, may be present in advanced cases and will tend to be focal and submacular in location.

The subretinal exudate is typically hyperintense compared to the vitreous on both T1 and T2W MR images. At times, the subretinal fluid may appear hypointense on T2W images when the cholesterol and lipid content is high. Similar to the imaging findings on CT scans, there is enhancement of the retina, but not the subretinal space after contrast administration. The conspicuous absence of a mass in the presence of retinal detachment helps to distinguish this disease from other ocular disorders such as retinoblastoma, toxocaral endophthalmitis, or persistent hyperplastic primary vitreous.[12,53,95–97]

Persistent Hyperplastic Primary Vitreous

Persistent hyperplastic primary vitreous (PHPV) refers to the persistence and proliferation of the primary retrolental fibrovascular mesodermal tissue including the hyaloid artery. This may lead to spontaneous cataracts, calcification, or ossification of the lens. Vitreoretinal traction caused by contraction of the retrolental mass eventually leads to retinal detachment, which is found in a third of the cases.

PHPV usually presents as unilateral leukocoria in the microphthalmic eye of a full-term infant. It may be associated with Norrie disease, trisomy 13, or Warburg disease (an autosomal recessive disease with hydrocephalus, lissencephaly, and mental retardation in addition to PHPV). In these cases, PHPV will typically be found bilaterally. It has also been reported in association with fetal alcohol syndrome, fetal hydantoin syndrome, and midline congenital cranial defects. If there is minimal involvement, surgery may be utilized to attempt to save vision. However, the usual course of the disease is progressive and leads to the eventual enucleation of a nonfunctional eye.

Imaging appearances depend upon the extent of ocular involvement and the presence of complications. Retinal detachment and/or intravitreal hemorrhage may be evident. CT scans may show microphthalmia in the affected globe, increased density of the vitreous usually from previous hemorrhage, absence of calcifications, and discrete intravitreal densities suggesting persistence of the fetal tissue and/or hyaloid artery. This tissue may appear in a range of shapes from a linear band or conical shape between the posterior lens and posterior globe to an intravitreal mass. There may be a small irregular lens and anterior chamber. In the decubitus position, subhyaloid or subretinal fluid with hemorrhagic byproducts may show dependent layering without enhancement. Moderate to marked enhancement of the abnormal vitreal tissue will be evident after contrast injection.

MR evaluation may show a microphthalmic eye, an abnormal lens, and retinal and posterior hyaloid detachment. The vitreous may be hyperintense owing to the repeated hemorrhages on both T1W and T2W images (**Fig. 2-47**). A retrolental soft-tissue mass that is hypointense to isointense on T1W images and enhances post contrast administration may be evident. A variable range of shapes of the retrolental soft tissues similar to that seen on CT scans is observed. In the more advanced stages of the disease, differentiation between Coats' disease, ROP, and retinoblastoma may be difficult.[12,53,95,96,98,99]

Choroidal Hemangioma

Choroidal hemangiomas are congenital vascular hamartomas of the eye. There are two types; a circumscribed and solitary lesion without other associated abnormalities or a diffuse lesion associated with Sturge-Weber syndrome (**Fig. 2-48**). Sturge-Weber disease is characterized by angiomatosis of the intracranial structures, typically the meninges, the face and the choroid. The facial angiomas or "nevus flammeus" typically involve

The choroidal hemangioma associated with Sturge-Weber syndrome has a similar intensity on imaging, but may show greater and more circumferential involvement of the globe.

Treatment of these lesions is not necessary unless complications develop such as retinal detachment, in which case surgical repair and/or laser photocoagulation may be performed. Glaucoma is a frequent complication of these lesions and may be the presenting symptom. Choroidal hemangiomas may be difficult to differentiate from choroidal melanomas and a significant number of involved eyes may be enucleated or treated with radiation therapy, if this distinction cannot be made.[91,100,101]

Choroidal Osteoma

Choroidal osteoma is a rare, benign tumor containing bone and vascular elements. It may be found unilaterally or bilaterally and there may be solitary or multiple lesions in a globe. Patients are typically young females who may present with central or paracentral scotomas, but are most commonly asymptomatic.

On CT scans the lesion appears plaque-like and calcified and is typically located in the posterior globe (**Figs. 2-49** and **2-50**). The MRI appearance is variable depending upon the amount of marrow and fat within the bony lesions. Some choroidal osteomas show the typical appearance of a bony lesion that contains marrow. The tumor appears to have high signal intensity on T1W images, show enhancement after contrast administration, and have low signal intensity on T2W images.

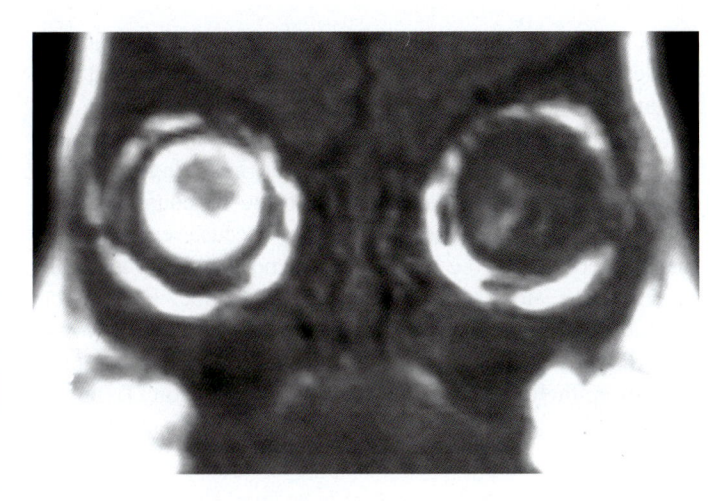

Figure 2-47 PHPV: Bilateral
Bilateral PHPV in an infant with cataracts. Coronal T1W image shows hyperintensity in the right globe, representing hemorrhage, and an abnormal retrolental hyperintensity within the left globe.

the region of the cutaneous distribution of the first and second divisions of the trigeminal nerve. There may also be seizures and mental deficiency. One third of patients with Sturge-Weber will have diffuse choroidal hemangiomas (**Table 2-21**). These lesions appear on fundoscopic exam as a "tomato catsup" fundus or a bright red-orange mass of the fundus. Associated retinal detachment is frequent.

CT scans reveal a dome shaped mass that enhances intensely (**Fig. 2-48**). The solitary choroidal hemangioma appears isointense to hyperintense to the vitreous on T1W images and isointense to the vitreous on T2W and proton-weighted MR images. The lesion most frequently will be located posterior to the equator of the globe and have a lenticular or dome shape. After administration of gadolinium the lesion will show intense enhancement.

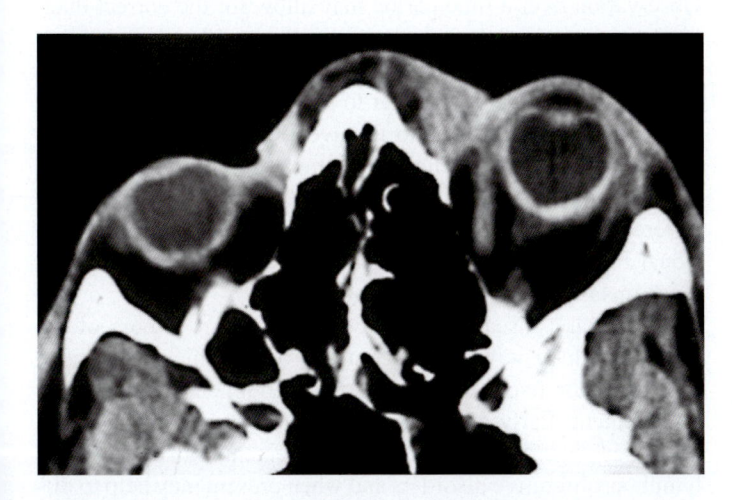

Figure 2-48 Choroidal Hemangioma Sturge-Weber
Choroidal hemangioma and Sturge-Weber disease. Axial CT scan with contrast shows thickening and enhancement of the left posterior globe in the region of the choroid suggesting a choroidal angioma. The left eye is also buphthalmic.

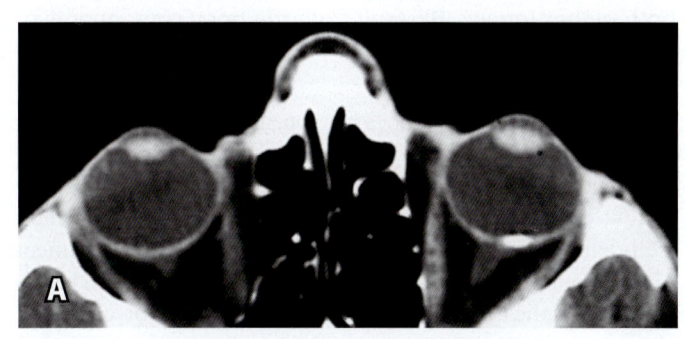

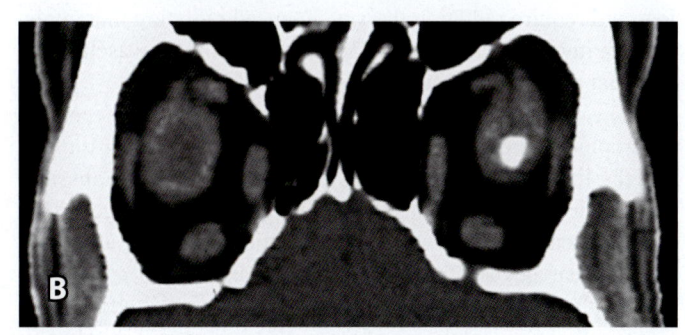

Figure 2-49 Choroidal Osteoma: Unilateral
Macular choroidal osteoma in a patient presenting with blurred vision in the left eye. Axial (**A**) and (**B**) coronal CT scans without contrast. There is a thickened choroid with an area of calcification temporal to the left optic nerve (**A**). In **B** there is a region of calcification in the area of the macula.

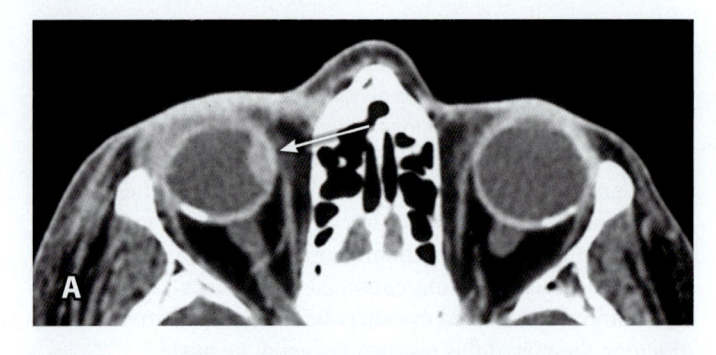

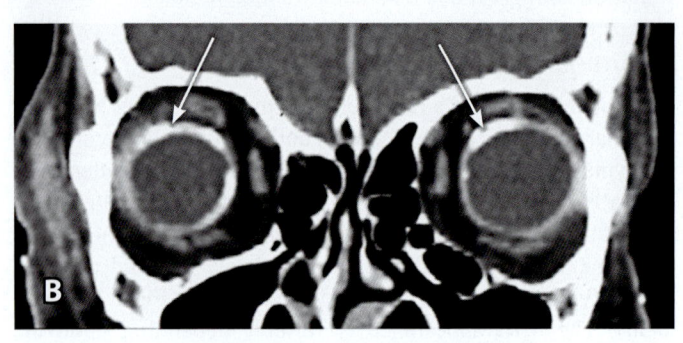

Figure 2-50 Choroidal Osteoma: Bilateral
Bilateral choroidal osteomas with subchoroidal hemorrhage in the right globe. Axial (**A**) and coronal (**B**) CT scans. There are hyperdense regions within the choroid that follow the contour of the globe wall. An area of moderate density in a "lens" shape on the medial wall of the right globe (*arrow*, **A**) represents subchoroidal hemorrhage. The calcified regions in both globes (*arrows*, **B**) result from the bony components of the choroidal osteomas.

A choroidal osteoma that does not appear as cortical bone is difficult to differentiate from a choroidal melanoma on MRI.

Fundoscopic examination of these patients shows a rounded, yellow-white-orange lesion with scalloped or geographically well-delineated margins in the juxtapapillary region. Treatment of a choroidal osteoma is usually not necessary unless the lesion causes complications such as retinal detachment or choroidal neovascularization. A tumor near the macula may lead to visual loss and require radiation therapy. Focused radiation therapy by gamma rays or protons will retard the choroidal neovascularization that can lead to blindness.

The differential diagnosis includes other lesions that contain dystrophic or metastatic calcifications, other intraocular tumors, and the linear nevus sebaceous syndrome or Jadassohn disease. The linear nevus sebaceous syndrome represents a congenital or developmental disease with characteristic findings of a midline facial linear nevus of Jadassohn, intracranial CNS anomalies, and ocular abnormalities including conjunctival lipodermoid, microphthalmos, coloboma of the eyelid and uvea, orbital angioma, and choroidal calcifications.[22,53,91,102–105]

Uveal Melanoma

Malignant melanoma is the most common tumor to involve the uveal structures in adult patients. In some cases, it may arise from pre-existing lesions including uveal nevi, congenital melanosis, ocular melanocytosis, or oculodermal melanocytosis. The incidence of melanoma increases with increasing age, and most tumors are diagnosed in middle-aged or elderly patients.

Fundoscopic examination of a uveal melanoma reveals a choroidal mass of varying pigmentation, including an amelanotic appearance that may extend into the vitreous in a characteristic "mushroom-like" manner and/or cause retinal detachment. Alternatively, the tumor may extend in a flat, plaque-like configuration along the structures of the globe. Factors that indicate a poor prognosis include older age, greater than 15-mm tumor basal diameter, anterior location in the ciliary body, presence of epithelioid cells, and extraocular extension. Treatment ranges from observation to enucleation. A thorough search to identify metastasis must be instituted in order to avoid unnecessary enucleation.

Although usually diagnosed on fundoscopic examination and fluorescein angiography, CT or MRI may be helpful when direct visualization of the lesion is not possible or in determining the extent of a lesion beyond the globe (**Fig. 2-51**). On CT scans, the lesion typically appears as an elevated, hyperdense (unless amelanotic) sharply marginated enhancing lesion.

Extension into the retrobulbar space is best diagnosed with MRI. An ocular melanoma will appear as a lesion with high signal intensity on T1W and proton-weighted images when compared to the vitreous. On T2W images the tumor has a low signal compared to the vitreous or may be hyperintense. Necrosis and hemorrhage within melanotic lesions is common. The shape of the tumor is highly variable from a flat lesion to a nodular mass. Some lesions may involve the entire ciliary body forming a ring like pattern. Lesions less than 1.8 mm in thickness may be difficult to detect with MR imaging, unless a surface coil is utilized. Post contrast administration these lesions usually show moderate enhancement on fat-saturated T1W images.

A congenital lesion, the choroidal nevus is typically diagnosed in late childhood. A choroidal nevus appears identical to a choroidal melanoma both fundoscopically and radiographically. Observation over a time period may allow for the correct diagnosis, but some of these lesions may eventually give rise to a melanoma anyway.

Lesions that appear similar to uveal melanoma on imaging studies include metastasis to the uveal tract, choroidal hemorrhage and detachment, choroidal lymphoma, leukemic infiltration, and nodular posterior scleritis and must be included in the differential diagnosis. The more irregular appearance and occasional bilateral involvement of the globes may help to distinguish metastasis from uveal melanoma.

Metastatic disease especially from primary tumors of the breast and lung is the most common ophthalmic malignancy. The posterior uveal tract is the most common site of ocular involvement. Early on patients are asymptomatic or may have decreased visual acuity. Bilateral involvement is also seen in the lymphoproliferative disorders and when present may help to differentiate these lesions as well.[22,100,106–108]

Retinal Angiomatosis

Retinal angiomatosis may also be referred to as retinal capillary angioma and may occur in association with von

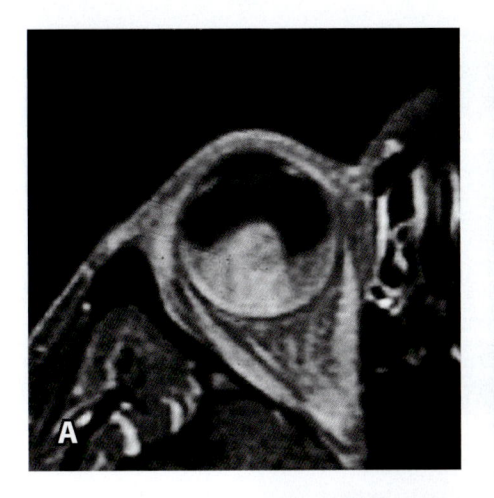

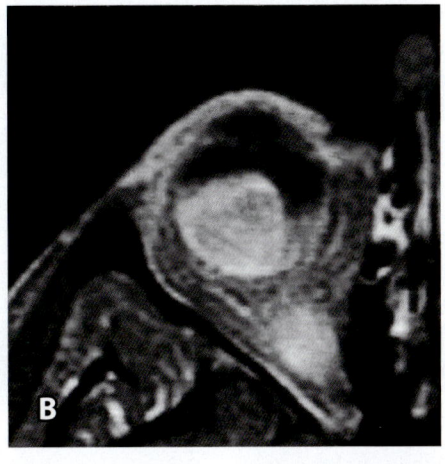

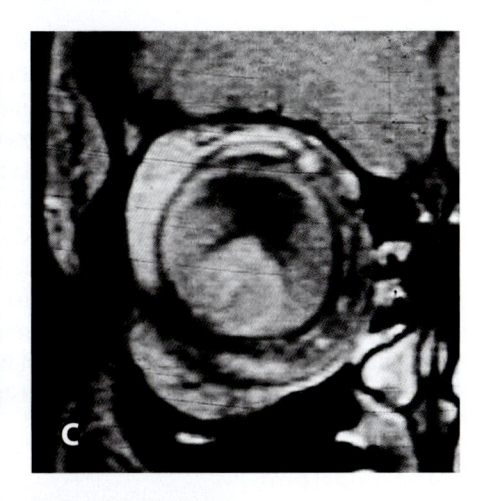

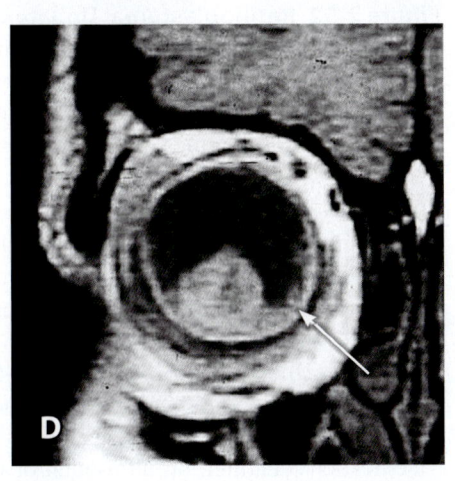

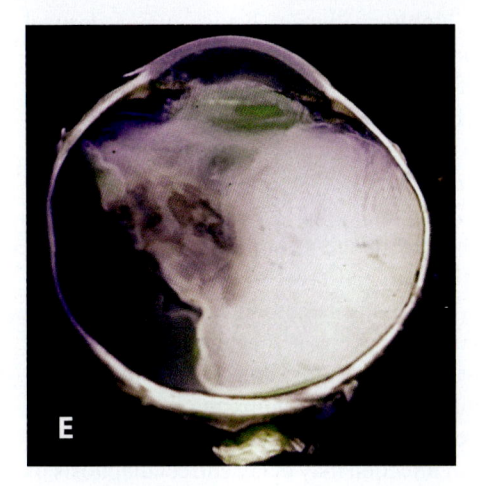

Figure 2-51 Uveal Melanoma
Uveal melanoma complicated by a total retinal detachment in a 38-year-old female. Axial T1-W MR scans with contrast. **A** shows a heterogeneously enhancing tumor in the posterior right globe. In **B** the lesion is still present, but is now bordered by slightly less intense areas on both the medial and lateral sides. Coronal T1-W MR without contrast (**C**) shows a moderately intense lesion filling most of the right globe with a slightly hypointense region inferiorly. Coronal T1-W MR scans with contrast. Compared to the noncontrast coronal view, in **D** there is enhancement of the region that was previously hypointense suggestive of tumor along with the detachment (*arrow*, **D**). Pathology specimen (**E**) shows the lesion with the associated retinal detachment. (Case courtesy of Ben J. Glasgow, MD.)

Hippel-Lindau syndrome (**Table 2-21**) or as an isolated tumor. When the lesions are multifocal and bilateral, they are most likely part of the von Hippel-Lindau syndrome, but are otherwise the same both clinically and histologically as an isolated lesion. Brain and body imaging must be performed in such patients to rule out cerebellar hemangioblastomas that are seen in von Hippel-Lindau syndrome along with renal cell carcinoma, pheochromocytoma, and cysts of the kidneys and pancreas. Von Hippel-Lindau syndrome is inherited in an autosomal dominant pattern with variable penetrance and typically does not present until young adulthood.

On fundoscopic examination, a retinal capillary angioma appears as a reddish-orange nodule with both a tortuous feeding artery and a draining vein. It tends to be located in the juxtapapillary region or in the temporal peripheral region. Fluorescein angiography is used to help confirm the diagnosis and differentiate the lesion from papilledema or optic neuritis.

MR imaging depicts a lesion that may be similar in appearance to the choroidal melanoma in adults and a retinoblastoma in children. The lesion is isointense to hyperintense compared to the vitreous on T1W images and isointense to hypointense to the vitreous on T2W lesions. There is moderate enhancement after contrast administration. Frequent episodes of vitreous hemorrhage may result in an exudative posterior retinal detachment leading to blindness.[22,53,107]

Retinal Astrocytoma

Retinal astrocytomas are benign, uncommon tumors that may occur in isolation or as phakomas in cases of tuberous sclerosis, NF-1 (**Table 2-21**). Tuberous sclerosis or Bourneville disease is an autosomal dominant disorder that is characterized by adenoma sebaceum, mental deficiency, and seizures. Retinal astrocytomas originate from the nerve fiber layer of the retina or the optic nerve itself and contain fibrillary astrocytes and sometimes "giant astrocytes." These tumors may present with visual loss and/or leukokoria. They appear as flat or finely nodular yellow-white to white lesions on the posterior retina during fundoscopic examination. The nodular lesions are sometimes referred to as "mulberry lesions" and may contain cysts or calcifications.

CT imaging of a retinal astrocytoma will show a mass along the retina. The lesion may contain calcifications and have variable enhancement after contrast administration. Necrosis, hemorrhage, and intravitreal fungating growths are not typical of a retinal astrocytoma and may help to distinguish the lesion from a retinoblastoma. Associated intracranial findings associated with tuberous sclerosis or NF-1 may also be visualized and assist in the diagnosis.[95,107]

Retinoblastoma

Retinoblastoma is a highly malignant ocular tumor derived from the primitive embryonal retinal cells. It is caused by the inactivation or loss of both alleles of the retinoblastoma 1 gene on chromosome 13q14. Only children under the age of three when affected by this genetic defect will develop a resulting tumor. Retinoblastoma is the most common intraocular malignancy in children. Most tumors occur sporadically, but approximately a third are inherited in an autosomal dominant pattern. Leukocoria is the most common presenting clinical sign of a retinoblastoma. Other presenting symptoms include strabismus, pain, glaucoma, pseudohypopyon, iris heterochromia, visual loss, proptosis, and preseptal cellulitis. Preseptal orbital cellulitis results from intratumoral ocular hemorrhage that may cause discomfort in the eye that is then rubbed by the child's nonsterile hand. Such as an infection may delay correct diagnosis of an intraocular tumor unless fundoscopic examination or imaging is carried out.

There are three growth patterns observed on fundoscopic examination of retinoblastomas. These include endophytic or anterior growth of the tumor into the vitreous, exophytic growth of the tumor into the subretinal space, and diffuse infiltrating growth or plaque-like growth within the retina. There is frequently retinal detachment that can be caused by all three different growth patterns and there may be multiple lesions within one globe. Seeding of the vitreous by tumor occurs in the endophytic growth pattern and may cause opacification of the vitreous and decreased visibility of the mass.

Most cases of retinoblastoma are diagnosed clinically and radiographic evaluation is performed in order to confirm the diagnosis, evaluate size and spread of the tumor, identify calcifications, and to look for additional lesions such as a pinealblastoma. A retinoblastoma can be demonstrated on 80% of ultrasound imaging studies, but assessment of the extent of the lesion is limited. Most endophytic and exophytic lesions have calcifications, but some of the diffuse infiltrating lesions do not. The lesions themselves appear as irregular and heterogeneous masses and may contain cystic appearing areas suggestive of necrosis.

On CT scanning, the pattern of the calcifications is variable, with both punctate and aggregate calcifications (**Fig. 2-52**). Vitreous hemorrhage and ocular lens and retinal detachments are common. The mass itself may be hyperdense and enhancing following administration of contrast.

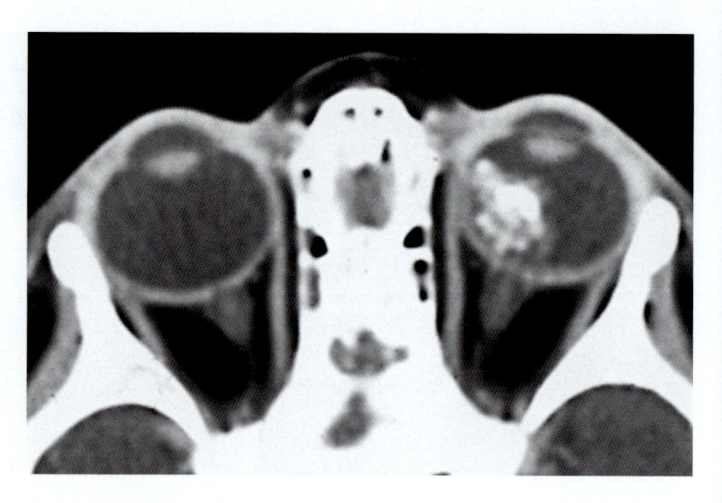

Figure 2-52 Retinoblastoma: Unilateral
Retinoblastoma in a 17-month-old infant presenting with leukocoria in the left eye. Axial CT scan with contrast shows an irregular highly calcified mass in the left globe. There is enhancing tissue around the calcifications.

MR imaging allows for accurate evaluation of the extent of retinoblastomas. The lesion must be approximately 2 mm thick in order to be recognizable on MR. Such lesions will appear isointense to hyperintense to the vitreous on T1W images and have a low signal on T2W images (**Fig. 2-53**). The lesion histology may correlate with the MR appearance of undifferentiated lesions being less hyperintense than well-differentiated lesions. Calcification identified on ultrasound or CT scans may not be evident on MR unless they are large and then will appear as areas of marked hypointensity on both T1W and T2W images and may cause a retinoblastoma to appear heterogeneous.

MR imaging is used to distinguish associated retinal abnormalities including retinal detachment with exudate or hemorrhage. Contrast administration will show a lesion with moderate to marked enhancement that is heterogeneous due to areas of calcification and necrosis. The globe will be normal in size, a factor that may be helpful in distinguishing retinoblastoma from other lesions that cause leukocoria such as PHPV. The remaining differential diagnosis for retinoblastoma is extensive. There are many intraocular calcified lesions that have a similar imaging appearance and the definitive diagnosis can be difficult (**Table 2-4**). A calcified ocular mass in a child less than three years old is considered to be a retinoblastoma until proven otherwise.

Common routes of spread of retinoblastoma include extension to the intracranial subarachnoid space via the optic nerve, to the systemic circulation via the ocular venous system, and to the extraocular orbit via the choroid and sclera. Bilateral tumors are present in a third of the cases and are usually the familial form of retinoblastomas (**Fig. 2-54**). Up to 3% of patients with bilateral retinoblastomas also have a pinealblastoma of the pineal gland or other primitive tumor of the supra or parasellar region; this combination is referred to as trilateral retinoblastoma.

Treatment options are varied and range from photocoagulation to enucleation with optic nerve excision. Patients with lesions confined to the eye have a 90% five-year survival and 90% of the eyes will maintain useful vision. For lesions extending

Chapter 2: The Orbit and Globe   67

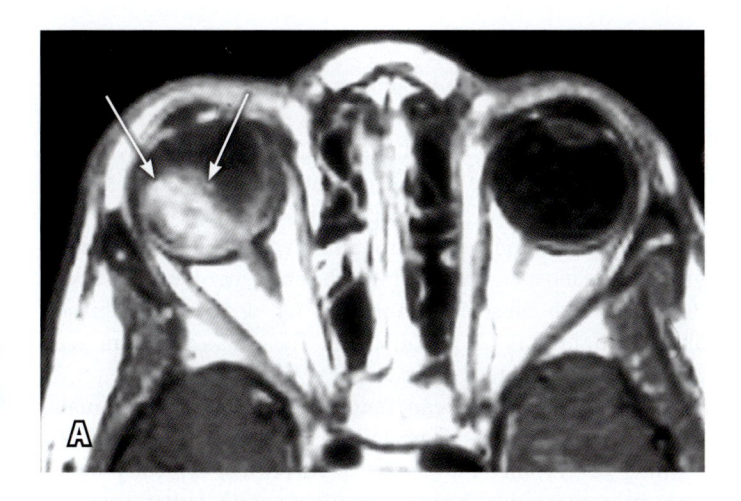

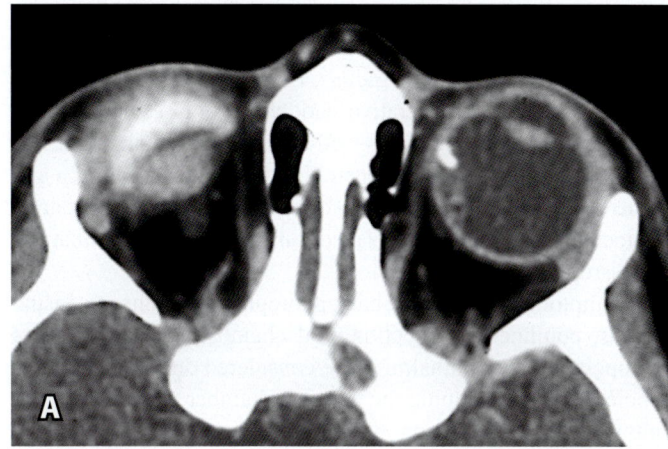

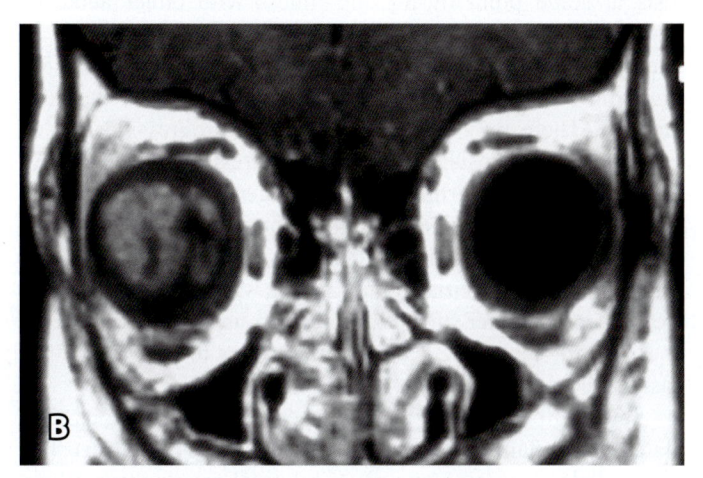

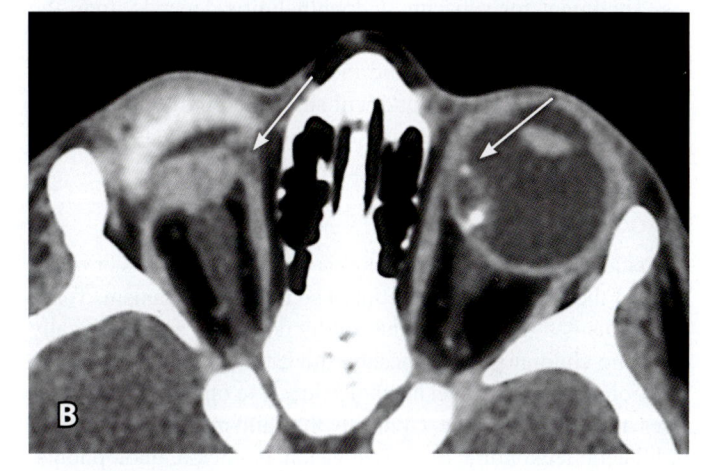

Figure 2-53 Retinoblastoma: Unilateral
Total retinal detachment in a three-year-old girl with retinoblastoma. T1W MR scans with contrast. In the axial view (**A**) there is a hemorrhagic mass in the right globe. The retina is fully detached and the "half moon" shape (*arrow*, **A**), representing the folds of the retina, are noted to be lifted into the vitreous. In the coronal view (**B**), there is a hemorrhagic irregular mass in the right globe. The findings are less specific in MR, as the calcifications cannot be detected.

Figure 2-54 Retinoblastoma: Bilateral
Bilateral retinoblastoma (previous resection of the tumor in the right globe with placement of an ocular prosthesis). Axial CT scans with contrast (**A** and **B**) demonstrate calcifications of the left globe with (*arrow on the right side of the image*) choroidal detachment and involvement of the posteromedial ocular prosthesis on the right side (*arrow on the left side of the image*).

beyond the globe or trilateral retinoblastoma, the prognosis is much worse. Patients with heritable retinoblastoma have a tendency to develop secondary cancers, especially osteosarcomas and a variety of other soft tissue sarcomas.[22,100,106,107,109,110]

OCULAR INFECTIONS AND INFLAMMATIONS

Ocular infections may involve the internal structures of the globe, termed endophthalmitis, or may predominantly affect a particular tissue layer of the globe, for example retinitis in reference to the retina. Primary infection of the globe may stem from a hematogenous source or from direct inoculation of the eye, e.g., penetrating trauma into the globe. The causative organisms are varied including bacteria, viruses, fungi, or parasites.

Infection of the extraocular orbit may secondarily involve the globe, which was discussed earlier in the section on extraconal lesions. Various systemic illnesses may cause inflammation of tissues of the eye including posterior scleritis seen in cases of idiopathic orbital pseudotumor and uveitis associated with sarcoidosis. Although the etiologies may differ, the imaging appearance of infectious lesions may be identical.

Endophthalmitis

Endophthalmitis describes intraocular infections involving the anterior chamber and vitreous that may be acute, subacute, or chronic (**Fig. 2-16**). The causes can be divided into three categories: postoperative (70%), post-traumatic (20%), and endogenous (8%). Postoperative causes can be further subdivided into acute (less than 6 weeks after surgery), delayed (more than 6 weeks after surgery), and filtering bleb-associated. The organisms responsible for acute and bleb-associated endophthalmitis are usually bacterial (coagulase-negative staphylococci, *Streptococcus* species, *Staphylooccus aureus*, *Haemophilus influenzae*). In contrast, delayed postoperative endophthalmitis can be caused by fungi (Candida species) as well as bacteria. The incidence of endophthalmitis following penetrating trauma is 3% to 7% and higher (30%) in rural settings. The risk increases with retained intraocular foreign body, delayed surgery, soil contamination, and disrupted artificial lens.

Symptoms may include pain, photophobia, discharge, visual deficits, conjunctival injection, and chemosis. Cases of acute postoperative endophthalmitis are considered ophthalmic emergencies requiring tapping the anterior chamber and vitreous for cultures and administering intravitreal and subconjunctival antibiotics, topical antibiotics and steroids, and possibly IV antibiotics. Treatment for subacute endophthalmitis depends upon the clinical situation, but are similar to acute cases. If patients have visual acuity worse than hand motion, then immediate vitrectomy is indicated. Ultrasound will show medium to high intensity echoes diffusely in the vitreous. The appearance is similar to vitreal hemorrhage, but the echoes are less mobile.

Toxocariasis

Parasitic toxocaral infections may cause endophthalmitis or infections of the temporal chorioretina. The infective organism, Toxocara canis is transmitted to the soil by dog feces and then orally to young children. After ingestion the larvae burrow to the liver and from there may travel hematogenously to other visceral structures including the globe. Clinically the child may have unilateral or bilateral leukokoria, decreased vision, erythema, photophobia, and pain caused by ocular larva migrans. The ophthalmologic examination may reveal anterior chamber flare, keratic precipitates, vitritis, vitreous synechia, retinal or choroidal mass, tractional or exudative retinal detachment and/or cataract. The organism causes an eosinophilic and granulomatous reaction.

Imaging is often performed in patients with suspected toxocariasis to rule out retinoblastoma in a child with leukokoria. The ultrasound imaging appearance is similar to retinoblastoma and may show a mass with medium to low signal echoes in the peripheral fundus, but the internal high-intensity echoes suggestive of calcifications often seen in retinoblastoma are usually absent. CT examination reveals a thickened sclera and/or focal uveoscleral thickening. A high attenuating intravitreal mass without calcifications in a normal sized eye may be present along with retinal detachment.

MR reveals a granulomatous intravitreal mass or ill-defined area that is isointense compared with the vitreous on T1W images and hyperintense or hypointense on T2W and proton density images. There is typically enhancement of the granuloma after contrast administration. With a retinal detachment there may be a subretinal exudate that is typically hyperintense on both T1W and T2W sequences. This appearance is similar to Coats' disease and along with retinoblastoma should be included in the differential diagnosis. The diagnosis can be confirmed by performing an enzyme-linked immunosorbent assay. The patient may also have associated convulsions and intracranial calcifications in cases of advanced disease.[12,30,53,95]

Sarcoidosis

Sarcoidosis is a disease of unknown etiology in which there are noncaseating granulomas found in multiple organ systems, but most commonly in the lungs, hilar lymph nodes, eyes, and skin. The orbit is the most frequent extrapulmonary system involved, and 25% to 50% of cases involve the eye. The uvea is the most common ocular structure involved, and the lacrimal gland is the most common orbital structure involved. However, the extraocular muscles, retrobulbar fat, optic nerve, chiasm, and radiations may also be affected. The classical patient is an African-American female under 40 years.

Clinically, patients can range from being asymptomatic to having multiorgan system failure. The disease may be self-limiting or chronic. Pulmonary involvement typically manifests at some point during the illness with either acute or chronic symptoms. In the eye there may be a rapid onset of uveitis with blurred vision, photophobia, and excessive lacrimation. Pale yellow nodules may be observed on the conjunctiva. There may be acute or chronic progressive loss of vision, pain, proptosis, and ophthalmoparesis. There is usually painless, bilateral lacrimal gland enlargement that is palpable in 10% of the cases. The triad of erythema nodosum, bilateral hilar adenopathy, and polyarthralgias is referred to as Lofgren's syndrome. When uveitis and parotiditis with facial nerve palsy are present together, this is referred to as uveoparotid fever or Heerfordt syndrome. Lupus pernio refers to the presence of nasal sarcoidosis.

Imaging of sarcoidosis is nonspecific and the lesions simulate other inflammatory or tumorous lesions (**Fig. 2-36**). The lacrimal glands may show diffuse bilateral enlargement. When the optic nerve is enlarged it is typically more pronounced intracranially and the nerve or nerve sheath may enhance postcontrast administration, simulating an optic nerve tumor. The extraocular muscles may also be involved and appear enlarged.

Diagnosis is made by biopsy, and there may be an associated increase in angiotensin converting enzyme in the blood or CSF. Patients are either observed or treated with steroids. The differential diagnosis includes lymphoma, leukemic infiltration, IOP, and meningioma, glioma or demyelinating disease of the optic nerve.[111-113]

CMV Retinitis

Although complications of acquired immunodeficiency syndrome (AIDS) may affect many parts of the globe, cytomegalovirus (CMV) retinitis is the most common ocular infection affecting up to 40% of patients with AIDS, especially when the CD4 falls below 50 cells/mm^3. CMV retinitis can lead to retinal necrosis and retinal detachments secondary to recurrent retinal hemorrhages. Treatment involves aggressive systemic antiviral treatment and local treatment of the retinitis and retinal detachments using antivirals, vitreoretinal surgery, and/or laser photocoagulation. Ganciclovir implants, or injections may be used to treat CMV retinitis. Such devices may be visible on CT or MR imaging as small focal hyperdense or hypointense lesions.

Episcleritis and Scleritis

Isolated episcleritis is diagnosed clinically and imaging studies are usually not performed. The illness is self-limiting and typically follows a viral infection. Scleritis is often divided into anterior scleritis or posterior scleritis. The anterior sclera is more commonly affected than the posterior, and when the posterior sclera is affected it is usually in conjunction with the anterior sclera. Some cases of posterior scleritis are considered to be on a continuum with IOP as was discussed in the section on extraconal lesions.

Scleritis rarely presents as an isolated phenomenon without an associated systemic illness. Both anterior and posterior scleritis may be the presenting manifestation of a variety of systemic diseases including rheumatoid arthritis, Wegener granulomatosis, sarcoidosis, inflammatory bowel disease among many others.[29]

Complications of scleritis are usually the result of further posterior scleral involvement. The presence of inflammation causes alterations in the vascular supply to the sclera. The anterior sclera with its rich vascular supply can usually compensate, but the posterior sclera will usually undergo ischemic changes. There will be scleral thinning, necrosis, and perforation (scleromalacia perforans). The patient may have proptosis, visual loss, and pain in these stages. In addition, uveal effusion, uveitis, retinal detachment, secondary glaucoma, and/or disc edema may complicate posterior scleritis.[22,100,114]

Focal, nodular, and/or diffuse scleral thickening are observed on imaging studies. The nodular form of posterior scleritis may resemble choroidal melanoma or metastasis and the more diffuse form may appear after trauma or surgery. On MR imaging, scleritis appears isointense to the vitreous on T1W images and hypointense on T2W images. The diffuse variety may show marked enhancement while the nodular variety little to no enhancement after contrast administration. It is important to note that the imaging appearance of scleritis may mimic the volume averaging of the sclerouveal rim and the scleral surface of the globe.

LACRIMAL GLAND AND NASOLACRIMAL APPARATUS

A variety of pathologic entities affect the lacrimal gland and lacrimal apparatus, but there are predominantly two patterns of involvement. There is either obstructive lesions of the drainage apparatus or infiltrating neoplasms or inflammations that lead to enlargement of the lacrimal gland (**Table 2-25**). The more common etiologies of both of these problems will be discussed in this section along with the unique imaging tools that may be used to evaluate this area.

Dacryocystography

Dacryocystography uses contrast material injected into the lacrimal apparatus to image the anatomy. Following injection of contrast, plain film or CT scans may be obtained (**Fig. 2-55**). The presenting indication is epiphora and the examination is utilized to determine patency of the canaliculi, lacrimal sac, and/or nasolacrimal duct. The site and degree of obstruction, presence of fistulae, diverticula, and concretions may also be identified. At times, there may be a physiological obstruction that is overcome by performing the cannulation of the duct followed by dacryocystography.

In some cases, dacryoscintography or MR with dacryocystography needs to be performed. These procedures differ from dacryocystography in that radioactive tracer or drops of gadolinium-based contrast material is allowed to drain from the eye naturally without direct injection into the nasolacrimal apparatus. If an area of obstruction is identified, the radioactive agent or gadolinium-based contrast fails to progress into and out of the nasolacrimal duct. These procedures are noninvasive alternatives to the standard dacryocystography.[2,3,115–119]

Nasolacrimal Sac and Duct

Pathology of the nasolacrimal drainage apparatus typically presents with epiphora that develops following an anatomic or functional obstruction. Anatomic obstruction may be due to congenital lesions, inflammatory or neoplastic lesions, dacryoliths, or idiopathic inflammation, and scarring. Obstruction in the adult population is more common in women and an exact etiology is usually not identified.

Congenital nasolacrimal duct obstruction presenting in neonates is usually due to an imperforate membrane within the lacrimal duct epithelium and nasal mucosa at the lower end of the duct. Most uncomplicated cases will resolve spontaneously with the aid of topical massage and/or antibiotics. The obstruction is usually complete and presents with clinical epiphora and/or a dacryocystocele or congenital lacrimal sac mucocele (**Figs. 2-56** and **2-57**). Approximately 2% of patients with distal

Table 2-25 Lacrimal Gland Enlargement

- Epithelial tumors (50%)
- Benign adenoma
- Carcinoma (adenocystic Ca most common)
- Lymphoid lesions (50%)
- Lymphoma
- Benign lymphoid hyperplasia
- Idiopathic orbital pseudotumor (IOP)
- Sjögren's syndrome
- Mikulicz's disease (benign, chronic dacryoadenitis)
- Dermoid
- Metastasis
- Sarcoidosis
- Wagener granulomatosis
- Amyloidosis
- Kimura's disease (inflammatory disorder characterized by triad of painless subcutaneous masses in head or neck region, eosinophilia, elevated serum immunoglobulin E)

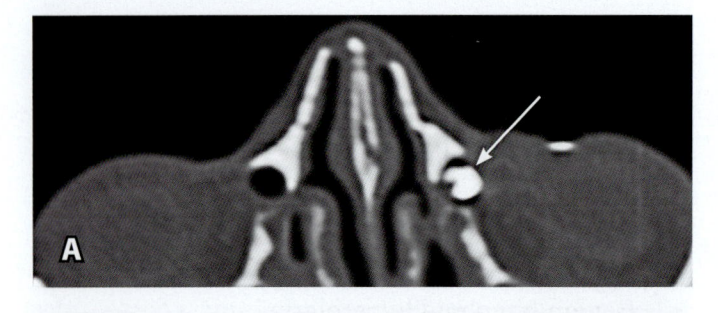

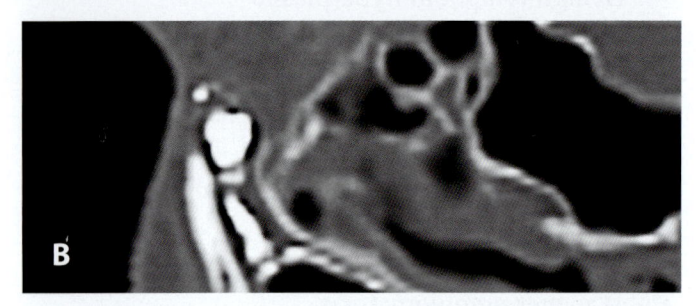

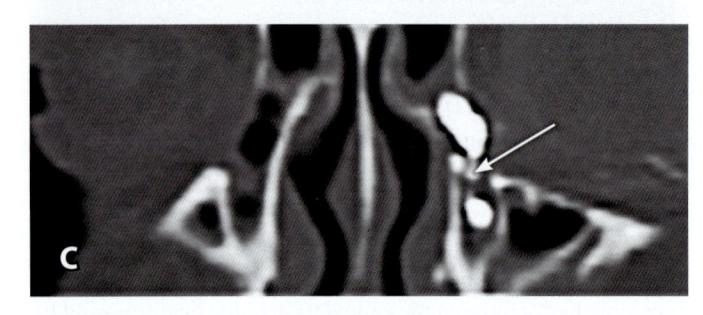

Figure 2-55 Nasolacrimal Duct Papilloma
Papilloma of the nasolacrimal sac and duct in a patient with chronic epiphora. CT-dacryocystogram obtained following cannulation and injection of contrast into the left nasolacrimal sac. Scan (**A**) demonstrates the left nasolacrimal sac filled with contrast (*arrow*). Reformatted sagittal scan (**B**) shows contrast in the lacrimal sac, but not in the lacrimal duct inferiorly. Coronal scan (**C**) demonstrates that contrast injected into the nasolacrimal puncta does go beyond the nasolacrimal sac in successive sections following the length of the drainage system, but with significant narrowing (*arrow*, **C**) at the junction of the nasolacrimal sac with the duct.

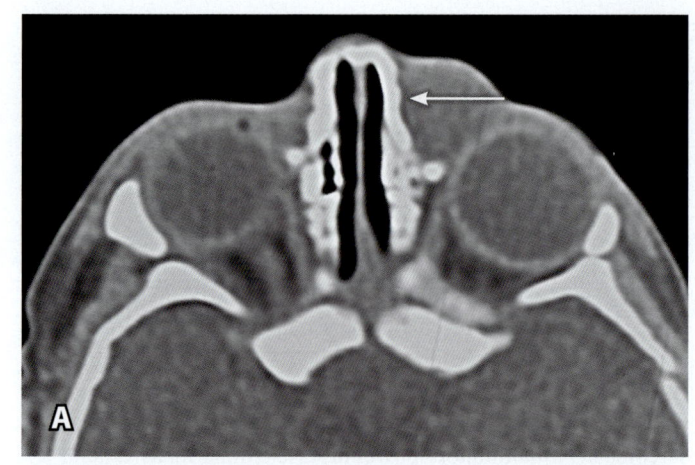

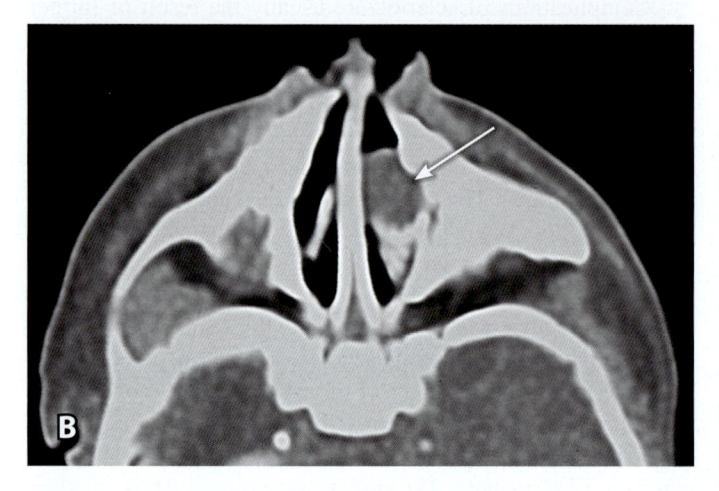

Figure 2-56 Nasolacrimal Sac Mucocele
Dacryocystocele (nasolacrimal sac mucocele) with a dysfunctional valve of Hasner. Axial CT scans (**A** and **B**) show a mass in the area of the left nasolacrimal sac and another mass in the left side of the nasal cavity (*arrows*, **A**, **B**). These findings are part of a classical triad found in infants with congenital obstruction of the nasolacrimal apparatus both superiorly and inferiorly and include a medial canthal mass, dilation (or mucocele) of the nasolacrimal duct, and a submucosal nasal mass. In this particular case, a dysfunctional valve of Hasner and subsequent mucocele formation caused the distal obstruction.

obstruction also have proximal obstruction leading to the formation of the dacryocystocele by distention of the lacrimal sac. If there is distention of the distal end of the nasolacrimal duct, this entity is referred to as a nasolacrimal mucocele. Such a lesion may be a significant cause of respiratory distress in the newborn. The reported incidence of secondary infection and formation of a dacryocystopyocele or mucopyocele is variable, but may be associated with orbital cellulitis as well.[2,116]

Although often diagnosed clinically, imaging is performed to confirm the diagnosis of a dacryocystocele or nasolacrimal mucocele. On CT scans, the lesion will appear as a thin-walled sac with lower density material within. There is associated lacrimal fossa and bony nasolacrimal canal enlargement suggesting the chronic nature of the lesion (**Figs. 2-56** and **2-57**).

On MR imaging, the material will have low to intermediate signal on T1W scans and high signal on T2W and proton density scans. If infection is present there may be thickening and enhancement of the walls along with the nearby soft tissues. Dacryocystography may be used to illustrate the site of obstruction and dilation. The differential diagnosis includes nasoethmoidal cephaloceles, hemangiomas, or other tumors.[120,121]

In adult patients, the differential diagnosis of a medial canthal mass includes both inflammatory and neoplastic processes such as primary tumor of the lacrimal sac, IOP, sarcoidosis, ethmoidal mucocele, basal cell carcinoma, and non-Hodgkin's lymphoma. Direct extension from squamous cell carcinoma of the ethmoid air cells can form a soft tissue mass with nasolacrimal duct or sac obstruction.[122]

Chapter 2: The Orbit and Globe   71

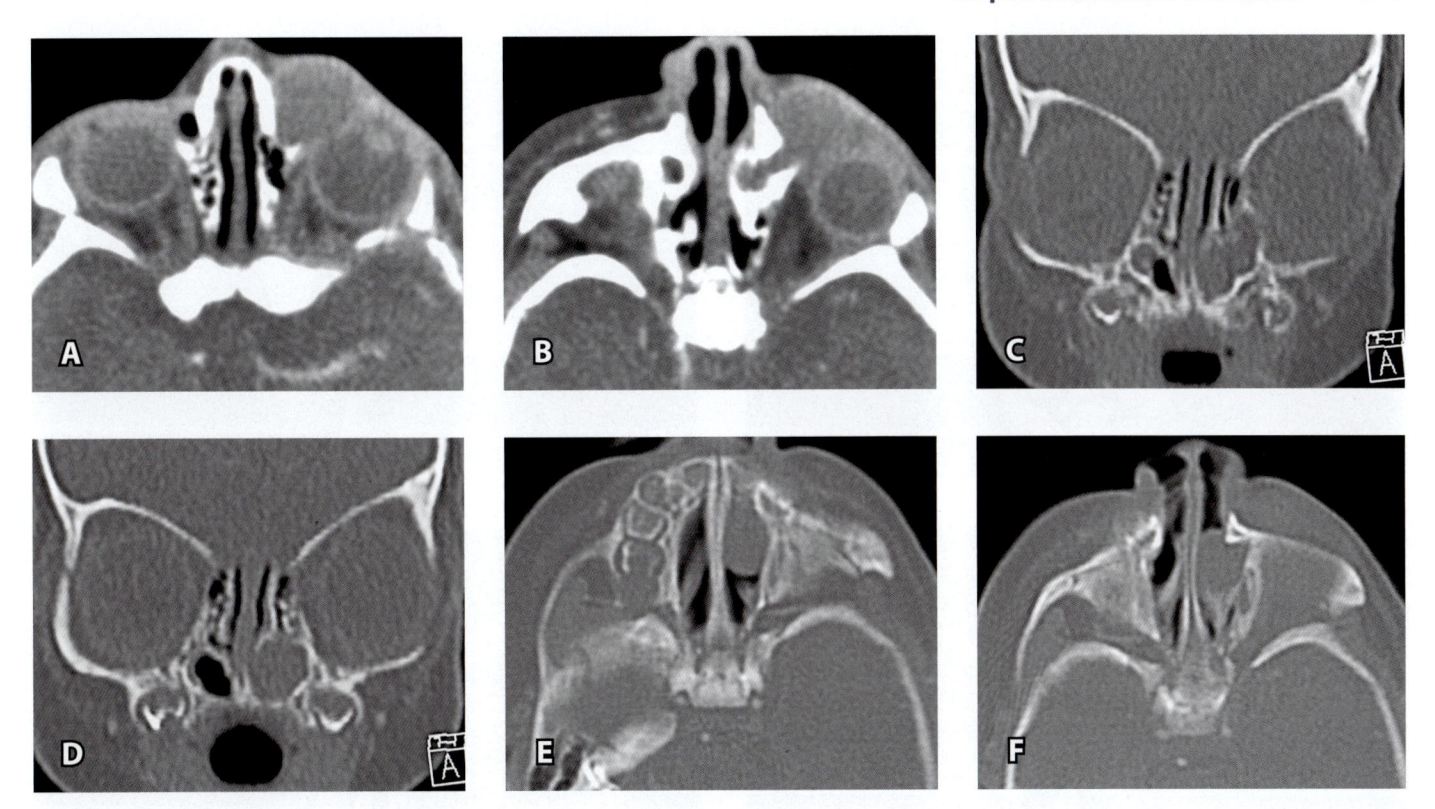

Figure 2-57 Nasolacrimal Sac Mucocele
Dacryocystocele (nasolacrimal duct mucocele) in a newborn infant. Axial CT scans with contrast (**A–B**) coronal CT bone windows (**C–D**) axial CT bone windows (**E–F**) show a dumbbell-shaped, lobulated, cystic mass filling both the nasolacrimal sac and the nasolacrimal duct, which is expanded throughout its course. This is due to incompetency of the valves of Hasner with associated dilatation of the nasolacrimal apparatus.

A complication of anatomic obstruction of the nasolacrimal apparatus is dacryoliths or concretions. Concretions may be formed from the presence of infectious organisms such as Actinomyces species or Staphylococus aureus, which produce filamentous aggregates. The patient may present not only with epiphora, but may also show signs of infection such as orbital swelling and erythema (**Figs. 2-58** and **2-59**). The stones or concretions may be identified on dacryocystography as prestenotic filling defects and may be removed via dacryoplasty, irrigation, and surgery or may pass spontaneously. Diverticula or fistula may also result from chronic obstruction and may be identified on imaging studies.[2]

Lacrimal Gland

Many disease processes involve the lacrimal gland. Diffuse infiltration of the gland causing palpable enlargement is a common presenting sign and represents a radiographically identifiable feature. Many lesions that affect other parts of the orbit cause diffuse enlargement of the lacrimal gland and cannot be

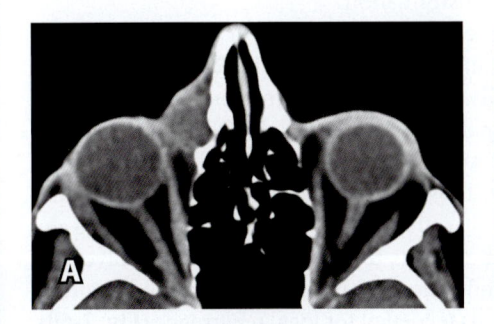

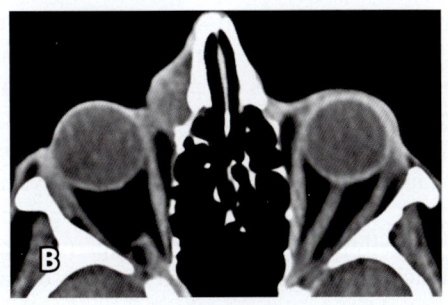

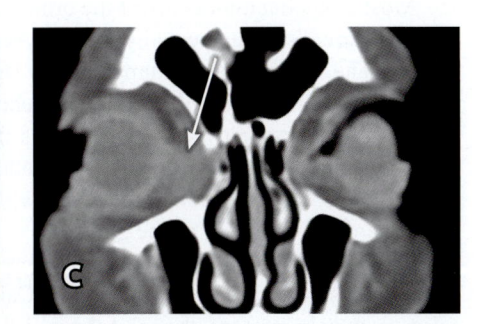

Figure 2-58 Dacryocystitis
Dacryocystitis of the right lacrimal sac. Axial (**A–B**) and coronal reformatted (**C**) CT scans with contrast demonstrate a soft tissue mass with a low density center expanding from the right nasolacrimal fossa in the region of the nasolacrimal sac. There is obscuration of the medial epicanthal folds with soft tissue extending into the medial portion of the right orbit (*arrow*, **C**).

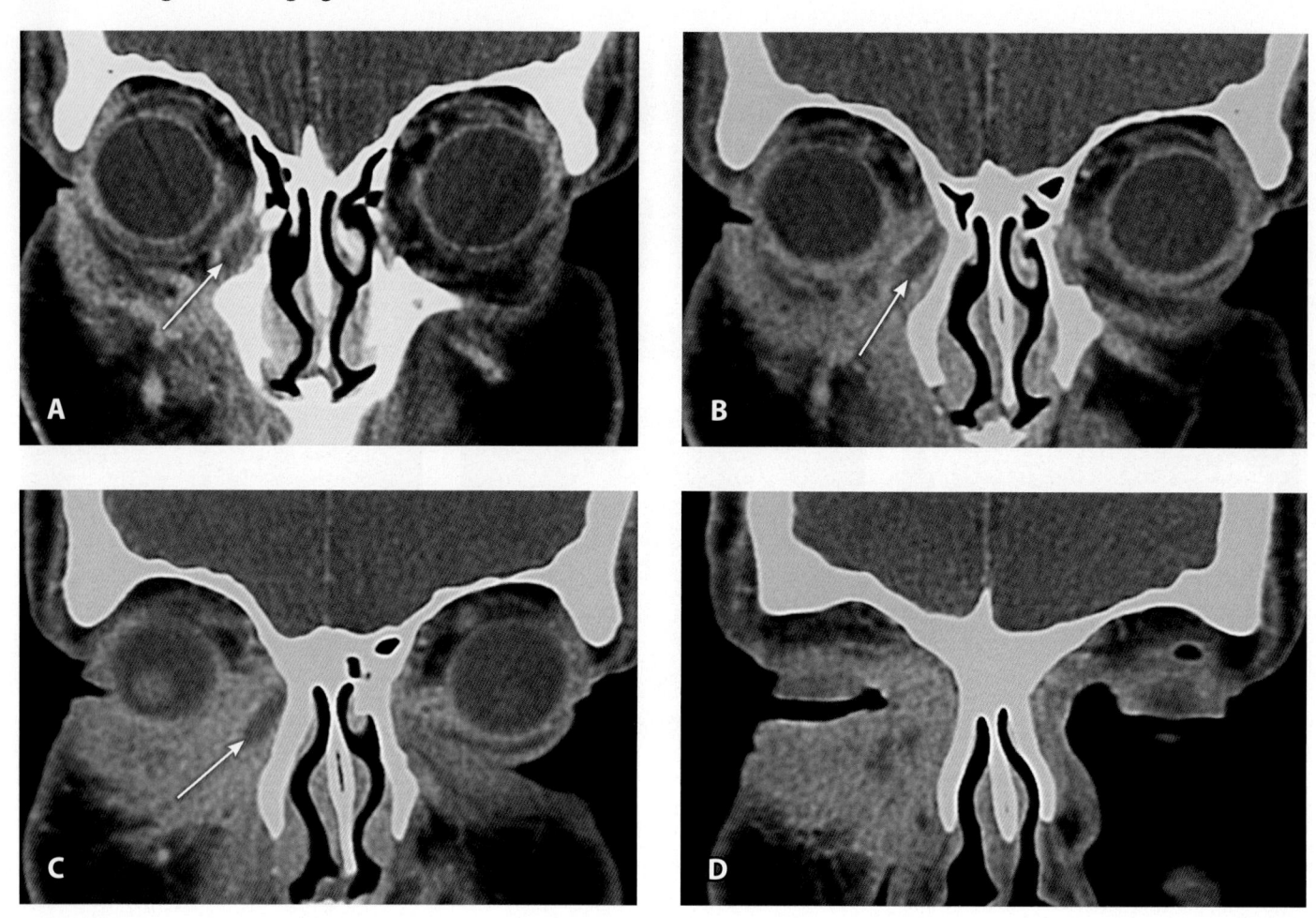

Figure 2-59 Lacrimal Sac Abscess
Lacrimal sac abscess with preseptal cellulitis in a 35-year-old male. Coronal CT scans. In **A** there is fatty streaking in the soft tissues below the left orbit. In **B** and **C**, a low-density oval shape is seen in the region of the right lacrimal sac representative of abscess (*arrows*, **A**, **B**, **C**). **D** shows the inflammation involving the cheek as well as the underlying soft tissues.

readily diagnosed by imaging alone (see **Table 2-9** for a list of causes of lacrimal gland enlargement). Half of all lacrimal gland masses are epithelial tumors and their classification is similar to that of salivary gland tumors. Many other lacrimal gland lesions are inflammatory or lymphoproliferative.

Most epithelial tumors affect the orbital lobe of the lacrimal gland and are distributed equally between benign and malignant lesions. The most common tumor of the lacrimal gland is the benign mixed tumor or pleomorphic adenoma. These tumors present as painless, slow-growing masses in the region of the lacrimal gland in middle-aged adults. Because the orbital lobe is usually involved, expansion of the tumor will cause a downward and inward displacement of the globe.

On CT examination, lacrimal gland tumors usually appear as well circumscribed round or oval lesions. Calcification and bony sclerosis may be present, though not typically. On MR imaging, the lesions have a low signal on T1W images and an increased signal on T2W images with a heterogeneous or nodular appearance in some cases. There is moderate to marked enhancement postcontrast administration.

Treatment is complete excision of the tumor. If an incisional biopsy is performed there is a high rate of recurrence and this must be avoided due to the incidence of malignant transformation occasionally observed in these tumors. Local invasion may occur with recurrences, but metastasis does not usually occur without malignant transformation.[22,123]

Adenoid cystic carcinoma is the most common primary malignant tumor or the lacrimal gland (**Fig. 2-60**). The clinical presentation is usually different from the presentation of a benign tumor and includes pain, blepharatosis, inhibited ocular motility, and the presence of a hard palpable mass that has been present for less than a year. These tumors occur in adults of a slightly younger age group than those with pleomorphic adenoma do. The aggressive nature of this lesion leads to early involvement of nerves, vessels, and bones accounting for the painful nature of this lesion as well as its tendency for local recurrence (**Fig. 2-60**).

CT scans reveal a rounded lesion with irregular borders. Calcifications are more common in these malignant lesions of the lacrimal gland than in the benign pleomorphic adenoma. MR imaging may reveal a mass that is heterogeneous and

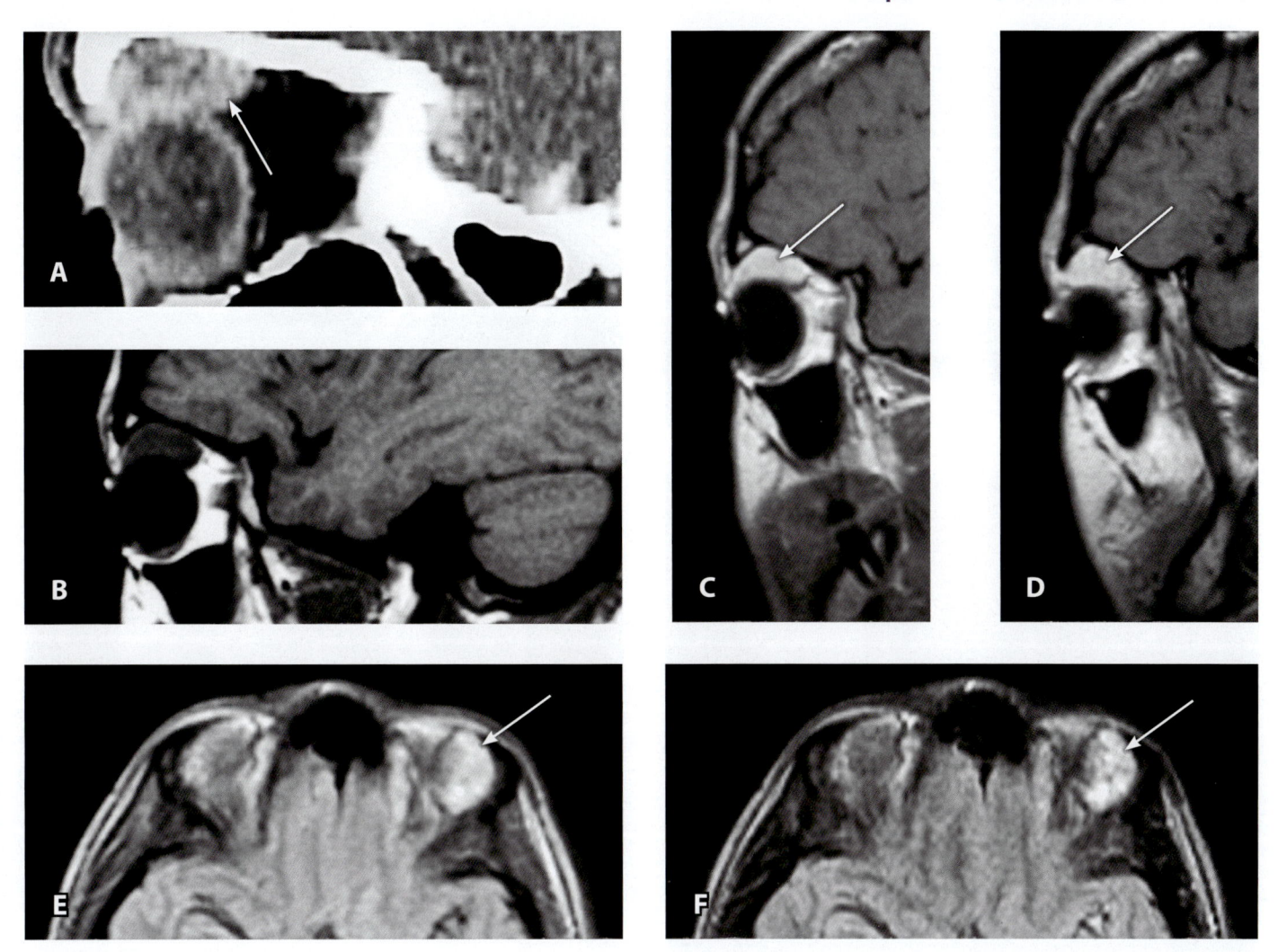

Figure 2-60 Adenoid Cystic Carcinoma of the Lacrimal Gland
Adenoid cystic carcinoma of the left lacrimal gland in a 24-year-old female. There is an enhancing mass superior to the left globe in this reformatted sagittal view CT scan (**A**). Sagittal T1W MR scan (**B**) shows a homogeneous mass of moderate intensity overlying the left globe (*arrow,* **A**). Sagittal T1W enhanced MR scans (**C–D**) show a homogeneous enhancing mass in the superior left orbit (*arrows,* **C, D**). There is remodeling of the orbital roof between the mass and frontal lobe of the brain. Axial proton density MR (**E**) shows the left lacrimal gland mass is hyperintense when compared with the normal lacrimal gland on the right side (*arrow,* **E**). In the axial T2W MR (**F**), the mass also appears hyperintense (*arrow,* **F**), but less than that in the proton density scan.

hyperintense to muscle, but hypointense to fat on T1W images. On T2W images, the lesion may appear hyperintense and heterogeneous compared to the muscles and fat. Enhancement is typically present on postcontrast CT or MR scans (**Figs. 2-60 and 2-61**).[22,123]

TRAUMA

Orbital trauma consists of fractures, soft tissue injury, and foreign body penetration. High-resolution CT is the method of choice for evaluating traumatic orbital lesions. It can demonstrate fractures, subperiosteal hematomas, ocular lacerations, orbital or ocular gas collections, hemorrhages, retroocular hematomas, optic nerve compression, and lacerations. Axial CT best demonstrates the medial and lateral walls of the orbit, and the anterior wall of the maxillary sinus. Coronal CT best demonstrates the orbital roof and floor. Due to its rapid scanning time and the ability to be rapidly converted into reconstructed images, spiral CT is the most useful technique to evaluate acute orbital trauma.

Once evidence of a metallic foreign body has been ruled out, orbital MR imaging may be needed in addition to CT, due to its superior ability to detect and differentiate edema from hematomas, soft tissue injuries, vascular injuries, and wooden foreign bodies. Although fractures with bony fragments produce a signal void on MR imaging, the associated displacement of fat around and through fractures can often lead to the correct diagnosis. MR images are particularly useful in cases of post-traumatic brain herniation into the orbit (**Fig. 2-62**).[22] Ultrasound imaging

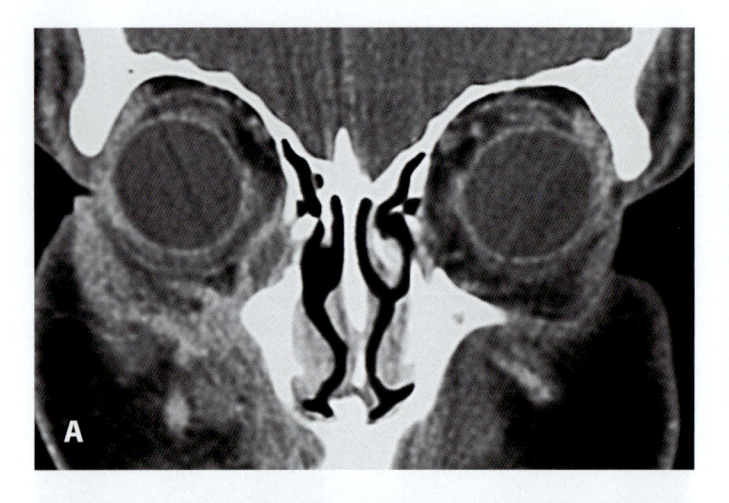

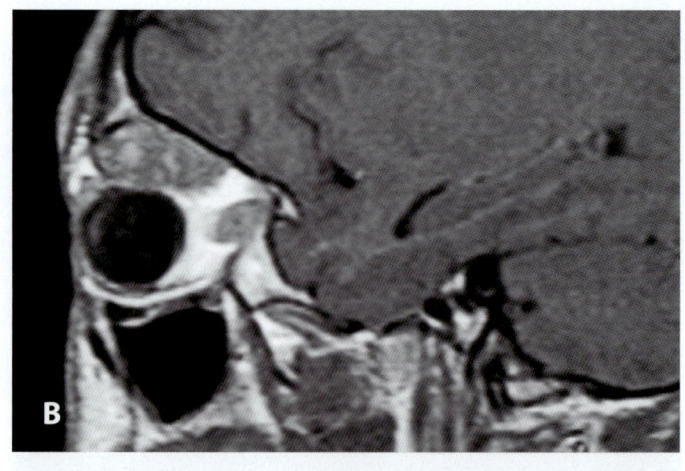

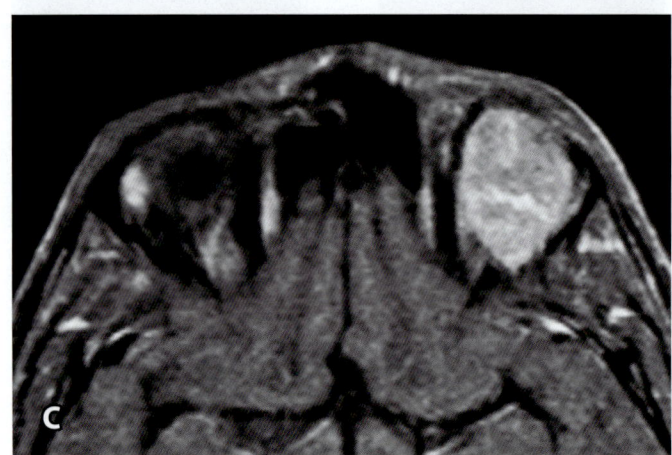

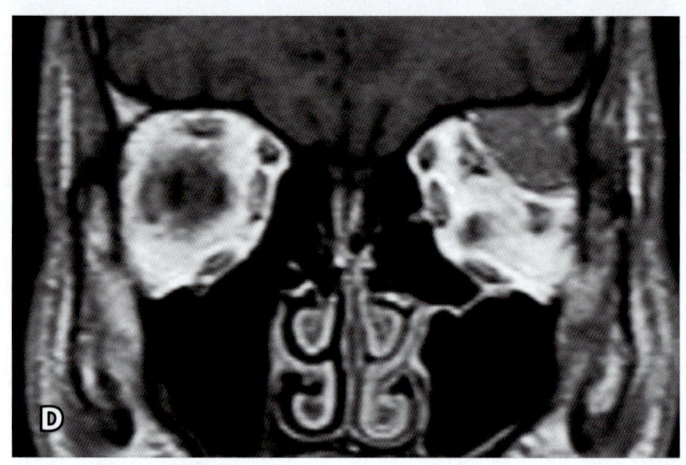

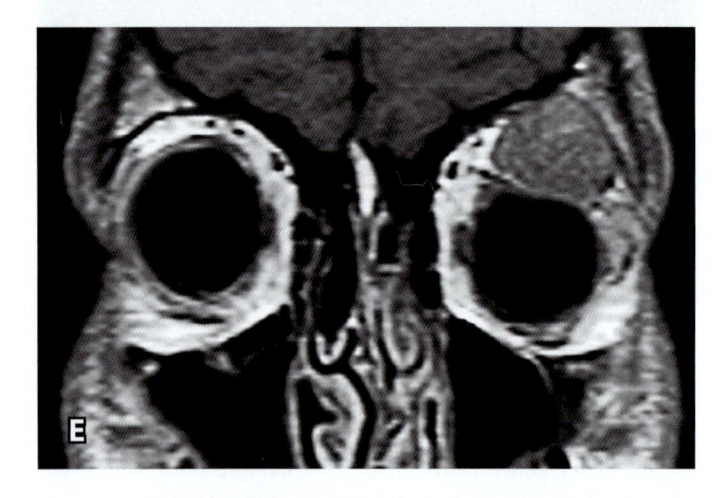

Figure 2-61 Mucoepidermoid Carcinoma
The axial T2-W scan (**A**) shows a moderately intense heterogeneous mass in the in the left orbit superior to the left globe. The sagittal T1-W scan (**B**) shows an intermediate intensity mass in the superior orbit with patchy areas of higher intensity within. The T1-W MR scans with contrast and fat suppression show that the lesion enhances with a slightly heterogeneous pattern in the axial view (**C**). Coronal views (**D** and **E**) show the mass in the superolateral portion of the orbit causing downward displacement of the superior rectus and superior oblique muscles.

may also be useful in the evaluation of suspected foreign bodies, but may be difficult to perform if the globe has been severely ruptured.[124,125]

Soft Tissue Injury

Injury to the soft tissues of the eye may or may not accompany fractures. Traumatic injury to the orbit may lead to changes in the orbital fat and hemorrhage into the orbital spaces. With acute trauma an increased linear and reticular pattern is seen in the fat, along with vascular engorgement and edema. With acute hemorrhage, MR will show low signal on both T1W and T2W images. Such hemorrhage may be difficult to identify if the lesion is small. When hemorrhage is subacute, the resultant increase in signal intensity can be appreciated on T1W images if fat suppression techniques are used. The signal intensity of chronic hemorrhage is hyper to hypointense on T1W sequences.[22]

Fractures

Isolated fractures of the orbital rims can occur, although they are usually associated with orbital wall fractures as well. Because

Chapter 2: The Orbit and Globe 75

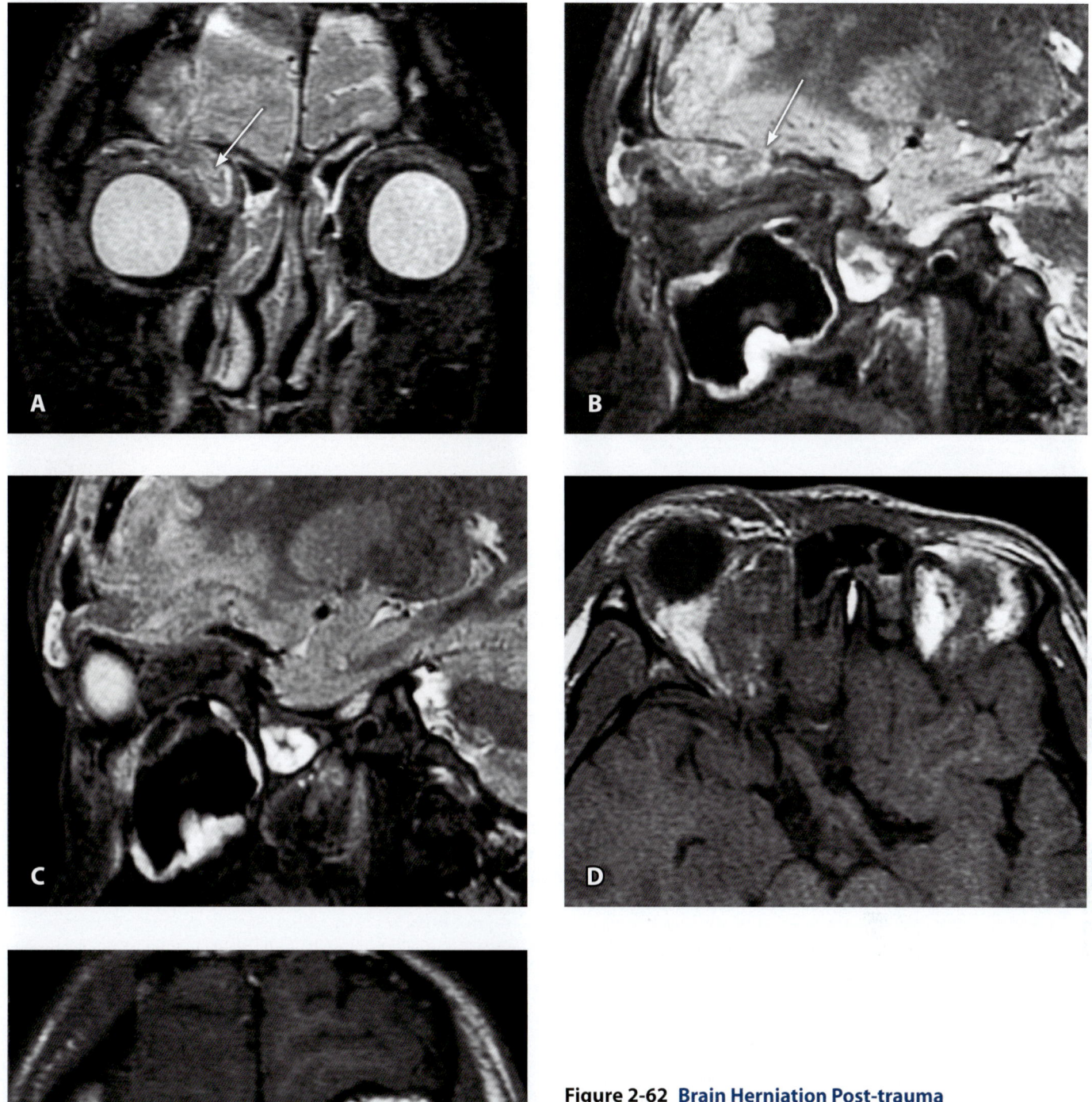

Figure 2-62 Brain Herniation Post-trauma
Comminuted fractures with entrapment and post-traumatic brain hernia in a 21-year-old male. Coronal T2W MR scan (**A**) shows a portion of brain recognized by the gyral markings in the superomedial portion of the right orbit squeezing through the orbital roof (*arrow*, **A**). Sagittal T2W MR scans (**B–C**) show a portion of hemorrhagic brain as it is passing through the defect in the orbital roof (*arrow*). Axial T1W MR scan (**D**) illustrates the defect in the medial portion of the orbital roof and proptosis of the right globe. In the coronal T1W MR (**E**), there is downward displacement of the globe into the right maxillary sinus indicating a secondary inferior blow-out fracture.

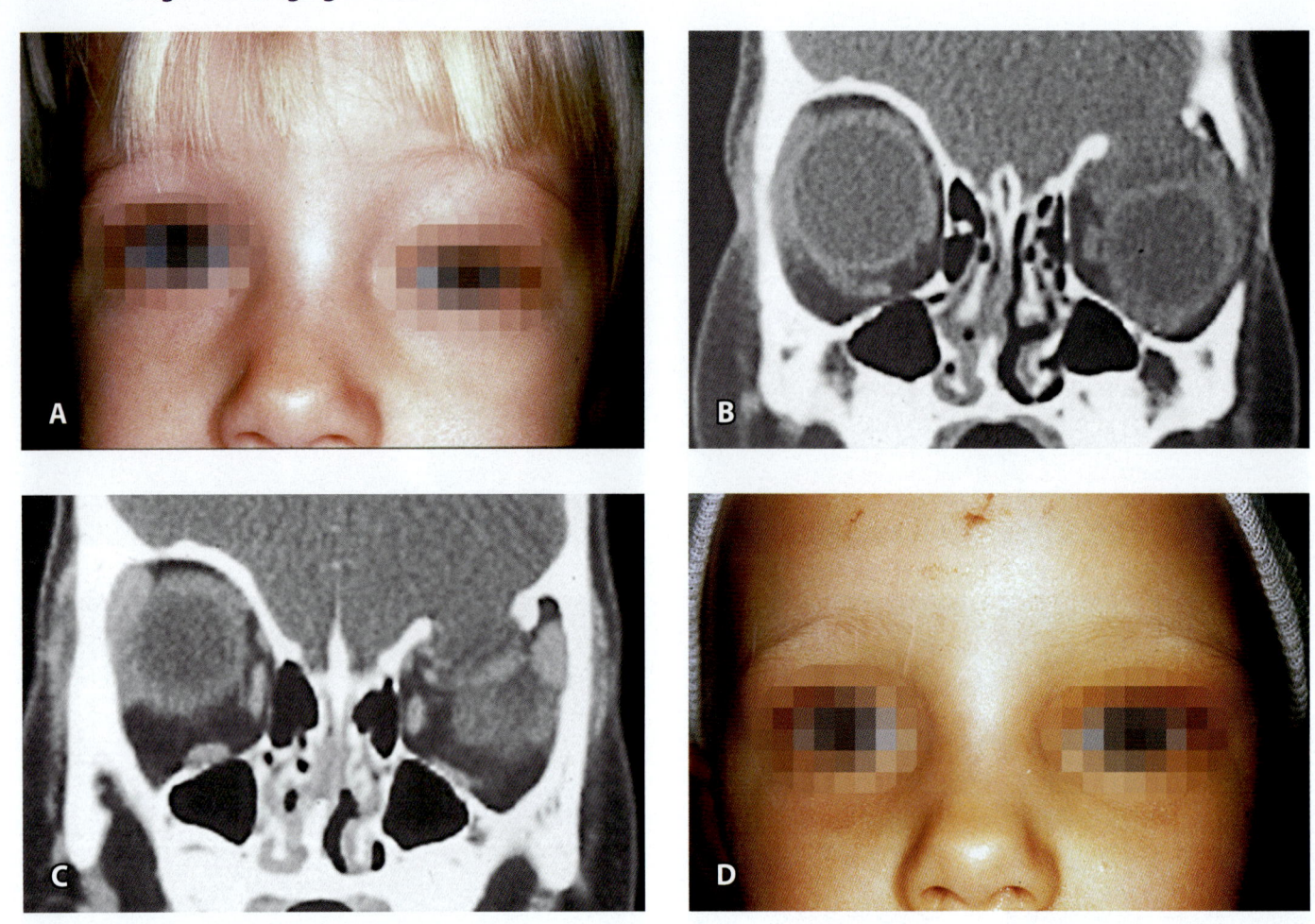

Figure 2-63 Blow-down (Blow-in) Fracture
Blow down fracture refers to an inferiorly displaced orbital roof fracture. (**A**) preoperative photo of a boy with a blow down fracture of the left orbit. Note that his left eye is displaced downward. A preoperative series of scans (**B** and **C**) show the fracture of the orbital roof and the severe downward displacement of the left globe. Postoperative photo of the same child (**D**) with marked improvement in cosmesis. (Case courtesy of Thomas Nadich, MD.)

the orbital rim is a circular structure, a search for a second fracture of the orbit should always be made. Surgical plating may be required if there is a free fragment or rim displacement. Orbital rim fractures should not be considered a form of the blowout or blow-in groups of fractures.[124,125]

Fractures of the orbital walls with an intact orbital rim can be separated into two different groups referred to as blow-in or blowout fractures. Blow-in fractures are much less common than blowout fractures and are characterized by displacement of orbital wall fragments into the orbit. The most common blow-in injuries involve the orbital roof (**Fig. 2-63**). These fractures are typically unilateral, are commonly associated with frontal sinus or skull fractures, and may extend into the orbital apex and cause injury to the optic nerve. Pneumocephalus or cerebrospinal fluid leaks may complicate these fractures. There is an acute decrease in orbital volume that may result in immediate proptosis and/or a compensatory blowout fracture as well. These injuries require urgent surgical intervention.[124–127]

Blowout fractures are typically the result of increased force to the orbital soft tissues resulting in fractures of the thin medial and/or inferior orbital walls with displacement of the fragments away from the orbit. These orbital floor and medial wall fractures result in bony fragmentation into the maxillary or ethmoid sinuses respectively (**Fig. 2-64**).

Blowout fractures can be complicated by herniation of the orbital fat and/or the extraocular muscles into the adjacent cavities. Orbital emphysema may be noted with medial wall fractures secondary to disruption of the ethmoid air cells. The extraocular muscles may have limited range of motion due to their new position against the intact or ragged edge of the wall resulting in entrapment, contusion, and/or laceration. Entrapment is likely to occur with smaller fractures, whereas enophthalmos may occur if the fractures are larger.[124,125] An air-filled space does not bind the lateral wall of the orbit, and therefore entrapment is less likely to occur laterally than medially or inferiorly. To test for muscle entrapment, forced ductions of the extraocular muscles may be performed to check for resistance to passive movement in any direction. If entrapment is suspected, surgery must be performed to relieve the impingement prior to muscle atrophy or necrosis or permanent nerve damage.

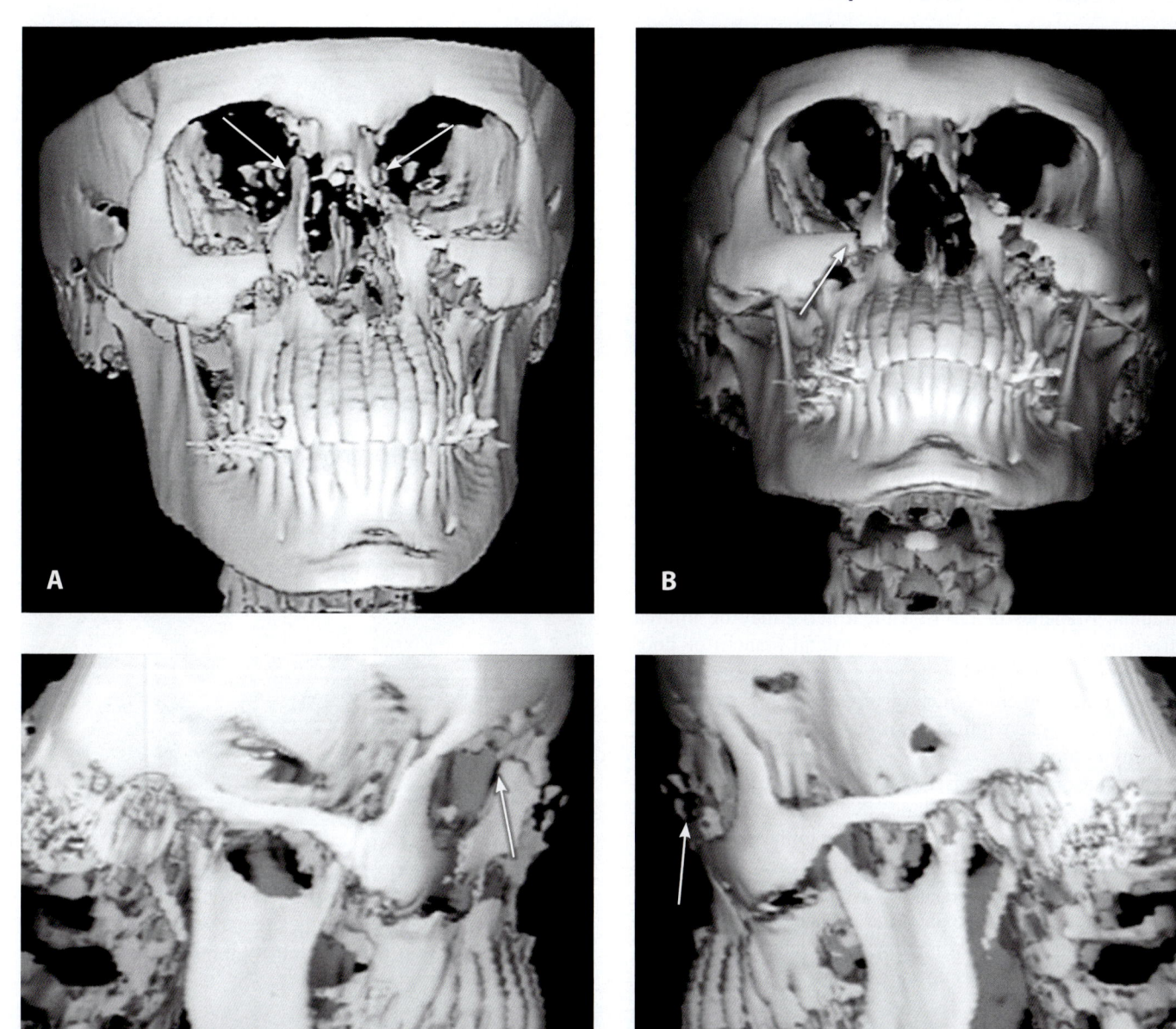

Figure 2-64 Naso-orbital-ethmoidal Fracture
3D reconstructions of axial CT scans (**A**–**D**). In **A** the right lacrimal bone (left *arrow*) and left lamina fractures (right *arrow*, **A**) are visible. In **B** there is a comminuted fracture of the left orbital rim and the left maxilla (*arrow*, **B**). Right lateral view (**C**) shows the fracture of the nasal bones and the right lacrimal bone (*arrow*, **C**). In **D** the left lateral view the naso-orbital-ethmoidal fracture is visible (*arrow*, **D**).

Neurovascular Injuries

A fracture of the superior orbital fissure or optic canal may cause injury to the optic nerve. Injury may result from direct penetration or laceration by bony fragments, mechanical tearing, stretching, avulsion, contusion, compression, and ischemia. Ischemia may result from hemorrhage within the optic nerve sheath, thrombosis, or compression of the arterial blood supply. Compression of the arterial supply can be either intrinsic or extrinsic to the optic nerve. Another process such as retrobulbar hemorrhage may compress the blood supply, or injury to the optic nerve itself may cause swelling and inhibition of local blood flow.

Injury to the optic nerve is typically intracanalicular, because here the nerve is immobile, unable to stretch or swell, and likely to be near bony fragments. Blindness following optic nerve injury is referred to as traumatic optic neuropathy (TON). It typically results from head trauma without direct effects on the globe or retina. Optimal treatment of this condition is highly controversial with steroids and surgical decompression having unconvincing results when compared with watchful waiting. Hemorrhage within the optic nerve sheath is identified as an asymmetry between the sizes of optic nerves on CT scan. Optic nerve avulsion is unlikely to be seen on CT but may be demonstrated by MR imaging as loss of the continuity of the nerve. Oblique sagittal MR sequences are most useful for the evaluation of optic nerve trauma.[124–126]

Nerve injuries involving cranial nerves other than the optic nerve may also be seen. Typical symptoms of CN III, IV, or VI damage include diplopia in primary gaze or with eye movement, and/or decreased eye movement, along with other findings consistent with the given nerve's functions. Isolated oculomotor nerve palsies due to injury are uncommon, whereas palsies of the trochlear nerve are common secondary to trauma. Branches of the trigeminal nerve may be injured in fractures of the orbital roof (supraorbital branch) or floor (infraorbital branch). Abducens nerve palsy is the most common post-traumatic cranial neuropathy. Because the abducens nerve has an extensive intracranial course, it has increased susceptibility to trauma.

The acute or delayed onset of diplopia may be caused by not only neuromuscular injury, but also by a direct carotid cavernous fistula. The fistula results from a tear in the carotid artery wall within the cavernous sinus. Diplopia may result from compression of the cranial nerves in the cavernous sinus by vascular engorgement, or from hypoxia of the extraocular muscles. The patients may also present with proptosis and chemosis from the resultant reversal of venous flow.[124]

Subperiosteal Hematoma, Hematic Cyst, and Cholesterol Granuloma

Extraocular orbital hemorrhage is most commonly the result of trauma or other hemorrhagic systemic illnesses (leukemia, thrombocytopenia, blood dyscrasia, and hemophilia). Such hemorrhage is given many different names depending upon the location and age of the blood collection. After trauma there is a tendency for blood to collect in the subperiosteal space superiorly and this is referred to as a subperiosteal hematoma. A hematic cyst is a collection of old blood products in the orbit, but not necessarily in the subperiosteal space or adjacent bone. Hemorrhage into a bony space within the walls of the orbit typically will give rise to a cholesterol granuloma, which likely results from a prior distant trauma. It is possible to differentiate these lesions from other masses based on their lack of enhancement post contrast administration on both CT and MR images.

An acute subperiosteal hematoma may present with painful unilateral proptosis. A chronic subperiosteal hematoma may have variable clinical presentations. This lesion is best appreciated on coronal CT scans and appears as a fusiform or biconvex nonenhancing mass against the bony orbit (**Fig. 2-65**). In the acute stage, it may appear hyperdense on CT, but in the chronic stage it will eventually appear heterogeneous and hypodense. Over time, there may be progressive expansion and erosion of the adjacent bone. Coronal MR scans are more useful in the chronic stage of a subperiosteal hematoma. These images reveal a similarly shaped lesion with variable signal intensity depending upon the age of the contained blood products.

Chronic hematic cysts result when a previous hemorrhage fails to resorb. They may present with painless proptosis and/or diplopia. The imaging appearance of this lesion may mimic a solid tumor on CT scans sometimes appearing isodense with muscle. Bone involvement will show well-defined defects without sclerosis as this lesion slowly erodes and expands the bony walls. The MR appearance will vary depending upon the age of the blood degradation products, but due to the chronic nature of the lesion is often reported as having an increased signal on both

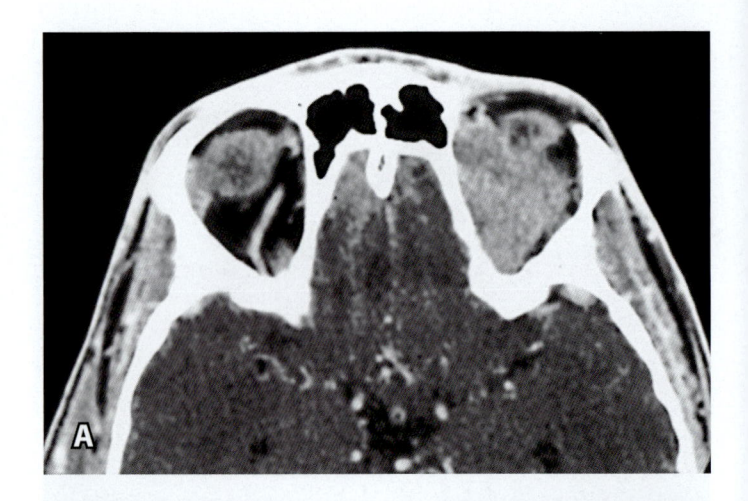

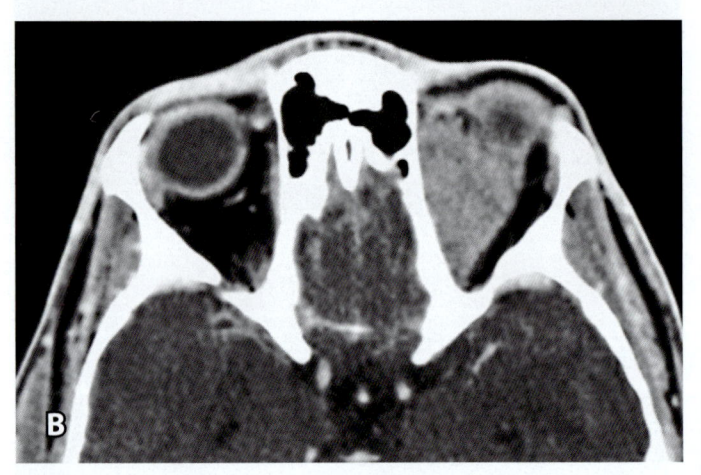

Figure 2-65 Subperiosteal Hematoma: Acute
Subperiosteal hematoma in the left orbit. This patient had a history of acute trauma. Axial CT scans with contrast (**A** and **B**) show a collection of high-density material above the left globe.

etration and/or rupture. With the extrusion of vitreous from the eye, there will be a resultant loss of internal volume. This is first evident by a flattening of the posterior wall of the globe known as the "flat tire" sign (**Fig. 2-68**). In addition, there may be deepening of the anterior chamber. This is best evaluated by comparison between the globes in which there is typically no greater than a 2 mm difference in the depth of the anterior chamber.[130] A penetration of the eye anteriorly may instead cause a decompression of both the anterior and posterior chambers and again is best evaluated by comparison between the globes.[124,125] In addition, there may be air or blood in any of the spaces of the eye. Over time, extensive ocular insult may lead to a shrunken, calcified, "end stage" eye referred to as phthisis bulbi (**Fig. 2-69**).

Intraocular air or hemorrhage may occur as a result of trauma. Hemorrhage into the various spaces or potential spaces of the eye may also cause detachment of the layers. Anterior chamber hemorrhage or hyphema is the most common ocular injury in children and is readily identified clinically. There may be hemorrhage into the vitreous secondary to trauma, surgery or arterial hypertension. On ultrasound, there is increased echogenecity of the vitreous if the hemorrhage is mild, and if severe there may be numerous, irregular, poorly defined, mobile, low-intensity echoes in the vitreous. With time, vitreous membranes may develop and their lack of attachment to the area of the optic nerve differentiate them from retinal detachments.

Retinal detachment can occur due to trauma, hemorrhage, exudative or inflammatory processes, or a scar. It results from the separation of the neurosensory retina from the retinal pigment epithelium. There are associated fluid collections in the newly formed space and their imaging appearance depends upon the content and composition of the fluid. The points of attachment left between the two layers of the retina allow for differentiation of a retinal detachment from a choroidal detachment or vitreous membranes. In a retinal detachment, the retina will remain attached to the optic nerve head due to the continuation of the neurosensory retina with the rest of the central nervous system. From the point of attachment at the optic cup, there may be detachment of the retinal layers in all directions, which will appear as a "V" or "gull wing" pattern on axial views (**Fig. 2-2**).

Choroidal detachment may be caused by trauma, surgery, or may be spontaneous. Similar to retinal detachments, these detachments result in or from the accumulation of fluid in the suprachoroidal space between the choroid and sclera. The imaging appearances of that fluid will depend upon the contents of the fluid. There are two types of choroidal detachments: hemorrhagic and serous (or choroidal effusion). Hemorrhagic choroidal detachments are caused by the rupture of choroidal vessels that lead to the accumulation of blood in the suprachoroidal space or within the choroid. They classically occur acutely during or up to one week after ocular surgery, but can also occur after trauma and rarely spontaneously. Patients typically experience pain, decreased vision, red eye, intraocular inflammation, and increased intraocular pressure. Serous choroidal detachments are caused by the transudation

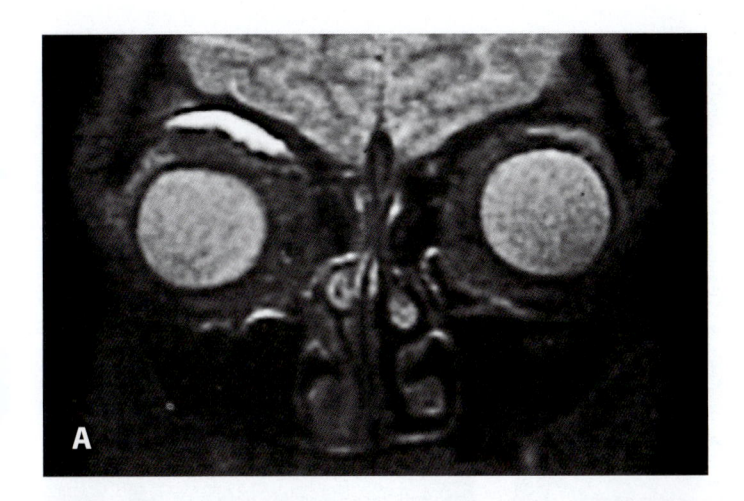

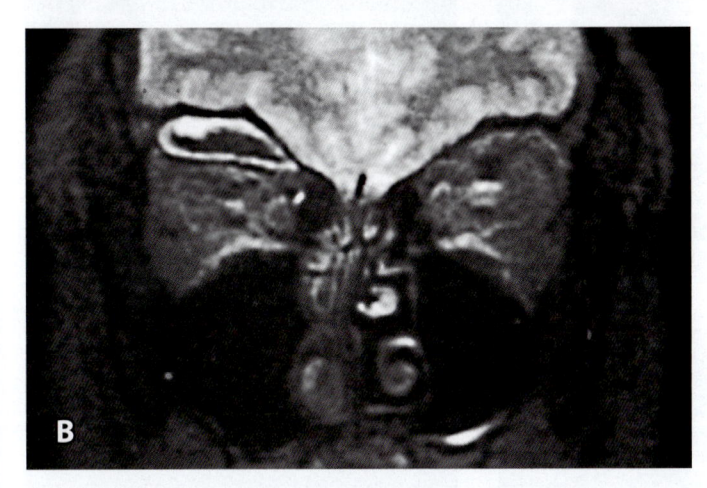

Figure 2-66 Subperiosteal Hematoma: Subacute
Subacute subperiosteal hematoma in the right orbit. Coronal T2-W MR scans (**A** and **B**) demonstrate a collection superior to the right globe. The collection is hypointense surrounded by an area of hyperintensity. This is consistent with a subacute acute bleed and there are no fractures.

T1W and T2W images (**Figs. 2-66** and **2-67**). A fluid–fluid level may also be observed.

Cholesterol granulomas first involve hemorrhage into the orbital walls and then may extend into the extraconal space and/or into the cranial fossa as an associated soft tissue mass. Extension into the extraconal space may cause proptosis and inferior displacement of the globe due to their common location near the lacrimal fossa. CT scans show the expansile bony lesions as lytic with irregular margins. The soft tissue component will appear homogeneous and isodense to brain. These lesions with blood products may appear hypointense to hyperintense on T1W and T2W images depending on the age of the hemorrhage.[17,22,33,128,129]

Ocular Injuries

Ocular injuries include rupture, perforation, and laceration. Several imaging findings have been associated with ocular pen-

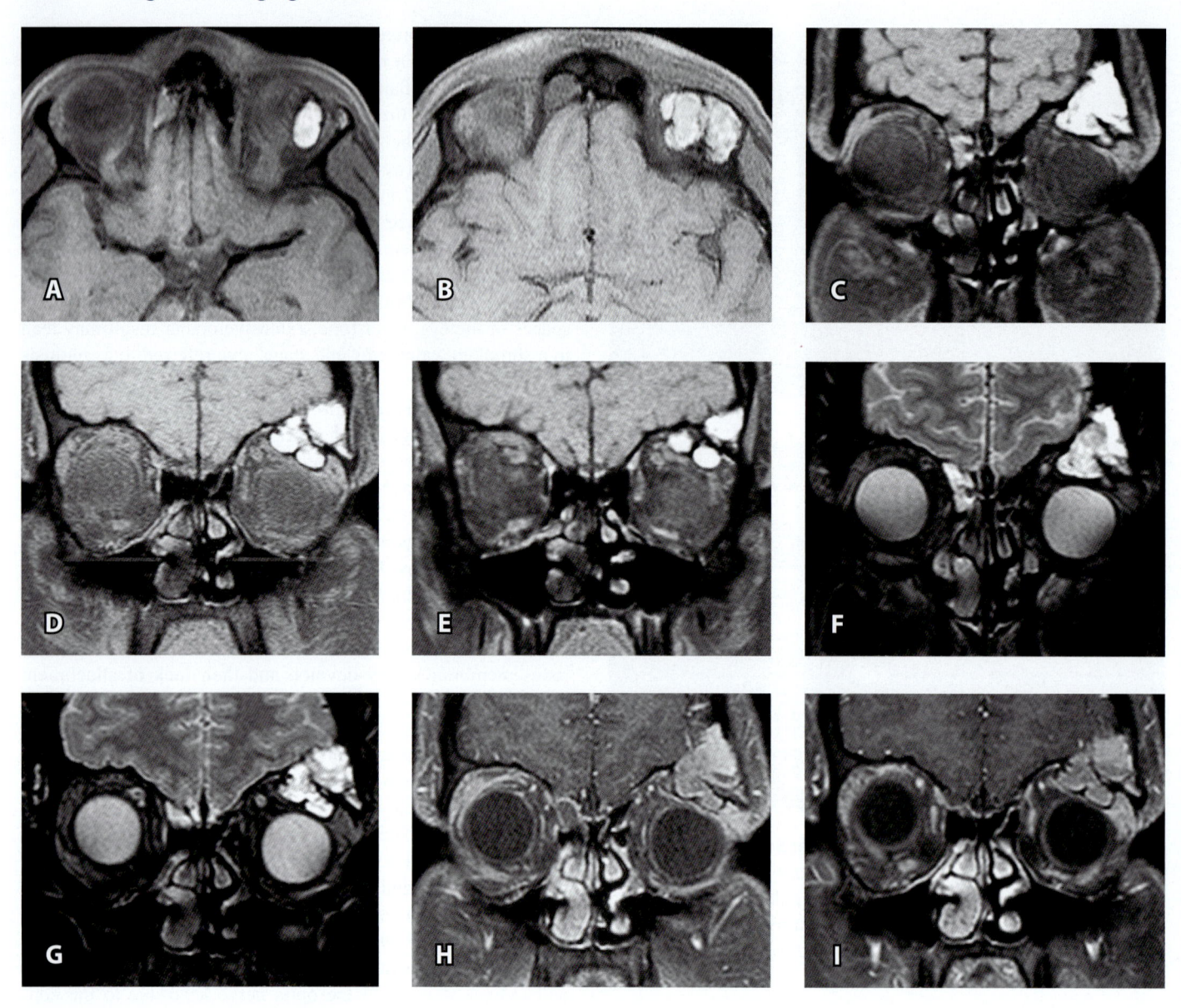

Figure 2-67 Chronic Hematic Cyst

Chronic hematic cyst due to remote orbital trauma, now presenting with increasing proptosis. Axial T1W (**A–B**) show a lobulated mass in the superior lateral portion of the orbit which contains bright blood products. Coronal T1W MR images (**C–E**) show similar findings expanding from the subperiosteal space of the orbit into the frontal bone. Note the downward displacement of the orbit. Coronal T2W MR images (**F–G**) show that the signal intensity of the lesion remains bright, consistent with old blood products. Coronal T1W enhanced images (**H–I**) show no enhancement with persistence of the high signal intensity, also consistent with blood products.

of serous fluid into the suprachoroidal space. This transudation may be secondary to acute ocular hypotony (which causes increased transmural pressure), trauma (open globe), ocular surgery, serum exudation (most frequently caused by posterior scleritis), Vogt-Koyanagi-Harada syndrome, intraocular tumors, or uveal effusion syndrome. Patients are often asymptomatic with decreased intraocular pressure and a shallow anterior chamber.

Choroidal detachment can be differentiated from retinal detachment by location. The choroidal detachment will not extend to the optic nerve, but will instead involve the area between the ciliary body to the macula and will have preserved attachments in the areas of penetration of the vortex veins (**Fig. 2-2**). The appearance of two biconvex fluid collections in the suprachoroidal space not involving the optic nerve is referred to as "kissing choroids." Fluid collections that are position-dependent on imaging studies are likely inflammatory, and those that aren't are more likely to be hemorrhagic. Ocular hypotony is a potential cause of choroidal detachment, but it can also mimic the appearance of a detachment without a true detachment.[131,132]

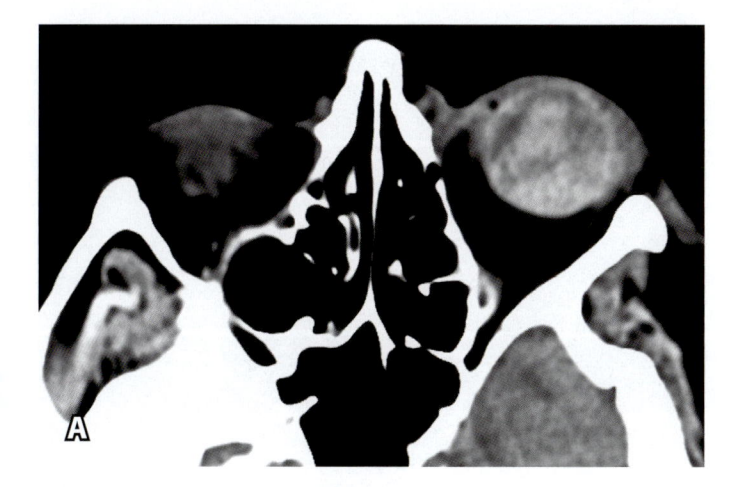

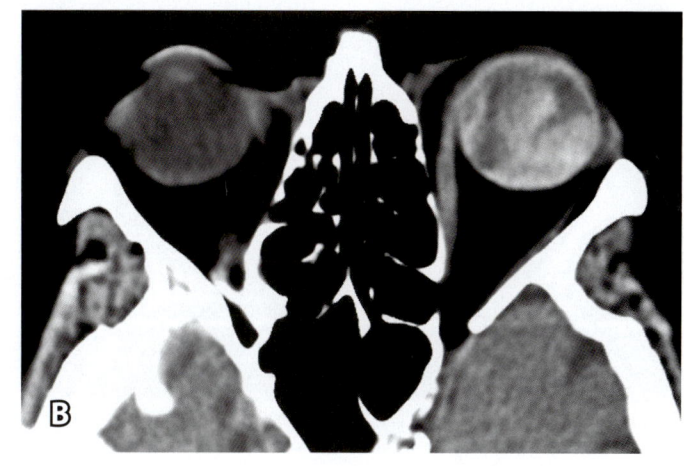

Figure 2-68 Ruptured Globe
Acute bulbar hemorrhages in an adult patient with a history of recent trauma. Axial unenhanced CT scans without contrast (**A–B**) show intravitreal hemorrhages, as well as subchoroidal and subhyaloid hemorrhages. The ocular lens is not visualized and is likely dislocated.

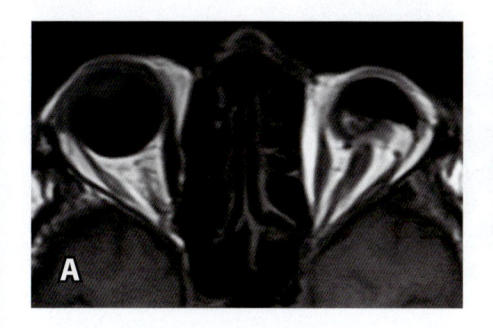

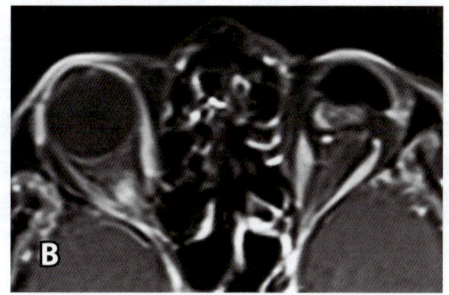

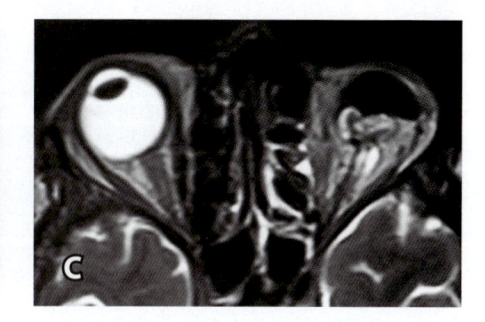

Figure 2-69 Phthisis Bulbi
Phthisis bulbi (shrunken globe) in an adult male with previous trauma and an ocular glass prosthesis. Axial T1W (**A**), FS (**B**) and T2W (**C**) MR images show shrunken and deformed posterior orbital contents due to associated granulation tissue. Note that the anterior glass portion of the eye is identical on all three sequences.

Lens injury can result in dislocation or subluxation of the lens, or traumatic cataract. The zonular fibers or suspensory apparatus of the lens hold the lens in place and transmit movements of the ciliary body to the lens to allow for accommodation. They are minute structures not visible with current imaging techniques. Subluxation results from partial tear of the zonular fibers. Dislocation results from complete tear of these fibers. With complete tear, the lens may sink through the vitreous to lie on the retina (**Fig. 2-70**). Traumatic cataract results from influx of fluid into the lens. This is observed as a lowering of the CT density from the usual hyperdense appearance.[6,124,125]

Foreign Body

Orbital foreign body evaluation is best performed with CT scan. Although ultrasound can detect 95% of foreign bodies in the globe, it can detect only 50% of those present in the orbit outside the globe. In addition, foreign bodies appear similar no matter their composition, hyperechoic with acoustic shadowing. MR

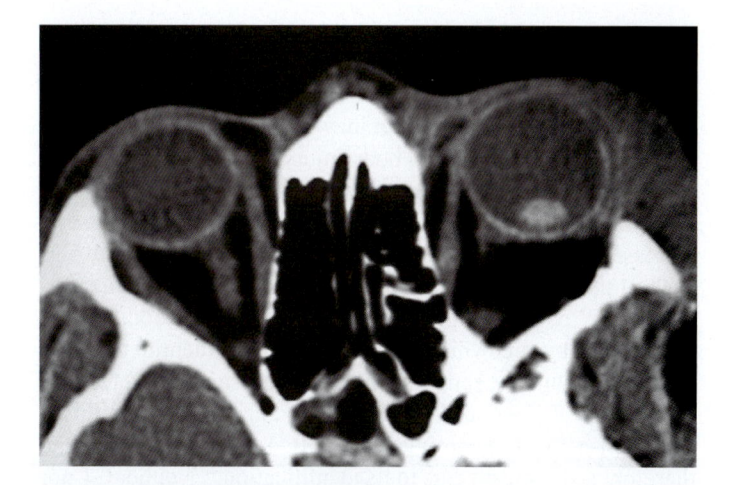

Figure 2-70 Lens Dislocation
Total lens dislocation in a male patient with a history of head trauma. Axial CT scan shows soft tissue swelling over the left eye. The lens has been dislocated and now rests on the retina in a dependent position in this supine study.

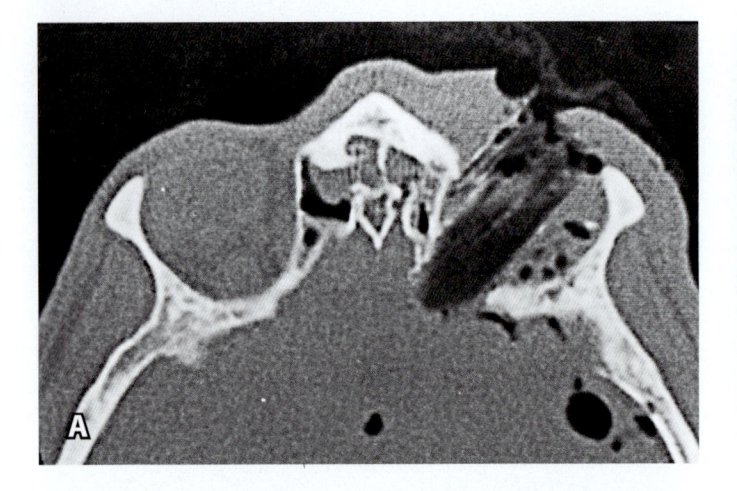

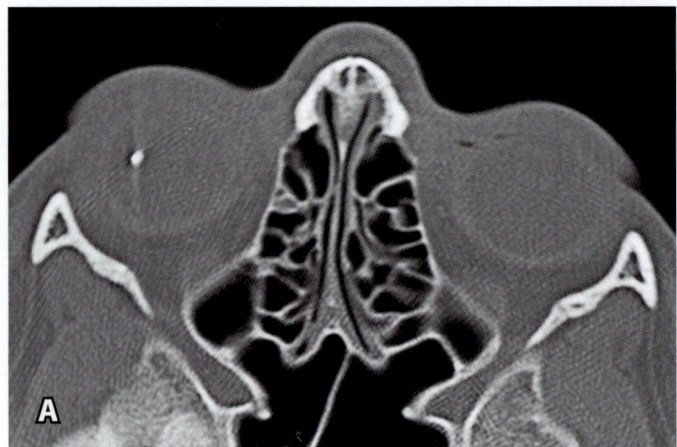

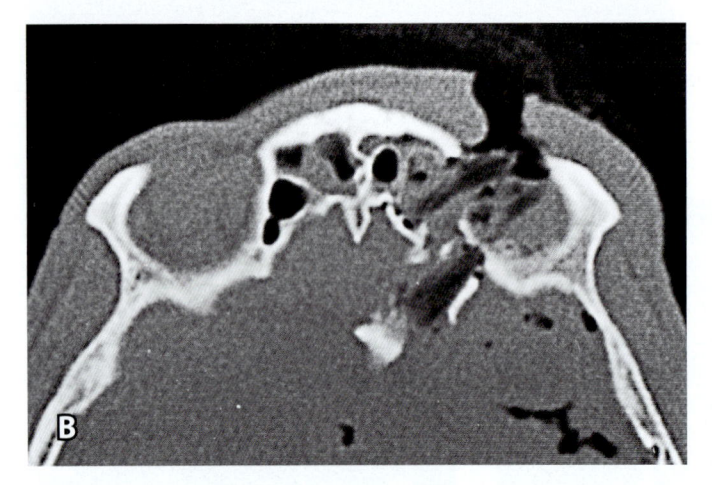

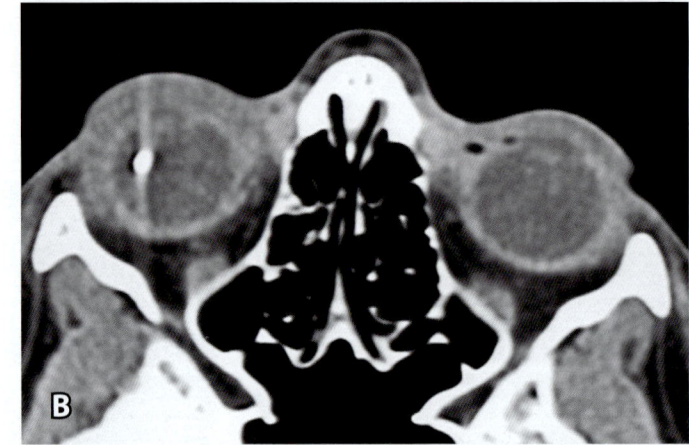

Figure 2-71 Wooden Foreign Body
Axial CT scans with wide window settings (**A** and **B**) show a large area of hypodense material with a fibrous appearance and multiple fractures of the left orbit. The fibrous or wood grain appearance is helpful to distinguish this as a wooden foreign body. Note the presence of pneumocephalus.

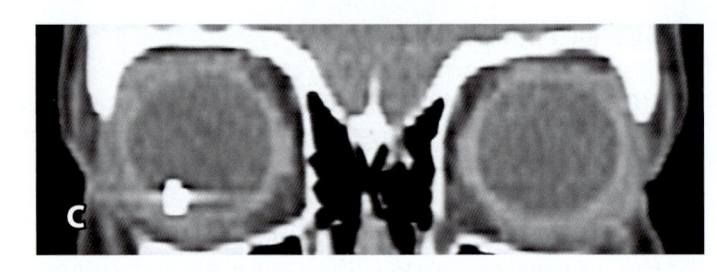

Figure 2-72 Intraocular Metallic Foreign Body
Axial CT bone window (**A**) shows a hyperdense, rounded structure located centrally in the right globe. Axial CT scan soft tissue window (**B**) shows the same hyperdense object with streak artifacts consistent with a metallic structure. Coronal reformatted CT (**C**) shows the metallic structure sitting in the inferior of the right globe in a dependent position consistent with a loose intraocular foreign body.

imaging is contraindicated until the presence of a ferromagnetic substance is ruled out, but may be helpful to determine the course and extent of foreign body injury.

If the foreign object is dry wood, it may appear isodense with air or fat on CT scans. The use of wide window CT and its increased soft tissue contrast may show an attenuation difference in the wood or the grain of the wood due to the alternating density pattern (**Fig. 2-71**). In addition, the wood may be surrounded by air, which may allow for its identification on wide bone window settings. MR imaging can also detect the presence of dry wood. Dry wood will appear as a low intensity, well-defined lesion with typically a geometric shape and therefore a significant clue to its identification.[22] Neither CT nor MR imaging can reliably detect the presence of wet or green wood.[126,127,133,134]

Bone window settings should be used to detect the presence of dense objects, e.g., metal and glass on CT scans, whereas plastic is best visualized on soft tissue windows. Metallic objects may cause beam-hardening streak artifacts, which can distort both the size and location of the foreign body (**Fig. 2-72**). This may be overcome by using spiral CT instead of conventional CT scanning. Glass particles appear hyperdense on CT scans and must be at least 1.88 mm in size to be detectable by CT scanning. Although some objects may be left in the eye without significant sequelae, copper and organic materials will usually cause a significant foreign body reaction and/or infection. Particles of copper must be at least 0.7 mm in size in order to be detected by CT scans.[124,125]

SURGICAL PROCEDURES AND IMAGING APPEARANCE OF SURGICAL MATERIALS

Procedures

Knowledge of the correct terminology to describe some of the basic surgical procedures that may be encountered on imaging studies is helpful when consulting with the ophthalmologist. Evisceration refers to the removal of the intraocular contents leaving the sclera intact. This procedure may be used to treat endophthalmitis. For a blind painful eye, malignancy, trauma or cosmesis the entire eyeball and anterior portion of the optic nerve may be removed. This is referred to as enucleation. When removal of the entire contents of the orbit is necessary, for example in cases of malignancy, exenteration is performed.

To access lesions that lie around the globe in the anterior of the orbit, various skin incisions may be performed leaving little residual radiographic findings due to the lack of disruption of the intraorbital structures. In order to access retrobulbar space lesions, a lateral orbitotomy with bone removal may need to be performed. This procedure consists of removal of a piece of bone by making two cuts: 1) the superior edge is 5 mm above the frontozygomatic suture, and 2) the inferior edge is at the level of the zygomatic arch. The transfrontal surgical approach is necessary for lesions of the orbital apex, optic canal, and adjacent cranial cavity. In this procedure the frontotemporal bone and the supraorbital rim may be removed. In cases of Grave's disease or other diseases requiring orbital decompression, the orbital walls (medial wall, ethmoid sinus, orbital floor, maxillary sinus, lateral wall, and/or temporalis fossa) and/or orbital fat may be surgically removed.[135]

Surgical Materials

A variety of materials and devices are used in surgical procedures of the eye. Being familiar with their imaging appearance is helpful in the evaluation of postoperative imaging studies. Lens implants are not consistently visualized on imaging studies. Several materials are used in scleral implants including silicone rubber, silicone sponge, and hydrogel. Silicone rubber is typically used for "banding" retinal detachments and is seen as areas of high attenuation on the outside edge of the globe on CT scans (Fig. 2-73). These silicone bands are not well visualized on MR studies. Silicone sponges will appear as air densities on CT scans. Hydrogel, although poorly visualized on CT scans, appears as an area of increased signal on both T1W and T2W MR scans.

Silicone oil may be injected into the vitreous space in the treatment of retinal detachment and proliferative vitreoretinopathy. On ultrasound, the oil produces significant artifact, but on MR it appears hyperintense. The tissue of a detachment would show an abrupt edge against an area of hyperintensity as the oil abuts the detached tissue.

When gases are injected into the vitreous space, their imaging appearance is similar to air. Sodium hyaluronate is used in cataract surgery and appears as an area of high attenuation on

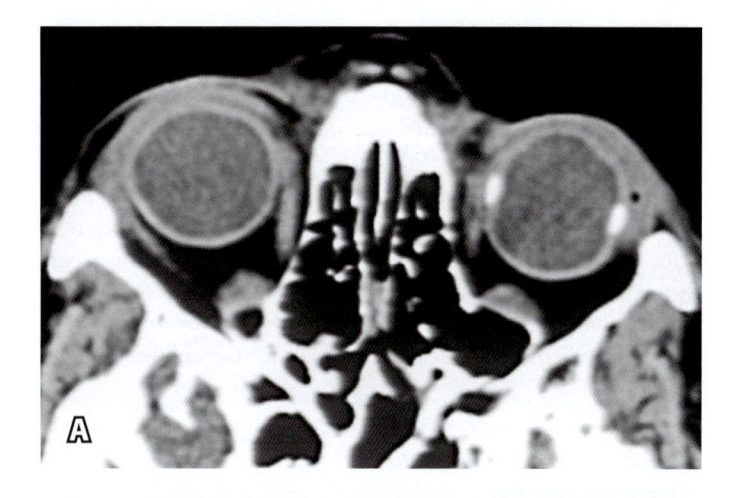

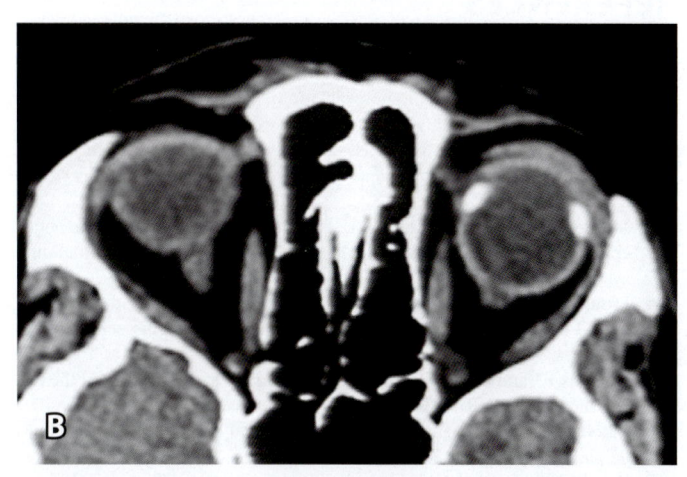

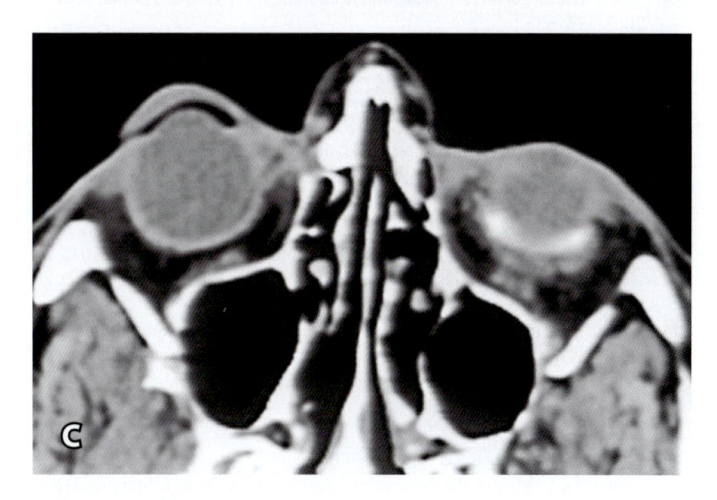

Figure 2-73 Surgical Banding
Surgical banding procedure using silicone to constrict ocular hypotony. Axial CT scans (**A–C**) show hyperintense material surrounding the left globe in a "tire" configuration.

CT scans and has an appearance similar to that of water on MR studies. Porus hydroxyapatite used in orbital reconstruction may appear as an irregular shaped calcified extraconal mass on CT scans. One may need to differentiate this material from similar appearing lesions such as a calcified subperiosteal hematoma, fibrous dysplasia, or bone tumor. The vascular ingrowth of an implant containing hydroxyapatite may need to be assessed prior to integration of an ocular prosthesis. This is best performed with contrast enhanced MR imaging. The amount of enhancement within the implant has been shown to be a reliable indicator of fibrovascular ingrowth for the ophthalmologic surgeon.[136-138]

REFERENCES

1. Weber AL, Romo LV, and Sabates NR: Pseudotumor of the orbit: clinical, pathologic, and radiologic evaluation. Radiol Clin North Am 1999; 37(1):151.
2. Wilhelm KE, Hofer U, Textor H, et al.: Dacryoliths: nonsurgical fluoroscopically guided treatment during dacryocystoplasty. Radiology 1999; 212:365.
3. Jansen AG, Mansour K, Krabbe GJ, et al.: Dacryocystoplasty: treatment of epiphora by means of balloon dilation of the obstructed nasolacrimal duct system. Radiology 1994;193:453.
4. Froula PD, Bartley GB, Garrity JA, et al.: The differential diagnosis of orbital calcification as detected on computed tomographic scans. Mayo Clin Proc 1993;68:256.
5. Bilaniuk LT and Farber M: Imaging of developmental anomalies of the eye and the orbit. AJNR 1992;13:793.
6. Jakobiec FA: Ocular anatomy, embryology, and teratology. 1st ed. Philadelphia, PA: Harper & Row; 1982:12–96.
7. Som PM and Curtin HD: Head and neck imaging. 4th ed. St. Louis: Mosby, 2003;533–535.
8. Newton TH, Hasso AN, and Dillon WP: Computed tomography of the head and neck. 1st ed. New York: Raven Press; 1988:8.1–9.64.
9. Braffman BH, Naidich TP, and Chaneles M: Imaging anatomy of the normal orbit. Semin Ultrasound CT MRI 1997;18(6):403.
10. Kaissar G, Kim JH, Bravo S, et al.: Histologic basis for increased extraocular muscle enhancement in gadolinium-enhanced MR imaging. Radiology 1991;179:541.
11. Amano Y, Amano M, and Kumazaki T: Normal contrast enhancement of extraocular muscles: fat-suppressed MR findings. AJNR 1997;18:161.
12. Hopper KD, Sherman JL, Boal DK, and Eggli KD: CT and MR imaging of the pediatric orbit. Radiographics 1992;12:485.
13. Levine RS, Powers T, Rosenberg HK, et al.: The cryptophthalmos syndrome. AJR 1984;143:375.
14. Smith M and Castillo M: Imaging and differential diagnosis of the large eye. Radiographics 1994;14:721.
15. Murphy BL and Griffin JF: Optic nerve coloboma (morning glory syndrome): CT findings. Radiology 1994;191:59.
16. Lanzieri CF: MRI of the optic nerves and visual pathways. Imaging Decis 1994; May/June:21.
17. Kaufman LM, Villablanca JP, and Mafee MF: Diagnostic imaging of cystic lesions in the child's orbit. Radiol Clin North Am 1998;36:1149.
18. El-Gharbawy FI: CT distinguishes Norrie's disease from retinoblastoma. Radiol Today 1989;September:23.
19. Taveras JM: Neuroradiology. 3rd ed. Baltimore, MD: Williams & Wilkins; 1996:165–166.
20. Dietrich RB, Glidden DE, Roth GM, et al.: The proteus syndrome: CNS manifestations. AJNR 1998;19:987.
21. Sanchez R, Weber AL, Alexander A, Swerdick S, and Vici G: Paraorbital lesions. Eur J Radiol 1996;22:53.
22. De Potter P, Shields JA, and Shields CL: MRI of the eye and orbit. 1st ed. Philadelphia, PA: J.B. Lippincott Company; 1995:45;55–61;93–97;131–132;145–146;160–161;213–214;283–284.
23. Bilaniuk LT and Rapoport RJ: Magnetic resonance imaging of the orbit. Top Magn Reson Imaging 1994;6(3):167.
24. Dalley RW: Fibrous histiocytoma and fibrous tissue tumors of the orbit. Radiol Clin North Am 1999;37:185.
25. Shrier DA, Wang AR, Patel U, et al.: Benign fibrous histiocytoma of the nasal cavity in a newborn: MR and CT findings. AJNR 1998;19: 1166.
26. Wenig BM, Mafee MF, and Ghosh L: Fibro-osseous, osseous, and cartilaginous lesions of the orbit and paraorbital region: correlative clinicopathologic and radiographic features, including the diagnostic role of CT and MR imaging. Radiol Clin North Am 1998;36:1241.
27. Peyster RG, Shapiro MD, and Haik BG: Orbital metastasis: role of magnetic resonance imaging and computed tomography. Radiol Clin North Am 1987;25:647.
28. Weber AL, Jakobiec FA, and Sabates NR: Pseudotumor of the orbit. Neuroimaging Clin North Am 1996;6:73.
29. Courcoutsakis NA, Langford CA, Sneller MC, et al.: Orbital involvement in Wegener granulomatosis: MR findings in 12 patients. JCAT 1997; 21(3):452.
30. Hershey BL and Roth TC: Orbital infections. Semin Ultrasound CT MRI 1997;18(6):448.
31. Osguthorpe JD and Hochman M: Inflammatory sinus diseases affecting the orbit. Otolaryngol Clin North Am 1993;26(4):657.
32. Tarazi AE and Shikani AH: Irreversible unilateral visual loss due to acute sinusitis. Arch Otolaryngol Head Neck Surg 1991;117:1400.
33. Eustis HS, Mafee MF, Walton C, et al.: MR Imaging and CT of orbital infections and complications in acute rhinosinusitis. Radiol Clin North Am 1998;36:1165.
34. Harris GJ: Subperiosteal abscess of the orbit: computed tomography and the clinical course. Ophthal Plast Reconstr Surg 1996;12(1):1.
35. Harril WC, Stewart MG, Lee AG, et al.: Chronic rhinocerebral mucormycosis. Laryngoscope 996;106:1292.
36. Eskey CJ, Whitman GJ, and Chew FS: Invasive aspergillosis of the orbit. AJR 1996;167:1588.
37. Mauriello Jr. JA, Yepez N, Mostafavi II R, et al.: Invasive rhino-orbital aspergillosis with precipitous visual loss. Can J Ophthalmol 1995;30:124.
38. Sperryn CW and Corr PD: CT evaluation of orbital hydatid disease: a review of 10 cases. Clin Radiol 1994;49:703.
39. Caparros-Lefebvre D, Pruvo JP, Remy M, Wallaert B, and Petit H: Neuroradiologic aspects of chester-erdheim disease. AJNR 1995;16:735.
40. Martinez R: Erdheim-Chester disease: MR of intraaxial and extraaxial brain stem lesions. AJNR 1995;16:1787.
41. Hidayat AA, Mafee MF, Laver NV, et al.: Langerhans' cell histiocytosis and Juvenile xanthogranuloma of the orbit: clinicopathologic, CT, and MR imaging features. Radiol Clin North Am 1998;36:1229.
42. Meyer JS, Harty MP, Mahboubi S, et al.: Langerhans cell histiocytosis: presentation and evolution of radiologic findings with clinical correlation. Radiographics 1995;15:1135.
43. Kim E, Choi J, Kim T, et al.: Huge Langerhans cell histiocytosis granuloma of choroid plexus in a child with Hand-Schuller-Christian disease. J Neurosurg 1995;83:1080.
44. Chaques VJ, Lam S, Tessler HH, and Mafee MF: Computed tomography and magnetic resonance imaging in the diagnosis of posterior scleritis. Ann Ophthalmol 1993;25:89.
45. Asao C, Korogi Y, Hotta A, et al.: Orbital pseudotumors: value of short inversion time inversion-recovery MR imaging. Radiology 1997; 202:55.
46. Cytryn AS, Putterman AM, Schneck GL, Beckman E, and Valvassori GE: Predictability of magnetic resonance imaging in differentiation of orbital lymphoma from orbital inflammatory syndrome. Ophthal Plast Reconstr Surg 1997;13(2):129.
47. Mombaerts I, Goldschmeding R, Schlingmann RO, et al.: What is orbital pseudotumor? Surv Ophthalmol 1996;41:66.
48. Valvassori GE, Sabnis SS, Mafee RF, et al.: Imaging of orbital lymphoproliferative disorders. Radiol Clin North Am 1999;37:135.
49. Gufler H, Laubenberger J, Gerling J, et al.: MRI of lymphomas of the orbits and the paranasal sinuses. JCAT 1997;21:887.
50. Weber AL, Jakobiec FA, and Sabates NR: Lymphoproliferative disease of the orbit. Neuroimaging Clin North Am 1996;6:93.
51. Smirniotopoulos JG and Chiechi MV: Teratomas, dermoids, and epidermoids of the head and neck. Radiographics 1995;15:1437.

52. Bilaniuk LT: Orbital vascular lesions. Radiol Clin North Am 1999;37:169.
53. Berrocal T, de Orbe A, Prieto C, et al.: US and color doppler imaging of ocular and orbital disease in the pediatric age group. Radiographics 1996;16:251.
54. Jansen BPW, Pillay M, de Bruin HG, et al.: 99mTc-SPECT in the diagnosis of skull base metastasis. Neurology 1997;48:1326.
55. Kim JW, Goldberg RA, and Shorr N: The inferomedial orbital strut: an anatomic and radiographic study. Ophthal Plast Reconstr Surg 2002;18:355.
56. Cruz AA and Leme VR: Orbital decompression: a comparison between trans-fornix/transcaruncular inferomedial and coronal inferomedial plus lateral approaches. Ophthal Plast Reconstr Surg 2003;19:440.
57. Weber AL, Dallow RL, and Sabates NR: Graves' disease of the orbit. Neuroimaging Clin North Am 1996;6:61.
58. Ohnishi T, Noguchi S, Murakami N, et al.: Levator palpebrae superioris muscle: MR evaluation of enlargement as a cause of upper eyelid retraction in graves disease. Radiology 1993;188:115.
59. Kendler DL, Lippa J, and Rootman J: The initial clinical characteristics of Graves' orbitopathy vary with age and sex. Arch Ophthalmol 1993;111:197.
60. Birchall D, Goodall KL, Noble JL, et al.: Graves ophthalmopathy: intracranial fat prolapse on CT images as an indicator of optic nerve compression. Radiology 1996;200:123.
61. Chang T, Huang K, Hsiao Y, et al.: Relationships of orbital computed tomographic findings and activity scores to the prognosis of corticosteroid therapy in patients with Graves' ophthalmopathy. Acta Ophthalmol Scand 1997;75:301.
62. Ohnishi T, Noguchi S, Murakami N, et al.: Extraocular muscles in Graves ophthalmopathy: usefulness of T2 relaxation time measurements. Radiology 1994;190:857.
63. Utech CI, Khatibnia U, Winter PF, et al.: MR T2 relaxation time for the assessment of retrobulbar inflammation in Graves' ophthalmopathy. Thyroid 1995;5:185.
64. Mafee MF, Pai E, and Philip B: Rhabdomyosarcoma of the orbit. Radiol Clin North Am 1998;36:1215.
65. Kodsi SR, Shetlar DJ, Campbell RJ, et al.: A review of 340 orbital tumors in children during a 60-year period. Am J Ophthalmol 1664;117:177.
66. Aletich V, Misra M, Shownkeen H, et al.: Evaluation and endovascular treatment of juxtaorbital vascular anomalies. Radiol Clin North Am 1999;37:123.
67. Barkovich AJ, Fram EK, and Norman D: Septo-optic dysplasia: MR imaging. Radiology 1989;171:189.
68. Gibby WA, Cohen MS, Goldberg HI, and Sergott RC: Pseudotumor cerebri: CT findings and correlation with vision loss. AJR 1993;160:143.
69. Jinkins JR, Athale S, Xiong L, Yuh WTC, Rothman MI, and Nguyen PT: MR of optic papilla protrusion in patients with high intracranial pressure. AJNR 1996;17:665.
70. O'Reilly GV, Hammerschlag SB, Bergland RM, et al.: Pseudotumor cerebri: computed tomography of resolving papilledema. JCAT 1983;7:364.
71. Kurz-Levin M and Landau K: A comparison of imaging techniques for diagnosing drusen of the optic nerve head. Arch Ophthalmol 1999;117:1045.
72. McNicholas MMJ, Power WJ, and Griffin JF: Sonography in optic disk drusen: imaging findings and role in diagnosis when fundoscopic findings are normal. AJR 1994;162:161.
73. Jackson A, Sheppard S, Laitt RD, et al.: Optic neuritis: MR imaging with combined fat- and water-supression techniques. Radiology 1998;206:57.
74. Kapoor R, Miller DH, Jones SJ, et al.: Effects of intravenous methylprednisolone on outcome in MRI-based prognostic subgroups in acute optic neuritis. Neurology 1998;50:230.
75. Sklar EML, Schatz NJ, Glaser JS, Post MJD, and Hove MT: MR of vasculitis-induced optic neuropathy. AJNR 1996;17:121.
76. Optic Neuritis Study Group: The 5-year risk of MS after optic neuritis: experience of the optic neuritis treatment trial. Neurology 1997;49:1404.
77. Brusaferri F and Candelise L: Steroids for multiple sclerosis and optic neuritis: a meta-analysis of randomized controlled clinical trials. J Neurol 2000; 247:435.
78. Beck RW, Arrington J, Murtagh FR, et al.: Brain magnetic resonance imaging in acute optic neuritis. Experience of the optic neuritis study group. Arch Neurol 1993;50:841.
79. Piquemal R, Cottier JP, and Arsène S, et al.: Radiation-induced optic neuropathy 4 years after radiation: report of a case followed up with MRI. Neuroradiology 1998;40:439.
80. Goldsmith BJ, Rosenthal SA, Wara WM, et al.: Optic neuropathy after irradiation of Meningioma. Radiology 1992;185:71.
81. Guy J, Mancuso A, Beck R, et al.: Radiation-induced optic neuropathy: a magnetic resonance imaging study. J Neurosurg 1991;74:426.
82. Hollander MD, FitzPatrick M, O'Connor SG, et al.: Optic gliomas. Radiol Clin North Am 1999;37:59.
83. Jinkins JR: Optic hydrops: isolated nerve sheath dilation demonstrated by CT. AJNR 1987;8:867.
84. Mafee MF, Goodwin J, and Dorodi S: Optic nerve sheath meningiomas. Radiol Clin North Am 1999;37:37.
85. Ortiz O, Schochet SS, Kotzan JM, and Kostick D: Radiologic-pathologic correlation: meningioma of the optic nerve sheath. AJNR 1996;17:901.
86. Carrol GS, Haik BG, Fleming JC, et al.: Peripheral nerve tumors of the orbit. Radiol Clin North Am 1999;37:195.
87. Webber JT, Osborn AG, Haas BD, and Hidayat AA: Orbital plexiform neurofibroma. Int J Neuroradiol 1995;1:102.
88. Zimmerman RA, Bilaniuk LT, Metzger RA, et al.: Computed tomography of orbital facial neurofibromatosis. Radiology 1983;146:113.
89. Biousse V, Mendicino ME, Simon DJ, et al.: The ophthalmology of intracranial vascular abnormalities. Am J Ophthalmol 1998;125:527.
90. Haik BG, Karcioglu ZA, Gordon RA, et al.: Capillary hemangioma (infantile periocular hemangioma). Surv Ophthalmol 1994;38:399.
91. Hammerschlag SB, Hesselink JR, and Weber AL: Computed tomography of the eye and orbit. Norwalk, Connecticut: Appleton-Century-Crofts; 1983:209–211.
92. Swayne LC, Garfinkle WB, and Bennet RH: CT of posterior ocular staphyloma in axial myopia. Neuroradiology 1984;26:241.
93. Anderson RL, Epstein GA, and Dauer EA: Computed tomographic diagnosis of posterior ocular staphyloma. AJNR 1983;4:90.
94. Lateef SS, Mukherji SK, Castillo M, et al.: Juvenile retinoschisis: imaging findings. AJNR 1999;20:1148.
95. Smirniotopoulos JG, Bargallo N, and Mafee MF: Differential diagnosis of leukokoria: radiologic-pathologic correlation. Radiographics 1994;14:1059.
96. Edward DP, Mafee MF, Garcia-Valenzuela E, et al.: Coat's disease and persistent hyperplastic primary vitreous. Radiol Clin North Am 1998;36:1119.
97. Sherman JL, McLean IW, and Brallier Dr: Coat's disease: CT-pathologic correlation in two cases. Radiology 1983;146:77.
98. Kaste SC, Jenkins III JJ, Meyer D, Fontanesi J, and Pratt CB: Persistent hyperplastic primary vitreous of the eye: imaging findings with pathologic correlation. AJR 1994;162:437.
99. Magill HL, Hanna SL, Brooks MT, et al.: Pediatric. Radiographics 1990; 10:515.
100. Mafee MF: Uveal melanoma, choroidal hemangioma, and simulating lesions: role of MR imaging. Radiol Clin North Am 1998;36:1083.
101. Griffiths PD, Boodram MB, Blaser S, Altomare, et al.: Abnormal ocular enhancement in sturge-weber syndrome: correlation of ocular MR and CT findings with clinical and intracranial findings. AJNR 1996;17:749.
102. Bryan RN, Lewis RA, and Miller SL: Choroidal osteoma. AJNR 1983;4:491.
103. Kadrmas EF and Weiter JJ: Choroidal osteoma. Int Ophthalmol Clin 1997;37:171.
104. Goodkens RH, Veiga-Pires JA, van Nieuwenhuizen O, et al.: CT of sebaceous nevus syndrome (Jadassohn disease). AJNR 1983;4:203.
105. Wilkes SR, Campbell RJ, and Waller RR: Ocular manifestations in association with ipsilateral facial nevus of Jadassohn. Am J Ophthalmol 1981;92:344.
106. Hosten N, Bornfeld N, Wassmuth R, et al.: Uveal melanoma: detection of extraocular growth with MR imaging and US. Radiology 1997;202:61.
107. Ozdemir H, Yucel C, Aytekin G, et al.: Intraocular tumors. The value of spectral and color doppler sonography. Clin Imag 1997;21:77.
108. Smith JA, Gragoudas ES, and Dreyer EB: Uveal metastases. Int Ophthalmol Clin 1997;37:183.
109. Kaufman LM, Mafee MF, and Song CD: Retinoblastoma and simulating lesions: role of CT, MR imaging and use of Gd-DPTA contrast enhancement. Radiol Clin North Am 1998;36:1101.
110. Girardot C, Hazebroucq VG, Fery-Lemonnier E, et al.: MR imaging and CT of surgica materials currently used in ophthalmology: in vitro and in vivo studies. Radiology 1994;191:433.
111. Mafee MF, Dorodi S, and Pai E: Sarcoidosis of the eye, orbit, and central nervous system: role of MR imaging. Radiol Clin North Am 1999;37:73.

112. Carmody RF, Mafee MF, Goodwin JA, et al.: Orbital and optic pathway sarcoidosis: MR findings. AJNR 1994;15:775.
113. Engelken JD, Yuh WTC, Carter KD, and Nerad JA: Optic nerve sarcoidosis: MR findings. AJNR 1992;13:228.
114. Johnson MH, DeFilipp GJ, Zimmerman RA, et al.: Scleral inflammatory disease. AJNR 1987;8:861.
115. Munk PL, Lin DTC, and Morris DC: Epiphora: treatment by means of dacryocystoplasty with balloon dilation of the nasolacrimal drainage apparatus. Radiology 1990;177:687.
116. Song H, Jin Y, Kim J, et al.: Nonsurgical placement of a nasolacrimal polyurethane stent. Radiology 1995;194:233.
117. Song H, Ahn H, Park C, et al.: Complete obstruction of the nasolacrimal system: part I: treatment with balloon dilation. Radiology 1993;186:367.
118. Lee J, Song H, Han Y, et al.: Balloon dacryocystoplasty: results in the treatment of complete and partial obstructions of the nasolacrimal system. Radiology 1994;192:503.
119. Ilgit ET, Yuksel D, Unal M, et al.: Transluminal balloon dilatation of the lacrimal drainage system for the treatment of epiphora. AJR 1995;165: 1517.
120. Naidich TP, Heier LA, Osborn RE, et al.: Facies to remember. Int J Neuroradiol 1996;2(4):389.
121. Rand PK, Ball Jr, WS, and Kulwin DR: Congenital nasolacrimal mucoceles: CT evaluation. Radiology 1989;173:691.
122. Friedman DP, Rao VM, and Flanders AE: Lesions causing a mass in the medial canthus of the orbit: CT and MR features. AJR 1993;160:1095.
123. Mafee MF, Edward DP, Koeller KK, et al.: Lacrimal gland tumors and simulating lesions. Radiol Clin North Am 1999;37:219.
124. Mauriello JA, Lee HJ, and Nguyen L: CT of soft tissue injury and orbital fractures. Radiol Clin North Am 1999;37:241.
125. Rhea JT, Rao PM, and Novelline RA: Helical CT and three-dimensional CT of facial and orbital injury. Radiol Clin North Am 1999;37:489.
126. Rothman M: Orbital trauma. Semin Ultrasound CT MR 1997;18(6):437.
127. Unger JM: Fractures of the nasolacrimal fossa and canal: a CT study of appearance, associated injuries, and significance in 25 patients. AJR 1992;158:1321.
128. Wiot JG and Pleatman CW: Chronic hematic cysts of the orbit. AJNR 1989;10:S37.
129. Dobben GD, Philip B, Mafee MF, et al.: Orbital subperiosteal hematoma, cholesterol granuloma, and infection: evaluation with MR imaging and CT. Radiol Clin North Am 1998;36:1185.
130. Weissman JL, Beatty RL, Hirsch WL, et al.: Enlarged anterior chamber: CT finding of a ruptured globe. AJNR 1995;16:936.
131. Mafee MF, Linder B, Peyman GA, et al.: Choroidal hematoma and effusion: evaluation with MR imaging. Radiology 1988;168:781–786.
132. Mafee MF and Peyman GA: Choroidal detachment and ocular hypotony: CT evaluation. Radiology 1984;153:697.
133. Dalley RW: Intraorbital wood foreign bodies on CT: use of wide bone window settings to distinguish wood from air. AJR 1995;164:434–435.
134. Ho VT, McGuckin JF, and Smergel EM: Intraorbital wooden foreign body: CT and MR appearance. AJNR 1996;17:134–136.
135. Rubin PAD and Remulla HD: Surgical methods and approaches in the treatment of orbital disease. Neuroimaging Clin North Am 1996;6(1):239.
136. Gross JG, Hesselink JR, Press GA, Goldbaum MH, and Freeman WR: Magnetic resonance imaging in the evaluation of vitreoretinal disease in eyes with intraocular silicone oil. Am J Ophthalmol 1990;110:366.
137. Weindling SM, Robinette CL, and Wesley RE: Porous hydroxyapatite in orbital reconstructive surgery: radiologic recognition. AJNR 1992;13:239.
138. Ainbinder DJ, Haik BG, and Mazzoli RA: Anophthalmic socket and orbital implants: role of CT and MR imaging. Radiol Clin North Am 1998;36:1133.

Sinonasal, Facial, and Mandibular Embryology, Anatomy, and Anomalies

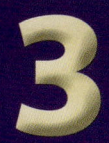

3

Mindy J. Kim-Miller, MD, PhD
Anton N. Hasso, MD, FACR

EMBRYOLOGY AND DEVELOPMENT

Midface

The primary events in the development of the cranial-oral-facial region occur between the fourth and eighth weeks of gestation. Three major sources of tissue contribute to the formation of the face and jaw: neural crest cells supply most of the facial mesenchyme, paraxial mesoderm evolve into the skeletal muscles and cartilage, and ectoderm provides the surface membranes (**Table 3-1**). The structures of the face develop from the frontonasal, maxillary, and mandibular prominences of the embryo (**Fig. 3-1**). By the end of gestational week 4, the maxillary prominences lie lateral to, and the mandibular prominences lie caudal to the stomodeum, which forms the center of the face or primitive mouth. Cranial to the stomodeum, the ectodermally derived frontonasal prominence and its two nasal placodes develop from the central mesenchyme ventral to the brain vesicles, and give rise to the midface structures. The first pharyngeal arch provides the neural crest-derived mesenchyme that develops into the maxillary and mandibular prominences, which contribute to the lateral facial structures.[1–3]

During week 5, the nasal placode invaginates to form a nasal pit as a ridge of tissue surrounding the pit forms medial and lateral nasal prominences. As the mesenchyme surrounding each nasal pit grows, the pit deepens to become a primitive nasal cavity or nasal sac. As the nasal cavity deepens, the posterior limiting membrane starts as a nasal fin but becomes the bucconasal membrane. About week 6, the bucconasal membrane dissolves to connect the primitive palate to the undersurface of the neurocranium, forming the primitive posterior choanae. Epithelial plugs within the primitive posterior choanae dissolve to form the permanent posterior choanae during the third trimester. Failure of the bucconasal membrane to dissolve may be the cause of choanal atresia.[4]

Five facial prominences will eventually form the nose: the frontal prominence gives rise to the bridge and nasal septum, the medial nasal prominences merge to form the crest and tip, and the lateral nasal prominences form the alae or wing. Overall, the medial nasal and frontal prominences give rise to the nasal septum, frontal bones, nasal bones, ethmoid sinus complexes, and upper incisors. By the end of the third month, the nasal capsule is well developed. The cartilaginous nasal capsule forms deep to the nasal and frontal bones. Its caudal border will give rise to the inferior nasal concha or turbinate, which ossifies to become a separate bone in the fifth month. The posterolateral portions of the nasal capsule will give rise to the ethmoid bone with its middle, superior, and supreme turbinates. Parts of the nasal capsule become the vomer and nasal bones while other parts remain cartilaginous and develop into the septal and alar cartilages of the nose.[4–7]

By the end of week 7, the ectoderm-covered mesenchyme of the maxillary prominence has grown medially and compressed the medial nasal prominence toward the midline (**Fig. 3-1**). The cleft between the maxillary and medial nasal prominences is lost as the two fuse to form the upper lip. The ectoderm along the nasomaxillary groove between the lateral nasal and maxillary prominences gives rise to a solid epithelial cord, which detaches from the overlying ectoderm and canalizes to form the nasolacrimal duct. After the epithelial cord detaches, the lateral nasal and maxillary prominences fuse, and the maxillary prominence produce the palatine process, maxilla, and cheek. As the maxillae grow medially, part of the medial nasal prominences fuse to form the intermaxillary segment, which gives rise to the philtrum of the upper lip, the median part of the maxillary bone with its four incisor teeth, and the triangular primary palate. The mandibular prominences develop into the lower lip and jaw.[2–7]

Palate

The fusion of the primary and secondary palates separates the nasopharynx from the oropharynx. The primary palate develops from fusion of the medial nasal and maxillary prominences. Concurrently, the secondary palate develops from the palatine shelves of the maxillary prominences, which appear on either side of the tongue at week 6. During week 7, the two shelves grow medially and ascend above the tongue to fuse, forming the secondary palate. The incisive foramen marks the midline between the primary and secondary palates. At week 8, a central

Table 3-1 Embryology and Development of the Nose, Paranasal Sinses, and Nasal Cavities

Embryonic Tissue Source	Contributes to Formation of
Entoderm	Epithelial lining of digestive tract (except part of mouth, pharynx, and terminal rectum, which are lined by ectoderm); lining cells of glands that open into digestive tract (including liver, pancreas); epithelium of auditory tube, tympanic cavity, trachea, bronchi, lung alveoli, urinary bladder, part of urethra, follicles of thyroid gland, and thymus
Mesoderm	Skeletal muscle; cartilage; connective tissue; circulatory system; urogenital system; gut wall; body wall; notochord; vertebral column dermis
Ectoderm	Nervous system/neural tube; skin epidermis; lining cells of sebaceous, sudoriferous, and mammary glands; hairs and nails; nasal turbinates, epithelium of nose, paranasal sinuses, and cheeks; roof of mouth; teeth enamel; anterior lobe of hypophysis cerebri; epithelium of cornea, conjunctiva, and lacrimal glands; neuroepithelium of sensory organs
Neural crest cells	Autonomic ganglia, chromaffin, neurolemma, integumentary pigment (facial mesenchyme)
Frontonasal prominence	Nasal capsule; nasal placode (from ectoderm)
Nasal capsule	Vomer; nasal bones; septal and alar cartilages
Caudal border	Inferior turbinate
Posterolateral border	Ethmoid bone; middle, superior, and supreme turbinates
Frontonasal prominence	Nasal turbinates; lateral nasal wall; paranasal sinuses; nasal septum and bridge
Medial nasal prominence	Nasal crest, tip; philtrum of upper lip; median part of maxillary bone with its four incisor teeth; triangular primary palate
Lateral nasal prominence	Nasal alae/wing
Maxillary prominence	Palatine process; maxilla; cheek; lateral part of upper lip
Mandibular prominence	Lower lip; jaw

ossification center appears to ossify the palatine bone in a membrane of connective tissue. By week 9, the primary and secondary palates separate the nasal and oral cavities, turbinates have appeared, and the definitive choanae are located at the junction of the oral cavity and the pharynx. By week 10, the nasal septum has grown down to fuse with the newly formed palate.[4–7]

Nasal Cavities and Paranasal Sinuses

The nasal capsule, which develops from the frontonasal prominence, will develop into two portions: the mesethmoid, which gives rise to the nasal septum; and the lateral ectethmoid, which gives rise to the turbinates and lateral nasal wall. The primitive nasal cavity begins as a single chamber. Ectoderm of the nasal sac grows toward and fuses with ectoderm of the mouth roof, forming the oronasal septum. Attenuation of the oronasal septum produces the oronasal membrane, which separates the nasal cavity from the pharynx. The oronasal membrane then undergoes degeneration, resulting in choanae formation. As the secondary palate develops and the primitive nasal chambers elongate, the final nasal chambers take shape, separated by the nasal septum.[8]

The nasal septum begins development at week 5 and forms from the frontonasal process, which grows in an anterior-to-posterior direction, eventually joining with the tectoseptal expansion, a median ridge of mesenchyme. The septum continues growing posteriorly, ultimately uniting with palatine processes. Fusion of the frontonasal process, tectoseptal expansion, and palatine processes results in separation of the oral and nasal cavities, as well as right and left nasal chambers (**Fig. 3-1**). The nasal septum subsequently undergoes chondrification and ossification of its various constituents. As the frontonasal prominence grows posteriorly from the cranium to the palate, it is joined by mesoderm from the maxilla called the tectoseptal extension. Together they form the primordia of the septum. The lateral nasal wall develops grooves that become the inferior and middle meati as the middle, superior, and supreme turbinates arise around week 8 of development. A cartilaginous capsule surrounds the developing nasal cavity.[9] At week 9 or 10, cartilaginous projections invade the developing turbinates, and a cartilaginous bud that will become the uncinate process appears. Lateral to this bud, a space that corresponds to the ethmoidal infundibulum appears around week 13 to 14.[4,7]

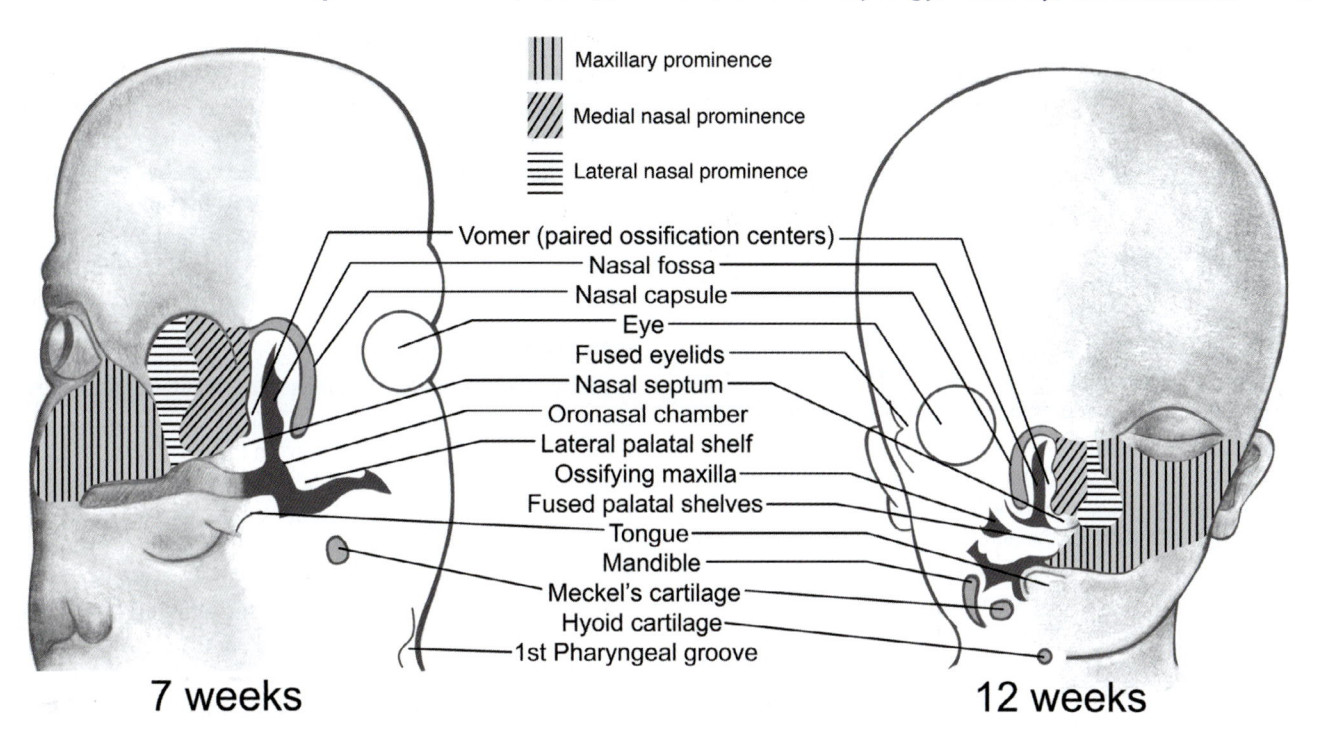

Chapter 3: Sinonasal, Facial, and Mandibular Embryology, Anatomy, and Anomalies

Figure 3-1 Early Embryology of the Face
Schematic illustration showing embryologic development of the midface at weeks 7 and 11. Superficial structures are shown on one half, and deeper structures are shown on the other half.

Paranasal sinuses arise from outgrowths or ridges (sometimes called ethmoturbinals) from the lateral cartilaginous nasal capsule. These outgrowths eventually extend into the maxillae, ethmoid, frontal, and sphenoid bones. Around the eighth week of gestation, 5 to 6 ethmoturbinals initially appear but eventually regress and fuse into 3 or 4 ridges. The first ethmoturbinal regresses to form the agger nasi and the uncinate process. The second ethmoturbinal develops into the middle turbinate, and the third develops into the superior turbinate. The fourth and fifth ethmoturbinals fuse to become the supreme turbinate. Inferiorly, another ridge, called the maxilloturbinal, contributes the inferior turbinate.[1-7] In the third trimester, there may be up to six turbinates, but after birth, the superior turbinates tend to coalesce and disappear by adulthood.[2] The supreme turbinate has been reported in 88% of fetuses, 73% of preadolescents, and 26% of adults.[3]

By the third to fourth month of gestation, mucous membrane infiltrates the cartilaginous structures of the lateral nasal wall by primary pneumatization. Later secondary pneumatization occurs into the bony structures of the sinuses. The paranasal sinuses continue to develop into puberty to contribute to the shape of the face.[10]

Maxillary Sinus

The maxillary sinus is the first sinus to appear in the third month of fetal development. It begins as an outgrowth in the lateral wall of the nasal capsule in a groove called the uncibullous groove, which lies posterior to the developing uncinate process. The sinus is fluid-filled at birth and measures 6 to 8 cm^3: about 8 mm in length, 3 mm in height, and 2 mm in width.[2] By the fourth to fifth postnatal month, the maxillary sinuses can be seen by plain film radiography. After birth, the sinus grows 2 mm vertically and 3 mm anterior/posteriorly each year for the first 3 years, then more slowly until the seventh year. From ages 7 until 12 years, there is rapid growth with pneumatization extending laterally to the lateral orbit and inferiorly to the floor of the nasal cavity. During the teen years, there is slower growth, and by adulthood, the floor of the sinus extends 4 to 5 mm inferior to the floor of the nasal cavity. In the average adult, the maxillary sinus measures 15 mm^3: 34 mm anteroposteriorly, 33 mm vertically, and 25 mm in width.[4] The maxillary sinuses are generally symmetric, but hypoplasia occurs in ~6%, and duplication can occur in 2.5% of patients.[7,11] Approximately 50% of maxillary sinuses have incomplete septi, and accessory ostia are found in 25% to 50% of adults and ~15% of children.[12]

Ethmoid Sinus

In the third month of gestation, the anterior and middle ethmoid cells begin as evaginations in the middle meatus of the lateral nasal wall. Later, the posterior cells arise from the superior meatus. The ethmoid sinus can have great variations as it can extend beyond the ethmoid bone itself. The anterior cells originate in the frontal recess of the middle meatus. At birth, the anterior sinus is 2 mm long, 4 mm high, and 2 mm wide; the posterior sinus 4 mm long, 5 mm high, and 2 mm wide. The ethmoid sinuses are fluid-filled at birth and are difficult to visualize by plain radiograph before one year of age.[2] In the early years, the ethmoid sinuses are spherical in shape but become flatter with age. By age 12 years, the ethmoids are nearly fully developed. The posterior ethmoids in the average adult measures 24 mm high, 23 mm long, and 11 mm wide.[12] As the ethmoids pneumatize adjacent bones, the resulting sinuses are named for the invaded bone. Therefore, the ethmoid cell that invades the frontal bone is called the frontal sinus. Due to pneumatization, the ethmoid bone becomes the lightest bone in the skull.[4]

Frontal Sinus

Development of the frontal sinus and recess varies greatly between individuals. During the fourth month of gestation, the frontal sinus may arise from several possible outgrowths in the frontal recess, the anterior ethmoid cells, or occasionally, the ethmoid infundibulum. In about 50% of cases, the frontal sinus develops from lateral extensions of anterior ethmoid cells within the frontal recess. Because such frontal sinuses essentially develop from displaced ethmoid cells, their drainage is either via an ostium into the frontal recess or via a nasofrontal duct into the anterior infundibulum. If the frontal sinus develops from an ethmoid cell within the ethmoid infundibulum, a true nasofrontal duct can develop. If it develops from extension of the anterior part of the frontal recess, or from the frontal furrow, then only a nasofrontal ostium without a duct occurs. In the least common approach, the frontal sinus arises as a direct extension of the entire frontal recess, resulting in a large communication between the frontal sinus and the middle meatus, depending on the size of the adjacent anterior ethmoid cells.[4-7] At birth, the sinus is small and indistinguishable from the adjacent anterior ethmoid cells. By 5 years of age, the frontal sinus begins to invade the vertical portion of the frontal bone and can be seen on plain radiograph by age 6. By late adolescence, the frontal sinuses reach adult size, measuring 28 mm high, 27 mm wide, and 17 mm deep.[11,12] In 4% to 15% of patients, one of the frontal sinuses fails to develop; asymmetry is common.[4]

Sphenoid Sinus

The sphenoid sinus begins as an outgrowth from the posterior portion of the cartilaginous nasal capsule. During the third gestational month, the nasal mucosa invaginates into the posterior nasal capsule to form a pouch called the cartilaginous cupolar recess of the nasal cavity.[13] Ossification centers appear around the ninth week of gestation. Until the seventh or eighth month of fetal development, the sphenoid consists of two main components: the presphenoid and postsphenoid. The presphenoid consists of the lesser wings, body, and tuberculum sella. The postsphenoid contains the dorsum sella, greater wings, and pterygoid plates. The first two ossification centers appear in the lesser wings of the sphenoid. The next two appear in the presphenoid part of the body. In the postsphenoid, ossification centers appear on the greater wings of the sphenoid. By birth, the sphenoid bone has three components: a central portion consisting of the body and lesser wing; and two lateral components, which contain the greater wings and pterygoid plates.

The sphenoid sinus at birth appears as an evagination of the sphenoethmoidal recess.[1-3] During the second and third years of age, the cartilage is resorbed, and the sinus begins to grow and pneumatize posteriorly, laterally, and inferiorly. By age 7, the sinus reaches the level of the sella turcica and the nerve of the pterygoid canal.[11] Pneumatization may involve the basisphenoid, extend into the greater and lesser wings of the sphenoid, and less commonly, the basilar process of the occipital bone. There are three major types of sphenoid sinuses based on pneumatization. In the sellar type, pneumatization extends beyond the tuberculum sella in 90% of cases. In the presellar type, pneumatization extends posteriorly to the sella turcica but not beyond the vertical plane of the tuberculum sella; this occurs in 10% of adults. Lastly, in the conchal type, pneumatization does not extend into the body of the sphenoid bone; this is found in 2.5% of adults. Asymmetry, incomplete septi, and various recesses are common. By adulthood, the sinus typically measures 20 mm high, 17 mm wide, and 23 mm deep.[4]

Nasofrontal Region

Initially, the fonticulus frontalis (nasofrontal fontanelle) separates the embryonic nasal and frontal bones, and a prenasal space separates the nasal bones from the cartilaginous nasal capsule.[14-17] As the nasal and frontal bones fuse, the fonticulus frontalis closes to form the nasofrontal suture. Concurrently, through the foramen cecum, a diverticulum of dura mater extends down from the anterior cranial fossa into a transient prenasal space and contacts the tip of the nose. As the surrounding bones develop, the dural diverticulum retracts back into the cranium, and the prenasal space regresses to the foramen cecum, which eventually fills with fibrous tissue[17,18] (**Fig. 3-2**).

Nasolacrimal Apparatus

By the end of the first gestational month, the surface ectoderm along the nasomaxillary (or nasooptic) groove involutes into an epithelial cord, which becomes canalized during the third to seventh gestational months to become the nasolacrimal duct.[1,2,17] The nasolacrimal duct opens below the middle turbinate bone via the Hasner membrane, which typically perforates to become the Hasner valve at birth or within the first year of life. At the other end of the duct, the lacrimal sac develops within the medial canthus.[17,19]

ANATOMY AND ANATOMIC VARIANTS

To understand the complex labyrinth of the paranasal sinuses and nasal cavities, it is important to appreciate the variability of the structures and drainage pathways of the sinuses (**Table 3-2**). Typically, the middle meatus receives drainage from the frontal sinus (via the frontal recess), maxillary sinus (via the maxillary ostium into the ethmoidal infundibulum), and the anterior ethmoid sinus (via the ethmoid ell ostia). The posterior ethmoids drain into the supreme and superior meati. The sphenoid sinus drains into the sphenoethmoid recess and subsequently into the superior meatus.

Ethmoid Sinus

The ethmoid bone consists of four parts: the horizontal cribriform plate (lamina cribrosa), which is part of the cranial base; the vertical perpendicular plate (lamina perpendicularis), which is part of the nasal septum; and the two lateral masses (labyrinths), which contain ethmoid air cells. The ethmoid sinus is very complex and variable between individuals. It can be divided into obliquely oriented lamellae based on their embryologic precursors. The first lamella is the *uncinate process*; the second is the *ethmoidal bulla*; the third is the *basal* or *ground*

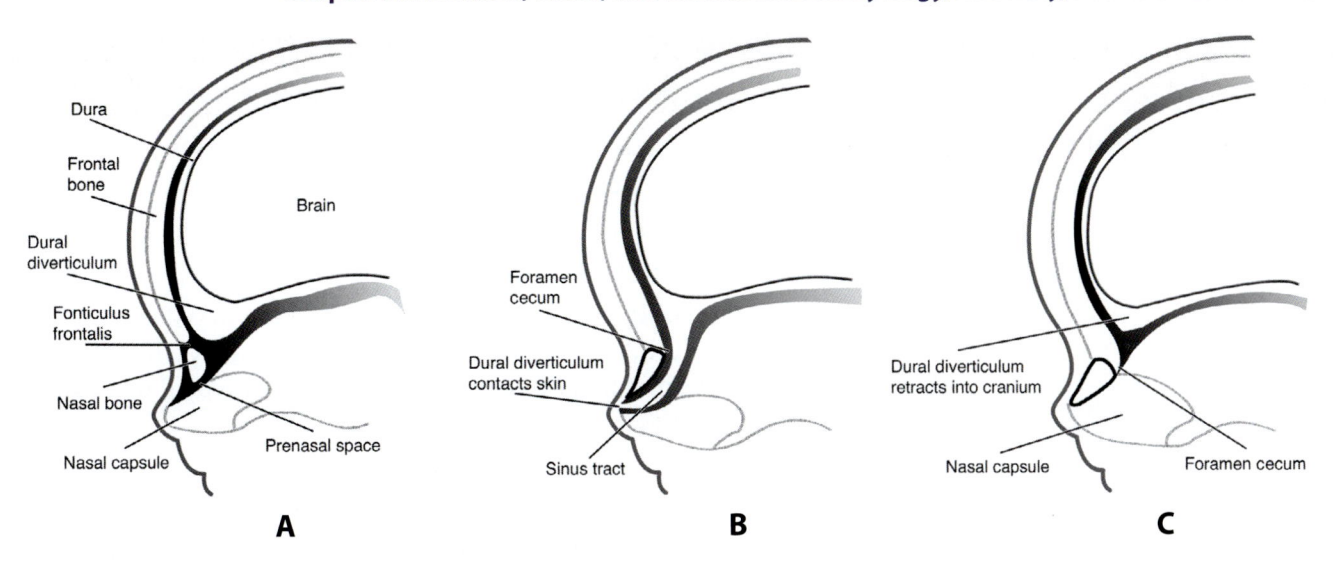

Figure 3-2 Normal Embryologic Development of the Craniofacial Region
Schematic illustration of normal embryologic development of the craniofacial region. (**A**) Fonticulus frontalis temporarily separates the nasal and frontal bones. Transient prenasal space separates the nasal bones and cartilaginous nasal capsule. (**B**) Nasal and frontal bones fuse; fonticulus frontalis closes to form the nasofrontal suture. Dural diverticulum extends through the foramen cecum into the prenasal space and transiently contacts the skin at the tip of the nose before retracting back through the anterior cranial fossa. (**C**) Dural diverticulum involutes back into the cranium. Prenasal space disappears; foramen cecum grows smaller and fills with fibrous tissue.

lamella of the middle turbinate; and the fourth is the *lamella of the superior turbinate*. The basal lamella of the middle turbinate divides the anterior and posterior ethmoids.

Agger Nasi

The agger nasi is a prominence located at and just anterior to the middle turbinate's insertion into the lateral nasal wall. Often, the agger nasi may be pneumatized by an anterior ethmoid cell, which is referred to as the agger nasi cell.

Agger Nasi Cell

Formed from pneumatization anteroinferiorly into the agger nasi, the agger nasi cell is the most anterior air cell of the ethmoid sinus (**Table 3-2**). It is bordered anteriorly by the frontal process of the maxilla, superiorly by the frontal recess/sinus, anterolaterally by the nasal bones, inferomedially by the uncinate process of the ethmoid bone, and inferolaterally by the lacrimal bone. Because the agger nasi cell forms part of the floor of the frontal sinus and anterior border of the frontal recess, it can play an important role in frontal sinusitis and frontal surgery. A large agger nasi cell may narrow the frontal recess, increasing the risk of frontal sinusitis. During surgery, if an agger nasi cell is mistaken for the frontal recess or sinus and dissected, the residual superoposterior wall of the agger nasi cell can scar posteriorly to the ethmoid roof, and iatrogenic stenosis of the nasofrontal connection can occur.[20]

Pneumatization may extend into the lacrimal bone. This close relationship to the lacrimal bone may cause epiphora in some patients with sinus disease.[21] Occasionally, pneumatization can extend inferomedially into the uncinate process to form a bulla of the uncinate.[22]

Uncinate Process

The uncinate process is a sickle-shaped, bony leaflet that attaches anterosuperiorly to the ethmoidal crest of the maxillae on the lateral nasal wall, and posteroinferiorly to the superior aspect of the inferior turbinate. It also has attachments to the perpendicular process of the palatine bone posterosuperiorly and lacrimal bone anteriorly. Its posterior margin is free without any bony attachments. Superiorly, it ascends to the lacrimal bone and most commonly bends laterally to attach to the lamina papyracea or lateral nasal wall. Superior and medial to this lies the floor of the frontal recess. The hiatus semilunaris lies directly behind the posterior margin of the uncinate.

The uncinate has no bony attachments anterior and posterior to its attachment to the inferior turbinate bone. These areas of the lateral nasal wall are referred to as the anterior and posterior fontanelles and are composed of mucosa and connective tissue rather than bone.[21] In 20% to 25% of patients, the maxillary sinus will often have an opening, the accessory ostium, into the posterior fontanelle, which can often be mistaken for the natural maxillary sinus ostia.[23]

Uncinate Process Variants

The superior aspect of the uncinate process most commonly attaches laterally onto the lamina papyracea at approximately 140 degrees.[24] But uncinate variants are common, including elongation and lateral and medial deviation of its superior attachment (**Table 3-2**). The most common variation is elongation of the superior aspect with insertion centrally into the skull base or floor of the anterior ethmoid air cells. In this variant, the semilunar hiatus may be absent or markedly narrowed.

Table 3-2 Important Anatomic Variants of the Paranasal Sinus Region

Anatomic Variations	Key Concepts
Agger nasi cell	Most anterior ethmoid cell; can narrow frontal recess
Uncinate process	
Attachment	Variants attach onto orbit, skull base, or middle turbinate
Displacement	Laterally – adheres to orbit; obstructs infundibulum; absent maxillary sinus ostium; predisposes to orbital injury in FESS; associated with MSH Medially – compresses middle turbinate; associated with polypoid disease
Bulla	Pneumatized uncinate; obstructs infundibulum
Ethmoidal infundibulum	Variable relationship to frontal recess and ethmoid ostium depending on attachment of uncinate process
Frontal recess	If uncinate attaches to ethmoid roof or medially on middle turbinate, frontal recess and infundibulum may be contiguous, infundibulum may link maxillary and ethmoid sinuses If uncinate attaches laterally to lamina papyraea, frontal recess drains medial to uncinate
Recessus terminalis	Blind terminal pocket of ethmoid infundibulum formed when uncinate inserts laterally on inferomedial floor of orbit
Prominent ethmoid bulla	Largest, most posterior anterior ethmoid cell; obstructs infundibulum
Torus lateralis	Bony projection of unpneumatized ethmoid
Frontal cell	Ethmoid cell extension into frontal sinus
Bulla frontalis	Ethmoid cell extension into frontal bone alongside frontal sinus
Supraorbital ethmoid cell	Pneumatized orbital plate of frontal bone
Maxillary sinus hypoplasia (MSH)	Hypoplastic maxillary sinus; thicker surrounding bone; hypoplastic uncinate adherent to inferior orbit
Haller's (infraorbital ethmoidal) cell	Ethmoid cell extension into roof of maxillary sinus; obstructs infundibulum
Paradoxical middle turbinate	Middle turbinate rotates laterally away from septum; obstructs middle meatus
Concha bullosa	Pneumatized middle turbinate; obstructs middle meatus, infundibulum
Onodi (sphenoethmoidal) cell	Most posterior ethmoid cell; can enclose optic nerve, carotid artery
Sphenoid sinus overpneumatization	Can cause dehiscence at optic canal, orbital apex, carotid groove
Incomplete intersinus septum	Between right and left sphenoid sinuses
Lamina papyracea dehiscence	Look for protrusion of orbital fat near insertion of basal lamella; increases risk of orbital injury during surgery
Cribriform plate dehiscence, low position, or deep olfactory fossa	Increases risk of skull base injury during surgery
Anterior ethmoid artery position	Can travel below ethmoid roof; increases risk of surgical complications
Nasal septal deviation	Can displace or compress middle turbinate

FESS = functional endoscopic sinus surgery.

In the lateral variant, the uncinate deviates more laterally to insert on the inferomedial floor of the orbit. In this case, the ethmoid infundibulum ends in a blind pocket, referred to as the recessus terminalis, which lies inferolateral to the superior aspect of the uncinate.[21]

In the medial variant, the uncinate attaches medially to the superior aspect of the vertical lamella of the middle turbinate near the turbinate's insertion to the cribriform plate.[25,26] The ethmoid infundibulum in medial variants may communicate directly with the ethmoid ostium, thereby directly linking the maxillary and ethmoid sinuses.[27]

In 3% of patients the uncinate may be significantly displaced, thereby impeding mucociliary drainage from the frontal, maxillary, and anterior ethmoid sinuses.[21,28] In lateral displacement or deviation, the uncinate rests against or fuses to the orbit or inferior aspect of the lamina papyracea (**Table 3-2**). As a result, the uncinate can obstruct the infundibulum. Additionally, the maxillary sinus ostium and the hiatus semilunaris may be absent; therefore, no communication occurs between the maxillary sinus and the middle meatus.[27] Awareness of lateral uncinate displacement is important in sinus surgery, because the usual incision in functional endoscopic sinus surgery (FESS) at the base of the uncinate would result in direct orbital injury. Lateral uncinate displacement is commonly seen in cases of maxillary sinus hypoplasia.

Medial uncinate displacement is often found in patients with extensive polypoid disease within the infundibulum. The uncinate may compress the mucosa of the middle turbinate and obstruct airflow into the middle meatus. Rarely the uncinate is displaced so medially that it recurves on itself and appears to be a duplicate of the middle turbinate.[21]

In some cases (0.4% to 2.5%), the uncinate process is pneumatized, resulting in an uncinate bulla, which can narrow the infundibulum and impede mucociliary drainage.[29,30]

Hiatus Semilunaris

The hiatus semilunaris usually refers to the hiatus semilunaris inferior, which is a crescent-shaped communication between the middle meatus and the ethmoid infundibulum. The borders of the hiatus semilunaris inferior are the posterior margin of the uncinate process and the anterior wall of the ethmoid bulla. The smaller hiatus semilunaris superior is the cleft formed between the posterior wall of the ethmoid bulla and the basal lamellae of the middle turbinate; it is the communication between the middle meatus and the sinus lateralis or suprabullar recess.

Ethmoidal Infundibulum

The ethmoidal infundibulum is a funnel-shaped passage that connects the anterior ethmoid cells, the maxillary sinus, and sometimes the frontal sinus, to the middle meatus via the hiatus semilunaris. It is bordered medially by the uncinate process, laterally by the lamina papyracea, anterosuperiorly by the frontal process of the maxilla, and superolaterally by the lacrimal bone. Sagittally it follows the curve of the uncinate process and ethmoid bulla. The inferior portion of the infundibulum typically contains the natural ostium of the maxillary sinus. The relationship of the superior aspect of the infundibulum to the frontal recess is largely determined by the uncinate process's insertion. In cases where the uncinate bends laterally to attach to the lamina papyracea to form the superior boundary of the infundibulum, the recessus terminalis, the frontal recess will drain medial to the uncinate. If the uncinate attaches to the ethmoid roof or inserts into the middle turbinate, the frontal recess will be contiguous with the ethmoidal infundibulum. Variations in the relationship of the infundibulum and the frontal recess are common (**Table 3-2**).

Ethmoid Bulla

The ethmoid bulla is the largest and most posterior of the anterior ethmoid air cells. It is located on the lamina papyracea and projects into the middle meatus directly posterior to the uncinate process and anterior to the basal lamella of the middle turbinate. Superiorly, the anterior wall of the ethmoid bulla can extend to the skull base and form the posterior limit of the frontal recess. Posteriorly, the bulla can blend with the basal lamella of the middle turbinate.

Ethmoid Bulla Variations

When highly pneumatized, the ethmoid bulla can be one of the largest ethmoid air cells and can lie in the lower aspect of the middle meatus (**Table 3-2**). If the bulla lies low enough, it can impede upon the ethmoidal infundibulum and impair mucociliary clearance. In about 8% of patients, the ethmoid remains unpneumatized, resulting in a bony projection from the lamina papyracea referred to as the torus lateralis.[25] Often, dehiscence or absence of the posterior wall of the ethmoid bullae results in an opening from the ethmoid bullae into the sinus lateralis.

Sinus Lateralis (Suprabullar and Retrobullar Recesses)

The sinus lateralis is an air space found posterior to the ethmoid bulla and anterior to the basal lamella of the middle turbinate. This space is also referred to as the suprabullar and retrobullar recesses. It is bordered superiorly by the ethmoid roof and laterally by the lamina papyracea. It communicates with the middle meatus via the hiatus semilunaris superior. If the ethmoid bulla does not extend to the skull base to form the posterior wall of the frontal recess, the sinus lateralis can communicate with the frontal recess and the hiatus semilunaris inferior.[25]

Ostiomeatal Unit/Complex

The ostiomeatal unit refers to a functional entity of middle meatal structures that represent the final common pathway for drainage of the frontal, maxillary, and anterior ethmoid sinuses. Although the anatomic margins are unclear, it is composed of the uncinate process, the ethmoid infundibulum, anterior ethmoid cells, and ostia of the anterior ethmoid, maxillary, and frontal sinuses.[31] The ostiomeatal unit plays a critical role in the pathophysiology of inflammatory sinus disease.

Frontal Recess and Sinus

The frontal sinus drains into the middle meatus via the frontal recess. Best seen on sagittal images, the structure resembles an hourglass whose upper portion is the sinus; the lower portion is the recess, and the waist of the hourglass is the frontal ostium.[21,32] The boundaries of the frontal recess are the posterosuperior wall of the agger nasi cell anteriorly, the middle turbinate medially, the lamina papyracea laterally, and the anterior wall of the ethmoid bulla posteriorly. If the anterior wall of the ethmoid bulla does not reach the skull base and form a complete posterior wall, the frontal recess may communicate with the suprabullar recess.[33]

Frontal Recess Region Variants

Approximately 50% of patients have anterior ethmoid cells that encroach into the frontal sinus, and about a third of these enter the area of the frontal ostium.[34] These cells are referred to as frontal cells (**Table 3-2**). Depending on their location, frontal cells can be classified as intersinus septal or intrasinus cells. With extensive pneumatization, frontal cells can appear to duplicate the frontal sinuses. If an anterior ethmoid cell from the frontal recess extends into the frontal bone alongside the frontal sinus, it is called a "bulla frontalis."[25] Pneumatization of the orbital plate of the frontal bone results in the supraorbital ethmoid cell. Drainage from this cell is variable depending on its origin.[21]

Maxillary Sinus

Depending on its size, its boundaries of the maxillary sinus are the orbital roof superiorly; the hard palate, alveolus, and dental portion of the maxilla inferiorly; the zygomatic process laterally; a thin plate of bone separating the cavity from the infratemporal and pterygopalatine fossa posteriorly; and the uncinate process, fontanelles, and inferior turbinate medially.[21] In most cases, the maxillary sinus ostium is located within the most posteroinferior one-third of the infundibulum. Occasionally, a bony or fibrous septum can divide the maxillary sinus into compartments, resulting in a septate maxillary sinus, which may drain separately into the middle meatus, or one compartment may drain into the other, with subsequent drainage into the middle meatus.[35]

Maxillary Sinus Hypoplasia

In maxillary sinus hypoplasia (MSH) or atelectasis, the sinus is smaller and nonaerated, the surrounding maxillary bone is thicker, and the uncinate process is hypoplastic and adheres to the inferomedial orbit or inferior lamina papyracea.[36] Additionally, the infundibulum is often atelectatic (**Table 3-2**).[37] On CT scans, the sinus may appear opacified, hypoplastic, with possibly orbital enlargement on the ipsilateral side. Due to the lateral displacement of the uncinate process, there is an increased risk of injury to the medial orbital wall during uncinectomies. Bilateral hypoplasia has been found in around 7% of patients with sinus complaints,[38] and unilateral MSH in 7% to 10% of symptomatic patients.[34,38] MSH may be misdiagnosed as chronic sinusitis.

Haller's Cell (Infraorbital Ethmoidal Cell)

Found in 10% to 18% of patients, Haller's cells or infraorbital ethmoidal cells are the most common anatomic variation in the maxillary sinus region.[30,39] Bilateral infraorbital ethmoidal cells are rare. These cells are extensions of ethmoid air cells into the orbital floor or medial roof of the maxillary sinus (**Table 3-2**). Haller's cells lie lateral to the uncinate process and inferolateral to the ethmoidal bulla. These cells often narrow the infundibulum. Other terms for Haller's cells include the maxillo-orbital cells, the maxilloethmoidal cells, and orbitoethmoidal cells.[21]

Middle Turbinate

The middle turbinate of the ethmoid bone lies medial to the ethmoid bullae and uncinate process. Anteriorly, the turbinate attaches with the medial wall of the agger nasi region at the crista ethmoidalis (ethmoidal eminence) of the maxilla. Superiorly and medially it attaches to the cribriform plate. As the turbinate extends posteriorly, it courses laterally and inferiorly to merge with the lamina papyracea and/or the medial wall of the maxillary sinus just posterior to the ethmoid bullae. This coronal portion is the basal or ground lamella, which divides the ethmoid sinus into its anterior and posterior components. Anteriorly the basal lamella is oriented almost coronally, and posteriorly it is almost horizontal. The most posterior aspect of the middle turbinate is attached inferiorly to the lateral wall of the perpendicular process of the palatine bone just anterior to the sphenopalatine foramen.[21]

Paradoxical Middle Turbinate

The major curvature of the middle turbinate is typically rotated medially toward the nasal septum. A paradoxical middle turbinate rotates laterally away from the septum, which may narrow the middle meatus and impede mucociliary clearance and ventilation.

Concha Bullosa

Posterior ethmoid cells can pneumatize into the middle turbinate anteriorly, and the anterior ethmoid cells and the sinus lateralis can pneumatize it posteriorly[25] (**Table 3-2**). Pneumatization of the inferior, bulbous portion of the middle turbinate is referred to as a concha bullosa. If the vertical portion or basal lamella is pneumatized, the cell is referred to as the interlamellar cell.[21] The pneumatization may be unilateral or bilateral and is found in 14% to 53% of cases.[40,41] An enlarged middle turbinate may obstruct the middle meatus, hiatus semilunaris, and/or the infundibulum.

Inferior Turbinate

The inferior turbinate develops from the maxilloturbinal of the lateral nasal wall as an independent bone and articulates with the palatine, maxillary, lacrimal, and ethmoid bones. The inferior turbinate is classified into four types: *type I* is the lamellar form characterized by a thin bony lamella; *type II* is the compact form due to its compact bony mass; *type III* is the combined form with compact and spongiosus aspects; and *type IV* is the bulbous type, which is pneumatized.[42] Anatomic variants are rare; pneumatization of the inferior turbinate is found in only 0.04% of cases.[43]

Posterior Ethmoid Sinus

The posterior ethmoid sinus is a collection of one to five ethmoid cells that drain into the superior and supreme meati. Anteriorly, it is bordered by the basal lamella of the middle turbinate, posteriorly by the anterior wall of the sphenoid sinus, laterally by the lamina papyracea, medially by the superior and supreme turbinates and their meati, and superiorly by the ethmoid roof.[21]

Onodi Cell (Sphenoethmoidal Cell)

Onodi or sphenoethmoidal cells are found in 9% to 12% of subjects and represent the most posterior ethmoid air cells, which are situated in close proximity to the skull base and optic nerve (Table 3-2).[44] Onodi described 38 variations in the relationship of the most posterior ethmoids to the optic nerves.[45] Extension of a posterior ethmoid cell along the lamina papyracea into the sphenoid bone can produce a sphenoethmoidal cell positioned adjacent to or surrounding the optic canal. If the sphenoethmoidal cell is large enough, the carotid canal can bulge into the cell as well. This proximity may result in inadvertent damage to the optic nerve or carotid artery during endoscopic surgery[46] (see Chapter 4).

Ethmomaxillary Sinus

The ethmomaxillary sinus is an enlarged posterior ethmoid air cell in the superior portion of the maxillary sinus that drains into the superior meatus. It is a rare anatomic variant found in 0.7% of patients with rhino-sinus symptoms, is usually bilateral (70%), and may be associated with concha bullosa (50%) or maxillary sinus hypoplasia (20%).[35] The ethmomaxillary sinus can be confused for Haller's cell (infraorbital ethmoidal cell), which is located more anteriorly and medially in the infraorbital wall and drains into the middle meatus.

Sphenoethmoidal Recess

The sphenoethmoidal recess is the cleft between the posterior wall of the posterior ethmoid cells and the anterior wall of the sphenoid sinus. The posterior ethmoid air cells drain into this recess and the superior meatus. The sphenoid ostia opens into the sphenoethmoidal recess as well.

Sphenoid Sinus

Located centrally within the skull, the sphenoid sinus is the most posterior paranasal sinus and is positioned superior to the nasopharynx, anteroinferior to the sella turcica, and posterior to the ethmoid cells. It borders laterally the carotid artery, optic nerve, cavernous sinus, and the third, fourth, fifth, and sixth cranial nerves.[47] In some cases, pneumatization of the sphenoid sinus will extend up to or surround the optic nerve anterosuperiorly and carotid artery posterolaterally, which are covered only by thin bone (Table 3-2). The bony covering around the optic nerve may be dehiscent in 4% of cases, and the bony covering around the carotid artery may be dehiscent in up to 22% of cases.[41,47] Due to their close proximity, dissection within the sphenoid sinus may result in inadvertent carotid and optic nerve damage (see Chapter 4).

Sphenoid Sinus Variants

Sphenoid sinus overpneumatization may lead to dehiscence at the optic canal, orbital apex, or carotid groove, increasing the risk of injury during sinus surgery (Table 3-2).

The intersinus septum, which separates the left and right sphenoid sinuses, can exhibit structural variability. It can be oriented obliquely rather than sagittally. Incomplete septations of the sphenoid sinus are common (Table 3-2). The septations and intersinus septum may also detach from the midline near or on the bony canal of the carotid artery.[21]

Dehiscence of the Lamina Papyracea

Dehiscence usually occurs near the site of insertion of the basal lamella into the medial orbital wall and may be congenital or secondary to nasal trauma or surgery.[28,48] On CT scans, it is often characterized by protrusion of orbital fat through the defect, which may be misdiagnosed as an infectious or tumoral process[49] (Table 3-2). Dehiscence of the lamina papyracea may increase the risk of orbital injury during sinus surgery.

Ethmoid Roof

An extension of the frontal bone forms the roof of the ethmoid. The ethmoid roof may vary in its orientation from being nearly horizontal to nearly vertical (Table 3-2). Most commonly, the ethmoid roof lies above the level of the cribriform plate.[21] The lateral lamellae of the cribriform plate (also known as the laminae lateralis of the lamina cribrosa) form the medial aspect of the ethmoid roof.

There are three types of skull-base conformations that have clinical relevance in sinus surgery. In *type 1*, the olfactory sulcus is 1 to 3 mm deep, the corresponding lateral lamella is short, and a significant portion of frontal bone backs the ethmoid roof, which contributes an extra 0.5 mm to the roof thickness, making it less penetrable. In *type 2*, the olfactory sulcus is 3 to 7 mm deep, and the lateral lamella contributes a significant portion of the structure of the medial ethmoid roof. In *type 3*, the olfactory sulcus is 7 to 16 mm deep, and the ethmoid roof lies above the cribriform plate. In this case, the thin lateral lamella (0.2 mm thick) contributes a much larger component to the roof and lacks backing by frontal bone, thereby increasing the risk of damage during sinus surgery.[50,51] The ethmoidal sulcus, which is the groove in the lateral lamella for the anterior ethmoidal artery, is only 0.05 mm thick.[48] Therefore, this is a common site for skull base injury and cerebrospinal fluid (CSF) leak during endoscopic sinus surgery.[42] Additionally, a low position or dehiscence of the cribriform plate may increase the risk of skull base injury during surgery (see Chapter 4).

Anterior Ethmoid Artery Variants

Appreciating the location of the anterior ethmoid artery is important for sinus surgery. After branching off the ophthalmic artery, the anterior ethmoid artery enters the ethmoid from the orbit through the anterior ethmoid foramen and crosses the ethmoid roof, typically in a bony canal at or just below the level of the roof. Occasionally the artery sits 1 to 3 mm below the roof on a mesentery (**Table 3-2**). It courses anteromedially to penetrate the lateral lamellae of the cribriform plate and enters the olfactory sulcus. An anterior ethmoid artery that lies below the ethmoid roof is vulnerable to dissection during endoscopic sinus surgery, which can result in a hemorrhage, orbital hematoma, and CSF leak.

Nasal Cavity

The nasal cavity is formed superiorly by the nasal and frontal bones, cribriform plate, sphenoid, alae of the vomer, and sphenoidal process of the palatine bone; inferiorly by the hard palate (palatine process of the maxilla and horizontal plate of the palatine bones); and laterally by the frontal process of the maxilla, lacrimal bone, ethmoid labyrinth, maxilla, inferior turbinate, perpendicular plate of the palatine, and medial pterygoid plate of the sphenoid. The maxillary spines mark the inferior margin of the pyriform aperture, or inlet of the nose. The nasal septum, composed of the perpendicular plate of the ethmoid, vomer, and septal cartilage, forms the medial wall of each cavity.[52,53] The posteroinferior vomer is usually around 0.23 cm in width and should not exceed 0.55 cm in children under 8 years old.[54] The posterior choanae, or openings between the nasal cavity and nasopharynx, should be at least 0.34 cm wide in adults, but should not exceed 0.34 cm in children less than 2 years old.[51]

Nasal Septal Deviation

Deviation of the nasal septum may be congenital or posttraumatic and may involve the cartilaginous or bony septum or both (**Table 3-2**). Septal deviation is found in 15% to 40% of the population and increases with age.[55] Significant septal deviation may laterally displace or compress the middle turbinate, narrowing the middle meatus and impeding drainage and ventilation through the ostiomeatal complex (OMC). Bony or cartilaginous septal spurs may further compromise the OMC.

Nasolacrimal Apparatus

The apparatus consists of the puncta, canaliculi, lacrimal sac, and nasolacrimal duct. The superior and inferior canaliculi meet at the common canaliculus, which leads into the lacrimal sac and then into the nasolacrimal duct. The nasolacrimal duct runs in the 1-mm-wide bony nasolacrimal canal for 12 mm, then runs in the nasal mucosa for 5 mm before draining into the inferior meatus via the Hasner valve.[56]

ANOMALIES OF THE PARANASAL SINUSES AND NASAL CAVITIES

Imaging patients with craniofacial, sinonasal, and maxillomandibular anomalies is important for accurate classification and differentiation of the various forms of developmental and congenital dysplasias and dysgenesis. Imaging is critical in

Table 3-3 Differential Diagnosis of Congenital Midline Frontonasal Masses
- Glioma
- Cephalocele
- Dermoid cyst
- Epidermoid cyst
- Hemangioma or lymphangioma
- Dacryocystocele, nasolacrimal duct cystocele
- Dacryocystitis

assessing the presence and extent of airway obstruction and in determining extracranial or intracranial approaches for surgical management. CT is the imaging modality of choice to evaluate possible pyriform aperture stenosis, choanal atresia, or anomalies of the nasolacrimal duct. MR imaging is the modality of choice for lesions with potential intracranial extension or associated intracranial anomalies such as congenital midface masses and craniofacial syndromes. Some anomalies, such as sinonasal dysplasias, are best evaluated using combined imaging studies (CT for the face and skull; MRI for the intracranial and soft-tissue anomalies). Midface anomalies are often categorized based on the degree of airway obstruction[57] or on embryogenesis and anatomic location.[58] We will discuss the anomalies based on the primary affected regions: craniofacial, sinonasal, and maxillomandibular. Then, we will discuss some syndromes associated with the following characteristic anomalies: orofacial clefting, hypertelorism, branchial arch anomalies and unusual facies.

Craniofacial Anomalies

Congenital midline nasofrontal masses are rare anomalies, occurring 1:20,000 to 40,000 live births.[59] They are usually obvious at birth, but may manifest at any age. They result from improper regression of the embryologic dural diverticulum from the prenasal space (**Fig. 3-1**). The location and type of mass depends on the nature of the improper regression. Masses can be located intranasally, extranasally, or a combination of both. Intranasal masses involve extension of the dura mater through the foramen cecum into the prenasal space and nasal cavity, whereas glabellar masses involved extension of the diverticulum through the fonticulus frontalis or the foramen cecum.[58] Intracranial extension should be suspected when imaging reveals widening of the foramen cecum and a bifid or dystrophic crista galli.[60] Common midline nasofrontal masses include cephaloceles, demoid/epidermoid cysts, and gliomas[61] (**Table 3-3**).

Cephaloceles

Cephalocele or encephalocele is a generic term for extracranial herniations of brain parenchyma, meninges, or ventricles. During embryonic development, failure of surface ectoderm to separate from the neuroectoderm leads to calvarial or skull base defects that can result in herniation of central nervous system elements (**Figs. 3-3** and **3-4**). In the calvarium, induction of bone formation may be defective, or an intracranial mass may cause pressure erosion. At the skull base, defects may result from

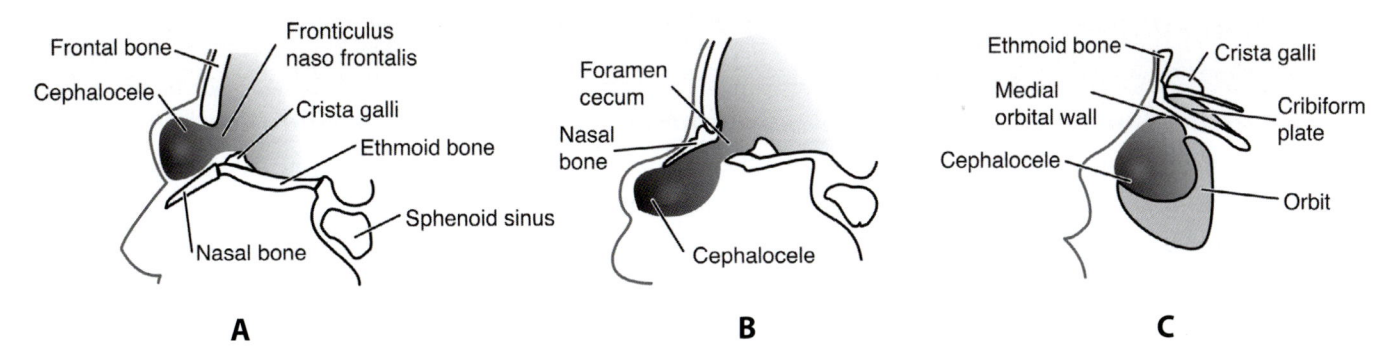

Figure 3-3 Sincipital Cephaloceles
Schematic illustration of sincipital cephaloceles. (**A**) Frontonasal cephalocele extends through the fonticulus frontalis anterior to the nasal bone and crista galli. (**B**) Nasoethmoidal cephalocele extends through the foramen cecum between the nasal bone and crista galli. (**C**) Nasoorbital cephalocele exits through a defect in the medial orbital wall.

faulty closure of the neural tube or failure of basilar ossification.[62] Approximately 90% of the cases are located along the midline. Cephaloceles are classified based on the contents of the herniated sac: *meningoceles* contain meninges; *meningoencephaloceles* (i.e., cephaloceles) contain neural tissue and meninges; and *encephalomeningocystoceles* contain neural tissue, meninges, and ventricular tissue.

Cephaloceles occur in 1:4,000 live births and are typically found in early childhood.[63] Most cases are sporadic, but some are familial or associated with other malformations[64] (**Table 3-4**). Nearly 30% to 40% of cases are associated with other congenital central nervous system anomalies such as microcephaly, micropthalmia, anophthalmia, dysgenesis of the corpus callosum, hydrocephalus, porencephaly, or colpocephaly.

Cephaloceles may be categorized into occipital (75%) (**Fig. 3-5**), frontoethmoidal (13% to 15%), parietal (10% to 12%), and sphenoidal.[62] Alternatively, cephaloceles may be categorized into occipital (75%) and frontal (aka, anterior, nasal) (25%).[65] Frontal types can be further divided into two types: sincipital and basal (**Table 3-5**). In this chapter we will focus on frontal cephaloceles.

Of the frontal cephaloceles, sincipital ones result from bony defects anterior to the cribriform plate in the region of the foramen cecum, producing external herniations subcategorized into three regions: frontonasal, nasoethmoidal, nasoorbital. Basal cephaloceles involve bony defects in the floor of the anterior fossa between the cribriform plate and the anterior clinoid process or through the superior orbital fissure, resulting in internal herniations subcategorized into transethmoidal, sphenoethmoidal, trans-sphenoidal, and sphenomaxillary (**Figs. 3-3, 3-4, and 3-6**).

Cephaloceles are typically soft, compressible, pulsatile masses that transilluminate, enlarge with crying and other Valsalva maneuvers, and have a positive Furstenburg test (bilateral compression of internal jugular veins) due to the intracranial connection. Clinically, patients may have a history of rhinorrhea, recurrent meningitis, a broad nose, or hypertelorism (dystopia canthorum).[66] The prenatal diagnosis of occipital cephaloceles in

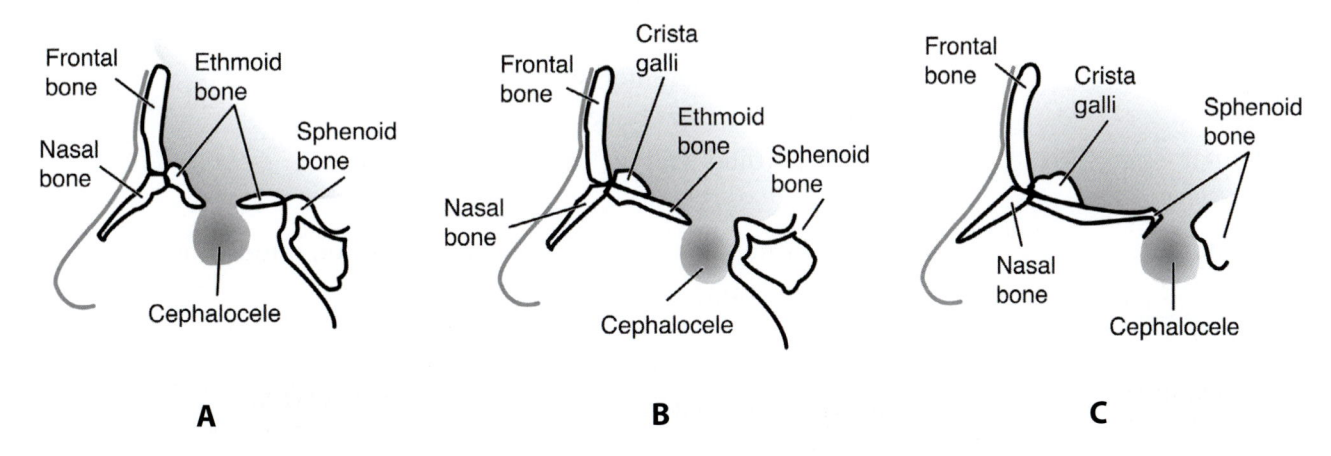

Figure 3-4 Basal Cephaloceles
Schematic illustration of three types of basal cephaloceles. (**A**) Transethmoidal cephalocele extends through the cribriform plate behind the crista galli. (**B**) Sphenoethmoidal cephalocele extends through the suture between the ethmoid and sphenoid sinuses anterior to the pituitary stalk. (**C**) Trans-sphenoidal cephalocele extends through the sella posterior to the pituitary stalk.

Table 3-4 Anomalies Associated with Cephaloceles

Anatomic Anomalies	Syndromes	In Utero Conditions
Dysgenesis of the corpus callosum Orofacial clefting Craniosynostosis (craniostenosis) Hypertelorism Optic nerve and ocular dysplasias Holoprosencephaly Aqueduct stenosis Arnold-Chiari II or III malformation Heterotropic gray matter and other brain migrational anomalies	Cryptophthalmos Dandy-Walker malformation/complex Ehlers-Danlos syndrome Fontonasal dysplasia/median cleft face syndrome Hypothalamic pituitary dysfunction Knobloch syndrome Meckel-Gruber syndrome Roberts syndrome (Roberts-SC phocomelia, hypomelia-hypotrichosis-facial hemangioma, pseudothalidomide syndromes) Trisomy 18 (Edwards syndrome) von Voss syndrome Walker-Warburg syndrome (Chemke, Pagan syndromes)	Amniotic band syndrome Gestational diabetes Maternal warfarin use Rubella

Table 3-5 Classification of Cephaloceles

Type	Site of Herniation	Location of Mass
Occipital (75%) and frontal/anterior/nasal (25%)		
Sincipital	Anterior to cribriform plate	
Frontonasal	Fonticulus nasofrontalis (anterior to crista galli and nasal bone)	Forehead or nasal bridge
Nasoethmoidal	Foramen cecum (anterior to crista galli, behind nasal bone)	Nasal bridge, nasal cavity
Naso-orbital	Medial orbital wall	Orbit
Basal		
Transethmoidal	Cribriform plate	Superior, middle meati
Sphenoethmoidal	Between ethmoid and sphenoid cells	Nasopharynx
Trans-sphenoidal	Sella and sphenoid sinus, craniopharyngeal canal	Nasopharynx
Sphenomaxillary	Ala of sphenoid, superior and inferior orbital fissure	Sphenomaxillary fossa
Spheno-orbital	Superior orbital fissure	Orbit

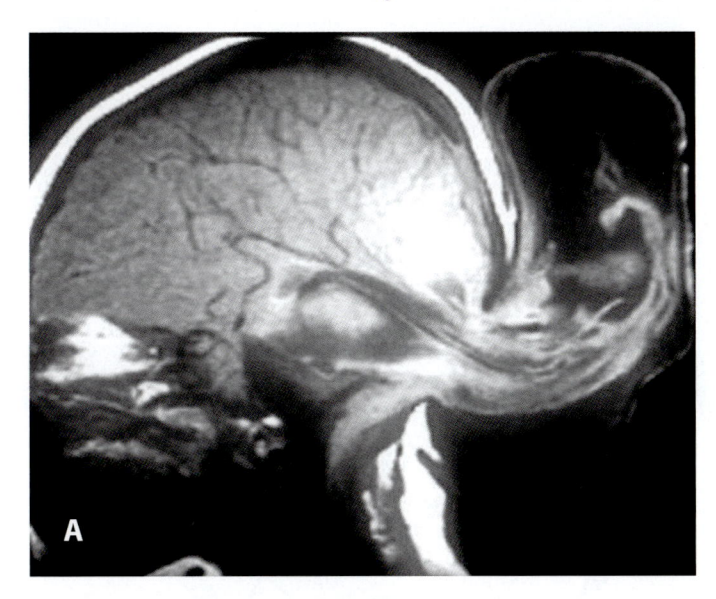

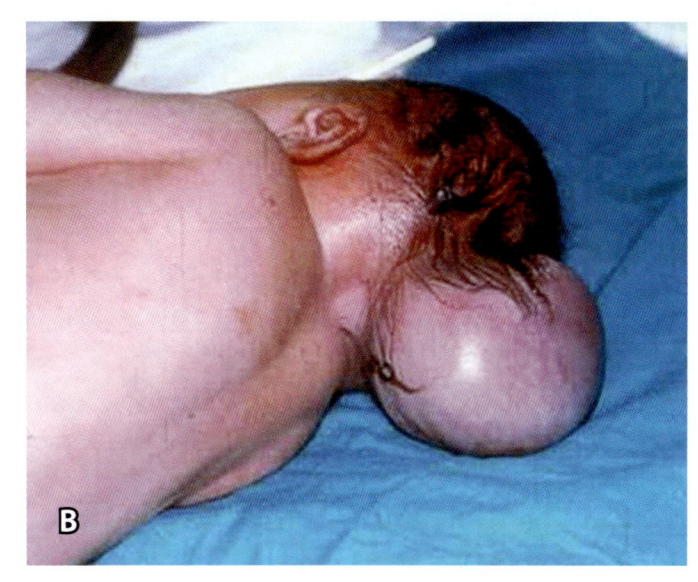

Figure 3-5 Occipital Cephalocele
Sagital T1W MR image (**A**) showing massive herniation of the posterior cerebral and cerebellar structures into a large extracranial cystic cavity. Posterior photograph (**B**) of an infant showing an occipital cephalocele.

the second and third trimester of pregnancy is relatively easy and accurate by ultrasound or MR. But prenatal diagnosis of frontal or parietal cephaloceles is more challenging. Prognosis depends on the location and contents of the herniated sac and the presence of other associated abnormalities. Treatment involves reduction of any herniated brain tissue, resection of protruding dura, closure of dural defects, and osseous repair of bony defects.[62,63]

MR is the imaging modality of choice for evaluating cephaloceles, but CT imaging can help assess the degree of bony defect (**Table 3-6**). The herniated sac typically contains disorganized brain matter, meninges, and/or ventricles and is covered by a CSF-filled space, which may communicate with the subarachnoid space or ventricles of the brain. Attenuation measurements may be used to differentiate brain tissue from CSF within the herniated sac. MR and CT can also be useful in demonstrating associated intracranial anomalies. A dermal defect is frequently present, such as a dermal sinus tract leading from the cranial defect, which may also be associated with an intracranial dermoid cyst. CT cisternography may be useful for identifying the communication with the intracranial subarachnoid space. The differential diagnosis includes tumors, infection, and trauma. Infection and tumors usually show destruction of bone, whereas encephaloceles have smooth, marginated cranial defects.[62]

Frontal Cephaloceles

Frontal (nasal, anterior) cephaloceles can be divided into two types: *sincipital* (60%), which involved the dorsum of nose, orbits, or forehead; and *basal* (40%), which involve the ethmoid and sphenoid sinuses, epipharynx, or orbit (**Table 3-5**).

Sincipital cephalocele
Sincipital cephaloceles typically present as soft compressible masses over the glabella. They can be divided into three subtypes: frontonasal (40% to 60%), nasoethmoidal (30% to 40%), and naso-orbital (5% to 20%).[63]

1. Frontonasal (nasofrontal) cephaloceles exit the cranium anterior to the crista galli and nasal bone through the fonticulus frontalis (between the frontal and nasal bones) into the forehead or nasal bridge. These are subdivided into two types: type I (extranasal) and type II (intranasal) (**Figs. 3-3A**, **3-6**, and **3-7**).
2. Nasoethmoidal cephaloceles exit the cranium through the cribriform plate/ethmoids at the foramen cecum anterior to the crista galli but behind the nasal bone (into the patent prenasal space) (**Figs. 3-3B**, **3-6**, and **3-8**). They can extend into the nasal bridge or nasal cavity.
3. Naso-orbital cephaloceles extend through a defect in the medial orbital wall between the frontal and lacrimal bones (**Figs. 3-3C**, **3-6**, **3-9**, and **3-10**).

Although rare, combinations of the subtypes of sincipital cephaloceles are possible. For example, there are cases of combined frontonasal and naso-orbital cephaloceles (**Fig. 3-3**).

Basal Cephalocele
Depending on their location and size, basal cephaloceles may remain asymptomatic for years. There are five subtypes: transethmoidal, sphenoethmoidal, trans-sphenoidal, and sphenomaxillary, and spheno-orbital. Transethmoidal, sphenoethmoidal, and trans-sphenoidal cephaloceles are sometimes classified as sphenopharygeal cephaloceles because they exit the cranium through or between the ethmoid and sphenoid bones.

Transethmoidal cephaloceles exit through the cribriform plate behind the crista galli into the nasal cavity, extending medial to the middle turbinate into the superior and middle meati (**Figs. 3-4A** and **3-6**).

Sphenoethmoidal cephaloceles exit the cranium through the cribriform plate at the suture between the ethmoid and sphenoid

100 Diagnostic Imaging of the Head and Neck

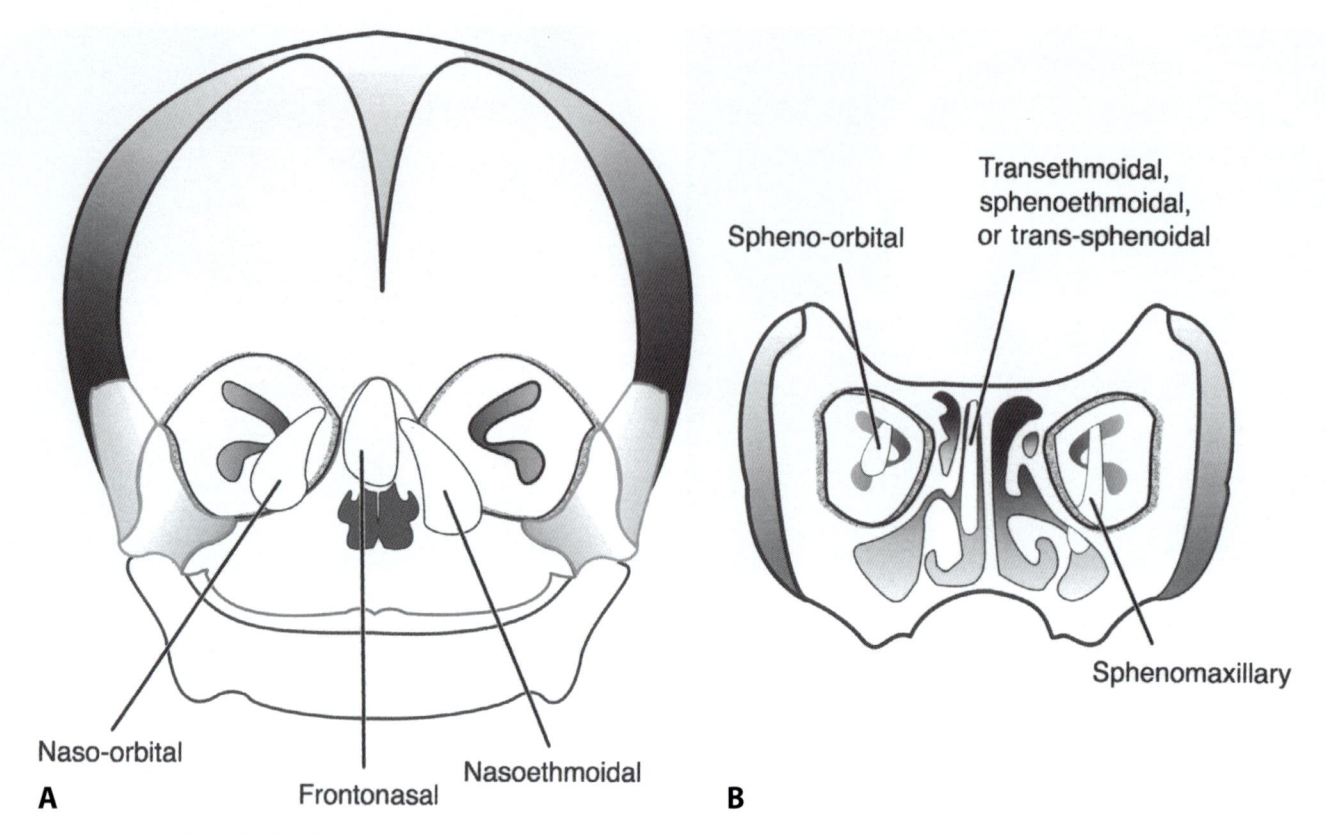

Figure 3-6 Frontal Cephaloceles
Schematic illustration of frontal cephaloceles. (**A**) Sincipital cephaloceles: transethmoidal rests in the forehead/nasal bridge; nasoethmoidal rests in the nasal bridge/cavity; naso-orbital rests in the orbit. (**B**) Basal cephaloceles: transethmoidal rests in the superior/middle meati; sphenoethmoidal rests in the mid nasopharynx; trans-sphenoidal rests in the posterior nasopharynx (not shown); sphenomaxillary (transalar) extends through the superior/inferior orbital fissure and rests in the pterygopalatine fossa; Spheno-orbital extends through the superior orbital fissure and rests in the orbit.

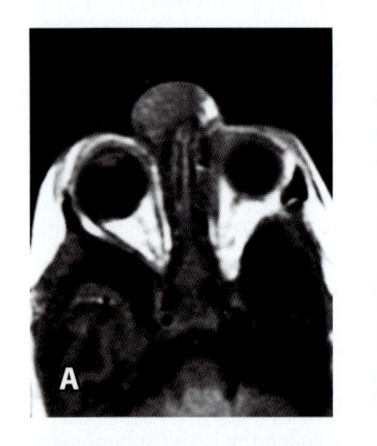

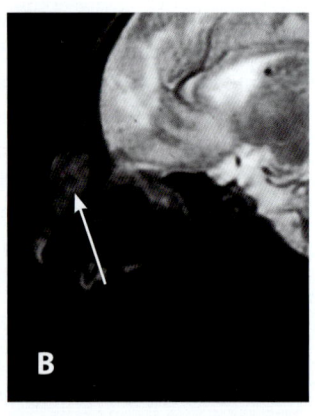

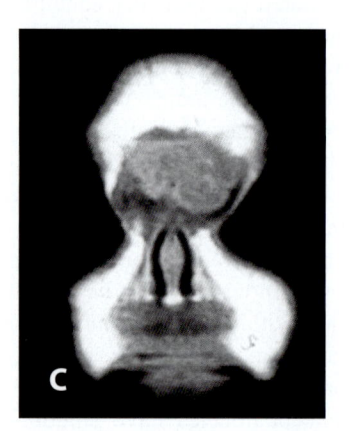

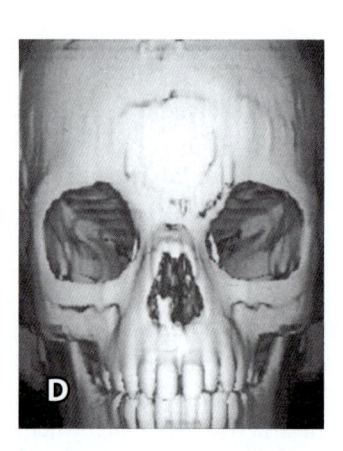

Figure 3-7 Frontonasal Cephalocele
Preop imges (**A–C**) and postop 3D surface rednered CT of a frontonasal cephalocele. Axial T1 MR (**A**) shows a mass bulging above the nasal bones, into the soft tissues of the face. Sagittal T2 MR scan (**B**) shows the contents of the mass to be similar to the intracranial contents. A tiny defect just beneath the frontal bone (*arrow,* **B**) can be seen, connecting the intracranial contents to the nasal mass. Coronal reformatted CT image (**C**) shows a defect in the frontal bone, filled with soft tissue. Postop 3D surface rendered CT (**D**) scan shows a mature skull repair with incorporation of the bone graft into the calvarium.

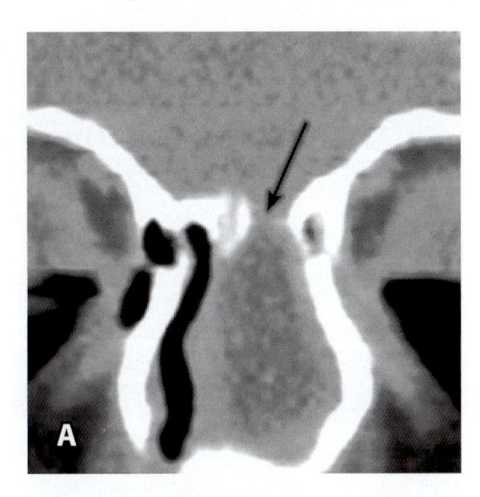

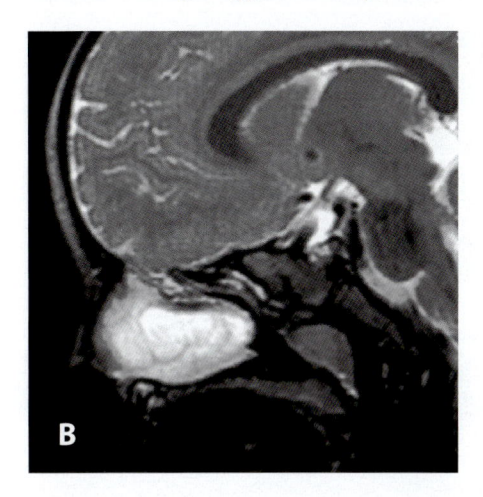

Figure 3-8 Nasoethmoidal Cephalocele
Coronal CT scan of the nasal region (**A**) shows a large defect in the left side of the cribriform plate (*arrow,* **A**) with herniation of the cranial contents into an expanded left nasal cavity. Left paramedian sagittal T2W MR scan (**B**) shows the contents of the cephalocele to be mainly meninges and CSF without any neural structures. (Images courtesy of C. Douglas Phillips, MD, FACR).

sinuses anterior to the pituitary stalk, and extend between the posterior ethmoid and sphenoid sinuses into the nasopharynx (**Figs. 3-4B, 3-6, 3-11**).

Trans-sphenoidal cephaloceles extend through the sella and sphenoid sinus posterior to the pituitary stalk, into the nasopharynx (**Figs. 3-4C** and **3-6**). In infants, it is worthwhile to record the defect in the skull base as well as to demonstrate any intracranial anomalies, both of which are readily detected with MRI (**Fig. 3-12**). Adults presenting with an intranasal mass are often examined by CT (**Fig. 3-13**).

Sphenomaxillary (transalar) cephaloceles exit the cranium through defects in the ala or greater wing of the sphenoid (typically at the superior or inferior orbital fissure) into the sphenomaxillary (pterygopalatine) fossa. There are two types: type I – defect occurs between membranous and cartilaginous portions of the sphenoid bone; type II – defect occurs in the membranous portion (**Figs. 3-6** and **3-14**).

Spheno-orbital cephaloceles extend through the superior orbital fissure into the orbit. This may cause exophthalmos (**Fig. 3-6**).

Nasal Gliomas (Nasal Cerebral Heterotopias)

Nasal gliomas are rare, sporadic, extracranial masses of dysplastic glial tissue from subarachnoid space that separated from the regressing dural diverticulum perhaps during abnormal closure of the fonticulus frontalis (**Fig. 3-15**). They may be cephaloceles that have lost their CSF connection. Nasal gliomas are classified as heterotopias and not neoplasias, because they resemble reactive gliosis in a connective tissue matrix and are benign.

Nasal gliomas can be intranasal (30% within the nasal cavities, mouth, or rarely in the pterigopalatine fossa), extranasal (60% external to the nasal bones and cavities), or both (10% with intra- and extra-nasal components communicating via a defect in the nasal bones or around its edges).[67,68] In 10% to 25% of cases, nasal gliomas are connected to intracranial structures by a stalk or pedicle of glial tissue, usually through a defect in the cribriform plate.[67,69] This helps distinguish it from cephaloceles, which almost always have pedicles[68] (**Table 3-6**).

Clinically, nasal gliomas are nonpulsatile, polypoidal masses that do not enlarge with crying (or other Valsalva maneuvers), do not transilluminate, and do not distend with ipsilateral jugular venous compression (negative Furstenberg sign). They are often unilateral to the right side. Extranasal gliomas are firm, smooth noncompressible masses located anywhere between the glabella and nasal tip, and may have telangiectasias on the overlying skin. Intranasal gliomas are usually attached to the lateral nasal wall near the middle turbinate bone and, less often, the nasal septum. Intranasal gliomas are soft, unencapsulated, pale masses situated between the nasal bones and nasal capsule, and may protrude from the nostril. They may grow in parallel with the brain.[58,60]

Nasal gliomas can cause remodeling of the adjacent bones, and may be associated with broadening of the nasal bridge or hypertelorism.[60,70] Rarely, nasal gliomas extend into the orbit, frontal sinus, nasopharynx, or oral cavity. Obstruction of the nasal passage and nasolacrimal duct can lead to respiratory distress and epiphora. Complications like CSF rhinorrhoea, meningitis, or epistaxis can also develop.[71] Treatment involves complete excision of the mass.

On imaging, nasal gliomas appear as nonenhancing soft-tissue masses at the glabella or nasal cavity (**Table 3-6**). On CT images, they are isodense. Cystic changes may occasionally occur, but calcifications are rarely present. Nasal gliomas can deform the bones of the nasal fossa and may extend into the glabella, nasal bones, cribriform plate, or foramen cecum. They rarely attach to the nasal septum. On MR images, they may appear isointense to hypointense, and occasionally hyperintense, to cerebral gray matter with T1-weighted sequences; and hyperintense with proton-density-weighted and T2-weighted sequences (**Fig. 3-16**). The presence of a pedicle and/or adjacent CSF space, which are more commonly found with cephaloceles, helps distinguish nasal gliomas from cephaloceles.

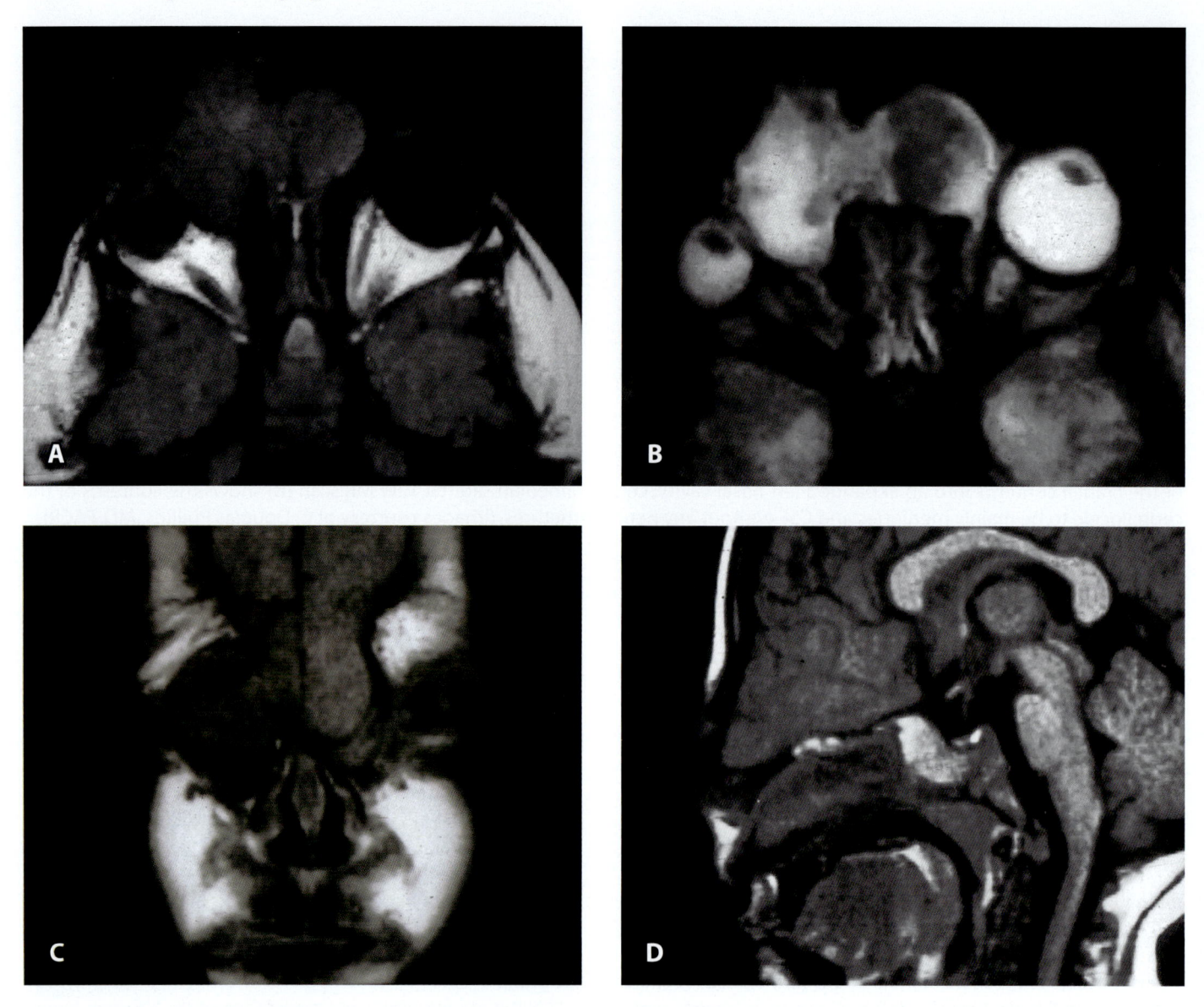

Figure 3-9 Combined Frontonasal and Naso-orbital Cephalocele
Axial T1W (**A**) and T2W (**B**) MR scans show a lobular mixed-intensity mass extending forward through the frontal region into the upper face and right orbit. The frontal lobe and meninges have both herniated out of the cranial cavity. Note the microophthalmia on the right side and the hypertelorism. Coronal T1 MR (**C**) clearly shows bilateral frontal lobe gyri herniating through the defect above the nose and into the right orbit. Sagittal T1W MR (**D**) shows the absent bony structures between the frontal bone and the planum sphenoidale, through which the brain has herniated.

CT cisternography may occasionally be required to show adjacent CSF space.[68]

Dermoid, Epidermoid Cysts, and Fistulas

Dermoids and epidermoids are epithelial-lined cavities or sinus tracts with variable numbers of skin appendages. They likely result from desquamation of cells from the dermis and epidermis lining the tract as the regressing dural diverticulum pulls skin elements into the prenasal space[72,73] (**Fig. 3-17**). Epidermoid cysts contain only ectodermal elements and are almost always superficial, producing a sessile, white or yellow-white nodule with or without a pore, located paramidline near the columella. Dermoid cysts (nasal dermal sinus cysts) and dermal fistulas can contain hair follicles, sebaceous glands, and eccrine glands, and usually present as a nasal pit or mass located at the midline near the glabella. A dermal sinus tract, cyst, or epidermoid cyst may form anywhere along the course of the dural diverticulum.[74,96,102] In 57% of cases, there is intracranial extension.[102]

Clinically, dermoid and epidermoid cysts appear as single or multiple firm, nonpulsatile lesions that do not transilluminate, do not change in size with crying or the Furstenberg test (compression of the jugular veins).[58,60] In up to 84% of dermoid or epidermoid cysts and dermal sinus tracts, the skin surface will have a dimple, tuft of hair, or opening that may discharge a

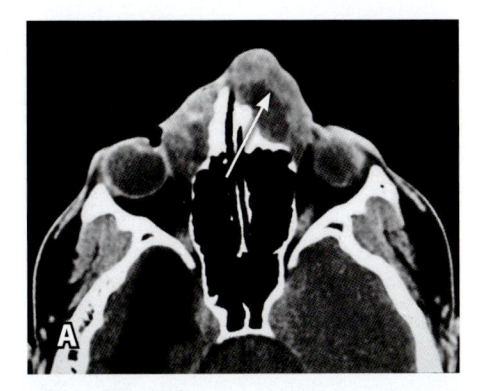

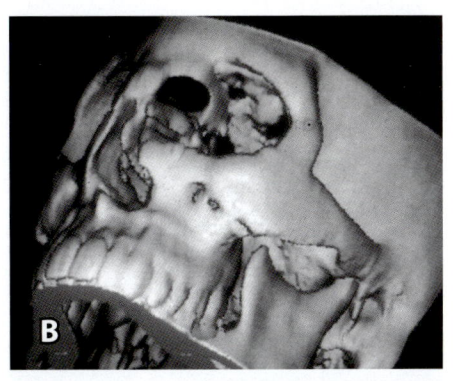

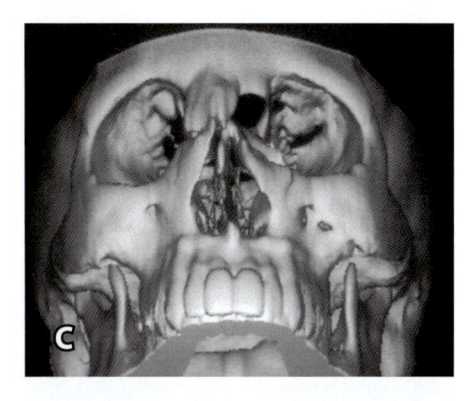

Figure 3-10 Nasoorbital Cephalocele
Axial NECT (**A**) shows herniation of a heterogenous lobular mass through the frontal region and into both orbits with a distinct fat–fluid level (*arrow*, **A**). Note the hypertelorism and the left microophthalmia, which are both commonly associated with the lesion. 3D CT reconstruction (**B–C**) show the large bony defect in the medial portion of the left orbit through which the herniation has occurred.

cheesy, sebaceous material.[61] Complications include infection of the sinus tract or cyst, orbital/periorbital cellulitis, osteomyelitis, meningitis, or brain abscess.[63] Treatment involves complete resection of the cyst, which may be delayed until 2 to 5 years of age if no complications arise.[58] Knowledge of any intracranial extension is critical in planning the surgical approach. Incomplete resection may lead to recurrence or meningitis in up to 15% of cases.[60]

Both MR and CT imaging can be helpful in evaluating dermoids and epidermoids (**Table 3-6**). Imaging may show fusiform swelling within the nasal septum, widening of the nasal vault, bifid septum, glabellar destruction, bony proliferation above cyst level, and large ethmoidal cystic spaces[63] (**Fig. 3-18**). Intracranial extension should be suspected if there is widening of the foramen cecum and crista galli involvement. CT demonstrating an intracranial mass, widened foramen cecum, and bifid crista galli is diagnostic for intracranial extension; nonetheless, MRI is recommended in all children with dermoid sinus cysts and those adults with suspected intracranial extension.[75]

Although dermoid and epidermoid cysts share some similar characteristics on imaging, there are some distinguishing features. Dermoid cysts are usually located in the midline and are more fatty, producing a strikingly hyperintense signal on T1-weighted and high signal intensity on fat-suppressed T2-weighted MR images. T1- and T2-hyperintense intralesional signals indicate fatty inclusions of dermoid cysts. Epidermoid cysts usually have fluid attenuation on CT and are

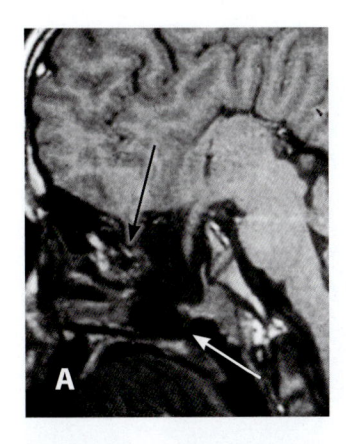

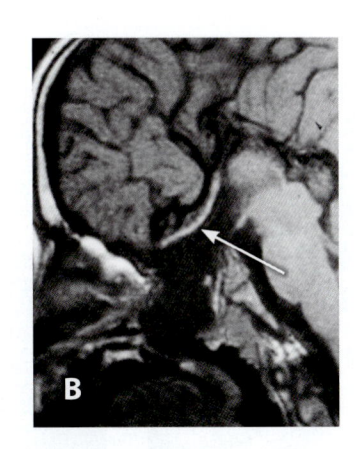

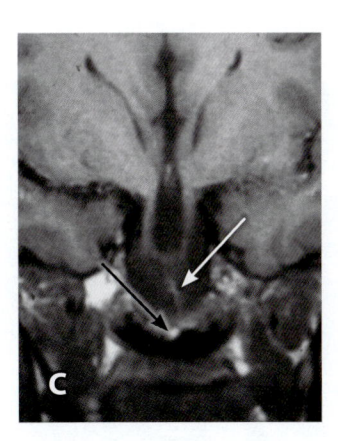

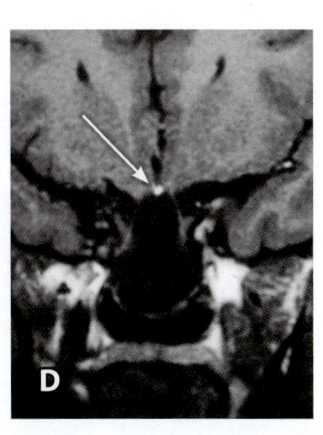

Figure 3-11 Sphenoethmoidal Cephalocele
Sagittal T1W MR images (**A** and **B**) show a defect between the sphenoid and ethmoid bone that incorporates the sella and sellar contents with downward extension of the hypothalamus and optic chiasm (*black arrow*, **A**). The cystic mass extends downward to the level of the hard palate (*white arrow*, **A**). Note the marked dysgenesis of the corpus callosum. Just beneath the anterior remnant of the corpus callosum, there is a curvilinear structure representing the anterior commisure (*arrow*, **B**). Coronal T1W images (**C** and **D**) show the marked downward displacement of the third ventricle, hypothalamus, and pituitary stalk (*white arrow*, **C**) with a remnant of the pituitary gland lying within the outline of the nasopharynx (*black arrow*, **C**). Note the pituitary bright spot lying superiorly between the downwardly displaced optic nerves and chiasm (*arrow*, **D**).

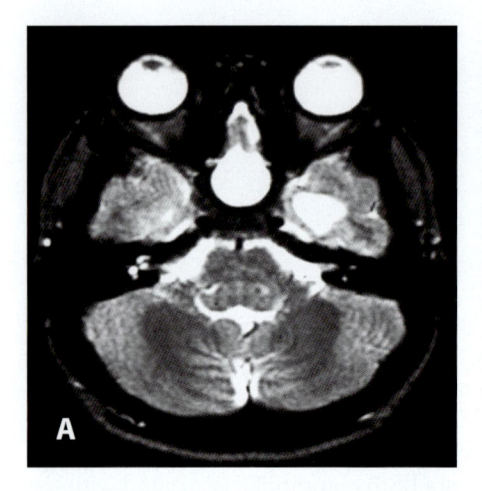

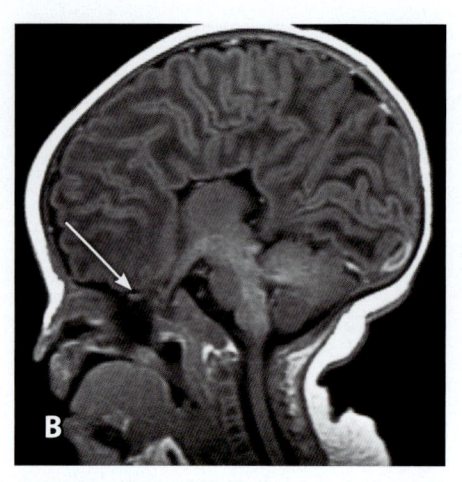

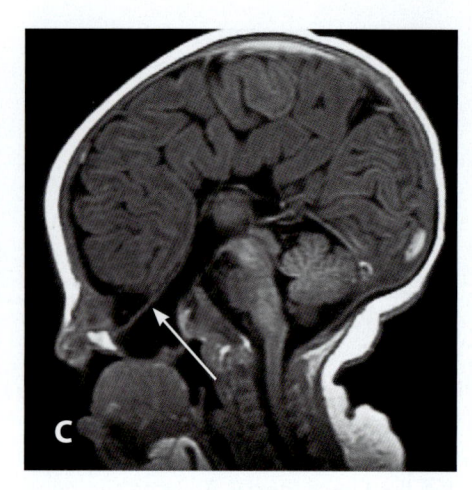

Figure 3-12 Trans-sphenoidal Cephalocele in an Infant
Axial T2W MR scan (**A**) shows a well-marginated heterogenous, high signal CSF in the sphenoid region with moderate hypertelorism. Sagittal T1W MR scans (**B** and **C**) show a downwardly-displaced optic chiasm (*arrow*, **B**) and a dark signal, sharply-demarcated CSF herniation through a large defect in the phenoid bone (**C**). Also note the downward displacement of the anterior commisure (*arrow*, **C**) and dysgenesis of corpus callosum.

iso- to marginally hyperintense to fluid on T1- and T2-weighted MR images. Bony erosion may or may not be present. Dermoid and epidermoid cysts are usually associated with dermal sinus tracts. Intracranial dermal sinus tracts have high signal intensity on T1-weighted and fat-suppressed T2-weighted MR images (**Table 3-6**).

Intracranial epidermoid lesions may pose a diagnostic challenge as they can mimic arachnoid cysts. Intracranial arachnoid cysts are solid masses that can be identified on MR imaging with diffusion-weighted or magnetization transfer sequences. Intracranial epidermoid cysts appear similar to brain matter and have characteristics of solid tissue on diffusion-weighted images. Magnetization transfer sequences will demonstrate magnetization transfer from the solid epidermoid cyst to adjacent free water, which is not seen in fluid-containing lesions such as arachnoid cysts.[58]

Orofacial, Midface Clefts

Orofacial clefts are defects in the upper lip, alveolar ridge, and/or palate due to failure of normal mesodermal migration or fusion of the maxillary and medial nasal processes and/or the palatal shelves around the fourth gestational week.[76,77] This heterogeneous group of defects include typical orofacial clefts such as unilateral or bilateral cleft lip, combined cleft lip and palate, and cleft palate; and atypical clefts including median, transverse, oblique, and other Tessier types of facial

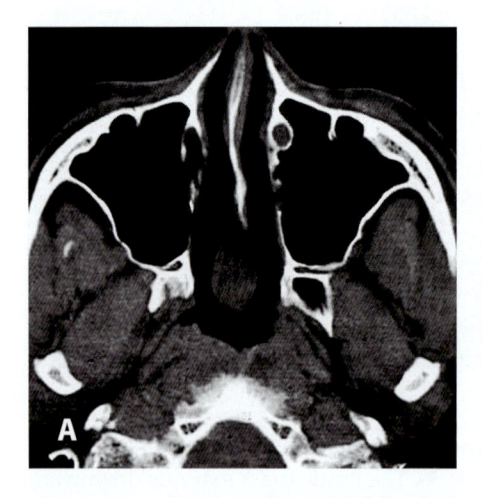

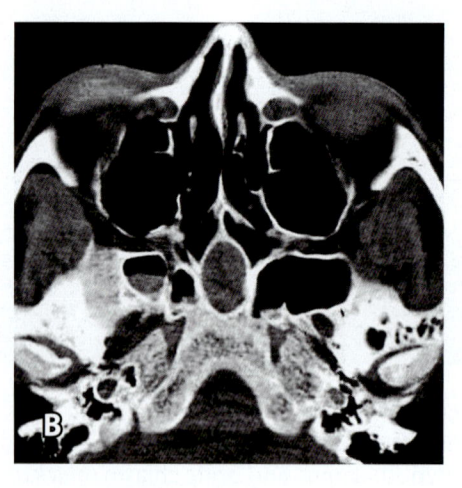

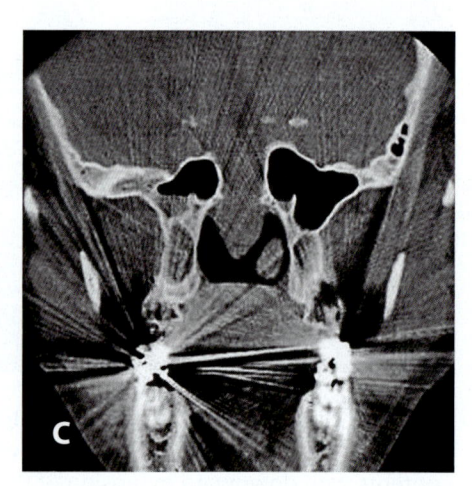

Figure 3-13 Trans-sphenoidal Cephalocele in an Adult
Axial CT scans (**A** and **B**) through the skull base a show a sharply demarcated mass lying within the nasopharynx, behind the nasal septum. The defect through the body of the sphenoid bone is well-corticated, without erosion or destruction, consistent with the congenital nature of the mass. Coronal CT scan (**C**) shows the separation of the lateral portions of the sphenoid sinuses, in between which lies herniated central brain contents. Again, note well-corticated bony margins.

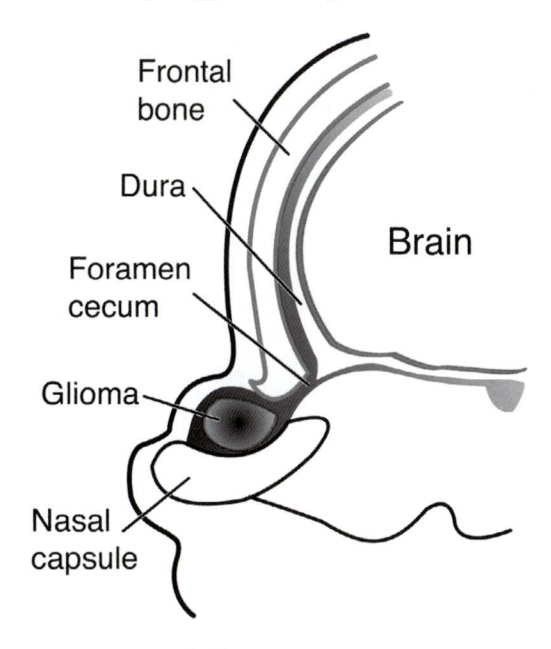

Figure 3-15 Nasal Gliomas
Nasal gliomas result when glial tissue separates from the regressing dural diverticulum. Gliomas may be intranasal, extranasal, or both. Occasionally, they are connected to intracranial structures by a pedicle that extends through the foramen cecum.

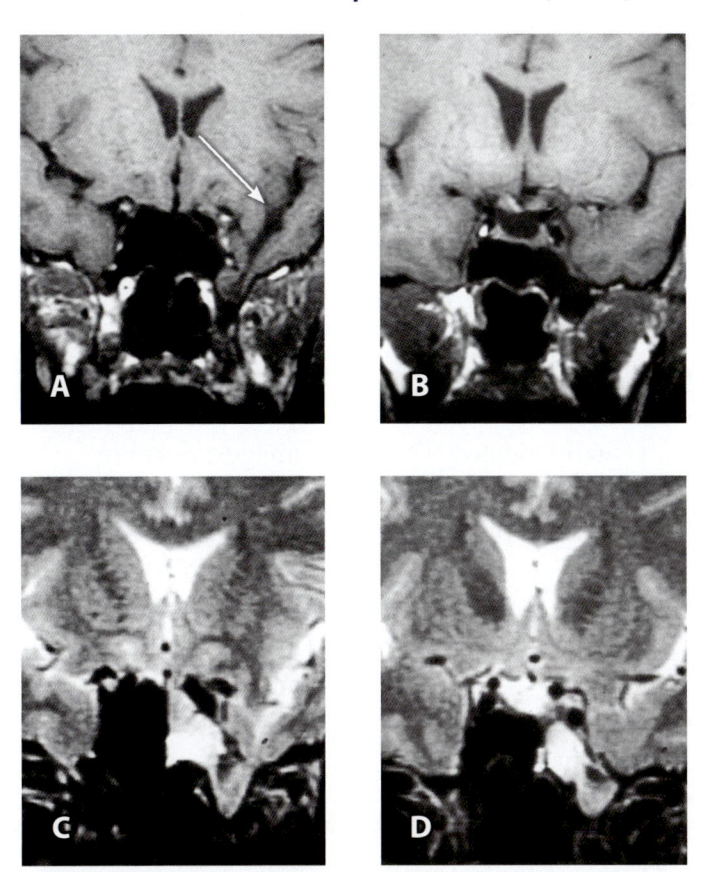

Figure 3-14 Transalar Cephalocele
Coronal T1W MR images (**A** and **B**) show a cystic lesion filling the left side of the sphenoid sinus and extending through a defect in the middle portion of the floor of the left middle cranial fossa, into the pterygoid region. T2W coronal scans (**C** and **D**) clearly show the contents of the cystic lesion to be cranial structures extending downward the defect in the medial portion of the floor of the left middle cranial fossa. Note the distortion of the left sylvian fissure towards the defect (*arrow*, **A**). (Case courtesy of Wally Peck, MD).

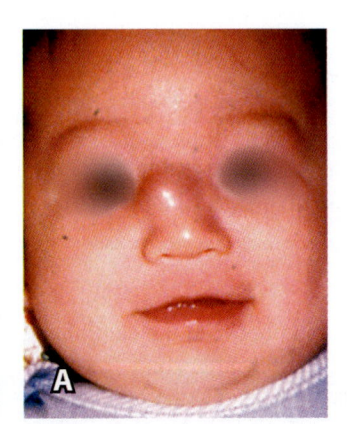

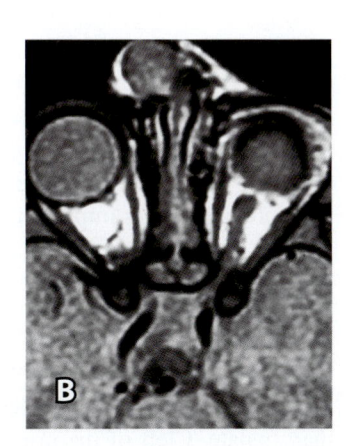

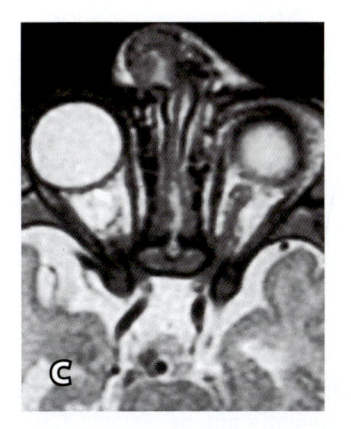

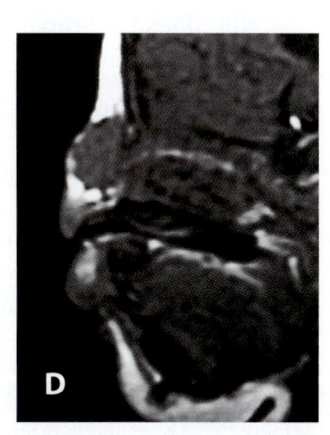

Figure 3-16 Nasal Glioma
Photograph of an infant (**A**) shows a soft-tissue mass located on the bridge of the nose. Axial T2W MR scans (**B–C**) show the soft-tissue mass immediately to the right of the nasal septum, showing signal and morphology characteristics identical to cortical gray matter. Midsagittal T1W MR (**D**) shows the location of the mass beneath the frontal bone and superior to the nasal bone.

Table 3-6 Comparison of Nasal Gliomas, Cephalocele, Dermoids, and Epidermoids

Gliomas	Cephalocele	Dermoids	Epidermoids
• Nonenhancing soft-tissue masses at glabella (extranasal), or nasal cavity medial to middle turbinate (intranasal), or both • MR: Hyperintense on T2-weighted and proton-density-weighted images; hypo-, iso- or hyper-intense to gray matter on T1-weighted images • CT: Isodense • May see cystic changes • Calcifications are rare • Stalk or pedicle is rare (15%) • May see bone remodeling, hypertelorism • Can extend into glabella, nasal bones, cribriform plate, or foramen cecum • Negative Furstenberg, firm, nonpulsatile, does not transilluminate	• Usually see adjacent CSF space and communication of herniated sac with intracranial subarachnoid space on MR and CT • MR: Contents of herniated sac may include CSF, brain tissue, ventricles • Usually connected to brain parenchyma via stalk/pedicle, dermal sinus tract • Sincipital: external herniations • Basal: internal herniations • May mimic nasal polyps, which are rare in infants • May see bone remodeling, hypertelorism • Positive Furstenburg, soft, pulsatile, expands with Valsalva, transilluminates	• MR: Markedly hyperintense on T1-weighted and fat-suppressed T2-weighted images • Fatty with fatty inclusions • Usually located midline near glabella with nasal pit or mass • Usually associated with dermal sinus tracts • Intracranial extension may be present • Bony erosion may be present • Firm, nonpulsatile, does not transilluminate, negative Furstenberg, negative Valsalva	• MR: Iso- to slightly hyperintense to fluid on T1-weighted and T2-weighted images; similar to brain matter, solid tissue on diffusion-weighted images; positive magnetization transfer • CT: Fluid attenuation • Usually located paramidline near columella • Usually associated with dermal sinus tracts • Intracranial extension may be present • Bony erosion may be present • Firm, nonpulsatile, does not transilluminate, negative Furstenberg, negative Valsalva

CSF = cerebrospinal fluid.

clefts.[78] Up to 70% of orofacial clefts are nonsyndromic and occur as isolated anomalies. About 30% are syndromic cases that can be divided based on etiology into one of three categories: 1) Mendelian syndromes (more than 350 known), 2) chromosomal anomalies, and 3) in utero exposure to teratogens (**Table 3-7**).[79]

In the United States, clefts occur in 1:500 to 1,000 live births, making it the one of the most common major birth defects.[78,80] They occur more frequently among Asians, Latinos, and Native Americans, and affect boys more often than girls. The causes include genetic and environmental factors. Cleft lip can be diagnosed using ultrasound (US) in the second trimester of pregnancy. Cleft palate is more difficult to diagnose by US unless the cleft is large. However, 3D imaging with prenatal US is improving the diagnosis of cleft palate in a fetus.[77]

Cleft Lip and Palate

Cleft lip usually occurs at the junction between the central and lateral parts of the upper lip. The cleft may affect only the upper lip, or it may extend more deeply into the maxilla and the primary palate. Cleft of the primary palate includes cleft lip and cleft of the alveolus.[77] *Cleft palate* is a partial or total lack of fusion of the palatal shelves or processes. Unilateral clefts are nine times more common than bilateral clefts and occur twice as frequently on the left side as on the right. Combined cleft lip

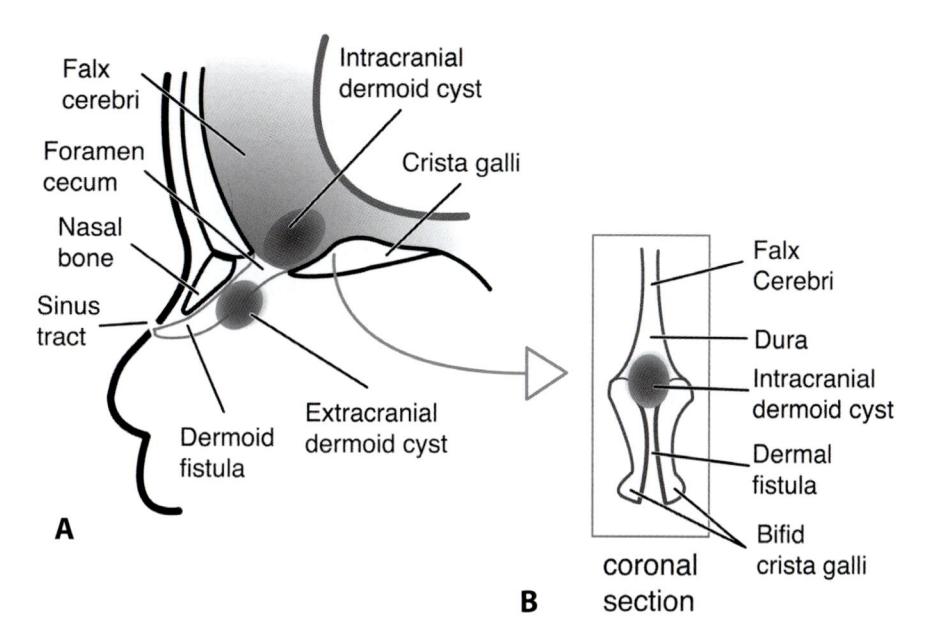

Figure 3-17 Nasal Dermoid, Epidermoid Cysts, Fistulas
Fistulas, dermoid and epidermoid cysts form when the regressing dural diverticulum pulls skin elements into the prenasal space. Dermoid and epidermoid cysts are usually associated with dermal sinus tracts. Epidermoid cysts (not shown) are typically superficial nodules located paramidline near the columella. (**A**) Dermoid cysts and fistulas or tracts may form anywhere along the course of the dural diverticulum, extracranial or intracranial. (**B**) Coronal view of an intracranial cyst with characteristic widening of the foramen cecum and bifid crista galli.

and palate is the most common presentation (50%), followed by isolated cleft palate (30%), and isolated cleft lip or cleft lip and alveolus (20%). Less than 10% of clefts are bilateral. Girls more often than boys have cleft palate without a cleft lip.[81,82] Of the multiple classification systems, the Kernohan system considers the lip, alveolus, and palate, and uses the incisive foramen as the boundary between clefts of the primary palate (lip and premaxilla) and those of the secondary palate.

Approximately 50% to 70% of cases of cleft lip/palate are not associated with a syndrome.[83] Clefts of the secondary palate alone are more likely to be associated with syndromes than are clefts involving the lip alone or the lip and palate. The most common associated syndrome is van der Woude syndrome (**Table 3-7**). An abnormal karyotype is found in 8% to 15% of cases of bilateral cleft lip and palate.[84,85] Trisomy 13 and 18 produce more severe clefts than those with normal karyotype.

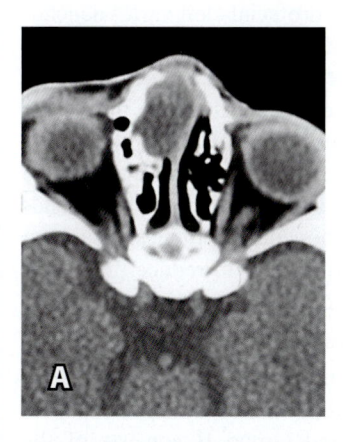

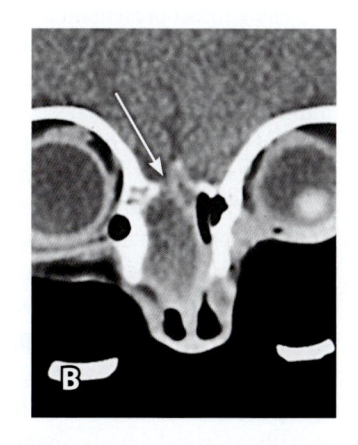

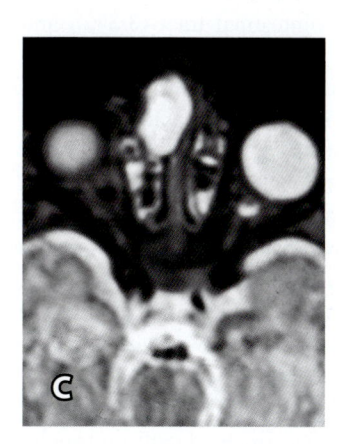

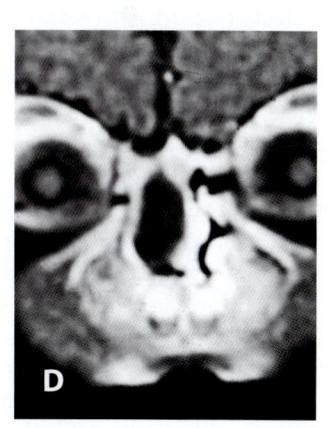

Figure 3-18 Nasal Dermoid Cyst
Axial NECT (**A**) shows a well-demarcated soft-tissue mass on the right side of the nasal cavity with displacement of the nasal septum to the left. Coronal NECT (**B**) show a soft-tissue mass extending through the right side of the cribriform plate. Note that the oriface is the size of a normal foramen cecum (*arrow*, **B**), whereas a nasoethmoidal cephalocele would expand the bony defect to approximate the size of the brain herniation. Axial T2 MR (**C**) shows a fairly intense signal within the soft-tissue mass, reflecting nonoily epidermal elements. Coronal postcontrast MR (**D**) showing nonenhancement of the contents of the cyst, reflecting its epidermal elements. Enhancement would suggest a neoplasm, such as a teratoma.

Table 3-7 Conditions Associated with Orofacial Clefting

Syndromes	Chromosomal Syndromes and Anatomic Anomalies
• Crouzon syndrome • Fraser syndrome • Fryns syndrome • Goldenhar syndrome [Oculo-auriculo-vertebral (OAV) dysplasia] • Orofacial-digital syndrome type I (Gorlin syndrome I, Gorlin-Psaume syndrome, Papillon-leage syndrome) • Orofacial-digital syndrome type II (Mohr syndrome, Mohr-Claussen syndrome) • Pai syndrome (with bifid nose) • Pierre-Robin sequence • Popliteal pterygium syndrome • Roberts syndrome • Treacher Collins syndrome (mandibulofacial dysostosis) • Van der Woude syndrome • Waardenburg syndrome	• Group A craniofacial dysraphisms • Median cleft syndrome (frontonasal dysplasia) • Bifid nose • Choanal atresia • Median mandibular defects • Orofacial clefts (typical, lateral, oblique) • Tetrasomy 9p • Trisomy 13 (Patau syndrome) • Trisomy 18 (Edwards syndrome) • Trisomy 4p
	Maternal Exposure
	• Retinoic acid • Phenytoin • Alcohol • Smoking

In cases with normal karyotype, the risk of an associated anatomic abnormality increases with the severity of the cleft. Twenty percent of patients with bilateral cleft lip/palate will have other anatomic abnormalities compared with 5% of those with unilateral cleft lip.[86] The most common associated anatomic abnormalities are facial (11.1%), central nervous system (8.5%), skeletal (7.8%), urogenital (6.3%), cardiovascular defects (e.g., ASD) (4.6%), gastrointestinal tract (3.3%), and eye anomalies (2.6%).[81,85]

The severity of clefting varies widely from microform, incomplete, to complete clefts. *Microform clefts* are characterized by a vertical groove and vermillion notching or a small coloboma in the lower portion of the lip with varying degrees of lip shortening. An *incomplete cleft* lip can have varying degrees of lip disruption with an intact nasal sill or a Simonart band (a band of fibrous tissue from the edge of the lip to the nostril floor). *Complete clefts* of the lip are characterized by disruption of the lip, alveolus, and nasal sill. The vermillion is distorted upward toward the nasal sill along the cleft. The upper lip muscle fails to decussate at the lip's midline but instead travels parallel to the cleft to insert at the alar base, resulting in the orbicularis bulge. Bilateral cleft lip usually involves the palate as well, with deficient vermillion and prolabial tissue, which lacks underlying muscle. The position of the premaxilla may vary. In *combined cleft lip and palate*, the cleft line continues from the foramen incisivum through the sutura palatina in the middle of the palate[77,82,87] (**Fig. 3-19**).

Unilateral or bilateral *cleft nose* is associated with varying degrees of bony deficiency of the maxilla with deflection of the nasal septum and bony pyramid toward the cleft side and displaced alar base(s).[87]

A transverse facial cleft (*macrostomia*) results from faulty union of the maxillary and mandibular processes in the formation of the corner of the mouth. It may be unilateral or bilateral and may be an isolated anomaly or part of a syndrome such as hemifacial microsomia.

The clinical presentation of an orofacial cleft varies depending on the degree of clefting. Feeding, speech, dental, and orthodontic problems may be present depending on the degree of midface deformity, dental occlusion, and eustachian tube function. Palatal clefts are often associated with persistent otitis media and middle ear effusions. Management approaches depend on the extent of clefting and displacement and involvement of surrounding structures. For wider clefts, orthopedic techniques or surgical lip adhesion may be used prior to surgery to reduce the width. Because each cleft is unique, surgical repair is individualized.[81,82]

Midline Cleft Lip and Craniofacial Dysraphisms

There are two groups of midline craniofacial dysraphisms: Group A includes midline clefts that involve the upper lip with or without nasal involvement; and Group B consists of the median cleft face syndrome, which involves clefts that affect the nose with or without upper lip and forehead involvement.[87] Numerous facial cleft classification systems exist, including the Sedano, DeMyer, and Tessier classifications.

Group A: Group A craniofacial dysraphisms are associated with basal cephaloceles, holoprosencephaly, agenesis (and less

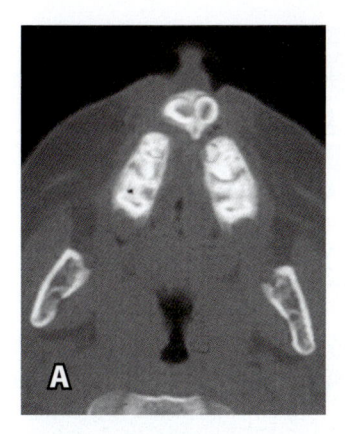

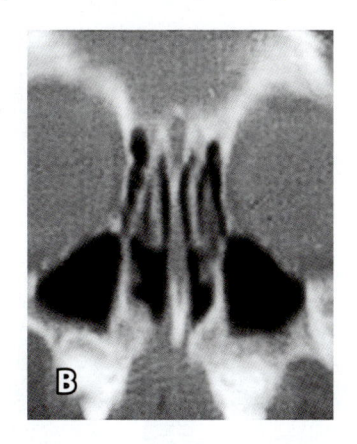

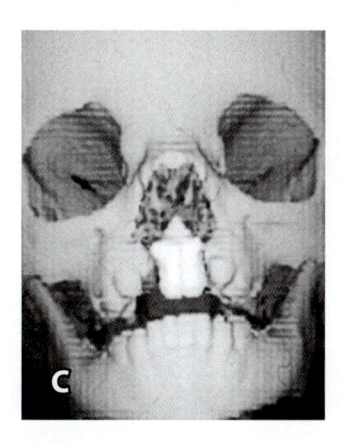

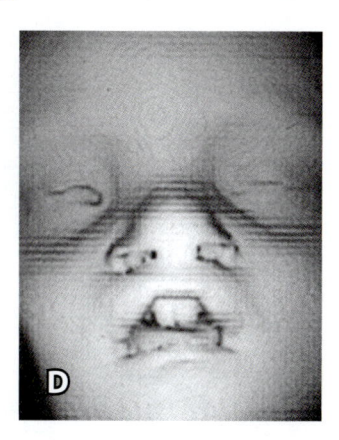

Figure 3-19 Cleft Palate and Paramedian Clefts of the Alveolar Ridges
Axial NECT (**A**) shows bilateral clefting between the premaxilla and alveolar ridges. Coronal reformatted NECT (**B**) shows a cleft palate with soft-tissue contiguity between the oral cavity and the nasal cavities. 3D NECT with surface rendering (**C**) shows excess bone structure extending upward in the midline of the nasal vestibule with associated widening of the nasal aperture. 3D NECT with bone and soft-tissue rendering (**D**) shows surface skin covering the defect. However, the thickening of the nasal frenulum and widening of the nasal apertures is aparent.

commonly lipomas) of the corpus callosum, and optic nerve dysplasias, such as optic pits, colobomas, and morning glory disc. Median cleft lip is a rare anomaly accounting for 0.4% of craniofacial clefts.[88] Characteristics include hypertelorism with an upper labial defect that can range from a small lip notch, to a triangular deficiency of the midline vermillion, to a complete linear cleft. This defect can occur as part of the orofacial-digital syndromes I or II.[87]

Group B: *Median cleft face syndrome (or frontonasal dysplasia)* is a rare form of dysraphism characterized by hypertelorism, median cleft nose (with or without midline cleft of the lip, premaxilla, and palate), broad nasal root, and cranium bifidum occultum frontalis (deficit in midline frontal bone). There may also be typical clefts of the lip and/or palate, nasal alar notching or clefting, low-set ears, telecanthus, ocular colobomas, microphthalmia, and meningoencephalocele. Associated malformations include lipoma or agenesis of corpus callosum, calcified falx, interhemispheric lipoma, tibial hypoplasia, polydactyly, epibulbar dermoids, ear tags, tetrology of Fallot, and syndromes such as Gorlin-Goldenhar and Pai[89–93,101] (**Table 3-7**).

Imaging features include hypertelorism, broad nasal root, and facial clefting (**Figs. 3-20** and **3-21**). There may also be intracranial calcifications related to interhemispheric lipomas and/or calcification of the anterior falx, which appears as a thick frontal crest.[89,94,102]

Bifid Nose

The bifid nose, or median cleft of the nose, is a rare anomaly within the spectrum of midline facial anomalies. It is frequently associated with other congenital malformations including brain anomalies, hypertelorism or pseudohypertelorism, and midline clefts of the lip. It may be associated with frontonasal dysplasia or Pai syndrome, but an autosomal dominant form of bifid nose without hypertelorism has also been proposed.[93,95] The presentation of a bifid nose ranges from a minimally noticeable central groove in a broadened nasal tip due to separation of the alar cartilage, to total clefting of the osteocartilaginous framework, resulting in two complete half noses. The nasal spine is typically absent or deficient, and the upper lip is commonly pulled upward with or without clefting.[96] Treatment involves reconstructive surgery.

Sinonasal Anomalies

Choanal Atresia and Stenosis

Choanal atresia is the most common congenital anomaly of the nasal cavity and the most common cause of neonatal nasal obstruction. Its incidence is 1:5,000 to 8,000 live births, with girls affected 2 to 5 times as often as boys.[58,97,98] In normal embryonic development, the fused palatal processes should rupture around day 38 to form the choanae (posterior nares). Because the primitive posterior choanae are located more anteriorly than the later, definitive choanae, choanal atresia may be positioned quite anteriorly. Some of the proposed theories regarding the etiology of choanal atresia include persistence of the buccopharyngeal membrane, failure of the bucconasal membrane of Hochstetter to rupture, medial outgrowth of vertical and horizontal processes of the palatine bone, abnormal mesodermal adhesions forming in the choanal area, and misdirection of mesodermal flow due to local factors.[99]

Choanal atresia is classified into three types. Type I is osseous or bony, which involves osseous fusion of the vomer and palatine plates due to incomplete canalization of the choanae. Type II is membranous, which results from incomplete resorption of epithelial plugs (**Fig. 3-22**). Type III is mixed or osseo-membranous atresia[100] (**Figs. 3-23** and **3-24**). The incidence of each type varies widely in the literature, but most atresias are at least partly bony.

Choanal atresia may be unilateral or bilateral. Bilateral choanal atresia (25% to 50% of cases of choanal atresias) can lead to acute respiratory failure in infants unless promptly diagnosed and the airway stabilized. Initial treatment options include

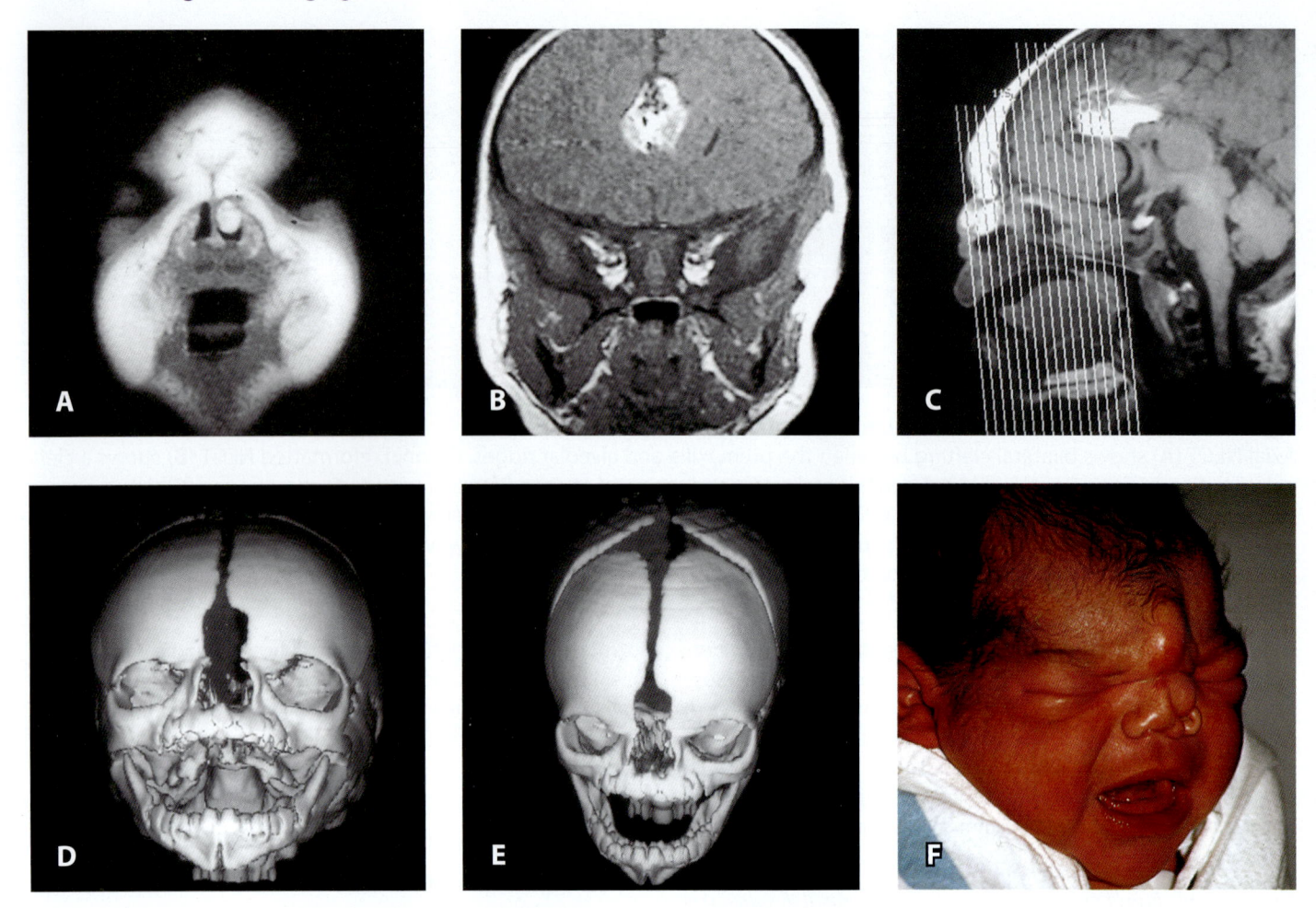

Figure 3-20 Median Cleft Face Syndrome in an Infant
Coronal (**A–B**) and sagittal (**C**) T1W MR images show a rounded soft-tissue mass extending into the left nasal vestibule (**A**). A separate similar intensity mass occupies the midline of both hemispheres in the region of the rostrum of the corpus callosum (**B–C**). Both of these lesions have fat intesity signal, characterstic of a dermoid with oily contents. There is severe callosal dysplasia (**B–C**). 3D NECT with surface rendering (**D–E**) shows wide cranioschisis of the midface with separation of the midline structures in contiguity with the meitopic and sagittal sutures. There is also partial separation of the midline of the mandible and a cleft palate, as well. Photograph of infant (**F**) shows a clefting of the nose and forehead with expansion of the cranial contents through the chranioschisis during crying. (Case courtesy of Mauricio Castillo, MD.)

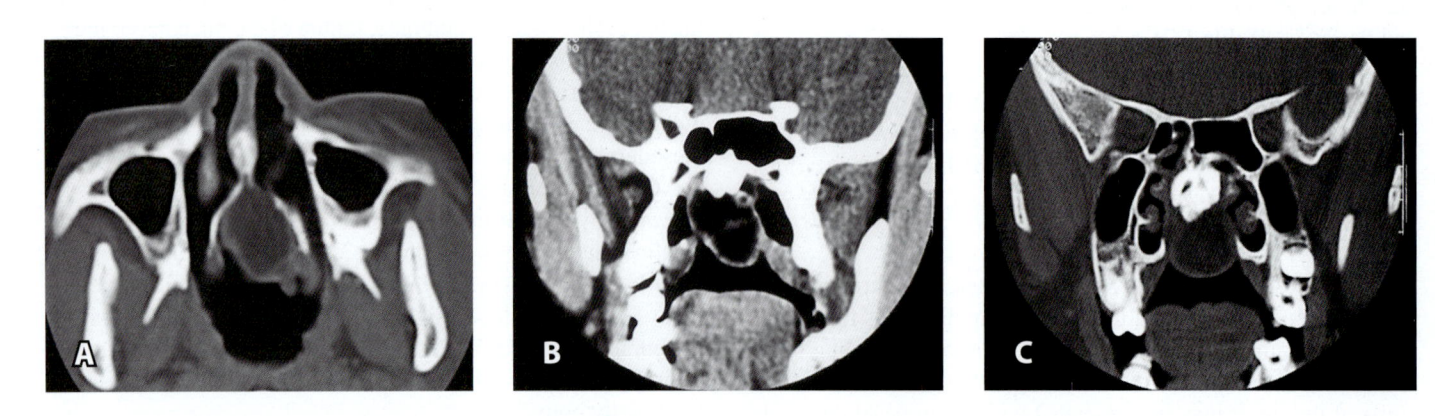

Figure 3-21 Median Cleft Face Syndrome in an Adult
Axial NECT (**A**) image shows splitting of the posterior portion of the nasal septum by a central cystic mass. Coronal NECT with soft-tissue windowing (**B**) shows a fat-filled midline mass protruding through a widely cleft hard palate. Coronal NECT with bone windowing (**C**) showing teeth remnants in the upper portion of the nasal cavity, just beneath the sphenoid sinus.

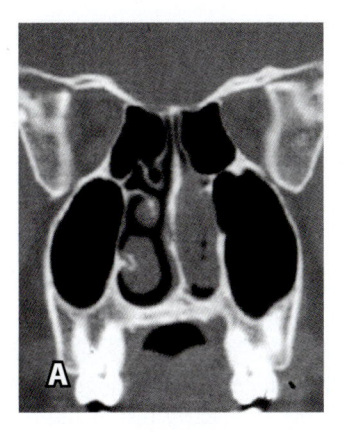

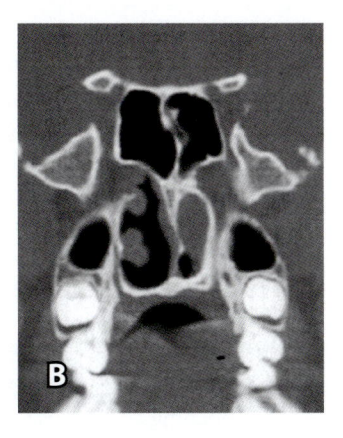

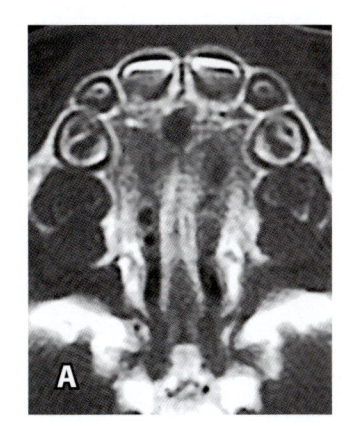

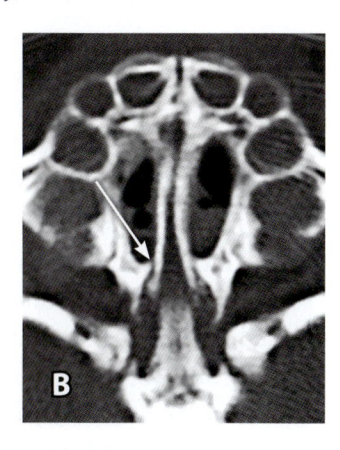

Chapter 3: Sinonasal, Facial, and Mandibular Embryology, Anatomy, and Anomalies

Figure 3-22 Membranous Choanal Atresia: Unilateral
Coronal NECT images (**A–B**) show a narrow left nasal cavity that is devoid of normal structures and filled by soft tissue. There is a small nasal passage just beneath the atretic left choanae. This teenager was noted to always breathe through the right nostril.

Figure 3-23 Osseos Choanal Atreseia: Bilateral
Axial NECT scans (**A–B**) show bilateral narrow air passages on both sides of the midline with fused widened vomer bones. There is complete absence of the nasal choanae with fusion of the laterally placed palatine bones to the posterior portions of the bifid vomer bone (arrow, **B**).

inserting an oral airway (moves the tongue away from the palate and secures an airway for up to several weeks), McGovern nipple, intubation, or tracheostomy.[58,97,99,100] Because neonates are obligate nose breathers for the first 2 to 6 months of life, they can sometimes relieve the respiratory distress by crying.[101,102] Bilateral choanal atresia is often seen with severe malformations of the midface. Choanal atresia may be seen in many syndromes, most commonly CHARGE, and is associated with systemic anomalies in 50% to 75% of cases[58,97,103] (**Table 3-8**).

Unilateral choanal atresia may not be diagnosed until later in life when patients present with nasal stuffiness, rhinorrhea, or recurrent infections. It usually presents on the right more than left side and may be found in children with a cleft lip or palate, or other mild midline facial anomalies. Treatment options for choanal atresia remain controversial but include choanal reconstruction with or without stent placement, transnasal or transpalatal endoscopic techniques, and carbon dioxide and potassium titanyl phosphate lasers.[58,90,99,103]

CT is the imaging modality of choice. Immediately prior to the scan, the patient should be suctioned and given a topical decongestant to minimize secretions. Images should be obtained in 1 to 1.5 mm section intervals with the patients in the prone

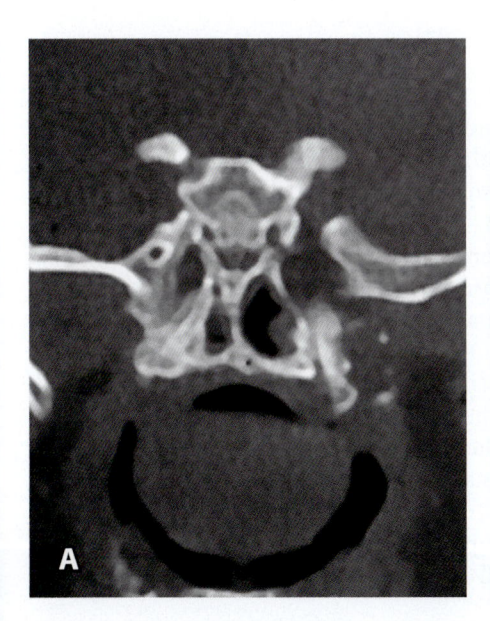

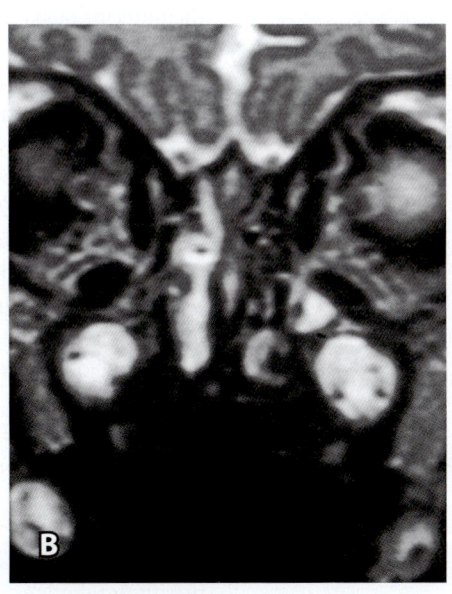

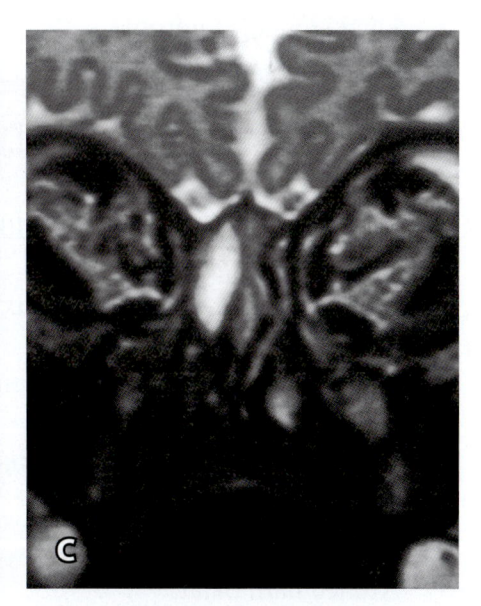

Figure 3-24 Osseomembranous Choanal Atresia: Unilateral
Coronal NECT (**A**) shows a narrow right nasal passage with a bony fusion between the right palatine bone and the vomer which narrows the nasal choanae. No air is detected, as there is soft-tissue membrane occluding the nonbony portion of the nasal choanae (**B**). Coronal T2 MR shows hyperintense tissue in the right nasal choanae obstructing the airway (**C**).

position and the gantry angled 5 to 10 degrees cephalad to the hard palate. Key imaging features are shown in **Table 3-9**.[58,103]

Choanal stenosis (narrowing) may appear similar to choanal atresia depending on the degree of narrowing. CT is the imaging modality of choice for diagnosis. If the stenosis is unilateral, treatment can be delayed until the child is 6 to 9 years old to allow time for normal growth of the nasal cavity. In neonates with bilateral obstruction, a secure airway must be established prior to considering treatment options.[58]

Pyriform Aperture Stenosis

Pyriform aperture stenosis is a rare, congenital narrowing of the osseous opening of the nose. It results from early fusion and/or hypertrophy of the medial nasal prominences. It is associated with other anomalies including a central megaincisor (75% of cases), alobar and semilobar forms of holoprosencephaly, facial hemangiomas, clinodactyly, central diabetes insipidus, and pituitary dysfunction.[58,97,103]

High-resolution CT images in planes angled along the hard palate should show a shelf of tissue extending across the nostrils just inside the nares, inward bowing of the maxillary spines, and narrowing of the pyriform aperture (**Fig. 3-25**). Although no standard measurements exist for the normal pyriform aperture, measurements should be taken at the level of the maximum transverse diameter of the pyriform aperture, posterior choanae, and posteroinferior os vomer. The general guidelines for diagnosing stenosis are when either the maximum transverse diameter of each aperture is less than or equal to 3 mm or when the total width is less than 8 mm.[104,105]

Treatment of pyriform aperture stenosis depends on the severity of the case. Mild cases may be treated with decongestants, which allow time for normal nasal growth. Severe cases may require surgical reconstruction with stent placement, sublabial resection of the anteromedial maxilla, or reconstruction of the anterior nasal passages.[57,58,103]

Arhinia

Arhinia is a very rare congenital absence of the external nose, nasal cavities, and olfactory apparatus due to the inversion and trisomy of chromosome 9 or reciprocal translocation of chromosomes 3 and 12.[106,107] There is typically midface hypoplasia with a depression instead of an external nose. CT imaging demonstrates the absence of nasal bones, nasal septum and turbinates, and a high arched palate. Additionally, there is often hypoplasia of the maxilla, hypertelorism, microphthalmia, coloboma of the iris, and hypoplastic or absent nasolacrimal ducts. It may also be associated with central nervous system anomalies, cleft palate, absent maxillary sinuses, low-set ears, and other eye anomalies.[108,109] Because neonates are obligate nose breathers, most experience respiratory distress. Treatment involves surgical repair to create an external nose and nasal cavities using local flaps and autologous cartilage grafts or prosthetic devices.[66,110]

Proboscis Lateralis (Congenital Tubular Nose)

Proboscis lateralis is a very rare anomaly (less than 1:100,000 live births) in which one side of the nose is replaced by a

---

Table 3-8 Conditions Associated with Choanal Atresia

Syndromes
- Acrophalyngosyndactyly (Apert syndrome)
- Antley-Bixter syndrome
- CHARGE syndrome/association
- Chromosome 18 anomaly
- Chromosome 12 anomaly
- Chromosome XO anomaly
- Crouzon syndrome (Craniofacial dysostosis)
- de Lange syndrome
- DiGeorge syndrome
- Treacher Collins syndrome

Anatomic Anomalies
- Colobomas
- Orofacial clefts
- Craniosynostosis
- Otocephaly, agnathia-holoprosencephaly, or agnathia-otocephaly complex
- Polydactyly
- Cardiac abnormalities
- Ventricular septal defect
- Patent ductus arteriosus
- Malrotation of the bowel
- Tracheoesophageal fistula

In Utero Conditions
- Amniotic band syndrome
- Fetal alcohol syndrome

Table 3-9 Radiologic Features of Choanal Atresia

Key Features
- Narrow posterior choanae (width <0.34 cm in children younger than 2 years)
- Inward bowing of posterior maxilla
- Fused or widened vomer
- Bone or soft-tissue septum extending across posterior choanae

Commonly Associated Findings
- Narrow nasopharynx
- Medialized lateral nasal wall
- Arched hard palate

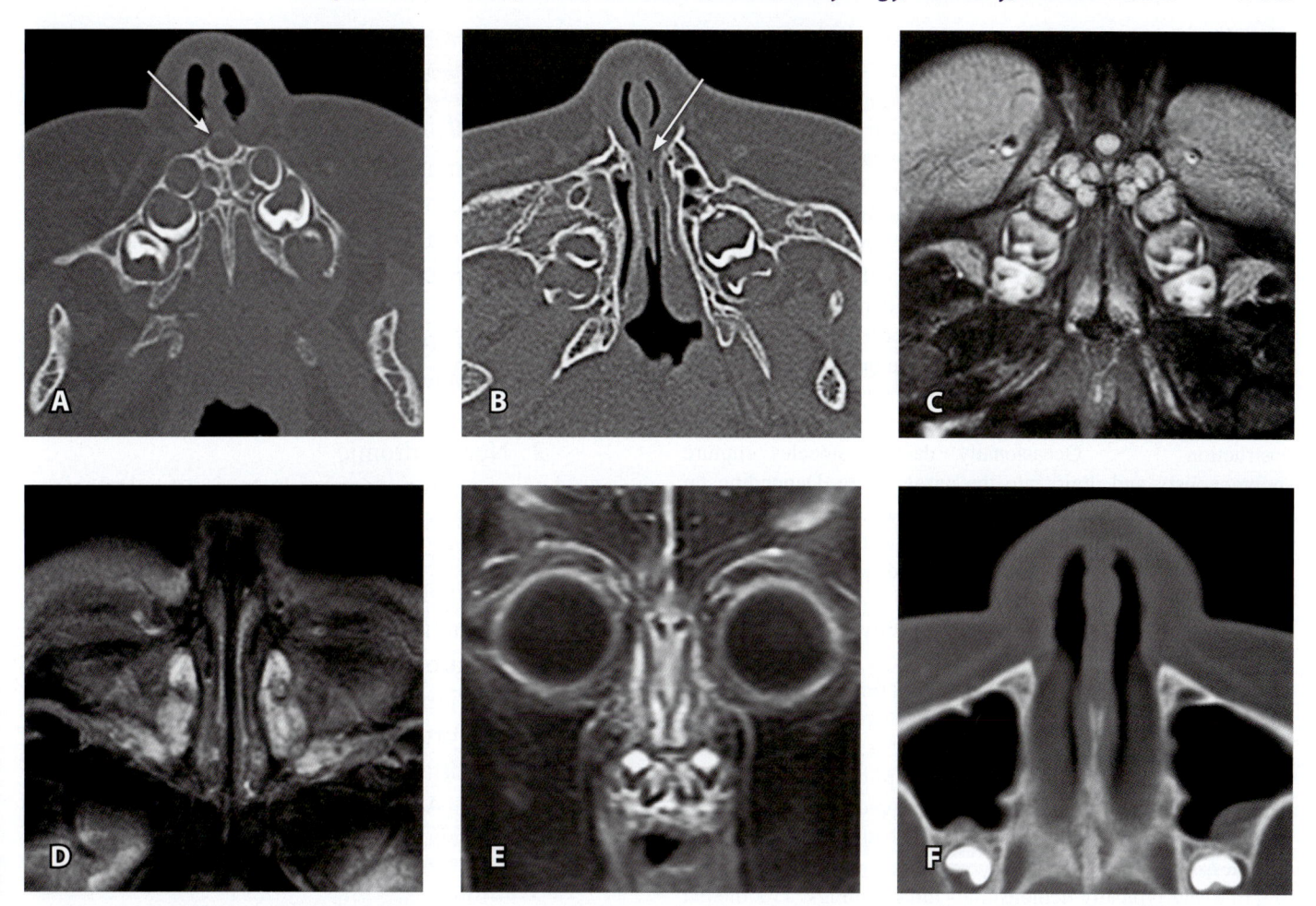

Figure 3-25 Pyriform Aperture Stenosis

Axial NECT with bone windowing through the hard palate and pyriform aperture (**A–B**). There is a triangular shaped palate and alveolar ridge with crowding of the tooth buds anteriorly. Note the fusion of the two incisors into a single megaincisor (*arrow*, **A**). The pyriform aperture is set at an obtuse angle at the vestibule and severely crowds the nasal airways at its narrowest point (*arrow*, **B**). Axial T2W MR (**C–D**) again shows the triangular alveolar ridge, the crowding of the tooth buds anteriorly, and the central megaincisor. Coronal T1W MR with contrast (**E**) shows enhancement of the mucosa of the nasal airways, demonstrating their slit-like appearance. Axial NECT with with bone window of a different patient showing a normal pyriform aperture with no stenosis for comparison. Notice the long, narrow appearance of the nasal passages in a stenosed pyriform aperture (**B, E**) compared to normal pyriform apeture (**F**).

tubular structure typically emanating from the medial canthus.[111,112] It is very rarely bilateral. This condition is caused by defective development or absence of the medial and lateral nasal processes, resulting in fusion of the maxillary process with the contralateral nasal processes. The club-shaped proboscis is typically 2 to 3 cm long, 1 cm in diameter, and may have a canal that traverses the entire proboscis to end in a cul-de-sac.[112] The nasal cavity and paranasal sinuses are absent on the affected side, so the nasolacrimal duct ends blindly. There is often an ipsilateral nasal wall anomaly that varies from absence to a small tissue defect in the wall. It may be associated with deformities of the ipsilateral eye, cleft lip/palate, and other anomalies, particularly those of the central nervous system. Surgical treatment involves excision of the tubular deformity and reconstruction of the external nose and nasal cavities.[66,110]

Polyrhinia

Polyrhinia (double nose) and supernumerary nostril (accessory nostril with a complete or partial ala nasi) are extremely rare duplication anomalies of the nose that are hypothesized to result from two pairs of nasal pits[113,114] or lateral nasal placodes.[115] The supernumerary nostril may be located lateral, medial, or superior to the normal nostrils. There may be up to two septae, four nostrils, and four nasal cavities. Typically, the supernumerary nostril does not have a connection to the lacrimal system.[116] Management consists of excising the medial halves of each nose to create one septum or resecting the supernumerary nostril.

Dacryocystocele

A dacryocystocele (nasolacrimal sac mucocele) is the cystic dilatation of the lacrimal sac at the medial canthal angle. Although congenital dacryocystocele is generally a benign condition, cases with bilateral involvement (10% of cases) or substantial intranasal extension can cause respiratory distress syndrome in neonates, who are obligate nose-breathers, making it the second most common cause of neonatal nasal obstruction after choanal atresia.[117–120] Dacryocystoceles result from obstruction of the proximal and distal ends of the nasolacrimal duct. The distal blockage is typically due to an imperforate Hasner membrane; the cause of the proximal blockage remains unclear.[121,122] A nasolacrimal duct mucocele occurs when a dacryocystocele extends into a dilated nasolacrimal duct and results in a cystic intranasal mass.[122]

Dacryocystoceles may be unilateral or bilateral. They typically present as a tense, bluish mass at the medial canthus or in the nasal cavity. They may cause persistent epiphora, conjunctivitis, dacryocystitis, facial cellulitis, and nasal or upper airway obstruction.[58,97,120,121] Occasionally, dacryocystoceles rupture spontaneously and drain into the nasal cavity. Depending on severity, treatment ranges from manual massage, to probing and irrigation, to endoscopic resection of the inferior turbinate, and rarely marsupialization (dacryocystorhinostomy) with silicone stenting.[102,123]

CT and MR imaging are equally sensitive at detecting dacryocystoceles. CT is the imaging modality of choice for evaluating possible bony changes of the nasolacrimal canal and possible choanal atresia. MRI has the advantage of characterizing the cystic contents and lack of radiation exposure; however, sedation may be required. Immediately prior to the scan, the patient should be suctioned and given a topical decongestant to minimize secretions. Images should be obtained with a section thickness of 3 mm.[58,124]

Imaging typically demonstrates three findings: 1) a medial canthus mass within an enlarged lacrimal sac, 2) an enlarged osseous nasolacrimal canal with an enlarged soft tissue nasolacrimal duct, and 3) an intranasal mass representing the inferior extension of the mucocele.[120,124] On CT, the nasolacrimal duct and canal appear dilated with a well-defined, homogeneous, thin-walled mass with fluid attenuation that may extend to the medial canthus or into the nasal cavity. The nasal septum may be shifted contralaterally, and the inferior turbinate bone may be displaced superiorly. Contrast administration may demonstrate slight enhancement of the cyst wall. With dacryocystitis, contrast enhancement is more pronounced, and adjacent soft-tissue enhancement and swelling are also common.[58] Dacryocystoceles may be diagnosed prenatally during the third trimester by sonography, which shows a cystic mass medial and inferior to the fetal orbit.[120]

Nasolacrimal Duct Stenosis

Nasolacrimal duct stenosis (dacryostenosis) results from obstruction of the nasolacrimal drainage system without distention of the nasolacrimal sac. It is usually caused by partial or complete persistence of the Hasner membrane.[117–120] Imaging findings may be normal or demonstrate an enlarged nasolacrimal duct containing secretions. Treatment begins with duct massage and possibly prophylactic antibiotics to prevent dacryocystitis and periorbital cellulitis. Ductal stenosis resolves spontaneously in 90% of children by age 1 year. If massage fails, then the Hasner membrane is perforated using duct probing and/or intubation.[121,123]

Table 3-10 Classification of Mandibular Hypoplasia

I. **Congenital**
  A. Malformational
    1. Syndromic
      a. Oculo-auriculo-vertebral (OAV) spectrum (Goldenhar syndrome)
        i. Hemifacial microsomia
        ii. Bifacial microsomia
      b. Mandibulofacial dystosis (Treacher Collins syndrome)
    2. Nonsyndromic
      i. Temporomandibular joint ankylosis
      ii. Aglossia, microglossia
      iii. Orofacial cleft
      iv. Isolated mandibular hypoplasia
  B. Deformational
    1. Syndromic or Nonsyndromic
      a. Pierre Robin sequence
      b. Torticollis
      c. Intrauterine constraint
        i. Amniotic band syndrome

II. **Acquired**
  A. Trauma
  B. Radiation
  C. Oncologic
  D. Hemifacial atrophy
  E. Teratogens
    1. Methotrexate

III. **Developmental**
  A. Etiology unclear

Maxillomandibular Anomalies

Mandibular Hypoplasia

Mandibular hypoplasia is highly variable in its presentation and etiology, which include congenital, acquired, and developmental[125] (**Table 3-10**). Congenital mandibular hypoplasia usually results from unilateral or bilateral maldevelopment of the first and second branchial arches. It is believed to result primarily from insufficient migration of neural crest cells into the first branchial arch, which gives rise to the mandibular and maxillary prominences.[126] The causes of acquired hypoplasia include trauma, radiation damage, oncologic defects, and hemifacial atrophy.[127] The etiology of developmental hypoplasia remains unclear.

Congenital mandibular hypoplasia can be subdivided into malformational or deformational forms.[125] Malformational mandibular hypoplasia involves intrinsic growth aberrations typically due to genetic mutations. Malformational hypoplasia can be syndromic or nonsyndromic, but most cases present as part of a syndrome such as oculo-auriculo-vertebral (OAV) spectrum and mandibulofacial dystosis. Deformational hypoplasia can be syndromic or nonsyndromic and result from extrinsic forces impeding normal growth, such as in cases of Pierre Robin sequence, torticollis, and intrauterine constraint.

Most cases of congenital mandibular hypoplasia are a component of one of more than 60 possible syndromes (**Table 3-11**).[128] The most common syndrome is *Goldenhar* or *oculo-auriculo-vertebral complex*, which usually presents with hemifacial or bifacial microsomia and hypoplasia of the mandible, maxilla, and/or cheekbones. The next most common is *Treacher Collins syndrome* or the mandibulofacial dysostosis group, which presents with a wide range of craniofacial abnormalities involving the cheekbones, jaws, mouth, ears, and/or eyes.

Nonsyndromic malformational mandibular hypoplasia can be subgrouped based on whether the hypoplasia is isolated or associated with other anomalies, which include temporomandibular joint ankylosis, aglossia or microglossia, and orofacial clefts. Those cases associated with other anomalies tend to have more severe micrognathia with a higher incidence of airway obstruction, feeding difficulties, and progressive retrognathia requiring multiple corrective procedures.[125]

Congenital mandibular hypoplasia usually results in bilateral deformity due to compensatory growth changes on the unaffected side. Presentations vary widely. In severe cases, the hypopharynx may be obstructed due to the reposition of the tongue into the posterior pharynx. This may cause airway obstruction and hinder feeding, resulting in hypoxic episodes and failure to thrive.[124] Speech development may also be affected. Initial treatment may involve endotracheal intubation or tracheotomy and gastric tube feedings.[129]

Hemifacial Microsomia

Hemifacial microsomia is the second most common facial birth defect after cleft lip and palate[130] (**Table 3-11**). The incidence is approximately 1:5,600 live births.[131] The patterns of inheritance may be autosomal dominant, autosomal recessive, or multifactorial. Due to varying severity and expression of the OAV spectrum anomalies, some classification systems consider hemifacial microsomia and Goldenhar syndrome as representing different severities of OAV spectrum and use the terms interchangeably.

Another classification system places hemifacial microsomia within the OMENS category. *OMENS* stands for each of the five major manifestations of hemifacial microsomia: orbital distortion, mandibular hypoplasia, ear anomaly, nerve involvement, and soft-tissue deficiency. The *OMENS-Plus* classification system expands the spectrum to include extracraniofacial anomalies: cardiovascular, central nervous system, gastrointestinal, pulmonary, renal, skeletal and limb anomalies. Grading is according to the degree of dysmorphology for each involved structure.

Using the OMENS classification system, studies have found that mandibular hypoplasia (97%) and auricular abnormalities (95%) are the most common clinical manifestations, followed

Table 3-11 Conditions Associated with Branchial Arch Anomalies or Unusual Facies

Syndromes	*Anatomic Anomalies*
• Binder syndrome	• Hemifacial microsomia
• Bixler syndrome	• Mandibular hypoplasia
• Branchio-oto-renal (Melnick-Fraser) syndrome	• Otocephaly/agnathia
• Branchio-oculo-facial syndrome	• Syngnathia
• Coffin-Siris syndrome	• Aglossia-adactylia syndrome
• Goldenhar syndrome [oculo-auriculo-vertebral (OAV) complex]	• Popliteal pterygium syndrome
• Miller syndrome	• Van der Woude syndrome
• Möbius syndrome	
• Nager syndrome	
• Noonan syndrome	
• Opitz BBB syndrome	
• Opitz G syndrome	
• Orofacial-digital syndromes (I–VIII)	
• Pierre Robin sequence	
• Robinow syndrome	*Other Malformations*
• Rubinstein-Tybi syndrome	• Corpus callosum dysgenesis
• Treacher Collins syndrome (mandibulofacial dysostosis group)	• Arnold-Chiari malformations
• Trisomy 18 (Edwards syndrome)	• Hypothalamic-pituitary dysfunction
• Wildervanck syndrome	

Table 3-12 Clinical Features of Hemifacial Microsomia using OMENS and OMENS-Plus Classifications

OMENS Classification System	OMENS-Plus Classification System
• Mandibular hypoplasia (97%) • Auricular anomalies (95%) • Middle ear hypoplasia or atresia (90%) • Conductive hearing loss (86%) • Ossicle malformation (75%) • Facial nerve weakness (45%–50%) • Macrostomia (23%–62%) • Unilateral aural atresia (50%) • Unilateral aural stenosis (30%) • Ear tags (40%) • Epibulbar dermoids (20%) • Palatal deviation towards normal side (39%) • Cleft lip/palate (10%–20%) • Bilateral aural atresia or stenosis (18%) • Sensorineural hearing loss (10%) • Horizontal asymmetry of orbits (15%) • Frontal plagiocephaly (5%)	• Right-sided microsomia (48%) • Left-sided microsomia (38%) • Bilateral microsomia (14%) • Normal orbits (77%) • Mild hypoplastic mandibular ramus-condyle, functioning TMJ (57%) • Normal facial nerve (76%) • Mild soft-tissue hypoplasia (73%) • Mild ear anomalies (53% grade 0 or 1) • Severe ear anomalies (47% grade 2 or 3) • Skeletal anomalies (40%–60%) • Cardiovascular anomalies (14%–47%) • Central nervous system anomalies (5%–15%) • Gastrointestinal (10%) • Pulmonary anomalies (10%) • Renal anomalies (10%)

TMJ = temporomandibular joint.

by conductive hearing loss (86%) and facial nerve weakness (45% to 50%) (**Table 3-12**). Unilateral aural atresia (50%) and unilateral aural stenosis (30%) were more common than bilateral anomalies (18%). Moderate hypoplasia or atresia of the middle ear, most commonly the oval window, was noted in 90% of cases, and ossicle malformation in 75% of cases.[132,133] Transverse oral clefting (macrostomia) is found in 23% to 62% of cases of hemifacial microsomia, and cleft lip/palate is found in 10% to 20% of cases. Additional associations include palatal deviation toward the normal side (39%) and epibulbar dermoids (20%).[134,135] Another study used the OMENS-Plus system and found that of 65 cases, 48% had right-sided microsomia (short transverse dimension), 38% had left-sided microsomia, and 14% had bilateral microsomia. The majority of patients had normal orbits (77%), mildly hypoplastic mandibular ramus-condyle with functioning temporomandibular joint (57% type M1 or M2a), normal facial nerve (76%), mild soft-tissue hypoplasia (73%)[136] (**Fig. 3-26**). The most common extracranial features associated with hemifacial microsomia include skeletal (40% to 60%), cardiovascular (14% to 47%), and central nervous system anomalies (5% to 15%).[137,138]

Mandibular deformity is graded into three types. *Type I* refers to a miniature mandible with identifiable anatomy. *Type II* is a functioning temporomandibular joint (TMJ) but with an abnormal shape and glenoid fossa. Type II is subcategorized into type IIA, which includes the glenoid fossa in an acceptable functional position; and type IIB, in which the TMJ is abnormally placed and cannot be incorporated in the surgical construction. *Type III* indicates an absent ramus and nonexistent glenoid fossa.[133]

The management of hemifacial microsomia depends on its severity. For severe hypoplasia of the ramus and condyle (type III), reconstruction using a bone graft taken from the ribs may be considered. Another possibility, used more often in types I and II, is to lengthen the involved bones using distraction osteogenesis. Additional staged surgeries include soft tissue reconstruction of the cheek to increase symmetry, excision of preauricular tags, closure of macrostomia, and transposition of the microtic ear lobule if it is located asymmetrically on the cheek.[133,139]

Syngnathia (Maxillomandibular Fusion)

Syngnathia is a rare congenital anomaly involving bony (synostosis), soft tissue (synechiae), or mixed adhesions between the maxilla and mandible. The etiology remains unclear. Proposed theories include persistence of the buccopharyngeal membrane, fusion of the gums due to aberrant ingrowth of ectoderm or other abnormal process in development, an abnormality of the stapedial artery, early loss of neural crest cells, amniotic constriction bands in the region of the developing branchial arches, environmental insults or trauma, and teratogens such as meclozine and vitamin A.[140,141] The embryologic basis of the defect appears to be failure of mesodermal migration into the midline structures of the mandibular portion of the first branchial arch (**Table 3-11**). There are two main types of synagnathia.[142]

Type 1 is *simple syngnathia* with no other head or neck anomalies.

Type 2 is complex syngnathia:
    2a: coexistent with aglossia.
    2b: coexistent with agenesis of hypoplasia of proximal mandible.

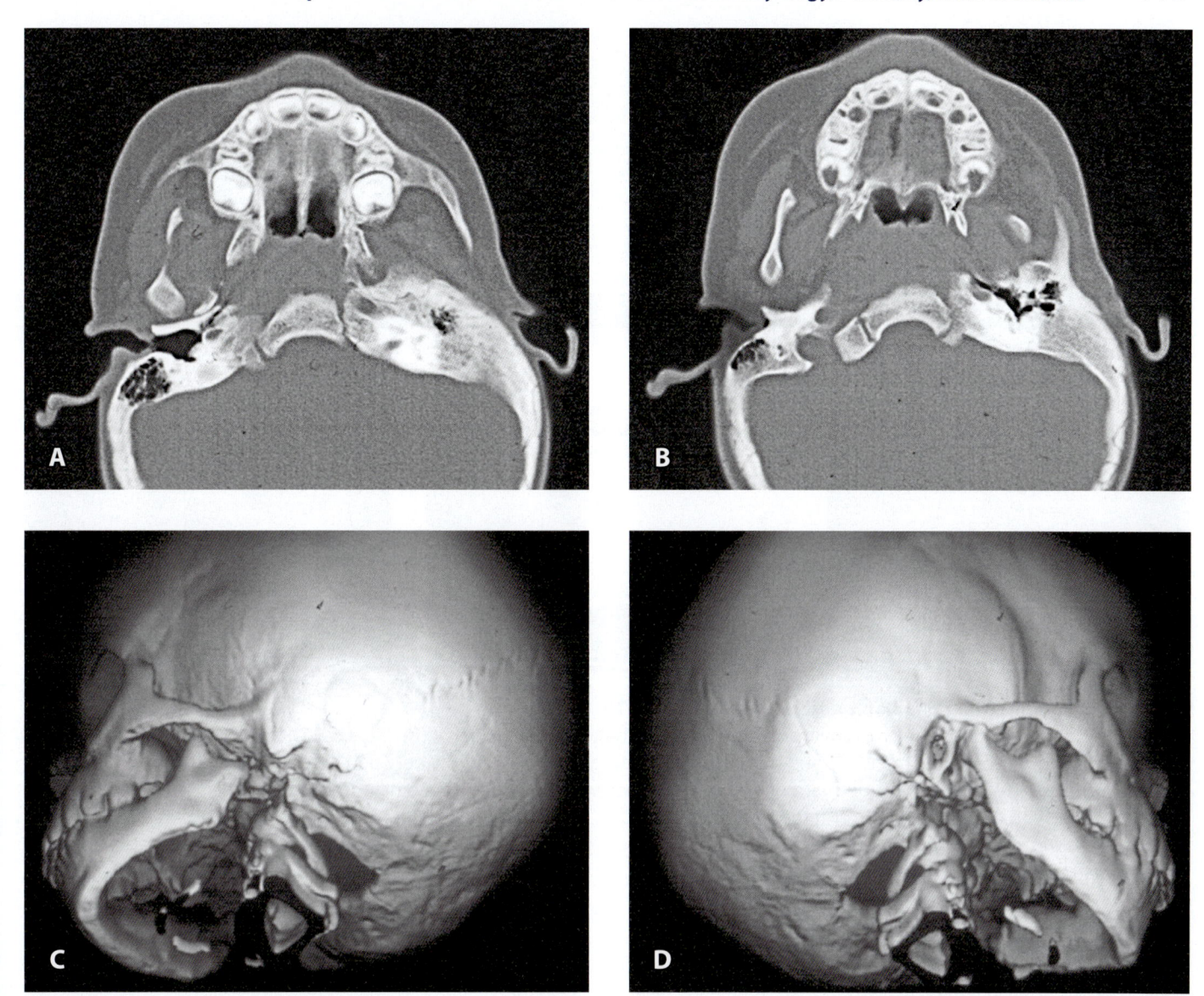

Figure 3-26 Hemifacial Microsomia
Axial bone window CT scans (**A** and **B**) demonstrate hypoplasia of both the mandibular ramus and the soft tissues of the left hemiface. There is complete absence of the internal auditory canal, no mastoid air cells, and a small tympanic cavity. These structures are normal on the right side. Left lateral 3D CT reconstruction with surface rendering looking upward (**C**) shows a hypoplastic left ramus compared to the normal ramus in figure (**D**) and the absence of the external auditory canal. Right lateral 3D CT reconstruction with surface rendering looking upward (**D**) shows completely normal structures, including visualization of the aperture of the external auditory canal.

A modified classification system has been proposed for bony syngnathia.[143]

- Type 1a is *simple anterior syngnathia*, characterized by bony fusion of only the alveolar ridge, without any other head or neck anomalies.
- Type 1b is *complex anterior syngnathia*, characterized by bony fusion of only the alveolar ridge, and associated with other congenital anomalies in the head or neck.
- Type 2a is *simple zygomatico-mandibular syngnathia*, characterized by bony fusion of the mandible to the zygomatic complex, resulting in only mandibular micrognathia.
- Type 2b is *complex zygomatico-mandibular syngnathia* characterized by bony fusion of the mandible to the zygomatic complex, and associated with clefts or temporomandibular joint ankylosis.

Fewer than 50 cases of syngnathia have been reported, and most cases are found in association with other oral and maxillofacial anomalies such as cleft lip/palate, aglossia, hypoplasia of the proximal mandible, hemifacial microsomia, cleft mandible, bifid tongue, small or absent tongue, temporomandibular (zygomaticomandibular) fusion, and other regional or systemic anomalies.[140,144–150] It also often presents as part of a syndrome, including *popliteal pterygium syndrome* (facial anomalies, cleft lip/palate, lip pits, syngnathia, popliteal pterygia, and genital anomalies), *van der Woude syndrome* (cleft lip/palate and lower lip pits or mounds), *aglossia-adactylia syndrome* (aglossia and

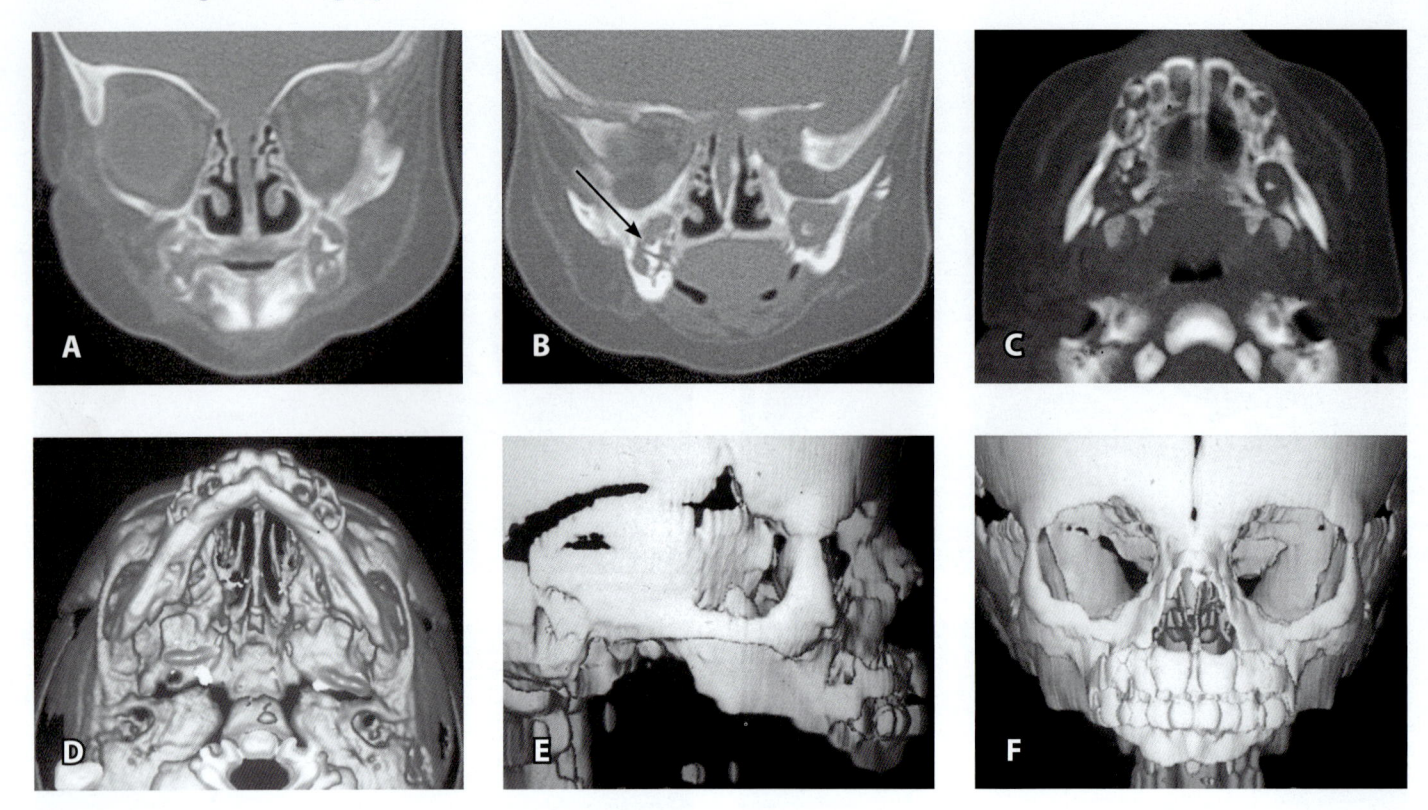

Figure 3-27 Syngnathia (Maxillomandibular Fusion) Type 1B
Newborn with a small mouth (microstomia) and hypoplasia of the tongue. Coronal (**A, B**) and axial (**C**) bone window CT scans show complete anterior fusion of the mandible and maxilla. There is merging of the marrow between these two structures with remnants of tooth buds intertwined within the marrow (*arrow*, **B**). Other types of fusion may include fusion of the zygomatic complex with mandible, with or without clefts or temporomandibular joint ankylosis. Axial (**D**), right lateral (**E**), and coronal (**F**) 3D CT with surface rendering show normal development of the zygomatic arches with a separation between the rami of the mandible and the zygomatic arches (**D**). The association of other congenital anomalies of the mouth and tongue classify these findings as type 1B.

variable limb deformities), and autosomal recessive *hypomandibular craniofacial dysostosis* (craniosynostosis, prominent eyes, deficient midface and zygomatic arches, short nose with anteverted nares, protruding lower face, small oral aperture, persistent buccopharyngeal membrane, and severe mandibular hypoplasia).[151–154] It has been proposed that some cases of van der Woude syndrome may in fact be mild variants of popliteal pterygium syndrome and that some genetic etiologic relationship exists between the two syndromes.[155]

Congenital synostosis of maxilla and mandible is less common than synechiae; most cases of synostosis involve incomplete unilateral fusion.[151] Syngnathia may be unilateral or bilateral (**Fig. 3-27**). Midline maxillomandibular bony fusion is extremely rare and has been associated with mandibular cleft, bifid tongue, severe mandibular hypoplasia, and class II malocclusion with temporomandibular and zygomaticomandibular fusion.[141,144]

The first piority in treating congenital maxillomandibular fusion is securing the airway, followed by placing a nasogastric or gastrostomy tube for nutrition. Surgical repair is urgent due to the high risk of aspiration pneumonia, feeding difficulties, and poor dentation and alignment. Treatment of synechiae may involve simple division of the bands. Surgical repair of synostosis may involve an osteotomy to separate the fused areas, temporomandibular joint reconstruction, and distraction osteogenesis to lengthen the affected mandible and maxilla.[141,155]

Agnathia (Otocephaly)

The term *agnathia* (mandibular aplasia) is often used interchangeably with the term *otocephaly* or *agnathia-synotia-microstomia syndrome*, which refers to a rare congenital syndrome whose findings are consistent with symmetrically deficient development of the first branchial arch (**Table 3-11**). Otocephaly is characterized by mandibular agenesis or atrophy, microstomia, aglossia or hypoplasia of the tongue, and ventromedially displaced or fused ears (synotia) (**Fig. 3-28**). It can occur in isolation or in combination with a variety of malformations such as holoprosencephaly and situs inversus.[156–159] Other associated findings may include central nervous system malformations, such as anterior cephalocele and Dandy-Walker cyst, bilateral bony syngnathia, cleft lip and palate, choanal atresia, narrowed dysplastic larynx, midline proboscis, tracheoesophageal fistula, cardiac anomalies, and adrenal hypoplasia.[156,160] The incidence is 1:60,000 to 70,000 live births and may be linked to a recessive gene.[158,161]

Agnathia-holoprosencephaly is a more severe form of agnathia complicated by holoprosencephaly, a reduction in the forebrain and frontonasal prominence. There are three forms of holoprosencephaly: alobar, semilobar, and lobar.[87]

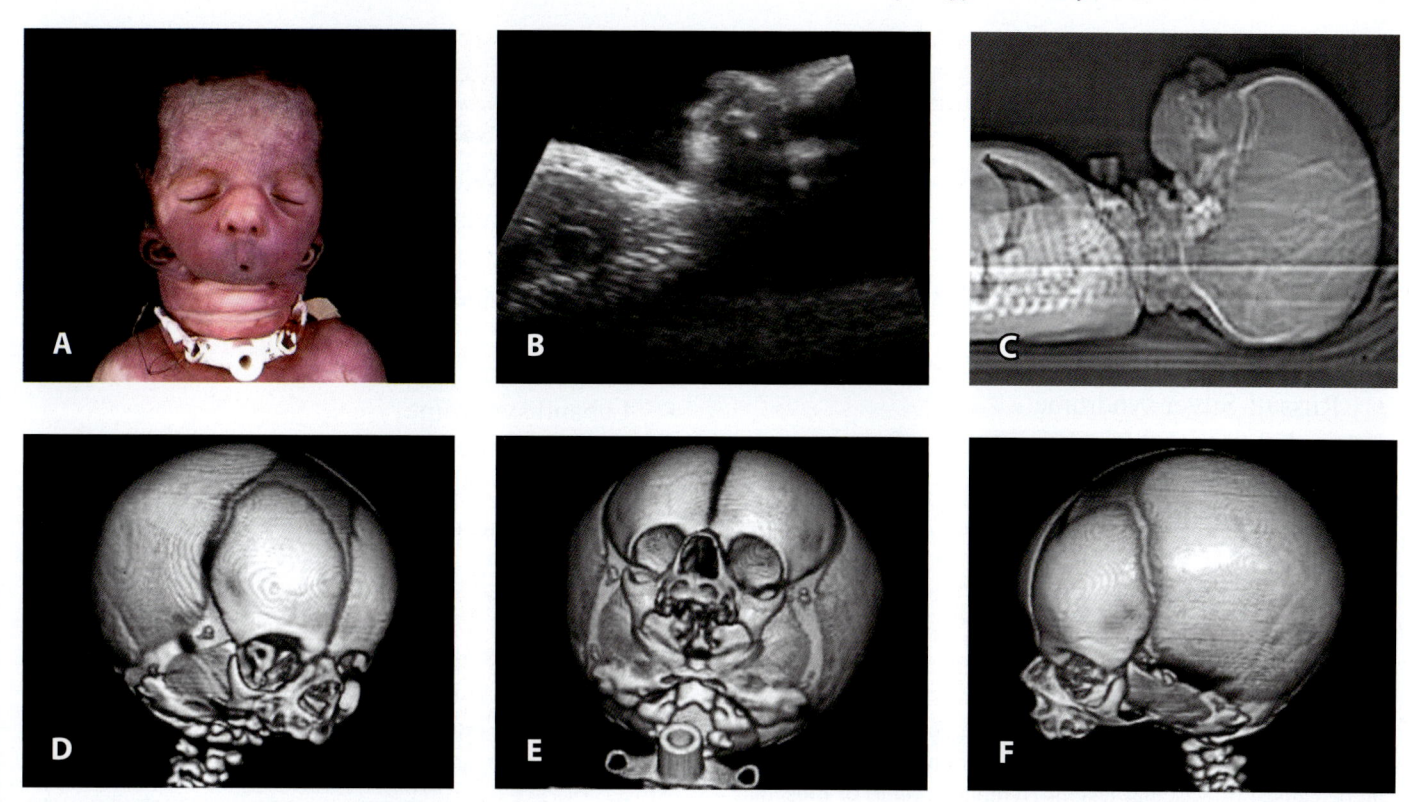

Chapter 3: Sinonasal, Facial, and Mandibular Embryology, Anatomy, and Anomalies

Figure 3-28 Oto-cephaly Agnathia Syndrome
Photograph (**A**) of a newborn cadaver. Note the abscence of the mandible and the microscopic oral aperture. Prenatal transverse ultrasound of the face (**B**) and postnatal sagittal CT scout view of the upper torso (**C**) demonstrate mandibular agnathia. Postmortem right oblique (**D**), AP (**E**) and left lateral (**F**) 3D CT scans with surface rendering show total agenesis of the mandible and marked hypoplasia of the midface with hypotelorism. Also note the bilateral absence of the external auditory canal. The patient had an absent oral cavity and bilateral osseos choanal atresia documented on postmortem pathological examination.

Alobar holoprosencephaly is the most severe form with the supratentorial brain showing no differentiation into hemispheres or lobes, absent falx, absent longitudinal fissure, absent superior and inferior sinuses, absent or rudimentary third ventricle, and an undivided monoventricle.

Semilobar holoprosencephaly is the most common form and shows partial development of two hemispheres, longitudinal fissure, falx, sagittal sinuses, and posterior and temporal ventricles.

Lobar holoprosencephaly shows nearly complete formation of the brain posteriorly but incomplete formation anteriorly, and complete formation of the longitudinal fissure, flax, and dural sinuses.

Alobar (83% to 90%) and semilobar (30%) holoprosencephaly are associated with facial anomalies including cyclopia, ethmocephaly, and cebocephaly.[162,163]

Diagnosis may be made prenatally by ultrasound, MRI, or in utero helical CT.[157,164,165] Due to oropharyngeal obstruction, otocephaly is typically lethal. Treatment involves securing the airway at birth. Without a swallowing mechanism and an underdeveloped larynx, oral feeding and speech are unlikely, and there is a predisposition to aspiration. There are no reported cases of total mandibular reconstruction in otocephalic patients partially due to the fact that the vast majority of these patients are stillborn. Nonetheless, reconstruction of the mandible followed by multiple osteodistraction interventions may allow for a more normal appearance and function.[156]

Micrognathia

Micrognathia is a relative term describing a small lower jaw. Its incidence is about 1:1,000 live births. In true micrognathia, the jaw is small enough to interfere with feeding, therefore the infant may require special equipment and feeding techniques for adequate nutrition.[166,167] Micrognathia may be an isolated anomaly, which is often self-correcting with growth, especially during puberty when the jaw grows significantly. It may also be associated with certain inherited disorders and syndromes such as Pierre-Robin sequence, Treacher-Collins syndrome, and Turner's syndrome (**Table 3-13**). Severe micrognathia is associated with polyhydramnios possibly because glossoptosis prevents swallowing. In severe cases, there may be airway obstruction requiring intervention.[167,168] Teeth misalignment is a common characteristic. Depending on severity, treatment may involve orthodontic appliances or surgical repair such as distraction osteogenesis.[166,169,223]

Macroglossia

Macroglossia refers to an abnormally large tongue in which the resting tongue protrudes beyond the teeth, alveolar ridge,

Table 3-13 Conditions Associated with Micrognathia

- Cri du chat syndrome
- Hallerman-Streiff syndrome
- Marfan's syndrome
- Oculodentodigital dysplasia
- Pierre-Robin sequence or syndrome
- Progeria
- Roberts syndrome
- Russell-Silver syndrome
- Seckel syndrome
- Smith-Lemli-Opitz syndrome
- Treacher-Collins syndrome
- Trisomy 13
- Trisomy 18
- Turner's (XO) syndrome

Table 3-14 Congenital Conditions Associated with Macroglossia

Syndromic/Systemic
- Beckwith-Wiedemann syndrome
- Behmel syndrome
- Blomstrand chondrodysplasia (Lethal dwarfism of Blomstrand)
- Down syndrome (trisomy 21)
- Gargoylism
- Laband syndrome
- Microcephaly-hamartoma of Wiedemann
- Skeletal dysplasia of Urbach
- Tollner syndrome
- Trisomy 22

Localized
- Ankyloglossia superior
- Congenital (autosomal dominant)
- Gland hyperplasia
- Muscle hypertrophy (idiopathic)
- Transient idiopathic

Metabolic/Endocrine
- Aspartylglucosaminuria
- Cretinism
- Mucopolysaccharidosis
- Ganglioside storage disease type I
- Lingual thyroid
- Neonatal diabetes mellitus (transient)

Neoplastic
- Hemangioma
- Lymphangioma
- Other neoplasms

or mandible. In some cases, macroglossia occurs as an isolated congenital condition with autosomal dominant inheritance. It can be caused by vascular lesions (lymphangioma) or muscular hypertrophy, or it can occur as part of a congenital syndrome such as Down syndrome or Beckwith-Wiedemann syndrome.[170] In rare cases, it is acquired as a result of trauma or conditions such as amyloidosis, neurofibromatosis, acromegaly, hypothyroidism, and chronic edema.[171,172] The prevalence of macroglossia depends on the underlying disorder. It is commonly found in *Down syndrome* (1:700 live births), in 97.5% of *Beckwith-Wiedemann syndrome* cases (0.73:10,000 live births), and in *congenital hypothyroidism* (2.5:10,000 live births)[173–178] (**Table 3-14**).

Clinical findings associated with macroglossia may include stridor, snoring, and/or feeding difficulties. Imaging can clarify the morphology of the tongue and assist with the diagnosis if the tip of the tongue extends past an imaginary line drawn between the mandible and maxilla on sagittal scans, or past the lower lip on axial scans. Associated features depend on the underlying disorder. In the case of *Beckwith-Wiedemann syndrome*, other features may include omphalocele, nephromegaly, gigantism (sometimes hemihypertrophy), hepatomegaly, genital anomalies, cystic adrenal glands, and heart defects.[179]

Microglossia

Microglossia is a rare congenital anomaly that usually presents in association with anomalies of the extremeties (especially the hands and feet), cleft palate, and dental agenesia as part of a syndrome. One example is Mobius syndrome, which may involve the hypoglossal nerve, causing paralysis and hypoplasia of the tongue.[180,181] The tongue appears small and rudimentary. *Aglossia* is microglossia with extreme glossoptosis.

Ankyloglossia

Ankyloglossia (tongue-tie) refers to tethering of the tongue tip due to a short, tight lingual frenulum attached more anteriorly and superiorly on the tongue than normal. Ankyloglossia may cause speech problems (50%) and mechanical limitations (57%).[182] It can also hinder breastfeeding. One study found that 3.2% of the inpatient and 12.8% of the outpatient infants with breastfeeding difficulties had ankyloglossia.[183] On examination, the lingual apex may appear bilobed with a midline cleft or septal limitation.[184] To diagnose ankyloglossia, one can measure the length of the frenulum and the interincisal distance during maximum opening of the mouth and with the tip of the tongue touching the palatal papilla. A frenulum length more than 2 cm and an interincisal distance more than 2.3 cm are normal.[185] Most cases of ankyloglossia resolve or are asymptomatic. If surgical intervention (frenotomy or frenuloplasty) is desired, it is typically performed around the age one year in order to prevent long-term effects of ankyloglossia.[182,186]

Cleft Mandible/Lower Lip/Neck

Clefts of the mandible and lower lip are extremely rare and vary widely in presentation from a small notch of the vermillion to complete clefting of the lower lip, tongue, mandible, medial neck, hyoid, and manubrium sterni. In some cases, the hyoid may be absent.[187] Typical presentations include a bifid anterior tongue, which may be bound to the cleft mandible. The cleft neck may be associated with cysts, chords, contractures, and dermoids. There may also be upper lip and palate clefting.[160,188]

Bifid Mandibular Condyle

A bifid mandibular condyle (double-headed condyle) is a rare condition characterized by duplicity of the head of the mandible. Possible causes include developmental abnormalities (e.g., persistence of fibrous septa), genetics, teratogens, endocrinological disorders, nutritional disorders, perinatal trauma (e.g., rupture of septal blood vessels), condylar fracture, surgical condylectomy, infection, and radiation damage.[189–191] Most cases of bifidism involve only one condyle; bilateral bifidism is very rare with less than ten known cases, and only one case of trifidism has been reported.[189,192] Although the majority of patients (67%) have no symptoms, some patients have nonspecific complaints such as articular sounds (clicking), pain, swelling, restricted mandibular movement, trismus, ankylosis, snoring, mandibular hypoplasia, and deviation toward the affected side.[189,193–195] It is usually diagnosed on routine radiographic examination. The degree of bifidism can range from a shallow groove to two distinct condyles with a separate neck, and the orientation of the head may be deviated mediolaterally (coronally) or anteroposteriorly (sagittally).[196,197] Treatment of symptomatic bifid condyle is usually conservative, but surgical intervention has been pursued in cases involving limited mouth opening and ankylosis.[198]

Syndromes Associated with Characteristic Anomalies

Syndromes Associated with Orofacial Clefting

See **Table 3-7**.

Van Der Woude Syndrome

Van der Woude syndrome is an autosomal dominant condition characterized by lower lip pit(s) and/or cleft lip and palate. It affects 1:75,000 to 100,000 infants and has been linked to mutations in the gene for interferon regulatory factor 6 located on chromosome 1.[199,200] The presentation is highly variable and may be associated with other anomalies such as lip mounds, syndactyly, ankyloblepharon, ankyloglossia, polythelia, and rarely syngnathia between different parts of the oral cavity.[128,155,201] Lip pits are typically bilateral and may contain mucous glands or salivary glands. Treatment typically involves repairing the cleft lip at around 3 to 4 months of age, cleft palate at 9 to 12 months of age, and removing any lip pits.

Trisomy 13 (Patau Syndrome)

Trisomy 13 is one of the most severe forms of the viable autosomal trisomies with an incidence of around 1:10,000 live births and mean survival time of 8.5 days.[202–204] Nearly 85% to 90% of patients die by one year of life, although one child has reportedly survived to 28 months.[205] Severe mental retardation and failure to thrive are commonly associated findings. Trisomy 13 generally presents with more severe craniofacial and midline defects than those found in trisomy 18 or 21 (**Table 3-7**). The major midline dysmorphic features are due to defective fusion of the midline prechordal mesoderm in the first three weeks of gestation. Major features include[204,206]:

- Predominantly median cleft lip and/or palate (60% of cases)
- Cardiac defects (80%, VSD, ASD, PDA, or dextrocardia)
- Holoprosencephaly (60%)
- Scalp defects (20%, cutis aplasia)
- Renal anomalies (30%)
- Omphalocele (10%)
- Microcephaly
- Microphthalmia
- Ear anomalies, hearing loss
- Polydactyly
- Scoliosis

Imaging studies may include echocardiography for cardiac anomalies, MR or CT imaging to evaluate suspected holoprosencephaly, cardiac, renal, and skeletal anomalies. Rapid aneuploidy testing and prenatal sonography can help diagnose trisomy 13. Sonographic findings include tachycardia, polyhydramnios, early onset intrauterine growth restriction, holoprosencephaly with associated facial anomalies, feet and/or hand anomalies, megalocystis, and omphalocele.[207,208]

Trisomy 18 (Edwards Syndrome)

Trisomy 18 is the second most common autosomal trisomy after trisomy 21 (Down syndrome) with an incidence of 1:3,000 to 8,000 live births and a 3:1 female:male predominance. Mean survival time is 6 days; 50% of patients die by one week of life, and 90% of patients die by one year of life.[202,203] The degree of essential organ involvement and severity of clinical features vary significantly; one mildly affected patients survived to be 19 years old.[209] Severe mental retardation and failure to thrive are commonly associated findings. Major features include[204,210]:

- Cardiac defects (90% of cases, VSD with polyvalvular heart disease, ASD, PDA)
- Cleft lip/palate (5% to 10%, larger clefts than those with normal karyotype)
- Multiple joint contractures (10%)
- Hearing loss (>50%), low-set ears
- Eye (10%)
- Radial bone aplasia (5% to 10%)
- Micrognathia
- Choanal atresia
- Microphthalmia
- Prominent occiput
- "strawberry-shaped" calvarium
- Clenched hand (with overlapped second and fifth digits over the third and fourth)
- Spina bifida
- Renal anomalies

(**Tables 3-4**, **3-7**, and **3-11**)

Diagnostic imaging studies include echocardiography for cardiac anomalies, barium swallow for gastrointestinal anomalies, ultrasonography for genitourinary anomalies, and CT to evaluate skeletal anomalies (absent radius, talipes equinovarus, short sternum, hemivertebrae, fused vertebrae, short neck, scoliosis, rib anomaly, and dislocated hip). Prenatal sonography can be utilized to diagnose trisomy 18 by detecting common major abnormalities including cardiac, central nervous system, gastrointestinal, and genitourinary anomalies, and intrauterine growth restriction; and minor abnormalities including short ear length, facial, and upper and lower extremities anomalies.[211]

Syndromes Associated with Hypertelorism

See Table 3-15.

Apert Syndrome (Acrocephalosyndactyly Type 1)

Apert syndrome (acrocephalosyndactyly type 1) is an autosomal dominant craniofacial dysostosis associated with mutations in the *FGFR2* (fibroblast growth factor receptor 2) gene found in approximately 1:65,000 live births.[212] The major features are craniosynostosis (most commonly involving the coronal sutures) and severe syndactyly of the hands and the feet (second, third, or fourth, or all digits).[213] The craniosynostosis of the coronal suture results in maxillary hypoplasia, retrusion of the midface, an acrocephalic skull that is shortened anteroposteriorly, brachycephaly, turribrachycephaly, flat occiput, and prominent forehead (Fig. 3-29). In approximately 4% of infants, there is scaphocephaly (cloverleaf skull). The pituitary fossa and the basiocciput are larger than normal. Central nervous system anomalies include malformations of the corpus callosum, limbic structures, or gyri; megalencephaly; hypoplasia of the white matter; and heterotropic gray matter. Mental retardation is found in 30% of affected patients. There are large fontanelles that exhibit delayed closure and a gaping midline defect.[133,213]

Facial features include hypertelorism, downward slanting palpebral fissures, shallow orbits, proptosis, exophthalmos, strabismus, amblyopia, optic atrophy, and rarely, luxation of the eye globes, keratoconus, ectopic lentis, congenital glaucoma, and lack of pigment in the fundi with occasional papilledema. The nose has a markedly depressed nasal bridge with a short and wide bulbous tip, parrot-beaked appearance, and choanal stenosis or atresia. The mouth area has a prominent mandible, down-turned corners (trapezoid mouth), high, narrow, arched palate (Byzantine arch palate), bifid uvula, crowded upper teeth, malocclusion, ectopic eruption, shovel-shaped incisors, supernumerary, ectopic teeth, V-shaped maxillary dental arch, and bulging alveolar ridges. Cleft palate occurs in up to 30% of cases. Anomalies of the ears include conductive hearing loss, fixation of the stapedial footplate, wide cochlear aqueduct, absence of the internal auditory canals, and enlarged subarcuate fossa. Other anomalies include fusion of one or more of the cervical vertebrae (typically involving C5 and C6), other skeletal and cartilaginous segmentation defects, and anomalies of the skin, cardiovascular, gastrointestinal, genitourinary, and respiratory systems.[128,133,213,214]

Crouzon Syndrome

Crouzon syndrome (acrocephalosyndactyly type II) is the most frequent craniofacial dysostosis with an incidence estimated to be approximately 16.5:1,000,000 live births.[215] It is an autosomal dominant disorder characterized by premature craniosynostosis due to multiple mutations in the fibroblast growth factor receptor 2 (FGFR2) on chromosome 10. In addition to premature fusion of the cranial sutures, it causes hypoplastic midface, exophthalmos, hypertelorism, and mandibular prognathism. Crouzon syndrome with acanthosis nigricans is due to a mutation in the *FGFR3* gene.[213]

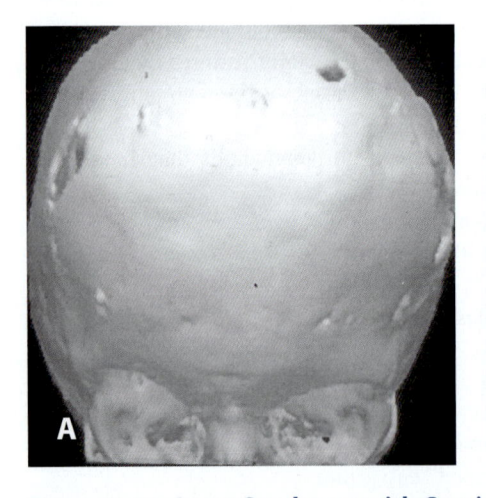

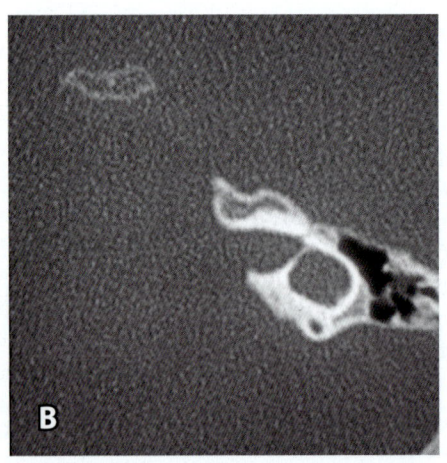

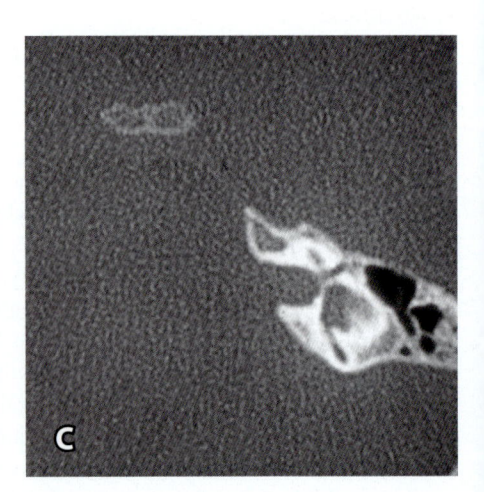

Figure 3-29 Apert Syndrome with Craniosynostosis and Temporal Bone Anomalies
AP 3D CT with surface rendering (**A**) of a six-year-old boy with Apert syndrome. Note the turribrachycephaly and prominent forehead secondary to the craniosynostosis. Axial thin section CT of the left temporal bone scans (**B–C**) show a large cystic cavity that contains the vestibule and semicircular canals. The visualized internal auditory canal is normal. The combination of craniosynostosis and other congenital anomalies is a common feature in syndromic synostoses.

Craniosynostosis of the coronal, sagittal, and lambdoid sutures may occur, giving the skull a brachycephalic or, occasionally, a scaphocephaly (cloverleaf) shape (**Figs. 3-30** and **3-31**). There is lateral and anteroposterior flattening of the skull with growth mostly in the vertical axis. The face appears to grow at a rate about a third that of normal, and forward growth appears to stop at about age 9.[216,217] The face is wide with maxillary hypoplasia, producing pseudoprognathism. The deepest part of the hypoplastic midface is usually at the top of a short, parrot-like nose. The patient may have a high and wide forehead, hypertelorism, divergent squint, and drooping upper eyelids ("frog face"). The upper lip is shortened and sometimes cleaved.[218] Intracranial findings include jugular venous obstruction, anomalous venous drainage and progressive hydrocephalus.[219] Chiari I malformation is seen in 71.4% of patients.[58]

One result of the hypoplastic midface is a high, arched palate, which can raise the nasal floor, crowding the nasal cavities. Additional anomalies of the palate can include lateral palatal swellings and cleft lip/palate. There may be deviation of the nasal septum, narrowed or obliterated anterior nares, and a wide, beaked nose. The maxillary teeth are often crowded, and an anterior open bite is usually present. Proptosis secondary to shallow orbits occurs in most cases and may result in exposure keratitis. Other ocular findings include optic nerve atrophy, strabismis, amblyopia, megalocornea, nystagmus, keratoconus, ectopia lentis, or colobomas of the iris. An estimated 30% to 55% of patients with Crouzon syndrome experience hearing loss (usually conductive). The external auditory canals may be atretic. Ossicular fixation and deformities have also been described.[213,215] Calcification of the stylohyoid ligament occurs most of the time. Anomalies of the cervical vertebrae usually involve C2 and C3; however, there may be other anomalies of the skull and spine.[218]

Carpenter Syndrome, Coffin-Lowry Syndrome, Jackson-Weiss Syndrome, Pfeiffer (Noack) Syndrome, Saethre-Chotzen Syndrome
See **Table 3-15**.

Syndromes Associated with Branchial Arch Anomalies and Unusual Facies
See **Table 3-11**.

Goldenhar Syndrome and Oculo-auriculovertebral Complex
Goldenhar syndrome and the oculo-auriculovertebral complex are rare congenital disorders characterized by a wide spectrum of symptoms and physical features involving the cheekbones, jaw, mouth, ears, eyes, and vertebrae. Originally, *Goldenhar syndrome* referred to mandibular dysostosis, epibulbar dermoids, and perauricular skin tags and pretragal fistulae.[220] Vertebral anomalies were later added to this triad, and the syndrome was renamed *OAV dysplasia*.[221] Then, microtia was added, and the condition was renamed the *OAV complex*.[222] Within the OAV spectrum of anomalies, hemifacial microsomia represents a milder condition, and Goldenhar syndrome represents a more severe form. The incidence of Goldenhar syndrome is 1:3,500 to 5,600 live births, and that of the OAV complex is 1:45,000 live births.[135]

Facial features include hemifacial (or bifacial) microsomia, facial asymmetry, malar hypoplasia, maxillary and mandibular hypoplasia, temporal hypoplasia, macrostomia, cleft palate, cleft lip, and/or teeth abnormalities. Most cases show mixed transverse and vertical hypoplasia. Most cases of hemifacial microsomia are unilateral, but approximately 16% to 35% of cases are bilateral, with typically the right side affected more severely than the left.[223,224] Eye anomalies may also be present, including epibulbar dermoids and lipodermoids, colobomas of the upper eyelids, microphthalmia, narrow palpebral fissures, and strabismus.[225] Ear anomalies include anotia and/or microtia, external auditory canal atresia, preauricular tags, and conductive and/or sensorineural hearing loss.[135] Vertebral malformations may involve hypoplasia, fusion, and agenesis of vertebrae. Cardiac anomalies include ventricular septal defect, patent ductus arteriosus, tetralogy of Fallot, and coarctation of the aorta. Other associated anomalies may involve the skeletal, neurologic, pulmonary, renal, and gastrointestinal systems. Mild mental retardation is found in approximately 5% to 15% of patients. Patients with cleft lip/palate and anophthalmia/microphthalmia seem to be at an increased risk for cerebral malformation and mental retardation.[133]

Pierre-Robin Sequence
Pierre-Robin sequence (syndrome, complex, or triad) refers to a series of anomalies caused by a cascade of events initiated by a single malformation (**Tables 3-7** and **3-11**). The characteristics include micrognathia (**Fig. 3-32**), glossoptosis (tongue rests far back in the oropharynx), and cleft soft palate (no cleft lip). Although there are several theories about the etiology of this condition, the most accepted theory proposes that the initial event, mandibular hypoplasia, begins between the seventh and tenth weeks of gestation, prevents the tongue from descending below the two halves of the palate. Because the tongue remains high in the oral cavity, it obstructs complete closure of the palatal shelves. This theory explains the high arched palate, the rounded, U-shaped cleft palate, and the absence of cleft lip.[226–228] The associated ear anomalies (abnormal auricles, abnormal stapes footplates, aplasia of the lateral semicircular canals, islands of cartilage in the expected position of Reichert's cartilage, and dehiscence of the fallopian canal) are consistent with improper development of the first and second branchial arches.[229]

The prevalence is approximately 1:8,500 live births (1:2,000 to 30,000, depending on how strictly the condition is defined).[228,230] Pierre-Robin sequence can occur as an isolated anomaly (17%) or as a feature of another syndrome such as Stickler syndrome (34% of cases have the syndrome), velocardiofacial syndrome (11%), or Treacher Collins syndrome (5%). It can also be caused by teratogens as in the case of fetal alcohol syndrome (10%) and fetal hydantoin syndrome. An X-linked variant which is associated with cardiac malformations and clubfeet.[231,232]

Posterior placement of the tongue may cause choking episodes, feeding difficulty, and upper airway obstruction, especially while sleeping. Three-dimensional CT with volume rendering can provide quantitative information about any airway

124 Diagnostic Imaging of the Head and Neck

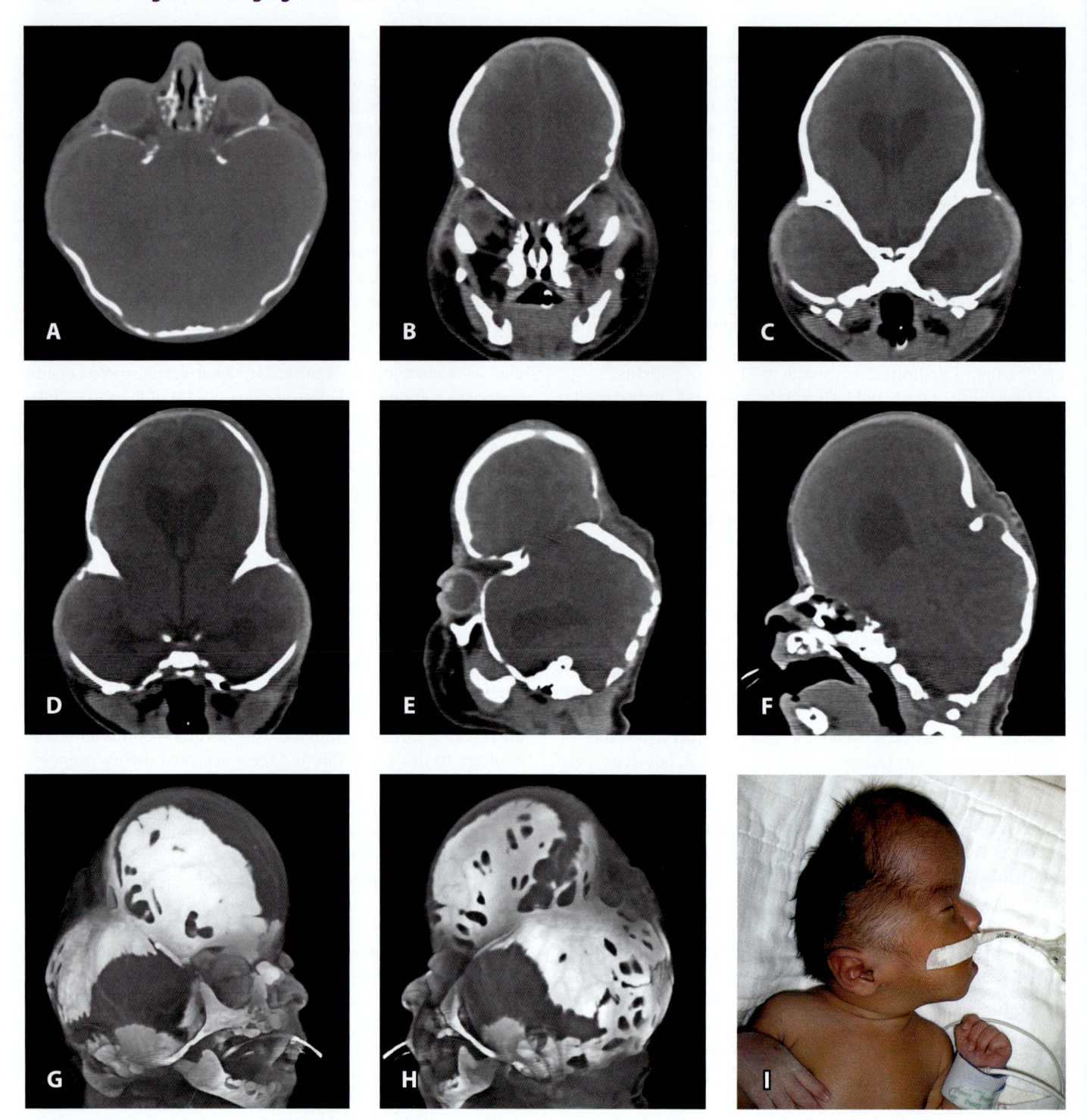

Figure 3-30 Crouzon Syndrome with "Cloverleaf" Skull
Newborn infant to a mother with Crouzon syndrome. The child has a profound cloverleaf deformity of the head, secondary to universal craniosynostosis, except for the sagittal and meitopic sutures. Axial (**A**), reformatted coronal (**B–D**), and reformatted sagittal (**E–F**) CT images show extensive bulging superiorly and laterally, with a disproportionately large skull, relative to the hypolastic midface. Note the shallow orbit with approximation of the globe to the posterior portion of the orbit (**E**) and the choanal atresia with bony constriction of the posterior nasal airway (**F**). Right lateral (**G**) and left lateral (**H**) 3D CT reconstructions with surface rendering show a discrepancy in development between the normal facial bones, including the maxilla and the mandible, that are preformed from cartilage from the remainder of the markedly deformed calvarium. The apparent defects in the skull result from areas of thin calvarium that are below the threshold set for the reconstruction sequence. Photograph (**I**) of the newborn depicted in (**A–H**) shows the gross appearance of the cloverleaf skull and the midface hypoplasia. There is an endotracheal tube in place to compensate for the choanal atresia. (Case courtesy of Christopher R. Trimble, MD).

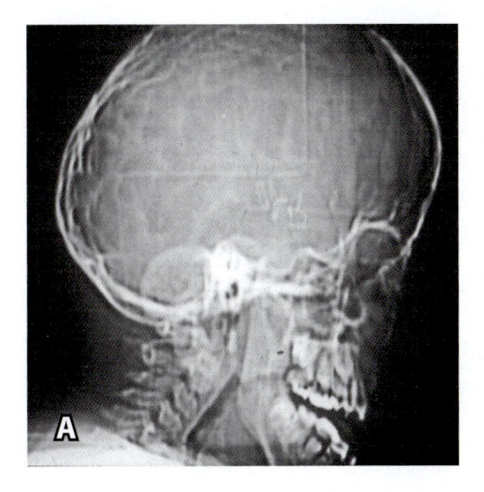

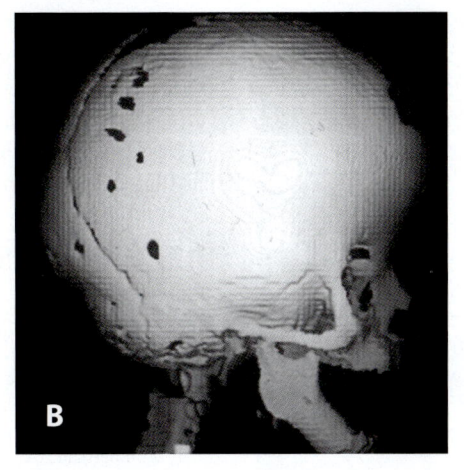

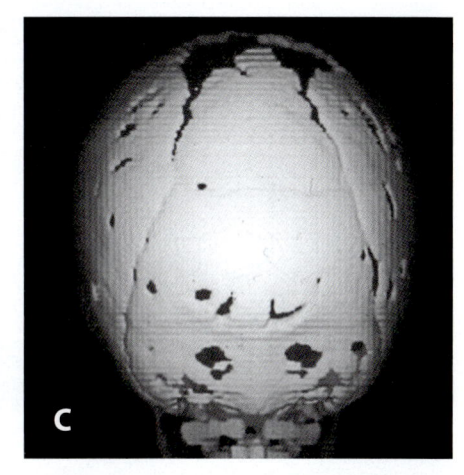

Figure 3-31 Crouzon Syndrome without "Cloverleaf" Skull
Sagittal plain film of the skull (**A**) shows increased convolution markings with alternating foci of thickened and thin calvarium. Also note the disproportionately large head, compared to a hypoplastic midface and maxilla with the associated underbite. The Sagittal (**B**) and PA (**C**) 3D CT reconstruction with surface rendering show the universal synostosis without the superior and lateral bulging seen with the "cloverleaf" variant of Crouzon syndrome.

obstruction and bony defects (Fig. 3-32). If airway obstruction is severe, a tracheotomy may be necessary. Neonatal distraction osteogenesis may be effective in treating micrognathia and tongue ptosis with airway obstruction without the need for tracheotomy.[233,234] In moderate cases, a nasopharyngeal airway may be sufficient. Bronchial aspiration, pulmonary infection, and gastroesophageal reflux are common complications. In many patients, the mandible grows rapidly during the first year of life and may grow within normal range by the time the child is four to six years old. Children who do not have sufficient growth may require surgical repair. The cleft palate, if present, should be repaired generally between 1 and 2 years of age.[228,235]

Branchio-oto-renal Syndrome
Branchio-oto-renal (BOR) syndrome (Melnick-Fraser syndrome) is an autosomal dominant disorder caused by mutations in the EYA1 gene that result in auricular malformations, deafness, branchial fistulae, and renal anomalies. The prevalence is estimated to be 1:40,000 in the general population.[236] The pathogenesis is presumed to be a deficiency in the differentiation of the first and second branchial arches. The anomalies of the renal system are the result of abnormal interaction between the ureteric bud and the metanephric blastema.

The renal malformations and hearing impairment can be significant. Renal dysplasia is reported in over two-thirds of patients and varies from tapered superior poles (duplication of the collection system) to agenesis of the kidney. The syndrome may include Potter sequence.[133] The auricular malformations include preauricular pits in the superior part of the pinna (75% to 85% of cases), preauricular tags, lop or bat ears, and microtia. The external auditory canals may be atretic. Anomalies of the middle ear include abnormalities of the ossicles, the facial nerve, and the fallopian canals. Hearing loss (75% to 90% of cases) is usually stable and may be conductive, sensorineural, or mixed. An estimated 2% of children with profound deafness have BOR syndrome.[133,236]

CT imaging of the temporal bone may show the most common characteristics of BOR syndrome: 1) hypoplastic apical turn of the cochlea, 2) facial nerve deviated to the medial side of the cochlea, 3) funnel-shaped internal auditory canal, and 4) patulous eustachian tube.[237] BOR patients with an enlarged endolymphatic

Table 3-15 Conditions Associated with Hypertelorism

Syndromes
- Median cleft syndrome / frontonasal dysplasia
- Tetrasomy 9p
- Syndromes with craniosynostosis
  - Antley-Bixler syndrome
  - Apert syndrome (acrocephalosyndactyly type 1)
  - Carpenter syndrome (Fig. 3-36)
  - Coffin-Lowry syndrome (Lowry's, Coffin-Siris-Wegienka)
  - Crouzon syndrome (acrocephalosyndactyly type II)
  - Jackson-Weiss syndrome
  - Lowry-Wood syndrome
  - Pfeiffer (Noack) syndrome
  - Saethre-Chotzen syndrome
  - Waardenburg syndrome

Anatomic Anomalies
- Frontal cephaloceles
- Dysgenesis of the corpus callosum
- Bifid nose

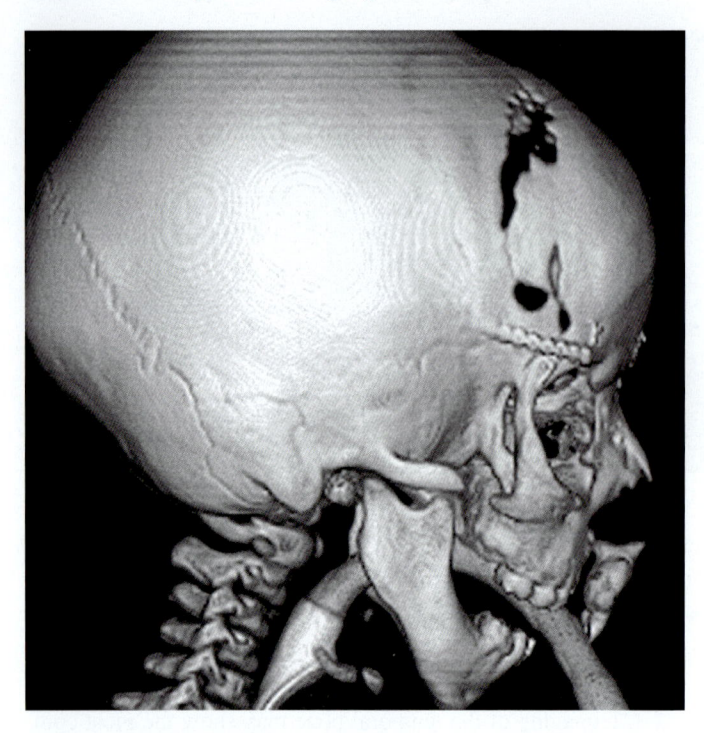

Figure 3-32 Pierre-Robin Sequence with Zygomatic Hypoplasia
3D CT reconstruction shows Pierre-Robin clefts with zygomatic hypoplasia in a newborn. An orotracheal tube is also visualized.

duct and/or sac on MR images seemed to be predisposed to developing more severe hearing impairment.[238] The branchial fistulae (63%) of BOR syndrome are usually bilateral and in the lower part of the neck with external openings on the medial border of the sternomastoid muscle. Other associated manifestations include aplasia or stenosis of the lacrimal ducts (8% to 9%), high-arched or cleft palate, and deep overbite. Some authors consider hemifacial microsomia to be a severe form.[133]

Branchio-oculo-facial Syndrome
Branchio-oculo-facial (BOF) syndrome (lip-pseudocleft hemangiomatous branchial cyst syndrome) is a rare autosomal dominant disorder with incomplete penetrance and variable expression affecting the eye, ear, oral, and craniofacial structures.[239] It is characterized by nonmidline pseudocleft of the upper lip, malformed nose with broad bridge and flattened tip, lacrimal duct obstruction, atresia of the external ear, maxillar and mandibular hypoplasia, branchial cleft sinuses/cysts, and/or linear skin lesions behind the ears.[240,241] Other anomalies include coloboma, microphathalmia, auricular pits, lip pits, high, arched palate, dental anomalies, subcutaneous, cysts of the scalp, stenotic external auditory canals, inner ear dysplasia associated with conductive or sensorineural hearing loss, hypertrichosis of the neck, and renal malformations.[231,242] Premature graying of hair has been reported in affected adults. Growth retardation, developmental delay, and hand anomalies are variable components of the syndrome.[229,230]

Although branchio-oculo-facial syndrome and branchio-oto-renal syndrome can both present with naso-lacrimal duct stenosis, hearing loss, prehelical pits, malformed pinna, and renal anomalies, BOF syndrome is not associated with the EYA 1 gene mutations responsible for BOR syndrome.[176,243] Furthermore, BOF syndrome is associated with the unusual areas of thin, erythematous, wrinkled skin of the neck and/or auricular region, which differs from the discrete, cervical pits, cysts, and fistulas of BOR syndrome.[187]

REFERENCES

1. Hamilton WJ and Mossman HW, eds.: Human Embryology. 4th ed. Baltimore: Williams & Wilkins, 1972:291–376.
2. Schaeffer JP: The Nose, Paranasal Sinuses, Nasolacrimal Passageways and Olfactory Organ in Man: A Genetic, Developmental, and Anatomico-Physiological Consideration. Philadelphia: P Blakiston's Son, 1920.
3. Zimmerman AA: Development of the paranasal sinuses. Arch Otolaryngol 1938;27:793–795.
4. Donald PJ, Gluckman JL, and Rice DH, eds.: The Sinuses. New York: Raven Press, 1995:15–23.
5. Som PM and Curtin HD, eds.: Head and Neck Imaging. 4th ed. St Louis: Mosby, 2003:3–147.
6. Mafee MF, Valvassori GE, and Becker M, eds.: Valvassori's Imaging of the Head and Neck. 2nd ed. New York: Thieme Medical Publishers, 2005:353–370.
7. Kennedy DW, Bolger WE, and Zinreich SJ, eds.: Diseases of the Sinuses. Hamilton: BC Decker, 2001:1–11.
8. Tewfik TL and Yoskovitch A: Congenital malformations, nose. Emedicine. www.emedicine.com/ent/topic320.htm; 2003.
9. Bingham B, Wang RG, Hawke M, and Kwok P: The embryonic development of the lateral nasal wall from 8 to 24 weeks. Laryngoscope 1991;101:912–997.
10. Libersa C, Laude M, and Libersa JC: The pneumatization of the accessory cavities of the nasal fossae during growth. Anat Clin 1981;2:265–273.
11. Maresh MM: Paranasal sinuses from birth to late adolescence. Am J Dis Child 1940;60:58–75.
12. Van Alyea OE: Nasal Sinuses: An Anatomic and Clinical Consideration. 2nd ed. Baltimore: Williams and Wilkins, 1951.
13. Vidic V: The postnatal development of the sphenoidal sinus and its spread into the dorsum sellae and posterior clinoid processes. Am J Roentgenol 1968;104:177–183.
14. Castillo M: Congenital abnormalities of the nose: CT and MR findings. Am J Roentgenol 1994;162:1211–1217.
15. Kennard CD and Rasmussen JE: Congenital midline nasal masses: diagnosis and management. J Dermatol Surg Oncol 1990;16:1025–1036.
16. Vogelzand PH, Babeel RW, and Harnsberger HR: The nose and nasal vault. Semin Ultrasound CT MR 1991;12:592–612.
17. Lowe LH, Booth TN, Joglar JM, and Rollins NK: Midface anomalies in children. RadioGraphics 2000;20:907–922.
18. Sadler TW: Langman's Medical Embryology. 5th ed. Baltimore: Williams & Wilkins, 1985.
19. Rand PK, Ball WS, and Kulwin DR: Congenital Nasolacrimal Mucoceles: CT Evaluation. Radiology 1989;173:691–694.
20. Kuhn FA, Bolger WE, and Tisdal RG: The agger nasi cell in frontal recess obstruction: an anatomic, radiologic and clinical correlation. Op Tech Otolaryngol Head Neck Surg 1991;2:226–231.
21. Kennedy DW, Bolger WE, and Zinreich SJ, eds.: Diseases of the Sinuses. Hamilton: BC Decker, 2001:1–27.
22. Bolger WE, Woodruff WW, and Parsons DS: CT demonstration of uncinate process pneumatization: a rare paranasal sinus anomaly. Am J Neurorad 1990;11:552.
23. Van Alyea OE: Ostium maxillare: anatomic study of its surgical accessibility. Arch Otolaryngol Head Neck Surg 1939;24:552–569.
24. Yousem DM: Imaging of sinonasal inflammatory disease. Radiology 1993;188:303–314.
25. Stammberger H: Functional Endoscopic Sinus Surgery: The Messerklinger Technique. Philadelphia: BC Decker, 1991.
26. Onishi T: Bony defects and dehiscences of the roof of the ethmoid cells. Rhinology 1981;19:195–202.
27. Lee C and Archer SM: CT scan, nasal cavity. Emedicine. www.emedicine.com/ent/topic386.htm; 2004.

28. Oliverio PJ, Benson ML, and Zinreich SJ: Update on imaging for functional endoscopic sinus surgery. Otolaryngol Clin North Am 1995; 28:585–608.
29. Bolger WE, Woodruff WW, and Parsons DS: CT demonstration of uncinate process pneumatization: a rare paranasal sinus anomaly. Am J Neurorad 1990;11:552.
30. Kennedy DW and Zinreich SJ: Functional endoscopic approach to inflammatory sinus disease: current perspectives and technique modifications. Am J Rhinol 1988;2:89–96.
31. Naumann H: Patholische anatomic der chronischen rhinitis und sinisitis. In: Proceedings VIII International Congress of Oto-rhinolaryngology. Amsterdam: Excerpta Medica;1965;12.
32. Moonis G: Imaging of sinonasal anatomy and inflammatory disorders. Crit Rev Comp Tomog 2003;44:187–228.
33. Stammberger HR, Bolger WE, Clement PAR, et al.: Anatomic terminology and nomenclature in sinusitis. Ann Otol Rhinol Laryngol 1995;104:7–19.
34. van Alyea OE: Frontal cells. Arch Otolaryngol 1941;34:11–23.
35. Sirikci A, Bayazit YA, Bayram M, and Kanlikama M: Ehtmomaxillary sinus: a particular anatomic variationof the paranasal sinuses. Eur Radiol 2004;14:281–285.
36. Bolger WE, Woodruff WW, Morehead J, and Parsons DS: Maxillary sinus hypoplasia: classification and description of associated uncinate hypoplasia. Otolaryngol Head Neck Surg 1990;103:759–765.
37. Bolger WE and Kennedy DW: Atelectasis of the maxillary sinus. J Respir Dis 1992;13:1448–1450.
38. Karmody CS, Carter B, and Vincent ME: Developmental anomalies of the maxillary sinus. Trans Am Acad Ophthalmol Otolaryngol 1977;84:723–728.
39. Kantarci M, Karasen RM, Alper F, et al.: Remarkable anatomic variations in paranasal sinus region and their clinical importance. Eur J Rad 2004; 50:296–302.
40. Lloyd GAS: CT of the paranasal sinuses: study of a control series in relation to endoscopic sinus surgery. J Laryngol Otol 1990;104:477–481.
41. Perez-Pinas I, Sabate J, Carmona A, et al.: Anatomical variations in the human paranasal sinus regions studied by CT. J Anat 2000;197:22–27.
42. Uzun L, Ugur MB, Savranlar A, et al.: Classification of the inferior turbinate bones: a computed tomography study. Eur J Radiol. 2004;51:241–245.
43. Ozturk A, Alatas N, Ozturk E, et al.: Pneumatization of the inferior turbinates: incidence and radiologic appearance. J Comput Assist Tomogr 2005;29:311–314.
44. van Alyea OE: Ehmoid labyrinth: anatomic study, with consideration the clinical significance of its structural characteristics. Arch Otolaryngol 1939;29:881–902.
45. Onodi A: The Optic Nerve and the Accessory Sinuses of the Nose. London: Bailliere, Tindall and Cox; 1910:1–26.
46. Maniglia AJ: Fatal and major complications secondary to nasal and sinus surgery. Laryngoscope 1988;99:276–283.
47. Wyllie JW, Kern EB, and Djalilian M: Isolated sphenoid sinusitis. Laryngoscope 1973;83:1252–1265.
48. Chen MC and Davidson TM: Clinical evaluation of postoperative sinonasal surgical patients. Semin Ultrasound CT MR 2002;23:466–474.
49. Moulin G, Dessi P, Chagnaud C, et al.: Dehiscence of the lamina papyracea of the ethmoid bone: CT findings. Am J Neuroradiol 1994;15:151–153.
50. Keros P: Uber die praktische beteudung der Niveau-Unterschiede der lamina cribrosa des ethmoids. In: Naumann HH, ed. Head and Neck Surgery. Vol 1. Face and Facial Skull. Philadelphia, PA: WB Saunders, 1980:392.
51. Kainz J and Stammberger H: The roof of the anterior ethmoid: a place of least resistance in the skull base. Am J Rhinol 1989;3:191–199.
52. Shankar L, Evans K, Hawke M, and Stammberger H: An Atlas of Imaging of the Paranasal Sinuses. Philadelphia: JB Lippincott Co, 1994:10.
53. Lowe LH, Booth TN, Foglar JM, and Rollins NK: Midface anomalies in children. Radiographics 2000;20:907–922.
54. Sadler TW: Langman's Medical Embryology. 5th ed. Baltimore, MD: Williams & Wilkins, 1985.
55. Yildirim I and Okur E: The prevalence of nasal septal deviation in children from Kahramanmaras, Turkey. Int J Pediatr Otorhinolaryngol 2003;67:1203–1206.
56. Kurihashi K, Imada M, and Yamashita A: Anatomical analysis of the human lacrimal drainage pathway under an operating microscope. Int Ophthalmol 1991;15:411–416.
57. Coates H: Nasal obstruction in the neonate and infant. Clin Pediatr 1992; 31:25–29.
58. Lowe LH, Booth TN, Joglar JM, and Rollins NK: Midface anomalies in children. Radiographics 2000;20:907–922.
59. Hughes GB, Sharpino G, Hunt W, and Tucker HM: Management of the congenital midline nasal masses: a review. Head Neck Surg 1980;2:222–233.
60. Fitzpatrick E and Miller RH: Congenital midline nasal masses: dermoids, gliomas, and encephaloceles. J La State Med Soc 1996;148:93–96.
61. Barkovich AJ, Vandermarch P, Edwards MSB, and Cogen PH: Congenital nasal masses: CT and MR imaging features in 16 cases. Am J Neuroradiol 1991;12:105–116.
62. Khan AN and Turnbull I: Encephalocele. Emedicine. http://www.emedicine.com/radio/topic246.htm, 2005.
63. Rahbar R, Resto VA, Robson CD, et al.: Nasal glioma and encephalocele: diagnosis and management. Laryngoscope 2003;113:2069–2077.
64. Cohen MM and Lemire RJ: Syndromes with cephaloceles. Teratology 1982;25:161–172.
65. Blumenfeld R and Skolnik EM: Intranasal encephaloceles. Arch Otolaryngol 1965;82:527–531.
66. Tewfik TL and Yoskovitch A: Congenital malformations, nose. Emedicine. http:/www.emedicine.com/ent/topic320.htm, 2003.
67. Gorenstein A, Kern EB, Facer GW, and Lows ER Jr.: Nasal gliomas. Arch Otolaryngol 1980;106:536–540.
68. Shah J, Patkar D, Patankar T, et al.: Pedunculated nasal glioma: MRI features and review of the literature. J Postgrad Med 1999;45:15–17.
69. Patterson K, Kapur S, and Chandra RS: Nasal gliomas and related brain heterotopias: a pathologist's perspective. Pediatr Pathol 1986;5:353–362.
70. Kennard CD and Rasmussen JE: Congenital midline nasal masses: diagnosis and management. J Dermatol Surg Oncol 1990;16:1025–1036.
71. Harley EH: Pediatric congenital nasal masses. Ear Nose Throat J 1991;70:28–32.
72. Pratt LW: Midline cysts of the nasal dorsum: embryologic origin and treatment. Laryngoscope 1965;75:968–980.
73. Sessions RB: Nasal dermal sinuses: new concepts and explanations. Laryngoscope 1982;92:7–28.
74. Vogelzand PJ, Babbel RW, and Harnsberger HR: The nose and nasal vault. Semin Ultrasound CT MR 1991;12:592–612.
75. Bloom DC, Cavalho DS, Dory C, et al.: Imaging and surgical approach of nasal dermoids. Int J Pediatr Otorhinolaryngol 2002;62:111–122.
76. Melnick M: Cleft lip and palate: Etiology and Pathogenesis. In Kenahan PA, Rosenstein SW and Dado DV, eds.: Cleft Lip and Palate: A System of Management. Baltimore: Williams and Wilkins, 1990:2.
77. Tolarova MM: Cleft lip and palate. Emedicine. http://www.emedicine.com/ped/topic2679.htm#target1, 2005.
78. Tolarova MM and Cervenka J: Classification and birth prevalence of orofacial clefts. Amer J Med Genet 1998;75:126–137.
79. Schutte BC: Genetic links to psychiatry: orofacial cleft gene a potential door to understanding brain development disorders. Currents. http://www.uihealthcare.com/news/currents/vol4issue2/cleftpalate.html, 2003.
80. Barbara P, Homeier BP, and Bartoshesky LE: Cleft lip and palate. KidsHealth. http://kidshealth.org/parent/medical/ears/cleft_lip_palate.html, 2005.
81. Kirschner RE and LaRossa D: Cleft lip and palate. Otolaryngol Clin North Am 2000;33:1191–1215.
82. Karmacharya J: Cleft lip. Emedicine. http://www.emedicine.com/ent/topic135.htm, 2005.
83. Murray JC: Face facts: genes, environment, and clefts. Am J Hum Genet 1995;57:227–232.
84. Berge SJ, Plath H, Reich RH, and Hansmann M: Significance of prenatal diagnosis of lip-jaw-palatal clefts. Mund Kiefer Gesichtschir 2002;2:85–90.
85. Stoll C, Alembik Y, Dott B, and Roth MP: Associated malformations in cases with oral clefts. Cleft Palate-Craniofac J 2000;37:41–47.
86. Babcock CJ: The fetal face and neck: facial clefts. In Callen, PW, ed. Ultrasonography in Obstetrics and Gynecology, 4th ed. Philadelphia: WB Saunders Company, 2000:324.
87. Naidich TP, Blaser SI, Bauer BS, et al.: Embryology and congenital lesions of the midface. In Som PM, Curtin HD, eds. Head and Neck Imaging, 4th ed. St Louis: Mosby, 2003:4–86.
88. Fogh-Andersen P: Rare clefts of the face. Acta Chir Scand 1965;129:275–281.

89. Naidich TP, Osborn RE, Bauer B, et al.: Median cleft face syndrome: MR and CT data from 11 children. J Comput Assist Tomogr 1988;12:57–64.
90. DeMyer W: The median cleft face syndrome: differential diagnosis of cranium bifidum occultum, hypertelorism, and median cleft nose, lip and palate. Neurology 1967;17:961–971.
91. Sedano HO, Cohen MM, Jirasek J, et al.: Frontonasal dysplasia. J Pediatr 1970;76:906–913.
92. Gupta H and Gupta P: Median cleft face syndrome. Indian Pediatr 2004;41:90.
93. Coban YK, Boran C, Omeroglu SA, and Okur E: Pai syndrome: an adult patient with bifid nose and frontal hairline marker. Cleft Palate–Craniofac J 2003;40:325–328.
94. Pascual-Castroviejo I, Pascual-Pascual SI, and Perez-Higueras A: Frontonasal dysplasia and lipoma of the corpus callosum. Eur J Pediatr 1985;144:66–71.
95. Anyane-Yeboa K, Raifman MA, Berant M, Frogel MP, Travers H, and Opitz JM: Dominant inheritance of bifid nose. Am J Med Genet 1984;17:561–563.
96. Miller PJ, Grinberg D, and Wang TD: Midline cleft. Treatment of the bifid nose. Arch Facial Plast Surg 1999;1:200–203.
97. Sadler TW: Langman's Medical Embryology, 6th ed. Baltimore: Williams & Wilkins, 1990.
98. Bhattacharyya AK and Lund VJ: Unilateral choanal atresia in siblings – a rare occurrence. J Laryngol Otol 1996;665–667.
99. Tewfik TL and Hagr AA: Choanal atresia. Emedicine. http://www.emedicine.com/ent/topic330.htm, 2005.
100. Brown OE, Pownell P, and Manning SC: Choanal atresia: a new anatomic classification and clinical management applications. Laryngoscope 1996;106:97–101.
101. Vogelzand PJ, Babbel RW, and Harnsberger HR: The nose and nasal vault. Semin Ultrasound CT MR 1991;12:592–612.
102. Paoli CH, Francois M, Triglia JM, Frydman E, Polonovski JM, and Narcy PH: Nasal obstruction in the neonate secondary to nasolacrimal duct cysts. Laryngoscope 1995;105:86–89.
103. Castillo M: Congenital abnormalities of the nose: CT and MR findings. Am J Roentgenol 1994;162:1211–1217.
104. Royal SA, Hedlund GL, and Wiatrak BJ: Single central maxillary incisor with nasal pyriform aperture stenosis-CT diagnosis prior to tooth eruption. Pediatr Radiol 1999;29:357–359.
105. Belden CJ, Mancuso AA, and Schmalfuss IM: CT features of congenital nasal pyriform aperture stenosis: initial experience. Radiology 1999;213:495–501.
106. Hou J-W: Congenital arhinia with de novo reciprocal translocation, t(3;12)(q13.2;p11.2). Am J Med Genet 2004;130:200–203.
107. Shino M, Chikamatsu K, Yasuoka Y, et al.: Congenital arhinia: a case report and functional evaluation. Laryngoscope 2005;115:1118–1123.
108. Olsen OE, Gjelland K, Reigstad H, and Rosendahl K: Congenital absence of the nose: a case report and literature review. Pediatr Radiol 2001;31:225–232.
109. Albernaz VS, Castillo M, Mukherji SK, and Ihmeidan IH: Congenital arhinia. Am J Neuroradiol 1996;17:1312–1314.
110. Zeitouni AG and Shapiro RS: Congenital anomalies of the nose and anterior skull base. In: Tewfik TL and Der Kaloustian VM, eds.: Congenital Anomalies of the Ear, Nose, and Throat. New York: Oxford University Press, 1997:189–200.
111. Belet N, Belet U, Tekat A, and Kucukoduk S: Proboscis lateralis: radiological evaluation. Pediatr Radiol 2002;32:99–101.
112. Abou-Elhamd KA and Al-Hewaige MT: Proboscis lateralis: clinical and radiological features. J Laryngol Otol 2005;119:158–160.
113. Lindsay B: A nose with supernumerary nostrils. Trans Pathol Soc Lond 1906;57:329–330.
114. Tawse HV: Supernumerary nostril and cavity. Proc R Soc Med 1920;13:28–30.
115. Nakamura K and Onizuka T: A case of supernumerary nostril. Plast Reconstr Surg 1987;80:436–441.
116. Williams A, Pizzuto M, Brodsky L, and Perry R: Supernumerary nostril: a rare congenital deformity. Inter J Ped Otorhinolaryngol 1998;44:161–167.
117. Mansour AM, Cheng KP, Mumma JV, et al.: Congenital dacryocele: a collaborative review. Ophthalmology 1991;98:1744–1751.
118. Hepler KM, Woodson GE, and Kearns DB: Respiratory distress in the neonate: sequela of a congenital dacryocystocele. Arch Otolaryngol Head Neck Surg 1995;121:1423–1425.
119. Teymoortash A, Hesse L, Werner JA, and Lippert BM: Bilateral congenital dacryocystocele as a cause of respiratory distress in a newborn. Rhinology 2004;42:41–44.
120. Sepulveda W, Wojakowski AB, Elias D, et al.: Congenital dacryocystocele: prenatal 2 and 3-dimensional sonographic findings. J Ultrasound Med 2005;24:225–230.
121. Ogawa GS and Gonnering RS: Congenital nasolacrimal duct obstruction. J Pediatr 1991;119:12–17.
122. Rand PK, Ball WS, and Kulwin DR: Congenital nasolacrimal mucoceles: CT evaluation. Radiology 1989;173:691–694.
123. Paoli CH, Francois M, Triglia JM, Frydman E, Polonovski JM, and Narcy PH. Nasal obstruction in the neonate secondary to nasolacrimal duct cysts. Laryngoscope 1995;105:86–89.
124. Koch BL: Case 73: nasolacrimal duct mucocele. Radiology 2004;232:370–372.
125. Singh DJ and Bartlett SP: Congenital mandibular hypoplasia: analysis and classification. J Craniofac Surg 2005;16:291–300.
126. Moore KL: The branchi apparati and the head and neck. The Developing Human. Philadelphia: WB Saunders, Harcourt Brace Jovanovich, Inc, 1988.
127. McCarthy JG, Kawamoto H, Grayson BH, et al.: Surgery of the jaws. In: McCarthy, ed. Plastic Surgery. Philadelphia: WB Saunders, Harcourt Brace Jovanovich Inc, 1990:1188–1474.
128. Gorlin RJ, Cohen MM, and Levin LS, eds.: Syndromes of the Head and Neck. 3rd ed. New York: Oxford University Press, 1990:738–740.
129. Morovic CG and Monasterio L: Distraction osteogenesis for obstructive apneas in patients with congenital craniofacial malformations. Plast Reconstr Surg 2000;105:2324–2330.
130. David DJ, Mahatumarat C, and Cooter RD: Hemifacial microsomia: a multisystem classification. Plast Reonstr Surg 1987;80:525–535.
131. Gorlin RJ, Cohen MM, and Levin LS, eds.: Syndromes of the Head and Neck. 3rd ed. New York: Oxford University Press, 1990:641–649.
132. Rahbar R, Robson CD, Mulliken JB, Schwartz L, Dicanzio J, Kenna MA, McGill TJ, and Healy GB: Craniofacial, temporal bone, and audiologic abnormalities in the spectrum of hemifacial microsomia. Arch Otolaryngol Head Neck Surg 2001;127:265–271.
133. Tewfik TL: Manifestations of craniofacial syndromes. Emedicine. http://www.emedicine.com/ent/topic319.htm#target1, 2003.
134. Fan WS, Mulliken JB, and Padwa BL: An association between hemifacial microsomia and facial clefting. J Oral Maxillofac Surg 2005;63:330–334.
135. Naidich TP, Smith MS, Castillo M, et al.: Facies to remember. Number 7. Hemifacial microsomia. Goldenhar syndrome. OAV complex. Int J Neuroradiol 1996;2:437–449.
136. Poon CC, Meara JG, and Heggie AA: Hemifacial microsomia: use of the OMENS-Plus classification at the Royal Children's Hospital of Melbourne. Plast Reconstr Surg 2003;111:1011–1018.
137. Horgan JE, Padwa BL, la Brie RA, and Mulliken JB: OMENS-plus: analysis of craniofacial and extracraniofacial anomalies in hemifacila microsomia. Cleft paltate-Craniofaci J 1995;32:405–412.
138. Kapoor S, Mukherjee SB, Paul R, and Dhingra B: OMENS-plus syndrome. Indian J Pediatr 2005;72:707–708.
139. Cascone P, Gennaro P, Spuntarelli G, and Iannetti G: Mandibular distraction: evolution of treatment protocols in hemifacial microsomy. J Craniofac Surg 2005;16:563–571.
140. Daniels JS: Congenital maxillomandibular fusion: a case report and review of the literature. J Craniomaxillofac Surg 2004;32:135–139.
141. Ugurlu K, Karsidag S, Huthut I, Yildiz K, and Bas L: Congenital fusion of the maxilla and mandible. J Craniofac Surg 2005;16:287–291.
142. Dawson KH, Gruss JS, and Myall RW: Congenital bony syngnathia: a proposed classification. Cleft Palate Craniofac J 1997;34:141–146.
143. Laster Z, Temkin D, Zarfin Y, and Kushmir A: Complete bony fusion of the mandible to the zygomatic complex and maxillary tuberosity: case report and review. Int J Oral Maxillofac Surg 2001;30:75–79.
144. Rao S, Oak S, Wagh M, and Kulkarni B: Congenital midline palatomandibular bony fusion with a mandibular cleft and a bifid tongue. B J Plastic Surg 1997;50:139–141.
145. Kamata S, Satoh K, Vemura T, and Onizuka T: Congenital bilateral zygomaticomandibular fusion with mandibular hypoplasia. B J Plastic Surg 1996;49:251–253.
146. Shah RM: Palatomandibular and maxillo-mandibular fusion, partial aglossia and cleft palate in a human embryo. Teratology 1977;15:261–272.

147. Agrawal K, Chandra SS, and Sreckumar NS: Congenital bilateral intermaxillary bony fusion. Ann Plast Surg 1993;30:163–166.
148. Salleh NM: Congenital partial fusion of the mandible and maxilla. Oral Surg Oral Med Oral Pathol 1965;20:74–76.
149. Gartlan MG, Davies J, and Smith RJ: Congenital oral synechiae. Ann Otol Rhinol Laryngol 1993;102:186–197.
150. Behnia H and Shamse MG: Congenital unilateral fusion of the mandibular and maxillary alveolar ridge, tempo romandibular joint, and coronoid process. J Oral Maxillofac Surg 1996;54:773–776.
151. Hamamoto J and Matsumoto T: A case of facio-genito-popliteal syndrome. Ann Plast Surg 1984;13:224–229.
152. Gartlan MG, Davies J, and Smith RJ: Congenital oral synechiae. Ann Otol Rhinol Laryngol 1993;102:186–197.
153. Johnsson GF and Robinow M. Aglossia-adactylia. Radiology 1978;128:127–132.
154. Knoll B, Karas D, Persing JA, and Shin J: Complete congenital bony syngnathia in a case of oromandibular limb hypogenesis syndrome. J Craniofac Surg 2000;11:398–404.
155. Puvabanditsin S, Garrow E, Sitburana O, Avila FM, Nabong MY, and Biswas A: Syngnathia and Van der Woude syndrome: a case report and literature review. Cleft Palate Craniofac J 2003;40:104–106.
156. O'neill BM, Alessi AS, and Petti NA: Otocephaly or agnathia-synotia-microstomia syndrome: report of a case. J Oral Maxillofac Surg 2003;61:834–837.
157. Yang SH, Seo YS, Lee YS, et al.: Prenatal sonographic diagnosis of isolated agnathia: a case report. Ultrasound Obstet Gynecol 2003;22:190–193.
158. Shermak MA and Dufresne CR: Nonlethal case of otocephaly and its implications for treatment. J Craniofac Surg 1996;7:372–375.
159. Bixler D, Ward R, and Gale DD: Agnathia-holoprosencephaly: a developmental field complex involving face and brain. Report of 3 cases. J Craniofac Genet Dev Biol Suppl 1985;1:241–249.
160. Buyse ML: Birth Defect Encyclopedia. Center for Birth Defects Information Service, Inc. Dover, MA: Blackwell Scientific Publications, 1990:64–65.
161. Clarke L, Hepworth WB, Carey JC, et al.: Chondrodystrophic mice with coincidental agnathia. Teratology 1988;38:565–570.
162. Kurokawa Y, Tsuchita H, Sohma, T, et al.: Holoprosencephaly with Dandy-Walker cyst: rare coexistence of two major malformations. Childs Nerv Syst 1990;6:51–53.
163. Osaka K and Matsumoto S: Holoprosencephaly in neurosurgical practice. J Neurosurg 1978;48:787–803.
164. Chen CP, Wang KG, Huang JK, et al.: Prenatal diagnosis of otocephaly with microphthalmia/anophthalmia using ultrasound and magnetic resonance imaging. Ultrasound Obstet Gynecol 2003;22:214–215.
165. Ebina Y, Yamada H, Kato EH, Tanuma F, Shimada S, Cho K, and Fujimoto S: Prenatal diagnosis of agnathia-holoprosencephaly: three-dimensional imaging by helical computed tomography. Prenat Diagn 2001;21:68–71.
166. Monasterio FO, Molina F, Berlanga F, Lopez ME, Ahumada H, Takenaga RH, and Ysunza A: Swallowing disorders in Pierre Robin sequence: its correction by distraction. J Craniofac Surg 2004;15:934–941.
167. Vettraino IM, Lee W, Bronsteen RA, Harper CE, Aughton D, and Comstock CH: Clinical outcome of fetuses with sonographic diagnosis of isolated micrognathia. Obstet Gynecol 2003;102:801–805.
168. Chigurupati R and Myall R: Airway management in babies with micrognathia: the case against early distraction. J Oral Maxillofac Surg 2005;63:1209–1215.
169. Steinbacher DM, Kaban LB, and Troulis MJ: Mandibular advancement by distraction osteogenesis for tracheostomy-dependent children with severe micrognathia. J Oral Maxillofac Surg 2005;63:1072–1079.
170. Vogel JE, Mullikan JB, and Kaban LB: Macroglossia: a review of the condition and a new classification. Plast Reconstr Surg 1986;78:715–723.
171. Smith A and Speculand B: Amyloidosis with oral involvement. Br J Oral Maxillofac Surg 1985;23:435–444.
172. Wang J, Goodger NM, and Pogrel MA: The role of tongue reduction. Oral Surg Oral Med Oral Pathol 2003;95:269–273.
173. de Miguel-Diez J, Villa-Asensi JR, and Alvarez-Sala JL: Prevalence of sleep-disordered breathing in children with Down syndrome: polygraphic findings in 108 children. Sleep 2003;26:1006–1009.
174. Pettenati MJ, Haines JL, Higgins RR, et al.: Wiedemann-Beckwith syndrome: presentation of clinical and cytogenetic data on 22 new cases and review of the literature. Hum Genet 1986;74:143.
175. Rump P, Zeegers MP, and van Essen AJ: Tumor risk in Beckwith-Wiedemann syndrome: A review and meta-analysis. Am J Med Genet A 2005;136:95–104.
176. LaFranchi S: Diagnosis and treatment of hypothyroidism in children. Compr Ther 1987;13:20–30.
177. Haeusler MCH, Hofmann HMH, Haberlik A, and Eyb H: Macroglossia. The Fetus.net. http://www.thefetus.net/page.php?id=210, 1992.
178. Thrasher RD and Allen GC: Macroglossia. Emedicine. http://www.emedicine.com/ent/topic746.htm, 2005.
179. Weksberg R, Shuman C, and Smith AC: Beckwith-Wiedemann syndrome. Am J Med Genet C Semin Med Genet 2005;137:12–23.
180. Kumar D: Moebius syndrome. J Med Genet 1990;27:122–126.
181. MacDermot KD, Winter RM, Taylor D, and Baraitser M: Oculofacialbulbar palsy in mother and son: review of 26 reports of familial transmission within the 'mobius spectrum of defects.' J Med Genet 1990;27:18–26.
182. Lalakea ML and Messner AH: Ankyloglossia: does it matter? Pediatr Clin North Am 2003;50:381–397.
183. Ballard JL, Auer CE, and Khoury JC: Ankyloglossia: assessment, incidence, and effect off frenuloplasty on the breastfeeing dyad. Pediatrics 2002;110:e63.
184. Hilton LM and Ayers FJ: Ankyloglossia: "Tongue Tie": An illustrated clinical case study. Retrieved February 11, 2003, from University of Nebraska at Kearney, College of Ed. Web site: http://coe.unk.edu/hiltonlm/AnkyloglossiaHiltonAyersFeb2003/.
185. Ruffoli R, Giambelluca MA, Scavuzzo MC, et al.: Ankylogossia: a morphofunctional investigation in children. Oral Dis 2005;11:170–174.
186. Heller J, Gabbay J, O'Hara C, et al.: Improved ankyloglossia correction with four-flap Z-frenuloplasy. Ann Plast Surg 2005;54:623–628.
187. Oostrom CAM, Vermeij-Keers C, Gilbert PM, and van der Meulen JC: Median cleft of the lower lip and mandible: case reports, a new embryological hypothesis and subdivision. Plast Reconst Surg 1996;97:313–320.
188. Surendran N and Varghese B: Midline cleft of the lower lip with cleft of the mandible and midline dermoid in the neck. J Pediatr Surg 1991;26:1387–1388.
189. Antoniades K, Hadjipetrou L, Antoniades V, and Paraskevopoulos K: Bilateral bifid mandibular condyle. Oral Surg Oral Med Oral Pathol Oral Radiol Endod 2004;97:535–538.
190. de Sales MA, do Amaral JI, de Amorim RF, and de Almeida Freitas R: Bifid mandibular condyle: case report and etiological considerations. J Can Dent Assoc 2004;70:158–162.
191. Shriki J, Lev R, Wong BF, Sundine MJ, and Hasso AN: Bifid mandibular condyle: CT and MR imaging appearance in two patients: case report and review of the literature. Am J Neuroradiol 2005;26:1865–1868.
192. Stefanou EP, Fanourakis IG, Vlastos K, and Katerelou J: Bilateral bifid mandibular condyles. Report of four cases. Dentomaxillofac Radiol 1998;27:186–188.
193. Loh FC and Yeo JF: Bifid mandibular condyle. Oral Surg Oral Med Oral Pathol 1990;69:24–27.
194. To EW: Mandibular ankylosis associated with a bifid condyle. J Craniomaxillofac Surg 1989;17:326–328.
195. Garcia-Gonzales D, Martin-Granizo R, and Lopez P: Imaging quiz case 4. Bifid mandibular condyle. Arch Otolaryngol Head Neck Surg 2000;126:795–799.
196. Szentpetery A, Kocsis G, and Marcsik A: The problem of the bifid mandibular condyle. J Oral Maxillofac Surg 1990;48:1254–1257.
197. Kahl B, Fischbach R, and Gerlach KL: Temporomandibular joint morphology in children after treatment of condylar fractures with functional appliance therapy: a follow-up study using spiral computed tomography. Dentomaxillofac Radiol 1995;24:37–45.
198. To EW: Supero-lateral dislocation of sagitally split bifid mandibular condyle. Br J Oral Maxillofac Surg 1989;27:107–113.
199. Cervenka J, Gorlin RJ, and Anderson VE: The syndrome of pits of the lower lip and cleft lip and/or palate: genetic considerations. Am J Hum Genet 1967;19:416–432.
200. Sander A, Schmelzle R, and Murray J: Evidence for a microdeletion in 1q32–41 involving the gene responsible for van der Woude syndrome. Hum Mol Genet 1994;3:575–578.
201. Shaw WC and Simpson JP: Oral adhesions associated with cleft lip and palate and lip fistulae. Cleft Palate J 1980;17:127–131.
202. Brewer CM: Survival in trisomy 13 and trisomy 18 cases ascertained from population based registers. J Med Genet 2002;39:e54.

203. Siberry G and Iannone R, eds.: The Harriet Lane Handbook, 16th ed. St Louis: Mosby, 2002:278–279.
204. Baty BJ, Blackburn BL, and Carey JC: Natural history of trisomy 18 and trisomy 13: I. Growth, physical assessment, medical histories, survival, and recurrence risk. Am J Med Genet 1994;49:175–188.
205. Duarte AC, Menezes AI, Devens ES, et al.: Patau syndrome with a long survival. A case report. Genet Mol Res 2004;3:288–292.
206. Best RG and Stallworth J: Patau syndrome. Emedicine. www.emedicine.com/ped/topic1745.htm, 2002.
207. Tongsong T, Sirichotiyakul S, Wanapirak C, and Chanprapaph P: Sonographic features of trisomy 13 at midpregnancy. Int J Gynaecol Obstet 2002;76:143–148.
208. Nicolaides KH and Wegrzyn P: Sonographic features of chromosomal defects at 11(+0) to 13(+6) weeks of gestation. Ginekol Pol 2005;76:423–430.
209. Petek E, Pertl B, Tschernigg M, et al.: Characterisation of a 19-year-old "long-term survivor" with Edwards syndrome. Genet Couns 2003;14:239–244.
210. Chen H: Trisomy 18. Emedicine. www.emedicine.com/ped/topic652.htm, 2005.
211. Yeo L, Guzman ER, Day-Salvatore D, et al.: Prenatal detection of fetal trisomy 18 through abnormal sonographic features. J Ultrasound Med 2003;22:581–590.
212. Cohen MM, Kreiborg S, Lammer EJ, et al.: Birth prevalence study of the Apert syndrome. Am J Med Genet 1992;42:655–659.
213. Carinci F, Pezzetti F, Locci P, et al.: Apert and Crouzon syndromes: clinical findings, genes and extracellular matrix. J Craniofac Surg. 2005;16:361–368.
214. Chen H: Apert Syndrome. Emedicine. http://www.emedicine.com/ped/topic122.htm, 2003.
215. Cohen MM and Kreiborg S: Birth prevalence studies of the Crouzon syndrome: comparison of direct and indirect methods. Clin Genet 1992;41:12–15.
216. Fearon JA: Halo distraction of the Le Fort III in syndromic craniosynostosis: a long-term assessment. Plast Reconstr Surg 2005;115:1524–1536.
217. Flores-Sarnat L: New insights into craniosynostosis. Semin Pediatr Neurol 2002;9:274–291.
218. Szybejko-Machaj G and Miklaszewska M: Crouzon syndrome. Emedicine. http://www.emedicine.com/derm/topic734.htm, 2005.
219. Collmann H, Sorensen N, and Krauss J: Hydrocephalus in craniosynostosis: a review. Childs Nerv Syst 2005;21:902–912.
220. Feingold M and Baum J: Goldenhar's syndrome. Am J Dis Child 1978;132:136–138.
221. Gorlin RJ, Jue KL, Jacobsen U, and Goldschmidt E: Oculoauriculovertral dysplasia. J Pediatr 1963;63:991–999.
222. Rollnick BR and Kaye CI: Hemifacial microsomia and variants: pedigree data. Am J Med Genet 1983;15:233–253.
223. Rollnick BR, Kaye CI, Nagatoshi K, Hauck W, and Martin AO: Oculoauriculovertebral dysplasia and variants: phenotypic characteristics of 294 patients. Am J Med Genet 1987;26:361–375.
224. Smahel Z: Craniofacial changes in hemifacial microsomia. J Craniofac Genet Dev Biol 1986;6:151–170.
225. Mansour AM, Wang F, Henkind P, et al.: Ocular findings in the facioauriculovertebral sequence (Goldenhar-Gorlin syndrome). Am J Ophthalmol 1985;100:555–559.
226. Cohen MM: Robin sequences and complexes: causal heterogeneity and pathogenetic/phenotypic variability. Am J Med Genet 1999;84:311–315.
227. Jones KL: Robin Sequence. Smith's recognizable patterns of human malformation, 5th ed. Philadelphia: WB Saunders, 1997:234.
228. Tewfik TL: Pierre Robin syndrome. Emedicine. http://www.emedicine.com/ent/topic150.htm, 2005.
229. Gruen PM, Carranza A, Karmody CS, and Bachor E: Anomalies of the ear in the Pierre Robin triad. Ann Otol Rhinol Laryngol 2005;114:605–613.
230. Elliott MA, Studen-Pavlovich DA, and Ranalli DN: Prevalence of selected pediatric conditions in children with Pierre Robin sequence. Pediatr Dent 1995;17:106–111.
231. Shprintzen RJ: The implications of the diagnosis of Robin sequence. Cleft Palate Craniofac J 1992;29:205–209.
232. Marques IL, Barbieri MA, and Bettiol H: Etiopathogenesis of isolated Robin sequence. Cleft Palate Craniofac J 1998;35:517–525.
233. Wittenborn W, Panchal J, Marsh JL, et al.: Neonatal distraction surgery for micrognathia reduces obstructive apnea and the need for tracheotomy. J Craniofac Surg 2004;15:623–630.
234. Denny A and Amm C: New technique for airway correction in neonates with severe Pierre Robin sequence. J Pediatr 2005;147:97–101.
235. Elluru RG: Treatment options for severe upper airway obstruction in Pierre-Robin sequence. J Pediatr 2005;147:7–9.
236. Rodriguez Soriano J: Branchio-oto-renal syndrome. J Nephrol 2003;16:603–605.
237. Propst EJ, Blaser S, Gordon KA, et al.: Temporal bone findings on computed tomography imaging in branchio-oto-renal syndrome. Laryngoscope 2005;115:1855–1862.
238. Kemperman MH, Koch SM, Kumar S, et al.: Evidence of progression and fluctuation of hearing impairment in branchio-oto-renal syndrome. Int J Audiol 2004;43:523–532.
239. Fujimoto A, Lipson M, Lacro RV, et al.: New autosomal dominant branchio-oculo-facial syndrome. Am J Med Genet 1987;27:943–951.
240. Lin AE, Gorlin RJ, Lurie IW, et al.: Further delineation of the branchio-oculo-facial syndrome. Am J Med Genet 1995;28:96–102.
241. Ozturk O, Tokmak A, Demirci L, et al.: Branchio-oculo-facial syndrome with the atresia of external ear. Int J Pediatr Otorhinolaryngol 2005;69:1575–1578.
242. Kulkarni ML, Deshmukh S, Kumar A, and Kulkarni PM: Branchio-oculo-facial syndrome. Indian J Pediatr 2005;72:701–703.
243. Legius E, Fryns JP, and Van Den Berghe H: Dominant branchial cleft syndrome with characteristics of both brancho-oto-renal and branchio-oculofacial syndrome. Clin Genet 1990;37:347–350.

Sinonasal Endoscopic Surgery, Infections and Neoplasms

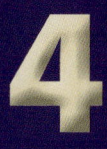

Michael Kim, MD
Mindy J. Kim-Miller, MD, PhD
Christopher R. Trimble, MD, MBA
Anton N. Hasso, MD, FACR

ENDOSCOPIC SINUS SURGERY

Principles

Developed in the 1970s from the work of Messerklinger[1] and Wigand et al.,[2] functional endoscopic sinus surgery (FESS) has become the standard surgical option for the treatment of uncomplicated inflammatory sinus disease. Some otolaryngologists also use the endoscopic approach to treat complicated conditions such as mucocele, allergic fungal sinusitis, and localized neoplasias such as inverted papilloma. In sinus surgery, as in other areas, endoscopic techniques facilitate a minimally invasive approach and reduce postoperative discomfort and recovery time. The goals of FESS are to restore the central drainage pathways of the sinonasal cavity and improve mucociliary clearance and sinus ventilation while preserving the mucosa of the paranasal sinuses.

FESS utilizes mucosa-sparing techniques to remove areas of chronic inflammation, diseased bony partitions, and sinus cells in the ostiomeatal complex, and to create patent sinus antrostomies that widen the sinus ostia and expose the sinus mucosa. It addresses the pathophysiologic mechanisms underlying sinusitis as proposed by Messerklinger, who demonstrated that contact between mucosal surfaces leads to disruption of mucociliary clearance of secretions with subsequent obstruction of the sinuses. Another important finding was that mucosal damage and mucociliary dysfunction are largely reversible if adequate drainage is established; therefore, removing the outflow tract obstruction should allow the diseased mucosa to recover function.[3–5] Obstruction of the ostiomeatal complex is believed to be a critical step in the pathogenesis of chronic sinus disease, and much of endoscopic procedures focuses on this region.[6–9]

Due to the complexity and variability of the paranasal sinuses, imaging (particularly CT) plays a critical role in endoscopic surgery. Systematic nasal endoscopy and high-resolution CT imaging provide complementary diagnostic information that can allow for precise localization of the disease processes and aid in planning the appropriate therapy. Three important functional units of the sinonasal cavity should be addressed: the frontal recess draining the frontal sinus; the ostiomeatal complex draining the frontal recess, anterior ethmoid air cells, and maxillary sinus; and the sphenoethmoidal recess draining the sphenoid sinus and posterior ethmoid air cells (**Table 4-1**). There are two main questions that the radiologist should address[10]:

1. Are there anatomic features on the CT scan that predispose the patient to impaired mucociliary clearance?
2. Are there anatomic features that pose a surgical hazard?

Imaging can provide critical information about potential hazards such as dehiscence of the lamina papyracea, the proximity of the orbit to diseased areas, a low-lying ethmoid fovea and cribriform plate, and adhesions of the uncinate process to the medial orbital wall.[11] Important anatomic landmarks in endoscopic sinus surgery include the middle turbinate, middle meatus, agger nasi cells, uncinate process, hiatus semilunaris, ethmoid infundibulum, frontal recess, bulla ethmoidalis, natural ostium of the maxillary sinus, basal lamella, superior meatus, sphenoethmoidal recess, and location of the internal carotid artery and optic nerve (**Fig. 4-1** and **Table 4-1**). Additionally, imaging can identify anatomic variants such as variations in frontal recess anatomy, the presence of sphenoethmoid (Onodi) and infraorbital (Haller) cells, and septation of the frontal or sphenoid sinuses.

In chronic or recurrent sinusitis, disease of the anterior ethmoids and ostiomeatal complex are the most common preoperative CT scan findings.[12] For standard FESS, a limited coronal view sinus CT scan may provide sufficient information, but a complete axial and coronal sinus CT scan may facilitate evaluation of the posterior ethmoid and sphenoid sinuses.

Table 4-1 Sinus CT Checklist

Note Anatomic Landmarks

- Turbinates (note attachments, position, symmetry, particularly of middle turbinate; Cor)
- Septum (alignment)
- Meati
- Frontal recess and sinuses (relationship, status, pneumatization; Cor)
- Agger nasi
- Uncinate process (attachment, position)
- Hiatus semilunaris
- Bulla ethmoidalis
- Ethmoid infundibulum (integrity, position, size, symmetry)
- Natural ostium of maxillary sinus
- Sphenoethmoidal recess
- Maxillary sinuses (status, size, pneumatization, distance to ethmoid roof; Cor)
- Ethmoid sinuses (status, size, pneumatization, position)
- Sphenoid sinuses (status, size, pneumatization, position of intersinus septae; Axi)
- Lamina papyracea (integrity, shape of medial orbital wall; Cor)
- Internal carotid artery
- Optic nerve

Note Anatomic Variants

- Septal deviation
- Onodi cell (relationship to internal carotid artery, optic nerve; Axi)
- Haller cell
- Agger nasi cell
- Concha bullosa
- Paradoxical middle turbinate (Cor)
- Uncinate process (attachment, position)
- Frontal sinuses septation or pneumatization
- Sphenoid anomalies (variable intersinus septae, septation, pneumatization, indentation of carotid artery or optic nerve)
- Dehiscence of bony covering of carotid artery or optic nerve (Axi)
- Dehiscence of lamina papyracea
- Dehiscence of cribriform plate
- Anterior skull base, ethmoid roof (integrity, position, slope, thickness; Cor)
- Anterior clinoid process pneumatization

Assess Functional Units

- Frontal recess
- Ostiomeatal complex
- Sphenoethmoidal recess

Note Depth of Olfactory Fossa (Distance from Cribriform Plate and Fovea Ethmoidalis; Cor)

Check for Nasal Polyps

Check for Herniation of Intraorbital or Intracranial Structures

Cor = best assessed in coronal CT sections; Axi = best assessed in axial CT sections.

Types of Endoscopic Sinus Surgery

Functional Endoscopic Sinus Surgery for Chronic Rhinosinusitis

The focal point of FESS is the ostiomeatal complex. Using an endoscope, the otorhinolaryngologist identifies the middle turbinate and uses it as a landmark. At the anterior end of the middle turbinate, the uncinate process is identified and removed, exposing the ethmoid bulla, hiatus semilunaris, and ethmoidal infundibulum. The surgeon then opens the anterior ethmoid air cells but leaves the bone covered with mucosa. If the maxillary ostium is obstructed, it is opened via a middle meatal antrostomy. Typically, the inflammation is confined to the ostiomeatal complex and anterior ethmoids. In such cases, this minimal surgery will often be sufficient to improve the function of the ostiomeatal complex and ventilation of the maxillary, ethmoid, and frontal sinuses. However, disease may extend into the posterior ethmoids and the sphenoid sinuses. If indicated, the surgeon can open the posterior ethmoid air cells by penetrating the ground lamella of the middle turbinate, and dissect into the posterior

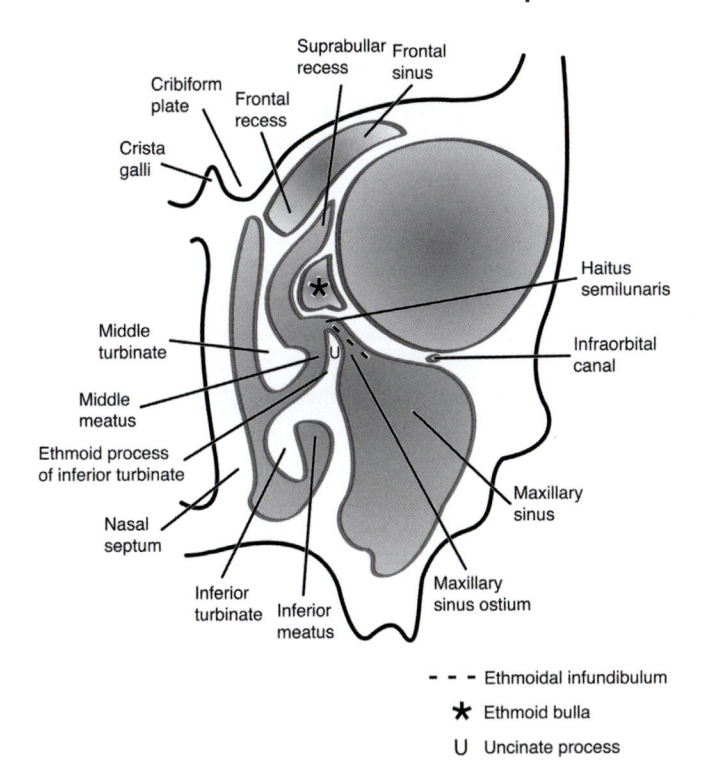

Figure 4-1 Paranasal Sinuses
Schematic of the paranasal sinuses depicting surgical landmarks and spaces in functional endoscopic sinus surgery.

ethmoid and sphenoid sinuses. Based on the findings that in addition to nasal mucosal involvement, adjacent bone involvement can be responsible for chronic or recurrent sinusitis, FESS may involve aggressive removal of all ethmoidal sinus partitions and wide drainage of the maxillary sinus in order to remove osteitic bone, thereby minimizing recurrence.[12,13]

Outcomes after FESS are most successful when utilized in conjunction with medical therapy. When compared with the previous standard for sinus surgery, the Caldwell-Luc procedure, both methods were found to be effective, but there was strong patient preference for FESS.[14] A study of adult patients undergoing FESS for chronic sinus disease found that 88% of the patients were symptom-free or improved, and 41.5% required some additional medical therapy during a mean follow-up period of 17 months. Minor complications developed in 8% of the patients, and a major complication occurred in one patient.[15] In another study of geriatric patients (older than 60 years) undergoing FESS for chronic rhinosinusitis, 64% of the patients reported improvement of symptoms at 3 months, 73% reported improvement at 6 months, and 75% at 12 months.[16] The outcomes for the use of FESS to remove nasal polyps are similar. A review of 33 studies found that overall symptomatic improvement ranged from 78% to 88% for FESS compared with 43% to 84% for similar techniques. Disease recurrence was 8% for FESS compared with 14% for the Caldwell-Luc technique. The percentage of overall complications was rare (1.4% for FESS versus 0.8% for conventional procedures). The case series studies reported overall symptomatic improvement for patients with nasal polyps ranging from 37% to 99% (median 89%). Total complications in the case series studies ranged from 22.4% to 0.3% (median 6%).[17] In long-term follow-up (average of 7.8 years) of 72 patients, 98.4% reported symptomatic improvement compared with before surgery, and 18% required subsequent surgical procedures.[18]

Results are similar in the pediatric population. A meta-analysis of retrospective studies found a beneficial outcome after FESS in 88.7% of children with less than 1% incidence of major complications.[19] Although there was concern regarding the effects of sinus surgery on midfacial growth, prospective studies indicate that midfacial growth is not significantly affected by sinus surgery in humans.[20,21]

The most common etiology for surgical failure following FESS is incomplete resection of the uncinate plate, which can impair mucociliary clearance through the maxillary sinus ostium and infundibulum. This problem has been called the missed ostium sequence.[22] Other common causes of failure include recurrence of nasal polyposis, synechial formation, infection, and persistent rhinitis. Persistent maxillary disease may result from bony foreign body dislodgement during maxillary antrostomy, and nasofrontal recess stenosis may occur in around 10% of patients undergoing nasofrontal sinus surgery.[23]

Minimally Invasive Sinus Technique

Developed in 1996,[24] the minimally invasive sinus technique (MIST) has the same goals as FESS for the treatment of chronic rhinosinusitis (CRS) but is more standardized, reduces mucosal trauma, and does not involve a middle meatal antrostomy. It is based on the assumption that the removal of the uncinate process and medial wall of the ethmoidal bulla with occasional removal of the posterior wall of the agger nasi cell will restore the frontal drainage pathway.[25]

The procedure involves a step-wise, anatomically based progression beginning with the identification of the uncinate process at the hiatus semilunaris.[26] Any polyps within the nasal cavity are removed for better visualization. The surgeon incises the uncinate process from the hiatus semilunaris toward the nasolacrimal duct and performs an uncinectomy to uncover the agger nasi cells superiorly and the primary maxillary sinus ostium inferiorly. The next landmarks are the posteromedial wall of the agger nasi cell and the nasofrontal recess that lies just behind it. Occasionally, the posterior wall of the agger dome must be removed to further enlarge the recess. The next landmark is the face of the ethmoid bulla. The entire medial wall of the bulla is removed, thereby exposing the basal lamella and enlarging the hiatus semilunaris transition space. If a posterior ethmoidectomy is required, the basal lamella is opened in the inferomedial quadrant. The superior meatus and sphenoethmoidal recess are examined, and any polyp in these areas are removed. The remainder of the medial corridor (that space between the middle turbinate and septum) is inspected and contact points are reduced with a freer. Upon completion of surgery, no nasal packing is placed. For all patients who have undergone middle meatal surgery, a Merogel stent is rolled in the shape of the number 9, and placed into the middle meatus to help prevent synechiae. A piece of Gelfilm can also be placed in the medial corridor to help prevent readhesion of contact points.

Outcome studies have shown that MIST is comparable to FESS in the treatment of CRS. In a formal comparison of MIST and FESS, MIST either equaled or surpassed conventional FESS with overall improvement in 78.8% of patients; many more patients after MIST were improved to a level that was better than the normative symptom data for a healthy individual in the general population; and the surgical revision rate following MIST was 5.9%, compared with an average of 10% following FESS. Furthermore, the results after MIST were consistent across the spectrum of disease severity (using CT grades I through IV), suggesting that the procedure is effective for severe as well as minimal disease.[27]

The advantages of MIST over FESS include a reduction in the potential for mucosal scarring, a smaller likelihood of mucosal stripping and complications of bone exposure, less time in surgery, and typically minimal postoperative care. Some physicians believe MIST should be the first surgical option considered for select patients with CRS.[26] Others believe that complete removal of bony partitions within the region of disease as in FESS results in greater success for severe or more complicated cases of CRS.[25] Long-term outcome studies (>2 years) on MIST have yet to be completed.

Frontal Sinusotomy

The extent of the procedures involved in endoscopic frontal sinus surgery, or frontal sinusotomy, varies depending on the extent and severity of the disease. The most limited of these procedures expands the inferior frontal recess with an uncinectomy and possibly a middle turbinate head reduction. This can be extended to include excision of the anterior ethmoid air cells that might obstruct the frontal recess, such as the agger nasi and frontal bulla cells. A more extensive procedure is referred to as the Draf IIB, which involves excision of the frontal sinus floor from the middle turbinate neck to the lamina papyracea. The most definitive endoscopic procedure of the frontal sinus has many names: the Draf III, the frontal sinus drill out, the transeptal frontal sinusotomy, and the endoscopic modification of the Lothrop procedure. The Draf III creates a large frontonasal opening with a complete anterior ethmoidectomy, excision of the anterior segment of the perpendicular ethmoid plate and intersinus frontal septation, and excision of the entire frontal sinus floor between the lacrimal bones.[22] Temporary stents are commonly placed after frontal sinus ESS and removed 4 to 8 weeks later. Nonetheless, restenosis of the outflow tract is common, especially when the surgical ostium is less than 5 mm in diameter.[28]

Sphenoethmoid Recess

ESS of the posterior ethmoid and sphenoid sinuses addresses obstruction or disease at the sphenoethmoid recess. The typical posterior FESS involves a posterior ethmoidectomy and anterior sphenoidotomy. However, a minimal version of this procedure involves only the removal of polyps and redundant musoca from the sphenoethmoid recess. This region is best evaluated in axial CT scans.[22]

Indications for ESS

Absolute indications for surgery in sinus disease include the development of complications from sinusitis, mucoceles, allergic or invasive fungal sinusitis, and suspected neoplasia. Relative indications include the presence of symptomatic nasal polyps that are unresponsive to medical therapy and symptomatic chronic or recurrent acute sinusitis that persists despite appropriate medical therapy.[29] Although there are no absolute indications for an endoscopic approach as opposed to other endonasal or external operations, several publications have demonstrated both improved results and lower morbidity with FESS.[30–32] There is no clear consensus regarding the timing of endoscopic surgery for sinus disease; however, the literature supports FESS

1. when maximal medical therapy, adenoidectomy (in the pediatric population), and culture-directed systemic antibiotics have all failed with persistence of sinonasal disease;
2. when anatomic abnormalities predispose to chronic rhinosinusitis by obstructing normal sinonasal drainage pathways;
3. in sinonasal polyposis to facilitate application of topical steroids or as an adjunct to desensitization in aspirin-sensitive patients;
4. when orbital or intracranial complications of sinonasal disease occur;
5. in selected cystic fibrosis patients to improve quality of life and facilitate application of topical antibiotics with activity against Pseudomonas.[19]

It is important to note that the role of FESS, particularly in the pediatric population, is still evolving.

In more complicated cases, computer-assisted endoscopic sinus surgery may be useful. The American Academy of Otolaryngology Head and Neck Surgery has published recommended indications for computer-assisted endoscopic sinus surgery (**Table 4-2**).

Complications

Complications of endoscopic sinus surgery can be divided into major and minor categories (**Table 4-3**).

In one study, the overall major complication rate of FESS was 0.23%, compared with 1.4% in patients having similar, nonendoscopic procedures.[33] One of the rare but most catastrophic complications is blindness resulting from damage to the optic nerve.[33,34] The most common route of injury is through the lamina papyracea during dissection of the ethmoid, but also maxillary and sphenoid sinuses. Prior surgery can result in scarring of the ethmoid. Guided imaging can help identify the roof of the ethmoid and the lamina papyracea, which is important in preventing penetration of the orbit.[35] If the periorbita or orbit are penetrated, orbital fat will bulge through the defect into the ethmoid air cell, and edema may develop in or around the medial rectus muscle.[22] Entrapment in the bone defect or direct damage to extraocular muscles can lead to diplopia. Injury to the central retinal branch of the ophthalmic artery within the orbit can cause blindness. An expanding hematoma or air dissecting into the orbit can increase the intraocular pressure and lead to ischemia and blindness.[36] To evaluate an orbital injury, an orbital CT with fine axial and coronal slices should be obtained.

Table 4-2 Indications for Computer-assisted Endoscopic Sinus Surgery
• Revision sinus surgery • Distorted sinus anatomy of development, postoperative, or traumatic origin • Extensive sinonasal polyposis • Pathology involving the frontal, posterior ethmoid, and sphenoid sinuses • Disease abutting the skull base, orbit, optic nerve, or carotid artery • Cerebrospinal fluid rhinorrhea or conditions where there is a skull-base defect • Benign and malignant sinonasal neoplasms • Choanal atresia

http://www.entlink.net/practice/rules/image-guiding.cfm

Table 4-3 Complications of FESS
Major Complications
• Optic nerve damage resulting in visual loss • Injury to extraocular muscles • Orbital hematoma • Severe hemorrhage • Dehiscence of lamina papyracea • Nasolacrimal duct injury or stenosis • Cerebrospinal fistula • Miningitis • Anosmia • Brain injury • Brain abscess
Minor Complications
• Minor hemorrhage • Synechiae • Infection • Epistaxis • Atrophic rhinitis • Crusting

The most common major complication of ESS is cerebrospinal fluid (CSF) leakage, which occurs in about 0.2% to 0.5% of cases.[33,37] CSF leaks usually occur from injuries to the cribriform plate and ethmoid plate (39%), frontal sinuses (15%), and the sella turcica through the sphenoid sinus (15%).[38] The lateral lamella of the cribriform plate is the weakest component of the anterior skull base and easily penetrated during dissection of the middle turbinate neck. CSF leaks are usually recognized at the time of surgery and can be repaired endoscopically with fascia and a mucosal flap. Small leaks recognized postoperatively as CSF rhinorrhea can heal spontaneously with conservative treatment. Large or persistent leaks require surgical repair before further complications such as meningitis develop. CT scans will typically show an anterior skull base defect. However, if a bone defect cannot be identified, then a CT cisternogram may help locate the leakage site. If the bone defect is large, brain and meninges may herniate into the nasal cavity or sinuses. Pneumocephalus may also accompany the skull base defect, especially after nose blowing.[22]

Massive hemorrhages may result from injury to the internal carotid artery during dissection of the sphenoid sinuses, particularly of the Onodi cells. In addition to subarachnoid hemorrhages, patients may develop pseudoaneurysms. Postoperative patients complaining of sudden onset headaches and/or photophobia should be evaluated for intracranial hemorrhage with a noncontrast head CT. If a subarachnoid hemorrhage is noted, then emergent angiography with balloon occlusion can locate and control the bleeding. Laceration of the anterior ethmoid artery can also lead to profuse bleeding. If transected, the proximal end of the anterior ethmoid artery may retract into the orbit, resulting in an orbital hematoma. A canthotomy may need to be performed to relieve the elevated intraocular pressure.

Postoperative Sinus CT

Patients may undergo a postoperative sinus CT if complications develop or if symptoms fail to resolve or recur. Key issues to consider include:

1. the intended surgical procedure;
2. the structures that were completely or partially removed;
3. the status of the natural sinus ostium and outflow tract;
4. if the outflow tract is opacified, whether it is because of bone or soft-tissue material;
5. whether there is a physiologic obstruction due to diseased sinuses.[22]

It is important to keep in mind that irrigation fluid, mucosal edema, and packing material will be present in the immediate postoperative period. Inflammation, edema, crusting, and debris may persist for 6 to 8 weeks. Therefore, evaluation of the mucosa and bones is best done after 8 weeks postoperatively and should include both coronal and axial CT slices. In reviewing the images, radiologists should consider the following issues:[23]

1. Patency of the frontal recess. Obstruction of this recess is a common cause of recurrent frontal sinus disease. Any remnants of agger nasi cells or the middle turbinate can lead to obstruction of the frontal recess.
2. Extent of resection of the ostiomeatal complex. Assess the extent of the uncinectomy and ethmoidectomy. If the middle turbinate has been resected, then its vertical attachment to the cribriform plate and basal lamella should be examined. Force applied during the turbinate resection can cause injuries in these regions.
3. Integrity of the sphenoid sinus. Look for dehiscence of the optic nerve or carotid artery and cephaloceles. Residual polypoid mucosal disease may hinder identification of a cephalocele.

4. Integrity of the lamina papyracea. Look for dehiscence or medial protrusion of orbital soft tissue.

FACIAL FRACTURES

Imaging of Facial Fractures

Facial fractures usually result from trauma such as impact during motor vehicle accidents, interpersonal violence, falls, sporting accidents, and work-related injuries. Immediately following the trauma, emergent issues should be addressed first, including maintaining an airway, breathing, hemodynamic stability, and the evaluation and treatment of other, more serious injuries. Once these problems have been managed, the evaluation and treatment of facial fractures may be addressed.

CT imaging has increased the sensitivity and accuracy of fracture detection, facilitating more detailed analysis and classification of facial fractures.[39–41] In some cases, a deformity from broken bones may be obvious. In other cases, it may be necessary to wait for swelling to subside before imaging can be acquired to diagnose a fracture. The main objectives of imaging following facial trauma are fracture detection, fracture classification, assessment of complications, and evaluation of structural displacement.

Imaging Techniques

High-resolution CT is currently the imaging modality of choice for most facial fractures. Soft-tissue complications as well as the anatomy and fractures of the facial bones are well demonstrated by CT. Helical CT technology permits multiple, sequential CT scans to be obtained quickly in multitrauma patients.[42] A standard protocol may include nonenhanced helical scanning of the face with 3 mm collimation, a pitch of 1 or 1.5, a soft-tissue reconstruction algorithm, and slice reconstruction at 0.5 or 1 mm intervals using a high-resolution algorithm for the bone. Thinner 1.0 mm collimation may be indicated for investigating areas of subtle trauma such as fractures of the optic canal.[43]

In acutely injured patients, unenhanced axial and/or coronal CT can provide effective, safe, and rapid diagnostic imaging, with transaxial CT being the most common modality.[44,45] Primary axial images are obtained parallel to the Frankfurt Horizontal (FH) plane (ear–eye plane) using 1.0 to 1.25 mm slice thickness from above the frontal sinuses to below the alveolar process of the maxilla. Coronal images are obtained from in front of the nasal bones to behind the sphenoid sinuses. In cases of suspected midfacial or mandibular fractures, the scan is usually extended to include the mandible in the axial plane, and the temporomandibular joints in the coronal plane.

Careful attention must be given to patient positioning within the CT scanner in order to obtain symmetric axial images parallel to the FH plane. If the patient cannot hyperextend the neck for coronal section acquisition, the coronal plane should be reconstructed strictly orthogonal to the axial images. Sagittal plane image reformation may be performed either relative to the coronal plane or as sagittal obliques parallel to the optic nerve. In cases where the face is not positioned symmetrically on the original axial CT images, reformation of the axial images parallel to the FH plane should be considered to aid side-to-side comparison of craniometric measurements.[46] Multiplanar reconstruction can help improve the representation of skeletal injuries, especially along the axial planes.[39] 3D-CT reconstruction can be very useful in the evaluation of fracture comminution, displacement, rotatory components, complex fractures involving multiple planes, asymmetries of the whole face, large craniofacial defects, as well as during treatment evaluation and surgical planning for facial injuries.[47,48]

Although CT imaging is highly accurate, one limitation is its inability to precisely show the magnitude of osseous fragmentation in complex fractures seen at surgery, regardless of CT technique.[46] Other considerations include the significant radiation dose that maxillofacial CT scanning delivers to the orbits, and radiation to the soft tissues of the neck (e.g., thyroid) during scans that include the mandible, an especially important consideration in the pediatric population.[49]

MR imaging of facial injuries is useful for assessing soft-tissue involvement but limited for fracture detection. MR is particularly useful in cases involving visual or extraocular muscle deficits, unexplained neurologic deficits, and fractures with a high probability of intracranial complications. Acquisition of MR images should start in the coronal plane and include the entire orbit, followed by images in the axial or oblique sagittal plane.[43]

Fracture diagnosis

Signs and symptoms of a facial fracture include pain or tenderness to touch, swelling, epistaxis, subcutaneous and periorbital hematomas, irregular or misshapen facial appearance, bone mobility, and rough sensation when the nose is moved. A careful history and clinical examination can help with the diagnosis[6,50–54] (**Tables 4-4** and **4-5**).

When describing facial injuries, each half of the face should receive a separate evaluation. In order to diagnose facial fractures by radiography, at least two views should be examined. The direct and indirect radiographic signs of facial fractures are listed in[55] **Table 4-6**.

Coronal and axial CT images are particularly useful for diagnosing blow-out fractures. The orbits require careful examination since 60% to 70% of all facial fractures involve the orbit in some way.[56] Fractures that do not involve the orbits include local nasal bone fractures, zygomatic arch fractures, and LeFort I fracture.

Midfacial Anatomy

"Crumple Zone" Buttress System

The midfacial skeleton is composed of several bones that form a lattice-like system of buttresses developed to withstand the masticatory forces transmitted from the teeth to the skull base. Therefore, the buttress system withstands significant force vertically, but is easily fractured by relatively mild forces applied from other directions. There are five vertical, four horizontal,

Table 4-4 Assessment of Traumatic Fractures of the Upper Face

Location	Clinical Findings	Clinical Indication
Orbit	Reduced eye movement	
	Subconjunctival hemorrhage	
	• Inferolateral segmental hemorrhage	Consider malar fracture
	• Bilateral complete subconjunctival hemorrhage	Usually indicative of anterior fossa fracture extending into the orbits
	Proptosis, ophthalmoplegia	Consider retrobulbar hemorrhage
	Enophthalmos (recessed eye), ptosis	Consider blow-out fracture; look for herniated soft tissue in maxillary sinus, "trapdoor" fragment of bone protruding down into sinus (often hinged on ethmoidal side)
	Diplopia, decreased visual acuity, or visual field loss	
	• Intercanthal distance >35 mm	Consider nasoethmoid fracture
	• Interpupillary distance >55 mm	
Nasoethmoid Region	Movement of nasal bones or displacement of nasal septum	
	Crepitus with manipulation	
	Epistaxis (often heavy)	
	Septal hematoma	
	Medial canthus displaced laterally and inferiorly with or without traction	
	Nasolacrimal apparatus injury	
	CSF rhinorrhea (can appear as clear fluid line with blood stained streaking at the margins, or tramlining)	Indicative of central middle third and nasoethmoid fractures with anterior cranial fossa fracture

and four sagittal sets of buttresses. The traumatic disruption of one buttress may weaken the lattice system and cause its collapse into reoccurring fracture patterns (e.g., zygomaticomaxillary and Le Fort fractures), which may actually serve to protect the delicate structures contained within the lattice.[46]

The vertical buttresses are composed of four paired buttresses (from anteromedial to posterolateral): 1. The nasomaxillary (or medial), 2. the zygomaticomaxillary (or lateral), 3. the pterygomaxillary (or posterior) buttresses, and 4. the posterior border of the ascending ramus of the mandible. The unpaired, midline, vertical buttress is the frontoethmoid vomerine or bony nasal septum. These buttresses diffuse vertical forces over the cranial base.

The nasomaxillary buttress passes along the lateral piriform aperture, up the frontal process of the maxilla, and into the frontal bone. The zygomaticomaxillary buttress passes laterally from the maxilla to the zygoma and attaches to the skull base at the zygomaticofrontal suture. The pterygomaxillary buttress rests posterior to the other two and connects the maxilla with the sphenoid bone.

The horizontal buttresses include the frontal bar (composed of the thickened portion of the frontal bone and superior orbital rim), the inferior orbital rim, the palato-alveolar ridge, and the horizontal portions of the mandible. The sagittal buttresses are composed of the frontal bone, the posterior part of the body and angle of the mandible, the zygomatic arch, and the hard palate.[46,57]

Trauma to the midface may involve important, nonosseous structures. The infraorbital nerve travels through the inferior orbital fissure and the infraorbital foramen. Damage to this nerve can result in hypesthesia of the cheek and upper teeth. The midface receives its vascular supply from the internal maxillary artery, which may need to be ligated in cases of extensive bleeding. Because of the proximity of the orbits, damage may also occur to the globe, optic nerve, extraocular muscles, medial and lateral canthi, and lacrimal system (**Table 4-7**).

Table 4-5 Assessment of Traumatic Fractures of the Middle and Lower Face

Location	Clinical Findings	Clinical Indication
Oral Cavity	Malocclusion	Fractured teeth common with fractures of the alveolar process of maxilla
	Loosened or displaced groups of teeth	
	Mobile palate	
	"Cracked pot" percussion note when teeth are tapped	
	Intraoral hematomas	
	Palpate integrity of nasomaxillary buttress, anterior maxillary sinus wall, zygomaticomaxillary buttress	
	Mucosal tear or anteroposterior linear bruise of palate	Consider palate fracture
Zygomaticomaxillary Complex (Tripod, Malar, Zygomatic)	Periorbital edema, hematoma	
	Flattened cheek prominence/step deformity	
	Segmental subconjunctival hemorrhage	
	Infraorbital sensory loss or hypesthesia	Consider damage to infraorbital nerve
	Unilateral epistaxis	
	Palpable displaced fracture of infraorbital margin and buccal sulcus	
	Enophthalmos	Consider blow-out fracture
	Diplopia	Consider extraocular muscle or orbital fat entrapment, nerve damage, or periorbital swelling
	Anesthesia in temporal area	Consider damage to zygomaticofacial and temporal nerves from displaced malar fractures
	Restricted jaw movement	Consider impingement of the malar/zygomatic arch fragment upon the coronoid process of the mandible or temporalis muscle
Mandible	Palpable or visible step-offs, mobile fracture	
	Sublingual hematoma	Characteristic of body fractures
	Crepitus, trismus, restricted jaw movement, malocclusion, pain	Condylar neck fractures can also present with these signs
	Mental anesthesia (lower lip and chin)	Consider fractures of the body and ramus
	Preauricular swelling, pain, restricted condylar movement, malocclusion	Consider condylar neck injury or fracture
	Bleeding from external auditory meatus	Lacerations of the inferior or anterior wall of the meatus are associated with TMJ injuries. Lacerations of the posterior or superior walls or the tympanic membrane +/− CSF leak are associated with middle fossa injuries.

TMJ = temporomandibular joint; CSF = cerebrospinal fluid.

Fracture Classification

To classify craniofacial fractures, the skull can be divided into three anatomic regions:

1. Upper third – frontal bones
2. Middle third (midfacial) – zygoma, nasal bones, and maxilla
3. Lower third – mandible and teeth

This section will focus primarily on midfacial fractures, which can be categorized into two groups: transfacial and limited. Limited fractures are further subdivided into complex (multiple) strut and single strut fractures (**Table 4-8**).

The most commonly used system for describing midfacial fractures remains that proposed by Rene Le Fort, who described "the great lines of weakness" according to fracture patterns he experimentally produced.[58] Some argue that the Le Fort classification is inadequate, because it does not describe the facial skeletal supports, the comminuted, incomplete, or combination maxillary fractures, nor fractures extending into the skull base.[59] The Le Fort classification can therefore underestimate the complexity of fractures and provide insufficient information for fracture description and treatment planning.

CT imaging has facilitated the development of new classification systems that more precisely define craniofacial fractures and treatment applications. Some authors have proposed classifying facial fractures based on the integrity of the horizontal and vertical buttress systems of the skull.[60,61]

Table 4-6 Radiographic Features of Facial Fractures

Direct Signs
- Nonanatomic linear lucencies
- Cortical defect or diastatic suture
- Bone fragments overlapping, causing a "double density"
- Asymmetry of face

Indirect Signs
- Soft-tissue swelling
- Opacification/fluid in a paranasal sinus
- Soft-tissue emphysema or periorbital/intracranial air

Table 4-7 Complications of Midfacial Fractures

Central Midface	Lateral Midface	Orbital Blow-out
CSF leak, intracranial infection or pneumocele	Superior orbital fissure syndrome (CN III, IV, V1, V2, VI)	Enophthalmos, diplopia
Optic nerve injury	Traumatic optic neuropathy, optic nerve injury	Extraocular muscle entrapment
Enophthalmos, diplopia	Extraocular muscle injury (lateral rectus, inferior rectus)	Ocular injury (ruptured globe, hyphema, traumatic cataract, lens dislocation, iris hernia, vitreous, and macular hemorrhage)
Extraocular muscle dysfunction (superior oblique tendon sheath syndrome)	Infraorbital nerve injury	Optic nerve injury
Medial canthal ligament injury	Carotid artery injury	Infraorbital nerve injury
Post-traumatic hypertelorism, telecanthus	Lateral canthal ligament injury	Epistaxis (vascular injury)
Orbital, periorbital hematoma	Orbital hematoma	Encephalocele and globe protrusion (orbital roof fractures)
Lacrimal system injury, epiphoria, chronic dacrocystitis	Ocular injury	
Epistaxis (vascular injury)	CSF leak, intracranial infection, pneumocele	
Sinus drainage dysfunction (frontal-maxillary)	Trismus	
Chronic sinusitis	Devitalized teeth	
Retention mucocele		
Nasal septal hematoma		
Devitalized teeth		

Table 4-8 Classification of Midfacial Fractures

Limited Fractures

Complex Strut Fractures

Central Midface
- Nasofrontoethmoidal
- Nasomaxillary buttress
- Maxillo-alveolar buttress

Lateral Midface
- Zygomaticomaxillary complex (tripod, trimalar, zygomatic)
- Sphenotemporal buttress

Single Strut Fractures
- Nasal bone
- Localized sinus wall
- Alveolar ridge
- Zygomatic arch
- Isolated orbital rim
- Orbital blow-out

Transfacial Fractures
- Le Fort I
- Le Fort II
- Le Fort III
- Complex Le Fort

One proposed system applies the AO/ASIF (Arbeitsgemeinschaft fur Osteosynthesefragen/Association for the Study of Internal Fixation) fracture classification system to the craniofacial region. Analogous to the AO scheme, the new system classifies midfacial/craniofacial fractures into hierarchical triads.[47] The midface is divided into three topographic units: I – the caudal or lower midface, II – the upper or cranial midface, and (III) the craniobasal facial unit.

In the new AO system, fractures are first localized to one of four vertical compartments, then categorized by fracture type, followed by the group and subgroup (**Table 4-9**). The subgroup refers to the topographic unit(s) involved. Group 1 can have sub-subgroups that further specify the location and type of fracture. For example, a lateral A1.2.2 is a nondisplaced, upper midfacial fracture involving two buttresses (zygomaticomaxillary and pterygomaxillary). A central C3.3 is a complex, complete fracture of the nasoethmoidal region with extension into the central alveolar process, frontal sinus, and frontobasal and centrobasal regions beyond the sphenoidal limbus. Fractures are categorized from the lowest severity (A1.1) to the highest (C3.3).

Transfacial Fractures

Because the Le Fort system is the most commonly used classification for describing midfacial fractures, we will describe transfacial fractures using that system.

All Le Fort fractures involve fracture of the pterygoid process. Additionally, almost all Le Fort fractures cause blood to collect in the maxillary sinus. However, each Le Fort type has a unique component that is easily recognizable on CT images. To classify these fractures, one should systematically evaluate the pterygoid process, anterolateral margins of the nasal fossa above the maxillary alveolar ridge, inferior orbital rims, and zygomatic arches.[62]

Features of each Le Fort type are listed in **Table 4-10**.[54,55,57,63] It is important to note that with the exception of Le Fort I fractures, pure Le Fort fractures are rarely seen. Fracture lines often diverge from the categorical pathways and can result in asymmetric, mixed-type, or atypical fractures.

Le Fort I Fractures (Transmaxillary / Low-Level / Guerin Type)

A Le Fort I fracture is a horizontal fracture of the maxilla just above the teeth and palate. It runs through the floor of the maxillary sinuses, extending from the nasal septum to the lateral pyriform rims, crossing below the zygomaticomaxillary junction, and traversing the pterygomaxillary junction to disrupt the lower portion of the pterygoid plates (**Fig. 4-2**).

Le Fort I fractures may occur as a single entity or in combination with Le Fort II and III fractures. It is infrequently present in association with a downwardly displaced fracture of the zygomatic complex. Clinically, Le Fort I fractures are characterized by malocclusion of the teeth with a "floating palate" displaced posteriorly (**Table 4-10**).

Imaging demonstrates a fracture extending horizontally across the inferior maxilla, sometimes including a fracture of the lateral sinus wall, extending into the palatine bones and pterygoid plates. The unique component of Le Fort I fractures is the involvement of the anterolateral margin of the nasal fossa, which is intact in Le Fort II and III types.[62]

Le Fort II Fractures (Pyramidal)

A Le Fort II fracture is a pyramidal fracture that extends from the dorsum of the nose at or below the nasofrontal suture, inferolaterally through the medial wall of the orbit (lacrimal bone) and orbital floor, through the zygomaticomaxillary suture, across the maxilla below the zygoma, and across the pterygomaxillary fissure into the upper pterygoid plates (**Fig. 4-2**). This results in widening of the inner canthus of the nasal bridge.

Le Fort II fractures are characterized by mobility of the nose relative to the dental arch. Because the fracture travels near or through the inferior orbital foramen, damage to the infraorbital nerve often results in hypesthesia. An extensive Le Fort II fracture can result in a flat, elongated face (dish face or pan face) (**Table 4-10**).

Imaging demonstrates fractures of the inferior orbital rim lateral to the infraorbital canal, orbital floor, medial orbital wall, and nasal bone with extension posteriorly into the pterygoid plates (**Figs. 4-3** and **4-4**). The unique component of Le Fort II fractures is the involvement of the inferior orbital rim, which is intact in Le Fort I and III types.[62]

Le Fort III Fractures (Craniofacial Dysjunction/Transverse/High Level/Suprazygomatic)

In Le Fort III fractures, the facial bones are detached from the anterior cranial base. The fracture line starts from the dorsum

Table 4-9 AO-Analogue Classification System of Midfacial/Craniofacial Fractures

Vertical Compartment	Group	Subgroup
Lateral (Right or Left)	1: Isolated involvement of a single unit	1.1: Caudal or lower midfacial fracture (Unit I)
		1.2: Cranial or upper midfacial fracture (Unit II)
		1.3: Craniobasal fracture (Unit III)
	2: Combined fractures of the midface and/or craniobasal-facial unit without skull base involvement	2.1: Complete midfacial (I + II)
		2.2: High craniofacial (II + III with frontotemporal calvarium involvement)
		2.3: Complete craniofacial (I + II + III with frontotemporal calvarium involvement)
	3: Combine fractures of the midface and/or craniobasal-facial unit with skull base involvement	3.1: High craniofacial/craniobasal (II + III with skull base involvement)
		3.2: Complete craniofacial/frontobasal (I + II + III with frontal skull base involvement)
		3.3: Complete craniofacial/frontolaterobasal (I + II + III with frontolateral skull base involvement)
Central (Right or Left)	1: Isolated involvement of a single unit	1.1: Maxillopalatinal fracture (Unit I)
		1.2: Maxillo-nasoorbitoethmoidal fracture (Unit II)
		1.3: Frontal sinus/craniobasal fracture (Unit III)
	2: Combined fractures of the midface and/or craniobasal-facial unit without skull base involvement	2.1: Complete maxillo-nasoorbitoethmoidal (I + II)
		2.2: High frontofacial (II + III with ventral frontal sinus wall / calvarium involvement)
		2.3: Complete frontofacial (I + II + III with ventral frontal sinus wall / calvarium involvement)
	3: Combined fractures of the midface and/or craniobasal-facial unit with skull base involvement	3.1: High frontofacial/craniofacial (II + III with skull base or dorsal frontal sinus wall involvement)
		3.2: Complete frontofacial/frontobasal (I + II + III with frontal skull base involvement)
		3.3: Complete frontofacial/craniobasal (I + II + III with rhinobasal and centrobasal involvement)
Fracture Type		

A: Nondisplaced
B: Displaced
C: Complex-defect fracture

Adapted from Buitrago-Tellez CH, et al.: A comprehensive classification of craniofacial fractures: postmortem and clinical studies with two- and three-dimensional computed tomography. Injury 2002;33(8):651–668.

of the nose at the nasofrontal and frontomaxillary sutures and the cribiform plate, and extends posteriorly along the medial orbital wall through the nasolacrimal groove and ethmoid bones. It stays below the optic foramen as it crosses the orbital floor along the inferior orbital fissure into the lateral orbital wall and through the zygomaticofrontal suture and zygomatic arch (**Fig. 4-2**). Intranasally, a fracture line crosses the ethmoid bone through the base of the perpendicular plate below the cribriform plate and through the vomer and pterygoid plates to the base of the sphenoid.

Table 4-10 Features of Le Fort Fractures

Le Fort I	Le Fort II	Le Fort III
• Transmaxillary fracture from piriform fossa to pterygoid fissure detaching palate and maxillary alveolus • Unique component: anterolateral margin of the nasal fossa • Mobile alveolar portion of maxilla • Palpable crepitation in upper buccal sulcus • Malocclusion • "Cracked pot" percussion note from upper teeth • Hematoma intraorally over root of zygoma, palate • Fractured cusps of cheek teeth • Bruising of upper lip and lower half of midface • Inadequate reduction can result in malunion and bony deformities (overlong face)	• Pyramidal fracture through sinus wall laterally and nasal bones medially • Unique component: inferior orbital rim involved • Mobile maxilla • Palpable step-offs – zygomatic buttress, infraorbital margin • Infraorbital nerve damage resulting in paresthesia of midface • Periorbital echymosis/hematoma • Eyes – diplopia, subconjunctival hemorrhage • Anterior open bite • Gagging on posterior teeth • Nose included or separate • Inadequate reduction can result in malunion and bony deformities (overlong face or flattening "dish face" deformity)	• Fracture through frontozygomatic sutures and orbits, detaching facial skeleton from base of skull • Unique component: zygomatic arch • Mobile middle third of face • Palpable step-offs – zygomatic buttress, infraorbital margin • Separation of frontozygomatic suture • CSF rhinorrhea • Infraorbital nerve damage • Periorbital ecchymosis/hematoma • Eyes – diplopia, visual defects, subconjunctival hemorrhage • Increased intercanthal distance (displaced frontomaxillary or lacrimal bones, or avulsion of medial canthal ligament) • Anterior open bite • Gagging on posterior teeth • Nose included or separate • Retrobulbar hemorrhage may occur following reduction surgery • Inadequate reduction can result in malunion and bony deformities (overlong face or flattening "dish face" deformity)

Common component: fracture of pterygoid process

Le Fort III fractures are characterized by mobility of the nose and dental arch without frontal bone movement. Due to the craniofacial detachment, the face appears long and flat (dish face or pan face). Because these fractures involve the zygomatic bone and orbital walls, disturbances in vision are common (Table 4-10).

Imaging demonstrates fractures of the zygoma, zygomaticofrontal suture, medial orbital wall, and nasal bone, with extension posteriorly through the orbit at the pterygomaxillary suture into the sphenopalatine fossa. Separation of the nasofrontal suture may be seen in either Le Fort II or III fractures. The unique component of Le Fort III fractures is the involvement of the zygomatic arch, which is intact in Le Fort I and II types.[62]

Complex Le Fort Fractures

Most cases of maxillary fractures involve a combination of the Le Fort types. Complex Le Fort fractures may include nasofrontoethmoidal or zygomaticomaxillary fractures. One of the most common combinations is the LeFort II – tripod fracture complex, which is usually caused by the large forces encountered in a motor vehicle accident. Other complex patterns include a mixed LeFort II/LeFort III or a LeFort II/LeFort III/tripod complex.

Complex Strut Fractures

Central Midface

Nasofrontoethmoidal fractures (nasoorbital/nasofrontal/nasoethmoidal)

Nasofrontoethmoidal or nasoorbital fractures result from trauma to the upper middle third of the face. These fractures involve the nasal bones, walls of the frontal sinuses, cribriform plate, ethmoid sinuses, frontal processes of the maxillae, lacrimal bones, and nasal septum (Fig. 4-5). Some classification systems distinguish

Chapter 4: Sinonasal Endoscopic Surgery, Infections and Neoplasms 143

Le Fort I Fracture
Le Fort II Fracture
Le Fort III Fracture

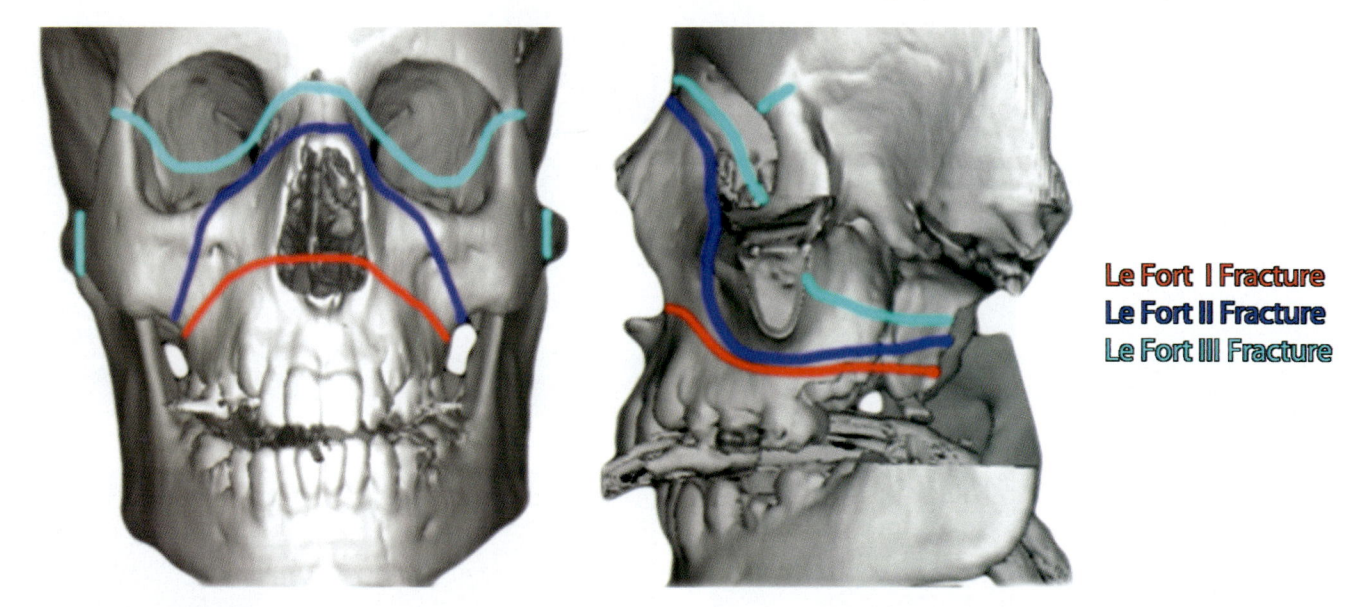

Figure 4-2 Le Fort Fracture Planes
Coronal and sagittal 3D CT reconstructions depicting fracture planes of Le Fort I (*red*), II (*blue*), and III (*turquoise*) fractures. Le Fort I fractures are characterized by transmaxillary and anterolateral nasal fossa fracture planes (*red line*), detaching the palate and maxillary alveolus. Le Fort II fractures involve the pyramidal process, inferior orbital rims, and nasal process (*blue lines*), detaching the maxilla. Le Fort III fractures comprise zygomatic arch, frontozygomatic suture, orbital, and nasal bone fractures (*turquoise line*), detaching the middle third of the face. Note that each type of Le Fort fracture involves the pterygoid process of the sphenoid (lateral view). (Images courtesy of Lindell Gentry, M.D., University of Wisconsin.)

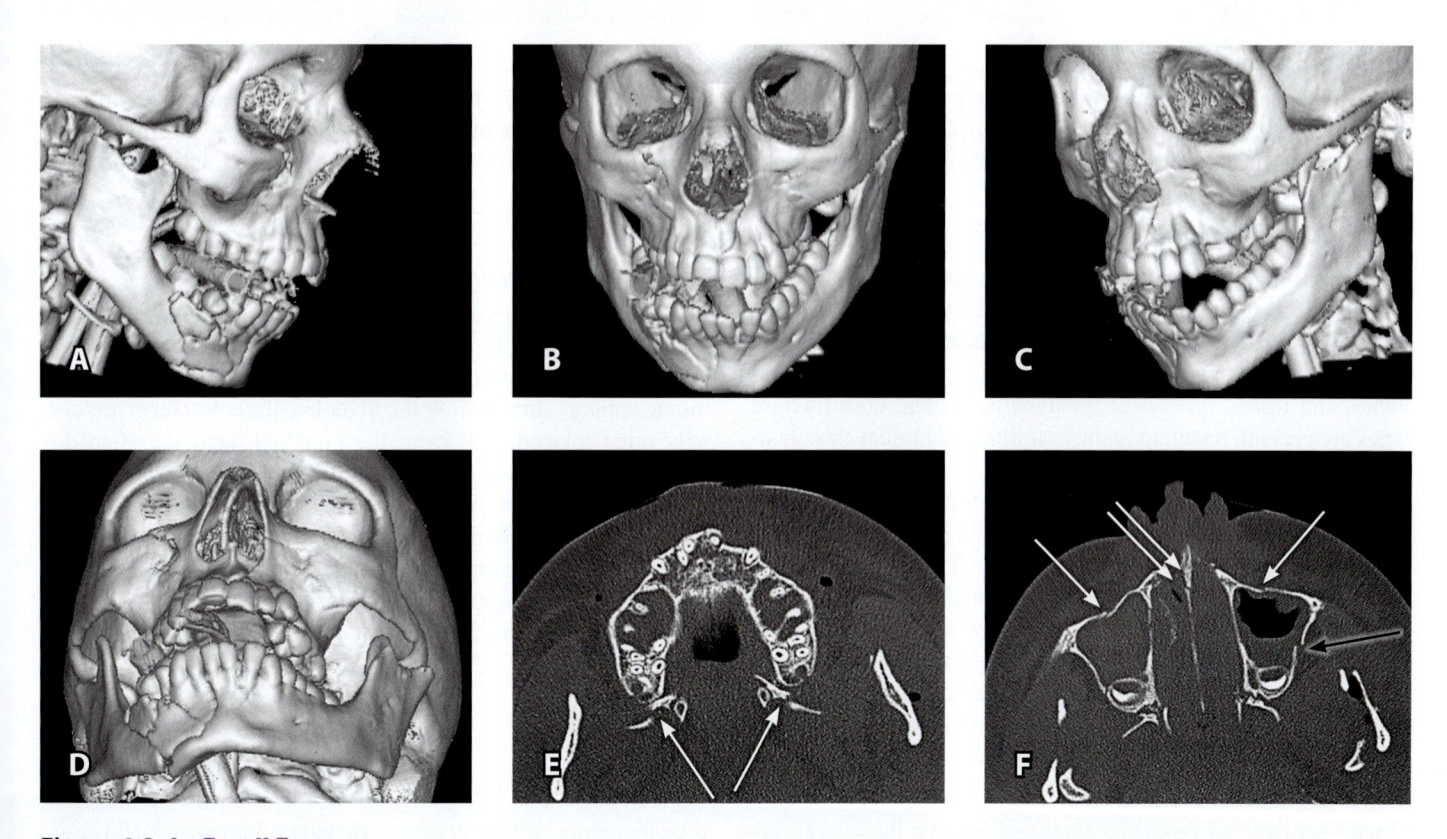

Figure 4-3 Le Fort II Fracture
Near-complete Le Fort II fracture resultant from a four-storey fall with direct impact on the chin. 3D CT reconstructions with surface rendering (**A–D**) and axial bone CECT images (**E, F**) depict bilateral fractures of the anterior maxillary sinus walls (*white arrow,* **F**), fracture of the left posterolateral maxillary sinus wall (*black arrow,* **F**), comminution of lateral pterygoid plates (*arrows,* **E**), bilateral fractures of the orbital rims (**B, D**), fracture of nasal septum (**D**, *double white arrows,* **F**), alveolar ridge (**B, C**), and nasal bones (**C**). Also note the comminuted fracture of the right mandibular body (**A, D**) and bilateral condylar fracture-dislocations of the jaw (**A, C**).

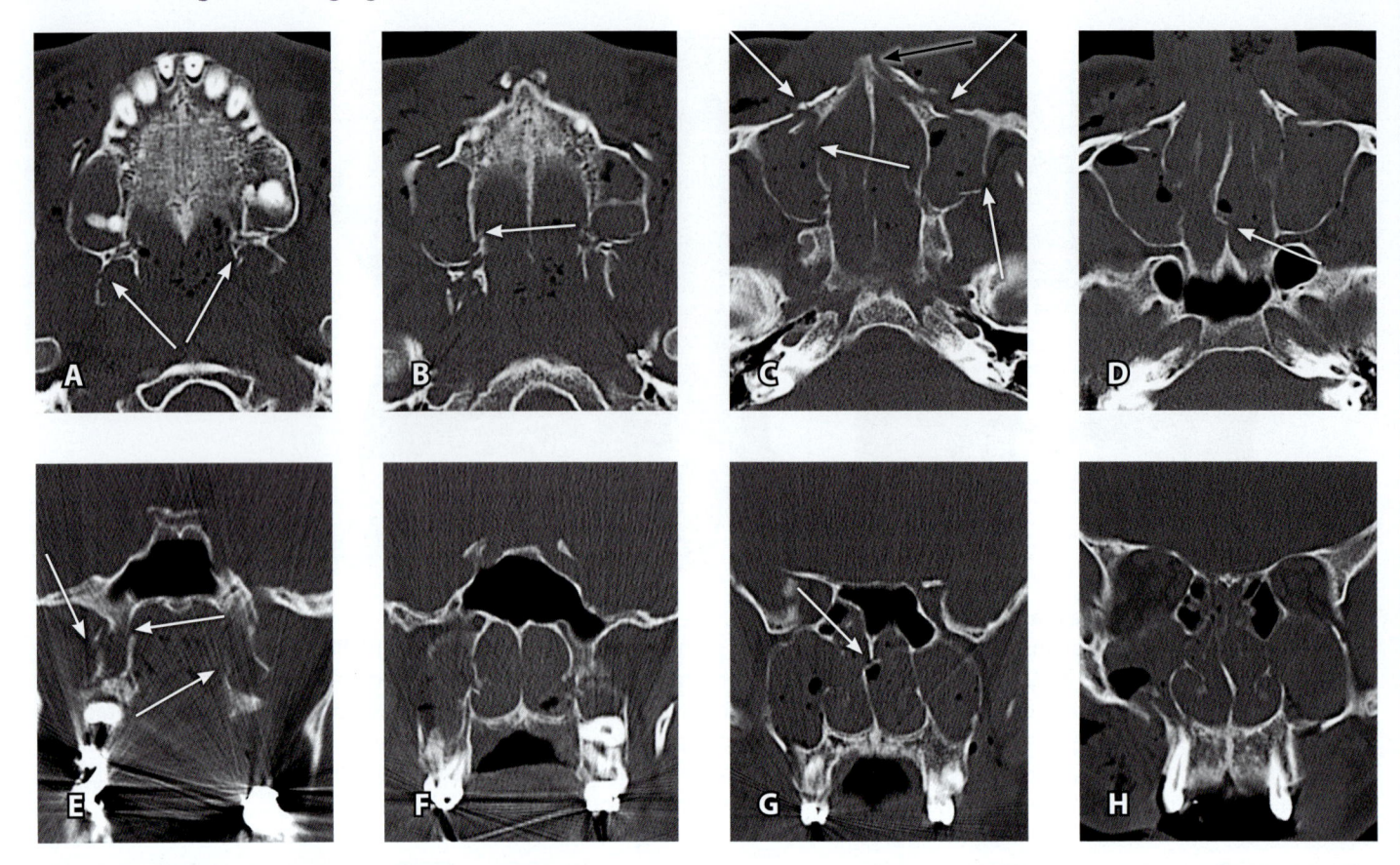

Figure 4-4 Le Fort II Fracture
Axial (**A–D**) and coronal (**E–H**) bone NECT images through the midface region show multiple midface fractures involving the alveolar ridges (**A, B**), the hard palate (*arrow,* **B**), the anterior, posterior, and medial walls of the maxillary sinuses (*arrows,* **B, C**), the nasal septum (*arrows,* **D, G**) and bilateral involvement of the pterygoid plates (*arrows,* **A, E**). Also note the fractured anterior nasal spine of the maxilla (*black arrow,* **C**).

nasofrontal fractures from nasoethmoidal fractures.[64] Nasofrontal fractures involve the superomedial orbital walls, frontal sinus, and cribiform plate. Nasoethmoidal fractures involve the lower two-thirds of the medial orbital walls, ethmoidal sinuses, nasal bones, and frontal process of the maxillae. Often, both fracture types are present, resulting in the nasofrontoethmoidal classification.

A nasofrontoethmoidal fracture should be suspected if a patient has evidence of a nasal fracture with telecanthus, hypertelorism with detached medial canthus, and/or CSF rhinorrhea.[54] On axial images, there is posterior displacement of the nasal pyramid with the ethmoid lamina fractured on itself in an accordion fashion. Because the dura of the anterior cranial fossa is thin and adherent to the bone, ethmoidal fractures can easily result in CSF leaks (**Table 4-7**). To find the site of a dural tear, a CT cisternogram may be required.

Nasomaxillary buttress fractures
Fractures of the nasomaxillary buttress involve the lateral piriform aperture, frontal process of the maxilla, and the frontal bone up to the superior orbital rim (**Fig. 4-5**). These fractures may occur from focal trauma to the center of the face. Potential complications may involve the medial orbital rim, frontal and maxillary sinuses, and nasal septum (**Table 4-7**).

Maxillo-alveolar buttress fractures
Alveolar fractures are common maxillary fractures (**Fig. 4-5**). The typical cause is an upward blow to the mandible, which pushes the maxillary teeth upward and outward. Because of the tissue support surrounding the alveolus, these fractures are usually nondisplaced. However, the involved teeth are often displaced and devitalized (**Fig. 4-6, Table 4-7**). Less commonly, a blow by a narrow object over the lower portion of the maxilla can result in partial fractures of the maxilla involving the anterior and lateral antral walls, extending toward the pyriform aperature and down into the maxillary alveolus.[65]

Potential complications from central midfacial fractures are listed in **Table 4-7**.[51,53,54,64–67]

Lateral Midface

Zygomaticomaxillary complex fractures (tripod, trimalar, zygomatic complex)
Zygomaticomaxillary complex or lateral buttress fractures are the second most common facial fracture, accounting for 40% of facial fractures.[45,66] The zygoma has four processes: frontal, maxillary, orbital, and temporal. Superiorly, the frontal process articulates with the frontal bone at the zygomaticofrontal suture. Inferiorly, the maxillary process articulates with the maxilla at

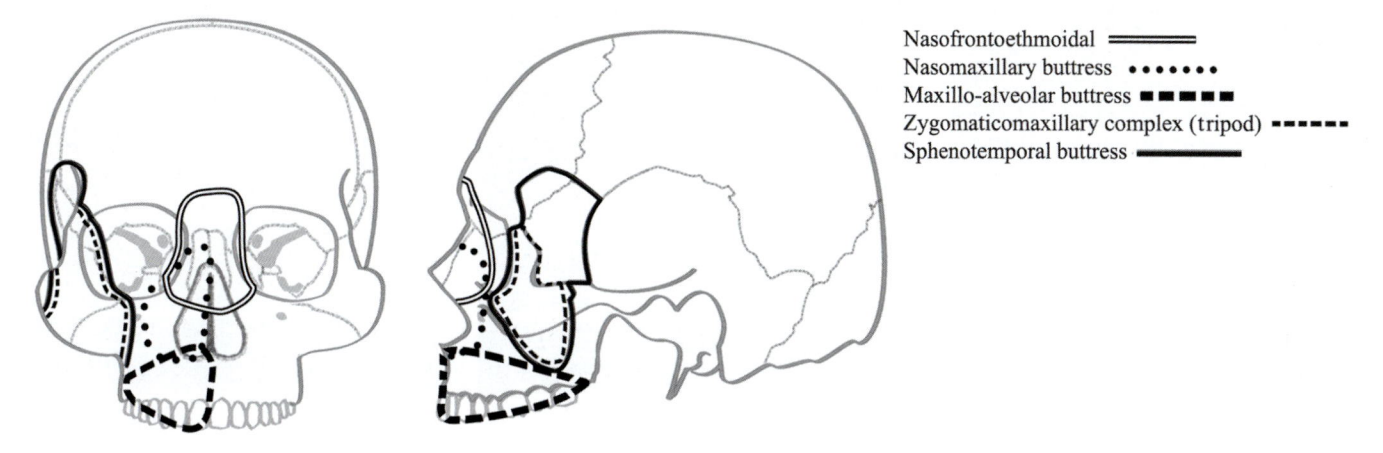

Figure 4-5 Midface Fractures
Schematic demonstrating common fracture planes of the face.

the zygomaticomaxillary suture. Medially, the orbital process articulates with the greater wing of the sphenoid. Laterally, the temporal process joins the temporal bone.

Zygomaticomaxillary fractures occur at the articulations of the zygoma with the frontal bone (lateral orbital wall), maxillae, and zygomatic arch, and often extends through the orbital floor. As the zygoma separates from its attachment points, there is widening of the zygomaticofrontal and zygomaticosphenoidal sutures, and disruption of the inferior orbital rim involving the posterolateral wall of the maxillary sinus (**Fig. 4-5**).

Because the infraorbital nerve passes through the orbital floor into the zygomaticomaxillary area where it exits, hypesthesia often occurs in the midface. Other findings include subconjunctival hemorrhage, ecchymosis, and flattening of the malar eminence, which may be obscured by periorbital edema. The lateral canthus may be depressed if the zygoma is displaced inferiorly. The patient may complain of cheek pain with jaw movement and trismus (difficulty opening the mouth) due to impingement of the temporalis muscle as it passes under the zygoma.[54] Step-offs may be palpated at the zygomaticomaxillary arch from

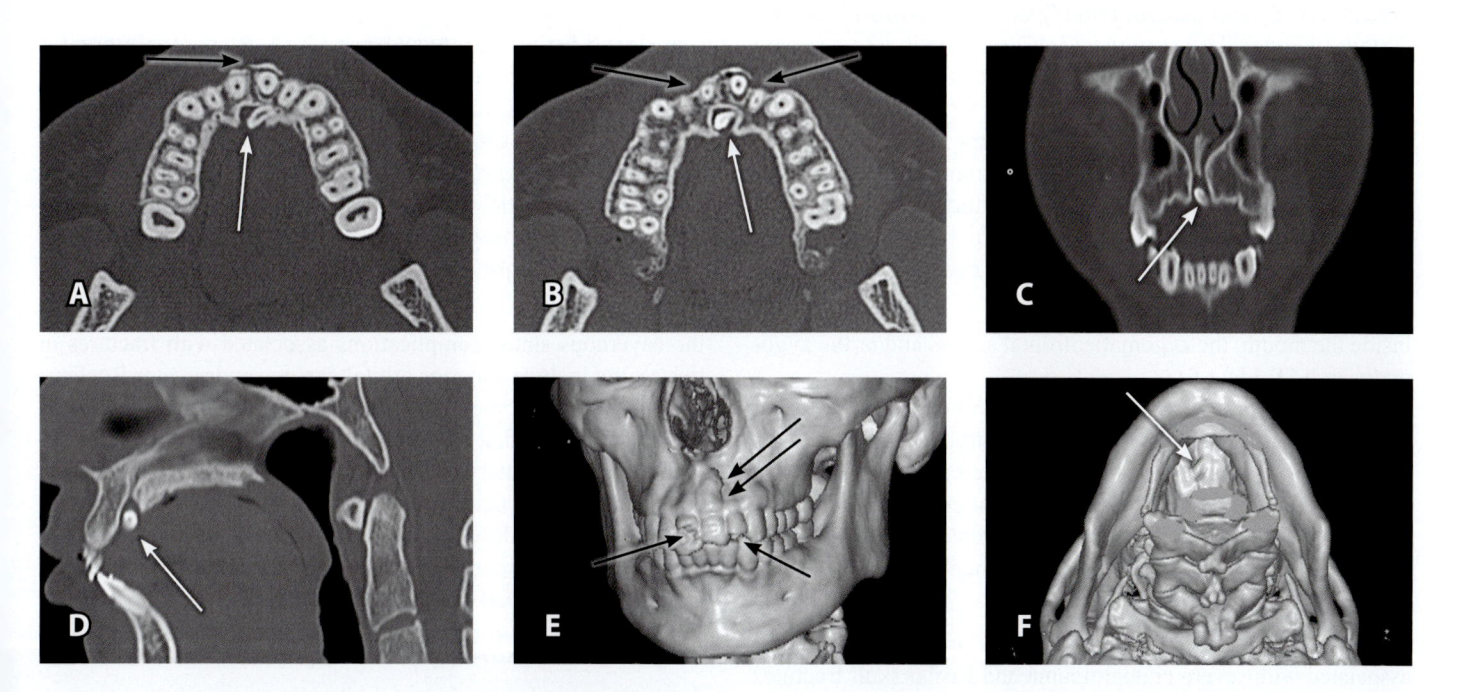

Figure 4-6 Maxillary Fracture with Incidental Mesiodent
Comminuted maxillary fracture with an overbite deformity and incidental mesiodent. Axial bone window CT (**A–B**), coronal bone window CT (**C–D**), and 3D reconstructed CT images with surface rendering (**D–F**) show a comminuted fracture in the premaxilla and right upper alveolar ridge (*black arrow*, **A**, *black arrows*, **B**, *double black arrows*, **E**), and disruption of upper right medial incisor and upper left lateral incisor (*black arrows*, **E**). Also note the mesiodent lying in the nasopalatine canal (*white arrows*).

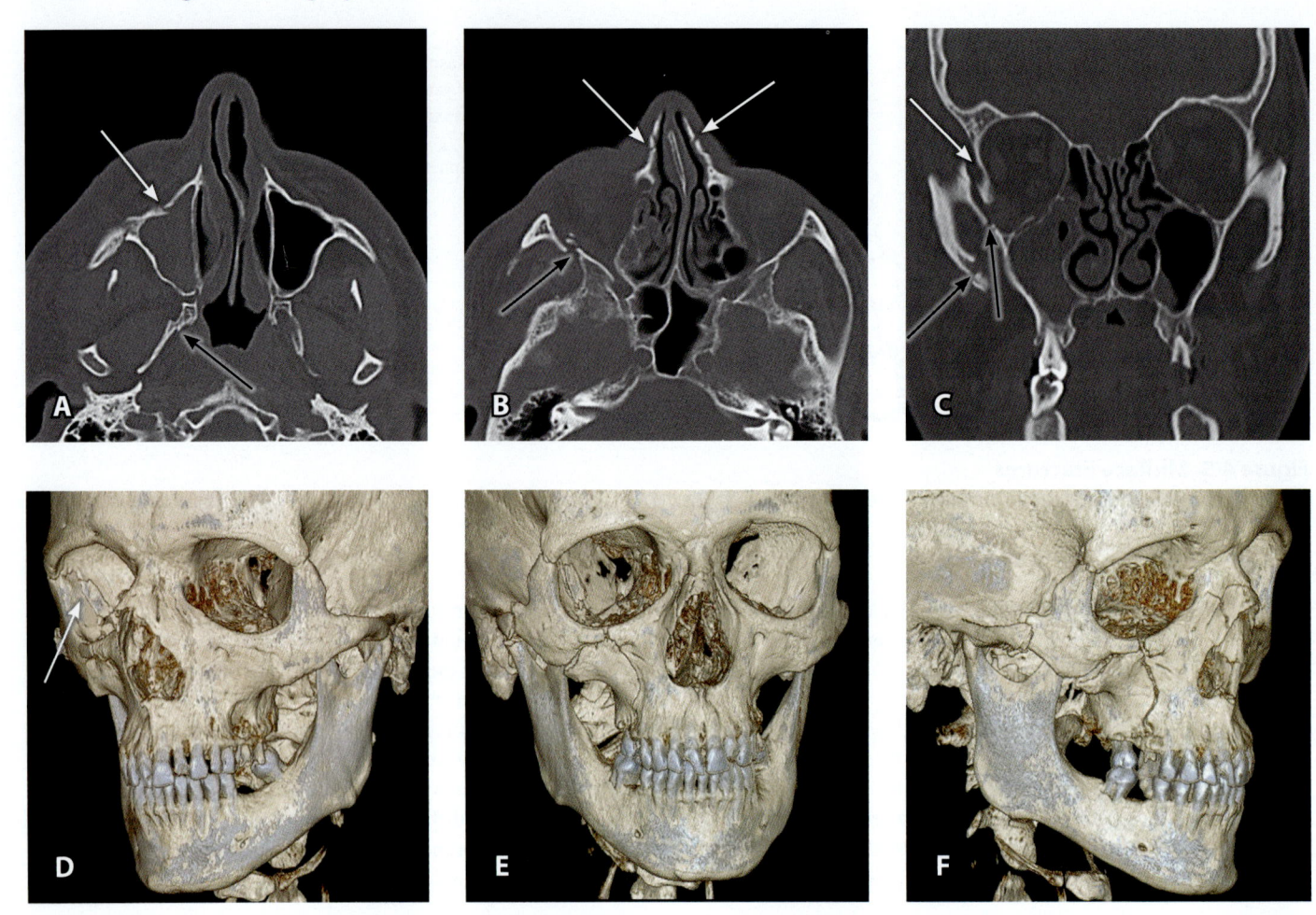

Figure 4-7 Zygomaticomaxillary Complex Tripod Fracture

Zygomaticomaxillary complex (ZMC) fracture in 47-year-old victim of closed-fist assault. Axial bone CT (**A–B**), coronal bone CT (**C**), and 3D reconstructed CT with surface rendering (**D–F**) scans show the several fracture planes of the assault. There is a fracture of the anterior wall of the right maxillary sinus (*white arrow,* **A**) with resultant hematoma occupying the lumen of the sinus. Also note the contralateral displacement of the nasal septum, as well as the fracture of the lateral pterygoid plate of the sphenoid (*black arrow,* **A**). There are bilateral comminuted fractures of the nasal bones (*white arrows,* **B, F**). The maxillary ZMC is fractured in three places, including 1) comminuted fractures of the right sphenozygomatic sutures and overhanging fragments of distracted frontozygomatic sutures in the region of the lateral orbital wall (*black arrow,* **B**, *white arrow,* **C**, *white arrow,* **D, E, F**), 2) the zygomatic arch (**F**), and 3) inferior orbital wall with inferior extension to the right alveolar ridge (*black arrows,* **C, E, F**).

inside the mouth, the zygomaticofrontal suture, and/or the zygomatic arch (**Table 4-5**).

Zygomaticomaxillary fractures are best evaluated on coronal CT images, especially with 3D reconstruction. After impact, the zygoma is usually displaced and often rotated around the vertical and/or horizontal axes. Posterior or medial displacement and/or medial rotation around the horizontal axis and lateral rotation around the vertical axis are common[65] (**Fig. 4-7**).

Sphenotemporal buttress fractures

Fractures of the sphenotemporal buttress are rare and usually associated with severe cranial trauma and basilar skull fractures (**Fig. 4-5**). Up to 24% of patients sustaining blunt head trauma have a skull base fracture.[68] Due to the complex anatomy of this area, fractures in this region may damage neighboring structures including the internal carotid artery, cranial nerves, and the cavernous sinus. Because the sphenoid and temporal bones border the cavernous sinus, complications associated with fractures in this region include superior orbital fissure syndrome or Rochon-Duvigneaud syndrome (retroorbital pain, restriction of eye motility, impairment of first trigeminal branches, and frequent involvement of the optic nerve), and other manifestations of injury to cranial nerves III (oculomotor), IV (trochlear), V1 (ophthalmic branch), V2 (maxillary branch of trigeminal), and VI (abducens). See Chapter 11 for more information. Potential complications from lateral midfacial fractures are listed in **Table 4-7**.

Single Strut Fractures

Nasal Bone Fractures

Simple nasal fractures are the most common of all facial fractures, accounting for half of all facial bone fractures.[45,66] Patients typically present with a history of trauma with swelling, tenderness, and crepitus over the nasal bridge. Epistaxis but no CSF

Table 4-11 Classification of Nasal Bone Fractures

Injury Type	Features
Plane 1	• Injury remains anterior to plane that extends from caudal tip of nasal bones to anterior nasal spine • Avulsion of upper lateral nasal cartilages occurs with posterior dislocation of septal and alar cartilages • Typically results from mild lateral or oblique impact, which medially displaces ipsilateral lower nasal bone, frontal process of maxilla, and possibly pyriform aperture margin
Plane 2	• Involves external nose, nasal septum, and anterior nasal spine • Splaying or flattening of nasal bones and septal cartilage • Results in medial displacement of ipsilateral nasal bone and lateral displacement of contralateral nasal bone and septum
Plane 3	• Orbital and possibly intracranial structures are damaged • Typically see comminuted nasal bone fractures with additional fractures of frontal processes of maxillae, lacrimal bones, and ethmoid labyrinth

leakage should be present. Nasal fractures must be distinguished from the more serious nasofrontoethmoidal fractures.

The majority of nasal bone fractures involve the thinner, distal third of the nasal bones, usually from lateral rather than frontal impact injuries.[67] One classification system for nasal fractures categorizes frontal injuries into three types: Plane 1, 2, and 3[65] (**Table 4-11**). Severe nasal septal injuries can extend upward to involve the cribriform plate and orbital roof.[66]

Lateral blows to the nose usually fracture only the ipsilateral nasal bone. Frontal blows usually result in bilateral nasal bone fractures with displacement and fracture of the nasal septum (**Fig. 4-5**). With greater force, the entire nasal pyramid including the frontal processes of the maxillae may become detached.[67] Posterior displacement of the nasal bones and septum results in a saddle nose deformity and splaying of the nose.[69] Severe fractures may also result in traumatic hypertelorism and telecanthus. Additionally, hemorrhage due to rupture of the anterior and posterior ethmoidal arteries may be severe.

In children, the internasal suture is not yet ossified, so the nasal bones act as separate, hinged units resting on the frontal processes of the maxillae. Consequently, the frontal processes do not usually fracture in childhood nasal injuries.[65,70] If a child's nose is struck from the side, the lateral cartilaginous walls may be displaced, which may not be demonstrated radiographically. Such an injury can result in cosmetic deformity and functional impairment that become more evident as the edema and hemorrhage resolve.[66]

In cases involving buckling of the nasal septal cartilage, the perichondrium may separate from the cartilage, allowing a hematoma to develop in that space. As the septal hematoma interrupts the overlying mucoperiosteal vascular supply, cartilage necrosis can occur. The septal hematoma can organize into a firm, thickened septum, or become infected. If a septal abscess develops, the cartilage can eventually necrose, resulting in a saddle nose deformity, and the infection may spread intracranially. Therefore, if imaging studies are performed, careful attention should be paid to the nasal septum for any localized septal swelling, septal bone fracture, and/or cartilage dislocation.[65,67]

Radiographic examination plays a minor role in the management of nasal bone fractures unless there is severe injury or extension to other facial bones. Imaging can be performed to confirm the clinical diagnosis or to determine the displacement of the fracture fragments.[40] It is important to note that fracture of cartilage may not be demonstrated by any imaging modality.[67]

Localized Sinus Wall

Fractures of the frontal sinuses may involve the anterior wall or both the anterior and posterior walls (**Fig. 4-5**). The fractures may be linear and nondisplaced or comminuted and depressed.

Isolated fractures of the maxillary sinus are uncommon (**Fig. 4-5**). There may be a fracture in the anterolateral wall or a depressed fracture of the anterior wall of the maxillary antrum.[43]

Ethmoid sinus fractures usually occur as part of complex strut or Le Fort III patterns, but may be isolated (**Fig. 4-2**). Localized fractures may occur in the roof of the ethmoid labyrinth in the region of the cribriform plate, which may be associated with pneumocephalus. If the fracture involves the medial orbital wall, it may result in orbital emphysema.[43]

Alveolar Ridge

Alveolar ridge fractures occur just above the level of the teeth through the alveolar process of the maxilla (**Fig. 4-5**). Usually a group of teeth is loose or fractured, and blood is noted at the gingival line. A chest film should be considered to look for any aspirated tooth fragments if all the fractured teeth are not located.[55]

Zygomatic Arch

Most zygomatic fractures result from lateral blows and involve the arch and a portion of the lateral orbital wall, but some fractures may be isolated to the arch.[71] Zygomatic arch fractures tend to occur in 2 to 3 places along the arch (**Fig. 4-5**). Often

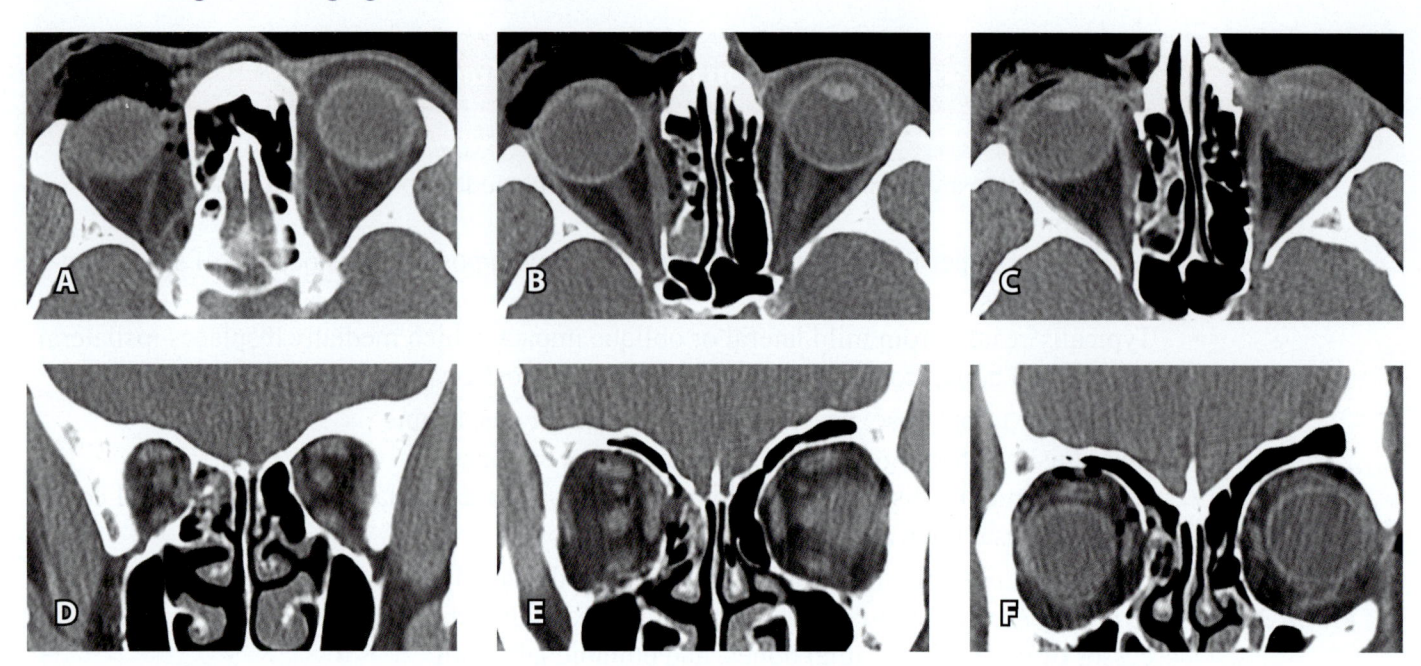

Figure 4-8 Medial Orbital Wall Blowout Fracture
Axial (**A–C**) and coronal (**D–F**) CT images show a blowout fracture of the left lamina papyracia with patchy opacification of the ipsilateral ethmoid air cells. Also note the massive right orbital emphysema with pockets of air tracking posteriorly toward the fractured medial orbital wall (lamina papryecia). The fracture fragments do not extend into the orbit or cause constriction of the extraocular muscles.

three breaks occur: one at each end of the arch and a third in the middle, forming a V-shaped depression, which often impinges on the temporalis muscle or coronoid process of the mandible below to cause trismus.[54,55]

Isolated Orbital Rim

The orbital rim is composed of several bones (**Fig. 4-5**). The frontal bone contributes the superior and upper medial portions of the orbital rim. The lateral orbital rim is part of the zygoma. The inferior and lower medial rims are part of the maxilla. Lastly, the lacrimal bone contributes the medial rim, which separates the orbit from nares.

There are three main types of orbital rim fractures that can occur in isolation or in conjunction with other craniofacial fractures: 1) superior orbital rim fractures, which are frontal bone/frontal sinus fractures; 2) zygomatic fractures, which involve the inferolateral rim/zygoma and usually occur as part of a tripod fracture; and 3) inferior orbital rim fractures.[64,72] Because a great deal of force is required to cause orbital rim fractures, they often occur with extensive craniofacial trauma. Orbital rim fractures can extend into the orbit, often the orbital floor. Superior orbital rim fractures can extend into the posterior wall of the frontal sinus and the cribriform plate, resulting in CSF leakage. Even in cases of isolated orbital rim fractures, one should consider potential

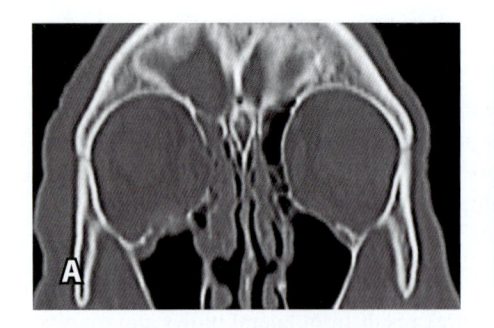

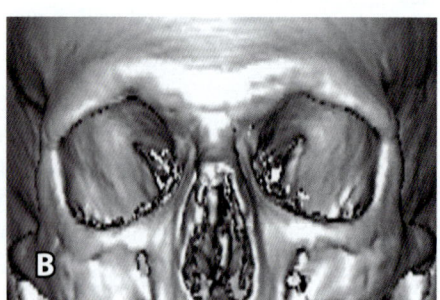

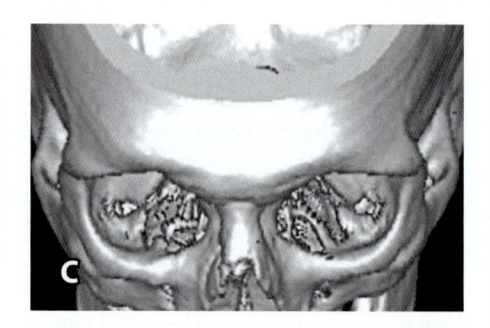

Figure 4-9 Combined Medial and Inferior Orbital Blowout Fractures
Coronal reformatted (**A**) and 3D surface rendered (**B–C**) CT images show destruction of the medial and inferior walls of the right orbit. The 3D images are of great help in reconstructing the symmetry of the face in order to ensure optimal cosmetic results.

Table 4-12 Classification of Mandibular Fractures by Anatomic Region

Fracture Type	Anatomic Region
Symphysis	• Region of central incisors that runs from alveolar process through inferior border of mandible
Parasymphyseal	• Region bounded by vertical lines distal to canine teeth
Body	• Region from distal symphysis to a line coinciding with alveolar border of masseter muscle, including third molar
Angle	• Triangular region bounded by anterior border of te masseter muscle to posterosuperior attachment of masseter muscle, distal to third molar
Ramus	• Region bounded by superior aspect of angle to two lines forming an apex at sigmoid notch
Condylar	• Posterior region superior to ramus and including condylar process
Coronoid process	• Anterior region superior to ramus and including coronoid process
Alveolar	• Region that normally contains teeth

injuries to the cranium, eye, optic nerve, extraocular muscles, infraorbital nerve, paranasal sinuses, and the lacrimal system.[73]

Orbital Wall "Blow-out"
Blow-out fractures occur when a blow to the eye causes a backward displacement of the globe, increasing the intraorbital pressure, causing the weak orbital floor (maxilla) or medial wall (lamina papyracea) to "blow out".[74] Typically, the posteromedial region of the orbital floor fractures, and the orbital rim remains intact (**Figs. 4-5**, **4-8**, and **4-9**). When periorbital fat, extraocular muscles, and most importantly, connective tissue septa herniate into the maxillary sinus or ethmoid bone, they can become entrapped, resulting in decreased ocular mobility, enophthalmos, and diplopia.[75,76] Potential complications from orbital blow-out fractures are listed in **Table 4-7**.[64,76] Diplopia, extraocular muscle limitation, and "trap-door" fractures (bone fragments are hinged and appear almost perfectly realigned) occur more frequently in children than in adults.[77]

Coronal and axial CT images of the orbit and facial bones are important in evaluating the degree of orbital wall displacement. MR imaging should demonstrate hyperintense, prolapsed orbital fat and the involvement of any extraocular muscles. See Chapter 2.

Mandibular Fractures
The mandible is one of the most commonly fractured bones in the facial skeleton along with the zygomatic complex and the nose.[78] The most common fracture location varies depending on the cause of the injury.[79] Mandibular fractures can be classified by anatomic region[80] (**Table 4-12**). Depending on the study, most fractures have been reported to occur in the angle (15% to 36%), body (21% to 29%), condyle (26%), and parasympyhseal (17% to 35%) regions; whereas the ramus (4%) and coronoid process (1%) have lower occurrence rates[81–83] (**Fig. 4-10**).

Angle fractures can be characterized in two ways: 1. vertically favorable or unfavorable and 2. horizontally favorable or unfavorable. In vertically and horizontally unfavorable fractures, the muscles attached to the ramus (masseter, temporal, medial pterygoid) displace the proximal segment upward and medially. Conversely, in horizontally and vertically favorable fractures, these same muscles tend to stabilize the bony fragments.[80]

In bilateral fractures of the cuspid region, the symphysis of the mandible is displaced inferiorly and posteriorly by the pull of the digastric, geniohyoid, and genioglossus muscles.

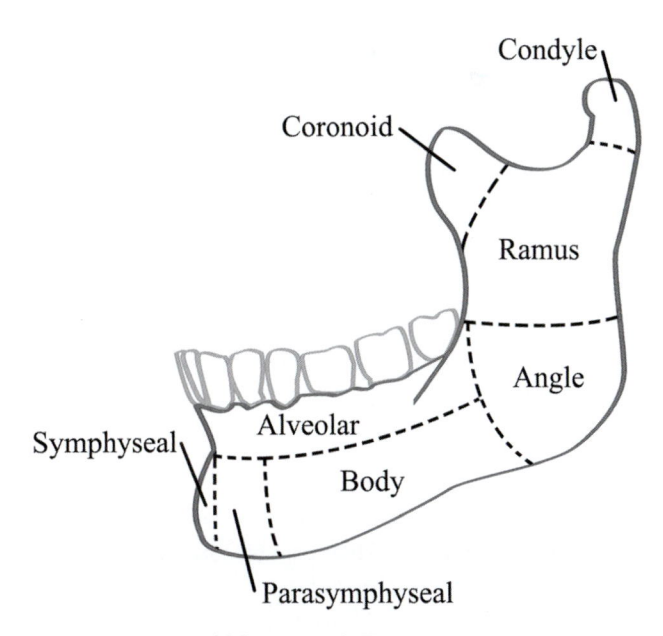

Figure 4-10 Mandible Lateral View
Schematic depicting the anatomic regions of the mandible from a lateral view.

Table 4-13 Features of Mandibular Fractures

- Multiple fractures are common and are typically bilateral.
- Most fractures occur in the angle, body, condyle, and parasymphyseal regions.
- Common combination fractures include mandibular angle plus contralateral condyle or body.
- Significantly displaced fractures may be associated with other fractures
  - Direct fractures in canine region are often associated with indirect condylar neck fractures.
  - Bilateral angle fractures are often associated with bilateral condylar neck fractures.
- Angle fractures are classified as vertically and horizontally favorable or unfavorable depending on stabilizing or destabilizing actions of masseter, temporal, and medial pterygoid muscles on the bony fragments.
- Condylar fractures are classified (extracapsular, subcondylar, or intracapsular) and typed (I–V) by severity.
- If fracture line enters root of a tooth, it is an open fracture by definition.
- CT: useful for evaluating condylar neck and complex fractures.
- MR: useful for evaluating intracapsular and condylar fractures, and temporomandibular joint (low-signal on T1-W and T2-W).
- An anteromedially displaced condylar fragment gives impression of an empty glenoid fossa.
- In bilateral fractures of cuspid region, symphysis of mandible is displaced inferiorly and posteriorly.
- If the trauma and level of injury are disproportionate, look for pathologic fractures (periapical abscess or mandibular tumor).

Condylar fractures are classified as extracapsular, subcondylar, or intracapsular.[80,84] They can be categorized into five types in order of increasing severity:

1. Type I is a fracture of the neck of the condyle with relatively minimal displacement of the head. The angle between the head and axis of the ramus varies from 10 to 45 degrees.
2. Type II fractures have an angle between the head and axis of the ramus from 45 to 90 degrees, resulting in tearing of the medial portion of the joint capsule.
3. Type III fractures contain fragments that are confined within the area of the glenoid fossa but are not in contact. The head is displaced medially and forward, resting outside of a torn capsule.
4. Type IV fractures articulate on or in a forward position with regard to the articular eminence.
5. Type V fractures consist of vertical or oblique fractures through the head of the condyle.

The lateral pterygoid muscle tends to cause anteromedial displacement of the condylar head, giving the impression of an empty glenoid fossa in diagnostic images.[51]

Most mandibular fractures are obvious on clinical exam (**Table 4-5**). Clinical findings include facial asymmetry or distortion, malocclusion of the teeth, or abnormal mobility of portions of the mandible or teeth.[81] Bilateral anterior mandibular fractures may allow the tongue to fall back and obstruct the airway. Spasm in the masseter and pterygoid muscles tend to force the condyles up the anterior slope of the articular eminence, restricting mouth closure.[55] Because the condyle is the growth center for the mandible, childhood injury to the condyle can cause significant deformity.

Panoramic views and plan films may be sufficient for evaluating solitary mandibular fractures. CT imaging is useful for complex fractures and those involving the condylar neck. In cases involving fractures of the condyle, the traction of the external pterygoid muscle displaces the condylar head anteromedially, giving the impression of an empty glenoid fossa.

MR imaging provides superior images of the temporomandibular joint (TMJ) and avoids ionizing radiation near the eyes.[64] T1-weighted (T1-W) images in the sagittal or sagittal-oblique plane are very helpful in evaluating intracapsular and condylar fractures. On sagittal views, the TMJ meniscus appears as a biconcave, low-signal structure on both T1-W and T2-W images, and has an anterior and posterior band at either end separated by a narrow intermediate zone.[85] At rest, the posterior band lies in a 12 o'clock position relative to the condylar head. As the mouth opens, the condylar head and meniscus shift forward as far as the temporal eminence. MR can demonstrate abnormal condylar and meniscal positions and movement (**Table 4-13**).

Because greater than 50% of mandibular fractures occur in two or more locations,[83] a second fracture site or dislocation should always be considered. When double fractures occur, they are usually on contralateral sides of the symphysis (**Table 4-14**). Common combinations include the angle or symphysis (typical points of impact) and the contralateral condyle or body (zone of force dissipation) (**Figs. 4-11–4-13**). Triple fractures are less common, but often involve both condyles plus the symphysis.[55,86]

Treatment of Facial Fractures

The goal of fracture treatment is to re-establish facial appearance and function including vision, breathing, mouth opening, and chewing. Nondisplaced or minimally displaced fractures resulting in minimal occlusal derangement may be treated conservatively. Minimally displaced Le Fort I fractures may require

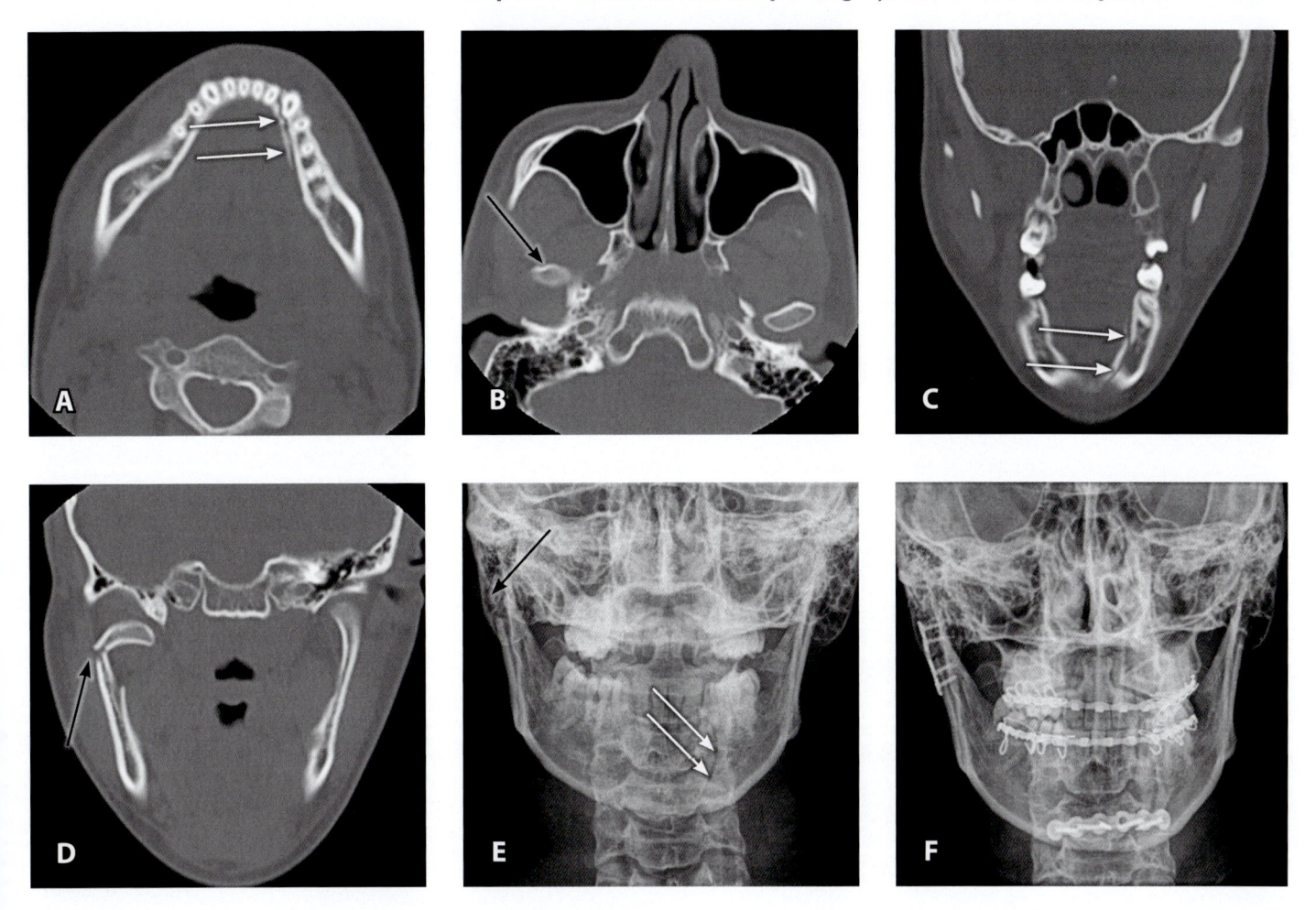

Chapter 4: Sinonasal Endoscopic Surgery, Infections and Neoplasms   **151**

Figure 4-11 Condylar and Body Fractures of the Mandible
Axial bone CT (**A–B**), coronal bone CT (**C–D**) and AP views pre (**E**) and post (**F**) ORIF show a transverse fracture of the left mandibular body (*white arrows*), as well as a fracture of the right mandibular angle with disarticulation of the right temporomandibular joint (*black arrows*).

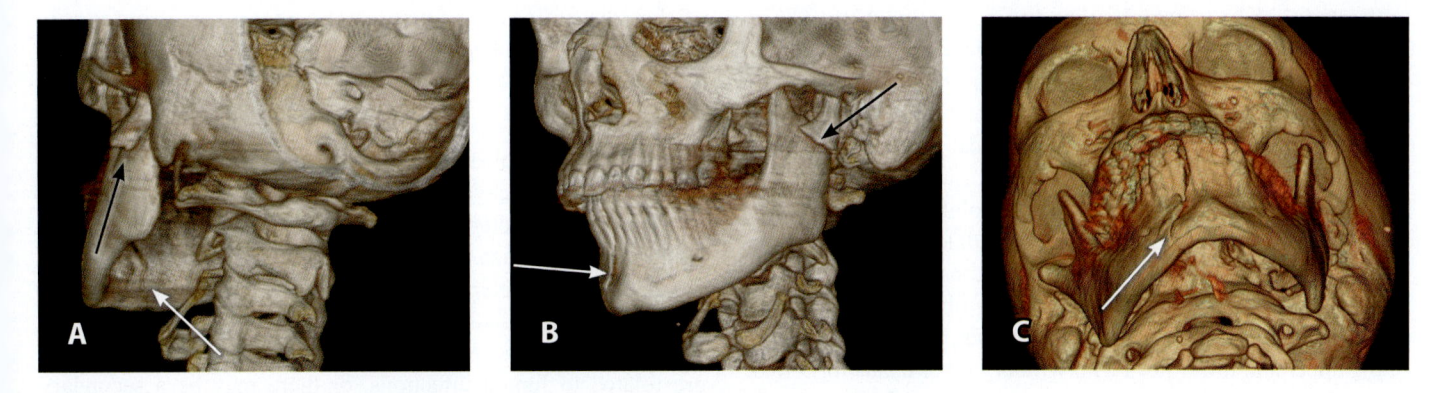

Figure 4-12 Mandibular Condylar and Parasymphyseal Fractures
Condylar and parasymphyseal mandibular fractures in a 19-year-old victim of assault. 3D CT reconstructions with surface rendering show a complete parasymphyseal fracture on the right (*white arrows*), as well as a complete fracture of the left mandibular condyle (*black arrows*).

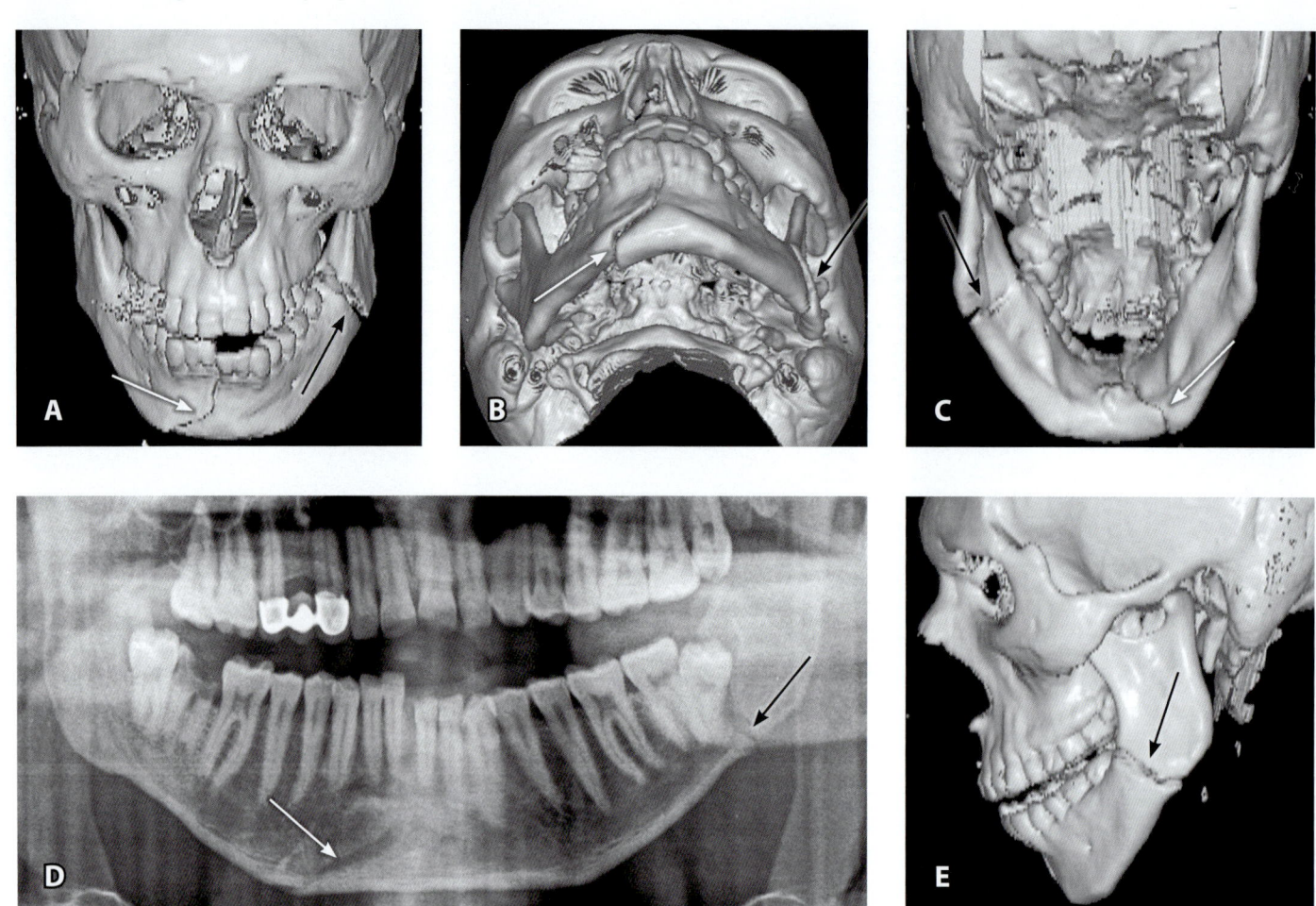

Figure 4-13 Mandible Body and Angle Fractures
Fractures of the body and angle of the mandible in a 28-year-old male victim of blunt trauma inflicted with fists. 3D CT reconstruction with surface rendering (**A–C, E**) and panorex (**D**) images show a complete right parasymphyseal (*white arrow*) and left angle (*black arrow*) fractures of the mandible.

3 weeks of intermaxillary fixation. Simple nasal fractures may be treated with an external splint and internal packing. Other fractures may require closed or open surgical repair.

Indications for operative intervention are asymmetry, displacement, comminution, malocclusion, and obstruction of the airway or paranasal sinus drainage. Surgical treatment of facial fractures consists of reduction and fixation, usually with mini and micro plates, braces, splints, or other immobilizing device. Most surgeons believe that surgical repair of midfacial injuries should be undertaken within 7 to 10 days of the time of injury, prior to the onset soft-tissue contraction and early fibrous tissue formation.[46] Some mandible fractures may require temporary locking of the upper and lower jaws with wire or rubber bands for 3 to 6 weeks. Some jaw fractures can be treated with arch bars or braces that stabilize the fracture without wiring shut the jaws.

INFECTIONS AND INFLAMMATION

Sinonasal infections and inflammations have a diverse appearance on imaging examinations ranging from benign-looking opacifications to destructive appearances. Imaging is particularly useful to detect the extent of disease including involvement of the adjacent orbit or intracranial compartments, and to rule out an unsuspected neoplasm.

Acute Sinusitis

Acute sinusitis typically follows acute inflammatory involvement of the nasal cavities, by obstructing the drainage orifices of the sinuses. Bacteria such as streptococcus pneumonia and hemophilus influenza account for about half the cases of sinusitis. Clinically, bacterial sinusitis presents with a suppurative discharge. Viral disease is seen in approximately 20% of cases with acute sinusitis. A significant percentage of sinus diseases are related to fungal infections, or there may be a secondary infection in an infected sinus caused by a mycotic agent.

Acute sinusitis usually presents with facial pain, a purulent nasal discharge, and a postnasal drip. These symptoms may last for 4 to 7 days and may be associated with headaches. Ethmoid sinusitis commonly presents with periorbital edema and increased lacrimation. Maxillary sinusitis usually occurs by itself, whereas infections of the frontal and sphenoethmoidal sinuses often occur simultaneously. Acute sinusitis usually necessitates antibiotic and decongestive treatments for several days to weeks. Orbital involvement is a frequent complication of acute ethmoid sinusitis, and may present with proptosis and swelling of the eyelids. This condition may be treated medically or with incision and drainage of a subperiosteal abscess that is typically seen in the medial or superior orbital walls. Serious intracranial complications such as meningitis, brain abscess, and epidural empyema may be related to untreated frontal sinusitis.

Chronic Sinusitis

Approximately 25% of cases of chronic maxillary sinusitis are related to dental disease. Chronic sinusitis associated with dental disease often contains mixed anaerobic infections. Chronic sinusitis manifests radiologically by mucoperiosteal thickening and sclerotic bony sinus walls, whereas acute sinusitis presents with edema of the lining epithelium. Chronic sinusitis may require surgical treatment with endoscopic or open surgical relief of the obstructed ostia.

About 95% of sinonasal secretions and interstitial fluids are water. Due to the presence of increased water (high density of mobile protons), the inflamed mucosa presents with a low signal intensity on the T1-W images, and intermediate signal intensity on the proton density weighted images, and high signal intensity on the T2-W images. Sinonasal tumors, that show intermediate signal intensity on the T2-W images, are thus easily distinguished from the intensely long T2 signal of inflamed tissues. A low to intermediate signal intensity on all imaging sequences may be seen with fibrosis that makes it more difficult to distinguish this entity from tumors. Other causes for low-intensity signal on T1-W images and high-intensity signal on T2-W images include several common entities such as retention cysts, polyps, or mucoceles of the sinonasal cavities.[87–89]

Nasal Cycle

On MR imaging, some asymptomatic patients appear to have a prominent unilateral increase in mucosal volume. This is known to be the normal cyclic edema of the mucosa of the nasal cavities, turbinates and ethmoid sinuses due to the physiologic nasal cycle. On the T2-W images, the increased mucosal volume and elevated signal intensities are shown to alternate from one to the other side of the nasal cavity at approximately 50 minutes to 6 hour intervals. These mucosal changes are not typically seen in the maxillary, frontal, or sphenoid sinuses. This cycle may be difficult to distinguish from inflamed mucosa, but is typically interrupted with topical vasoconstrictors. Awareness of such normal cyclic changes in patients without history of sinonasal disease will help to distinguish normal mucosa from pathologic mucosa.[90]

Retention Cysts and Polyps

Retention cysts and polyps are common complications of inflammatory sinusitis. Mucous retention cysts are the most common and may be found in 10% of patients. These retention cysts develop following obstruction of seromucinous glands and are mostly filled with mucous. The less common form of retention cysts develops from the accumulation of serous fluid in the submucosa. The mucosa becomes a wall of serous retention cysts – a distinguishing characteristic from the mucous retention cyst, whose wall consists of the epithelium of the obstructed duct of a mucous gland.

Polyps result from a local upheaval of mucosa, not unlike the serous cysts. The polyps increase in size by accumulating intracellular fluid. The presence of collagen synthesis within the stroma represents an attempt of the stroma to limit growth of the polyp. Polyps in the paranasal sinuses and nasal cavities appear to be similar histologically, although located in different places.

Unique forms of polyps include the antrochoanal polyp and the sphenochoanal polyp, the former being the most common type (**Figs. 4-14** and **4-15**). Each consists of hyperplastic, edematous submucosa that herniates from the maxillary or sphenoid sinus into the ostium of the adjacent nasal cavity. The angiomatous polyp is a special type of fibrous nasal polyp that arises as a reaction to minor trauma. Clinically, angiomatous polyps may be easily confused with nasopharyngeal angiofibromas. The angiomatous polyps are located primarily in the nasal fossa (not in the nasopharynx as in the typical angiofibromas), and rarely extend into the pterygopalatine fossa, sphenoid sinuses, or cranial cavity. Angiographically, angiomatous polyps have few, if any, feeding vessels. There is no evidence of profound enhancement and no evidence of vascular flow channels on MR images. Such angiomatous polyps are readily removed surgically by a "shelling out procedure." Aggressive surgery or embolization procedures are not needed.[91]

Mucoceles

A mucocele can form as a complication of mucosal edema of the sinus ostia, leading to their obstruction. The sinus expands as the obstruction persists, whether with or without an associated infection. The presenting symptoms are mass effect with proptosis, obstructed breathing, or a nasal sound to the voice. The mucocele expands the sinus cavity, causing pressure necrosis and subsequent erosion of the sinus walls. The periosteum will then produce new bone that is characterized as remodeled (**Figs. 4-16–4-20**).

Both CT and MR imaging appear to be excellent imaging techniques for the diagnosis of mucoceles. There is an important correlation between the signal intensity on MR imaging and the density on CT. Mucoceles with hypointense signal intensities on the T1- and T2-weighted images correlate with hyperdense mucoceles on CT. Mucoceles with hyperintense signal intensities on the T1- and T2-weighted images correlate with hypodense mucoceles on CT. Markedly inspissated secretions with few available hydrogen ions result in hypointense signal intensities or signal void on MR imaging, which may be mistaken for normal aerated sinuses. Whenever the water content of a mucocele is increased, a brighter signal is seen on the T2-weighted image. The use of gadolinium-enhanced MR imaging may help to distinguish between certain tumors and mucoceles (**Fig. 4-21**). Only the rim of infected mucoceles (pyoceles) will enhance. In some cases, the rim enhancement does not represent infection but may be related to crowding of the surface mucosa around the mass lesion.[92,93]

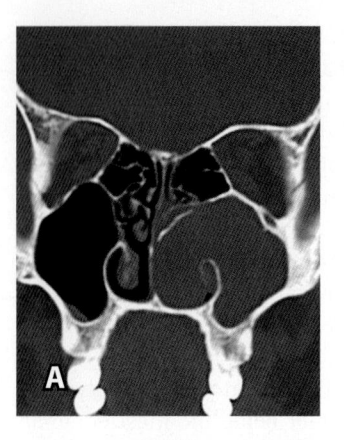

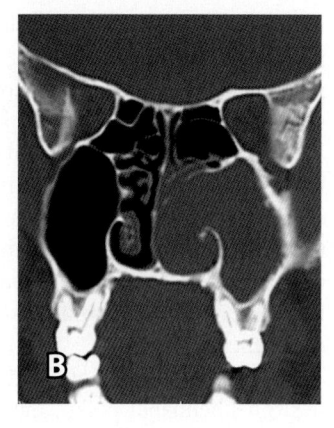

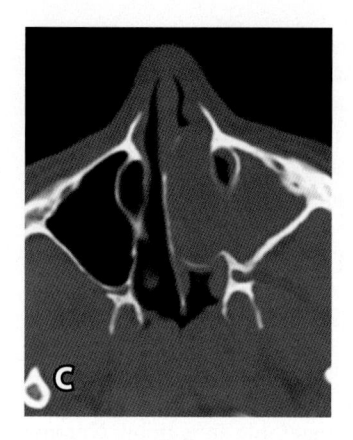

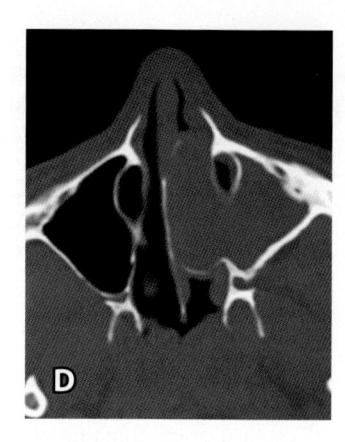

Figure 4-14 Antrochoanal Polyp
Coronal (**A–B**) and axial (**C–D**) bone window CT images show a soft-tissue mass in the left nasal cavity with expansion through a markedly enlarged maxillary ostium into the maxillary sinus. There are some chronic sinus changes in the walls of the left maxillary sinus, evidenced by osteitis. These findings are consistent with an antrochoanal polyp.

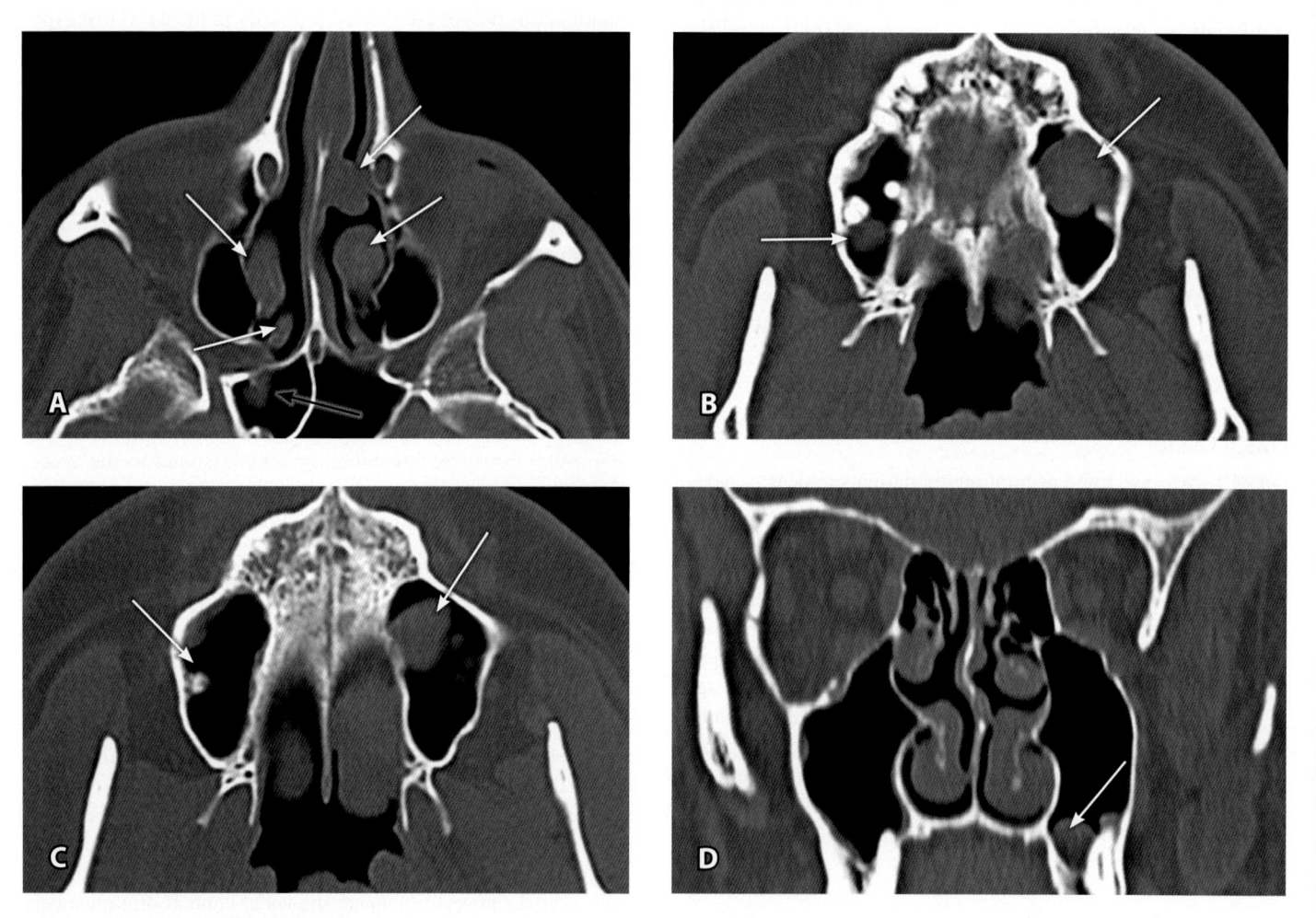

Figure 4-15 Sinonasal Polyposis
Axial (**A–C**) and coronal (**D**) NECT images show multiple polyps in the nasal cavity (*white arrows,* **A**), sphenoid sinus (*black arrow* **A**), and maxillary sinus (*white arrows,* **B, C, D**). There is no evidence of obstructive sinus disease.

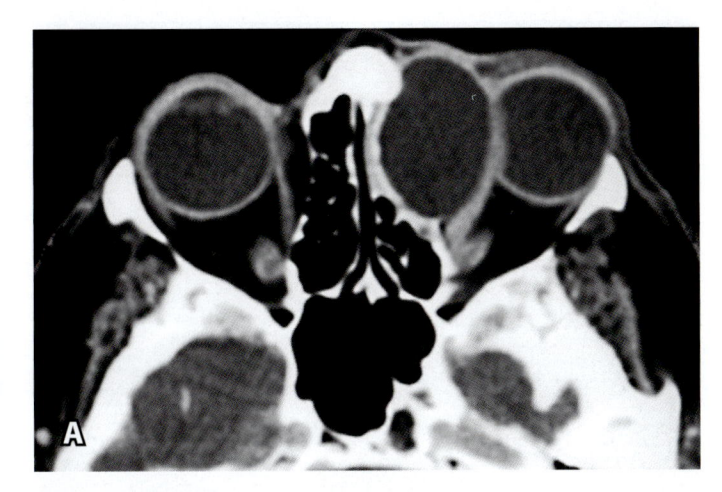

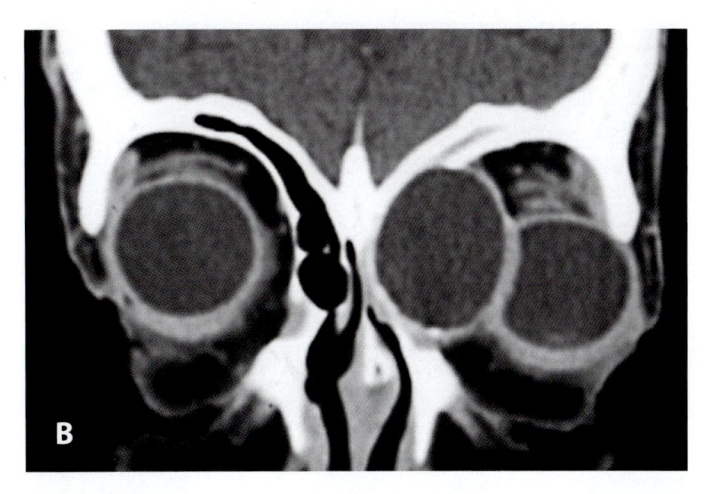

Chapter 4: Sinonasal Endoscopic Surgery, Infections and Neoplasms 155

Figure 4-16 Ethmoid Sinus Mucocele
Axial (**A**) and coronal (**B**) CECT images show smooth expansion of the left ethmoid air cells with erosion through the lamina papyracia into the left orbit. The left globe is proptotic and displaced downward by the expansion. The appearance of the mucocele lying between the two globes simulates a triclops.

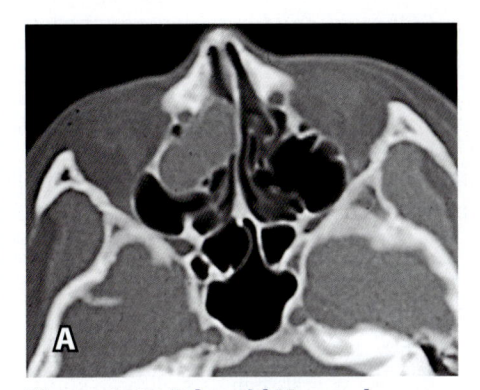

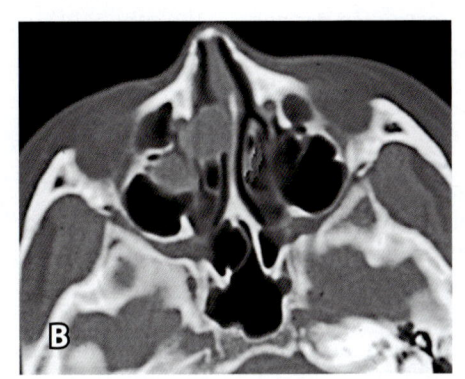

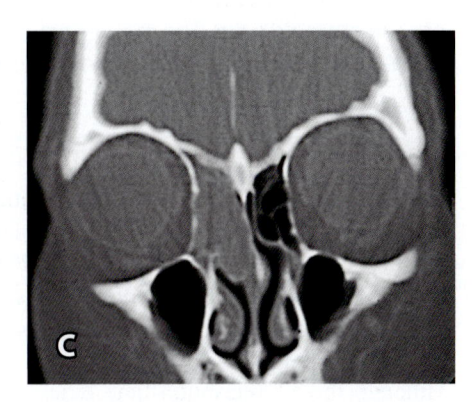

Figure 4-17 Ethmoid Mucocele
Ethmoid mucocele obstructing the right nasolacrimal duct in a patient presenting with epiphora. Axial (**A–B**) and coronal (**C**) NECT images of the sinuses show a lobular mass selectively involving the medial and anterior right ethmoid air cells with expansion in the nasal cavity. The expanding mass is causing obstruction of nasolacrimal duct, manifesting as epiphora.

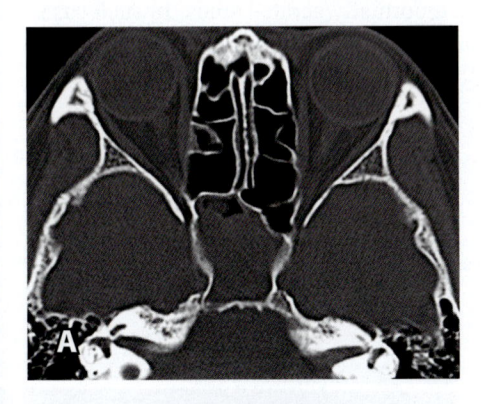

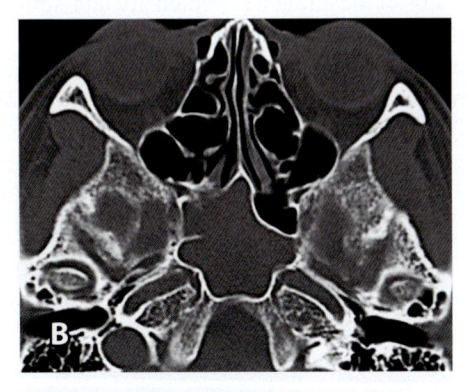

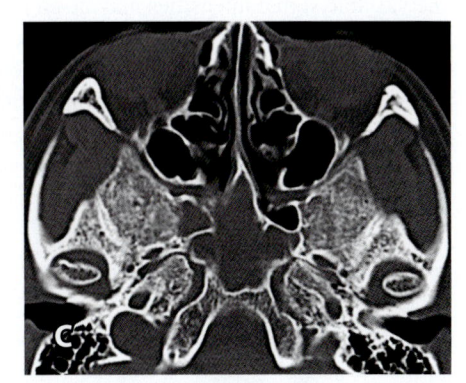

Figure 4-18 Sphenoid Mucocele
Axial bone CT images (**A–B**) showing a large fluid intensity almost completely occupying the sphenoid sinus. Also note the remodeling and outward bowing of the lateral walls of the sphenoid sinus.

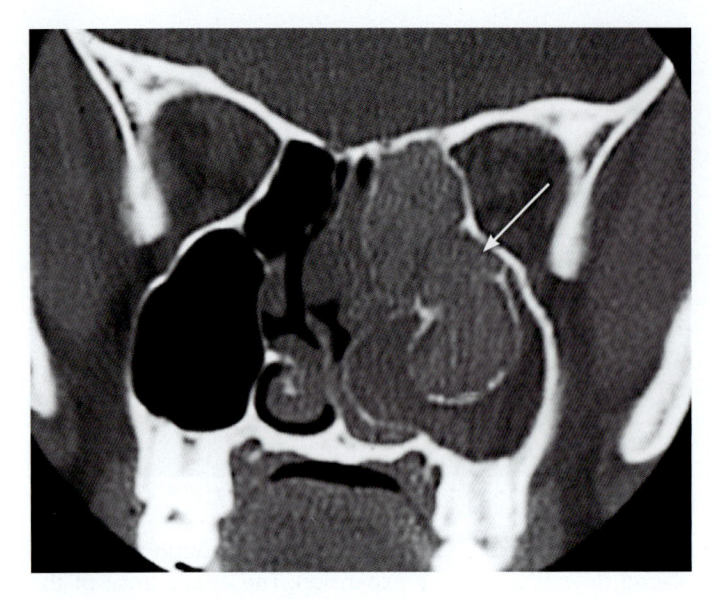

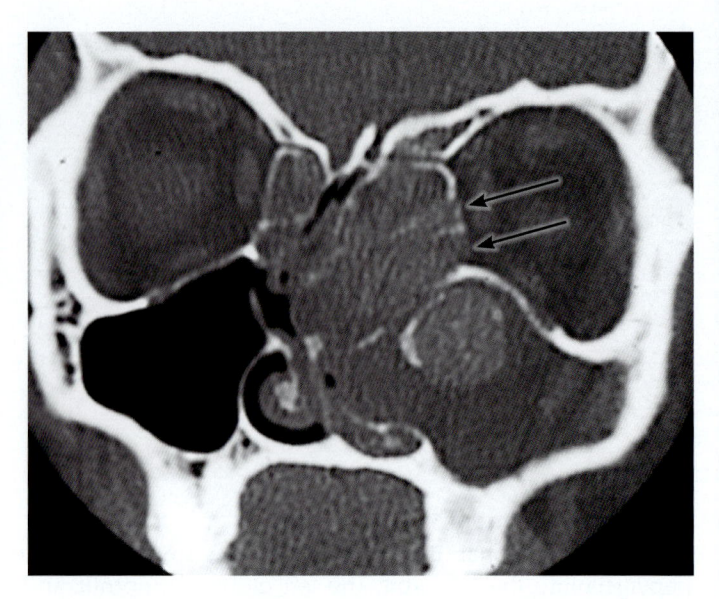

Figure 4-19 Haller Cell Mucocele
Mucocele of infraorbital ethmoid cell or Haller cells. Coronal CT scans through the maxillary sinus show uniform density cystic expansion originating from the left Haller cells (*white arrow*) with extension inferiorly into the left maxillary sinus and superiorly into the ethmoid sinus. The mass effect has obstructed drainage of the sphenoid, maxillary, ethmoid, and frontal sinus on the left side. Also note the smooth erosion of the left lamina papyracia (*black arrows*).

Chronically Inspissated Secretions

MR imaging has some significant limitations in patients with chronic inflammatory sinonasal disease. For example, the signal intensity of highly concentrated mucoceles may resemble the signal of a normal aerated sinus. As sinonasal secretions get older, the protein concentration increases while the water content decreases, and the viscosity of the secretion increases. Although the T1 relaxation time is less sensitive than the T2 relaxation time, both are shortened with an increase in protein content. A decrease in free water content of the secretion results in decreased signal intensity on the T2-weighted images. Therefore, protein and water content appear to be the major factors that cause variations in the T1 and T2 signal intensities. Whereas the variable signal intensities may be an indicator of the amount of protein in the secretion and thus determine the age of the specimen, it may be impossible to differentiate the signal void of a normally aerated sinus from a chronically inspissated mucocele. In such cases, CT scanning is diagnostic.[94] As previously discussed, certain fungal infections can also appear predominantly low in signal intensity on MRI and simulate a normally aerated sinus.[95]

Noninvasive Fungal Sinusitis

Fungal sinusitis is much less common than bacterial or viral sinusitis. Typically, the disease is first seen as a chronic sinusitis that does not resolve with antibiotic therapy or sinus irrigation. Sometimes, the true identity of the disorder is not recognized until surgery or afterwards when there is subsequent pathologic evaluation of a fungus ball or mycetoma. On MRI, fungal infections may appear with predominantly low signal intensity and simulate a normally aerated sinus. In such cases, CT will show an intrasinus soft-tissue abnormality with scattered calcifications that can confirm the presence of a mycetoma[96,97] (**Fig. 4-22**).

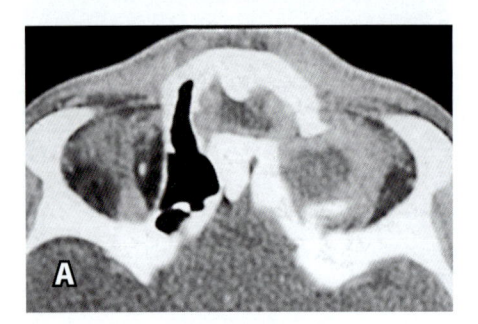

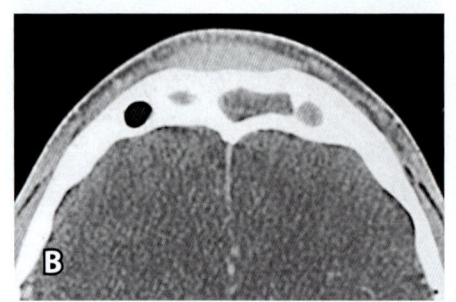

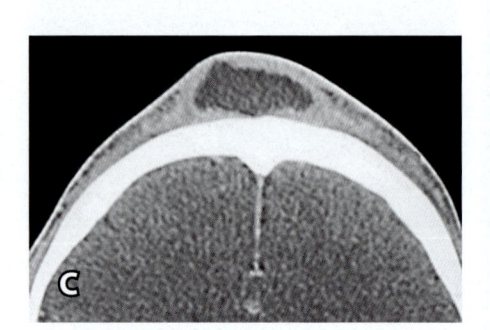

Figure 4-20 Frontal Mucocele
Axial NECT scans at the level of the frontal sinus (**A–C**) show low attenuation opacification of the frontal sinus, especially on the left side. There is mild smooth expansion of the bones of the sinus (**B**), consistent with chronic sinonasal mucocele.

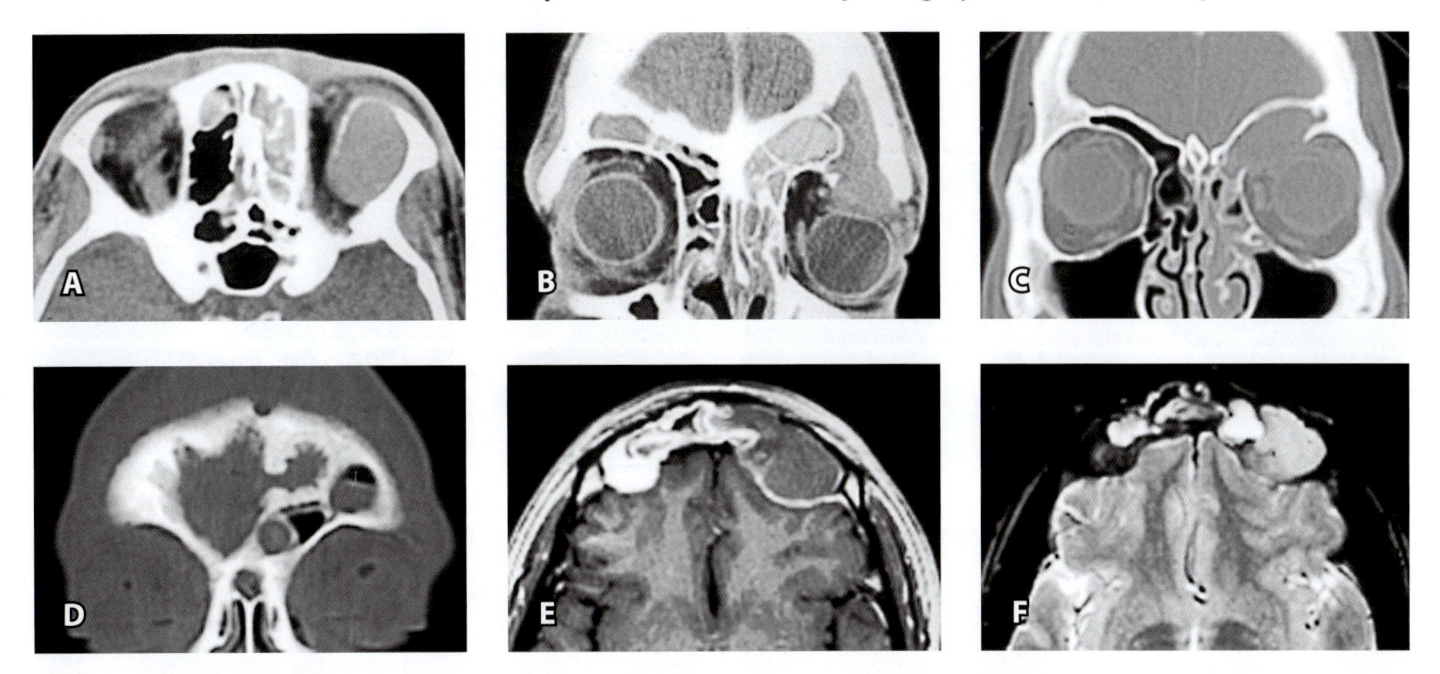

Figure 4-21 Obstructed Frontal Mucocele
Axial (**A**) and coronal (**B–D**) NECT scans show a dilated left frontal sinus filled with pockets of low-attenuating fluid in the superior aspect of the left orbit, with inferior displacement of the left globe and superior expansion of the anterior skull base. Axial MR scans show low T1 signal (**E**) and high T2 signal (**F**), confirming the cystic nature of the encapsulated mucocele contents.

Allergic Fungal Sinusitis

It is now clear that many patients with chronic sinus disease are suffering from allergic fungal sinusitis (AFS). Such patients are immunocompetent and often have asthma, eosinophilia, and elevated total fungus-specific immunoglobulin E concentrations. The pathology of the sinus contents reveals greenish black or brown material (allergic mucin), which has the consistency of peanut butter mixed with sand and glue. Allergic mucin and polyps may form a partially calcified expansile mass that obstructs sinus drainage. Growth of the mass may cause pressure-induced erosion of bone, rupture of sinus walls, and occasional leakage of the sinus contents into the orbit or brain. Antibiotics are ineffective against AFS and antihistamines neither relieve nor reverse the symptoms of AFS. Antifungal agents have been effective against allergic fungal sinusitis; however, surgery is generally considered the treatment of choice. Goals of surgical therapy are conservative debridement of the allergic mucin and polyps (if present) from the involved sinuses and restoration of sinus aeration. Goals may be achieved endoscopically if possible. An external approach can be considered if the lesion is not accessible endoscopically. Adequate ventilation of the sinus is essential to prevent relapse or recurrence of the disease once the disease is exenterated. The MRI scans on patients with AFS will show decreased signal intensity on T1-weighted images and markedly decreased signal intensity on the T2-weighted images. This is partially due to the presence of calcium and ferromagnetic elements such as iron and manganese within the mycetomas. Contrast enhancement should always be used to rule out unsuspected intrasinus tumors. In patients with renal problems, such as diabetic nephropathy, or in patients that are undergoing treatment with the nephrotoxic amphotericin-B drug, MR imaging with gadolinium contrast is the preferred imaging modality over CT with iodinated contrast material[98,99] (**Fig. 4-23**).

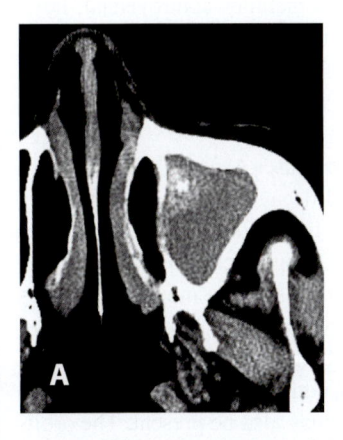

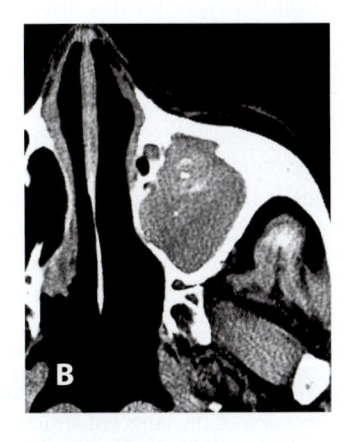

Figure 4-22 Mycetoma of the Left Maxillary Sinus
Axial CT of the left maxillary sinus (**A–B**) shows an expansile process of the left maxillary sinus with focal calcifications anteriorly. At surgery, a calcified mycetoma was removed.

Rhinocerebral Mucormycosis

Rhinocerebral mucormycosis is a deadly infection caused by a fungus of the genus called zygomycetes. Commonly found in bread mold, zygomycete spores are inhaled and may cause rhinocerebral disease in the mildly immunosuppressed individual with conditions such as acidosis, hyperglycemia, severe leukopenia, malnutrition, cancer, cirrhosis, and in the severely immunosuppressed patients

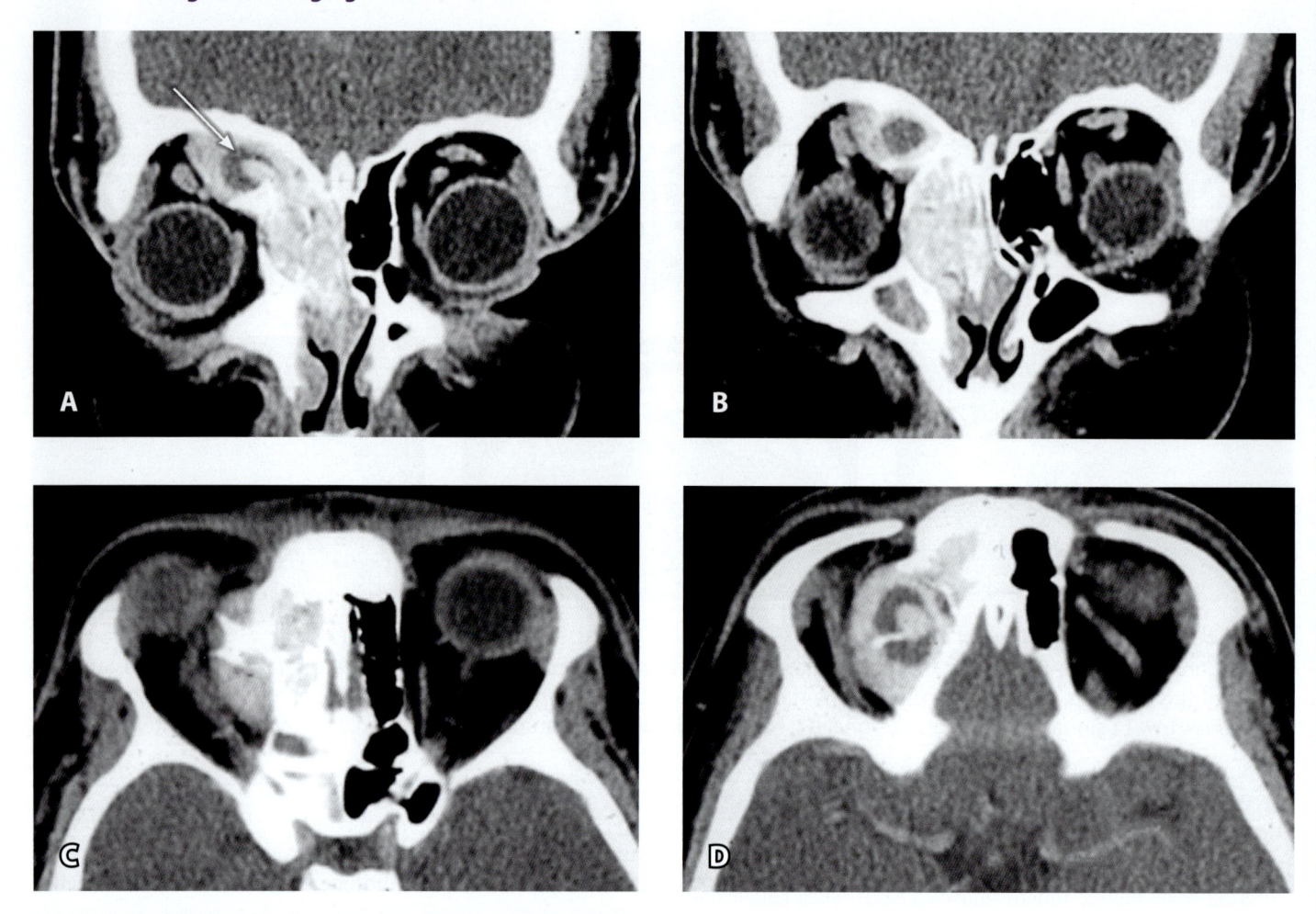

Figure 4-23 Allergic Fungal Sinusitis with Aspergillous Mycetoma
Coronal (**A–B**) and axial (**C–D**) postcontrast images showing a dense, expansile process in the ethmoid air cells extending superior to the right orbit. The central area of nonenhancement located in the medial portion of the right orbit was a well-defined fungus ball (aspergilloma).

on prolonged antibiotic or steroid therapy. Commonly involved organs include the lungs, skin, gastrointestinal tract, and the paranasal sinuses, particularly the ethmoid air cells. Histologically, zygomycetes stain well with hematoxylin and eosin, show pleomorphic and nonseptate hyphae and right-angle branching. Zygomycetes produce a necrotizing infection that easily invades adjacent structures causing vasculitis, thrombosis, and erosion of the orbits and extension into the cranial cavity. Clinical manifestations commence with symptoms such as headache, nasal stuffiness, eye irritation, infraorbital numbness with proptosis, and loss of vision. Extension into the intracranial cavity may cause poor mentation, and extension into the sphenoidal region may result in ophthalmoplegia. On examination, the nasal turbinates, nasal septum and soft palate are necrotic and covered with a black crust. As fungal infections predispose to septic thrombosis, MRI studies may demonstrate complications such as septic thrombosis of the carotid artery or cavernous sinuses. There may be a hyperintense rim of inflammation around the vessel walls in cases of septic thrombosis of the carotid artery or cavernous sinus.[100] Imaging of mucormycosis is not always specific for a fungal infection. There may be expansion and destruction of the bony walls as the infection spreads from the nose to the anterior cranial fossa. As previously discussed, a finding associated with mycotic infection, but not with bacterial infection, is the hypointensity of an abscess or a mycetoma on T2-W MR scans. Ideal treatment for this disease is sometimes controversial; however, both surgical and Amphotericin B medical therapies are typically utilized with variable results.[100,101]

Aspergillosis

The organism aspergillus fumigatus causes Aspergillosis. This fungus is frequently found in soil and decaying foods. It commonly contaminates the human respiratory tract and occasionally involves the paranasal sinuses. Both immunosuppressed and healthy people may become afflicted with aspergillosis. If the infection involves the paranasal sinuses, it typically starts in the maxillary sinus. Clinically, sinus pain and foul-smelling nasal discharge are usually evident. Similar to mucormycosis, additional symptoms related to invasion of the adjacent structures may also be present. The orbits and adjacent anterior skull base may be involved secondary to direct extension from the paranasal sinuses.[102]

Imaging findings show characteristics of an invasive infection with bone destruction and dense calcifications in a heterogeneous mass similar in density to muscle on CT scans and a low-signal or no-signal mass on MR T1-W and T2-W images. This mass will enhance after contrast administration. Cavernous sinus involvement may be identified in some patients. Invasive aspergillosis requires emergent aggressive antibiotic and surgical therapies.

CNS Complications of Sinonasal Infections

The common intracranial complications of untreated or undertreated sinonasal infections include meningitis, subdural empyema, frontal lobe abscesses, interhemispheric abscesses, osteomyelits, thrombophelibits, and cavernous or superior sagittal sinus thrombosis. There may be perineural or perivascular spread of a sinonasal infection into the cavernous sinus or brain stem, particularly with mucormycosis. Such complications require aggressive medical and surgical intervention to prevent excessive morbidity and mortality.[103,104] Complications of sinusitis have been recognized to be a more common problem in AIDS patients; unlike the immunocompetent host, the majority of HIV-infected patients with advanced immunodeficiency develop posterior sinus disease. Although bacterial infections are more common, fungal infections are also more prevalent in AIDS patients.

Granulomatous Lesions

Infectious granulomatous diseases include actinomycosis, nocardiosis, coccidiomycosis and tuberculosis. Noninfectious granulomatous processes include Wegener granulomatosis and sarcoidosis. Wegener granulomatosis is a rare multisystemic necrotizing granulomatous vasculitis that characteristically involves the upper or lower respiratory tracts and kidneys. The clinical manifestations and symptoms are nonspecific and include systemic findings such as fever, malaise, weight loss, arthralgia, and myalgia. Although most patients initially present with upper airway illness, ophthalmic, neurologic and dermatologic involvement are relatively common.[105] When there is involvement of the upper respiratory tract with Wegener granulomatosis, imaging will show sinonasal opacifications with mucosal erosions, most commonly involving the nasal septum with concomitant involvement of the maxillary and ethmoid sinuses. Involvement of the frontal sinus is rare, but there may be extension into the orbit, with or without bony destruction.[106] Sarcoidosis is a multisystem disorder resulting in noncaseous granulomas. Nasal sarcoidosis occurs in up to 10% to 20% of patients with other organ involvement and commonly involves the nasal septum, turbinates, and intracranial structures. Imaging shows permeative destruction of the nasal bridge and adjacent sinus walls.

Amyloidosis

Amyloidosis presents with submucosal deposits of abnormal proteinaceous materials. This disease can involve any organ singly or in conjunction with other organs and can do so in the form of a focal, tumor-like lesion or as an infiltrative process. These findings may be limited to the central airways including the tracheobronchial tree, larynx, and sinonasal cavities.[107] The imaging findings with amyloidosis are problematically nonspecific and diverse. This lack of specificity is compounded by the fact that amyloidosis is strongly associated with and frequently coexists with many other chronic disease states that have their own imaging findings. In the sinonasal passages, the imaging findings are of smooth concentric thickening of the mucosal surfaces. In some cases, patchy or prominent calcifications may be seen, but the nasal septum and cartilages are normal without destructive or erosive lesions.[108]

SINONASAL NEOPLASMS

Clinical Features

Sinonasal tract neoplasms are extremely rare. In the United States, the incidence is reported to be 1 per 100,000 people. Only 3% of all head and neck cancers are located in the paranasal sinuses, with 80% of them originating in the maxillary antrum. There is a wide spectrum of neoplasms that can invade into the sinonasal tract. Approximately 60% of all sinonasal cavity tumors are squamous cell carcinomas. The remaining 30% comprise a diverse population of tumors that include but are not limited to papillomas, adenomas, angiofibroma, vasoformative lesions, fibro-osseous and odontogenic lesions, esthesioneuroblastoma, sinonasal undifferentiated carcinoma, melanoma, minor salivary gland tumors, lymphomas, sarcomas, and metastatic disease.[109,110]

A variety of occupational hazards have been associated with malignancies of the sinonasal cavities. Elevated risks have been observed in a number of occupations and industries, including textile workers, farm workers, construction workers, metal industry, workers exposed to chromium and nickel compounds, formaldehyde, and asbestos.[111]

Many sinonasal tract neoplasms are unexpected because their clinical presentation overlaps with that of benign sinus disease. Tumors arising in the sinonasal cavities have an abundant place to grow without causing many symptoms. Neoplasms in these locations often remain silent until they reach an advanced stage. The diagnosis of a sinonasal neoplasm is often delayed due to nonspecific symptoms that are often confused with inflammatory disease. Patients may be treated with antibiotics for long periods of time before the true nature of their disease is known. The time interval from the onset of symptoms to diagnosis has been found to average about 6 months. Nasal complaints include stuffiness, obstruction, rhinorrhea, and epistaxis. Oral complaints include tooth pain, tooth loosening, ulceration, and swelling of the palate. Visual symptoms may include tearing, visual deficits, and proptosis. Extension through the ventral maxillary wall may include swelling and asymmetry of the face. Neurological manifestations from invasion of CN V may cause numbness, pain, or paresthesias, or atrophy of the masticator muscles. However, direct invasion into the masticatory walls can cause trismus. The constellation of potential symptoms is diverse[112] (**Table 4-14**).

Characterizing the extent of the tumor is of paramount importance. The assessment of tumor extension has an integral role in deciding whether to attempt curative rather than palliative treatment. The intricately complex and compact anatomy of the sinonasal region, make surgical resection and radiotherapy a perilous endeavor. Craniofacial resection is frequently disfiguring and morbid, and the proximity of

Table 4-14 Potential Presenting Symptoms of Sinonasal Neoplasms

Nasal	• Stuffiness • Obstruction • Sinusitis • Rhinorrhea • Epistaxis
Oral	• Tooth pain • Tooth loosening • Ulceration • Fistula • Swelling of the palate
Visual	• Tearing • Visual deficits • Swelling • Proptosis
Facial	• Swelling • Asymmetry • Skin changes
Neurological	• Numbness • Pain • Paresthesias • Atrophy of masticator • Trismus

important structures limit the margins of resection and radiotherapy dose. Resection margins are extremely difficult to evaluate in sinonasal neoplasms, since resection is often not in one piece and important aesthetic and functional structures preclude wide limits of excision.[113]

The surgeon is most interested in whether a tumor is resectable and if so, which vital structures can be salvaged and which ones cannot (i.e., externation of orbit). The radiation oncologist is also dependent on the radiologist's assessment of tumor extension. Accurate tumor bed mapping also facilitates a more precise delivery of radiation, with the obvious goal of avoidance of radiation-induced sequelae. (i.e., blindness).

The combination of delayed presentation and the limitations of surgical and radiotherapy due to proximal vital structures, make the overall prognosis of sinonasal malignancies poor. Most series report 5-year local control and overall survival rates between 40% and 60%. Prognostic factors include T classification, invasion to the orbit, and presence of positive lymph nodes. T classification is the most significant prognostic factor. In addition, patients with orbital and neural invasion are at significantly greater risk of poorer local control and cause-specific survival.[113,114]

Imaging Characteristics

There are no pathognomonic imaging features that can lead to a radiological diagnosis of a sinonasal neoplasm. The goals of imaging are to characterize the mass and extension into neighboring structures (**Table 4-15**). The exact location and precise extent of the tumor are of critical importance because many vital structures of the skull base and orbita may be affected. Thus, distinguishing tumor from infection, obstructed secretions, granulation tissue, and fibrosis is essential. CT scanning and MRI play complementary roles. Subtle bony erosion signifying early tumor extension is best seen on CT. Aggressive, rapidly growing lesions tend to invade bone and cause irregular destruction, which can be detected on either CT or MRI. Slowly growing lesions tend to remodel bone, although this is not a steadfast rule. MRI is superior in precisely delineating soft-tissue extension and characterizing invasion of tissues such as the brain, dura, nerves; and distinguishing neoplasm from sinonasal secretions.

Most sinonasal cancer usually displays intermediate signal intensity on both T1-weighted and T2-weighted sequences. Spin echo T2-weighted sequences are the optimal technique to detect signal differences between the neoplasm (exhibiting intermediate signal), from adjacent structures and retained secretions (generally hyperintense). Only approximately 5% of tumors that have high signal intensity on T2-weighted images cannot be confidently differentiated from inflammatory tissue, and is mainly seen with tumors from salivary gland origin or neuromas (**Table 4-16**). In these few cases, differentiation from inflammatory changes can be difficult. Ideally, variable enhancement of neoplastic tissue obtained by Gd-DTPA infusion can accentuate discrimination of tumor from adjacent tissues on spin-echo T1-weighted images. Most sinonasal neoplasms enhance more intensely than normal muscle or brain. Retained secretions do not enhance and are encompassed by inflamed mucosa that demonstrates a characteristic pattern of peripheral enhancement. Tumors generally show a diffuse enhancement pattern except for areas of central necrosis.

Methodical inspection of critical neighboring structures should include the anterior cranial fossa, the orbit, and the pterygopalatine and superior orbital fissures (**Table 4-17**). Tumor can

Table 4-15 Checklist of Items to be Reviewed for Sinonasal Neoplasms

Tumor Mass Characteristics
- Bone erosion or remodeling at tumor margins
- Calcifications in tumor
- Signal characteristics
- Differentiation from inflammatory tissue

Tumor Extension
- Perineural spread
- Skull base
- Intracranial
- Orbit
- Neck
- Lymph nodes

Table 4-16 Differentiating Sinonasal Tumors from Inflammatory Tissue

Inflammatory	Tumor
• High intensity on T2-weighted sequences	• Intermediate signal intensity on T2-weighted (95% of lesions) • High intensity signal on T2-weighted (only 5% of lesions)

gain access to the anterior cranial fossa by invading superiorly through the nasoethmoidal roof, and is best studied on coronal and sagittal sections. The earliest sign of invasion of the anterior cranial fossa is bony erosion of the interface between the nasoethmoidal roof and floor of the anterior cranial fossa. Invasion into the anterior cranial fossa may have several different characteristics: the lesion may displace and erode the cribriform plate but not involve the dura (hyperintense thickened dura), it may extend beyond the dura but leave the CSF unmolested (hypointense CSF), or extend beyond the dura and invade CSF and brain.[88,89]

Invasion of the orbit usually occurs through the medial or inferior wall. Coronal sections are the best plane to detect orbital involvement. The orbital walls appear hypointense on all MR sequences. The surfaces of the lamina papyracea appear as hypointense lines adjacent to hyperintense signals of orbital fat. The first signs of orbital involvement is erosion of the delicate borders of bone (lamina papyracea and floor of orbit). The index of suspicion of orbital invasion should be raised when the interface between tumor and orbital fat is diminished. Fat-saturated and STIR sequences are useful to delineate orbital fat from extrinsic muscle. Distortion and displacement of orbital walls by ethmoidal neoplasms is a common finding.[115]

Extension toward the infratemporal fossa occurs through the posterior wall of the maxillary sinus, which serves as a conduit to the infratemporal, pterygopalatine fossa and orbital floor. Particular attention should be focused on the bony-periosteal barrier at this location, which will show erosion as an early sign of invasion and is best visualized on axial slices. From here, the pterygopalatine fossa may become involved from extension from the posterior wall of the maxillary sinus. A normal pterygopalatine fossa is seen as a small fatty "cleft" lying between the posterior bony wall of the maxillary sinus and the pterygoid plates. On MR images, the sphenopalatine artery is a useful landmark within the pterygopalatine fossa. It is best identified on T1- and T2-weighted images because of the presence of hyperintense fat. It is usually bilaterally symmetric and contains tiny flow voids from branches of the internal maxillary artery. Neoplastic invasion should be suspected if fat surrounding the vessel has been replaced by soft-tissue intensity, or if the vessel is encased or unrecognizable, or if there is abnormal enhancement or widening of the pterygopalatine fossa.[116]

From the pterygopalatine fossa, tumor has access to grow superiorly into the inferior orbital fissure and the orbital apex. Further superior extension provides route to the superior orbital fissure. From here, the tumor can easily gain access to the cavernous sinus via posterior extension along the maxillary nerve in the foramen rotundum.

The complex and extensive neural anatomy of the head and neck makes perineural extension along nerves an insidious conduit for tumor invasion and extension to other extra- and intracranial structures. Perineural spread has a significantly grave impact on treatment and prognosis, including increased tumor recurrence and decreased long-term survival, with a reduction of more than 30% of local control rate being reported. Squamous cell carcinoma is the most common tumor with perineural extension. Adenoid cystic carcinoma, although less prevalent, has a particular penchant for perineural extension. Other tumors types include basal cell carcinoma, melanoma, mucoepidermoid tumor, lymphoma, neurinoma, and neurofibroma. Clinical evidence of perineural tumor infiltration may include pain, paresthesias, or denervation of the masticator muscles. However, most clinical presentations of perineural invasion is nonspecific. Most patients who have perineural involvement do not have symptoms unless there is extensive nerve invasion.[117–122]

CT scanning and MRI play complementary roles in assessing perineural tumor spread. MR is less accurate than CT in the

Table 4-17 Signs of Tumor Extension

Anterior Cranial Fossa
- Bony erosion of nasoethmoidal roof or floor of anterior cranial fossa
- Erosion or displacement of cribriform plate
- Invasion into dura (hyperintense thickened dura)

Orbit
- Bony erosion of lamina papyracea
- Bony erosion of floor of orbit
- Diminished interface of mass and orbital fat

Pterygopalatine Fossa
- Bony erosion of posterior maxillary sinus wall
- Displacement of perivascular fat signal of sphenopalatine artery with soft-tissue intensity of tumor
- Widening of pterygopalatine fossa

Table 4-18 Signs of Perineural Invasion

- Widening, destruction, abnormal enhancement in neural foramina (rotundum, ovale, palatine, stylomastoid, vidian)
- Expansion or abnormal enhancement of cavernous sinus or Meckel's cave
- Displacement of perivascular fat signal of sphenopalatine artery with soft-tissue intensity of tumor, widening of pterygopalatine fossa
- Denervation atrophy of masticator muscles (V3)

assessment of focal bone erosions, since the calcium content cannot be adequately detected. Nevertheless, the most effective barrier to spread of aggressive lesions, neoplastic or inflammatory – beyond sinusal walls does not depend on the mineral content of bone, but on the periosteum. CT scanning shows the bony changes quite well, which is important because a substantial portion of the trigeminal and facial nerves are surrounded by or contained within bony structures. However, MRI is superior to CT scanning in evaluation of soft-tissue tumors and in its ability to discriminate between normal tissue and secretions from tumor. Imaging signs of perineural spread are foraminal enlargement and replacement of normal fat within the neural foramina (Table 4-18). Contrast-enhanced MR images show enhancement of the nerve, which cannot be imaged with CT.[89,123]

Head and neck cancers can leave the primary tumor mass and travel retrogradely along nerves to re-emerge at deeper intracranial destinations. Cranial nerves V2 and V3 and the descending facial nerve are most commonly involved because of their extensive distribution. Tumors can invade into any of these extensive nerve branches and use them as a conduit to invade into other locations, in both centripetal and centrifugal fashion. Lesions can also directly expand and destroy the posterior wall of the maxillary sinuses and gain direct access to the pterygopalatine fossa. From the pterygopalatine fossa, the vulnerable sphenopalatine ganglion is wide open for perineural invasion. Here, the lesion can spread in antegrade or retrograde fashion and easily extend into the cavernous sinus through the foramen rotundum. Tumors that extend to the cavernous sinus can then disseminate among the abundant nerves at this region, with the oculomotor nerve being most commonly involved. It is important to evaluate suspected lesions in their entire course, because perineural spread may be discontinuous, with "skip areas."[124]

Although V2 and V3 are the most common routes of perineural tumor spread, other less common routes of invasion have been characterized. Perineural tumor spread from the pterygopalatine fossa posteriorly along the vidian nerve may result in enlargement and erosion of the pterygoid canal, which is a bony duct that lies between the sphenoid sinus and the pterygoid process. Extension from the vidian nerve to the greater superficial petrosal nerve, which runs under Meckel's cave, provides route to the geniculate ganglion.[125,126]

The neural foramina of the skull base should be examined for signs of destruction, widening, or abnormal enhancement. (foramen rotundum, ovale, palatine, stylomastoid, vidian). It is important to remember that a tilted head position can result in asymmetric skull base foramina, and result in a false positive finding. The cavernous sinus and Meckel's cave should also be carefully examined with high resolution MR imaging to exclude tumor involvement. The MR findings of cavernous sinus invasion include enlargement and lateral bulging of the sinus and replacement of the high intensity venous signal by the intermediate intensity tumor tissue on both T2- and T1-enhanced weighted sequences. Neoplastic encasement of the internal carotid artery at the cavernous sinus with thickened vessel wall enhancement is a tenable indication of internal carotid invasion.[127,128]

Although a malignant neoplasm is the most common and most grave of the tissue types that can spread in a perineural fashion, it is important to remember that benign pathology, such as hemangioma, meningioma, juvenile angiofibroma, infectious processes, and pseudotumor, can also spread by this route. Lesions involving the trigeminal and facial nerves are not necessarily malignant tumors.

Tumors of the sinonasal cavities may also extend via the rich lymphatic network present in the head and neck region. Lesions that are able to destroy the basement membrane and subdermal extracellular matrix can gain access to the local lymphatic networks of the sinonasal cavity. The lymph collectors of the sinonasal cavities are organized into a superficial and deep network. The anterior nasal collectors travel with the facial artery vessels and drain into the submental node (level I). The posterior efferent collectors travel through the pharyngeal fornix, and drain into the lateral retropharyngeal lymph nodes and into the deep jugular lymph nodes (level II). A few lymph collectors will drain into the subdigastric lymph node (level II). Eventually, drainage of a metastatic embolus through the regional lymphatic network will provide access to the vascular system. The incidence of cervical nodal involvement at diagnosis of sinonasal tract tumors ranges from 3.3% to 26%.[129]

Lymph nodes appear on CT as oval, circumscribed masses of soft-tissue density. Intravenous contrast is useful to distinguish lymph nodes from blood vessels. On MR, lymph nodes appear as low-intensity masses on T1-weighted sequences, and intermediate-intensity masses on T2-weighted sequences, and are easily differentiated from blood vessels. The characteristics of metastatic lymph nodes that can be depicted are increased size, rounder shape, and presence of noncontrast enhancing parts or irregular contrast enhancement caused by tumor necrosis, keratinization, or cystic areas of tumor. Whereas positron emission tomography (PET) has a higher sensitivity than MR for detecting cervical node metastasis, neither modality currently has sufficient resolution to detect microscopic invasion. Several new imaging techniques are being developed to achieve finer detail of the cervical lymph nodes in the head and neck, such as lymphoscintigraphy and dynamic MR lymphangiography.[129–131]

Metastatic tumors seeding to the sinonasal cavities is an uncommon finding. The majority of instances that occur are from renal cell carcinoma. Other tumors may also metastasis

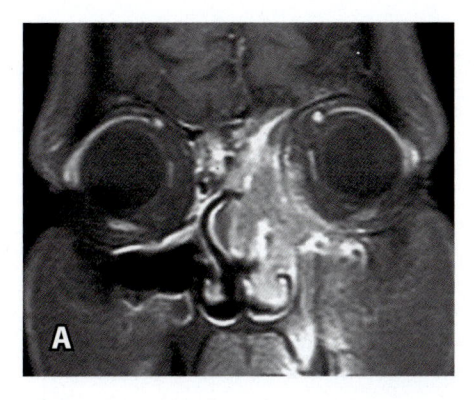

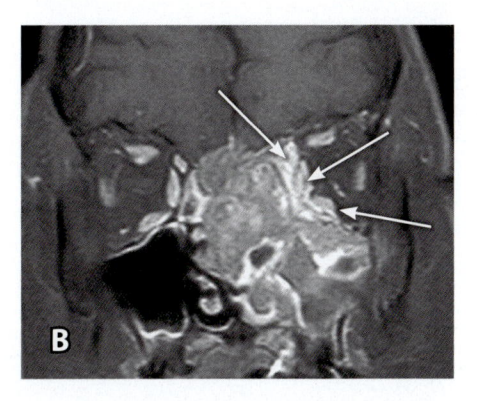

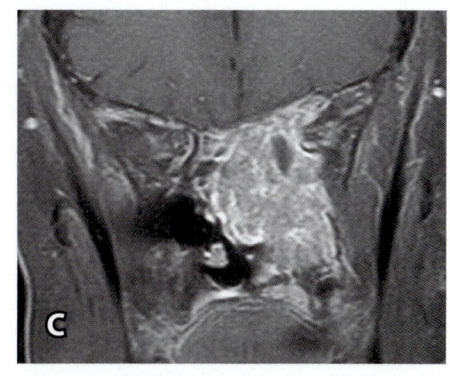

Figure 4-24 Sinonasal and Orbital Undifferentiated Cancer Metastasis
Extensive sinonasal and orbital undifferentiated cancer metastases. Coronal T1W MR images with contrast show heterogeneously enhancing, locally destructive masses in occupying the sphenoid, ethmoid, and maxillary sinuses. There is infiltration and partial destruction of the turbinates and nasal septum, as well as infiltration of the posterior nasopharynx on the left (**C**). Also note the involvement of the lateral portion of the intraconal and extraconal left orbit. Infiltration of the left lateral rectus, medial rectus, and superior oblique muscles is suggested by their enlarged size and near complete envelopment by the tumor (*arrows*, **B**). The tumor extends to the level of the anterior skull base, though there is no definite evidence of intracranial extension.

to the paranasal sinuses, in decreasing frequency: breast, lungs, testes, and thyroid. The most common sinus involved are the maxillary sinuses, followed by the ethmoid and frontal sinuses (**Fig. 4-24**).

Renal cell carcinoma is an abundantly vascularized tumor. Renal cell carcinoma metastasis in the sinonasal cavities have a propensity to bleed, as such, epistaxis is a common symptom for these patients. In addition to renal cell carcinoma, sinonasal melanoma metastasis tend to present with epistaxis.

On CT, most metastatic lesions to the sinonasal cavities are aggressive and demonstrate bone destruction and erosion. These imaging features are nonspecific and indistinguishable from squamous cell carcinoma. Few exceptions may be noted: prostate cancer may show osteoblastic, sclerotic features, while renal cell carcinoma and melanoma can display brisk enhancement due to their rich vascularity. Multifocal lesions argue for metastasis rather than a local primary lesion, which is more likely to have a unifocal, contiguous path of destruction.[132]

Benign Lesions

Papillomas

Inverted papilloma is an uncommon lesion constituting 0.5% to 4% of all nasal tumors, and constitute 75% of all sinonasal papillomas. It is characterized by hyperplasia of the basal cells and invagination of the epithelium in the underlying stroma. The inverted papilloma is a benign tumor that may become locally aggressive. The incidence of inverted papilloma is highest in middle age. There is evidence that human papilloma virus may contribute to the development of inverted papillomas. HPV DNA occurs in 32% of inverted papillomas and may play a role in malignant transformation. Several growth factors have been implicated in the progression of inverted papillomas. Epidermal growth factor receptor (EGFR) and transforming growth factor-α are frequently increased in expression. Overexpression of these growth factors has also been demonstrated in squamous cell carcinoma. The association between inverted papilloma and squamous cell carcinoma necessitates the complete excision and histological examination of this lesion.[133]

Inverted papillomas are most frequently located in the nasal cavity. Here, most inverted papillomas develop from the lateral wall of the nose, whereas exophytic papillomas usually develop from the nasal septum (**Fig. 4-25**). Papillomas may cause obstruction of ostia and secondary sinusitis. As they expand in size, they can cause bowing of the nasal septum; however, this structure usually remains intact. Inverted papillomas that affect the paranasal sinuses usually reach this location by extension from lesions that originate in the nasal cavity. The predominant sinonasal cavities involved are the maxillary and ethmoid sinuses, less frequently, extension into the sphenoid and frontal sinuses can occur. Most inverted papillomas do not show signs of intracranial extension; however, expansive growth can cause significant bone destruction of the sinonasal tract. Areas of bony destruction along the margins of the inverted papilloma should raise the suspicion of an associated carcinoma.[128,134,135]

There are no distinctive MR imaging characteristics that may help differentiate inverted papilloma from malignancy. However, MR compared to CT more accurately defines the limit of the lesion. This is due to the superiority of MR in distinguishing inflammatory tissue from neoplasm. The precise description of the localization and extension of the tumor are important for the surgeon's plan of approach and method of excision. Radical en bloc resection is traditionally considered the treatment of choice. However, with the advent of modern endoscopic techniques, an increasing number of cases are managed with a minimally invasive approach. The high recurrence rate and the association of malignancy with inverted papillomas necessitate routine clinical follow-up.

Pleomorphic Adenoma

Tumors of the salivary gland are very uncommon and represent only 2% to 3% of head and neck neoplasms. The glands

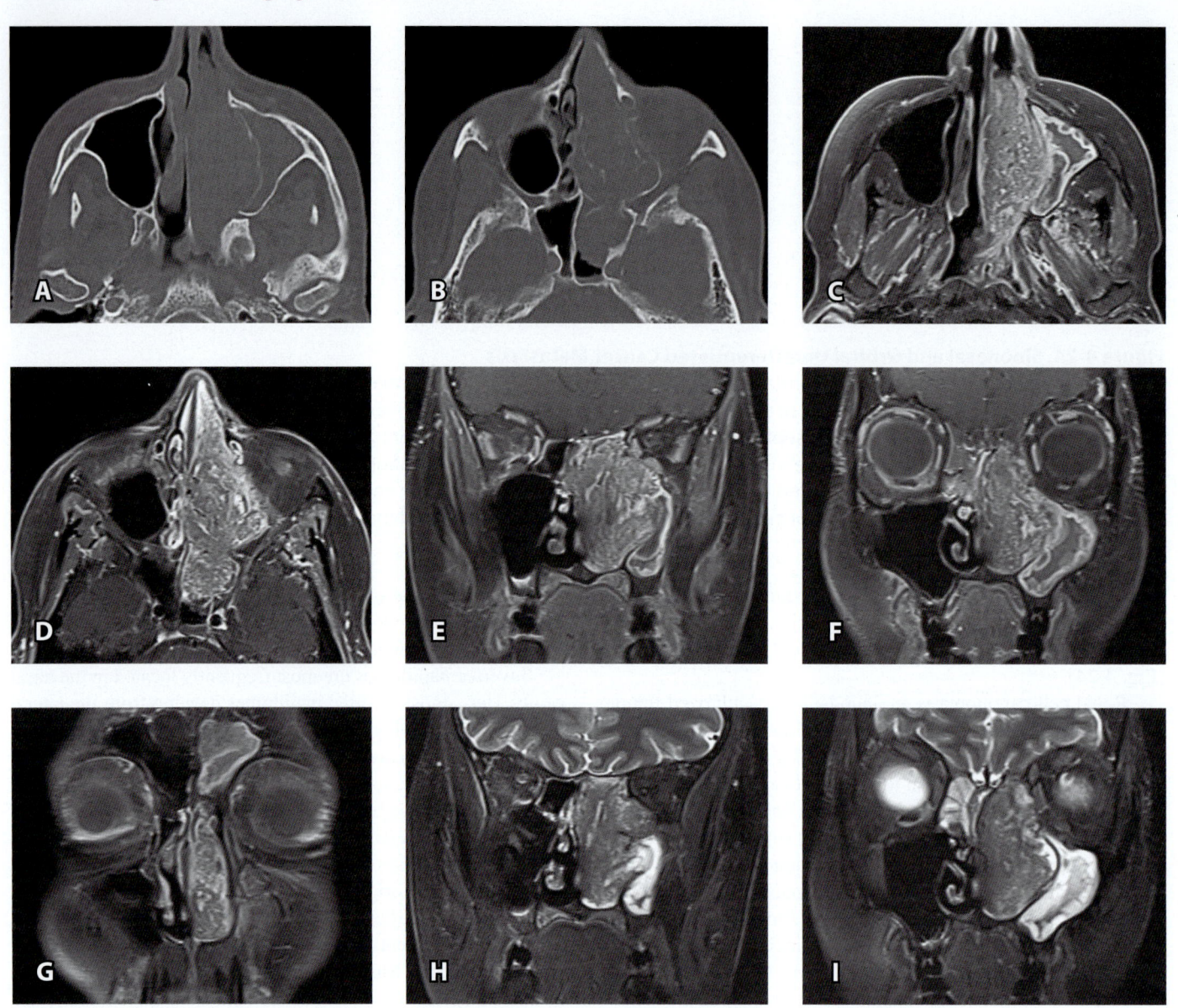

Figure 4-25 Inverted Papilloma

Inverted papilloma in a 54-year-old female presenting with progressive congestion and nasal obstruction over several years. Axial bone NECT images (**A–B**) show a soft-tissue density mass completely occupying the left nasal cavity, left maxillary sinus, and ethmoid sinuses, with partial extension into the left sphenoid sinus. The mass extends superiorly to the cribriform plate and inferiorly to the level of the uvula. There is also remodeling and lateral bowing of the medial wall of the left maxillary sinus. Axial (**C–D**) and coronal (**E–G**) T1W contrast-enhanced MR images show the characteristic cerebriform tumor mass. Coronal T2W MR images (**H–I**) show a definite distinction between the tumor mass and the high signal postobstructive retained secretions in the left maxillary sinus. There is also increased T2 signal at the level of uvula, which may indicate reactive mucosal inflammation or necrosis. There is no distinct evidence of orbital or intracranial infiltration. Pathologic examination confirmed inverted papilloma with squamous cell carcinoma in situ.

are divided into major and minor salivary gland categories. The major glands are parotid, submandibular, and sublingual, whereas the minor glands are dispersed throughout the upper aerodigestive submucosa (i.e., palate, lip, pharynx, nasopharynx, larynx, parapharyngeal space). Pleomorphic adenomas most often arise in the hard and soft palates, with the upper lip being the second most frequented site. Pleomorphic adenomas infrequently may arise in the sinonasal cavities. In this region, pleomorphic adenomas originate from the mucosa of the nasal septum (90%), while 10% arise from the lateral nasal walls. Histologically, this is perplexing because the majority of the salivary glands reside in the lateral nasal walls.

The maxillary sinus is the second most often affected region of the sinonasal cavities.

Pleomorphic adenomas are benign tumors that contain both mesenchymal and epithelial components. Although histologically

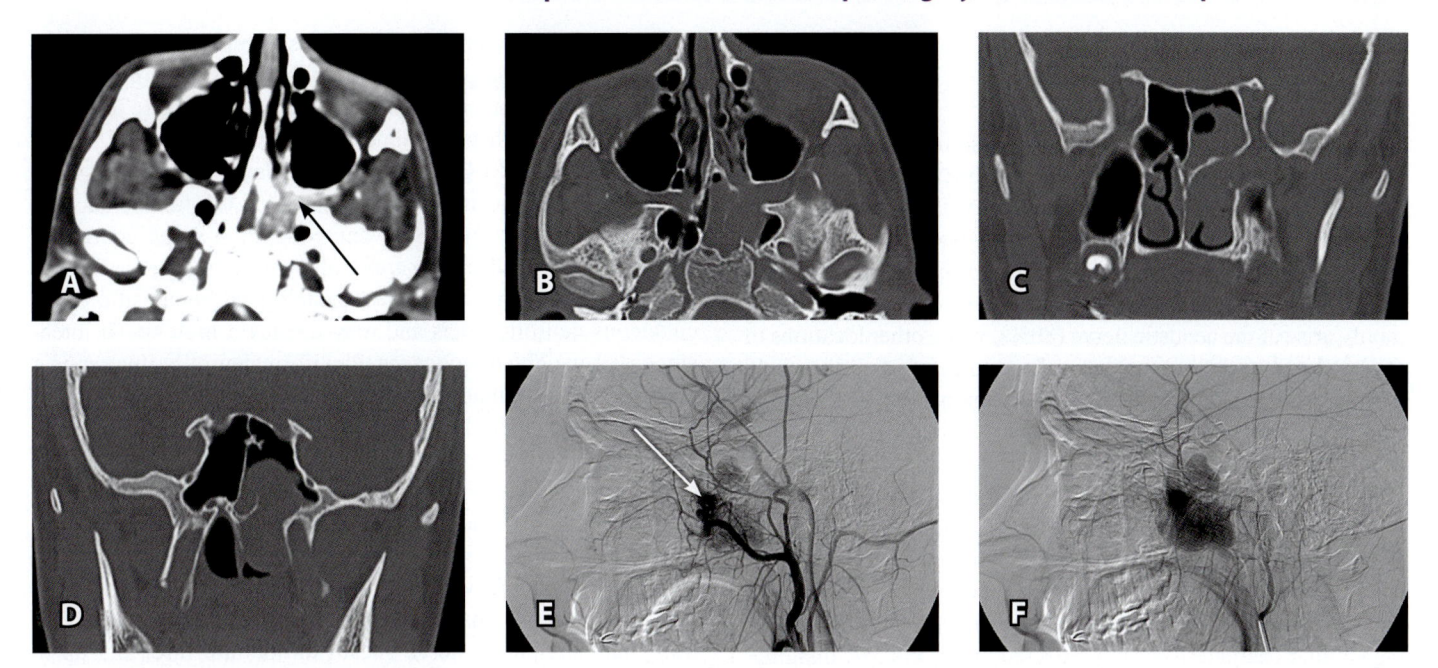

Figure 4-26 Juvenile Angiofibroma
Juvenile Angiofibroma in a 15-year-old male presenting with a nasal mass. Axial soft tissue NECT image (**A**) shows a heterogeneous, intermediate density mass occupying the left sphenoid sinus with extension into the left sphenopalatine foramen (*arrow*). Axial (**B**) and coronal (**C–D**) bone algorithm NECT images show the extension of the mass inferiorly into the left nasal cavity (**C**), superoposteriorly into the left sphenoid sinus (**B–C**) and inferiorly into the left nasopharynx (**D**). Note the marked expansion of the left sphenopalatine foramen by the infiltrating mass. Sagittal views of early (**E**) and late phase (**F**) angiograms of the left external carotid artery shows an intense blushing in the region of the left sphenoid sinuses, fed by the internal maxillary artery (*arrow*, **E**), demonstrating the highly vascular nature of this lesion. Perioperative embolization was performed prior to surgical resection.

similar to the more commonly seen pleomorphic adenoma arising from the major salivary glands, there is increased cellularity in sinonasal pleomorphic adenomas. This variability in cellular density is the reflected in pleomorphic adenomas imaging characteristics. Less dense tumors have more of a heterogeneous appearance on CT, and display a high signal on T2-weighted sequences on MR. Conversely, more dense tumors displays as a homogenous mass on CT, and display an intermediate signal on T2-weighted sequences on MR.[136–139]

Angiofibroma

Juvenile nasopharyngeal angiofibroma (JNA) are benign, non-encapsulated, highly vascular tumors that almost exclusively occur in adolescent males. Although histologically benign, these tumors show aggressive growth behavior. JNA comprises only 0.5% of all head and neck lesions. The histological characteristic of angiofibromas consists of numerous endothelial lined vascular spaces with little or no smooth muscle layers. Biopsy is discouraged due to the abundant vascularity of these tumors. Angiofibroma can be diagnosed by using CT, MR imaging, and angiography with such a high degree of certainty that preoperative biopsy will usually not be needed.[140–142]

Common presenting symptoms include recurrent epistaxis, nasal obstruction, nasal speech, and deformity of the face. In advanced cases, invasion into the orbits or intracranial extension can lead to proptosis, loss of vision and other cranial nerve deficits. In the majority cases, the tumor arises in the region of the posterior choanae and expands into the pterygopalatine fossa. The preferential direction and route of JNA expansion nearly always involves the sphenopalatine foramen. Erosion of the medial pterygoid plate and widening of the sphenopalatine foramen are early imaging findings. MR imaging will often reveal anterior bowing of the posterior wall of the adjacent maxillary sinus (Holman-Miller sign) and is a characteristic sign of this tumor. The tumor may extend into the nasal cavities and subsequently through the roof of the nasopharynx into the sphenoid sinuses (**Fig. 4-26**). The lesion has intermediate signal intensity on T1- and T2-weighted images. Multiple flow void channels represent major tumor vessels and are characteristic features of this highly vascular tumor. There is typical prominent enhancement following contrast infusion, which signifies the markedly vascular nature of angiofibromas.[141]

Surgery is the treatment of choice. Preoperative embolization and cell saver techniques are frequently used in the management of these tumors because of their tendency to bleed during surgery. Postsurgical irradiation may help unresectable intracranial spread of the disease. Radiation therapy is particularly useful if the tumor has extended intracranially, invaded the orbit, or has acquired a massive blood supply such that blood loss would be massive during surgery. There is a 15% recurrence rate after surgical resection. Involvement of the orbit, middle cranial fossa and base of the pterygoid by the primary JNA results in a higher incidence of recurrent tumor.[143,144]

Neurogenic Tumors

Schwannoma

Schwannomas are benign tumors that arise from Schwann cells at the peripheral nerve sheath. Sinonasal tract schwannomas are rare, representing 4% of schwannomas of the head and neck. Infrequently, schwannomas may be associated with neurofibromatosis type 1 (NF1), and in these cases they usually present with multiple or plexiform lesions. Schwannomas most commonly arise at the acoustic nerve (80%), while other locations in the head and neck can uncommonly occur, including the neck, parotid gland, cheek, tongue, scalp, and sinonasal cavities. In the sinonasal cavities, schwannomas most commonly originate, in descending order: the nasal fossa, ethmoid, maxillary, and sphenoid sinuses. Sinonasal schwannomas present with nonspecific features such as nasal congestion and epistaxis.[145,146]

Histologically, schwannomas are composed of two major components; Antoni A displaying a more compact region of cells, while Antoni B having more loose myxoid stroma. These varying cellular characteristics are reflected in CT and MR imaging, and may have a heterogeneous appearance that include degeneration and cystic cavitation. On MR, schwannomas usually display an intermediate signal intensity on both T1-weighted and T2-weighted sequences. Signal intensities may vary depending on the cellular characteristics of the lesion, and are best seen on T2-weighted sequences. CT is useful for showing bone displacement as the tumor expands, whereas bone erosion is not a common feature and if detected should raise the suspicion of an alternative, more aggressive lesion.[147]

Schwannomas most frequently affect patients who are in the second through fourth decades of life. The prognosis of sinonasal schwannomas is good, with nearly all patients cured by surgical resection. Local recurrences are rare, and malignant transformation is usually limited to patients with NF1 or who have undergone prior radiation therapy.[147,148]

Neurofibromas

Neurofibromas are benign nerve-sheath tumors consisting of axons, schwann cells, fibro blasts, perineural cells, mast cells, and collagen fibrils surrounded by extracellular myxoid matrix. These lesions are most commonly associated with neurofibromatosis. Neurofibromatosis is divided into two variants, type 1 and type 2. Neurofibromatosis type 1 (von Recklinghausen's disease) is one of the most common genetically transmitted diseases and occurs in 1 in 4000 births. NF1 is an autosomal dominant genetic disorder with 70% to 80% penetrance. The genetic lesion is located on chromosome 17, and up to 50% of cases originate from a spontaneous mutation. Neurofibromatosis type 2 is much less common (1 in 50,000), and primarily affects the central nervous system, with occurrence of bilateral acoustic neuromas, gliomas, or meningiomas.[149,150]

The most common tumors found in patients with NF1 are neurofibromas and optic gliomas. Neurofibromas can be either the plexiform or cutaneous variety. Plexiform neurofibromas are pathognomonic of NF1. These lesions usually occur in early childhood and precede cutaneous neurofibromas. Plexiform neurofibromas are benign, locally invasive tumors that have more endoneurial matrix and schwann cells compared to cutaneous neurofibromas. A large proportion of plexiform neurofibromas originate in the head and neck (50%), and usually arise along the distribution of the trigeminal nerve.[149,150]

On CT and MR, neurofibromas have variable displays that depend on the histologic features of the tumor, such as the myelin content from Schwann cells, high water content of myxoid tissue, and cystic areas of hemorrhage and necrosis. Plexiform often have a different histological composition than cutaneous neurofibromas and may display a high signal intensity on T2-weighted sequences. Plexiform neurofibromas appear as large, multilobulated masses, often described as the "bag of worms" appearance. Plexiform neurofibromas may also sometimes display a characteristic target sign, with a hypointense center with a hyperintense ring peripherally, on T2-weighted images. Cutaneous neurofibromas on the other hand are usually ovoid shaped with intermediate intensity signal on both T1-weighted and T2-weighted sequences.[149,151,152]

There is a 4% chance of malignant transformation in NF1. Malignant peripheral nerve sheath tumors are rare, and up to 50% are associated with neurofibromatosis. Aggressive bone destruction is not commonly seen in neurofibromas, and its presence should raise the suspicion of malignant transformation or alternative diagnosis.[147,152]

Meningioma

Meningiomas are benign, gradually growing tumors that derive from neoplastic arachnoid cap cells that form the dural membranes. Meningiomas account for nearly 20% of all intracranial neoplasm, and are the second most common tumors of the central nervous system. Although benign, meningiomas may exhibit aggressive behavior and cause significant symptoms depending on their anatomical location.

Extracranial meningiomas are rare tumors, comprising 1% to 2% of all meningiomas. Primary extracranial meningiomas are not associated with an intracranial mass, whereas secondary extracranial meningiomas represent extensions of an intracranial lesion. Most extracranial meningiomas occur in the head and neck, and the majority of reported cases are secondary extracranial meningiomas representing regional extension of an intracranial meningioma. A variety of unusual locations of extracranial meningiomas have been described, but very rarely it appears as an extracranial tumor secondarily extended into the paranasal sinuses.[153–156]

The clinical presentation of paranasal sinus meningiomas are nonspecific, and may include signs of nasal obstruction, sinusitis, epistaxis, proptosis, facial deformity, and pain.

Adequate evaluation should include both CT and MR. Meningiomas usually compress adjacent soft tissue without infiltration and induce hyperostosis of surrounding bone. CT is useful for detecting hyperostotic changes that are associated with this tumor; however, the bony changes can be confused with fibrous dysplasia. CT in axial and coronal scans is useful to define the destruction of the ethmoid-sphenoid plane and the walls of the invaded sinuses and the orbital cavities. On MR, tumors have similar signal intensities to the brain on all imaging sequences, and enhance with contrast. The evaluation of tumor extension into the sinonasal cavities is best displayed mainly in postcontrast coronal and sagittal T1-weighted sequences.[155,157]

The current treatment of choice for accessible benign meningiomas is complete surgical excision with long-term tumor control in the region of 72% to 100%. Complete surgical resection of meningiomas located in the region of the sinonasal cavities is difficult to achieve due to the inherent complexity of this region. Patients with inoperable or incompletely excised meningiomas are offered postoperative radiation therapy. The reported tumor control following subtotal resection and postoperative irradiation is 70% to 80% at 10 years for skull base meningiomas.[153,154]

Osseous Tumors

Osteoma

Osteomas are the most common benign neoplasm of the nose and paranasal sinuses. The most common sinuses involved are the frontal sinus, followed by the ethmoidal and maxillary sinuses. Osteomas may also less frequently develop in other craniomaxillofacial bones, including the mandible, orbita, sphenoid, external auditory canal, occipital and temporal bones.[158]

Clinically, the peripheral osteoma is usually asymptomatic. Symptoms vary depending on their location, and can present as pain, deformity, facial asymmetry, headache, rhinorrhea, anosmia, nasal obstruction, sinusitis, or ocular symptoms. Nearly all osteomas are asymptomatic and remain locally in the sinuses. Osteomas are most often detected incidentally, and generally, conservative treatment is recommended.[159]

The pathogenesis of osteomas is unclear. Neoplastic, infectious, traumatic, and developmental etiologies have been proposed. There are two major histologic subtypes of osteomas. The "ivory" or compact osteoma, is composed of dense, mature bone. The "fibrous" or cancellous osteoma contains greater amounts of fibrofatty tissue and marrow. These differences are reflected in their radiologic appearance. On CT, the compact osteoma has a very dense and sclerotic appearance, whereas the cancellous osteoma has a less dense and less ossified display (Fig. 4-27). CT is an effective method for determining the extent of osteomas and bony invasion. On MR imaging, both compact and cancellous osteoma display a heterogeneous, low to intermediate signal intensity on all imaging sequences. MR is particularly helpful in differentiating inflammatory lesions from neoplasm.[65,160]

Osteomas are distinct from exostosis in that they develop within the bone, while exostosis develop on the surface of the bone. Exostoses are bony excrescences that occur on the palate, mandible, and external auditory canal. The etiology of exostoses are reactive, and have no malignant potential. The radiographic features of osteomas can be confused with odontomas and focal sclerosing osteomyelitis. Though very rare, Gardner's syndrome should be considered in patients that present with osteomas and abdominal complaints. Gardner's syndrome is an autosomal dominant disorder characterized by familial polyposis of the large bowel, with supernumerary teeth, fibrous dysplasia of the skull, osteomas, fibromas, and epithelial cysts. Malignant transformation of the colon polyps occurs in nearly 100% of patients affected by Gardner's syndrome by the age of 40 years.[161,162]

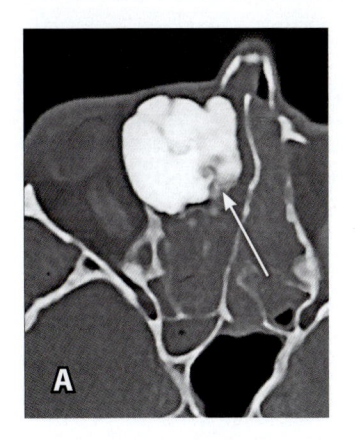

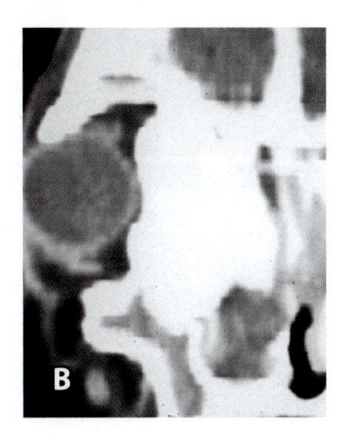

Figure 4-27 Ethmoid Osteoma
Compact ethmoid osteoma. Axial (**A**), coronal reconstructed (**B**) bone NECT images show a large, well-marginated calcified mass originating in the right lamina papyracea, with medial extension into the ethmoid sinuses, lateral extension into the right orbit and anterolateral displacement of the right globe. With the exception of a small cancellous portion of tumor posteromedially (*arrow*, **A**), the mass is highly calcified, consistent with the ivory or compact osteoma variant.

Definitive treatment of the osteoma consists of complete surgical removal at the base where it unites with the cortical bone. Varying surgical techniques have been advocated depending on the location and extent of the osteoma. Osteomas Recurrence is extremely rare, and there is no potential for malignant transformation.[158]

Fibrous Dysplasia

Fibrous dysplasia is an idiopathic skeletal disorder where normal bone is replaced by poorly organized, structurally deranged fibro-osseous tissue. Besides congenital fibrous dysplasia (cherubism), there is no hereditary basis for this disease, with the etiology remaining unclear. Fibrous dysplasia is organized into three categories: monostotic fibrous dysplasia, polyostotic fibrous dysplasia, and Albright's syndrome. Monostotic fibrous dysplasia comprises 75% to 80% of all cases of fibrous dysplasia, and is the designation used when the lesion is confined to one bone. Polyostotic fibrous dysplasia is the term used when more than two bones are affected by disease, and accounts for 20% to 25% of all cases. The unique triad of polyostotic fibrous dysplasia coexisting with cutaneous pigmentation and precocious sexual development is known as Albright's syndrome. Albright's syndrome contributes to 1% to 3% of all cases of fibrous dysplasia and is more common in females.[139]

Monostotic fibrous dysplasia is the most likely type of fibrous dysplasia to affect the head and neck. In general, 20% to 25% of monostotic fibrous dysplasia arise in the head and neck and most commonly arise in the maxilla, followed by the mandible. Pathologically distinguishing fibrous dysplasia from ossifying fibroma can be quite difficult, and nearly impossible radiographically. The term, "benign fibro-osseous lesion" has been advocated by many authorities instead. The radiological display is dependent on the proportion of fibrous tissue present in the lesion. Fibrous dysplasia usually have

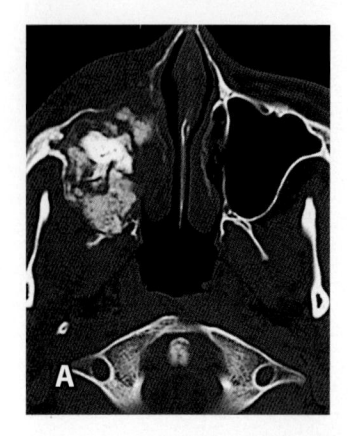

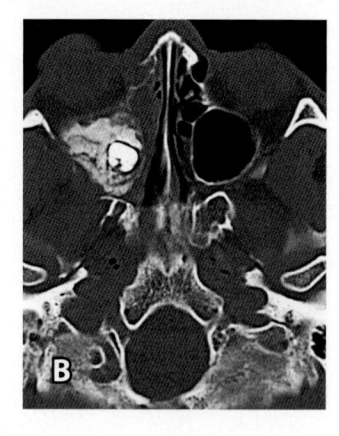

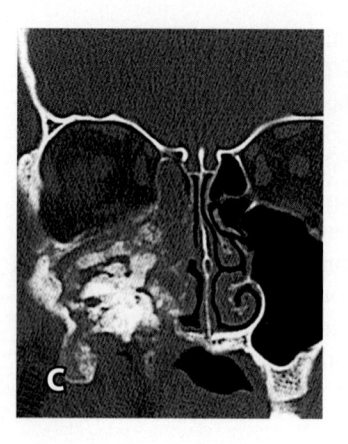

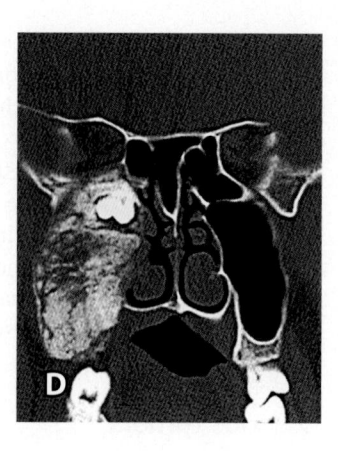

Figure 4-28 Fibrous Dysplasia
Fibrous dysplasia in the right maxillary sinus. Axial (**A–B**) and coronal (**C–D**) bone CT scans show an ill-defined enlargement of the diploic space of the right zygomatic process that has expanded into and completely obliterated the right maxillary sinus. Note the ground glass appearance of the fibrous tissue with interspersed cystic areas. Though the cortex is thinned at some places as the dysplastic tissue expands, cortical bone is usually not directly affected.

a "ground-glass" appearance on CT (**Fig. 4-28**). On MR, fibrous dysplasia display low to intermediate signal intensity on T1-weighted and T2-weighted sequences. Cystic components or associated mucoceles will display a high intensity on T2-weighted images. Tissue biopsy for a histopathological diagnosis is mandatory for these lesions due to their nonspecific imaging features.[163,164]

Fibrous dysplasia has an associated rate of malignancy of 0.5%, with most reported cases being associated with irradiation. Definitive treatment of fibrous dysplasia is surgical resection. Advances in minimally invasive techniques have led to the increased use of endoscopic approaches in the management of fibrous dysplasia.[163,165]

Ossifying Fibroma

Ossifying fibroma is a rare, expansile, benign tumor that is presumed to originate from primitive mesenchymal cells. This tumor is histologically characterized by a demarcated proliferation of cellular fibrous connective tissue with variable quantities of osseous products. Ossifying fibroma usually develops in the mandible (75%) or maxilla (15%), where it is usually slow growing and asymptomatic. Rarely, this lesion can develop in the midface and paranasal sinuses, and in these locations the tumor tends to behave more aggressively. Ossifying fibroma most commonly presents between the second through fourth decades, and occurs more frequently in females. Patients may present with nonspecific symptoms that are dependent on the anatomic location of the lesion.[166,167]

CT imaging displays an eggshell-thin rim of bone surrounding a lytic area. The attenuation of the lesion is usually lower than that of neighboring soft tissues, and older lesions may have striations of calcifications (**Figs. 4-29** and **4-30**). MR imaging demonstrates low to intermediate signal intensity on T1-weighted images and variable signal intensity on T2-weighted images, with some ossified areas having low signal intensity and certain regions having high signal intensity (e.g., associated cysts, mucoceles, nonossified regions). Varying enhancement of the outer wall may be seen: in some cases the lesion may display a brisk, thick enhancement of the outer wall of the lesion, whereas in other cases there may be incomplete enhancement outlining a thin outer shell. Fluid–fluid levels within a sinonasal ossifying fibroma has been recently reported.[163,168,169]

Ossifying fibroma and fibrous dysplasia are extremely difficult to distinguish radiographically. Ideally, there may be certain imaging features that can assist in differentiating ossifying fibroma from fibrous dysplasia. Ossifying fibroma may display a crisp demarcation of the tumor from adjacent bone, whereas fibrous dysplasia tends to have more diffused margins. In addition, ossifying fibromas usually are more aggressive and cause greater displacement and mass effect of normal bone, whereas fibrous dysplasia growth tends to be self-limiting with skeletal maturation and ceases once adulthood is reached.[170]

Radiotherapy is contraindicated as treatment of ossifying fibroma because it may increase malignant transformation rates. Simple curettage ostectomy is the treatment of choice to treat this lesion in uncomplicated cases in the mandible, but the more aggressive nature and higher recurrence rates of this tumor outside of the mandible necessitate wide local excision.[170,171]

Juvenile Active Ossifying Fibroma

Juvenile active ossifying fibroma is a fibro-osseous neoplasm that arises within the craniofacial bones in children and adolescents. In most cases, juvenile active ossifying fibroma involves the maxilla, the paranasal sinuses, the orbit, the frontoethmoid complex, and mandible. Ninety percent of these lesions involve the sinuses, particularly the maxillary sinus. The tumor has an expansile nature, often extending into adjacent structures including the ethmoid and sphenoid sinuses, nasal cavity, and orbital walls. Males and females are equally affected. Presenting symptoms are nonspecific and variable. Symptoms may include nasal obstruction, facial swelling, proptosis, teeth displacement, and pain.[172]

Histologically, there is no general agreement among pathologists with regard to the proper terminology of this tumor. The

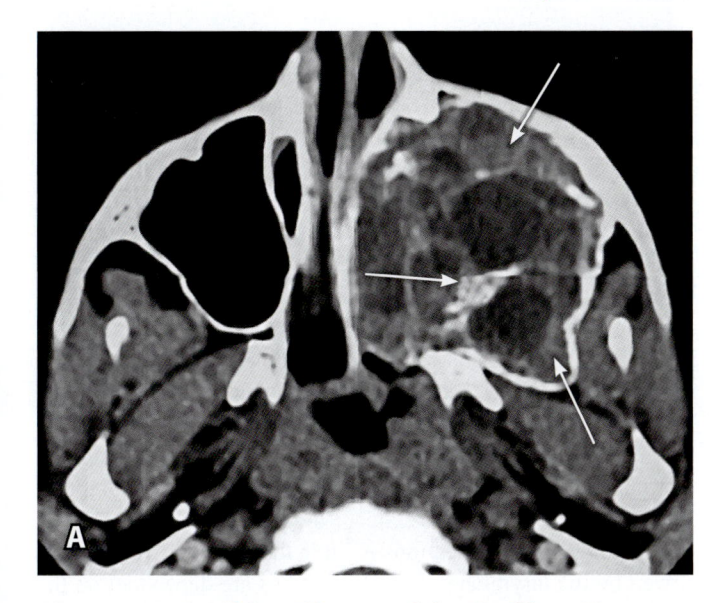

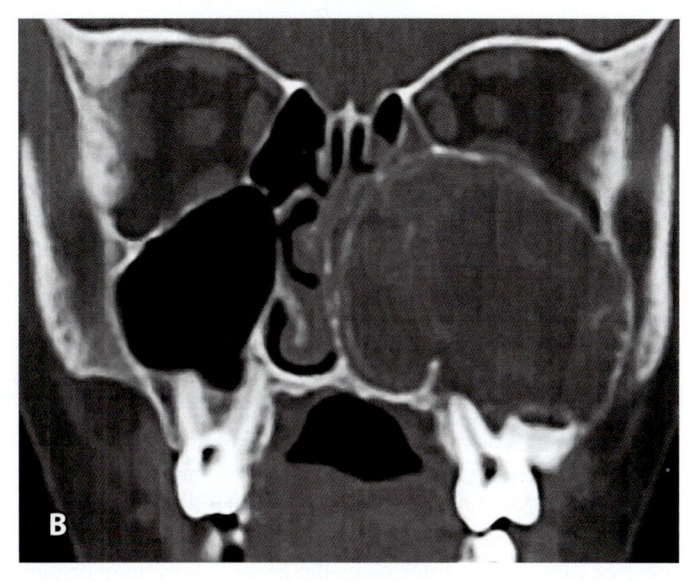

Chapter 4: Sinonasal Endoscopic Surgery, Infections and Neoplasms   169

Figure 4-29 Ossifying Fibroma of the Maxillary Sinus
Axial soft tissue window (**A**) and coronal bone window (**B**) NECT images show a large expansile mass completely occupying the left maxillary sinus with soft-tissue density fibrous areas surrounded by distinct peripheral ossifications (*arrows,* **A**), consistent with an ossifying fibroma. The mass has also completely invaded the left nasal cavity and has infiltrated the ethmoid sinuses (**B**). Note the significant remodeling of the left inferior orbital wall and the mass effect on the left inferior rectus muscle.

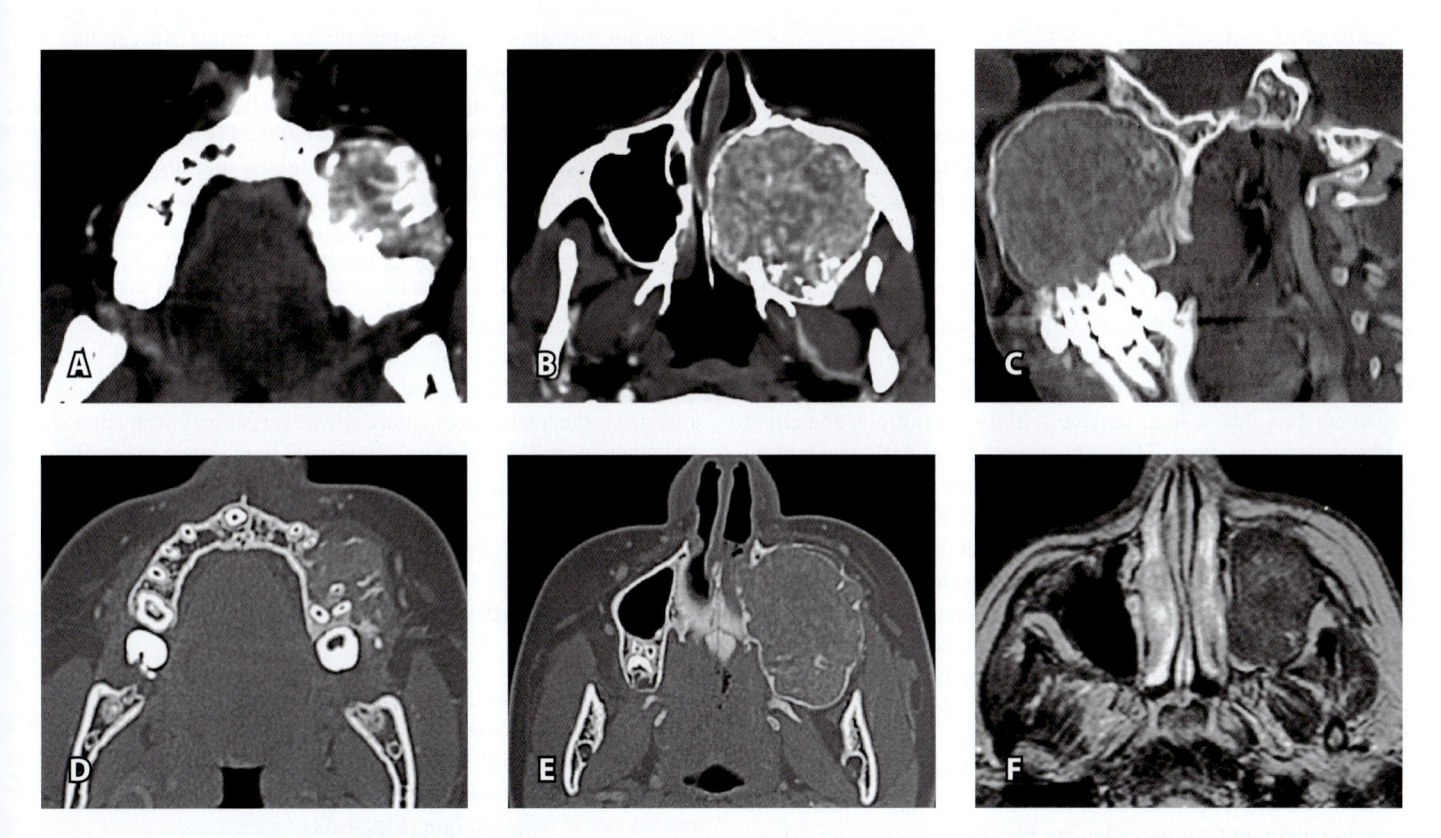

Figure 4-30 Cementing Ossifying Fibroma
Cementing variant of ossifying fibroma occupying the left maxillary sinus. Axial CT images (**A–B**), sagittal CT image (**C**) axial bone CT (**D–E**) and axial T1W MR image (**F**) show a large lesion filling the left maxillary sinus. The heterogeneous matrix of the tumor, peripheral rim of ossification (**B, E**), continuity with the space around the roots of the molars of the left alveolar process (**C, D**), and pathologic confirmation of cementum are typical of cementing ossifying fibroma, a benign tumor of the periodontal ligament.

World Health Organization describes the tumor as an actively growing lesion mainly affecting individuals below the age of 15 years, which is composed of a cell-rich fibrous tissue containing bands of cellular osteoid without osteoblastic rimming, together with trabeculae of more typical woven bone. Small foci of giant cells may also be present. In general, the more aggressive nature, increased recurrence, and earlier age of presentation, distinguish juvenile active ossifying fibroma from the conventional form of ossifying fibroma.[172]

CT imaging of juvenile ossifying fibroma are similar to those of the conventional form. CT imaging shows an expansile mass, with sclerotic rimming and well-defined borders. Internal calcifications are also commonly seen in the tumor. MR imaging is similar to the conventional form, and displays low to intermediate signal intensity on T1-weighted images and variable signal intensity on T2-weighted images. The conventional and juvenile forms of ossifying fibroma share very similar imaging characteristics; however, in some cases the juvenile form may display more aggressive behavior with cortical destruction. In addition, the conventional form may demonstrate relatively more sclerotic components.[173–175]

Although simple curettage has been considered as a conservative potential treatment option for juvenile active ossifying fibroma, due to the more aggressive nature and propensity for recurrence of this tumor, en bloc resection is advocated as the treatment of choice.[170,176]

Benign Fibrous Histiocytoma

The sinonasal tract is the most common site of origin of fibrous histiocytomas from the head and neck, accounting for one-third of all cases. Most fibrous histiocytomas are malignant, and will be addressed in a later section of this chapter. Benign fibrous histiocytomas most commonly arise in the skin of the extremities in children and young adults. Benign fibrous histiocytomas include: fibrous histiocytoma, juvenile xanthogranuloma, reticulohistiocytoma, and xanthoma. Benign fibrous histiocytoma most commonly occurs on the skin of the extremities of young to middle aged persons. The lesions may be solitary or multiple, and either subcutaneous or deep. They are composed of cells resembling histiocytes and fibroblasts with a storiform pattern of growth, likened to a cartwheel. Juvenile xanthogranuloma is a superficial histiocytic tumor composed of multinucleated giant cells, often with an eosinophilic infiltrate. This lesion most commonly occurs in the skin of children. Reticulohistiocytoma is a rare, benign cutaneous histiocytic proliferation. A multicentric form of this occurs and is associated with destructive arthritis accompanied by multiple skin lesions. Xanthoma is an accumulation of lipid-laden histiocytes that most commonly arise in association with different types of hyperlipidemias. They most commonly arise in the skin and tendons of the hands and feet. There are no specific imaging features of benign fibrous histiocytomas. These lesions are very uncommon in the sinonasal tract.[177]

Fibromatosis

Aggressive fibromatosis (desmoid tumor, grade I fibrosarcoma) is an uncommon, benign group of tumors characterized by fibroblastic proliferation. Although aggressive fibromatosis is a nonmetastasizing tumor with benign histological features, it has a significant potential for local invasiveness and recurrence. The etiology of aggressive fibromatosis is unknown, but there is an association with pregnancy, soft-tissue trauma, osteoma, Gardner's syndrome, and familial adenomatous polyposis. The incidence of aggressive fibromatosis is remarkably higher in families with familial adenomatous polyposis and Gardner's syndrome, and has been associated with different sites of germline mutations in the adenomatous polyposis coli (APC) gene.[178,179]

Aggressive fibromatosis is more common in women and has a peak incidence in the second through fourth decades of life. However, an aggressive presentation occurs at a young age in the rare germline APC-mutation associated faction. Aggressive fibromatosis most often occur in the lower extremities and trunk, whereas approximately 15% occur in the head and neck. In this region, the common locations include the sinonasal region, followed by the larynx and neck. Symptoms are dependent on the anatomical location and are nonspecific.[178–180]

The diagnosis of aggressive fibromatosis is based on histology. They demonstrate interdigitating and infiltrative growth and have poorly defined margins, which contributes to their high recurrence rate (30%). Fortunately, despite frequent recurrence, cause-specific mortality is extremely low, with overall survival rates in the high ninety percent range. Aggressive fibromatosis does not metastasize to regional nodes or distant sites so that a metastatic evaluation is unnecessary. The imaging findings are nonspecific. On CT, aggressive fibromatosis are usually homogenous and minimally enhancing with contrast (**Fig. 4-31**). MR is useful to determine the extent of the tumor, and displays a low to intermediate signal intensity on all imaging sequences and enhance minimally. Due to the high recurrence rate, the radiological assessment of tumor extent is very important. On MR, an association between a low signal intensity band as a marker for recurrence rate and extension may be observed.[181]

Local control is equivalent to cure. Treatment should be tailored to the locality and extent of tumor. Surgical excision with free margins is the treatment of choice. However, surgery with adjuvant radiotherapy and radiotherapy alone have been shown to be efficacious treatment alternatives in advanced or unresectable cases.[179]

Odontogenic Cysts and Tumors

Odontogenic Cysts

Periapical Cysts

Periapical (radicular) cysts are the most common odontogenic cysts and arise as toxins from an infected tooth pulp leak through the apex of the tooth and cause irritation of epithelial cells of the periodontal ligament. Eventual necrosis of this epithelium causes cystic degeneration (**Fig. 4-32**).

Dentigerous Cysts

A dentigerous cyst arises from the crown of an unerupted tooth. Such cysts are thought to arise during amelogenesis as fluid accumulates between the enamel epithelium and the enamel surface. Seventy-five percent of such lesions arise from the mandible and are clinically asymptomatic. CT typically shows a

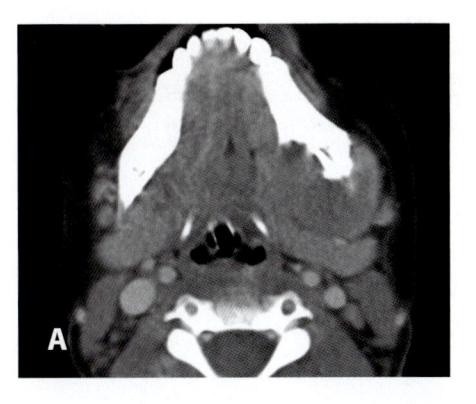

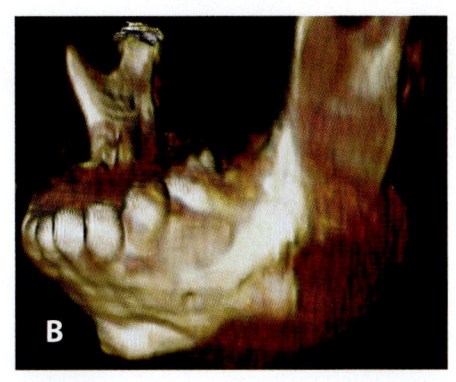

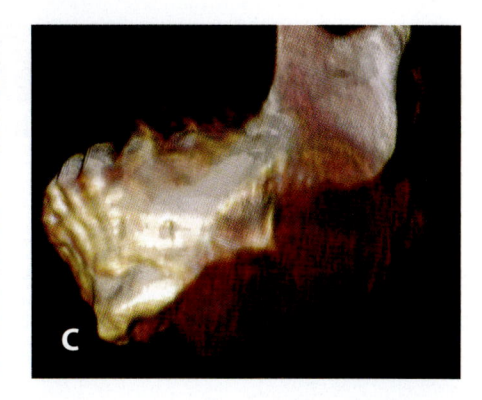

Figure 4-31 Aggressive Mandibular Fibromatosis
Axial CECT (**A**) shows a heterogeneously enhancing, poorly marginated mass originating from the junction between the angle and body of the mandible, expanding into the floor of the mouth, and displacing the parapharyngeal space surrounding the mandible. 3D CT reconstruction with surface rendering (**B–C**) show the extent of infiltration of this tumor and is utilized to reconstruct a mandibular prosthesis following the reconstruction of the mass. (Case courtesy of Wende K. Smoker M.D., University of Iowa.)

unilocular radiolucent cyst with well-defined margins surrounding the crown of an unerupted tooth (**Fig. 4-33**). Treatment of odontogenic cysts involves enucleation tooth extraction.[184]

Odontogenic Keratocysts

Odontogenic keratocysts are aggressive developmental jaw cysts thought to arise from the dental lamina. Seventy-five percent are located in the posterior mandible, but may also involve the maxillary process. Odontogenic keratocysts may mimic dentigerous cysts if located near unerupted teeth. Odontogenic keratocysts, however, are not associated with tooth crowns and are more likely to be multiloculated (**Table 4-19**). Treatment of odontogenic cysts involves enucleation and curettage.[184]

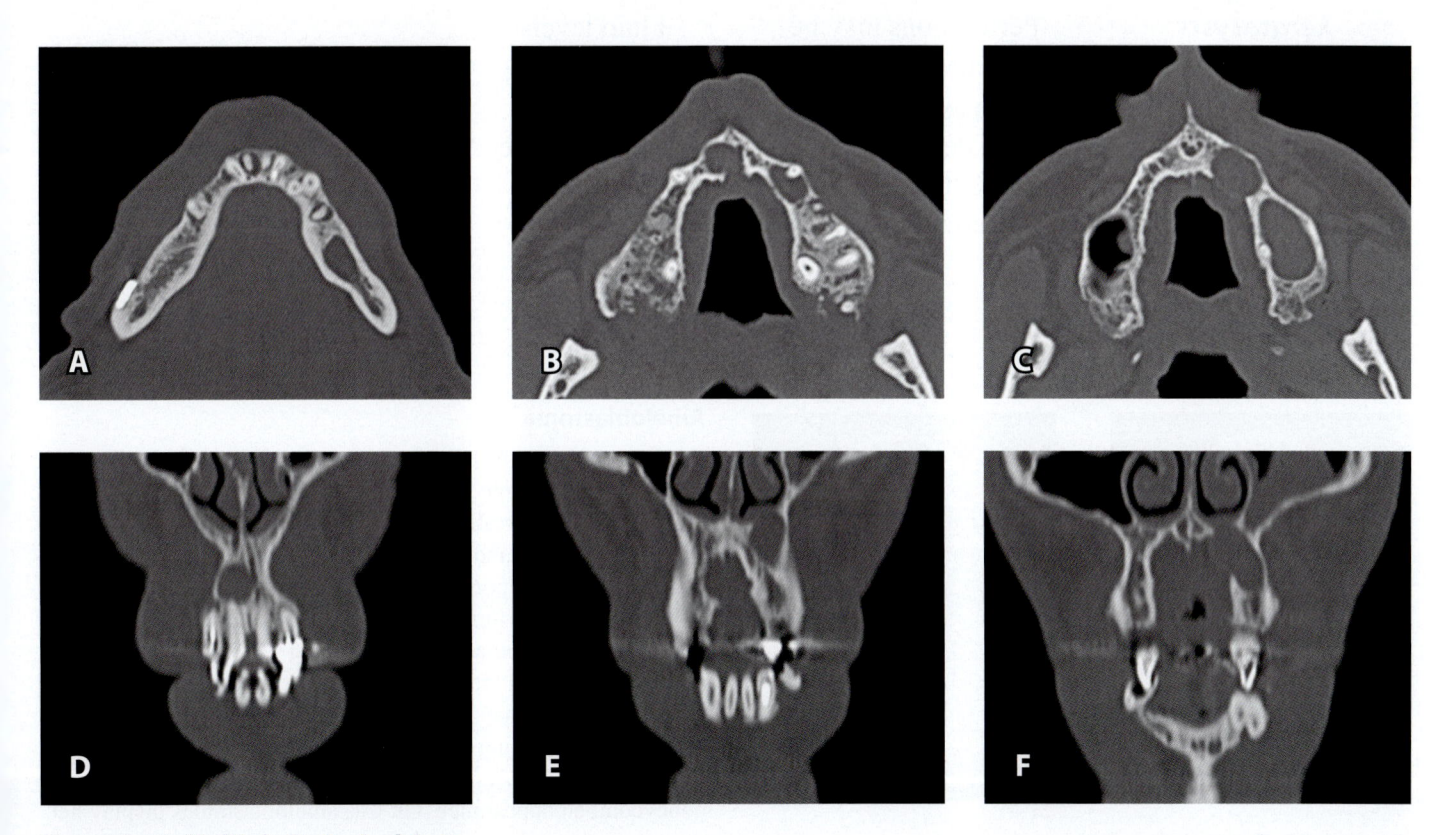

Figure 4-32 Multiple Periapical Cysts
Periapical cysts presenting with evidence of oronasal fistula. Axial (**A–C**) and coronal (**D–F**) bone CT images show multiple large periapical cysts in the alveolar ridge. The alveolar ridge is nearly completely eroded in some areas (**C**). There is also expansion and erosion into the left nasal meatus. Also noted is opacification of the left maxillary sinus, which may be related to an occult oroantral fistula (**F**).

Table 4-19 Characteristics of Lesions of the Jaw

Lesion	Computed Tomography	Magnetic Resonance Imaging
Ameloblastoma	• Bone expansion with cortical destruction and soft tissue extension	• Multilocular • Cystic and solid components • Papillary extensions • Irregular thick margins • High intensity signal spots on T1 • Enhancement
Pindborg tumor	• Bone expansion with sharp margins and cortical thinning • Radio-opacities • Multilocular, tooth embedded	• High signal on T2 • Low signal on T1 • Low signal areas representing bony septations
Myxoma	• Bone expansion with thinning • Trabeculated and cystic • Soft tissue extension	• High signal on T2 • Cystic and solid components
Odontogenic keratocysts	• Well-defined margin • Cortical thinning • Perforations may be present	• Multiloculated • Fluid levels
Aneurysmal bone cyst	• Bone expansion with no bone destruction • Smooth margins • Septations	• Multiloculated • Fluid levels

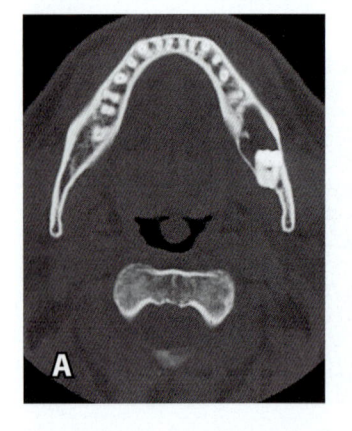

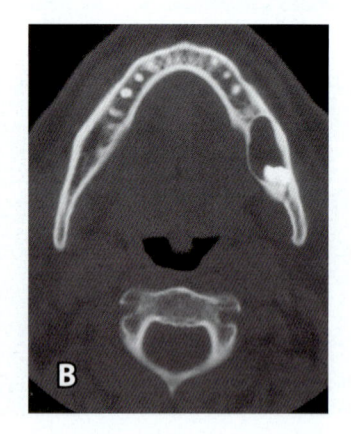

Figure 4-33 Dentigerous Cyst
Dentigerous cyst of the left mandibular molar tooth. Axial bone window CT images show a nondestructive cystic expansion surrounding the crown of a molar tooth, consistent with a dentigerous cyst.

Ameloblastoma

Ameloblastomas are benign tumors that derive from the remnants of odontogenic epithelium, lining of odontogenic cysts, and the basal layer of the overlying mucosa. These lesions are locally aggressive and have a tendency for recurrence. Approximately 80% of reported cases occur in the mandible and the remaining 20% originate in the maxilla. The overwhelming majority of ameloblastomas involving the sinonasal cavities secondarily extend from the maxilla. Less commonly, primary ameloblastomas may originate within the sinonasal cavities without a pre-existing lesion originating from the maxilla.[182,183]

On plain film, ameloblastoma has a multilocular, cystic, honeycombed appearance. On CT, ameloblastomas display heterogeneously and show minimal enhancement. On MR, they display mixed signal intensities, representing solid and cystic components of the lesion. These tumors display a low to intermediate signal intensity on T1-weighted images, and have variable intermediate and high signal intensities on T2-weighted images, with enhancement of the solid portions[184–186] (**Fig. 4-34, Table 4-19**).

Ameloblastomas most commonly occur in younger patients between the second and fourth decades of life. However, primary sinonasal ameloblastomas typically occur in older patients between 60 and 80 years old. The treatment of ameloblastomas include curettage, enucleation plus curettage, or radical surgery. Recurrence rates are much higher with conservative surgery, ranging around 30%. Wide surgical excision has a much lower recurrence rate, down to 7.1% after radical surgery. The involvement of sinonasal extension of an ameloblastoma precludes conservative management because lesions in this location are more likely to present with invasion of soft tissue and have a higher risk of skull base and intracranial extension.[182,183]

Pindborg Tumor (Calcifying Epithelial Odontogenic Tumor)

Pindborg initially described the calcifying epithelial odontogenic tumor in 1956. Pindborg tumors are rare lesions, and account for approximately 1% of all intraosseous odontogenic tumors. Pindborg tumors are benign, slow-growing lesions, often asymptomatic and identified incidentally. Pindborg tumors usually occur in patients in the fourth to fifth decades of life and occur in both sexes equally. Approximately 70% of cases arise from the mandible, while 30% of cases arise in the maxilla. Most lesions arise in the bicuspid-molar area. Usually, the neoplasm is not painful and is detected incidentally.[187]

Pindborg tumors are characteristically multilocular. On CT, the tumor displays as a well-defined mass of soft-tissue attenuation, and may contain thick bony trabecula and scattered high-density foci. On MR, they display a low signal intensity on T1-weighted images, and high signal intensity on T2-weighted images. An accompanying unerupted tooth can been seen in approximately 50% of Pindborg tumor cases (**Table 4-19**). The majority of Pindborg tumors are intraosseous, expansile lesions that do not breach the cortex or have extraosseous soft-tissue components. However, although rare (5%), extraosseous Pindborg tumors may display significant bone destruction and soft-tissue invasion.[188,189]

Treatment of Pindborg tumors is dependent on the size of the lesion. Smaller lesions can be treated with enucleation. The reported local recurrence for enucleation ranges from 10% to 14%. Larger lesions may require en bloc resection. Metastatic disease is extremely rare, with only several reported cases described in the literature.[190]

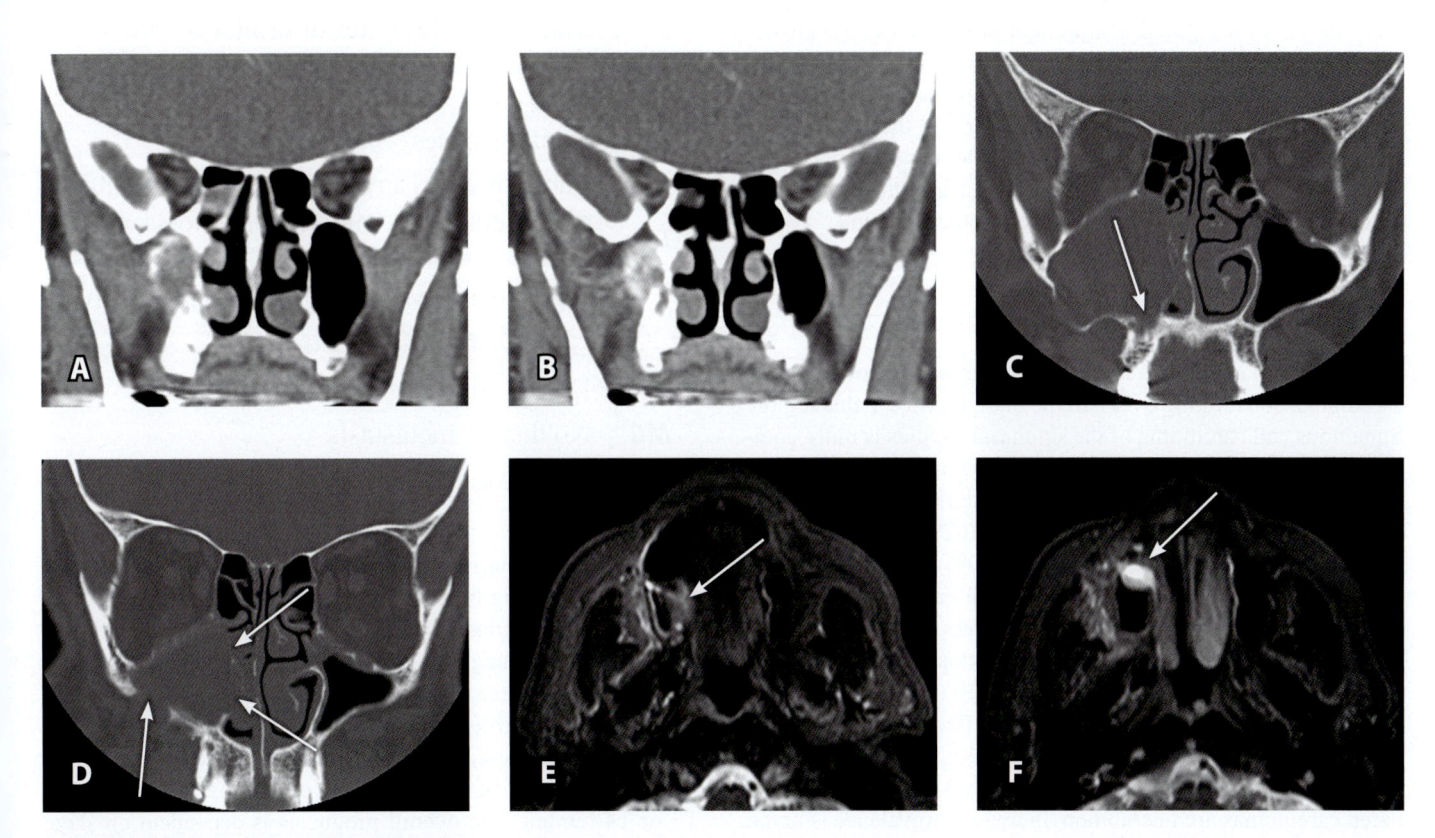

Figure 4-34 Maxillary Ameloblastoma

Coronal NECT (**A–B**) and coronal bone CT (**C–D**) images show a large mass completely occupying the right maxillary sinus. The soft tissue density mass shows areas of sclerosis along the posterior maxillary sinus wall (*arrows,* **A–B**) with some invasion of the sphenoid sinus. Bone algorithm show evidence of tumor expansion surrounded by scalloped and thinned cortex superiorly into the orbit, medially into the nasal cavity, and through the lateral maxillary wall (**C–D**). Lack of cortex along the right maxillary ridge suggests this as the site of origin (*arrow,* **C**). Also note the focal areas of dehiscence (*arrows,* **D**). Axial T2W MR images at the level of the maxillary sinus highlight the cystic heterogeneity of the lesion and confirm its origin in the premolar space of the right maxilla (*arrow,* **E**), with extension into the anterior portion of the maxillary sinus (*arrow,* **F**).

Myxoma and Fibromyxoma

Myxoma is a rare neoplasm of mesenchymal origin that is composed of undifferentiated stellate cells in a myxoid stroma. Myxomas are slow-growing, expansile lesions that usually present in the second and third decades of life. Myxomas most commonly derive mainly from soft-tissue areas such as heart, subcutaneous tissue, aponeurotic tissue, bone, genitourinary system, and skin. In the head and neck region, myxomas are usually interosseous.[191]

The most common location of myxoma in the head and neck region are the jaws. In this location, the tumor is derived from dental mesenchmye and are called odontogenic myxoma. Odontogenic myxoma of the jaws arise 45% of the time in the maxilla, and 55% of the time in the mandible. Odontogenic myxomas located in the maxilla can locally expand and invade into the maxillary sinus and nasal cavity. Myxomas in this region are usually undetected for many years. When the tumor becomes advanced, symptoms such as nasal congestion, epistaxis, and facial distortion may occur.

On CT, odontogenic myxoma of the sinonasal cavities display as a multilocular soft-tissue mass with bone destruction and thinning. Teeth may be displaced or their roots absorbed. Lesions in the maxillary sinus may extend upward to involve the orbit and intracranial cavity. On MR, they display intermediate signal intensity on T1-weighted images, and intermediate to high signal intensity on T2-weighted images (**Table 4-19**). These lesions may attain a considerable size prior to diagnosis because of their insidious growth characteristics, particularly in the maxilla. The treatment of choice is surgical excision. Odontogenic myxomas recur 26% of the time, most often due to inadequate resection by curettage. Larger lesions may require en bloc resection.[192]

Malignancies

Squamous Cell Carcinoma

Squamous cell carcinoma is the most common type of sinonasal carcinoma, constituting over half the malignancies in this region. Squamous cell carcinoma of the sinonasal cavities is more common in males (2:1 male to female ratio), and usually occurs within the fifth to seventh decades of life. The most common site of involvement is the maxillary sinus (62%) followed by the nasal cavity (26%), the ethmoid sinus (10%), and the sphenoid sinus (2%). Histologically, squamous cell carcinoma has infiltrating beds, nested islands, or small clusters of malignant cells, with variable amounts of eosinophilic cytoplasm. Keratin formation within cells and nested between cells (keratin pearls) signify a mucosal origin; however, poorly differentiated squamous cell carcinoma has little or no keratin present. Most lesions are moderately to well-differentiated tumors, while poorly differentiated carcinomas are uncommon. Increased prevalence is noted in patients with exposure to tobacco, ionizing irradiation, occupational exposure to wood dust, nickel, and chromates, boot shoe manufacturing, textile manufacturing, presence of inverted papilloma, asbestos, formaldehyde exposure, and infection with human papillomavirus types 16 and 18.[139,193]

The most common paranasal sinus to be afflicted is the maxillary sinus. Ohngren's line, which is drawn from the medial canthus to the angle of the mandible, divides the maxillary sinus

Table 4-20 American Joint Committee on Cancer (AJCC) Maxillary Sinus TNM Definitions 2002

Primary Tumor (T)	
TX	Primary tumor cannot be assessed
T0	No evidence of primary tumor
Tis	Carcinoma in situ
T1	Tumor limited to maxillary sinus mucosa with no erosion or destruction of bone
T2	Tumor causing bone erosion or destruction including extension into the hard palate and/or the middle of the nasal meatus, except extension to the posterior wall of maxillary sinus and pterygoid plates
T3	Tumor invades any of the following: bone of the posterior wall of maxillary sinus, subcutaneous tissues, floor or medial wall of orbit, pterygoid fossa, ethmoid sinuses
T4a	Tumor invades anterior orbital contents, skin of cheek, pterygoid plates, infratemporal fossa, cribriform plate, sphenoid or frontal sinuses
T4b	Tumor invades any of the following: orbital apex, dura, brain, middle cranial fossa, cranial nerves other than maxillary division of trigeminal nerve (V2), nasopharynx, or clivus
Distant Metastasis (M)	
MX	Distant metastasis cannot be assessed
M0	No distant metastasis
M1	Distant metastasis

into an inferior-anterior portion from a superior-posterior portion. Tumors arising from the superior-posterior portion usually have a worse prognosis than tumors that arise in the inferior-anterior portion. Ohngren's line was incorporated into the American Joint Committee on Cancer TMN guidelines for maxillary tumors in 1976 (**Table 4-20**). The delayed presentation of maxillary sinus squamous cell carcinoma results in dire consequences, with 60% to 97% of these patients presenting with advanced T3 or T4 tumors. The overall prognosis is dependent on stage and not on the particular anatomical origin of the tumor (**Table 4-21**). The overall 5-year survival rate for maxillary sinus squamous cell carcinoma has a 5-year overall survival rate of 42%. Local recurrence is seen in 45% of cases. During the course of the disease, 22% will develop positive regional lymph nodes and 18% will develop distant metastasis.[139,194,195]

Squamous cell carcinoma of the nasal cavity arises most often from the lateral wall of the middle turbinate or nasal septum.

Table 4-21 AJCC Stage Groupings	
Stage 0	• Tis, N0, M0
Stage I	• T1, N0, M0
Stage II	• T2, N0, M0
Stage III	• T3, N0, M0 • T1, N1, M0 • T2, N1, M0 • T3, N1, M0
Stage IVA	• T4a, N0, M0 • T4a, N1, M0 • T1, N2, M0 • T2, N2, M0 • T3, N2, M0 • T4a, N2, M0
Stage IVB	• T4b, any N, M0 • Any T, N3, M0
Stage IVC	• Any T, any N, M1

Nasal cavity lesions have an earlier clinical presentation compared to lesions located in the paranasal sinuses because they are more likely to have earlier symptoms such as nasal obstruction and epistaxis, while sinus lesions have more vague presentations such as sinusitis. The figures for nasal cavity squamous cell carcinoma fares better than the maxillary sinus; with 5-year overall survival rates at 60%. However, local recurrence occurs in 24%, positive regional nodes in 24%, and 20% will eventually develop distant metastasis. In both nasal cavity and maxillary sinus squamous cell carcinomas, local recurrence usually occurs within one year and is the most common cause of treatment failure and death. Patients who present with distant disease still most often succumb to local failure.[139,194,195]

On CT, squamous cell carcinoma appears as a soft-tissue mass with bone destruction and erosion. The soft-tissue mass is usually homogenous unless there is necrosis present (Fig. 4-35). The compact cellular density with little free water of squamous cell carcinoma is reflected in the MR appearance. These lesions display a low to intermediate intensity on T1-weighted images, and intermediate to slightly high intensity on T2-weighted images. Slight heterogeneous contrast enhancement can be present on both CT and MR. The characteristic feature of these lesions is its propensity to aggressively destroy bone; however, these imaging findings are nonspecific.[195]

The treatment of choice is surgical excision. Most lesions will require craniofacial resection. Surgery can be the sole treatment plan, depending on the tumor extent. However, due to the preponderance of advanced stage presentations, surgery with adjuvant radiation therapy has become a standard treatment strategy. The surgical management of orbital involvement is controversial. Many surgeons perform orbital exenteration if there is evidence of invasion into the orbital periosteum. There is evidence that orbital exenteration may not have any added survival benefit over ethmoidectomy for lesions involving the orbit. Curative surgery is usually not attempted when there is extension to the central skull base, pterygopalatine fossa, nasopharynx, or regional and distant metastasis[194,196] (Table 4-22).

Adenoid Cystic Carcinoma

Adenoid cystic carcinoma is a malignant tumor of salivary tissues that most commonly arises in the parotid gland. This neoplasm can also originate in other salivary tissues, including the minor salivary glands, lacrimal glands, and ceruminous glands. Adenoid cystic carcinoma has an insidious and prolonged clinical course, with numerous recurrences over a span of many years that often lead to demise. This protracted clinical course is reflected in the overall survival rates for adenoid cystic carcinoma of the head and neck, which are fairly good (89%) at 5 years, but down to 39% at 15 years.[197]

Lesions involving the sinonasal tract usually arise from the palate and then extend upward into the nasal cavity and paranasal sinuses. Due to the delayed presentation common to tumors that arise sinonasal cavities, and the proximity to vital structures at the sinonasal cavities, adenoid cystic carcinoma of the sinonasal tract have an increased frequency of local recurrence and lower survival rates compared to other tumor site locations.[197]

Adenoid cystic carcinoma is classified into three grades based on their cellular pattern and density: tubular, cribriform, or solid. The different cellular densities of the various grades are reflected in their display on MR. On T2-weighted images, lesions with low signal intensity correspond to highly cellular tumors (solid), while lesions with high signal intensity correspond to less cellular tumors (tubular and cribriform). However, these imaging features are nonspecific, and biopsy is mandatory for diagnosis.[198]

Adenoid cystic carcinoma has a propensity for perineural invasion, and this feature has been implicated in its ability to generate "skip lesions" and proclivity for recurrence. Imaging signs of perineural spread are foraminal enlargement and replacement of normal fat within the neural foramina. Contrast-enhanced MR images show enhancement of the nerve, which cannot be imaged with CT.[123,198]

Prognostic factors have been identified in adenoid cystic carcinoma: with nodal metastasis, major nerve invasion, solid histological features negatively affecting survival. About half of sinonasal adenoid cystic carcinomas have distant metastasis that can spread to the lungs, brain, cervical lymph nodes, and bone. In most cases, treatment requires multimodality therapy. Even with the incorporation of aggressive skull base surgery with adjuvant radiation therapy, survival rates for sinonasal ACC remain grim and are associated with high morbidity.[197]

Esthesioneuroblastoma

Esthesioneuroblastoma, also known as olfactory neuroblastoma, is a rare malignant tumor of neuroectodermal origin that arises from the basal layer of the olfactory mucosa, either above or below the cribriform plate in the course of the olfactory nerves. Histologically, esthesioneuroblastoma are composed of small, round malignant cells that have cytogenetic features and patterns of protooncogene expression similar to the Ewing sarcoma family of peripheral primitive neuroectodermal tumors.[199–201]

Table 4-22 Nasal Cavity and Ethmoid Sinus

	Primary Tumor (T)		
TX	Primary tumor cannot be assessed		
T0	No evidence of primary tumor		
Tis	Carcinoma in situ		
T1	Tumor restricted to any one subsite, with or without bony invasion		
T2	Tumor invading two subsites in a single region or extending to involve an adjacent region within the nasoethmoidal complex, with or without bony invasion		
T3	Tumor extends to invade the medial wall or floor of the orbit, maxillary sinus, palate, or cribriform plate		
T4a	Tumor invades any of the following: anterior orbital contents, skin of nose or cheek, minimal extension to anterior cranial fossa, pterygoid plates, sphenoid or frontal sinuses		
T4b	Tumor invades any of the following: orbital apex, dura, brain, middle cranial fossa, cranial nerves other than (V2), nasopharynx, or clivus		
	Regional Lymph Nodes (N)		
NX	Regional lymph nodes cannot be assessed		
N0	No regional lymph node metastasis		
N1	Metastasis in a single ipsilateral lymph node, ≤3 cm in greatest dimension		
N2	Metastasis in a single ipsilateral lymph node, >3 cm but ≤6 cm in greatest dimension, or in multiple ipsilateral lymph nodes, ≤6 cm in greatest dimension, or in bilateral or contralateral lymph nodes, <6 cm in greatest dimension	N2a	Metastasis in a single ipsilateral lymph node >3 cm but ≤6 cm in greatest dimension
		N2b	Metastasis in multiple ipsilateral lymph nodes, ≤6 cm in greatest dimension
		N2c	Metastasis in bilateral or contralateral lymph nodes, ≤6 cm in greatest dimension
N3	Metastasis in a lymph node >6 cm in greatest dimension		

In clinical evaluation, the actual size of the nodal mass should be measured, and allowance should be made for intervening soft tissues. Most masses over 3 cm in diameter are not single nodes but confluent nodes or tumors in soft tissues of the neck. There are three stages of clinically positive nodes: N1, N2, and N3. The use of subgroups a, b, and c is not required but is recommended. Midline nodes are considered homolateral nodes.

Esthesioneuroblastoma usually arises high in the nasal vault near the cribriform plate and usually presents with locally advanced disease that involves the paranasal sinuses and anterior cranial fossa. This neoplasm comprises 3% of all intranasal neoplasms and has a wide range in age in incidence, and peaks between the fourth and sixth decades of life. Metastasis is present in 10% to 33% of patients upon presentation. The most common locations of metastasis are the cervical lymph nodes, lungs, brain, and osseous sites.[202,203]

Since the incorporation of craniofacial resection as a main treatment modality for esthesioneuroblastoma in 1970, overall survival rates have improved dramatically. Multimodality therapy has resulted in an improvement of 5-year overall survival rates, which are now are 89% to 93%, in contrast to 40% for squamous cell carcinomas in the paranasal sinuses. The Kadish staging system is a useful system that correlates well with the prognosis of esthesioneuroblastoma. Kadish stage A are tumors confined to the nasal cavity, stage B are limited to the nasal cavity and paranasal sinuses, while stage C have tumor extension beyond the nasal cavity and paranasal sinuses, including the cribriform plate, base of skull, orbit, or intracranial cavity. Most patients present with Kadish stage B and stage C lesions and require adjuvant chemoradiation after craniofacial resection.[203,204]

Imaging plays a critical role in the tumor mapping of esthesioneuroblastoma. On MR, the lesion displays an intermediate intensity signal on both T1-weigthed and T2-weighted images, with the

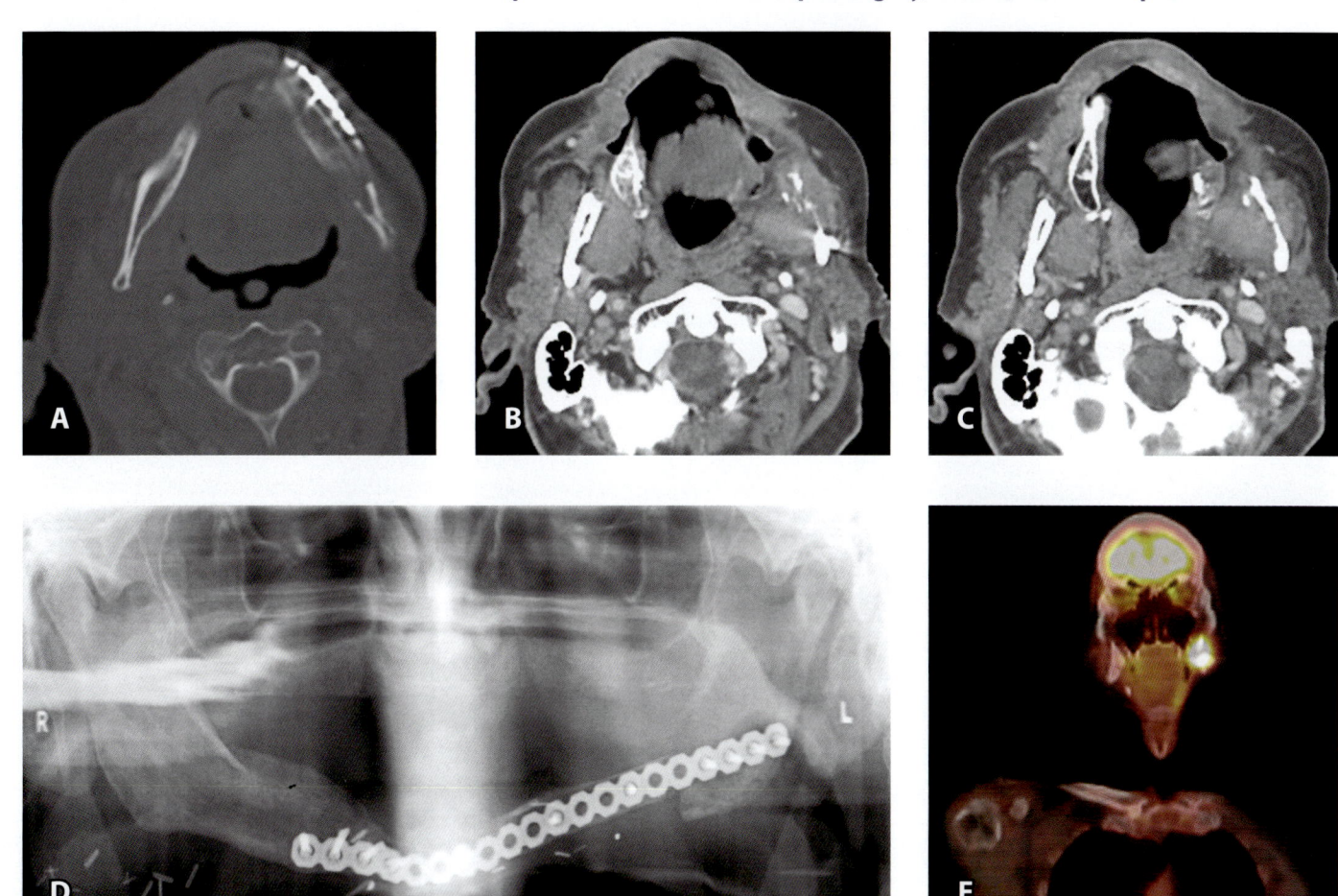

Figure 4-35 Mandibular Squamous Cell Carcinoma Recurrence
Recurrent squamous cell carcinoma following left hemimandiblectomy post ORIF. Bone window (**A**) soft tissue CECT (**B–C**) images show a soft tissue mass around destroyed fragments of the left mandibular ramus. Panorex views (**D**) shows the continuity of the reconstruction device from the angle to contralateral side of the body of the mandible. There is a haziness surrounding the left side of the surgical site. Fused PET/CT (**E**) shows marked increased metabolic activity in the region, which was confirmed by pathologic analysis to recurrence of the squamous cell carcinoma.

T2-weighted images being slightly brighter. On CT, esthesioneuroblastoma commonly appear as homogenous soft-tissue masses that enhance with contrast. In addition, bone erosion and displacement is commonly seen in these lesions. While these bony changes are better seen on CT, esthesioneuroblastoma usually present at a stage where detecting these findings on MR are easily performed. MR is superior to CT in defining tumor extension and distinguishing the lesion from inflammatory tissue[205,206] (**Figs. 4-36** and **4-37**).

Melanoma

Malignant melanoma is a common skin neoplasm, and its incidence is increasing at a faster rate than any other cancer. The head and neck region comprise 15% to 33% of cutaneous malignant melanomas. Melanoma in the sinonasal cavities is very rare, however, and account for approximately 1% of all malignant melanomas and 4% of those in the head and neck. Malignant melanomas arising in the sinonasal cavities originate from melanocytes derived from neural crest tissue, which are distributed throughout the mucosa of the upper respiratory tract and oral cavity. The pathologic differential diagnosis of sinonasal mucosal melanomas is broad, and the use of immunohistological markers S-100, HMB-45, and tyrosinase distinguish this malignancy.[207]

Sinonasal mucosal malignant melanomas most often originate from the middle and lower turbinates, and nasal septum. The paranasal sinuses are rarely the sites of origin of malignant melanomas. Rather, most melanomas affecting the paranasal sinuses reach this location by extension from a lesion that originates in the nasal cavity. Symptoms are nonspecific and include nasal obstruction, epistaxis, and pain.

Melanomas have significant vascularity, which facilitates strong enhancement observable on CT and MR. On MR, these tumors usually display intermediate signal intensity on T1-weighted and T2-weighted sequences. In some lesions, paramagnetic effects of blood products (hemosiderin) and melanin may display as high signal intensity on T1-weighted and low signal intensity T2-weighted sequences (**Figs. 4-38** and **4-39**). These lesions may demonstrate bone erosion and remodeling, which is best seen on CT; however, MR is superior in mapping soft-tissue extension, differentiating from inflammatory tissue, and detecting perineural invasion.[208,209]

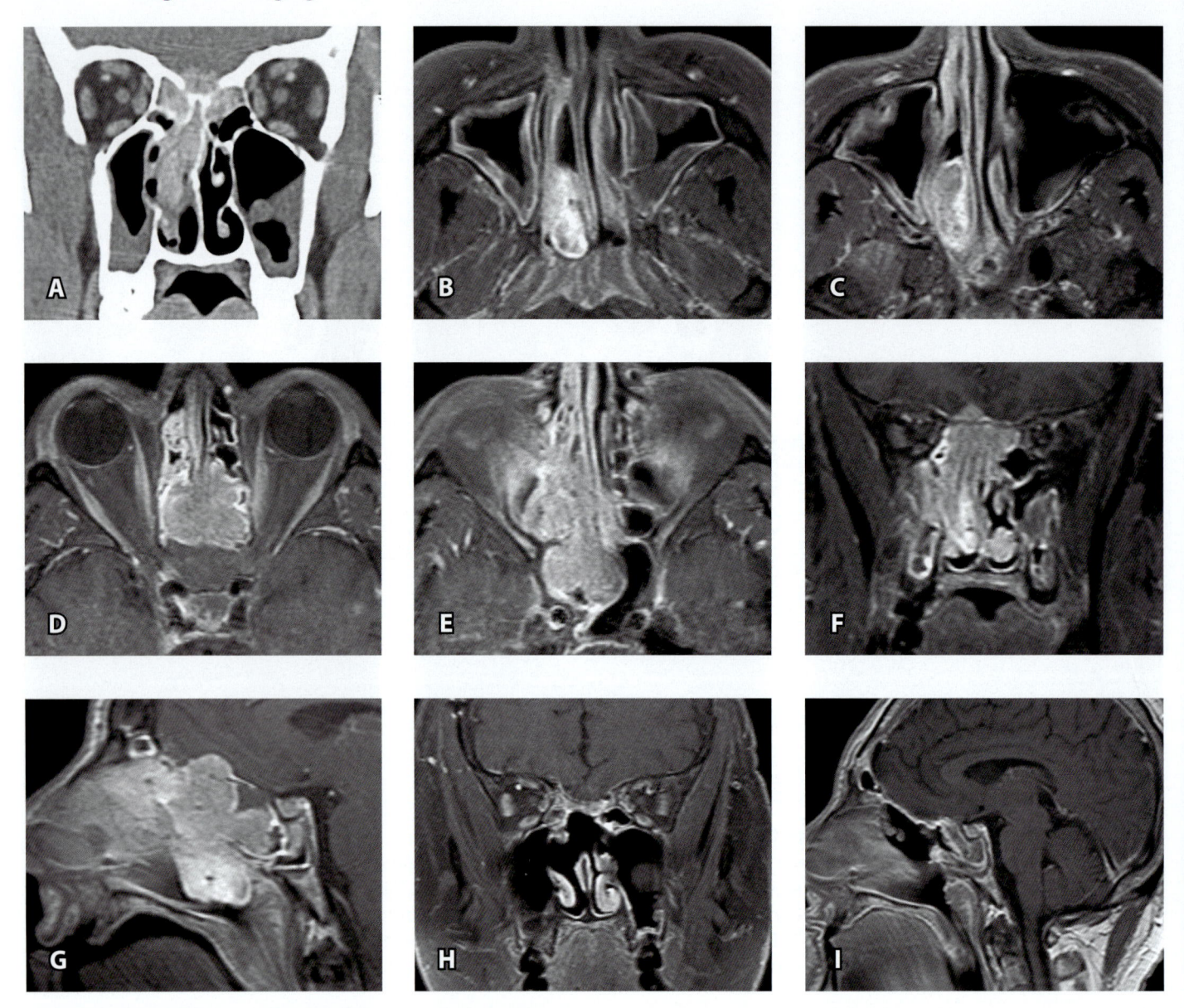

Figure 4-36 Esthesioneuroblastoma Preop and Postop
Coronal CECT image (**A**) shows an enhancing lesion occupying the right superior portions of the nasal cavity with superior extension through the anterior skull base into the cranial fossa. Axial T1W MR images with contrast (**B–E**) show a heterogeneous, yet diffusely enhancing lesion extending inferiorly from the lower portions of the right nasal cavity (**B–C**) to the level of the cribriform plate (**E**). There is diffuse infiltration of the ethmoid (**D**) and sphenoid (**E**) sinuses, though the orbits have been spared. Coronal (**F**) and sagittal (**G**) T1W MR images with contrast show a well-marginated lesion extending into the right maxillary sinus and superiorly through the cribriform plate into the anterior cranial fossa. T1W MR images (**H–I**) showing postoperative changes after extensive tumor resection, without evidence of residual tumor.

Sinonasal mucosal malignant melanoma arises most commonly in the fifth to eighth decades of life, and affect both sexes equally. The prognosis is dismal, with a 20% 5-year overall survival, which differs dramatically from the 88% 5-year overall survival rate for cutaneous malignant melanoma. Lesions that originate in the paranasal sinuses have an even more dismal prognosis (<1% 5-year overall survival) because they usually present later than lesions arising from the nasal cavity. Surgery offers the best probability of local control, and the benefit of chemoradiation has not been clearly established for this grim disease. Local failure is common (>50%), and often heralds metastatic disease, which most commonly are located in the lungs, lymph nodes, and brain.[207,210]

Adenocarcinoma

Adenocarcinoma account for 10% to 20% of all primary malignant neoplasms of the sinonasal cavities and is the third most common epithelial malignancy after squamous cell carcinoma and adenoid cystic carcinoma. Adenocarcinomas include the

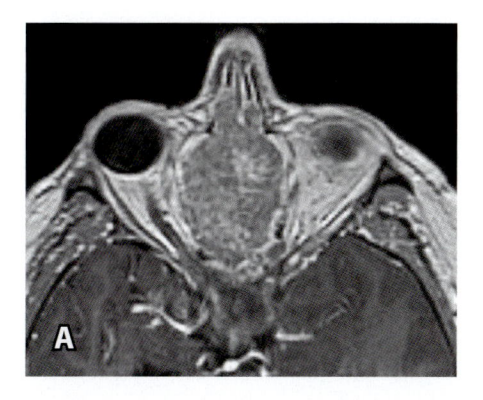

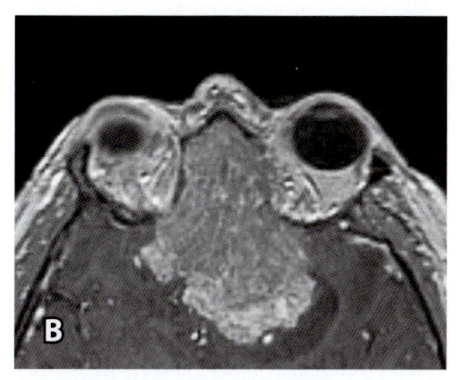

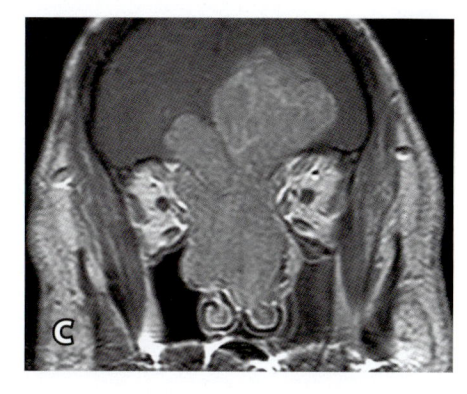

Figure 4-37 Esthesioneuroblastoma Eroding the Anterior Skull Base
Axial (**A–B**) and coronal (**C**) postcontrast MR images show a multilobular mass that fills the nasal cavities bilaterally, completely expands the ethmoid sinuses, and erodes into the medial portion of both orbits. There is impressive intracranial extension into both frontal lobes following growth of the tumor through the cribriform plate.

minor-salivary gland tumors, intestinal-type adenocarcinomas, or sinonasal neuroendocrine carcinomas.[211]

Intestinal-type adenocarcinoma (ITAC) have histological characteristics resembling colonic carcinomas, and represent for about 4% of the total malignancies in this region. There are five histological subtypes of intestinal-type adenocarcinoma: papillary, colonic, solid, mucinous, and mixed. The histological appearance of intestinal-type adenocarcinoma to colonic adenocarcinoma is very similar, and may be confused with a metastatic lesion from the gastrointestinal system. Although there are strong histological similarities, there are cytogenetic differences between these lesions. K-ras-2 mutation is commonly found in

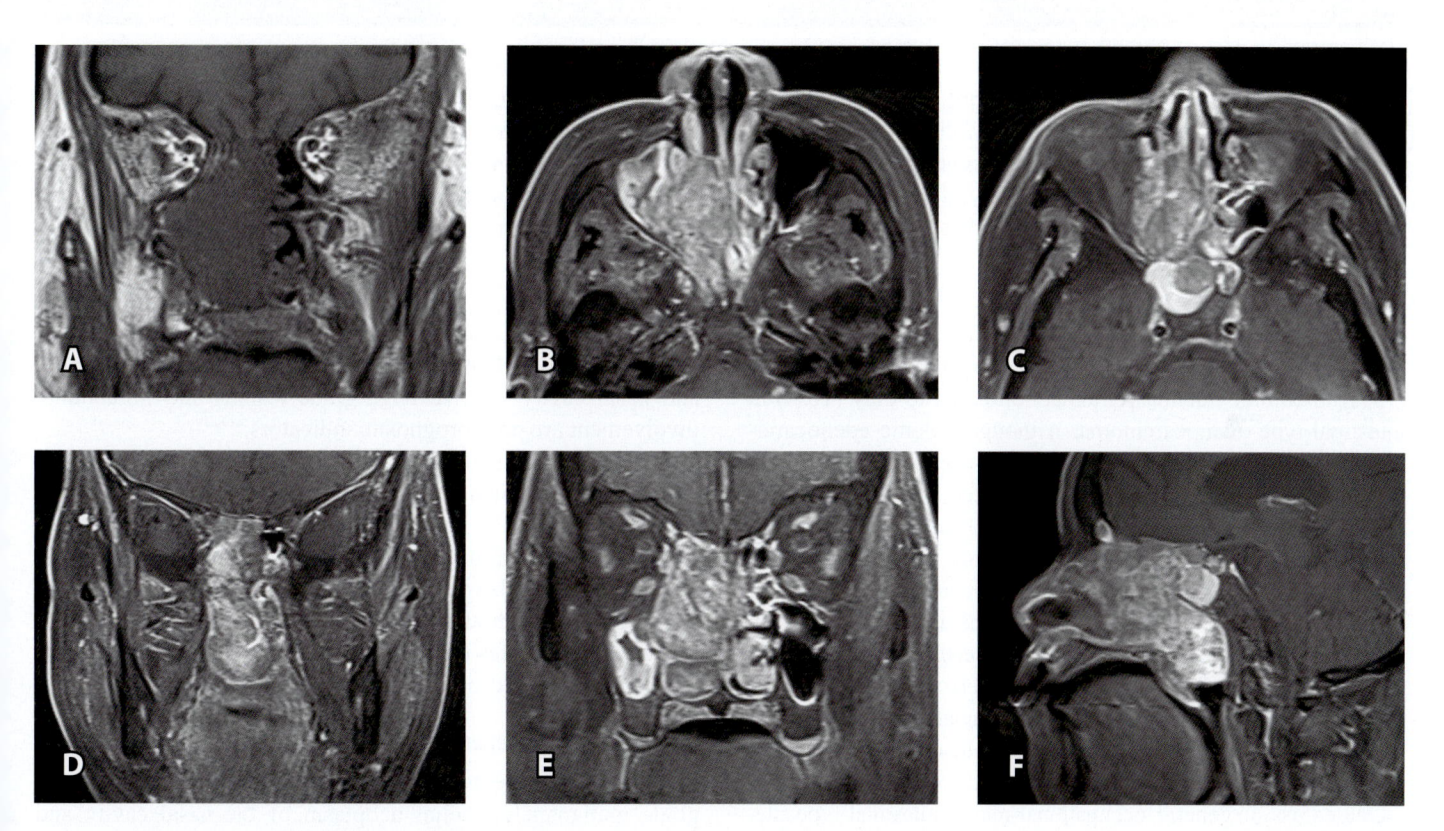

Figure 4-38 Sinonasal Malignant Melanoma
Sinonasal Malignant Melanoma in a 77-year-old female. Coronal T1 MR image without contrast (**A**), axial postcontrast MR images (**B–C**), coronal postcontrast MR images (**D–E**), and sagittal postcontrast MR image (**F**) show an enhancing lobulated mass centered in the right posterior ethmoid air cells with posterior extension into the right sphenoid sinus, lateral extension into the right maxillary sinus and inferior medial aspect of the right orbit, and superior extension to the cribriform plate. There is slight elevation and enhancement of the dura covering the posterior portion of the cribriform plate, which is most likely reactive inflammation, as there is no evidence of intracranial extension of the above described posterior ethmoid mass (**F**). Precontrast image shows no evidence of hemorrhage (**A**).

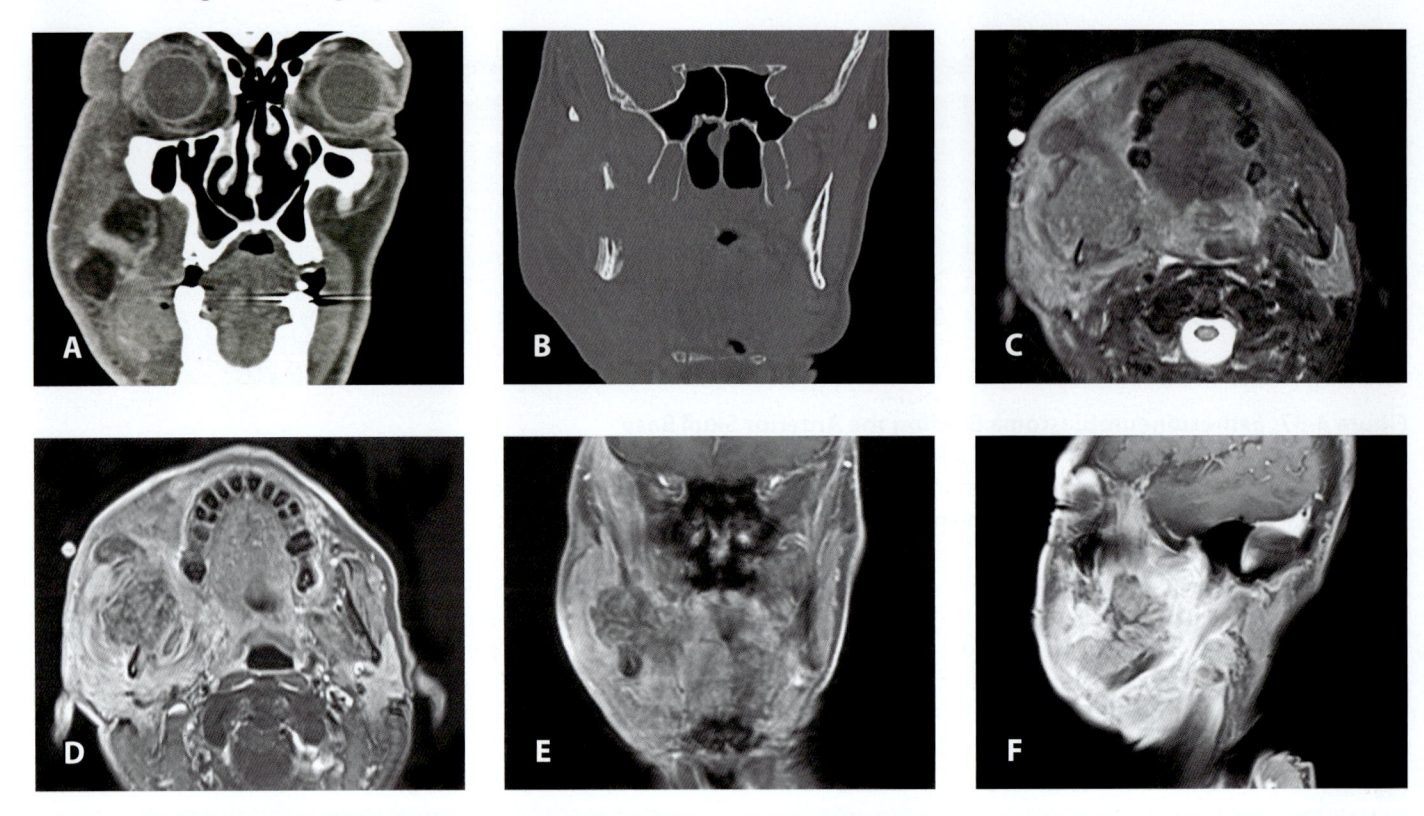

Figure 4-39 Masticator Space Abscess in an Orofacial Squamous Cell Carcinoma
54-year-old male with nonresectable right orofacial squamous cell carcinoma. Following two weeks of radiation therapy, the patient developed progressive facial swelling over a 5-month period. Despite antibiotic treatment, the patient developed purulent drainage from the right submandibular region. Coronal soft tissue (**A**) bone windows (**B**) NECT scans show two pockets of lucency surrounding a partially destroyed right mandibular ramus. Axial (**C–D**), coronal (**E**) and sagittal (**F**) T1 contrast enhanced MR scans showing intense enhancement surrounding a mass within the right mandibular ramus. Following drainage of the abscess, the mass decreased in size.

colonic adenocarcinoma, and is never found in intestinal-type adenocarcinoma. In addition, p53 is more frequently mutated (75%) in colonic adenocarcinoma, compared to only (18%) in intestinal-type adenocarcinoma. Although colonic adenocarcinoma metastasis to the sinonasal tract is uncommon, examination of the gastrointestinal tract is warranted due to the fact that some patients may initially present with head and neck symptoms from a gastrointestinal-located primary neoplasm.[212]

Intestinal-type adenocarcinoma may occur sporadically or associated with an occupational hazard. The association between sinonasal adenocarcinoma and wood or leather dusts has been widely documented, with industry workers having 900 times greater relative risk of acquiring this malignancy. Other occupational hazards have been identified as well: occupational exposure to formaldehyde and women exposed to textile dust are at increased risk. In general, occupational-related intestinal-type adenocarcinoma predominately occur in males in the fifth and sixth decades of life, while sporadic cases tend to arise in women.[111,211]

Intestinal-type adenocarcinoma most commonly occurs in the ethmoid sinuses (40%), nasal cavity (28%), and maxillary antrum (23%). Sporadic lesions most commonly arise in the maxillary sinuses, while occupational related cases most commonly occur in the ethmoid sinuses. Sporadic cases tend to have a delayed presentation with a more advanced stage of tumor compared to occupational-related ITAC because maxillary lesions do not become symptomatic as early as ethmoid and nasal cavity lesions. High-grade lesions and intracranial involvement are poor prognostic indicators.[213,214]

The imaging features of sinonasal adenocarcinomas are nonspecific and indistinguishable from squamous cell carcinoma (**Figs. 4-40** and **4-41**). Treatment is mainly craniofacial resection with adjuvant radiation therapy. Prognosis varies depending on the histological subtype, with the papillary subtype having the best prognosis with an 82% 3-year overall survival. Five-year overall survival rates have improved with modern multimodality therapy, with recent studies showing near 60%.[213,215]

Sinonasal Undifferentiated Carcinoma

Sinonasal undifferentiated carcinoma (SNUC) is a rare, high-grade malignant epithelial neoplasm of the nasal cavity and paranasal sinuses of uncertain histogenesis with or without neuroendocrine differentiation but without evidence of squamous or glandular differentiation.

SNUC is classically composed of small to medium-sized undifferentiated cells and is characterized by high mitotic rates, significant cellular pleomorphism, and high nuclear to cytoplasmic ratios, necrosis, and vascular invasion. There are three recognized types of SNUCs: (a) the Western type, the most common type

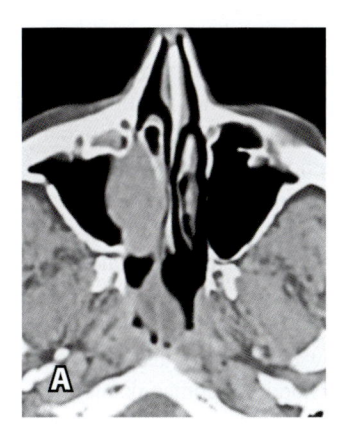

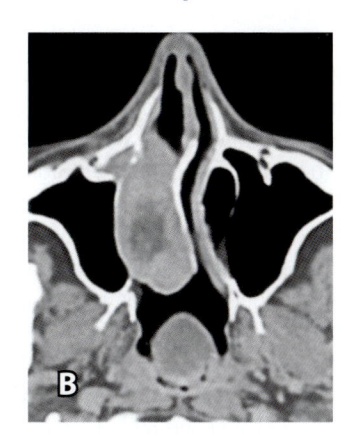

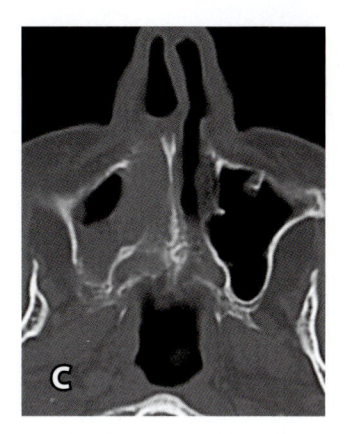

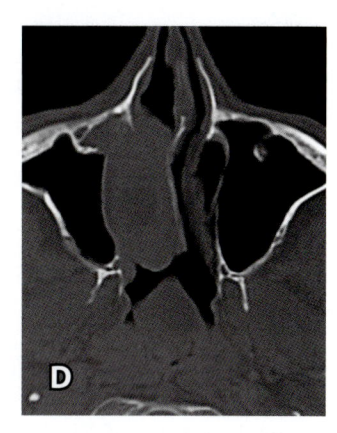

Figure 4-40 Polypoid Adenocarcinoma of the Nose
Polypoid mass in the right nasal cavity with expansion into the anterior right maxillary sinus. Soft tissue (**A–B**) and bone windows (**C–D**) CT images following contrast administration show an expansile tumor, simulating benign polypoid masses. However, the bony erosion into the adjacent anterior portion of the maxillary sinus should raise likelihood of a neoplasm. Biopsy confirmed the diagnosis of adenocarcinoma of the nasal cavity. Also note the incidental rounded mass in the nasopharynx which was a benign polyp.

found in Western countries including the United States, (b) a type identical with undifferentiated nasopharyngeal carcinoma, found mainly in Asian patients, (c) a large-cell type similar to large-cell carcinoma of the lung, also found largely in Asian patients. SNUC is a distinct entity that must be distinguished from other sinonasal malignancies, including esthesioneuroblastomas, small-cell carcinomas, nasopharyngeal-type carcinomas, and large-cell lymphomas. It is useful to conceptualize these neuroendocrine sinonasal malignancies into two groups, esthesioneuroblastomas and nonesthesioneuroblastoma neuroendocrine carcinomas. This categorization is useful because esthesioneuroblastomas can often be managed with local treatment alone, which is not the case for their counterparts. Pathologically, the tumors most commonly confused with SNUC are esthesioneuroblastoma and nasopharyngeal carcinoma (undifferentiated type). Immunohistochemistry plays an important role in distinguishing these tumors.[204]

These tumors are highly aggressive, with frequent invasion and extension into adjacent structures. Typically, SNUC presents generally as a large tumor involving multiple sinonasal tract sites and may extend into the nasopharynx. Symptoms typically present relatively acutely compared to other sinonasal malignancies (order of weeks to months), and include nasal obstruction, epistaxis, proptosis, visual disturbances, pain, and cranial nerve involvement. Significant bone destruction is common, and is best displayed on CT. On MR, they usually have an intermediate intensity signal on T1-weighted images, and intermediate to high intensity signal on T2-weighted images, with heterogeneous contrast enhancement.[204,216,217]

The prognosis of SNUC has historically been very grave. The tumor has anaplastic histologic features and usually presents at an advanced stage. The tumor also has a high tendency for distant metastasis and local recurrence. The original report on SNUC by Frierson et al, in 1986 showed a median survival of only 4 months. Many other series on the treatment of SNUC have also been very unfavorable.[107,109] However, better results have been shown by several recent studies, with Rischin et al. showing 64% 2-year overall survival, and Rosenthal et al. showing a 62.5% 5-year overall survival with multimodality therapy for SNUC.[216,218–220]

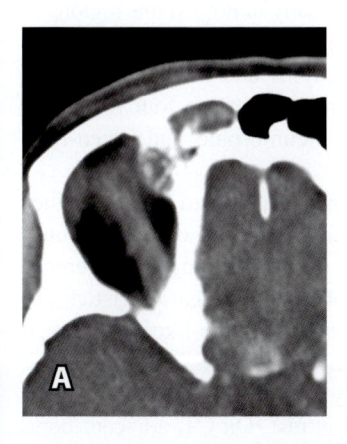

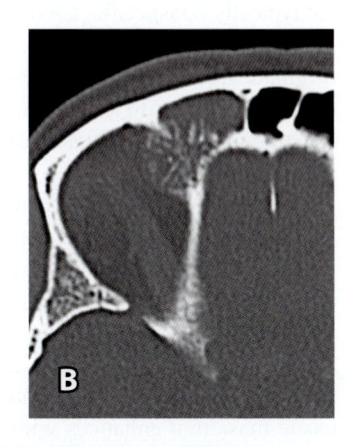

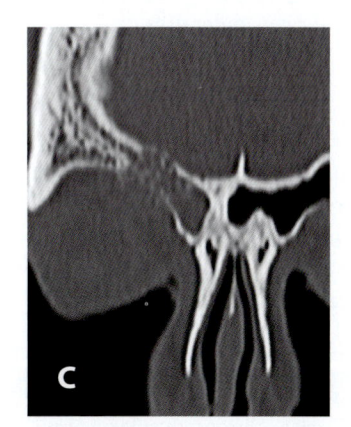

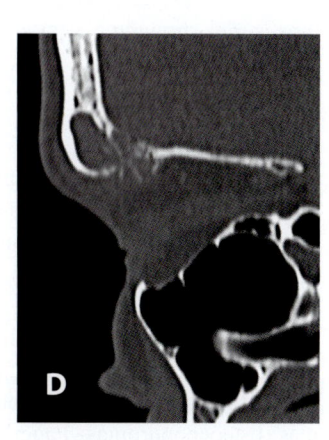

Figure 4-41 Atypical Carcinoid of the Frontal Sinus
Axial soft tissue (**A**), axial bone (**B**), coronal bone (**C**) and sagittal bone (**D**) NECT show a nonspecific expansile lesion in the lateral aspect of the fright frontal sinus with local bony destruction and spiculated calcifications throughout (**B–D**). Biopsy confirmed the diagnosis of carcinoid.

Lymphomas

Although nearly half of all patients with malignant lymphoma present with disease in the head and neck; disease in this region are mainly limited to the cervical lymph nodes. Lymphomas of the sinonasal cavities are almost exclusively non-Hodgkin lymphomas (NHL). Non-Hodgkin lymphoma comprises 3% to 5% of all malignancies, and only about 1% of these arise in the sinonasal cavities. NHL accounts for 5.8% to 8% of paranasal sinus malignancies. The sinonasal cavities are the second most frequent site of NHL after Waldeyer's ring. Sinonasal lymphomas have nonspecific clinical presentations, similar to most sinonasal neoplasms.[221]

Sinonasal lymphomas occur most frequently in the sixth to eighth decades of life. Sinonasal lymphoma is more common in Asian countries, where it is the second most frequent site of extranodal lymphomas. In the United States and Europe, the predominant NHL subtype is diffuse large b-cell lymphoma (DLBCL); whereas in Asia and Latin America, the predominant form is nasal NK/T-cell lymphoma.[222]

Nasal NK/T-cell lymphoma is an Epstein-Barr virus (EBV) associated neoplasm. In Asia, NHL commonly presents at a younger age and commonly arises in the nasal cavity compared to the paranasal sinuses; whereas in western countries, NHL arises more frequently in the paranasal sinuses. DLBCL more commonly presents in the elderly, usually in patients over the age of 60 years. DLBCL is much more likely to present with eye or orbital involvement compared to NK/T-cell lymphoma. Of the paranasal sinuses, the maxillary sinus is the most commonly involved, followed by the ethmoid, frontal, and sphenoid sinuses.[221,223]

Of the sinonasal cavities, the maxillary sinuses are most frequently involved, followed by the sphenoid, ethmoid, and frontal sinuses and nasal cavity. On CT, these lesions display bone remodeling and erosion that is common in paranasal sinus lymphoma. Soft-tissue resolution and delineation of intracranial extension is best seen on MR, and is a superior modality in detecting small lesions. Lymphomas typically have an intermediate signal intensity on all imaging sequences[222] (**Fig. 4-42**).

Sinonasal lymphomas are treated with chemoradiation, with 5-year survival rates varying widely for DLBCL (range of 29% to 80%). NK/T-cell lymphoma have a poorer prognosis, with most series showing 5-year survival rates under 40%.[223–225]

Sarcomas

Chondrosarcoma

Chondrosarcoma is a malignant tumor composed of a chondroid matrix without osteoid. Osteosarcoma, which can also produce chondroid, is discriminated from chondrosarcoma by the presence of osteoid. Chondrosarcoma is the second most common primary malignancy arising from bone after osteosarcoma. Primary chondrosarcoma originate from normal tissue such as cartilage, bone, or soft tissue, whereas secondary chondrosarcoma derive from preexisting benign cartilaginous neoplasm such as enchondromas, osteochondromas, Paget's disease, fibrous dysplasia, multiple hereditary exostosis, or multiple enchondromatosis.[205,226,227]

Approximately 1% to 12% of chondrosarcoma emanate in the head and neck, most commonly in the jaw bones, sinonasal cavities, maxilla, and cervical vertebrae. Approximately 12% of head and neck chondrosarcoma arise in the sinonasal cavities. Chondrosarcomas arising from laryngotracheal and soft tissue usually occur in adults aged 50 years or older, while sinonasal chondrosarcoma more frequently occurs in women aged 50 years or younger. Symptoms are nonspecific, similar to other tumors in the sinonasal region.[227]

On CT, bone erosion and bony displacement is usually present, and may display with or without calcifications depending on the amount of tumor matrix mineralization in the tumor. These tumors usually present as a soft-tissue mass, with expansion and bone destruction that frequently show areas of nodular or plaque-like calcification on CT. On MR, chondrosarcomas display low T1-weighted and high T2-weighted signal intensities and enhance with contrast. The contrast enhancement is usually seen in the periphery of the lesion, whereas the central chondromatous core does not. These imaging findings are nonspecific and can be similar to osteosarcoma. Osteosarcoma tends to have more aggressive bony erosion and may demonstrate reactive periosteal thickening.[228]

Surgery is the primary treatment modality, although the specific procedure varies greatly with the specific location and extent of disease. The role of multimodality therapy is unclear, and should be reserved for advanced stage, metastatic disease, higher grade, or aggressive histological subtypes. Five-year disease-specific survival is 87.5% for sinonasal chondrosarcoma, quite good when compared to other sinonasal malignancies. In addition, the overall survival from head and neck chondrosarcoma is higher than other lesions from other regions of the body. The finding of better survival in the head and neck region is surprising because the anatomical constraints of the head and neck would be expected to decrease the ability to achieve optimal tumor excision and increase the rate of local recurrence while reducing survival.[227,229,230]

Rhabdomyosarcoma

Rhabdomyosarcoma is the most common soft-tissue sarcoma in children and adolescents, but is rare in adults. Nearly half occur in the head and neck, including the orbit, nasopharynx, paranasal sinuses, and middle ear. In children, the most common location is in the orbit, in adults however, the sinonasal tract is the most common site of origin. The symptoms of paranasal rhabdomyosarcoma are typically nonspecific, similar to many tumors in this region.

Rhabdomyosarcomas are highly malignant tumors that originate from embryonal mesenchyme and have the potential of differentiating to striated muscle. There are four histological subtypes: embryonal, alveolar, pleomorphic, and mixed-type rhabdomyosarcoma.[231,232]

On MR, rhabdomyosarcoma has a similar to slightly higher signal on T1-weighted images, and high signal on T2-weighted images, with postcontrast images showing strong enhancement of the tumor (**Figs. 4-43** and **4-44**). These characteristics are nonspecific. However, a characteristic grape-like appearance (botyryoid sign) on contrast-enhanced MR has been described. The CT findings display a poorly defined, heterogeneous soft-tissue mass that enhances with contrast. On CT, adjacent bone erosion is evident as the tumor expands. In addition, the extent of bone erosion has been suggested as an important prognostic factor in nonorbital rhabdomyosarcomas of the head and neck. Necrosis, hemorrhage, or calcifications are not prominent

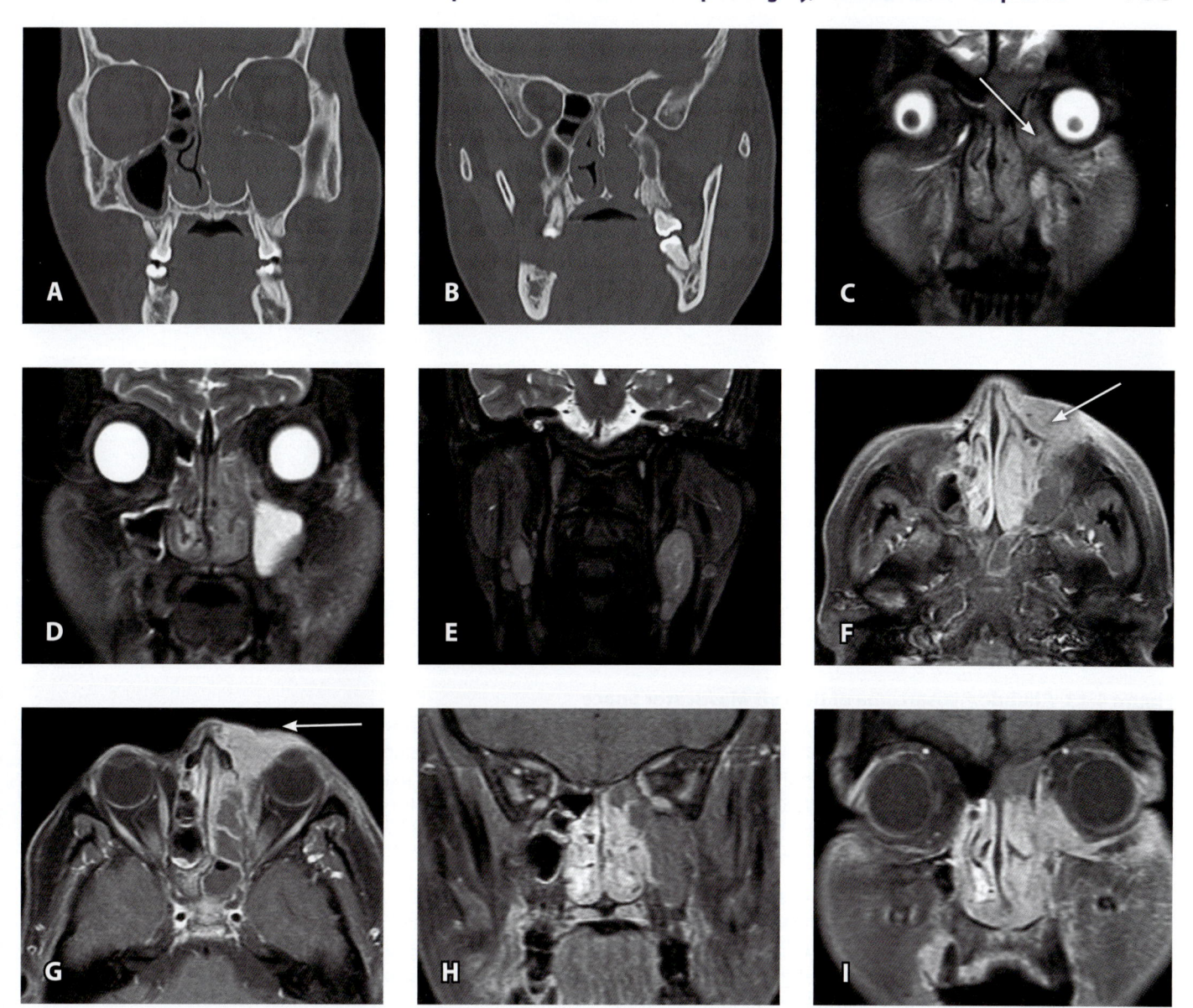

Figure 4-42 Natural Killer T Cell Lymphoma
Young adult female with rapid onset soft tissue mass in the left nasolabial region with skin penetration. Coronal CECT bone windows (**A–B**) show bony destruction of the left side of the face, involving the nasal cavity, maxillary sinus, ethmoid air cells, and medial orbital wall. Coronal T2W MR images (**C–E**) show definite extension beyond the nasal cavity into the medial left orbit (*arrow,* **C**). Postcontrast axial MR images (**F–G**) and coronal (**H–I**) show contiguous tumor from the skin surface of the left midface (*arrows,* **F, G**), expanding into the left orbit, nasal cavity, and ethmoid air cells. Also note bilateral submandibular lymphadenopathy (**E**). Biopsy confirmed natural killer T cell lymphoma.

features of this tumor. Liposarcomas usually have a component of fat/density/intensity. Chordoma, chondrosarcoma, and osteosarcoma usually have areas of calcification. Rhabdomyosarcomas imaging features are indistinguishable from SCC. However, the difference in age of presentation between these tumors is useful in ranking the differential diagnosis.[100,233–236]

Prognosis is markedly worse for adult patients compared to pediatric patients who present with rhabdomyosarcoma. This is because adults more commonly present with lesions in the sinonasal tract, and have a higher proportion of unfavorable histological subtypes (alveolar and pleomorphic). Survival statistics have significantly improved with the incorporation of multimodality therapy, with earlier studies showing 8% to 20% 5-year overall survival, compared to more recent studies demonstrating over 60% 5-year overall survival for rhabdomyosarcoma of the head and neck. However, the statistics for rhabdomyosarcoma of the sinonasal tract do not fare as well, with 5-year survival rates at 46% for this location.[237,238]

Fibrosarcoma

In the past, the term fibrosarcoma was often applied indiscriminately to any malignant-appearing spindle cell tumor associated

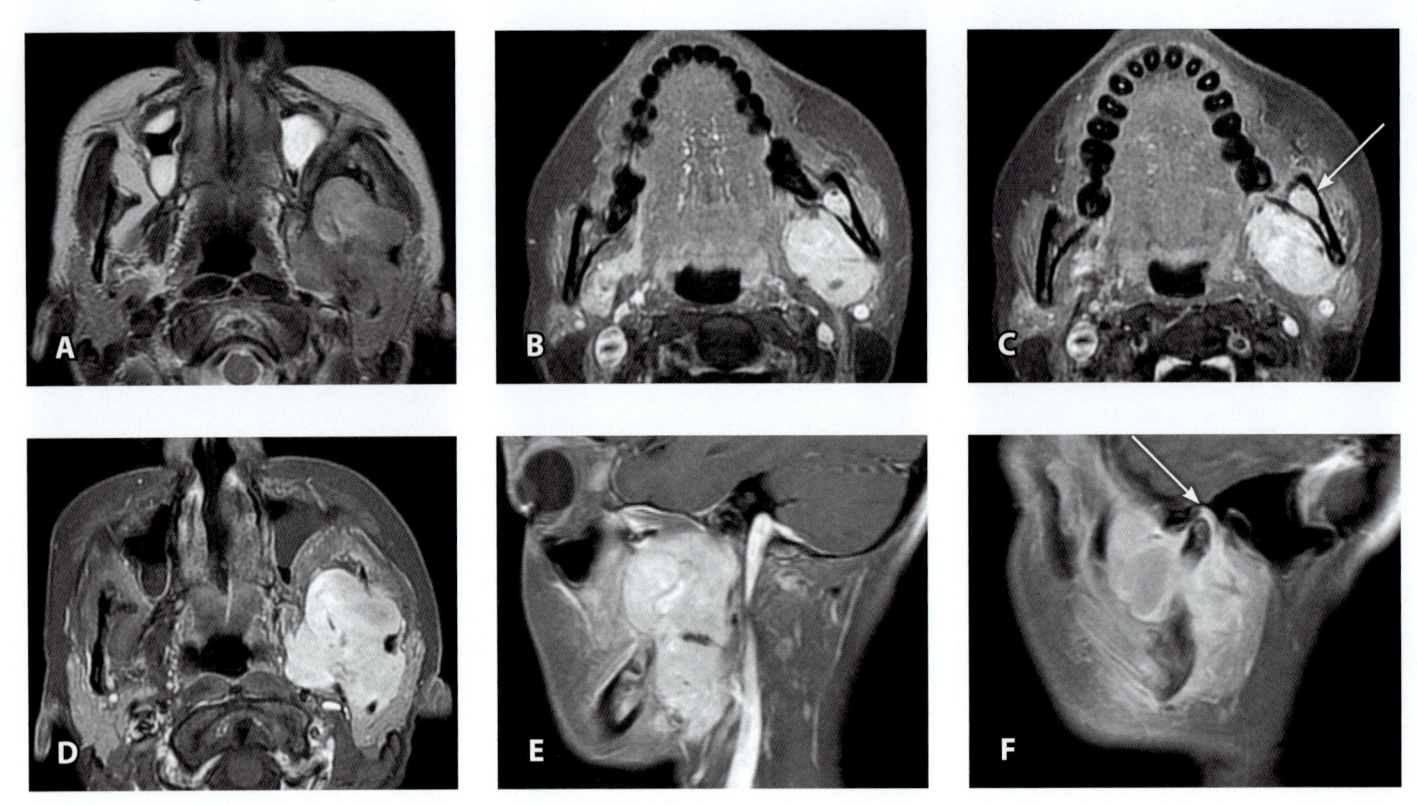

Figure 4-43 Rhabdomyosarcoma of the Left Masticator Space
T2 axial MR (**A**) shows a multilobular mass centered in the left masticator space, showing intermediate signal intensity. Axial (**B–D**) and sagittal (**E–F**) postcontrast MR images show well a well-marginated lesion with intense enhancement. Note also extension into the marrow of the left mandibular angle (*arrow*, **C**), as well as superior extension into the left temporomandibular joint (*arrow*, **F**). (Case courtesy of Wende N. Gibbs MD, Department of Radiology, Baylor University, Dallas.)

with collagen production, and hence was considered to be one of the most frequent soft-tissue sarcomas. With the improvement in pathological techniques, many of these tumors have now been recognized to be other lesions such as malignant fibrohistiocytoma, schwannoma, fibromatosis, and others. Fibrosarcoma is now considered to be a relatively uncommon tumor.

Fibrosarcoma is a tumor of mesenchymal origin that is composed of malignant fibroblasts in a collagen stroma. These malignant lesions can occur as a primary or secondary bone tumor. Secondary fibrosarcomas are malignancies associated with risk factors such as prior radiation exposure, Paget's disease, neurofibromatosis, fibrous dysplasia, and osteomyelitis. When these pre-existing risk factors are absent these lesions are called primary fibrosarcomas. Symptoms of sinonasal fibrosarcoma are nonspecific, just like most other tumors in this anatomical location.[139,239]

Fibrosarcomas most often occur in the lower extremities in middle age adults. Approximately 2% to 10% of fibrosarcomas arise in the head and neck. Of this region, fibrosarcoma most commonly arises in the sinonasal cavities and neck. On CT, sinonasal fibrosarcomas enhance and display aggressive destruction of bone. On MR, these lesions display low to intermediate signal on T1-weighted and T2-weighted images. These imaging features are nonspecific and cannot be distinguished from the more common squamous cell carcinoma.

Fibrosarcomas of the sinonasal region has a very grim prognosis, with a reported 21% 5-year overall survival rate. Because of the rarity of these tumors and paucity of documented cases, treatment remains experimental, most often with multimodality regimens.[230,239,240]

Malignant Fibrous Histiocytoma

Of the head and neck region, the sinonasal cavities is the most common site of origin of fibrous histiocytomas, accounting for one-third of all cases. Most fibrous histiocytomas that arise in the soft tissues and bone are malignant. Malignant fibrous histiocytoma is a pleomorphic sarcoma characterized by partial fibroblastic and histiocytic differentiation. Malignant fibrous histiocytoma has five histologic subtypes: including storiform-pleomorphic, myxoid, inflammatory, giant cell, and angiomatoid. This neoplasm is now recognized as the most common soft-tissue sarcoma in adults. Most lesions arises de novo, however, malignant fibrous histiocytoma is considered to be one of the most common postirradiation-associated sarcomas.[139,177,241]

Malignant fibrous histiocytoma is most commonly located in the abdomen and extremities and only about 3% occur in the head and neck. In the head and neck, the most common location involved is the sinonasal tract. Sinonasal malignant fibrous histiocytoma is slightly more common in men (56%) with peak incidence in the sixth decade. Symptoms are nonspecific and are

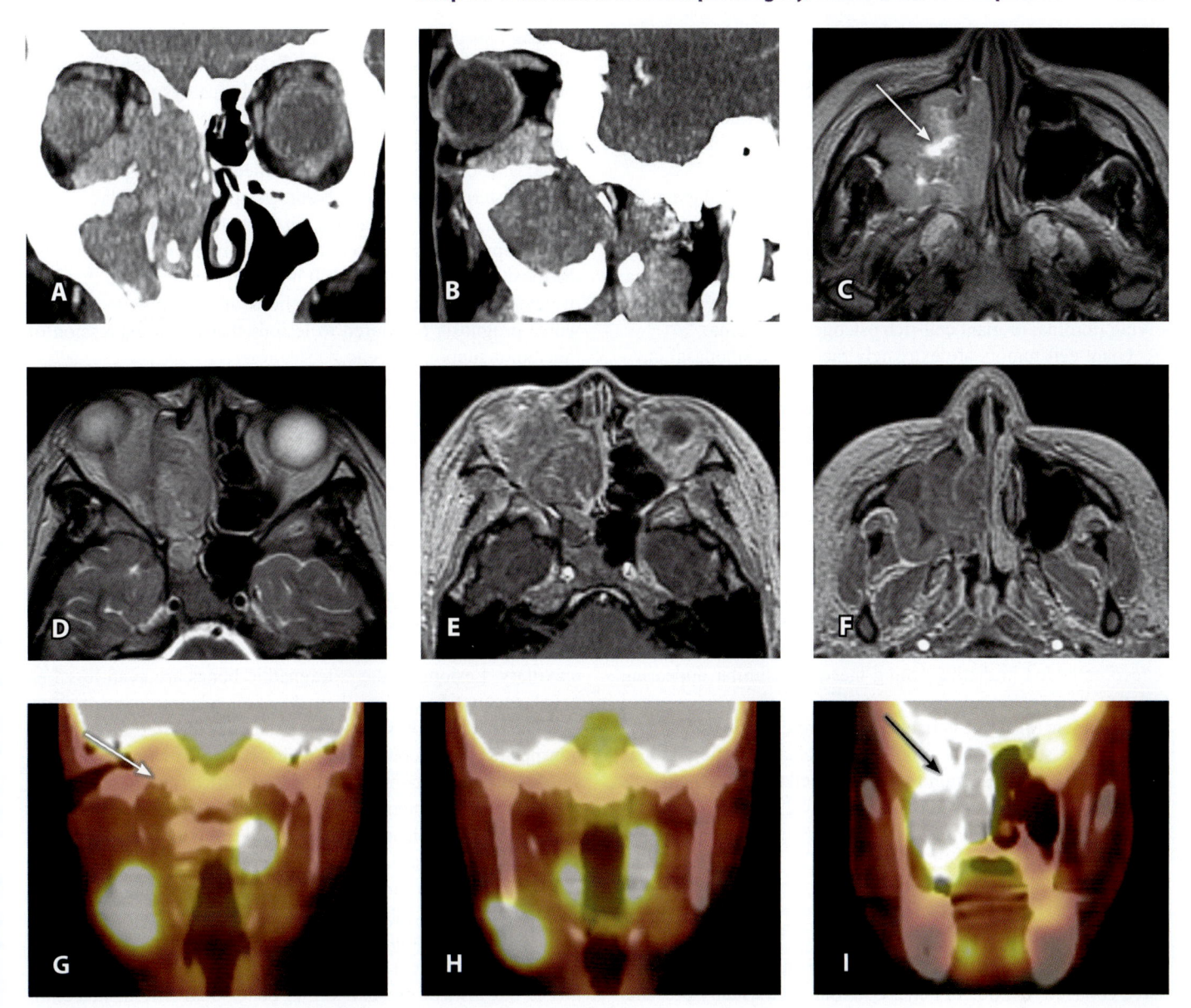

Chapter 4: Sinonasal Endoscopic Surgery, Infections and Neoplasms 185

Figure 4-44 Alveolar Rhabdomyosarcoma of the Sinonasal Cavity
Coronal and sagittal reformatted CECT images (**A–B**) show a large contiguous mass involving the right maxirry sinus, the right nasal cavity, the right ethoid sinus, and the right medial orbit. Axial T2 MR scans (**C–D**) show an intermediate-density tumor mass with slight central necrosis (*arrow,* **C**). Axial postcontrast MR images (**E–F**) show heterogeneous enhancement along all of the tumor margins. Coronal fused PET/CT images (**G–I**) show increased metabolic activity at the sight of the primary tumor (*arrow,* **I**). Also note increased activity in the right submandibular region due to secondary nodal metastasis (**G–H**).

similar to other locally aggressive tumors affecting this area, and include pain, epistaxis, and facial asymmetry.

The radiological features of malignant fibrous histiocytoma are nonspecific. On CT, bone remodeling and bone destruction can be observed, with moderate enhancement. On MR, they usually display low to intermediate intensity on T1-weighted images, and heterogeneous signal intensities on all T2-weighted images.

Sinonasal malignant fibrous histiocytoma has a poorer prognosis compared to other sites. The overall 5-year survival is 48% in the head and neck group compared to 77% for malignant fibrous histiocytoma of the trunk and extremities. Surgical excision is the treatment of choice. The complex anatomy of the sinonasal tract often limits adequate tumor free margins. Local recurrences are commonly observed, approximately 10% of patients develop cervical node metastases, while 30% develop systemic metastasis, most often to the lungs. Multimodality therapy is subsequently necessary due to these reasons.[200,241–243]

Osseous Malignancies

Giant Cell Tumor

Giant cell tumor is a relatively common skeletal tumor, accounting for 4% to 9.5% of all primary osseous neoplasms and 18% to 23% of benign bone neoplasms. These lesions most commonly occur in the third and fourth decades of life, with a female preponderance. Giant cell tumors are typically benign. However, multiple lesions have been described and can be associated with Paget's disease, while 5% to 10% of giant cell tumors may be malignant. The majority of these tumors are located in the long bones, and is very uncommon in the head and neck (<1%).[244,245]

Giant cell tumors contain a prominent osteoclastic giant cell component, however this feature may be present in many other lesions. Diagnosis requires radiologic correlation to exclude these other entities, such as giant cell reparative granuloma, osteoblastoma, chondroblastoma, aneurysmal bone cyst, nonossifying fibroma, or giant cell-rich osteogenic sarcoma.[244]

Giant cell tumors are extremely rare in the sinonasal cavities. Most reported cases involving the skull involve the sphenoid and temporal bones of the middle cranial fossa. On CT, the tumor displays as a lytic, homogeneous soft-tissue mass with moderate enhancement. Bone destruction and erosion may be present, whereas calcification is generally absent. On MR, the tumor displays a low to intermediate signal intensity on T1-weighted images and T2-weighted images, and enhance on postcontrast images. The brown tumor of hyperparathyroidism (giant cell reparative granuloma) can occur in the mandible and maxilla and has radiological features very similar to giant cell tumor. Obtaining calcium and parathyroid hormone levels is recommended in distinguishing these two similar appearing lesions.[244,246,247]

Treatment of giant cell tumor is surgical excision. Local recurrence is seen in 40% to 60% of marginal resection, and as low as 7% in wide resection for all giant cell tumors. Metastasis are infrequent, and occur in approximately 2% of cases. Malignant transformation is almost always associated with prior radiation treatment for giant cell tumor. Radiation therapy should be reserved only for inoperable tumors.[244,245]

Osteosarcoma

Osteosarcoma is a malignant neoplasm arising from undifferentiated connective tissue of bone. Osteosarcoma usually presents in the extremities, most frequently between the ages of 10 to 25 years. However, the average age of presentation for craniofacial osteosarcoma is about a decade later than osteosarcoma of the long bones. The exact cause of osteosarcoma is still undetermined. Several risk factors have been reported, including prior radiation exposure, Paget's disease, fibrous dysplasia, multiple osteochondromatosis, and osteomyelitis. When these risk factors are present, these lesions are called secondary osteosarcoma; and conversely, they are called primary osteosarcoma when these risk factors are absent. Osteosarcoma display a large variety of genetic alterations, in particular, mutations of the tumor-suppressor genes p53 and Rb (retinoblastoma) gene are the most frequently reported. It has been demonstrated that loss of heterozygosity or DNA alterations of the Rb gene confer a worse prognosis compared to lesions that retain expression of this tumor suppressor gene.[230,248,249]

Production of osteoid is a key feature of osteosarcoma, and distinguishes it from fibrosarcomas and chondrosarcomas. Osteosarcoma can present with a variety of matrix components, and these differences are reflected in the large numbers of histological subtypes that exist for this tumor, including, osteoblastic, chondroblastic, telangiectatic, fibroblastic, fibrohistiocytic, and round cell osteosarcomas.[226] Lesions in the craniofacial complex, account for fewer than 10% of osteosarcomas.

Craniofacial osteosarcoma constitutes only 9% of all cases. Of this region, the jaw is by far the most common site. Approximately 50% of craniofacial lesions are mandibular, and 25% are maxillary. Lesions in the extragnathic bones are even less frequent, accounting for less than 2% of all osteosarcomas.[226,248]

The clinical presentation of sinonasal osteosarcomas is nonspecific and depends on their anatomical location. Most sinonasal osteosarcomas present as a soft-tissue mass with or without bone destruction. On CT, the presence of tumor matrix mineralization, with aggressive bone destruction and soft-tissue extension, is strongly suggestive of osteosarcoma (**Fig. 4-45**). Radiological differentiation between osteosarcoma and chondrosarcoma can be difficult. Typically, chondrosarcoma have less bony destruction than osteosarcoma. Osteosarcoma may also have the typical "sunburst" periosteal reaction, although this is not always present. CT is better than MR in detecting tumor matrix mineralization and bony destruction and periosteal reaction. However, MR is superior in demonstrating tumor extension into soft tissue. Signal intensities may vary depending

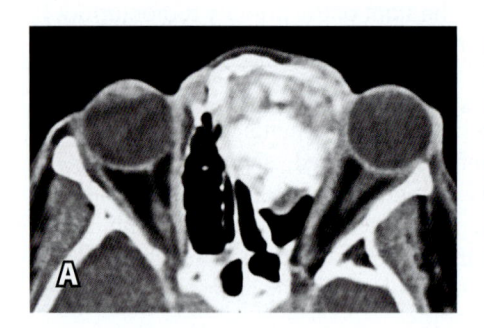

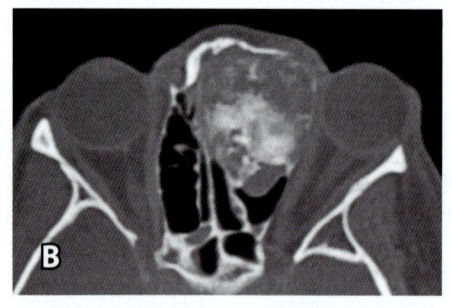

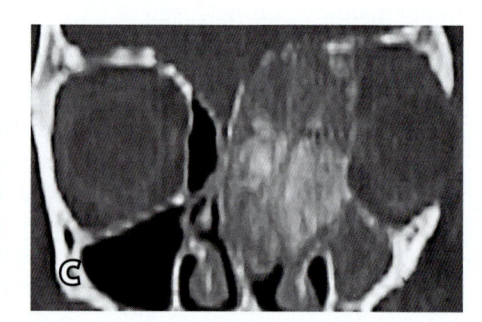

Figure 4-45 Osteosarcoma
Young boy presenting with left proptosis. Axial soft tissue (**A**), axial bone (**B**) and reconstructed coronal (**C**) CECT images show dense bony matrix within the left ethmoid air cells, expanding into the adjacent orbit and left side of the nasal cavity. The combination of mild enhancement and dense bony matrix is consistent with a tumor of fibro-osseous origin. Biopsy confirmed osteosarcoma.

on the bone content of the tumor. On MR, they usually display low signal intensity on T1-weighted images, and intermediate signal intensity on T2-weighted images.[248,250]

Most sinonasal osteosarcoma lesions present at an advanced stage and have a poor prognosis. The pattern of failure of osteosarcoma in the sinonasal cavities is different from that of the extremities. Historically, surgical resection with negative surgical margins was the treatment of choice for these lesions. Because of the difficulty in carrying out complete excisions in this anatomical region, local recurrences are commonly observed with surgery alone. Multimodality therapy is playing a major role in the treatment of these aggressive tumors and has resulted in improvements in overall and disease-free survival.[230,251,252]

Ewing Sarcoma

Ewing sarcoma most commonly arises in the skeleton of children and young adults. Ewing sarcoma has a peak incidence between 10 and 15 years of age and has a 1.5:1 male to female ratio. The most common locations are from the long bones, pelvis, and chest wall, and only arise in the head and neck region in 2% to 3% of all cases. The most common locations in the head and neck region are the mandible, maxilla, calvaria and cervical vertebrae. Sinonasal Ewing sarcoma is extremely rare, with only several cases of Ewing sarcoma in this location reported in the literature.[139,192,253,254]

Ewing sarcoma is a poorly differentiated small, round, blue cell tumor that is part of the peripheral primitive neuroectodermal tumors (PNET). PNET and Ewing sarcoma are associated with the t(11:22)(q24:q12) chromosomal translocation. The essential diagnostic test is the specific immunocytochemical CD99/013 marker. Ewing sarcoma is less differentiated from PNET, and this difference is what distinguishes it from PNET.

MR is the imaging modality of choice to evaluate the extent of the primary lesion, to monitor the response to neoadjuvant chemotherapy and to follow up nonresected Ewing sarcomas. On MR, Ewing sarcoma appears as a homogenous soft-tissue mass, displaying high signal on T2-weighted sequences. CT is useful for showing periosteal changes associated with Ewing sarcoma, but is limited in showing soft-tissue definition and tumor volume (Fig. 4-46). The rarity of a primary Ewing

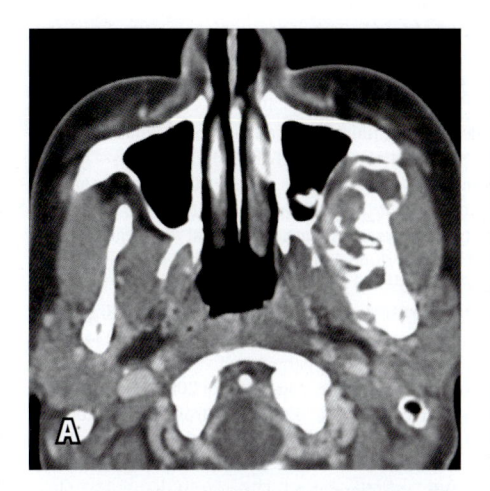

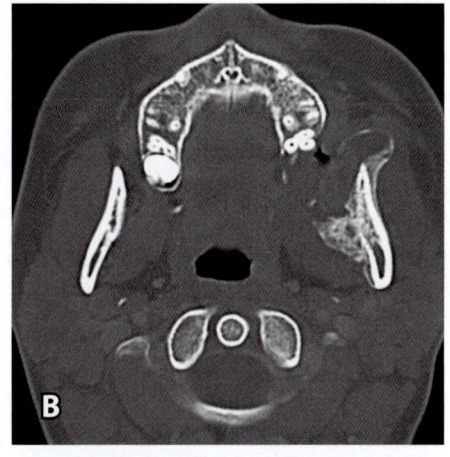

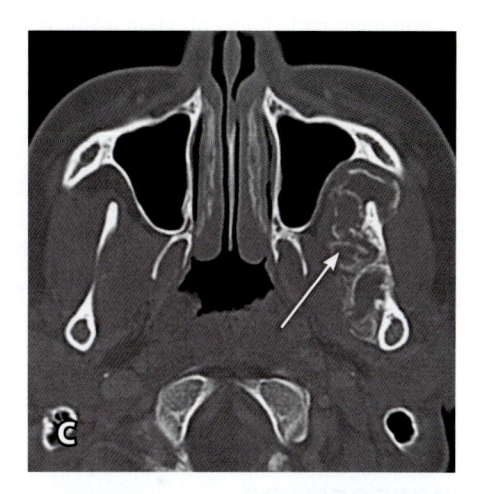

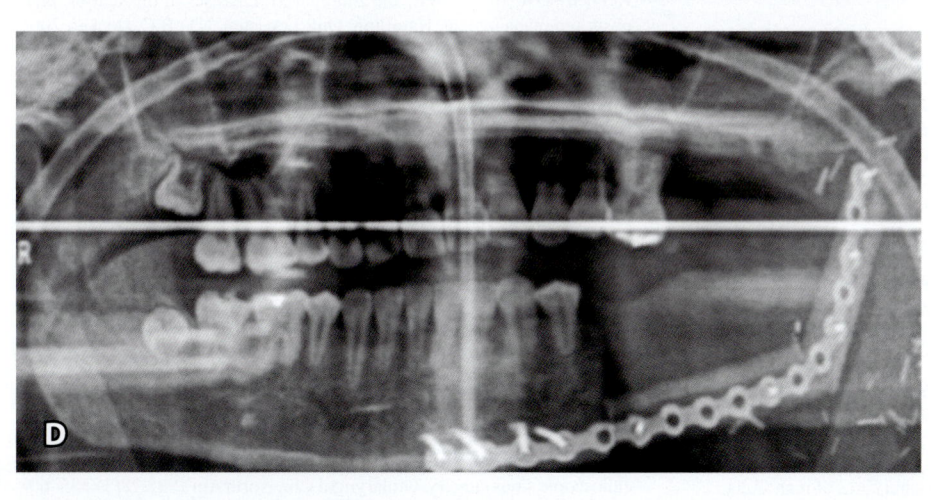

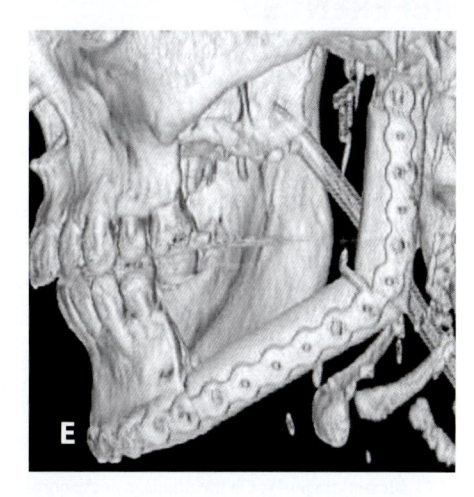

Figure 4-46 Ewing Sarcoma Pre- and Post-Op
Soft tissue (**A**) and axial bone (**B–C**) NECT images show an expansile, thin-walled osseous lesion originating from the ramus of the left mandible. The thinly expansile, bubbly lesions (*arrow*, **C**) may also be seen in aneurysmal bone cysts. Surgical resection confirmed the diagnosis of Ewing sarcoma. Wide spread excisions and ORIF surgical changes are visible in panorex (**D**) and 3D CT reconstruction with surface rendering (**E**).

sarcoma in the sinonasal cavities warrants a metastatic survey for a possible site of origin. Full-body MR has been shown to be more sensitive than skeletal scintigraphy, but less sensitive than positron emission tomography.[254–256]

Prognosis is mainly contingent on the presence or absence of metastasis upon presentation, age, location, and tumor volume. Patients free of metastasis have a 5-year survival around 55%, while those with metastasis are approximately 22%. In addition, tumors with lower volume have a better prognosis. Neoadjuvant chemotherapy followed by surgical excision is the treatment of choice. Radiotherapy is reserved for cases where adequate surgical excision is compromised.[257,258]

Odontogenic Malignancies

Malignant odontogenic tumors are quite rare, comprising only 1.6% odontogenic tumors. Malignant odontogenic tumors most commonly arise from transformation of a benign odontogenic tumor. Malignant odontogenic tumors include malignant ameloblastomas, ameloblastic carcinomas, primary intraosseous carcinomas, clear cell odontogenic carcinomas, malignant calcifying epithelial odontogenic tumors (Pindborg), odontogenic ghost cell carcinomas, and tumors of odontogenic mesenchymal origin.[179,259]

Diagnosis of these tumors may be complicated by the fact that they often histologically resemble their benign counterparts. In addition, diagnostic imaging of these tumors can be confused with benign odontogenic tumors for the following reasons: firstly, imaging is most often nonspecific; secondly, benign odontogenic lesions such as Pindborg and ameloblastoma can have aggressive extension features that may resemble malignant behavior. CT is useful to demonstrate bone erosion and displacement, while MR is effective in displaying soft-tissue extension.

The treatment of choice for malignant odontogenic tumors depends on the specific subtype, and for the most part requires multimodality therapy.

REFERENCES

1. Messerklinger W: Endoscopy of the nose. Baltimore: Urban & Schwarzenberg; 1978:180.
2. Wigand ME, Steiner W, and Jaumann MP: Endonasal sinus surgery with endoscopical control: from radical operation to rehabilitation of the mucosa. Endoscopy 1978;10(4):255–260.
3. Asai K, Haruna S, Otori N, et al.: Saccharin test of maxillary sinus mucociliary function after endoscopic sinus surgery. Laryngoscope 2000;110(1):117–122.
4. Elwany S, Hisham M, and Gamaee R: The effect of endoscopic sinus surgery on mucociliary clearance in patients with chronic sinusitis. Eur Arch Otorhinolaryngol 1998;255(10):511–514.
5. Min YG, Yun YS, Song BH, et al.: Recovery of nasal physiology after functional endoscopic sinus surgery: olfaction and mucociliary transport. ORL J Otorhinolaryngol Relat Spec 1995;57(5):264–268.
6. Becker SP: Anatomy for endoscopic sinus surgery. Otolaryngol Clin North Am 1989;22(4):677–682.
7. Messerklinger W: On the drainage of the normal frontal sinus of man. Acta Otolaryngol 1967;63(2):176–181.
8. Rice D: Endoscopic sinus surgery: Anterior approach. Oper Tech Otolaryngol Head Neck Surg 1990;(1):99–103.
9. Winther B and Gross C: Introduction and indications for functional endonasal (endoscopic) sinus surgery. Oper Tech Otolaryngol Head Neck Surg 1990;(1):92–93.
10. Moonis G: Imaging of sinonasal anatomy and inflammatory disorders. Crit Rev Comput Tomogr 2003;44(4):187–228.
11. Shankar L: An atlas of imaging of the paranasal sinuses. London/Philadelphia: Martin Dunitz; J.B. Lippincott 1994:208.
12. Giacchi RJ, Lebowitz RA, Yee HT, et al.: Histopathologic evaluation of the ethmoid bone in chronic sinusitis. Am J Rhinol 2001;15(3):193–197.
13. Kennedy DW, Senior BA, Gannon FH, et al.: Histology and histomorphometry of ethmoid bone in chronic rhinosinusitis. Laryngoscope 1998;108(4 Pt 1):502–507.
14. Penttila MA, Rautiainen ME, Pukander JS, et al.: Endoscopic versus Caldwell-Luc approach in chronic maxillary sinusitis: comparison of symptoms at one-year follow-up. Rhinology 1994;32(4):161–165.
15. Smith LF and Brindley PC: Indications, evaluation, complications, and results of functional endoscopic sinus surgery in 200 patients. Otolaryngol Head Neck Surg 1993;108(6):688–696.
16. Colclasure JC, Gross CW, and Kountakis SE: Endoscopic sinus surgery in patients older than sixty. Otolaryngol Head Neck Surg 2004;131(6):946–949.
17. Dalziel K, Stein K, Round A, et al.: Systematic review of endoscopic sinus surgery for nasal polyps. Health Technol Assess 2003;7(17):iii,1–159.
18. Senior BA, Kennedy DW, Tanabodee J, et al.: Long-term results of functional endoscopic sinus surgery. Laryngoscope 1998;108(2):151–157.
19. Lieser JD and Derkay CS: Pediatric sinusitis: when do we operate? Curr Opin Otolaryngol Head Neck Surg 2005;13(1):60–66.
20. Bothwell MR, Piccirillo JF, Lusk RP, et al.: Long-term outcome of facial growth after functional endoscopic sinus surgery. Otolaryngol Head Neck Surg 2002;126(6):628–634.
21. Senior B, Wirtschafter A, Mai C, et al.: Quantitative impact of pediatric sinus surgery on facial growth. Laryngoscope 2000;110(11):1866–1870.
22. Zeifer B: Sinusitis: postoperative changes and surgical complications. Semin Ultrasound CT MR 2002;23(6):475–491.
23. Chen MC and Davidson TM: Clinical evaluation of postoperative sinonasal surgical patients. Semin Ultrasound CT MR 2002;23(6):466–474.
24. Setliff RC, IIIrd: Minimally invasive sinus surgery: the rationale and the technique. Otolaryngol Clin North Am 1996;29(1):115–124.
25. Chiu AG and Kennedy DW: Disadvantages of minimal techniques for surgical management of chronic rhinosinusitis. Curr Opin Otolaryngol Head Neck Surg 2004;12(1):38–42.
26. Catalano PJ: Minimally invasive sinus technique: what is it? Should we consider it? Curr Opin Otolaryngol Head Neck Surg 2004;12(1):34–37.
27. Catalano P and Roffman E: Outcome in patients with chronic sinusitis after the minimally invasive sinus technique. Am J Rhinol 2003;17(1):17–22.
28. Hosemann W, Kühnel T, Held P, et al.: Endonasal frontal sinusotomy in surgical management of chronic sinusitis: a critical evaluation. Am J Rhinol 1997;11(1):1–9.
29. Kennedy DW, Bolger WE, and Zinreich SJ: Diseases of the sinuses: diagnosis and management. Hamilton, Ont./Lewiston, NY: B.C. Decker; 2001: xvii, 430.
30. Kennedy DW: Prognostic factors, outcomes and staging in ethmoid sinus surgery. Laryngoscope 1992;102(12 Pt 2 Suppl 57):1–18.
31. Levine HL: Functional endoscopic sinus surgery: evaluation, surgery, and follow-up of 250 patients. Laryngoscope 1990;100(1):79–84.
32. Stammberger H: Endoscopic endonasal surgery: concepts in treatment of recurring rhinosinusitis. Part II. Surgical technique. Otolaryngol Head Neck Surg 1986;94(2):147–156.
33. Cumberworth VL, Sudderick RM, and Mackay IS: Major complications of functional endoscopic sinus surgery. Clin Otolaryngol Allied Sci 1994;19(3):248–253.
34. Kennedy DW, Shaman P, Han W, et al.: Complications of ethmoidectomy: a survey of fellows of the American Academy of Otolaryngology-Head and Neck Surgery. Otolaryngol Head Neck Surg 1994;111(5):589–599.
35. Lusk R: Computer-assisted functional endoscopic sinus surgery in children. Otolaryngol Clin North Am 2005;38(3):505–513, vii.
36. Oliverio PJ, Benson ML, and Zinreich SJ: Update on imaging for functional endoscopic sinus surgery. Otolaryngol Clin North Am 1995;28(3):585–608.
37. May M, Levine HL, Mester SJ, et al.: Complications of endoscopic sinus surgery: analysis of 2108 patients–incidence and prevention. Laryngoscope 1994;104(9):1080–1083.
38. Clatterbuck R and Tamargo R: Intracranial emergencies. In: Eisele DW and McQuone SJ, eds. Emergencies of the Head and Neck. St. Louis: Mosby; 2000:4400–4403.

39. Laine FJ, Conway WF, and Laskin DM: Radiology of maxillofacial trauma. Curr Probl Diagn Radiol 1993;22(4):145–188.
40. Luka B, Brechtelsbauer D, Gellrich NC, et al.: 2D and 3D CT reconstructions of the facial skeleton: an unnecessary option or a diagnostic pearl? Int J Oral Maxillofac Surg 1995;24(1 Pt 2):76–83.
41. Manson PN, Markowitz B, Mirvis S, et al.: Toward CT-based facial fracture treatment. Plast Reconstr Surg 1990;85(2):202–214.
42. Novelline RA, Rhea JT, Rao PM, et al.: Helical CT in emergency radiology. Radiology 1999;213(2):321–339.
43. Salvolini U: Traumatic injuries: imaging of facial injuries. Eur Radiol 2002;12(6):1253–1261.
44. Kassel EE, Noyek AM, and Cooper PW: CT in facial trauma. J Otolaryngol 1983;12(1):2–15.
45. Noyek AM, Kassel EE, Wortzman G, et al.: Contemporary radiologic evaluation in maxillofacial trauma. Otolaryngol Clin North Am 1983;16(3):473–508.
46. Linnau KF, Stanley RB Jr, Hallam DK, et al.: Imaging of high-energy midfacial trauma: what the surgeon needs to know. Eur J Radiol 2003;48(1):17–32.
47. Buitrago-Tellez CH, Schilli W, Bohnert M, et al.: A comprehensive classification of craniofacial fractures: postmortem and clinical studies with two- and three-dimensional computed tomography. Injury 2002;33(8):651–668.
48. Cavalcanti MG, Haller JW, and Vannier MW: Three-dimensional computed tomography landmark measurement in craniofacial surgical planning: experimental validation in vitro. J Oral Maxillofac Surg 1999;57(6):690–694.
49. Brenner D, Elliston C, Hall E, et al.: Estimated risks of radiation-induced fatal cancer from pediatric CT. Am J Roentgenol 2001;176(2):289–296.
50. Hodgkinson DW, Lloyd RE, Driscoll PA, et al.: ABC of emergency radiology. Maxillofacial radiographs. BMJ 1994;308(6920):46–51.
51. Moos KF: Diagnosis of facial bone fractures. Ann R Coll Surg Engl 2002;84(6):429–431.
52. Surgical-tutor.org.uk: Facial and orbital fractures. 2009 25 January 2009 [cited 2009 30 January 2009]; Available from: http://www.surgical-tutor.org.uk/default-home.htm?core/trauma/facial_fractures.htm~right.
53. Swinson B and Lloyd T: Management of maxillofacial injuries. Hosp Med 2003;64(2):72–78.
54. Widell T: Fracture, face. 2009 6 Mar 6 2008 [cited 2009 30 January]; Available from: http://emedicine.medscape.com/article/824743-overview.
55. Richardson M: Facial and mandibular fractures 2009 [cited 2009 30 January]; Available from: http://www.rad.washington.edu/academics/academic-sections/msk/teaching-materials/online-musculoskeletal-radiology-book/facial-and-mandibular-fractures.
56. Dolan KD and Jacoby CG: Facial fractures. Semin Roentgenol 1978;13(1):37–51.
57. Kim D and Tawfilis A: Facial trauma, maxillary and Le Fort fractures. 2005 [cited 2005]; Available from: http://www.emedicine.com/plastic/topic481.htm.
58. Le Fort R: Etude Experimentale sur les fractures de la machoire superieure. Rev Chir Paris 1901;(23):208–227.
59. Manson PN: Some thoughts on the classification and treatment of Le Fort fractures. Ann Plast Surg 1986;17(5):356–363.
60. Donat TL, Endress C, and Mathog RH: Facial fracture classification according to skeletal support mechanisms. Arch Otolaryngol Head Neck Surg 1998;124(12):1306–1314.
61. Manson PN, Hoopes JE, and Su CT: Structural pillars of the facial skeleton: an approach to the management of Le Fort fractures. Plast Reconstr Surg 1980;66(1):54–62.
62. Rhea JT and Novelline RA: How to simplify the CT diagnosis of Le Fort fractures. Am J Roentgenol 2005;184(5):1700–1705.
63. Signs and symptoms of Le Fort fractures. 12/01/07 [cited 2009 30 January]; Available from: http://www.maxfaxsho.co.uk/index_files/Page4472.htm.
64. Gillespie James E and Gholkar A: Magnetic resonance imaging and computed tomography of the head and neck. 1st ed. New York: Chapman & Hall Medical, 1994:6, 233.
65. Som PM and Curtin HD: Head and neck imaging. 4th ed. St. Louis. MO: Mosby, 2003:xvi, 2322, 2357.
66. Muraoka M and Nakai Y: Twenty years of statistics and observation of facial bone fracture. Acta Otolaryngol Suppl 1998;538:261–265.
67. Arden RL and Crumley RL: Cartilage grafts in open rhinoplasty. Facial Plast Surg 1993;9(4):285–294.
68. Brawley BW and Kelly WA: Treatment of basal skull fractures with and without cerebrospinal fluid fistulae. J Neurosurg 1967;26(1):57–61.
69. Stanley RB, Jr. and Nowak GM: Midfacial fractures: importance of angle of impact to horizontal craniofacial buttresses. Otolaryngol Head Neck Surg 1985;93(2):186–192.
70. Stanley RB Jr.: Use of intraoperative computed tomography during repair of orbitozygomatic fractures. Arch Facial Plast Surg 1999;1(1):19–24.
71. Ellis E, IIIrd, el-Attar A, and Moos KF: An analysis of 2,067 cases of zygomatico-orbital fracture. J Oral Maxillofac Surg 1985;43(6):417–428.
72. Katzen JT, Jarrahy R, Eby JB, et al.: Craniofacial and skull base trauma. J Trauma 2003;54(5):1026–1034.
73. Marin MI, Tejero TR, Dominguez FM, et al.: Ocular injuries in midfacial fractures. Orbit 1998;17(1):41–46.
74. Smith B and Regan WF Jr.: Blow-out fracture of the orbit: mechanism and correction of internal orbital fracture. Am J Ophthalmol 1957;44(6):733–739.
75. Koornneef L and Zonneveld FW: The role of direct multiplanar high resolution CT in the assessment and management of orbital trauma. Radiol Clin North Am 1987;25(4):753–766.
76. Long J and Tann T: Orbital trauma. Ophthalmol Clin North Am 2002;15(2):249–253, viii.
77. Kwon JH, Moon JH, Kwon MS, et al.: The differences of blowout fracture of the inferior orbital wall between children and adults. Arch Otolaryngol Head Neck Surg 2005;131(8):723–727.
78. Chrcanovic BR, Freire-Maia B, Souza LN, et al.: Facial fractures: a 1-year retrospective study in a hospital in Belo Horizonte. Braz Oral Res 2004;18(4):322–328.
79. Fridrich KL, Pena-Velasco G, and Olson RA: Changing trends with mandibular fractures: a review of 1,067 cases. J Oral Maxillofac Surg 1992;50(6):586–589.
80. Tawfilis A and Byrne P: Facial trauma, mandibular fractures. 2006 [cited 2006; Available from: http://www.emedicine.com/plastic/topic227.htm.
81. Ellis E, IIIrd, Moos KF, and el-Attar A: Ten years of mandibular fractures: an analysis of 2,137 cases. Oral Surg Oral Med Oral Pathol 1985;59(2):120–129.
82. King RE, Scianna JM, and Petruzzelli GJ: Mandible fracture patterns: a suburban trauma center experience. Am J Otolaryngol 2004;25(5):301–307.
83. Ogundare BO, Bonnick A, and Bayley N: Pattern of mandibular fractures in an urban major trauma center. J Oral Maxillofac Surg 2003;61(6):713–718.
84. Loukota RA, Eckelt U, De Bont L, et al.: Subclassification of fractures of the condylar process of the mandible. Br J Oral Maxillofac Surg 2005;43(1):72–73.
85. Fulmer JM and SE Harms: The temporomandibular joint. Top Magn Reson Imaging 1989;1(3):75–84.
86. Hermans R, Van der Goten A, De Foer B, et al.: Imaging of maxillo-facial trauma. J Belge Radiol 1997;80(1):25–29.
87. Rak KM, Newell JD IInd, Yakes WF, et al.: Paranasal sinuses on MR images of the brain: significance of mucosal thickening. AJR Am J Roentgenol 1991;156(2):381–384.
88. Sievers KW, Greess H, Baum U, et al.: Paranasal sinuses and nasopharynx CT and MRI. Eur J Radiol 2000;33(3):185–202.
89. Som PM, Shapiro MD, Biller HF, et al.: Sinonasal tumors and inflammatory tissues: differentiation with MR imaging. Radiology 1988;167(3):803–808.
90. Zinreich SJ, Kennedy DW, Kumar AJ, et al.: MR imaging of normal nasal cycle: comparison with sinus pathology. J Comput Assist Tomogr 1988;12(6):1014–1019.
91. Hasso A and Vignaud J: Pathology of the paranasal sinuses, nasal cavity and facial bones. In: Newton TH, Hasso AN, and Dillon WP, eds. Computed tomography of the head and neck. New York: Raven Press; 1988:7.1–7.31.
92. Lanzieri CF, Shah M, Krauss D, et al.: Use of gadolinium-enhanced MR imaging for differentiating mucoceles from neoplasms in the paranasal sinuses. Radiology 1991;178(2):425–428.
93. Van Tassel P, Lee YY, Jing BS, et al.: Mucoceles of the paranasal sinuses: MR imaging with CT correlation. Am J Roentgenol 1989;153(2):407–412.
94. Som PM, Dillon WP, Curtin HD, et al.: Hypointense paranasal sinus foci: differential diagnosis with MR imaging and relation to CT findings. Radiology 1990;176(3):777–781.
95. Som PM, Som PM, Dillon WP, et al.: Chronically obstructed sinonasal secretions: observations on T1 and T2 shortening. Radiology 1989;172(2):515–520.
96. Dillon WP, Som PM, and Fullerton GD: Hypointense MR signal in chronically inspissated sinonasal secretions. Radiology 1990;174(1):73–78.
97. Som P and Curtin H: Sinuses. In: Stark DD and Bradley WG, eds. Magnetic resonance imaging. St. Louis: Mosby-Year Book, 1992:1113–1134.

98. Klapper SR and Patrinely JR: Orbital involvement in allergic fungal sinusitis. Ophthal Plast Reconstr Surg 2001;17(2):149–151.
99. Manning SC, Merkel M, Kriesel K, et al.: Computed tomography and magnetic resonance diagnosis of allergic fungal sinusitis. Laryngoscope 1997;107(2):170–176.
100. Yousem DM, Galetta Sl, Gusnard DA, et al.: MR findings in rhinocerebral mucormycosis. J Comput Assist Tomogr 1989;13(5):878–882.
101. Press GA, Weindling SM, Hesselink JR, et al.: Rhinocerebral mucormycosis: MR manifestations. J Comput Assist Tomogr 1988;12(5):744–749.
102. Zinreich SJ, Kennedy DW, Malat J, et al.: Fungal sinusitis: diagnosis with CT and MR imaging. Radiology 1988;169(2):439–444.
103. Harril WC, Stewart MG, Lee AG, et al.: Chronic rhinocerebral mucormycosis. Laryngoscope 1996;106(10):1292–1297.
104. Som PM, Lawson W, and Lidov MW: Simulated aggressive skull base erosion in response to benign sinonasal disease. Radiology 1991;180(3):755–759.
105. Hoffman GS, Kerr GS, Leavitt RY, et al.: Wegener granulomatosis: an analysis of 158 patients. Ann Intern Med 1992;116(6):488–498.
106. Provenzale JM and Allen NB: Wegener granulomatosis: CT and MR findings. Am J Neuroradiol 1996;17(4):785–792.
107. Georgiades CS, Neyman EG, and Fishman EK: Cross-sectional imaging of amyloidosis: an organ system-based approach. J Comput Assist Tomogr 2002;26(6):1035–1041.
108. Kim HY, Im JG, Song KS, et al.: Localized amyloidosis of the respiratory system: CT features. J Comput Assist Tomogr 1999;23(4):627–631.
109. Kondo M, Horiuchi M, Shiga H, et al.: Computed tomography of malignant tumors of the nasal cavity and paranasal sinuses. Cancer 1982;50(2):226–231.
110. Som PM, Shugar JM, and Biller HF: The early detection of antral malignancy in the postmaxillectomy patient. Radiology 1982;143(2):509–512.
111. Luce D, Leclerc A, Bégin D, et al.: Sinonasal cancer and occupational exposures: a pooled analysis of 12 case-control studies. Cancer Causes Control 2002;13(2):147–157.
112. Hasso AN and Vignaud J: Computed and conventional tomography of the paranasal sinuses. In: Littleton JT and Durizch ML, eds. Sectional imaging methods: a comparison. Baltimore: University Park Press, 1983:xx, 402.
113. Carrillo JF, Güemes A, Ramírez-Ortega MC, et al.: Prognostic factors in maxillary sinus and nasal cavity carcinoma. Eur J Surg Oncol 2005;31(10):1206–1212.
114. Porceddu S, Martin J, Shanker G, et al.: Paranasal sinus tumors: Peter MacCallum Cancer Institute experience. Head Neck 2004;26(4):322–330.
115. Lenz M: Computed tomography and magnetic resonance imaging of head and neck tumors: methods, guidelines, differential diagnoses, and clinical results. New York: Georg Thieme Verlag/Thieme Medical Publishers, 1993:8, 206.
116. Chong VF, Fan YF, Khoo JB, et al.: Comparing computed tomographic and magnetic resonance imaging visualisation of the pterygopalatine fossa in nasopharyngeal carcinoma. Ann Acad Med Singapore 1995;24(3):436–441.
117. Nemzek WR, Hecht S, Gandour-Edwards R, et al.: Perineural spread of head and neck tumors: how accurate is MR imaging? Am J Neuroradiol 1998;19(4):701–706.
118. Batsakis JG: Tumors of the head and neck: clinical and pathological considerations, 2nd ed. Baltimore: Williams & Wilkins, 1979:30–34,78–79, 177–187.
119. Conley J and Dingman DL: Adenoid cystic carcinoma in the head and neck (cylindroma). Arch Otolaryngol 1974;100(2):81–90.
120. Ballantyne AJ, McCarten AB, and Ibanez ML: The extension of cancer of the head and neck through peripheral nerves. Am J Surg 1963;106:651–667.
121. Dodd GD, Dolan PA, Ballantyne AJ, et al.: The dissemination of tumors of the head and neck via the cranial nerves. Radiol Clin North Am 1970;8(3):445–461.
122. Laccourreye O, N Bély, P Halimi, et al.: Cavernous sinus involvement from recurrent adenoid cystic carcinoma. Ann Otol Rhinol Laryngol 1994;103(10):822–825.
123. Laine FJ, Braun IF, Jensen ME, et al.: Perineural tumor extension through the foramen ovale: evaluation with MR imaging. Radiology 1990;174(1):65–71.
124. Catalano PJ, Sen C, and Biller HF: Cranial neuropathy secondary to perineural spread of cutaneous malignancies. Am J Otol 1995;16(6):772–777.
125. Ginsberg LE, De Monte F, and Gillenwater AM: Greater superficial petrosal nerve: anatomy and MR findings in perineural tumor spread. Am J Neuroradiol 1996;17(2):389–393.
126. Blandino A, Gaeta M, Minutoli F, et al.: CT and MR findings in neoplastic perineural spread along the vidian nerve. Eur Radiol 2000;10(3):521–526.
127. Tang T and Lee Y: CT and MR imaging evaluation of adenoid cystic carcinoma of the head and neck: emphasis on its perineural extension. Radiology 1995;197(Suppl P):173.
128. van Olphen AF, Lubsen H, and van't Verlaat JW: An inverted papilloma with intracranial extension. J Laryngol Otol 1988;102(6):534-537.
129. Fernandez JM, Santaolalla F, Del Rey AS, et al.: Preliminary study of the lymphatic drainage system of the nose and paranasal sinuses and its role in detection of sentinel metastatic nodes. Acta Otolaryngol 2005;125(5):566–570.
130. Nason RW, Torchia MG, Morales CM, et al.: Dynamic MR lymphangiography and carbon dye for sentinel lymph node detection: a solution for sentinel lymph node biopsy in mucosal head and neck cancer. Head Neck 2005;27(4):333–338.
131. Yen TC, Chang JT, Ng SH, et al.: Staging of untreated squamous cell carcinoma of buccal mucosa with 18F-FDG PET: comparison with head and neck CT/MRI and histopathology. J Nucl Med 2005;46(5):775–781.
132. Batsakis JG: The pathology of head and neck tumors: the occult primary and metastases to the head and neck, Part 10. Head Neck Surg 1981;3(5):409–423.
133. Lubsen H: Squamous hyperplasia of the larynx and inverted papilloma of the nose and paranasal sinuses. Thesis, Amsterdam: Free University Amsterdam, 1980.
134. Abildgaard-Jensen J and Greisen O: Inverted papillomas of the nose and the paranasal sinuses. Clin Otolaryngol Allied Sci 1985;10(3):135–143.
135. Hyams V: Papillomas of the nasal cavity and paranasal sinuses: a clinicopathologic study of 315 cases. Ann Otol Rhinol Laryngol 1971;80:192–206.
136. Hirai S, Matsumoto T, and Suda K: Pleomorphic adenoma in nasal cavity: immunohistochemical study of three cases. Auris Nasus Larynx 2002;29(3):291–295.
137. Motoori K, Takano H, Nakano K, et al.: Pleomorphic adenoma of the nasal septum: MR features. Am J Neuroradiol 2000;21(10):1948–1950.
138. Jackson LE and Rosenberg SI: Pleomorphic adenoma of the lateral nasal wall. Otolaryngol Head Neck Surg 2002;127(5):474–476.
139. Barnes L: Surgical pathology of the head and neck, 2nd ed. New York: M. Dekker; 2001.
140. Beranek JT and Masseyeff R: Hyperplastic capillaries and their possible involvement in the pathogenesis of fibrosis. Histopathology 1986;10(5):543–551.
141. Schick B and Kahle G: Radiological findings in angiofibroma. Acta Radiol 2000;41(6):585–593.
142. Ungkanont K, Byers RM, Weber RS, et al.: Juvenile nasopharyngeal angiofibroma: an update of therapeutic management. Head Neck 1996;18(1):60–66.
143. Cummings CW: Otolaryngology—head and neck surgery, 3rd ed. St. Louis: Mosby Year Book, 1998:1514.
144. Hosseini SM, et al.: Angiofibroma: an outcome review of conventional surgical approaches. Eur Arch Otorhinolaryngol 2005;262(10):807–812.
145. Buob D, Wacrenier A, Chevalier D, et al.: Schwannoma of the sinonasal tract: a clinicopathologic and immunohistochemical study of 5 cases. Arch Pathol Lab Med 2003;127(9):1196–1199.
146. Heffner DK and Gnepp DR: Sinonasal fibrosarcomas, malignant schwannomas, and "Triton" tumors. A clinicopathologic study of 67 cases. Cancer 1992;70(5):1089–1101.
147. Lin J and Martel W: Cross-sectional imaging of peripheral nerve sheath tumors: characteristic signs on CT, MR imaging, and sonography. Am J Roentgenol 2001;176(1):75–82.
148. Quesada JL, et al.: Sinonasal schwannoma treated with endonasal microsurgery. Otolaryngol Head Neck Surg 2003;129(3):300–302.
149. Khong PL, et al.: MR imaging of spinal tumors in children with neurofibromatosis 1. Am J Roentgenol 2003;180(2):413–417.
150. Wise JB, et al.: Management of head and neck plexiform neurofibromas in pediatric patients with neurofibromatosis type 1. Arch Otolaryngol Head Neck Surg 2005;131(8):712–718.
151. Arazi-Kleinmann T, et al.: Neurofibromatosis diagnosed on CT with MR correlation. Eur J Radiol 2002;42(1):69–73.
152. Visrutaratna P, Oranratanachai K, and Singhavejsakul J: Clinics in diagnostic imaging (96). Plexiform neurofi bromatosis. Singapore Med J 2004;45(4):188–192.

153. Daneshi A, Asghari A, and Bahramy E: Primary meningioma of the ethmoid sinus: a case report. Ear Nose Throat J 2003;82(4):310–311.
154. Jovanovic MB, et al.: Huge extracranial asymptomatic frontal invasive meningioma: a case report. Eur Arch Otorhinolaryngol 2006;263(3):223–227.
155. Maiuri F, et al.: Olfactory groove meningioma with paranasal sinus and nasal cavity extension: removal by combined subfrontal and nasal approach. J Craniomaxillofac Surg 1998;26(5):314–317.
156. Swain RE, Jr., et al.: Meningiomas of the paranasal sinuses. Am J Rhinol 2001;15(1):27–30.
157. Weingarten K, et al.: Detection of residual or recurrent meningioma after surgery: value of enhanced vs unenhanced MR imaging. Am J Roentgenol 1992;158(3):645–650.
158. Huang HM, Liu CM, Lin KN, et al.: Giant ethmoid osteoma with orbital extension, a nasoendoscopic approach using an intranasal drill. Laryngoscope 2001;111(3):430–432.
159. Sayan NB, Uçok C, Karasu HA, et al.: Peripheral osteoma of the oral and maxillofacial region: a study of 35 new cases. J Oral Maxillofac Surg 2002;60(11):1299–1301.
160. Lin CJ, Lin YS, and Kang BH: Middle turbinate osteoma presenting with ipsilateral facial pain, epiphora, and nasal obstruction. Otolaryngol Head Neck Surg 2003;128(2):282–283.
161. Jones K and Korzcak P: The diagnostic significance and management of Gardner's syndrome. Br J Oral Maxillofac Surg 1990;28(2):80–84.
162. Richardson P, Arendt DM, Fidler JE, et al.: Radioopaque mass in the submandibular region. J Oral Maxillofac Surg 1999;57:709–713.
163. Kendi AT, Kara S, Altinok D, et al.: Sinonasal ossifying fibroma with fluid-fluid levels on MR images. Am J Neuroradiol 2003;24(8):1639–1641.
164. Som PM and Lidov M: The benign fibroosseous lesion: its association with paranasal sinus mucoceles and its MR appearance. J Comput Assist Tomogr 1992;16(6):871–876.
165. Ikeda K, Suzuki H, Oshima T, et al.: Endonasal endoscopic management in fibrous dysplasia of the paranasal sinuses. Am J Otolaryngol 1997;18(6):415–418.
166. Marvel JB, Marsh MA, and Catlin FI: Ossifying fibroma of the midface and paranasal sinuses: diagnostic and therapeutic considerations. Otolaryngol Head Neck Surg 1991;104(6):803–808.
167. Tobey JD, Loevner LA, Yousem DM, et al.: Tension pneumocephalus: a complication of invasive ossifying fibroma of the paranasal sinuses. Am J Roentgenol 1996;166(3):711–713.
168. Engelbrecht V, Preis S, Hassler W, et al.: CT and MRI of congenital sinonasal ossifying fibroma. Neuroradiology 1999;41(7):526–529.
169. Sterling KM, Stollman A, Sacher M, et al.: Ossifying fibroma of sphenoid bone with coexistent mucocele: CT and MRI. J Comput Assist Tomogr 1993;17(3):492–494.
170. Post G and Kountakis SE: Endoscopic resection of large sinonasal ossifying fibroma. Am J Otolaryngol 2005;26(1):54–56.
171. Chong VF and Tan LH: Maxillary sinus ossifying fibroma. Am J Otolaryngol 1997;18(6):419–424.
172. Williams HK, Mangham C, and Speight PM: Juvenile ossifying fibroma. An analysis of eight cases and a comparison with other fibroosseous lesions. J Oral Pathol Med 2000;29(1):13–18.
173. Khoury NJ, Naffaa LN, Shabb NS, et al.: Juvenile ossifying fibroma: CT and MR findings. Eur Radiol 2002;12(Suppl 3):S109–S113.
174. Kuta AJ, Worley CM, and Kaugars GE: Central cementoossifying fibroma of the maxillary sinus: a review of six cases. Am J Neuroradiol 1995;16(6):1282–1286.
175. Yonetsu K and Nakamura T: CT of calcifying jaw bone diseases. Am J Roentgenol 2001;177(4):937–943.
176. Zama M, Gallo S, Santecchia L, et al.: Juvenile active ossifying fibroma with massive involvement of the mandible. Plast Reconstr Surg 2004;113(3):970–974.
177. Damjanov I and Linder J: Anderson's pathology, 10th ed. St. Louis, MI: Mosby; 1996:2490.
178. Bertario L, Russo A, Sala P, et al.: Genotype and phenotype factors as determinants of desmoid tumors in patients with familial adenomatous polyposis. Int J Cancer 2001;95(2):102–107.
179. Mendenhall WM, Zlotecki RA, Morris CG, et al.: Aggressive fibromatosis. Am J Clin Oncol 2005;28(2):211–215.
180. Buitendijk S, van de Ven CP, Dumans TG, et al.: Pediatric aggressive fibromatosis: a retrospective analysis of 13 patients and review of literature. Cancer 2005;104(5):1090–1099.
181. Tanaka H, Harasawa A, and Furui S: Usefulness of MR imaging in assessment of tumor extent of aggressive fibromatosis. Radiat Med 2005;23(2):111–115.
182. Nakamura N, Higuchi Y, Mitsuyasu T, et al.: Comparison of long-term results between different approaches to ameloblastoma. Oral Surg Oral Med Oral Pathol Oral Radiol Endod 2002;93(1):13–20.
183. Schafer DR, Thompson LD, Smith BC, et al.: Primary ameloblastoma of the sinonasal tract: a clinicopathologic study of 24 cases. Cancer 1998;82(4):667–674.
184. Minami M, Kaneda T, Ozawa K, et al.: Cystic lesions of the maxillomandibular region: MR imaging distinction of odontogenic keratocysts and ameloblastomas from other cysts. Am J Roentgenol 1996;166(4):943–949.
185. Minami M, Kaneda T, Yamamoto H, et al.: Ameloblastoma in the maxillomandibular region: MR imaging. Radiology 1992;184(2):389–393.
186. Weissman JL, Snyderman CH, Yousem SA, et al.: Ameloblastoma of the maxilla: CT and MR appearance. Am J Neuroradiol 1993;14(1):223–226.
187. Franklin CD and Pindborg JJ: The calcifying epithelial odontogenic tumor. A review and analysis of 113 cases. Oral Surg Oral Med Oral Pathol 1976;42(6):753–765.
188. Ching AS, Pak MW, Kew J, et al.: CT and MR imaging appearances of an extraosseous calcifying epithelial odontogenic tumor (Pindborg tumor). Am J Neuroradiol 2000;21(2):343–345.
189. Cross JJ, Pilkington RJJ, Antoun NM, et al.: Value of computed tomography and magnetic resonance imaging in the treatment of a calcifying epithelial odontogenic (Pindborg) tumour. Br J Oral Maxillofac Surg 2000;38(2):154–157.
190. Veness MJ, Morgan G, Collins AP, et al.: Calcifying epithelial odontogenic (Pindborg) tumor with malignant transformation and metastatic spread. Head Neck 2001;23(8):692–696.
191. Stout AP: Myxoma, the tumor of primitive mesenchyme. Ann Surg 1948;127(4):706–719.
192. Chiodo AA, Strumas N, Gilbert RW, et al.: Management of odontogenic myxoma of the maxilla. Otolaryngol Head Neck Surg 1997;117(6):S73–S76.
193. Furuta Y, Takasu T, Asai T, et al.: Detection of human papillomavirus DNA in carcinomas of the nasal cavities and paranasal sinuses by polymerase chain reaction. Cancer 1992;69(2):353–357.
194. Ganly I, Patel SG, Singh B, et al.: Complications of craniofacial resection for malignant tumors of the skull base: report of an International Collaborative Study. Head Neck 2005;27(6):445–451.
195. Kubal WS: Sinonasal imaging: malignant disease. Semin Ultrasound CT MR 1999;20(6):402–425.
196. Carrau RL, Segas J, Nuss DW, et al.: Squamous cell carcinoma of the sinonasal tract invading the orbit. Laryngoscope 1999;109(2 Pt 1):230–235.
197. Fordice J, Kershaw C, El-Naggar A, et al.: Adenoid cystic carcinoma of the head and neck: predictors of morbidity and mortality. Arch Otolaryngol Head Neck Surg 1999;125(2):149–152.
198. Sigal R, Monnet O, de Baere T, et al.: Adenoid cystic carcinoma of the head and neck: evaluation with MR imaging and clinical-pathologic correlation in 27 patients. Radiology 1992;184(1):95–101.
199. Appelblatt NH and McClatchey KD: Olfactory neuroblastoma: a retrospective clinicopathologic study. Head Neck Surg 1982;5(2):108–113.
200. Sabesan T, Xuexi W, Yongfa Q, et al.: Malignant fibrous histiocytoma: outcome of tumours in the head and neck compared with those in the trunk and extremities. Br J Oral Maxillofac Surg 2006;44(3):209–212.
201. Sorensen PH, Wu JK, Berean KW, et al.: Olfactory neuroblastoma is a peripheral primitive neuroectodermal tumor related to Ewing sarcoma. Proc Natl Acad Sci USA 1996;93(3):1038–1043.
202. Dias FL, Sa GM, Lima RA, et al.: Patterns of failure and outcome in esthesioneuroblastoma. Arch Otolaryngol Head Neck Surg 2003;129(11):1186–1192.
203. Diaz EM Jr., Johnigan RH III, Pero C, et al.: Olfactory neuroblastoma: the 22-year experience at one comprehensive cancer center. Head Neck 2005;27(2):138–149.
204. Ejaz A and Wenig BM: Sinonasal undifferentiated carcinoma: clinical and pathologic features and a discussion on classification, cellular differentiation, and differential diagnosis. Adv Anat Pathol 2005;12(3):134–143.
205. Burke DP, Gabrielsen TO, Knake JE, et al.: Radiology of olfactory neuroblastoma. Radiology 1980;137(2):367–372.
206. Schuster JJ, Phillips CD, and Levine PA: MR of esthesioneuroblastoma (olfactory neuroblastoma) and appearance after craniofacial resection. Am J Neuroradiol 1994;15(6):1169–1177.

207. Thompson LD, Wieneke JA, and Miettinen M: Sinonasal tract and nasopharyngeal melanomas: a clinicopathologic study of 115 cases with a proposed staging system. Am J Surg Pathol 2003;27(5):594–611.
208. Chang PC, Fischbein NJ, McCalmont TH, et al.: Perineural spread of malignant melanoma of the head and neck: clinical and imaging features. Am J Neuroradiol 2004;25(1):5–11.
209. Hammersmith SM, Terk MR, Jeffrey PB, et al.: Magnetic resonance imaging of nasopharyngeal and paranasal sinus melanoma. Magn Reson Imaging 1990;8(3):245–253.
210. Manolidis S and Donald PJ: Malignant mucosal melanoma of the head and neck: review of the literature and report of 14 patients. Cancer 1997;80(8):1373–1386.
211. Barnes L: Intestinal-type adenocarcinoma of the nasal cavity and paranasal sinuses. Am J Surg Pathol 1986;10(3):192–202.
212. Wu TT, Barnes L, Bakker A, et al.: K-ras-2 and p53 genotyping of intestinal-type adenocarcinoma of the nasal cavity and paranasal sinuses. Mod Pathol 1996;9(3):199–204.
213. Orvidas LJ, Lewis JE, Weaver AL, et al.: Adenocarcinoma of the nose and paranasal sinuses: a retrospective study of diagnosis, histologic characteristics, and outcomes in 24 patients. Head Neck 2005;27(5):370–375.
214. Sklar EM and Pizarro JA: Sinonasal intestinal-type adenocarcinoma involvement of the paranasal sinuses. Am J Neuroradiol 2003;24(6):1152–1155.
215. Claus F, Boterberg T, Ost P, et al.: Postoperative radiotherapy for adenocarcinoma of the ethmoid sinuses: treatment results for 47 patients. Int J Radiat Oncol Biol Phys 2002;54(4):1089–1094.
216. Enepekides DJ: Sinonasal undifferentiated carcinoma: an update. Curr Opin Otolaryngol Head Neck Surg 2005;13(4):222–225.
217. Phillips CD, Futterer SF, Lipper MH, et al.: Sinonasal undifferentiated carcinoma: CT and MR imaging of an uncommon neoplasm of the nasal cavity. Radiology 1997;202(2):477–480.
218. Musy PY, Reibel JF, and Levine PA: Sinonasal undifferentiated carcinoma: the search for a better outcome. Laryngoscope 2002;112(8 Pt 1):1450–1455.
219. Rischin D, Porceddu S, Peters L, et al.: Promising results with chemoradiation in patients with sinonasal undifferentiated carcinoma. Head Neck 2004;26(5):435–441.
220. Rosenthal DI, Barker JL Jr, El-Naggar AK, et al.: Sinonasal malignancies with neuroendocrine differentiation: patterns of failure according to histologic phenotype. Cancer 2004;101(11):2567–2573.
221. Quraishi MS, Bessell EM, Clark D, et al.: Non-Hodgkin's lymphoma of the sinonasal tract. Laryngoscope 2000;110(9):1489–1492.
222. Gufler H, Laubenberger J, Gerling J, et al.: MRI of lymphomas of the orbits and the paranasal sinuses. J Comput Assist Tomogr 1997;21(6):887–891.
223. Cuadra-Garcia I, Proulx GM, Wu CL, et al.: Sinonasal lymphoma: a clinicopathologic analysis of 58 cases from the Massachusetts general hospital. Am J Surg Pathol 1999;23(11):1356–1369.
224. Li CC, Tien HF, Tang JL, et al.: Treatment outcome and pattern of failure in 77 patients with sinonasal natural killer/T-cell or T-cell lymphoma. Cancer 2004;100(2):366–375.
225. Rodriguez J, Romaguera JE, Manning J, et al.: Nasal-type T/NK lymphomas: a clinicopathologic study of 13 cases. Leuk Lymphoma 2000;39(1–2):139–144.
226. Unni KK and Dahlin DC: Dahlin's bone tumors: general aspects and data on 11,087 cases, 5th ed. Philadelphia: Lippincott-Raven. 1996:xi, 463.
227. Koch BB, Karnell LH, Hoffman HT, et al.: National cancer database report on chondrosarcoma of the head and neck. Head Neck 2000;22(4):408–425.
228. Lloyd GA, Phelps PD, and Michaels L: The imaging characteristics of naso-sinus chondrosarcoma. Clin Radiol 1992;46(3):189–192.
229. Knott PD, Gannon FH, and Thompson LD: Mesenchymal chondrosarcoma of the sinonasal tract: a clinicopathological study of 13 cases with a review of the literature. Laryngoscope 2003;113(5):783–790.
230. Koka V, Vericel R, Lartigau E, et al.: Sarcomas of nasal cavity and paranasal sinuses: chondrosarcoma, osteosarcoma and fibrosarcoma. J Laryngol Otol 1994;108(11):947–953.
231. Enzinger FM and Weiss SW: Soft tissue tumors, 2nd ed. St. Louis: Mosby; 1988:448–488.
232. Nayar RC, Prudhomme F, Parise O Jr, et al.: Rhabdomyosarcoma of the head and neck in adults: a study of 26 patients. Laryngoscope 1993;103(12):1362–1366.
233. Hagiwara A, Inoue Y, Nakayama T, et al.: The "botryoid sign": a characteristic feature of rhabdomyosarcomas in the head and neck. Neuroradiology 2001;43(4):331–335.
234. Hasso AN: CT of tumors and tumor-like conditions of the paranasal sinuses. Radiol Clin North Am 1984;22(1):119–130.
235. Lee JH, Lee MS, Lee BH, et al.: Rhabdomyosarcoma of the head and neck in adults: MR and CT findings. Am J Neuroradiol 1996;17(10):1923–1928.
236. Mandell LR, Massey V, and Ghavimi F: The influence of extensive bone erosion on local control in non-orbital rhabdomyosarcoma of the head and neck. Int J Radiat Oncol Biol Phys 1989;17(3):649–653.
237. Crist W, Gehan EA, Ragab AH, et al.: The third intergroup rhabdomyosarcoma study. J Clin Oncol 1995;13(3):610–630.
238. Wurm J, Constantinidis J, Grabenbauer GG, et al.: Rhabdomyosarcomas of the nose and paranasal sinuses: treatment results in 15 cases. Otolaryngol Head Neck Surg 2005;133(1):42–50.
239. Frankenthaler R, Ayala AG, Hartwick RW, et al.: Fibrosarcoma of the head and neck. Laryngoscope 1990;100(8):799–802.
240. O'Connell TE, Castillo M, and Mukherji SK: Fibrosarcoma arising in the maxillary sinus: CT and MR features. J Comput Assist Tomogr 1996;20(5):736–738.
241. Singh B, Shaha A, and Har-El G: Malignant fibrous histiocytoma of the head and neck. J Craniomaxillofac Surg 1993;21(6):262–265.
242. Mahajan H, Kim EE, Wallace S, et al.: Magnetic resonance imaging of malignant fibrous histiocytoma. Magn Reson Imaging 1989;7(3):283–288.
243. Nakayama K, Nemoto Y, Inoue Y, et al.: Malignant fibrous histiocytoma of the temporal bone with endocranial extension. Am J Neuroradiol 1997;18(2):331–334.
244. Murphey MD, Nomikos GC, Flemming DJ, et al.: From the archives of AFIP. Imaging of giant cell tumor and giant cell reparative granuloma of bone: radiologic-pathologic correlation. Radiographics 2001;21(5):1283–1309.
245. Stolovitzky JP, Waldron CA, and McConnel FM: Giant cell lesions of the maxilla and paranasal sinuses. Head Neck 1994;16(2):143–148.
246. Rimmelin A, Roth T, George B, et al.: Giant-cell tumour of the sphenoid bone: case report. Neuroradiology 1996;38(7):650–653.
247. Tang JY, Wang CK, Su YC, et al.: MRI appearance of giant cell tumor of the lateral skull base: a case report. Clin Imaging 2003;27(1):27–30.
248. Lee YY, Van Tassel P, Nauert C, et al.: Craniofacial osteosarcomas: plain film, CT, and MR findings in 46 cases. Am J Roentgenol 1988;150(6):1397–1402.
249. Wadayama B, Toguchida J, Shimizu T, et al.: Mutation spectrum of the retinoblastoma gene in osteosarcomas. Cancer Res 1994;54(11):3042–3048.
250. Park HR, Min SK, Cho HD, et al.: Osteosarcoma of the ethmoid sinus. Skeletal Radiol 2004;33(5):291–294.
251. Deo SV, Shukla NK, Khazanchi RK, et al.: Multimodality management of a case of primary osteogenic sarcoma of the zygoma. J Postgrad Med 1995;41(1):13–15.
252. Kohanawa R, Tabuchi K, Okubo H, et al.: Primary osteogenic sarcoma of the ethmoid sinus: a case report. Auris Nasus Larynx 2005;32(4):411–413.
253. Hanna SL, Fletcher BD, Kaste SC, et al.: Increased confidence of diagnosis of Ewing sarcoma using T2-weighted MR images. Magn Reson Imaging 1994;12(4):559–568.
254. Howarth KL, Khodaei I, Karkanevatos A, et al.: A sinonasal primary Ewing's sarcoma. Int J Pediatr Otorhinolaryngol 2004;68(2):221–224.
255. Daldrup-Link HE, Franzius C, Link TM, et al.: Whole-body MR imaging for detection of bone metastases in children and young adults: comparison with skeletal scintigraphy and FDG PET. Am J Roentgenol 2001;177(1):229–236.
256. Mentzel HJ, Kentouche K, Sauner D, et al.: Comparison of whole-body STIR-MRI and 99mTcmethylene-diphosphonate scintigraphy in children with suspected multifocal bone lesions. Eur Radiol 2004;14(12):2297–2302.
257. Cotterill SJ, Ahrens S, Paulussen M, et al.: Prognostic factors in Ewing's tumor of bone: analysis of 975 patients from the European Intergroup Cooperative Ewing's Sarcoma Study Group. J Clin Oncol 2000;18(17):3108–3114.
258. Sandoval C, Meyer WH, Parham DM, et al.: Outcome in 43 children presenting with metastatic Ewing sarcoma: the St. Jude Children's Research Hospital experience, 1962 to 1992. Med Pediatr Oncol 1996;26(3):180–185.
259. Daley TD, Wysocki GP, and Pringle GA: Relative incidence of odontogenic tumors and oral and jaw cysts in a Canadian population. Oral Surg Oral Med Oral Pathol 1994;77(3):276–280.

The Larynx 5

David Floriolli, MD
Anton N. Hasso, MD, FACR

EMBRYOLOGY AND DEVELOPMENT

The laryngeal apparatus is derived from the pharyngeal arch system which begins to develop in the fourth week of gestation.[1,2] At the same time neural crest cells migrate to the area that will become the head and neck region, and a median ventral outgrowth of the foregut known as the laryngotracheal groove arises just below the level of the fourth arch. Toward the end of the fourth week the laryngotracheal groove evaginates and forms the respiratory diverticulum. As this elongates, tracheoesophageal grooves develop and grow toward each other until they eventually fuse, forming the tracheoesophageal septum. The result of the formation of this septum is the formation of a laryngotracheal tube which is now separate from the primordial pharynx and esophagus but still connected by a laryngeal inlet.[1,2]

The endoderm of the laryngotracheal tube forms the epithelial lining of the larynx. Neural crest cells form the mesenchyme of the fourth and sixth paryngeal arches. The cartilaginous structures that form the skeleton of the larynx develop from this mesenchyme, with the exception of the epiglottis which develops from the hypopharyngeal eminence, a derivative of the mesenchyme of the third and fourth arches. In approximately the fifth to sixth week of gestation, bilateral swellings at the base of the fourth arches known as the arytenoid swellings begin to grow toward the primordial epiglottis. Along with rapid proliferation of the laryngeal epithelium this results in temporary occlusion of the laryngeal lumen. Recanalization of the lumen, which normally occurs by the 10th week, results in the formation of the laryngeal ventricles. The intrinsic muscles of the larynx also develop from the fourth and sixth arches. As a result, the muscles are innervated by the recurrent laryngeal nerve, a branch of the vagus nerve.[1,2]

ANATOMY

Laryngeal Skeleton

In the adult the larynx is located at approximately the level of C4, 5, and 6. The skeleton of the larynx mainly consists of cartilage, with the hyoid bone being the only true bony structure. The hyoid bone is an important site of attachment for the external laryngeal muscles and some membranes and ligaments of the larynx. It is a U-shaped structure with three anatomic structures of the hyoid bone identified: the body, bilateral greater cornu, and bilateral lesser cornu. The body comprises the anterior curved portion of the hyoid and on either side of the body on the upper portion are the lesser cornu, two small tubercles which serve as the attachment site for the stylohyoid ligament. The body itself serves as the attachment point for the strap muscles (sternohyoid, thyrohyoid, and omohyoid), the genioyoid and genioglossus muscles, and the mylohyoid muscle.[3,4]

Located inferior to the hyoid bone is the thyroid cartilage. Two quadrangular plates known as the laminae of the thyroid cartilage meet anteriorly at an acute angle ranging from 90 degrees in males to 120 degrees in females.[4] The prominence that is formed by this meeting creates what is commonly called the "Adam's apple." The thyroid notch is created by an indentation at the midline where the two laminae meet. Rising superiorly from the posterior aspect of the laminae bilaterally are the greater cornua of the thyroid cartilage. The lesser cornua extend inferiorly and form an articulation with the lateral surface of the cricoid cartilage.

The cricoid cartilage is the only cartilaginous structure in the larynx which forms a complete ring. It is shaped like a signet ring, with a narrow anterior arch and a wide posterior lamina. Bilaterally, the lateral superior aspect of the posterior cricoid cartilage articulates with the inferior aspect of the arytenoid cartilages. The lateral aspect of the posterior arch of the cricoid cartilage articulates with the lesser cornua of the thyroid cartilage.

The arytenoid cartilages are two pyramid-shaped structures that, as mentioned above, are located atop the posterior lamina of the cricoid. They have three surfaces (medial, posterior, and anterolateral) and a base. At the bases of the arytenoids are the vocal and muscular processes. The vocal process extends anteriorly and serves as the attachment for the vocal ligament. The muscular process extends laterally and is the attachment of the lateral and posterior cricoarytenoid muscles. At its apex, the arytenoid articulates with the corniculate cartilage. The arytenoids are capable of rotating on the vertical axis and also are able to slide laterally along the cricoid cartilage.

The corniculate cartilages articulate with the apex of the arytenoids and serve to support the posterior aspect of the aryepiglottic folds on either side. The cuneiform cartilages are sesamoid cartilages that rest withing the aryepiglottic folds and also help to support this structure.[3]

The final cartilaginous structure of the larynx is the epiglottis. Of note, the epiglottis is composed of elastic cartilage, unlike the majority of structures in the larynx which are made of hyaline cartilage, and therefore does not calcify with age.[4] The epiglottis is a leaf-shaped structure that connects to the hyoid bone via the hyoepiglottic ligament and the thyroid cartilage via the thyoepiglottic ligament. Its connection to the arytenoids, the aryepiglottic folds, form the lateral borders of the laryngeal inlet and separate the opening of the piriform sinuses from the laryngeal inlet bilaterally. The posterior aspect of the epiglottis is dotted with indentations and perforations which contain mucous glands. The epiglottis rises superiorly and projects backward over the laryngeal inlet, assisting in prevention of aspiration during swallowing.

Ligaments and Membranes

The ligaments and membranes of the larynx (**Fig. 5-1**), while not often visualized with radiologic imaging, still play an important role in defining laryngeal spaces and affecting the route of tumor spread.

The thyrohyoid membrane attaches along the superior aspect of the thyroid cartilage and runs superiorly to attach to both the body and greater horns of the hyoid bone. The posterior aspect of this membrane thickens on either side to form the thyrohyoid ligament, which runs from the greater horn of the hyoid to attach to the apex of the superior horn of the thyroid cartilage. There is also a thickening of the median aspect of the thyrohyoid membrane which forms the median thyrohyoid ligament. The median cricothyroid ligament attaches at the midline to the superior border of the cricoid cartilage and extends to the inferior border of the thyroid cartilage. It is considered by some to be a part of the cricovocal membrane.[3–5]

The cricovocal membrane (or conus elasticus) attaches inferiorly to the superior surface of the cricoid cartilage and extends superiorly and medially. Anteriorly, it attaches to the thyroid cartilage near midline and posteriorly to the vocal process of the arytenoid cartilages. Its free upper margin runs between these two attachments and forms the vocal ligament.

Running from the lateral aspect of the epiglottis to the body and apex of the arytenoid is the quadrangular membrane. Its upper free margin forms the aryepiglottic fold while its inferior margin forms the vestibular fold or false vocal cord.

Table 5-1 summarizes the anatomic courses of the laryngeal ligaments.

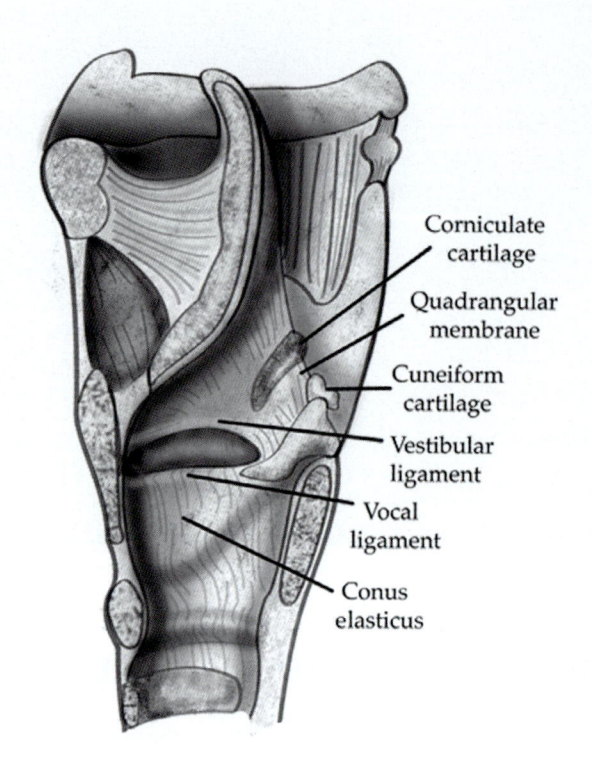

Figure 5-1 Ligaments and Membranes of the Larynx
A sagittal view of the larynx is shown, with most of the soft tissue removed in order to emphasize the ligaments. Note the conus elasticus and the upper fold which forms the vocal ligament. Note also the corniculate cartilage, suspended within the quadrangular membrane.

Table 5-1 Ligaments and Membranes of the Larynx

Ligament	Course
Thyrohyoid membrane	Superior thyroid to body and greater horns of hyoid
Median Cricothyroid ligament	Superior cricoid to inferior thyroid cartilage
Cricovocal membrane	Superior cricoid to midline of the thyroid cartilage and vocal process of arytenoid cartilages
Vocal ligament	Thickened free margin of the cricovocal membrane
Quadrangular ligament	Lateral epiglottis to arytenoid
Vestibular ligament	Inferior free margin of the quadrangular membrane
Thyroepiglottic ligament	Inferior aspect of the epiglottis to the thyroid cartilage

Spaces and Sinuses

The spaces and sinuses of the larynx are important structures when it comes to patterns of tumor spread and the variable contents of these spaces can also be used to aid in determination of tumor location.

While considered part of the hypopharynx, the pyriform sinuses remain an important structure in relation to the larynx. They are located lateral to the aryepiglottic folds on either side of the laryngeal inlet.

The laryngeal ventricles are the space between the true and false vocal folds. At the anterior end of this space is a pouch of mucosa called the saccule which contains mucous glands, the secretions of which help to lubricate the vocal cords.

There are three anatomically defined spaces in particular that play an important role in defining tumor location and helping one understand possible routes of spread. The first of these is the pre-epiglottic space. It is bounded by the hyoepiglottic ligament superiorly, thyrohyoid membrane anteriorly, and epiglottis and thyroepiglottic ligament posteriorly (**Fig. 5-2**). It contains mostly fat and is continuous with the paraglottic space inferolaterally which allows for tumor spread between these two spaces. Perforations in the epiglottis also put this space in contact with the mucosa of the laryngeal surface of the epiglottis. As a result, tumors from the mucosal surface can invade the preepiglottic fat.[4,6]

The second major space is the paraglottic space. Bounded laterally by thyroid cartilage, inferomedially by conus elasticus, medially by the vestibule, and superomedially by the quadrangular ligament, the paraglottic space is an important route of tumor spread, allowing supraglottic tumors to reach the glottic and subglottic spaces or giving access outside of the larynx (**Fig. 5-3**).

Finally, the third major space of the larynx is the subglottic space. This space is bounded superiorly by the vocal cords, laterally by the conus elasticus, and medially by the subglottic mucosa.

Table 5-2 summarizes the properties and boundaries of the laryngeal spaces.

Muscles of the Larynx

The larynx contains multiple intrinsic muscles and one extrinsic muscle (the cricothyroid). Arising from the posterior aspect of the lamina of the cricoid cartilage and attaching to the muscular process of the arytenoids are the posterior cricoarytenoid muscles. As the only abductors of the vocal cords the posterior cricoarytenoids are necessary to maintain patency of the airway.[3]

The interarytenoid muscle consists of both transverse and oblique fibers. The transverse fibers attach to the muscular process and lateral border of each arytenoid, respectively, and extend horizontally between the two cartilages. The oblique fibers of the interaytenoid originate at the muscular processes of the arytenoids and cross the midline to attach to the apex of the opposite arytenoid (the oblique fibers from either side form an "X"). Together, these fibers serve to pull the arytenoids toward each other and help close the laryngeal inlet during swallowing.[3]

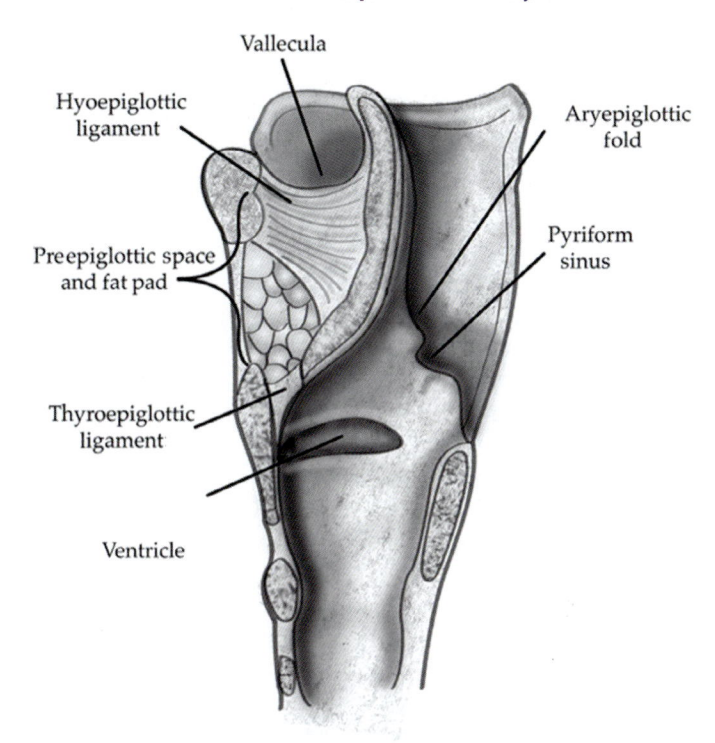

Figure 5-2 Spaces and Sinuses of the Larynx
A diagrammatic sagittal view of the larynx is shown. In this view, the ventricle is readily seen including the relationship to the midthyroid cartilage. Of greater significance is the pre-epiglottic space, bounded by the hyoepiglottic ligament superiorly, thyrohyoid membrane anteriorly, and epiglottis and thyroepiglottic ligament posteriorly. This space is an important route of laryngeal tumor spread.

Table 5-2 Spaces of the Larynx

Space	Contents	Boundaries
Preepiglottic	Mostly fat; rich lymphatics	Hyoepiglottic ligament, thyrohyoid membrane, epiglottis, and thyroepiglottic ligament
Paraglottic	Mostly fat	Thyroid cartilage, conus elasticus, vestibule, and quadrangular ligament
Subglottic	–	Vocal cords, conus elasticus, and subglottic mucosa

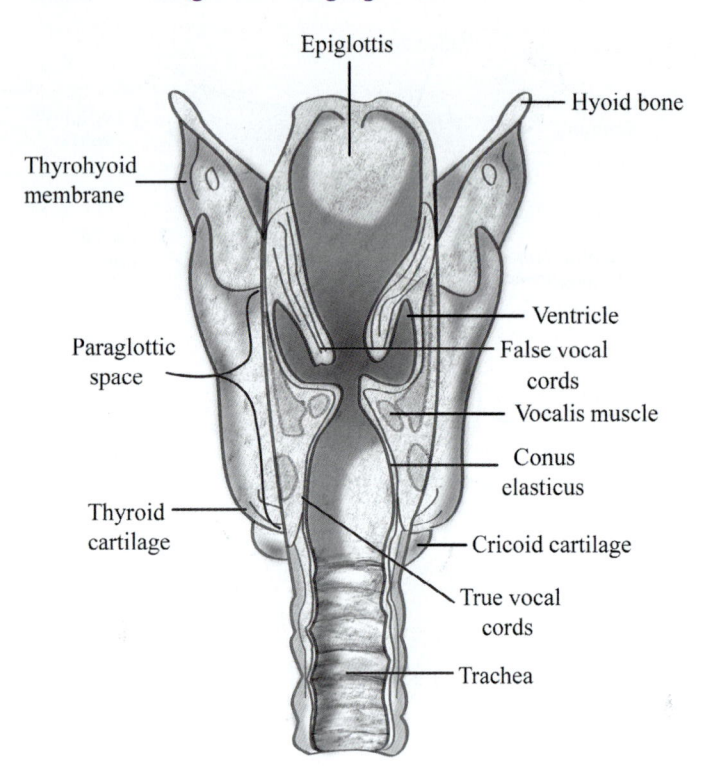

Figure 5-3 Mid-coronal View of the Larynx
A diagrammatic coronal view of the larynx is shown, as viewed from a posterior aspect. In this view, the relationship of the true and false vocal folds, forming the ventricles, can be seen. Of primary importance in this view is the paraglottic space which extends from the hyoid to the subglottic region. Similar to the preepiglottic space, this area is an important route of tumor spread.

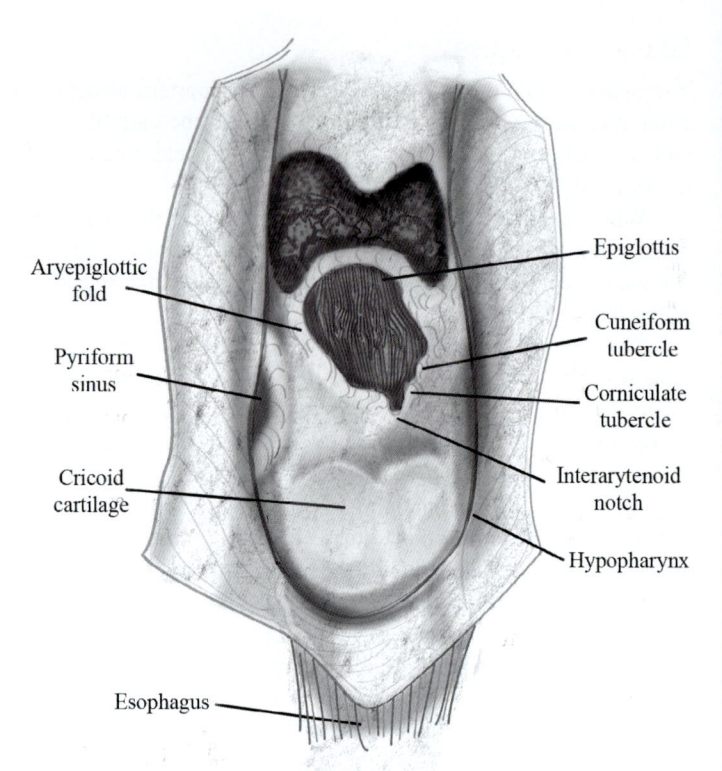

Figure 5-4 Posterior View of the Larynx
A posterior diagram of the larynx. The aryepiglottic folds can readily be seen, along with their relationship to the pyriform sinuses and the epiglottis. The aryepiglottic muscles aid in closing this opening in purse string fashion during deglutition. Note also the posterior aspect of the cricoid cartilage. It is the only laryngeal cartilage that makes a complete ring.

These oblique fibers then continue from the apex of the arytenoid to run within the aryepiglottic fold, forming the aryepiglottic muscles. In conjunction with the interarytenoid muscle, the aryepiglottic muscles serve to close the laryngeal inlet in purse-string fashion during swallowing (**Fig. 5-4**).

Also attaching to the muscular process of the arytenoid are the lateral cricoarytenoid muscles, which arise from the superior aspect of the arch of the cricoid cartilage. This muscle serves to adduct the vocal cords.

Location of the thyroarytenoid muscles on imaging serves as a useful landmark for the level of the true vocal cord.[7] The thyroarytenoid originates on the posterior aspect of the thyroid lamina in the midline and inserts on the lateral aspect of the arytenoid cartilage. The innermost fibers of the thyroarytenoid muscle, often referred to as the vocalis muscle, run within the vocal fold and along the vocal ligament to attach to the vocal process of the arytenoid. This muscle serves to decrease the tension of the vocal ligament and in turn changes the pitches made during phonation.

The last of the intrinsic muscles are the thyroepiglottic muscles. These originate superior to the thyroarytenoid muscle on the posterior aspect of the thyroid cartilage and insert on the lateral margin of the epiglottis. The thyroepiglottic muscles serve to pull the epiglottis over the laryngeal inlet during swallowing.

The cricothyroid muscle is the only muscle innervated by the external branch of the superior laryngeal nerve and is important for increasing tension in the vocal cords by tilting the cricoid cartilage posteriorly, making it an important muscle for phonation. It is made of both straight and oblique parts.

Blood Supply

The larynx is supplied by two main arteries: the superior laryngeal artery and the inferior laryngeal artery. These arteries form an anastamosis not only with their corresponding artery on the other side, but also with each other. The superior laryngeal artery is a branch of the superior thyroid artery and part of the external carotid system. The inferior laryngeal artery, on the other hand, is a branch of the thyrocervical trunk.

Innervation

The intrinsic muscles of the larynx are innervated by the right and left recurrent laryngeal nerves, branches of the 10th cranial nerve. The only exception is the cricothyroid muscle which is supplied by the external branch of the superior laryngeal nerve. The superior laryngeal nerve is also a branch of the vagus nerve and supplies the sensory innervation of the larynx above the level of the vocal fold. Below the vocal fold sensation is provided by the recurrent laryngeal nerves.

Table 5-3	Laryngeal Lymph Node Levels
Level I	Submadibular and submental nodes
Level II	Upper jugular nodes
Level III	Middle jugular nodes
Level IV	Lower jugular nodes
Level V	Posterior triangle nodes
Level VI	Anterior triangle nodes

Lymphatic Drainage

Lymphatic drainage in the larynx occurs in a cephalad direction. Another important note is that drainage is unilateral, meaning that malignant cells will not spread to the contralateral side until the tumor has invaded bilaterally.[7] Drainage of the supraglottic larynx is to the upper jugular nodes (levels II and III). The subglottic larynx drains to the nodes of the anterior triangle (level VI). The glottis and true cords have little to no lymphatic drainage.[7] A summary of the lymph node levels can be seen in **Table 5-3**.

Tumors of the glottic and subglottic larynx may cause enlargement of the Delphian node, located anterior to the cricothyroid membrane. Enlargement of this node has been suggested to be an early indication of tumor.[7]

Divisions

The larynx is divided into three main areas: the supraglottic, glottic, and subglottic larynx. The supraglottic larynx is defined as the area from the aryepiglottic folds to the lower margin of the false cords. Contained within this area are the supra- and infrahyoid portions of the epiglottis, arytenoids, aryepiglottic folds, and the false cords.

The area containing the true vocal cords and including the anterior and posterior commissures is known as the glottic larynx. Finally, the subglottic larynx extends 1 cm below the true cords.

PHYSIOLOGY AND FUNCTION

Airway Provision and Protection

The cartilaginous structures of the larynx serve to maintain patency of the airway. The mucoperichondrium is also tightly adherent in this area, which helps prevent airway obstruction due to edema.[4]

In humans, the airway is in communication with the esophagus and as a result protection of the airway during swallowing must be provided. During swallowing, the epiglottis serves to direct food away from the airway while contraction of the aryepiglottic and interarytenoid muscles result in purse string closure of the larynx to further protect the airway. Swallowed material is directed toward the piriform sinuses and into the esophagus.[6]

Phonation

The complex functions required for phonation are carried out largely by the larynx. Thoracic muscles serve to move air through the larynx causing vibration of the vocal folds. The muscles of the larynx change the length, tension, and thickness of the vocal cords which then results in changes in pitch.[8]

Subglottic Pressure Gradient

The shape and location of the false vocal folds allows them to serve as a one-way valve which prevents the outflow of air when the folds are brought together during muscular contraction.[6] This causes an increase in pressure to develop below the level of the false vocal folds allowing one to cough or to perform a Valsalva maneuver. The true vocal folds are capable of acting as a valve in the opposite direction and prevent the inspiration of air.[6]

IMAGING

Laryngoscopy Versus CT/MRI

Laryngoscopy allows for dynamic imaging of the larynx (**Fig. 5-5**). As a result, abnormalities in function, such as fixation of the vocal cords, may be seen. Mucosal lesions can also be identified using laryngoscopy. The limitation of this imaging modality is its inability to provide submucosal information, thus the extent of tumors and other lesions cannot be evaluated by this means. Computed tomography (CT) and/or magnetic resonance imaging (MRI), on the other hand, lack the ability to evaluate dynamic function but are excellent modalities for evaluating a lesion's submucosal extent. In general, CT is the modality of choice for imaging a laryngeal lesion preoperatively, whereas MRI is

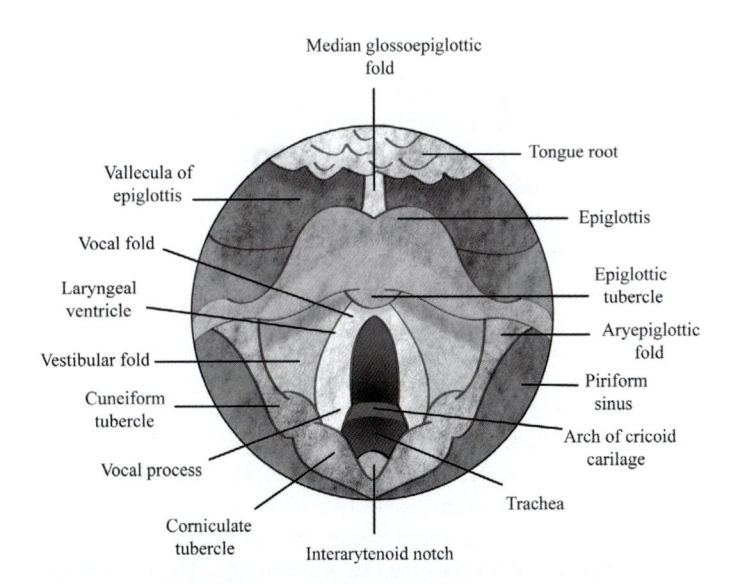

Figure 5-5 Superior View of the Larynx
View of the larynx from above. This view is similar to what would be seen when viewing through a laryngoscope. Note the appearance of the true vocal folds, the movement of which can be important for tumor staging.

superior in the postoperative or postradiation therapy patient as diffusion-weighted MRI aids in distinguishing radiotherapy-induced changes from tumor recurrence.[9] PET/CT is emerging, however, as the posttreatment examination of choice. Further discussion can be found in the section on tumor staging.

Computed Tomography

Important anatomic areas of the larynx can be distinguished based on their characteristic appearances on CT. The preepiglottic space, due to its fat content, will appear as an area of hypoattenuation, as will other fat containing areas such as the paraglottic space, the false folds, and the aryepiglottic folds.[10] The appearance of cartilage on CT varies depending on the amount of ossification. Nonossified areas will appear isodense to soft tissue whereas ossified cartilage will have a hyperattenuated core, a hypoattenuated marrow space and a hyperattenuated outer lining.[10] The thyroarytenoid muscles are a useful landmark for locating the level of the glottis. Another important CT characteristic of note is that laryngeal mucosa generally does not enhance with administration of contrast.

With sensitivity of 95% to 100%, contrast enhanced CT is excellent for evaluating tumor involvement of the preepiglottic and paraglottic spaces. Specificity for the preepiglottic space is also high at 90% to 93% but falls to 50% for the paraglottic space as the paraglottic space is often affected by inflammatory changes due to either tumor itself or as a result of systemic causes.[10]

Evaluation of cartilaginous involvement of tumor is important as it plays a role in prognosis, staging, and treatment. The modality of choice remains an area of controversy. This is discussed further in the section on evaluation of cartilaginous invasion.

Multidetector acquisition of imaging and spiral CT scanning are superior to conventional CT scanning when evaluating laryngeal trauma. Image acquisition is twice as fast which reduces motion artifact, and three-dimensional (3D) image reconstructions are greatly improved using multidetector scanners.[10] This is extremely important in the evaluation of arytenoid dislocation and subluxation as 3D imaging is imperative. Thin slices are also necessary in the evaluation of trauma as this will aid in visualization of fractures of the various cartilages. The value in reconstruction is illustrated in **Fig. 5-6**.

In order to obtain the best quality scan, it is recommended that the angulation be taken parallel to the laryngeal ventricle or parallel to C3/4 or C4/5 if the ventricle is not well visualized. Spiral scanning is preferred as this allows for the larynx to be scanned quickly, thereby reducing swallowing and other motion artifacts. The field of view can be adjusted depending on the size of the neck, though generally a view of 16 to 19 cm will be sufficient. The scan should cover the region from the hyoid bone to below the level of the cricoid cartilage. The images can then be reconstructed in order to provide coronal, sagittal, or 3D images. Contrast administration is also an important component of laryngeal CT imaging. Proper administration is important and a sufficient wait time must be given so that the contrast is able to diffuse into the tissues. In cases of significant airway compromise a tracheostomy may be a necessary prologue to iodinated contrast injection as there is risk of allergic reaction and significant mucosal edema which could be devastating in a patient with a compromised airway. If necessary, CT is also capable of taking images during dynamic maneuvers. Prolonged phonation allows for evaluation of arytenoid mobility, cord mobility, and a better view of the ventricles. Also, forcing air against closed lips expands the hypopharynx and allows better visualization of the pyriform sinuses.[9] **Table 5-4** illustrates the preferred protocol.

Magnetic Resonance Imaging

MRI has the benefit of superior soft tissue imaging when compared to CT and can obtain images in multiple planes (**Fig. 5-7**). A significant drawback to MRI is that it requires relatively long image acquisition times resulting in artifacts due to breathing, swallowing, and carotid artery pulsations. While improvements in scanning times have been made these issues along with questions of cost and patient comfort must still be considered.

When obtaining images a neck surface coil must be used and T1- and T2-weighted spin echo images should be acquired. In order to facilitate imaging of the larynx, hyperextension of the neck is used. This helps to reduce swallowing artifact by making swallowing difficult. By lying on their back the patient's airway is made parallel to the table. Sagittal images can be used as a localizer and then images in the coronal, axial, and sagittal planes can be obtained. Axial images are obtained with an angulation parallel to the vocal cords or to C3/4 or C4/5. T1 and T2-weighted images should be obtained with 3 to 5 mm thickness. Intravenous contrast is imperative in the evaluation of laryngeal neoplasms (**Table 5-5**).

Detection of Neoplastic Invasion of Cartilage: CT and MRI vs Histology

Detection of cartilaginous involvement of tumor spread has proven difficult; however, such detection is important in that cartilaginous involvement reduces the chances of successful radiotherapy and often precludes conservative surgical approaches. MRI is both more sensitive and specific than CT in the detection of cartilaginous involvement of tumor spread; however, CT is still often used in the evaluation of laryngeal tumors. Detection is made difficult by the characteristic appearance of cartilage on CT. As stated earlier, laryngeal cartilage slowly ossifies as a patient ages but shows a highly variable pattern of ossification. As a result, calcification due to tumor cannot be distinguished from a normal variant. On CT, ossified cartilage will show highly attenuating inner and outer cortical bone layers with a low-attenuating core containing marrow. Nonossified cartilage has a similar appearance to soft tissue and will have an attenuation much like that of tumor tissue.

In the past, CT has shown poor sensitivity compared with histology ranging from 44% to 66%.[11,12] Extralaryngeal tumor involvement on the outside of the laryngeal cartilage was previously the only criteria that could reliably predict cartilaginous involvement. Such spread, however, is only present in advanced

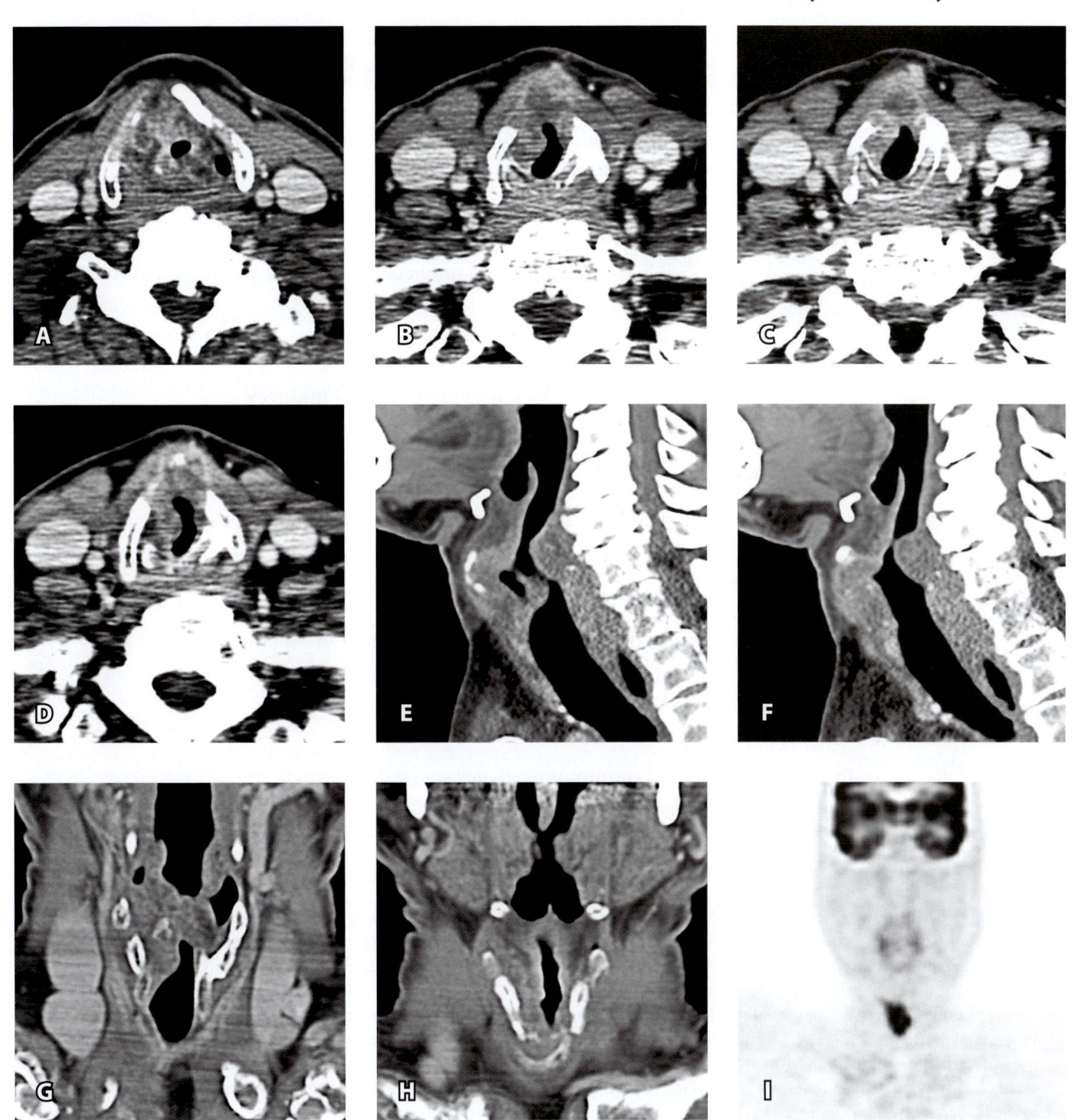

Figure 5-6 CT Imaging of the Larynx

(**A, B, C, D**) Axial contrast enhanced CT of the neck showing a right-sided T4 transglottic squamous cell carcinoma (SCC) involving the glottic and supraglottic spaces. Invasion of the laryngeal cartilage, strap muscles, and surrounding soft tissues is well shown, as is the narrowing of the airway. (**E, F**) Sagittal reconstructions of original axial images. Note the resulting improvement in the ability to view anterior and posterior involvement. Invasion of the pre-epiglottic space as well as destruction of the cartilages is easily seen. (**G, H**) Coronal reconstructions again showing a large right-sided lesion extending into and beyond the laryngeal cartilage. In image (**G**), the lesion crosses the midline. In (**H**), the narrowing of the airway by the nodular mass is well seen due to increased ability to evaluate inferior and superior extent. (**I**) Solitary coronal PET image following injection of FDG18 showing a well-circumscribed mass, but lacks morphologic detail to show extralaryngeal extension. In this case, the PET shows that there is no evidence of nodal metastasis. In certain cases, PET is highly sensitive for differentiating enlarged nodes that are reactive from those that contain metastasis.

Table 5-4 Laryngeal CT Protocol	
Indication:	Tumor, trauma, infection
Scanner settings:	kV(p): 140; mA: 220–260 upper and mid neck; 300 per 2 sec for lower neck and thoracic inlet
Oral contrast:	None
Phase of respiration:	Quiet breathing
Rotation time:	0.5–0.8 sec for upper and midneck; 2 sec for lower neck and thoracic inlet
Acquisition slice thickness	1.0–1.25 mm through upper and midneck; 2.5–3 mm through lower neck and thoracic inlet
Pitch:	0.75–1.0 (HQ = 3:1) through upper and midneck
	1.0–1.5 (HS = 6:1) through lower neck and thoracic inlet
	If the scanner is unable to perform the multislice helical imaging mode with the gantry in angled position, change the gantry angle to 0 degrees and reconstruct the images in the desired plane or use the multislice axial imaging mode.
Mulitplanar reconstruction slice thickness/interval for filming:	2.0–3.0 mm/2.0–3.0 mm
IV contrast — Concentration:	LOCM 300–320 mg iodine/ml or HOCM 282 mg iodine/ml 60% solution
Rate:	1 ml/sec
Scan delay:	100 sec
Total volume:	100 ml (minimum catheter size = 22 G)

LOCM = low osmolar contrast media; HOCM = high osmolar contrast media.
Modified with permission from Silverman, RM. Multislice Computed Tomography: A Practical Approach to Clinical Protocols. Philadelphia: Lippincott Williams & Wilkins; 2002:93–94.

disease (Fig. 5-8). A study by Becker et al. looked to improve upon this by introducing other criteria that could be used to increase sensitivity and allow for earlier detection of involvement. In this study, eight different criteria were evaluated for usefullness: extralaryngeal tumor spread, sclerosis of cartilage, tumor adjacent to nonossified cartilage, serpiginous contour of cartilage, erosion or lysis of cartilage, obliteration of marrow space, cartilaginous blowout, and bowing. These criteria were applied to 111 cases of laryngeal carcinoma and compared to histopathologic findings.

When compared to the histopathology, extralaryngeal spread showed high correlation with cartilaginous tumor involvement. Sclerosis showed correlation not necessarily with cartilage involvement (found in approximately 50% of cases) but rather with inflammatory changes within the cartilage related to products released by the nearby tumor cells. It was found that these changes can occur even before the tumor has invaded the cartilage. Serpiginous contour showed similar findings in that it can result from nearby tumor alone, without direct invasion. In addition, it may be a normal variant.

Due to the similarities in attenuation between nonossified cartilage and tumor tissue, tumor adjacent to nonossified cartilage was not found to be useful. Bowing and obliteration of the marrow space were similarly ineffective for differentiating between inflammation and tumor involvement.

Overall, the criteria of extralaryngeal spread, erosion or lysis, and sclerosis (except in the thyroid cartilage) are recommended by the authors as a means of improving sensitivity and specificity. This combination showed a sensitivity of 82%, specificity of 79%, and negative predictive value of 91%. CT appears to be capable of evaluating cartilaginous spread as its high negative predictive value makes it useful in the exclusion of cartilaginous involvement.[12]

In the case of MRI imaging, the area is less controversial in that criteria for identifying tumor have largely been established. When evaluating hyaline cartilage on T1-weighted images one should look for low signal intensity as an indication of tumor involvement. Proton density and T2-weighted images should show high signal intensity. Postcontrast T1 images may show areas of enhancement within the cartilage and adjacent to the tumor. Finally, as with CT, tumor seen on both sides of the cartilage should be considered evidence for cartilaginous involvement. Using these criteria, a sensitivity of approximately 92%

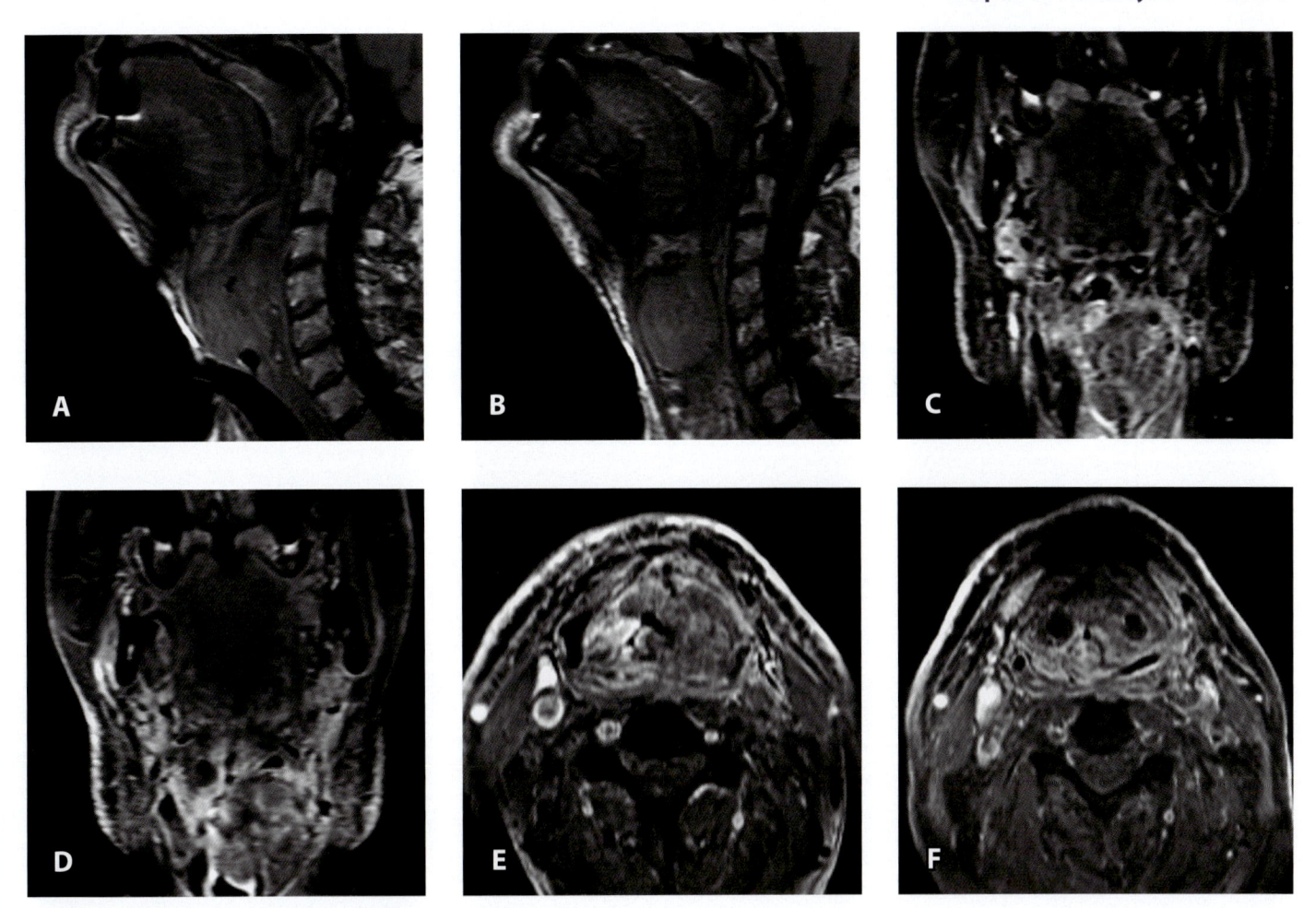

Figure 5-7 MR Imaging of the Larynx
MRI images with and without contrast. (**A, B**) Precontrast T1 sagittal images showing marked airway obstruction due to a large glottic tumor. There is a tracheostomy present. (**C, D**) Postgadolinium T1 fat saturation coronal images again showing the large left-sided glottic tumor, now with postcontrast enhancement of the lesion. There is extensive enhancement of the mucosal surfaces and facial planes likely secondary to mucositis with postradiation changes. There is a well-circumscribed mass that is primarily submucosal along the left side of the supraglottic portion of the larynx. (**E, F**) Postgadolinium T1 fat saturation axial images again illustrating a large left-sided enhancing lesion in the region of the glottis. The airway is extremely deformed by the mass which is seen to cross the midline superiorly at the level of the hyoid bone.

Table 5-5 Laryngeal MRI Protocol	
Angulation	Parallel to C3/4 or C4/5
Sagital T1	Use as localizer from SCM to SCM
Coronal T1	3–5 mm sections from anterior vocal cords to posterior larynx
Axial T1	Thin sections; midmandible to lower cricoid
Axial T2	Fast spin echo with fat saturation
Slice thickness	3–5 mm
FOV	16–18 cm for T1-weighted; 18–20 for T2-weighted
Pixel size	<1 × 1 mm
Matrix	256 × 256–512 × 512
IV contrast	Obtain pre- and postcontrast T1-weighted images

SCM = sternocleidomastoid; FOV = field of view.

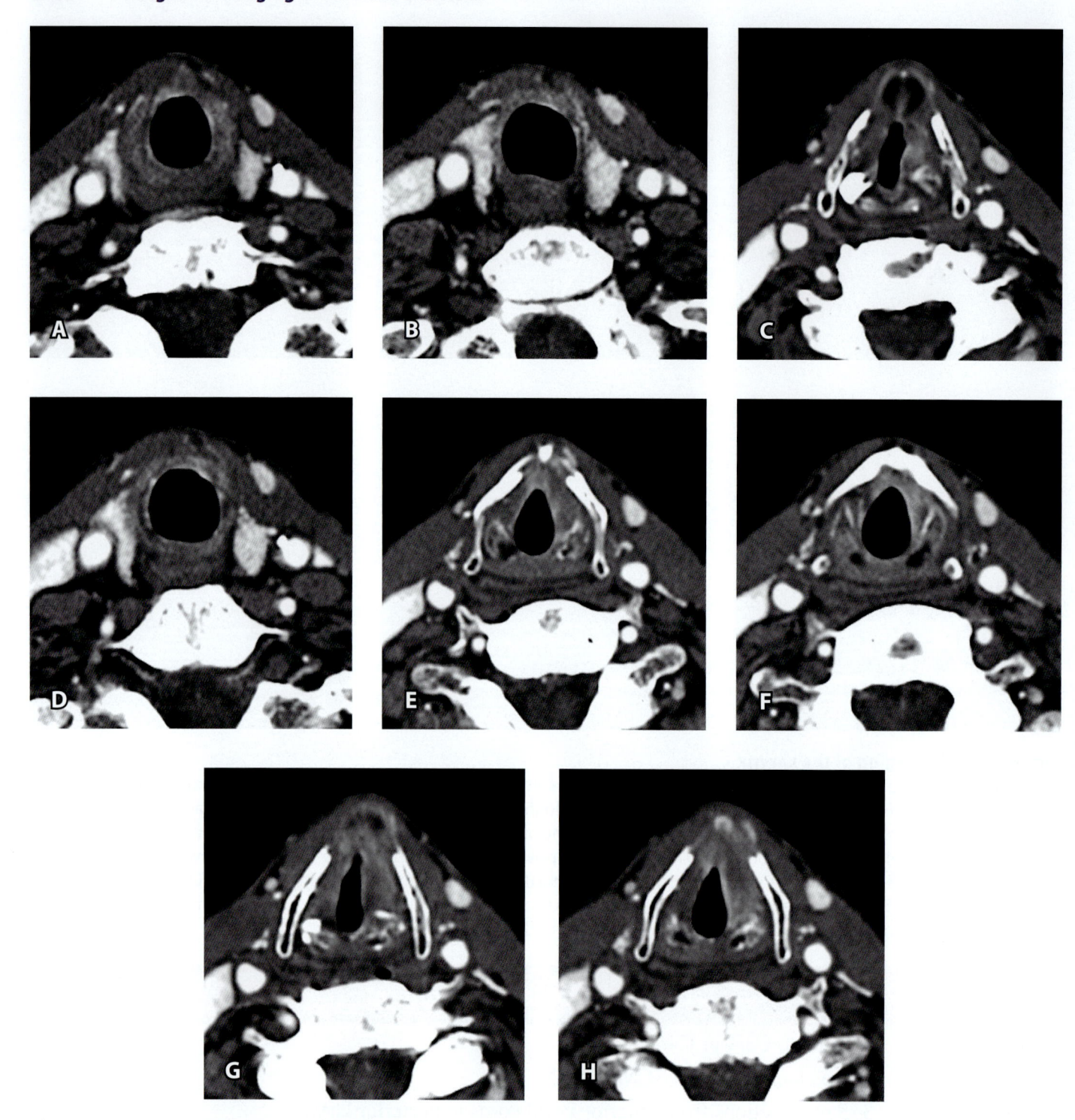

Figure 5-8 T4 Laryngeal Cancer CT Findings
(**A–H**) Postcontrast CT images showing a large T4 glottic heterogeneously enhancing mass abutting and eroding the thyroid cartilage with surrounding edema. The mass can be seen to extend beyond the true larynx into surrounding soft tissues accounting for the T4 classification. Size criteria are not included in the TNM staging in all laryngeal tumors including glottic, supraglottic, or infraglottic. See **Table 5-6**.

Table 5-6 Laryngeal Tumor Staging

	Supraglottis		Nodal Staging
T1	Limited to one subsite of supraglottis with normal vocal cord mobility	NX	Regional nodes cannot be assessed
T2	Invades more than one adjacent subsite of supraglottis or glottis or region outside the supraglottis without vocal cord fixation	N0	No regional lymph node metastasis
T3	Fixation of the vocal cord or invasion of postcricoid area, preepiglottic and/or paraglottic space, and/or minor thyroid cartilage erosion	N1	Metastasis in a single ipsilateral lymph node <3 cm in greatest dimension
T4a	Invasion through thyroid cartilage and/or soft tissues beyond the larynx (e.g., strap muslces, trachea, esophagus, thyroid gland)	N2a	Metastasis in a single ipsilateral lymph node >3 cm but <6 cm
T4b	Tumor invades prevertebral space, mediastinal structures, or encases carotid artery	N2b	Metastasis in multiple ipsilateral lymph nodes, all <6 cm
	Glottis	N2c	Metastasis in bilateral or contralateral lymph nodes, all <6 cm
T1	Tumor limited to vocal cord(s) with normal mobility, may involve anterior or posterior commissure	N3	Metastasis in any node >6 cm in greatest dimension
T1a	Limited to one vocal cord		Distant Metastasis
T1b	Involves both vocal cords	MX	Distant metastasis cannot be assessed
T2	Impaired vocal cord mobility and/or tumor extension into the supraglottis or subglottis	M0	No distant metastasis
T3	Vocal cord fixation and/or tumor invasion of paraglottic space, and/or minor thyroid cartilage erosion	M1	Distant metastasis
T4a	Tumor invades through thyroid cartilage or tissues beyond the larynx		
T4b	Tumor invades prevertebral space, mediastinal structures, or encases carotid artery		
	Subglottis		
T1	Tumor limited to subglottis		
T2	Tumor extends to vocal cord(s) with normal or impaired mobility		
T3	Tumor limited to larynx with vocal cord fixation		
T4a	Tumor invades through thyroid cartilage or tissues beyond the larynx		
T4b	Tumor invades prevertebral space, mediastinal structures, or encases carotid artery		

can be achieved, though specificity is low at approximately 83%. With a negative predictive value of 94%, however, MRI is excellent for exclusion of cartilaginous disease.[11] In addition, MRI has shown a superior ability to detect intracartilaginous invasion when compared to CT, detecting 91% of such lesions.[13] When examining lesions of this type, however, a high rate of false positives was also noted.

The low specificity on MRI is a result of physiologic changes that take place within the cartilage due to products released by nearby tumor cells. In another study by Becker et al. these changes of fibrosis, inflammation, and bone resorption were found in all histopathologic specimen which showed neoplastic invasion of cartilage, but were also seen in 44% of specimen which did not.[13] These changes will result in MRI findings that appear similar to the criteria used for evidence of cartilaginous invasion, including high signal intensity on T2-weighted images and postcontrast enhancement on T1-weighted images. This can result in a significant number of false positive results and explains the low specificity of MRI.

These physiologic changes were found to be much more common in thyroid cartilage than in cricoid or arytenoid cartilage. In fact, specificity of MRI for detection of cartilaginous invasion of the thyroid cartilage alone was found to be approximately 56%. This is in stark contrast to values of 87% and 95% found for the cricoid and arytenoid cartilages, respectively.[11] These findings would indicate that MR imaging of the cricoid and arytenoid cartilages is quite accurate and specific, whereas caution must be exercised when diagnosing involvement of the thyroid cartilage on MRI. Extralaryngeal tumor spread, however, remains an effective diagnostic criterion.

With the criteria put forth by Becker et al. the sensitivity of CT imaging appears to be essentially equivalent to that of MRI though this comes at the cost of sacrificing specificity. While MR shows higher specificity than CT, it too is prone to false positive results due to physiologic changes that occur in cartilage as a result of nearby tumor cells. The negative predictive values of both modalities are high and as a result both studies can be considered effective in pretherapeutic staging of disease as they are quite capable of ruling out cartilaginous involvement.

Positron Emission Tomography

In the initial evaluation of laryngeal lesions, PET alone does not appear to add significant value in regard to the primary tumor itself but is important with regard to evaluating occult metastases or distant metastases.[14] Pretreatment PET is also useful to help evaluate tumor response to chemotherapy or radiotherapy. When following treatment response it is recommended that PET images be obtained at least 8 to 12 weeks posttreatment if radiotherapy is used.[14] This is due to increased radiation changes being present in the early weeks after treatment which can increase the number of false positives.

PET scans play an important role in postoperative imaging as findings that may be related to postoperative change or granulation are better distinguished with PET. These findings can then be correlated with the previous imaging modalities. With tumor follow up PET is a highly sensitive modality though the level of anatomic detail is inferior to that of CT or MRI. The use of combined PET and CT scanners shows promise at overcoming this limitation and further adding to the usefulness of PET scanning in the posttreatment patient.[15]

Radiation therapy is often used in the treatment of laryngeal carcinoma as some believe it offers the best chance of preserved vocal quality. Surgical salvage therapy can be used in cases of treatment failure; however, due to tissue changes that take place as a result of radiation treatment, such as swelling and contrast enhancement, early diagnosis of tumor recurrence can be difficult, often resulting in detection being too late to allow conservative surgery. There is clearly a need for a method that allows for earlier detection of recurrence and PET has shown promise at filling that role.

A study by Kubota et al. compared the effectiveness of PET in detecting the recurrence of head and neck cancer as compared to MRI or CT. Thirty-six patients with a history of squamous cell carcinoma or undifferentiated carcinoma of the head and neck were evaluated. All had been treated previously with radiotherapy with a range from conclusion of therapy from 25 days to 5 years, with the median being 4 months. After imaging, diagnosis was confirmed with biopsy or surgical specimen in patients who showed evidence of recurrence. Patients with no evidence of recurrence were followed clinically.[16]

Sensitivity of PET scanning was found to be 87.5% compared to 75% for MRI/CT; however, this difference was not found to be statistically significant. Statistically significant differences were found in specificity, positive predictive value, and negative predictive value. In all cases PET was found to be superior. Specificity was 77.8% for PET and 29.6% for MRI/CT, positive predictive value was 70% for PET and 38.7% for MRI/CT, and negative predictive value was 91.3% for PET and 66.7% for MRI/CT.[16] Specificity for MRI/CT was poor due to a high number of false positives, illustrating well the point that postradiation changes can easily mimic tumor recurrence. Reasons for false diagnosis on PET were also examined. In two cases, recurrences were missed. Both times this appeared to be due to the small size of the lesion. Both patients were approximately 1.5 months posttreatment, a period of time which shows less specificity when compared to 6 to 11 months posttherapy (71% versus 100%, respectively). Of the false positive diagnosis, half were due to inflammation with the rest due to various other causes.[16]

Further accuracy in diagnosis and improvement in localization of disease can be obtained through the combination of PET and CT. A study by Fakhry et al. compared combination PET/CT with PET alone for detection of recurrence of head and neck squamous cell carcinoma. This study looked at 32 patients who had previously been considered cured of disease and later developed suspicion of recurrence based on new symptom onset or a local equivocal lesion.[17] Conventional workup was performed in all cases, including CT and/or MRI, physical examination, and nasofibroscopy. In all cases, the conventional workup was equivocal. Of the 32 patients examined, 15 were confirmed on biopsy to have local recurrence of disease. On analysis, PET/CT was found to reduce false positive rates and therefore enable the avoidance of unnecessary invasive procedures in 57% of patients.[17]

PET/CT is also developing a role in pretreatment evaluation of laryngeal neoplasms. Along with studying PET/CT in the evaluation of head and neck cancer posttreatment, a study by Connell et al. also evaluated the utility of PET/CT versus standard CT/MRI imaging for pretherapeutic staging. In that study, 34% of patients had a restaging of disease as a result of PET/CT imaging with two patients downstaged and ten upstaged. This had a clinically significant impact in 30% of patients.[18]

PATHOLOGY

Malignant Neoplasms

Squamous Cell Carcinoma

Squamous cell carcinoma forms the vast majority of malignant laryngeal neoplasms, accounting for approximately 95% of cases.[8] Men are affected more than women though a significant increase in the number of cases in women in recent years has been noted.[19,20] Overall survival is good at approximately 66%. The disease typically affects older individuals with incidence peaking in the sixth and seventh decades of life.[8,19]

Multiple factors have been identified as being associated with the development of laryngeal cancer, and first and foremost among them is cigarette smoking. A smoking habit consisting of more than two packs a day has shown a 10.4 times greater risk of developing squamous cell carcinoma of the larynx.[8] Alcohol is another important risk factor as it appears to act synergistically with tobacco and further increase risk. Alcohol alone also seems to be a risk factor for developing laryngeal cancer.[15] Other environmental factors may contribute to development of disease, including some occupations that carry risks of exposure to harmful chemicals. Patients exposed to therapeutic levels of radiation also show increased risk. Gastroesophageal reflux disease is another risk factor for laryngeal carcinoma.[8]

Tumor spread, prognosis, and treatment can vary depending on which compartment of the larynx is the site of tumor origin.[6,19,20]

Tumor Origin and Spread

Supraglottic Carcinoma

Tumors of this site are often able to grow to a larger size relative to glottic tumors as they are less likely to cause symptoms early on.[20] Perhaps as a result of this, coupled with a relatively rich lymphatic network, they are also more likely to have lymphatic spread.[6,20] Hoarseness is less commonly a symptom of supraglottic tumors compared to glottic tumors. Supraglottic tumors tend to present with lymphadenopathy or airway obstruction.

Embryologically, the supraglottis is mainly derived from the third and fourth branchial arches while the sixth arch serves as the origin of the glottis. This embryologic distinction plays an important role in tumor spread as the resulting lymphatics and blood supply are separate.[8] Studies using injection of traceable dye into the false vocal fold have shown only late entry of dye into the vocal fold, with early spread being directed instead into the paraglottic space, aryepiglottic folds, and pre-epiglottic space.[8] Entry of supraglottic tumors into the pre-epiglottic space is possible through the multiple fenestrations present in the epiglottis. From there, spread to the paraglottic space can occur.

The specific subsite of origin within the supraglottic space can also give the physician clues as to the expected pattern of spread.[11] Ventral supraglottic carcinomas are those which arise from the epiglottis. These tumors can be subdivided again into suprahyoid and infrahyoid tumors. Infrahyoid tumors of the epiglottis are able to spread to the pre-epiglottic space either directly through the epiglottic fenestrations or through cartilaginous invasion.[11] Invasion into this space changes tumor stage to T3 and is therefore important to diagnose. It is best seen with T1-weighted MRI, where differentiation between the high signal intensity of fat and the intermediate intensity of tumor can be seen, along with tumor enhancement on administration of contrast.[15] Suprahyoid epiglottic tumors arising at the junction of the aryepiglottic folds also have a general pattern of spread, tending to invade the pre-epiglottic space by going around the epiglottis rather than through the fenestrations. Invasion of the thyroid cartilage may also occur.[9,11]

Tumors of the ventricles, false vocal cords, or aryepiglottic folds spread submucosally and often have paraglottic invasion by the time they are diagnosed. The invasion of this space allows the tumor access to both glottic and subglottic spread. Similar to pre-epiglottic invasion, MRI and CT will show replacement of paraglottic fat with tumor tissue.[11,15]

Due to the rich lymphatic network of the supraglottis lymphadenopathy often occurs. Approximately 50% to 60% of patients will have lymphadenopathy on presentation.[9]

Glottic Carcinoma

The glottis is the most common site of tumor origin in the larynx. Tumors here tend to cause symptoms earlier than either supraglottic or subglottic tumors as smaller lesions can have an effect on function.[19] Symptoms can vary depending on the area or areas involved with hoarseness being the most common presenting symptom, though throat pain, dysphagia, and the presence of an obvious neck mass can also occur.[19,20] They most often arise on the free margin of the membranous cord.[6,15] Initially, tumor spread is inhibited superiorly due the different embryologic origin of the supraglottis and inferiorly by the vocal ligament, the anterior commissure, the thyroglottic ligament, and the conus elasticus, which serve as barriers to the spread of tumors. This leads to greater rates of cure in early stage glottic cancer.[8] Access to the paraglottic space can still be gained, however, resulting in transglottic spread. This access can be achieved by spread along the vocal cord or inferiorly through the conus elasticus.[8]

Tumors most commonly arise along the anterior half of the true vocal cord and spread toward the anterior commissure (**Fig. 5-9**). Early stage lesions are best seen endoscopically and in fact may be missed with CT or MRI.[11,15] Upon reaching the anterior commissure, however, access to the supraglottis and subglottis is possible and therefore CT and MRI remain necessary tools in evaluation in order to determine the amount of tumor extension.[11] In addition to access to these spaces, direct invasion of the thyroid cartilage may occur after spread to the anterior commissure, along with extralaryngeal spread through the cricothyroid ligament. Subglottic extension is detected through abnormal thickening of the soft tissue with a thickness greater than 1mm considered abnormal.[15]

While tumor spread along the vocal cord is most common, lateral spread into the theyroarytenoid muscle or posterior spread through the posterior commissure and into the cricoarytenoid joint can occur. Both may result in vocal cord fixation resulting in a tumor staging of T3 regardless of tumor size according to

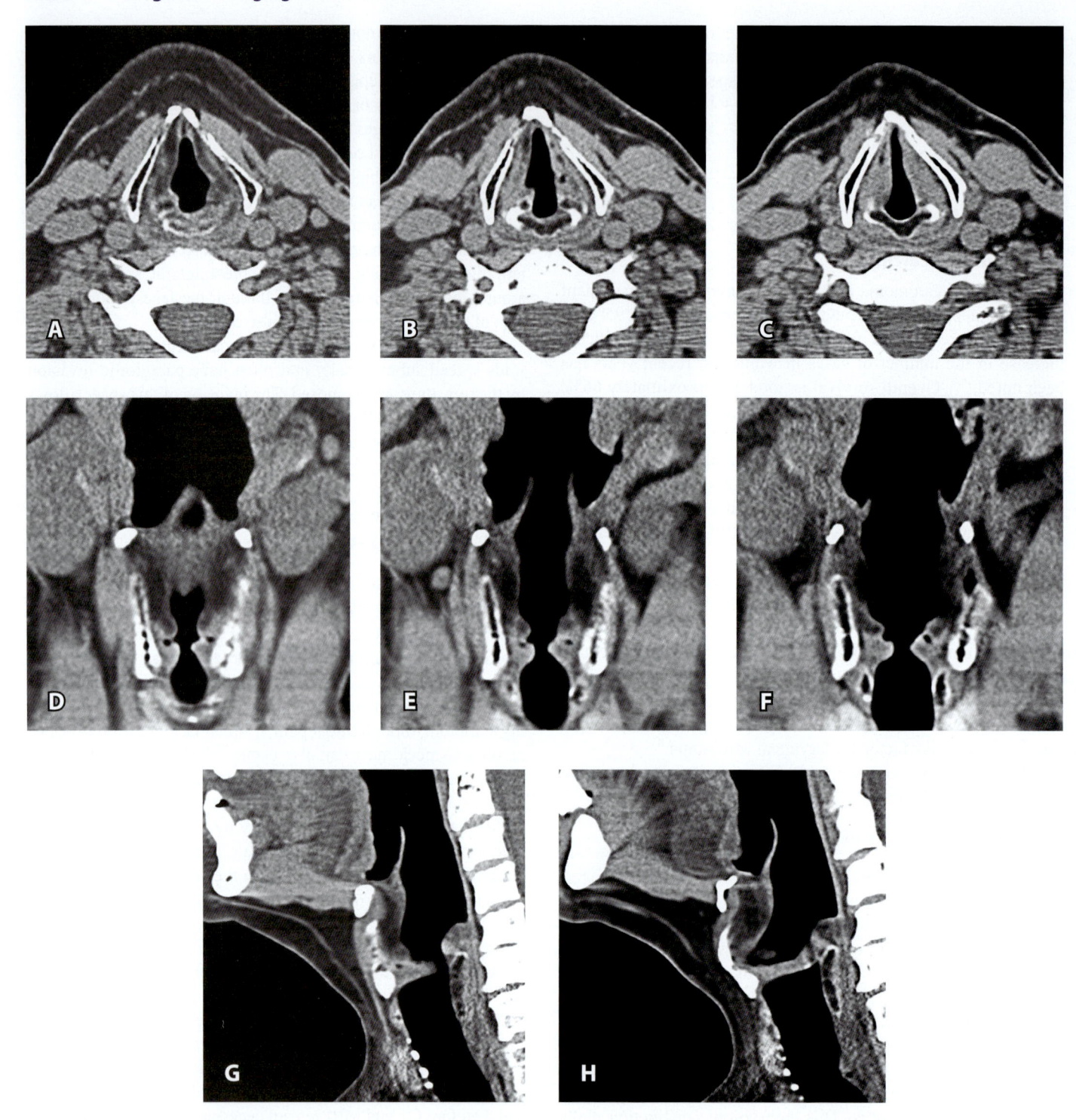

Figure 5-9 Glottic Carcinoma
NECT of the larynx, showing the value in T1 tumors of the glottis. While most head and neck CT imaging is performed with contrast, in some small tumors of the true cord, it may be worthwhile to avoid the natural tendency of swallowing and excess breathing following contrast infusion. Axial images (**A–C**) show a small tumor of the left true cord with extension into the left ventricle and false cord. Coronal reformatted images (**D–F**) confirm deformities of the left true cord ventricle with slight extension into the fat of the left false cord, which merges into the fat-filled paralaryngeal space. Reformatted sagittal images (**G–H**) show a thickened left true cord and a rounded bulge of the anterior portion of the false cord (**G**) and the normal right true cord for comparison (**H**).

the American Joint Committee on Cancer (AJCC).[11] Further lateral spread again gives access to the paraglottic space and thyroid cartilage. Early on the thyroid cartilage may serve as a barrier to force tumor spread into the paraglottic space or inferiorly into the subglottis, either through mucosal spread or through direct invasion of the conus elasticus.[9] Posterior spread into the retrocricoid hypopharynx and esophagus may also occur.

Cartilaginous invasion is an important aspect of glottic carcinoma that must be evaluated. CT and MRI are both useful in this regard though MRI is more specific.[15] Whether T1- or T2-weighted images are preferred depends on the state of ossification of the cartilage in question. Ossified cartilage will have high signal intensity on T1 and as a result tumor infiltration will show a decrease in intensity. On the other hand, nonossified cartilage is best evaluated with T2-weighted imaging wherein the tumor appears hyperintense compared to the cartilage. Edema may complicate this picture, however, as it also appears hyperintense on T2.[15] See the section on evaluation of cartilaginous invasion for more information.

Lymphatic spread in the case of glottic carcinoma is rare due to the relative paucity of lymphatics. However, once the tumor has spread beyond the glottic region, the risk of lymphatic spread increases greatly.[11,15]

Subglottic Carcinoma

Tumors of subglottic origin are the least common.[6,20] In fact, tumor in the subglottic region is more likely to be a result of tumor spread of glottic or supraglottic origin as opposed to a primary subglottic tumor. Spread tends to be caudad but tumors often show circumferential growth beneath the anterior commissure (**Fig. 5-10**).[6] While the conus elasticus often forces tumor growth medially, this structure can be destroyed by the tumor, making spread to many areas possible including the cricoid cartilage, other areas of the larynx, or extralaryngeal spread such as to the thyroid gland.[11,15] Whereas with supraglottic and glottic carcinoma cartilaginous involvement is only generally seen late in the disease progression, subglottic carcinoma can show early involvement of the cricoid cartilage.[9] Lymphatic drainage is generally to paratracheal nodes. Because these tumors tend to have late presentation, enlargement of the Delphian node (located anterior to the cricothyroid membrane) may be an important early clinical indication of subglottic disease.

Transglottic Carcinoma

Opinions differ regarding the definition of a "transglottic carcinoma" but it is generally accepted as a term referring to tumors that involve both the glottis and the supraglottis.[11] Transglottic invasion of tumor is a sign of advanced disease and as such carries a poorer prognosis and greater risk for lymph node metastasis and invasion of the laryngeal framework and skeleton.[11] Because submucosal spread is often a factor in such tumors CT and MRI are important tools for evaluation as such spread may not be visible on endoscopic examination.

Lymphatic Spread

Lymphatic tumor spread has been shown to be associated with poorer outcome.[7,8] As stated earlier in the section on lymphatic anatomy, lymphatic drainage of the larynx is generally to the ipsilateral side of the neck only. The result of this is that nodal tumor spread is limited to the ipsilateral side unless the primary tumor has spread to the contralateral side.[7,8] In the case of supraglottic carcinomas, lymph node levels I and V are only rarely involved in nodal spread, therefore it is generally accepted that dissection of these nodes during surgical treatment is unnecessary for tumors less than T4 and nodal disease of N0 or N1.[8] The relatively sparse lymphatics of the glottis as compared to the supraglottis results in a much lower incidence of nodal metastasis in glottic carcinoma.

Examination of nodal metastasis is challenging as discerning nodes with metastatic involvement from reactive nodes that are enlarged due to inflammation is difficult. Current criteria consist of an axial diameter larger than 10 mm or a hypodense center indicative of necrosis being accepted as signs of metastatic involvement (**Fig. 5-11**).[9] The decision to use 10 mm as a cutoff point balances sensitivity and specificity. If the criteria were raised, specificity would be gained but more cases would be missed, resulting in a loss of sensitivity. With these criteria CT is approximately 90% sensitive and 73% specific.[9]

The evaluation of distant metastasis plays an important role in prognosis and treatment. The most frequent site of metastasis is the lung, followed by bone and liver. When bone and liver metastasis are present they are nearly always associated with lung metastasis.[9] Findings associated with an increased risk of distant metastasis include: advanced disease (N2 or N3 nodal disease), extranodal tumor spread, neoangiogenesis, and perineural or vascular invasion.[9] In the interest of cost, a chest X-ray may be the primary screening modality looking for lung metastasis, but chest CT should be considered if other risk factors are present. PET imaging also plays an important role as it is capable of whole body imaging.

Tumor Classification and Staging

Accurate staging of laryngeal tumors is important as the recommended methods of treatment used can change dramatically based on tumor staging information (**Table 5-6**). As discussed in the section on laryngeal imaging, laryngoscopy is an important clinical tool in the evaluation of tumor stage. As the majority of laryngeal neoplasms have a mucosal component they will be easily seen on laryngoscopy, as will changes in function such as vocal cord paralysis or fixation. The limitation of laryngoscopy is its inability to evaluate submucosal spread, along with the fact that large exophytic tumors may obscure the view of important anatomic structures such as the anterior commissure. The anterior commissure is an important path of spread, allowing glottic tumors access to the paraglottic space. It is important that this area be evaluated when staging laryngeal neoplasms.

A study by Zbären et al. examined the accuracy of clinical examination including laryngoscopy as compared to laryngoscopy in conjunction with CT, and laryngoscopy in conjunction with MRI. In that study, laryngoscopy alone was found to correctly stage disease 57% of the time. When used in conjunction with CT or MRI, an accurate staging was reached 80% and 87.5% of the time, respectively.[21] The difference between CT and MRI was not statistically significant. These findings were similar to other studies. This shows that CT and MRI play an indispensable role in pretherapeutic staging of laryngeal neoplasms and that both modalities are equally reasonable choices.

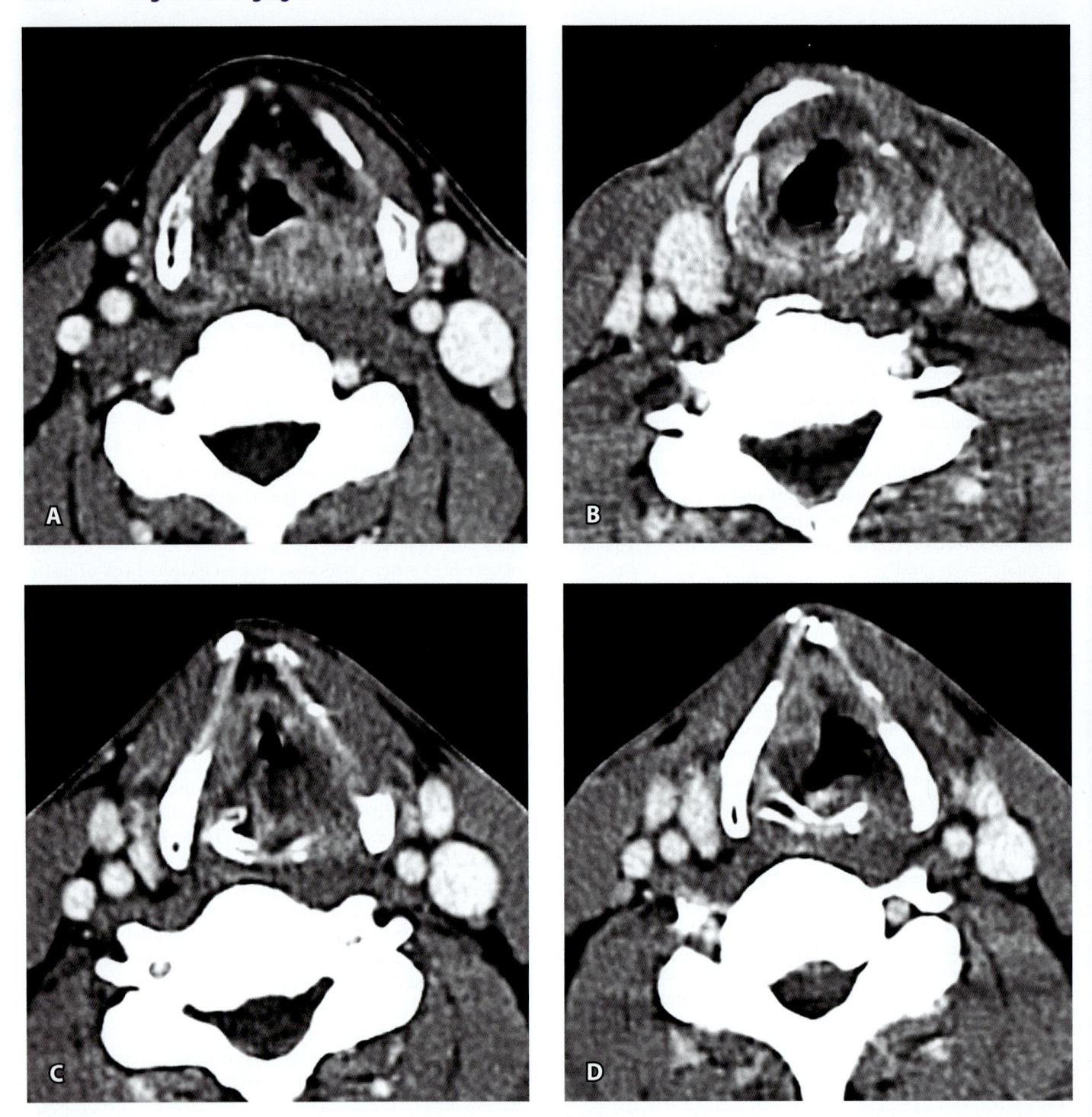

Figure 5-10 Subglottic Carcinoma
(**A–D**) Postcontrast axial CT showing a large transglottic mass that originates from the subglottic space. These images illustrate the characteristic circumferential growth often seen with tumors of subglottic origin. Invasion of the extralaryngeal space is often associated with extension of the tumor both upward and downward. On these images the precise direction of growth is difficult to determine.

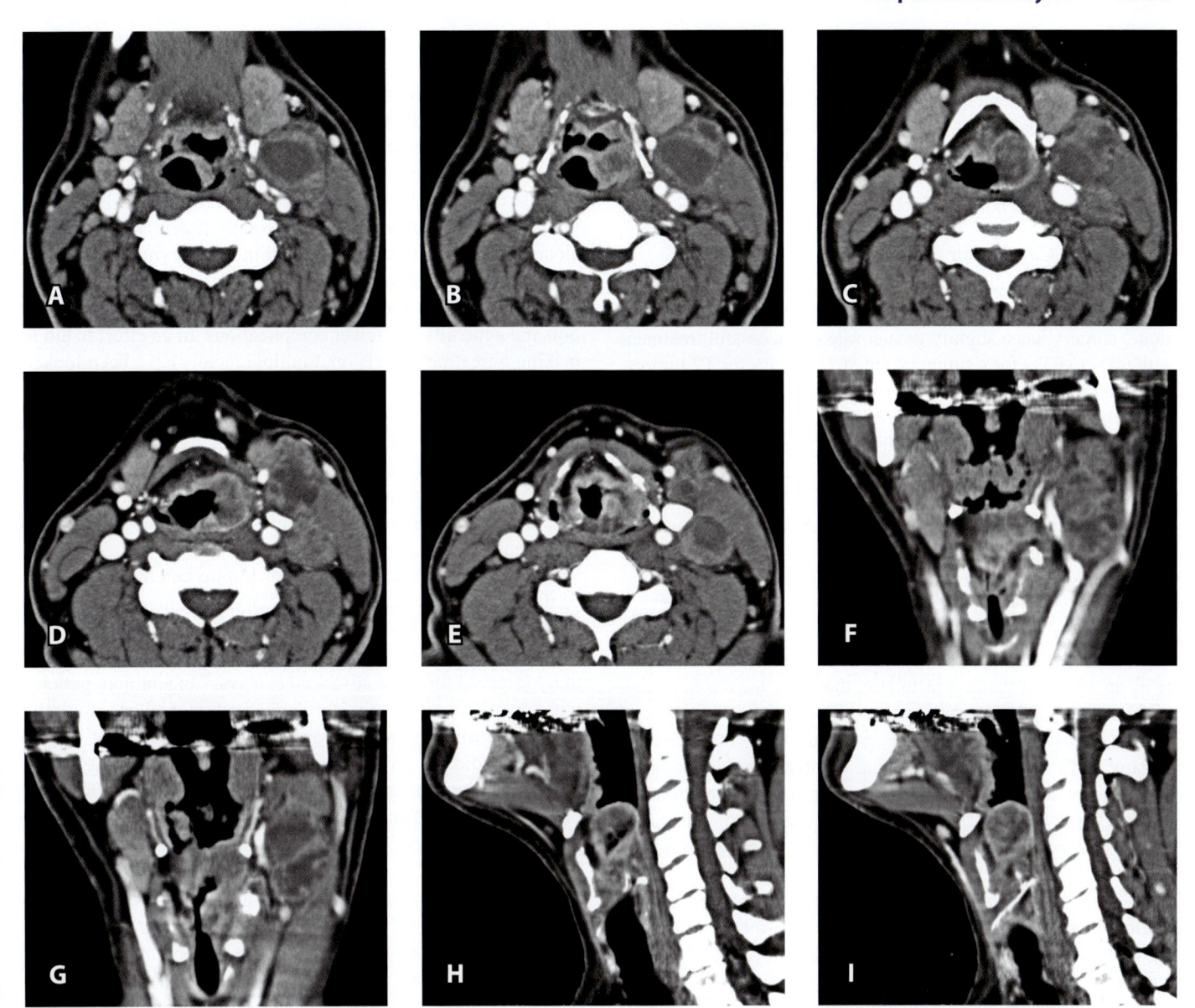

Figure 5-11 T3 Supraglottic Carcinoma
Improved staging based on imaging that defines the true extent of a tumor and metastasis. (**A–E**) Postcontrast axial CT showing a large, bulky, combined mucosal and submucosal supraglottic tumor. The tumor mass is originating from the left aryepiglottic fold and extending upward to the level of the hyoid bone and epiglottis with distortion and displacement of the epiglottis toward the right side. There is tumor extension downward toward the false cords but no apparent involvement of the true cords. Clinically, there is no evidence of cord paresis. This T3 tumor shows multilevel varying sized lymph nodes with a large confluent nodal mass on the left side at levels II and III, which makes this not only a T3 tumor but an N3 metastasis as well. It is clear that these are metastatic nodes not only by size criteria but also by noting the presence of differential enhancement. (**F, G**) In these coronal reconstructions of the original images, the tumor extension along the left side of the supraglottic larynx is well seen with an indentation on the airway. The confluent nodal mass elevates and distorts the left submandibular gland with medial displacement of the internal jugular vein and lateral displacement of the carotid artery. (**H, I**) With sagittal reconstruction the relationship to the laryngeal cartilages is quite clear with distortion of the epiglottis and primary location cephalad to the arytenoid and cricoid cartilages.

Treatment Based on Staging

There are many options for treatment of squamous cell carcinoma of the larynx including radiation, chemotherapy, surgery, laser resection, or various combinations of these modalities. The treatment of choice varies depending on many factors including tumor size, tumor stage, the overall health of the patient, and the patient's personal choice.

Supraglottic Carcinoma

Early stage supraglottic cancers tend to be treated with radiotherapy, supraglottic laryngectomy, or laser excision. When taken alone, surgery has a slightly greater rate of successful treatment with 90% to 95% for T1 tumors and 80% to 90% for T2 tumors. For radiation therapy alone the success rates are 80% to 90% and 70% to 80% for T1 and T2, respectively.[8] When surgery is used as a rescue therapy after radiation treatment, however, success rates become equal for both methods.[8] Radiation is often the treatment method desired by patients as it offers the best chance of maintaining laryngeal function. It should be noted, however, that detection of recurrence in a patient who has been treated with radiation therapy becomes more difficult and therefore may result in detection too late to perform conservative surgery.[8]

Radiation can also be used in conjunction with surgery, either as a first step in treatment in an attempt to shrink a tumor or as an adjuvant therapy in tumors that may have a high risk of recurrence after surgery.[22] More recently, chemotherapy has developed an important role in conjunction with radiation therapy, with some studies showing combination chemoradiation therapy having similar survival rates to surgery with adjuvant radiation therapy.[22] Chemotherapy makes tumor cells more susceptible to radiation treatment along with carrying the added benefit of reducing the incidence of distant metastasis.

Carbon dioxide laser therapy, while previously used mainly in glottic cancers, has emerged as an effective means of resecting early stage T1 and T2 lesions, and use for T3 and T4 stage tumors is increasing as well. Surgery is performed via a laryngoscope and has showed comparable rates of effectiveness to transcervical partial laryngectomy.[22] This is discussed further in the section on endoscopic laser surgery.

In general, advanced lesions (T3 or T4) are treated with total laryngectomy, but treatments consisting of combinations of radiotherapy and surgery or chemotherapy may still be considered.[22]

Because of the rich lymphatic network involved in supraglottic carcinoma, occult metastasis must be considered. Node involvement relates to tumor size with T1 and T2 tumors showing occult metastasis 16% of the time while T3 and T4 tumors may have occult nodal involvement up to 62% of the time.[22] Consideration of nodal dissection should be given even in N0 cancers.

Glottic Carcinoma

The use of endoscopic laser surgery for early stage (T1 or T2) treatment of lesions is quite effective and can be done as an outpatient for some lesions. Laser surgical treatment of more extensive lesions is in its early stages and shows promise.[23] A further discussion can be found in the section on laser excision.

While laser resection of favorable lesions is the mainstay of treatment, traditional treatment methods remain an important aspect of care. Early stage treatment of glottic carcinoma is similar to that of supraglottic carcinoma. T1 and T2 tumors can be treated with surgery, radiation therapy alone or with combination chemoradiation. Combination therapy has been shown to be more effective but carries an increased incidence of side effects.[23] Rescue therapy with surgery also remains an option after radiation treatment.

The decision of whether to treat with surgery or radiation can be difficult. Recurrence rates are slightly higher with radiation alone and salvage therapy may require total laryngectomy if the recurrence is detected late (**Fig. 5-12**). On the other hand, radiation therapy offers the best outcomes as far as voice conservation and generally has fewer complications. In an effort to aid in making a treatment decision, multiple factors have been looked at for signs of correlation with radiation failure. Decreased vocal cord mobility appears to be one such sign and should be factored into the decision.[8] Tumors with subglottic extension also show a poorer response to radiotherapy.[8] Cartilaginous involvement is also generally a contraindication to radiotherapy as these tumors tend to be less responsive, in addition to increasing the risk of radiation-induced chondronecrosis.[12]

Traditional surgical options for glottic carcinoma are vertical hemilaryngectomy and total laryngectomy. Tumors that show only limited involvement of the anterior commissure may be treated with a vertical hemilaryngectomy with total laryngectomy reserved for more advanced cancers.[23] In addition, patients with unilateral arytenoid cartilage fixation and/or subglottic tumor extension to the level up the upper border of the cricoid may be candidates for an extended partial laryngectomy.[9]

Unlike the supraglottis the glottis does not have a rich lymphatic network and as a result is less likely to have lymph node involvement in early stage disease with stage I and II cancers having an incidence of nodal involvement of only 1% to 8%.[23] This incidence rises to 20% to 30% with T3 and T4 tumors.[23] As mentioned in the section on lymphatic spread, the nodal levels involved are generally II, III, and IV. As a result, neck dissection and removal of these nodes is commonly a part of the treatment plan. If the tumor is confined to one side of the larynx, then unilateral dissection remains an option. Radiotherapy is an alternative to neck dissection. Because it can play an important role in guiding treatment with little added morbidity, unilateral neck dissection should also be considered for patients with N0 tumors.[8]

Survival rates for T1 and T2 tumors are approximately 85% to 95% regardless of treatment modality. For T3 tumors without nodal metastasis 5-year survival is 65% but this rate falls to 50% when nodes are involved. Likewise, T4 tumors show 5-year survival rates of 40% if there is no nodal disease, or 10% to 30% if nodal metastasis is present.[23]

Subglottic Carcinoma

Due to the rarity of subglottic carcinoma, there is a lack of studies comparing treatment methods. Some studies looking at primary radiation therapy have shown some effectiveness but generally poor outcomes regardless of treatment modality. Surgical therapy carries considerable morbidity but is generally the treatment of choice with total laryngectomy with thyroidectomy and paratracheal node dissection being the method used.[8] Adjuvant radiation therapy should be used for more advanced lesions.

Chapter 5: The Larynx   **211**

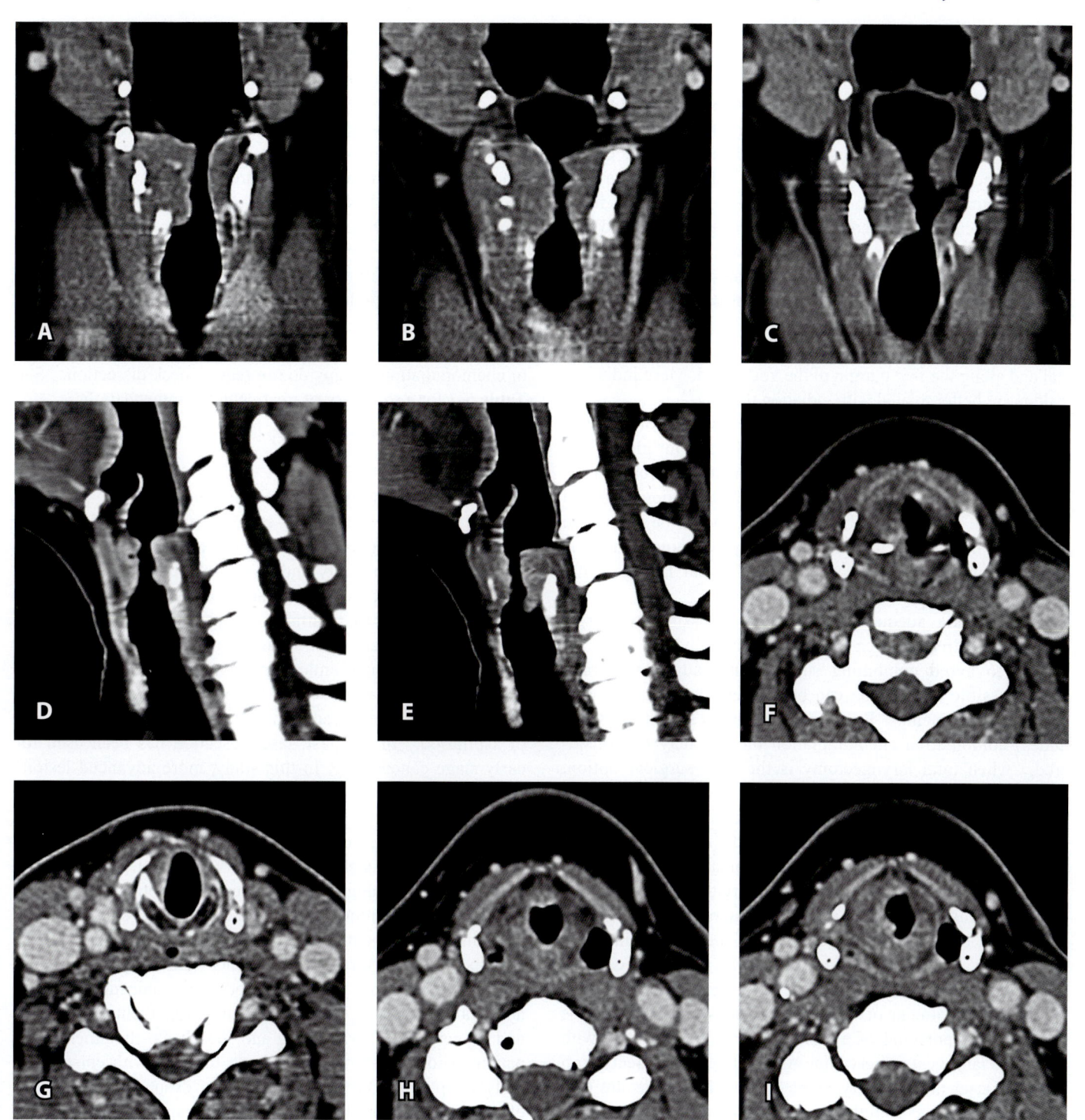

Figure 5-12 T2 Glottic Carcinoma Failed Laser Treatment
This patient underwent laser resection treatment of a T2 glottic tumor nine months prior to this study. (**A–C**) Postcontrast CT with coronal reconstruction showing transglottic spread of a right-sided mass secondary to recurrence of disease. (**D, E**) Postcontrast CT with sagittal reconstruction again showing the right-sided recurrent mass. (**F–G**) Postcontrast CT axial images showing the right-sided recurrent glottic mass with significant subglottic extension. (**H–I**) Postcontrast axial CT images showing supraglottic extension of the mass resulting in narrowing of the airway and compromise of the piriform sinus on the right. A lesion of this size would require total laryngectomy, regardless of a previous history of treatment failure.

American Society of Clinical Oncology Recommendations for Laryngeal Preservation

The American Society of Clinical Oncology (ASCO) has released recommendations for treatment of laryngeal cancer based on an analysis of prospective and retrospective cohort studies. Recommendations are based not only on best survival outcome but also take into consideration preservation of function, cost, local–regional control, disease-free survival, and toxicity of therapy.[24]

An overriding premise of their recommendations is that laryngeal preservation should be a goal of treatment for all T1 and T2 lesions. Endoscopic resection is the preferred modality of treatment in appropriate tumors such as those that are superficial and along the free margin of the vocal cord. More indistinct lesions are better treated with radiation therapy.[24]

T2 lesions have been noted by some investigators to have poor outcomes after failure of radiation therapy for glottic carcinomas.[24] Because of this, treatment remains an area of controversy as a balance between adequate local–regional control versus voice quality must be weighed. It should be left to the patient to decide the treatment modality of choice with the options being radiation or supracricoid partial laryngectomy with cricohyoidoepiglottopexy.[24]

Considering adequate outcomes are possible with single-modality treatment care should be taken with T1 and T2 tumors to avoid combining surgery and radiation therapy when possible as function can be further compromised with combined treatments.[24] For stage III tumors (T2 with positive nodes) combination chemoradiation therapy may be considered, "when total laryngectomy is the only surgical option, when the functional outcome after larynx-preservation surgery is expected to be unsatisfactory, or when surgical expertise in such procedures is not available."[24] A definite algorithm for treatment of early stage laryngeal carcinoma is not available as consideration must be made for each individual patient. These considerations include tumor size, node status, patient age and preference, overall medical condition of the patient, involvement of the anterior commissure, history of previous head and neck malignancy, and the expertise of the treating physician.[24]

For the treatment of T3 and T4 lesions, current methods allow for the potential of a more conservative approach with respect to laryngeal preservation. As discussed in the section on transoral laser microsurgery, some T3 and T4 lesions are currently being treated with that method. According to the ASCO, another potential treatment method is chemoradiation therapy or radiation therapy alone. When surgical salvage is used in conjunction with these methods overall survival is not compromised and there is a gain in the chance that the larynx may be preserved.[24] The choice to treat with either of these previous methods or with total laryngectomy will vary greatly among different patients and physicians.

Some signs may help the physician decide when laryngeal sparing treatment may be employed over traditional total laryngectomy; however, no definitive signs have been found. That said, cartilaginous involvement and involvement of the strap muscles makes patients poor candidates for this approach.[24]

Currently, the ASCO states that there is insufficient evidence for the use of induction chemotherapy in the treatment of T3 or T4 lesions and do not recommend that such treatment be used outside of clinical trials.[24]

Neck dissection is routinely recommended only for patients with N2 or N3 disease. Even patients who respond well to combination chemoradiation therapy are recommended to undergo neck dissection with N2 or N3 disease as outcomes after salvage surgery for recurrent neck disease are generally poor. In contrast, T1 and T2 lesions of the glottis with clinically N0 nodes do not require treatment of the neck. All supraglottic lesions and advanced glottic lesions should have treatment of the neck, however, even if clinically N0. Finally, patients with N1 lesions who have a complete response to definitive radiation therapy or chemoradiation therapy do not require neck dissection.[24] See **Table 5-7** for a summary of treatment recommendations.

Transoral Laser Microsurgery

Supraglottic

Endoscopic laser surgery has largely emerged as the preferred method of treatment for early stage glottic tumors. The precision of this procedure allows for conservative voice sparing treatment, low morbidity and mortality, and reduced hospital stays.[25] In a recent study by Grant et al., the effectiveness for laser microsurgery for treatment of supraglottic laryngeal carcinoma was evaluated. Contraindications to laser resection were listed as, "inadequate endoscopic access, extension of tumor to involve the great vessels of the neck, and tumor extension such that a complete resection puts the patient at serious risk of aspiration." In the past, laser resection has been used for early stage cancer only. In this study, more advanced lesions were treated with laser resection, including 8 T3 lesions and 8 T4 lesions.[25]

Postoperative complications were rare but included hemorrhage, supraglottic stenosis, upper airway obstruction following adjuvant radiation therapy, and one case of carotid artery rupture after radiotherapy related to wound complications at the site of neck dissection, not at the site of the laser surgical site.[25]

Six months posttreatment, patients were evaluated for preservation of function, measuring both communication function and swallowing function. Pretreatment most patients had normal and asymptomatic swallowing and speech. Posttreatment most patients showed normal swallowing function with episodic or daily symptoms of dysphagia and minor dysphonia. These side effects are comparable even to radiotherapy, which has been considered the preferred method of treatment when preservation of function is the main concern. Overall, laryngeal preservation rate was reported to be 97%, and overall 2- and 5-year survival estimates, including T3 and T4 lesions, were found to be 85% and 61%, respectively.[25] Another study by Motta et al. showed a 5-year survival rate of 97% for T1 tumors, 94% for T2 tumors, and 81% for T3 tumors.[26]

Similar to traditional surgical methods the inclusion of neck dissection is dependent on tumor size, nodal status, patient preference, and whether adjuvant radiation therapy is planned. The decision to treat with adjuvant radiotherapy is similarly unchanged compared to traditional surgical methods.

Table 5-7 American Society of Clinical Oncology Treatment Guidelines

Stage	Description	Recommended Treatment	Other Options
T1 and T2 Glottis Cancer			
T1	Tumor limited to the vocal cord(s) (may involve anterior or posterior commissure) with normal mobility	Endoscopic resection (selected patients) OR radiation therapy	Open organ preservation surgery
T1a	Tumor limited to one vocal cord		
T1b	Tumor involves both vocal cords		
T2	Tumor extends to supraglottis and/or subglottis, or with impaired vocal cord mobilty		
T2-favorable	Superficial tumor, on radiographic imaging, with normal cord mobility	Open organ preservation surgery OR radiation therapy	Endoscopic resection (selected patients)
T2-unfavorable	Deeply invasive tumor on radiographic imaging, with or without subglottic extension, with impaired cord mobility (indicating deeper invasion)	Open organ preservation surgery OR concurrent chemoradiation therapy (selected patients with node-positive disease)	Radiation therapy OR endoscopic resection (selected patients)
T1 and T2 Supraglottis Cancer			
T1	Tumor limited to one subsite of supraglottis with normal vocal cord mobility	Open organ preservation surgery OR radiation therapy	Endoscopic resection (selected patients)
T2	Tumor invades mucosa of more than one adjacent subsite of supraglottis or glottis or region outside the supraglottis (e.g., mucosa of base of tongue, vallecula, medial wall of pyriform sinus) without fixation of the larynx		
T2-favorable	More locally advanced and invasive T2 supraglottic lesions		
T2-unfavorable	Deep tissue inolvement	Open organ preservation surgery OR concurrent chemoradiation therapy (selected patients with node-positive disease)	Radiation therapy OR endoscopic resection (selected patients)
T3 and T4 Glottis and Supraglottis Cancer			
T3 glottis cancer	Glottis – tumor limited to the larynx with vocal cord fixation, and/or invades paraglottic space, and/or minor thyroid cartilage erosion (e.g., inner cortex)	Concurrent chemoradiation therapy OR open organ preservation surgery (in highly selected patients)	Radiation therapy
T3 supraglottis cancer	Supraglottis – tumor limited to larynx with vocal cord fixation and/or invades any of the following: postcricoid area, pre-epiglottic tissues, paraglottic space, and/or minor thyroid cartilage erosion (e.g., inner cortex)		
T4a glottis or supraglottis cancer	Tumor invades through the thyroid cartilage and/or invades tissues beyond the larynx (e.g., trachea, soft tissues of neck including deep extrinsic muscle of the tongue, strap muscles, thyroid, or esophagus)		
T4b glottis or supraglottis cancer	Tumor invades prevertebral space, encases carotid artery, or invades mediastinal structures		

Modified with permission from Pfister, et al.: American society of clinical oncology clinical practice guideline stategies in the treatment of laryngeal cancer. J Clin Oncol 2006;22:3693–3704.

Glottic

Another study by Grant et al. evaluated transoral laser microsurgery for treatment of glottic cancer as well. Contraindications for treatment were similar. Complications included one patient who developed supraglottic stenosis after treatment of a T4 tumor and required a tracheotomy until a disease recurrence prompted a total laryngectomy. A second patient developed persistent aspiration, also after resection of a T4 lesion, and local repair was performed.

Laryngeal preservation was 95% overall with a functional laryngeal preservation of 89%. A larynx was considered functional if adequate communication in social settings was possible and effective swallowing could be performed with no aspiration or weight loss.[27] Overall, 2- and 5-year survival rates were 95% and 89%, respectively. For T1 lesions, 2- and 5-year survival was 97% and 94%, 93%, and 93% for T2, and 90% and 60% for T3 and T4 lesions. The median hospital stay posttreatment was 1 day with an average stay of 2 days.[27]

Laser resection continues to improve the treatment of laryngeal neoplasms and with drastically reduced hospital stays compared to traditional surgery and functional sparing effectively equal to that of radiation therapy. As techniques and surgical experience improve, the use of transoral laser microsurgery will likely increase.

Squamous Cell Carcinoma Variants

There are distinct subsets of squamous cell carcinoma that show different properties histopathologically along with carrying different prognosis, treatment options, and diagnostic methods. Approximately 2% to 7% of laryngeal neoplasms are a variant form of squamous cell carcinoma.[11]

Verrucous Squamous Cell Carcinoma

Verrucous carcinoma accounts for approximately 3% of all laryngeal cancers.[19] The human papilloma virus (HPV) serotype 16 clearly plays an etiologic role in development of this disease.[11,19] Lesions of this type appear as broad-based, exophytic masses on endoscopy. Recurrence rates as high as 71% have been reported with radiation therapy whereas surgery alone has a recurrence rate of only 7%.[11] It is important, therefore, that care be taken to distinguish these lesions from squamous cell carcinoma as the treatment is different. Lymph node metastasis is extremely rare and as a result neck dissection need not be included in treatment. Pathologically, these lesions may at times appear benign so multiple biopsies should be taken when endoscopic or radiologic imaging suggests a malignant lesion.

Imaging will show an exophytic lesion with deep fingerlike projections and moderate enhancement upon administration of contrast.[11]

Spindle Cell Carcinoma

Spindle cell carcinoma is a biphasic carcinoma with both an epithelioid and spindle-shaped component. It affects males far greater than females with a ratio of approximately 11:1.[19] These lesions are described as exophytic, polypoid masses most often arising from the supraglottic larynx. Endoscopically, they appear as pedunculated masses attached by a stalk. Surgery is the treatment of choice. On radiologic imaging, these masses appear as exophytic, pedunculated masses with a thin stalk and show nonhomogeneous enhancement with administration of contrast.[11]

Basaloid Cell Carcinoma

Basaloid cell carcinoma is a variant of squamous cell carcinoma that consists of both basaloid and squamous carcinoma components. It is a high-grade lesion with a tendency to aggressively invade locally and commonly has regional and distant metastasis.[11,19] Macroscopically, this tumor appears as a solid, lobulated mass. This lends to identification on MRI as T1-weighted images show a lobulated enhancement pattern.[11] Treatment is generally with surgical resection and adjuvant radiotherapy, with some physicians recommending adjuvant chemotherapy due to the relatively high rate of distant metastasis.[11]

Adenosquamous Carcinoma

Adenosquamous carcinoma is another biphasic tumor composed of both adenocarcinoma and squamous cell carcinoma. This disease carries a poor prognosis as 65% of patients have nodal involvement on presentation.[19] Even with aggressive treatment with surgery and neck dissection, 2-year survival remains poor at 55%.[19]

Other Malignant Neoplasms

Chondrosarcoma

Chondrosarcoma is the most frequent sarcoma of the larynx.[11] The majority of chondrosarcomas (50% to 70%) arise from the cricoid cartilage while 20% to 35% arise from the thyroid cartilage.[28] Chondrosarcoma will have a similar appearance to chondroma on CT and MRI and is often difficult if not impossible to distinguish (see chondroma).

Adenoid Cystic Carcinoma

Unlike squamous cell carcinoma, adenoid cystic carcinoma does not appear to be associated with smoking and shows no difference in incidence between men and women.[11,28] The tumor origin tends to be in the subglottic larynx and tumor spread is generally submucosal. Perineural spread is a common component of this lesion and as a result recurrent laryngeal nerve paralysis and subsequent vocal cord paralysis can occur.[11]

Characteristics on CT and MRI are similar to squamous cell carcinoma. Cartilaginous involvement and submucosal spread is often present at the time of diagnosis.[11] Because of a lack of characteristic findings on imaging clinical correlation can help narrow a differential. This diagnosis should be considered in a nonsmoking patient with a primary subglottic tumor.[11]

Mucoepidermoid Carcinoma

Another tumor that occurs predominantly in males in their seventh decade, mucoepidermoid carcinoma occurs primarily in the supraglottic larynx.[8] It is a tumor of the minor salivary glands. Radiation therapy in generally ineffective when used alone, so treatment should be with surgery with consideration for postoperative radiation therapy.[8] As occult neck disease is often present, neck dissection is generally performed even for clinically N0 disease.[6]

Adenocarcinoma

The larynx contains several minor salivary glands and as a result can be a site of origin for adenocarcinoma, though this type

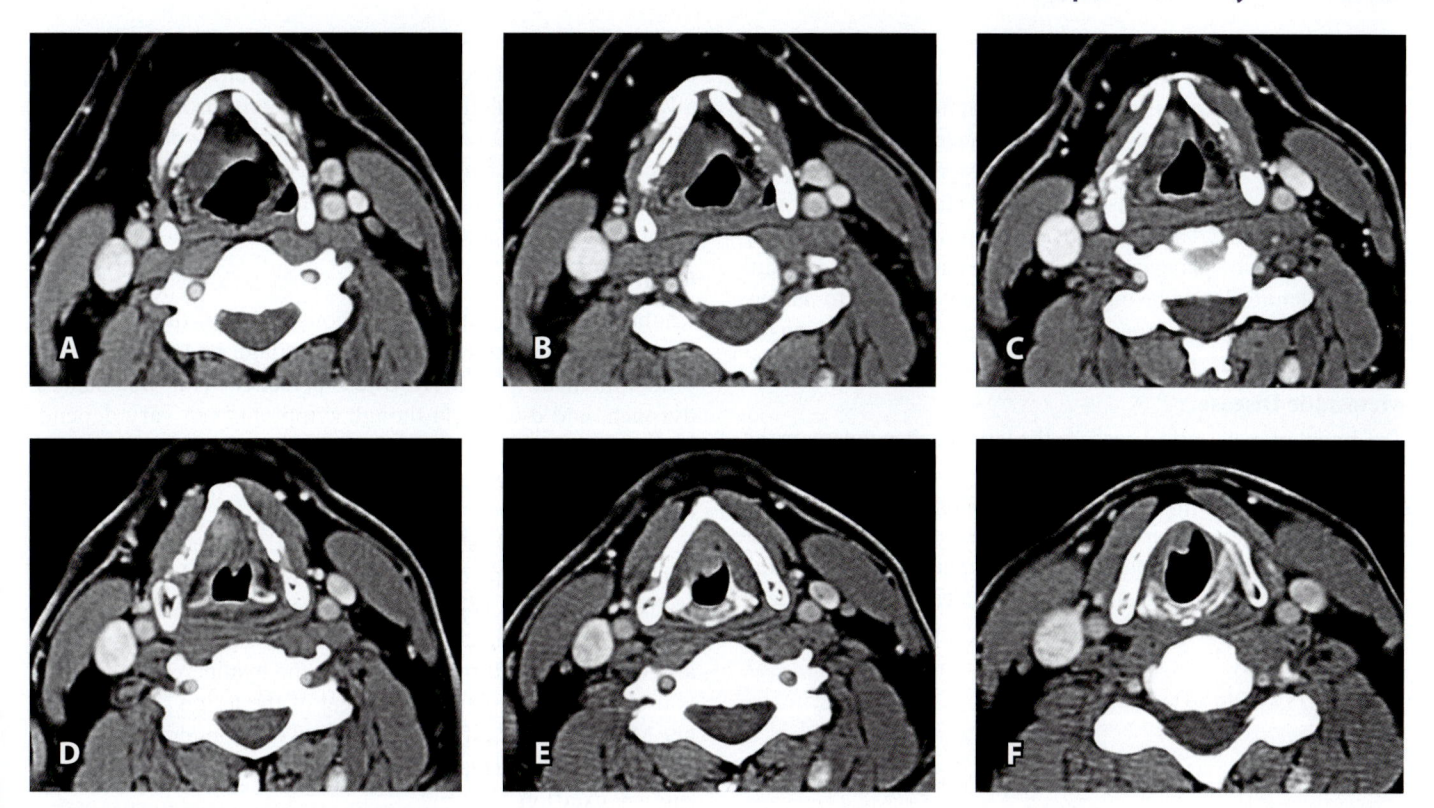

Figure 5-13 Leiomyosarcoma of the Larynx
This is a leiomyosarcoma of the larynx. Such lesions can only be diagnosed on histologic evaluation, as there are no specific imaging characteristics to differentiate rare laryngeal tumors from the typical squamous cell carcinoma. Size of lesion, patient's age, and other known malignancies may be helpful in the differential diagnosis. (**A–F**) Postcontrast axial CT images showing a large mass originating in the region of the right anterior larynx with extension downward into the subglottic region, crossing the midline with upward extension into the contralateral false cords, anterior commissure, and AE fold going to the level of the epiglottis.

of cancer remains very rare. The most common laryngeal site involved is the supraglottic larynx with symptoms corresponding to tumor size and location. Like squamous cell carcinoma, it is most common in the fifth to seventh decade and predominantly occurs in males. Cross-sectional imaging will often show extensive submucosal tumor spread, often with invasion of the laryngeal cartilage.[11]

Leiomyosarcoma

Leiomyosarcoma is an extremely rare tumor of the larynx with very few cases reported in the available literature. It is a tumor of smooth muscle cells that is most often found in the uterus or intestinal tract.[29] When these tumors do occur in the larynx they are more common in men than women and tend to occur in middle age.[29] Of the cases reported, the majority have been of supraglottic origin. Leiomyosarcoma has presenting symptoms similar to other laryngeal malignancies. Contrary to squamous cell carcinoma, there does not appear to be an association with tobacco or alcohol.[29] As this tumor shows poor response to chemotherapy or radiation therapy treatment is with functional preservation surgery if possible. Metastasis is hematogenous and does not appear to depend on tumor size.[29] The tumor is often slow growing and prognosis depends on the amount of tumor differentiation. **Figure 5-13** illustrates a case of laryngeal leiomyosarcoma.

Liposarcoma

Liposarcoma has a similar appearance to lipoma, though it may show increased contrast uptake (see section on lipoma).

Kaposi's Sarcoma

Kaposi's sarcoma of the larynx has become more common with the increased prevalence of acquired immune deficiency syndrome (AIDS), though there are two other types of Kaposi's sarcoma apart from the AIDS related disease. The other forms are the classic or Mediterranean form and the Central African form. The type most frequently seen in the United States is AIDS related Kaposi's sarcoma.

Laryngeal involvement is generally a late occurrence in the disease progression and as a result patients have generally been diagnosed with Kaposi's sarcoma from the characteristic skin lesions associated with the disorder.[28] The epiglottis is the most common area affected. AIDS-related Kaposi's sarcoma is usually a late manifestation of disease and often patients already have nodal and visceral involvement. Prognosis is usually poor. African Kaposi's of the larynx progresses rapidly and is usually fatal. In contrast, laryngeal involvement of the classic type shows a slow progression and patients may live for many years with the disease.[28]

On imaging, Kaposi's sarcoma will appear as a soft tissue mass, often well circumscribed, with enhancement upon administration of contrast. MRI will show high signal on T2-weighted images. Flow voids may also be present, characteristic of vascularized tumors.[28] The appearance of Kaposi's sarcoma is very similar to that of paragangliomas and hemangiomas. The full clinical picture should be taken into account in order to narrow a diagnosis, such as the presence of characteristic skin lesions of Kaposi's sarcoma.

Metastatic Disease

Treatment of metastatic disease to the larynx is dependent on the primary tumor but as it tends to be a late occurence in the disease course, treatment is often palliative. The most common tumors to metastasize to the larynx are, in order of incidence: melanoma, renal cell carcinoma, breast carcinoma, colon cancer, and lung cancer.[8,11] If the metastasis is a single lesion, treatment can be attempted though prognosis is generally very poor.[11]

Benign Neoplasms

Papilloma

Squamous papillomas are the most common benign neoplasm of the larynx,[6,19,20] representing 84% of benign lesions.[19] Molecular studies have shown the causative agent to be the HPV, specifically serotypes 6 and 11. Recurrent respiratory papillomatosis shows a bimodal age distribution, affecting children and young adults. The mode of transmission in children is likely perinatal. In adults, it is unclear whether infection represents reactivation of a perinatal infection or newly acquired infection.[6,19,20] Clinical presentation in adults is typically hoarseness, though in children presentation can be much more severe including stridor and respiratory distress.[6,19]

Laryngoscopy will show mucosal nodules, the extent of which are best evaluated with CT.[30] Contrast enhancing lesions are seen extending to the airway.[28]

Laser ablation has become the first line method of treatment though recurrence is common. Cidofovir has recently become an important tool for adjuvant therapy. Severe cases may be treated with tracheotomy.[31]

Neuroma

Schwannomas and nuerofibromas represent 0.1% to 1.5% of benign laryngeal tumors.[32] Schwannomas are a benign tumor of Schwann cells that are only very rarely associated with malignant transformation.[6]

Neurofibromas, which are associated with neurofibromatosis type I, have been known to become malignant.[6] They also differ from schwannomas in that they are unencapsulated.[33,34]

These neurogenic tumors generally arise from the superior laryngeal nerve and are found within the aryepiglottic fold, often near the apex of the arytenoid cartilage. Neurogenic tumors (including schwannoma, neurofibromas, and granular cell tumors) have similar features on MRI with signal intensity similar to the spinal cord on T1-weighted spin echo and high signal intensity on T2-weighted images. Contrast enhancement is variable though nearly all show some level of enhancement.[11,35] Due to encapsulation, schwannomas generally appear well delieated whereas neurofibromas are more diffuse lesions. On CT, schwannomas may show a lower attenuating outer ring with a higher attenuating inner area correlating with Anoni B and Antoni A areas, respectively.[28] Treatment is with surgical excision.[20,36]

Chondroma

Chondromas are a rare cartilaginous tumor of the larynx that generally arise from the cricoid cartilage and show a male predominance.[6,11,19,37,38] It often presents with hoarseness, dyspnea, and dysphagia though symptoms can vary depending on the location of the lesion.[6,19] Histologic distinction between chondroma and low grade chondrosarcoma may be difficult.[6,8]

This lesion is best visualized with CT as these lesions contain coarse or stippled calcifications which are best visualized with this modality. The masses are often well circumscribed and hypodense.[11,28,39] Signal intensity on T2-weighted MRI is generally high as a result of water within the hyaline cartilage. MRI is useful for determining the extent of the lesion.[19] Neither CT nor MRI allow for differentiation between chondroma or chondrosarcoma.[11,19,28] Treatment is typically with voice conserving surgical excision.[6,20,37,39]

Granular Cell Tumor

Granular cell tumors most commonly arise at the base of the tongue and are rare in the larynx. Due to the presence of the S-100 marker in these tumor cells, general opinion is that they originate from Schwann cells.[6,11,40] Patients may present with dysphagia, dysphonia, and foreign body sensation.[19,41,42]

CT and MRI findings are generally nonspecific but may be similar to those seen with other neurogenic tumors such as schwannomas and neurofibromas.[28,40,42] Treatment is generally with surgical or laser excision.[19,20,40–42]

Lipoma

Lipomas are rarely found in the larynx and mainly affect men over the age of 50.[11] Symptoms range from dyspnea, foreign body sensation, hoarsness, and dysphagia, to death from asphyxiation.[11,43] The tumors are composed of fatty tissue containing mature adipocytes and are usually encapsulated.[11,43,44]

Both CT and MRI are excellent modalities for diagnosing a lipoma. CT will show a homogeneous nonenhancing mass and will appear consistent with fat. On MRI, the lesion will show signal intensity that is equal to that of the subcutaneous fat regardless of the type of image acquisition – high signal intensity on T1-weighted images, very low signal on fat suppressed T1-weighted images, and decreased intensity on T2-weighted images.[11,28] Differentiation between lipoma and liposarcoma with CT or MRI is difficult; however, if areas of the lesion are isointense relative to soft tissue and the connective tissue shows contrast enhancement, liposarcoma should be considered.[11,28]

Treatment varies with the size and location of the tissue. Small lesions can be removed endoscopically with no increased risk of recurrence. Larger or more difficult lesions may be removed via an external approach.[11,20,43,44]

Paraganglioma

Paragangliomas arise from pairs of neuroendocrine tissue that are located at the anterior aspect of the false vocal cords and in the subglottic region, which are designated as the superior and inferior groups respectively. Lesions of the superior group are the most common.[6,20,28,45,46] Symptoms differ depending on location, with supraglottic tumors producing hoarseness and dysphagia while subglottic tumors causing symptoms of airway obstruction when they reach significant size.[45,46]

Diagnosis with CT or MRI is aided by the hypervascular nature of these lesions, which causes them to show high contrast enhancement.[28,47] MRI may show flow voids if a high flow vessel is present.[28] On T1-weighted imaging, they show intermediate intensity and high signal intensity on T2-weighted images.[7] Care must be taken when performing a biopsy of these lesions as severe hemorrhage can occur.[6] Immunohistochemical markers are an important tool in differentiating these tumors from other neuroendocrine neoplasms which may have a worse prognosis.[46]

Treatment is with local surgical excision and prognosis is excellent.[20,46,47]

Rhabdomyoma

Rhabdomyoma, while most commonly found in the heart, can occur in the head and neck. Rhabdomyoma of the larynx are generally of the adult type, though a fetal type can affect children under four years.[48–50] It is a benign tumor of skeletal muscle that typically presents with hoarseness, dysphagia, dyspnea, or foreign-body sensation. The duration of symptoms can be very long due to the slow growing nature of this tumor.[49,51]

On imaging, the lesions tend to be homogeneous and well circumscribed and may be slightly hyperintense when compared to nearby muscle on T1- and T2-weighted images.[28,49,52] Treatment is with careful surgical excision as local recurrence is common with incomplete excision.[11,49]

Amyloidosis

Amyloidosis is the deposition of extracellular protein in the body. The source and types of protein can be many and varied, with prognosis related to the underlying condition.[19,53] Amyloid deposition to the head and neck is rare, but the larynx is the most common area affected when it does occur.[53,54] Progressive dysphonia is the most common presenting symptom.[55]

Amyloid may deposit in any region of the larynx. On CT imaging, amyloidosis appears as a well-defined homogeneous submucosal mass of soft tissue density, or may appear as circumferential soft tissue thickening.[28,54] Appearance on MRI can be variable but has been reported to have signal intensity similar to skeletal muscle.[54] Treatment is with laser resection or focal surgical resection.[28,53]

Congenital Lesions

Laryngocele

Laryngoceles are dilations of the ventricular saccule that are generally believed to be caused by increases in laryngeal pressure against a congenitally weak mucosa.[6,11,19,56] They contain air and communicate with the lumen of the larynx.[6] Symptoms can be of variable severity as decompression of the air in the lesion may occur and thereby temporarily relieve symptoms. Care must be taken to rule out neoplasm as a cause of obstruction of and increased pressure in the ventricle.[28]

On CT or MRI, laryngoceles appear as air or fluid containing masses that are nonenhancing with contrast administration.[11,28,57] Three types of laryngocele are identified by degree of extension, with internal laryngoceles being contained within the paraglottic space and external laryngoceles showing extension through the thyrohyoid membrane into the soft tissues of the neck and a mixed laryngocele showing both characteristics.[11,56] Treatment is with marsupialization.[19,20]

Vasoformative Tumors

Congenital subglottic hemangioma often presents with stridor and infants may have a cough resembling croup.[6,58] The lesions are highly vascular and may be classified as capillary, cavernous, or mixed.[28]

On CT, these lesions generally show a well-demarcated mass with strong contrast enhancement. On MRI, T2-weighted images show high signal intensity, with low to intermediate intensity on T1. Enhancement after administration of gadolinium is high.[11,28]

While these lesions will generally involute later in life, the potential for significant complications generally warrants treatment.[6] Treatment is controversial, with many different management strategies being employed. Treatments include, close monitoring, corticosteroids, interferon, laser ablation, and tracheotomy.[28,58–60] Currently, the most common treatment is CO_2 laster ablation with steroid administration.[20]

Trauma

Laryngeal trauma is relatively rare as the larynx is protected by the cervical spine posteriorly, the mandible superiorly, and the sternum inferiorly. The most common cause of blunt laryngeal injury is motor vehicle accidents, with sports injuries and assaults contributing as well.[6,11,61–63] However, the most common cause of laryngeal injury overall is iatrogenic.[28] Airway management in the setting of laryngeal trauma is paramount, though the method of securing the airway is controversial as intubation may be difficult or impossible in the setting of laryngeal trauma and may lead to further injury, whereas tracheostomy has the potential to damage surrounding tissues.[61,63]

Management is controversial but if a patient is stable enough to undergo imaging, it is a necessary component of care. In cases where the patient is unable to undergo imaging, acute diagnostic evaluation should not be delayed any more than necessary. Treatment can range from conservative therapy to surgery with plates used for internal fixation.[61–64]

CT has proven to be a cost-effective method of evaluating laryngeal trauma as it can visualize the laryngeal skeleton along with showing evidence of edema or hematoma.[11,28] The radiologist must look for evidence of fracture of the hyoid, thyroid, or cricoid cartilage. Vertical fractures can be seen well on CT as they are perpendicular to the plane of imaging. These fractures are generally created when the thyroid cartilage is compressed against the spine.[7] Horizontal fractures, however, are in the plane of imaging and can be difficult to see without multidetector reconstruction allowing multiplanar analysis.[7]

In evaluation of cricoid cartilage fractures, the shape of the airway is an important evaluation tool. Fractures of the cricoid are often multiple and result in deformation of the airway as the anterior fragment is pushed posteriorly.[7] A normal airway is slightly oval; as a result, a round airway may be a sign of fracture. Subglottic swelling is another key factor. Treatment of these fractures generally requires surgical intervention.

More subtle signs such as rotation of the cricoid cartilage may be present as well indicating cricothyroid dislocation. In actuality such a dislocation is rare, with fracture of the inferior horn of the thyroid cartilage instead allowing the cartilages to separate and giving the appearance of dislocation.[7]

The cricoarytenoid joint may also become dislocated. Abnormal positioning relative to the cricoid cartilage suggests arytenoid dislocation. Comment on the position of the arytenoid relative to the articular tubercle should be made.[7]

Avulsion of the epiglottis is possible if the thyroepiglottic ligament is torn.[11,28] MRI may be a more effective method of visualization in a young patient where calcification of the cartilage has not begun to occur.[11] Edema and/or rounding of the normally ovoid airway may be a subtle indication of underlying trauma.[7]

Inflammation/Infection

Abscess

Abscess formation is as much a factor in the larynx as it is in other areas of the body (**Fig. 5-14**). As is occasionally the case with children, abscesses can form secondary to complicated and suppurative involvement of lymph nodes during infection.[65] Another common etiology is secondary to trauma, such as during a difficult intubation or other foreign body trauma that may cause perforation of the pharynx or upper esophagus.

Clinical presentation and patient history may aid in the diagnosis of an abscess as patients will often complain of severe pain with swallowing and may show evidence of mass effect, such as changes in voice or difficulty with swallowing or breathing. Imaging plays an important role in diagnosis as well. On CT, abscesses will appear hypodense. Other evidence such as soft tissue thickening may also be present. On MRI, T1-weighted images will show hypoattenuation, whereas T2-weighted imaging will show hyperattenuation secondary to the liquefaction that occurs within abscesses. Air bubbles may also be present.[65]

Tuberculosis

In the age of antibiotics, laryngeal involvement of tuberculosis has fallen to less than 1% of cases; however, with the resurgence

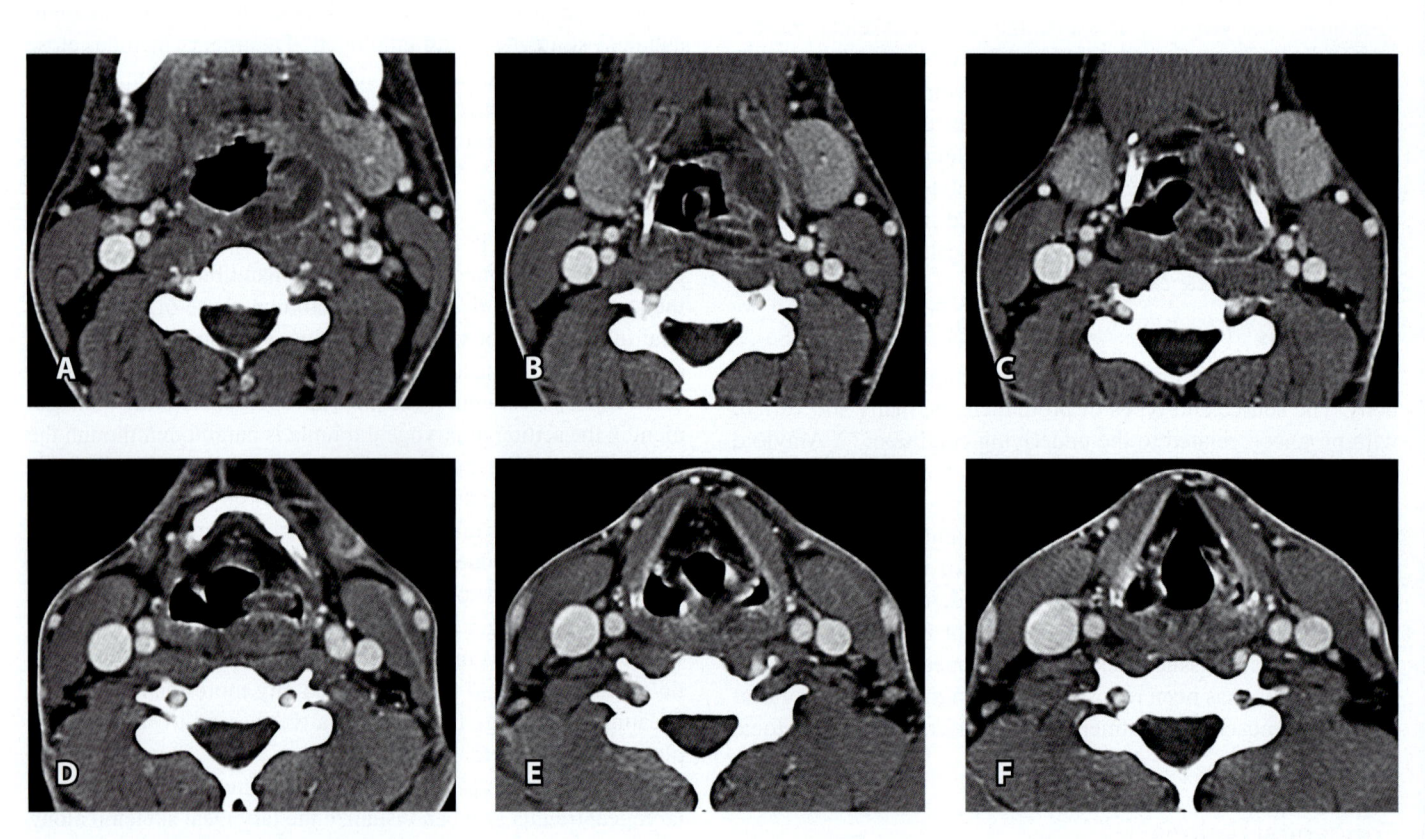

Figure 5-14 Supraglottic Abscess
Multilocular abscess of the supraglottic larynx. (**A–F**) Axial CT scans with contrast. The scans are oriented from top to bottom beginning at the level of the oropharynx (**A**) extending down into the vallecula (**B**) and then into the hypopharynx and piriform sinus (**C–D**) and then into the aryepiglottic fold (**E–F**). There is mucosal enhancement and thickening with loculations of nonenhancing puss that deform the airway and extend anteriorly and laterally into the paraglottic space. Note that the involvement of the paraglottic space enables the puss to migrate down into the larynx.

of tuberculosis in some countries, the emergence of multidrug resistant strains, and with the advent of AIDS and other immunocompromised states laryngeal tuberculosis continues to be a concern. A retrospective study by Wang et al. looked into the modern-day presentation of laryngeal tuberculosis. In the study, 26 cases of laryngeal tuberculosis were reviewed, with the criteria for diagnosis consisting of the presence of acid-fast bacilli on biopsy or the presence of caseating granulomas that showed response to antituberculosis therapy. The incidence showed a male preference with a male-to-female ratio of 2.7:1 and a mean age of 47, though patients ranged from 17 to 77 years old.[66]

Presenting symptoms were most often hoarseness and cough. The high incidence of hoarseness correlated with the most common anatomic area of invasion, with disease involving the true vocal fold in 81% of cases. The next most commonly involved area was the posterior commissure and false vocal folds with 39% involvement each. Vocal fold paralysis was relatively rare however, occurring in 10% of patients.[66] An important point to note is that the presenting symptoms are essentially identical to the presentations of any number of laryngeal pathologies. In this study, it was found that the initial impression based on symptoms and clinical picture was malignancy 80% of the time. This illustrates the importance of other methods of diagnosis, including chest X-rays, direct laryngoscopy and biopsy, and MRI.

The treatment of laryngeal tuberculosis involves multidrug treatment, usually with isoniazid, rifampin, pyrazinamide, and ethambutol. In the study by Wang et al., response to treatment was good and most experience complete resolution of symptoms, including all patients with vocal cord immobility regaining function. Of 26 patients, four reported persistent change in quality of voice secondary to scar formation on the vocal fold mucosa.

Findings on laryngoscopy can be nonspecific. Chest X-ray appears to be the most sensitive for diagnosis tuberculosis, but in the presence of vocal changes further diagnostic methods such as MRI may be employed to evaluate disease extent and/or to rule out concomitant diseases.

Rheumatoid Arthritis

As a true synovial joint, it is possible for the cricoarytenoid joint to be affected by rheumatoid arthritis. Symptoms can include dysphagia, dysphonia, and choking.[28,67] CT can show evidence of cricoarytenoid prominence, luxation, or erosion, along with abnormal positioning of the true vocal cord.[67] Rheumatoid nodules may also develop and be visible on CT.[28,68]

Vocal Cord Paralysis

Paralysis of the vocal cords (**Fig. 5-15**) can result from neurologic damage or dysfunction, or damage to the cricoarytenoid joint. Neurogenic paralysis of the vocal cords is associated with deficit of the superior laryngeal nerve, the recurrent laryngeal nerve, or a total vagal nerve deficit. Dysphonia is the most common presenting symptom but other symptoms including dysphagia and shortness of breath. These symptoms result from glottal incompetence. This inability to fully close the glottis can lead to aspiration during swallowing, especially of liquids. Also, patients lose the ability to create subglottic pressure and close the glottis during phonation. This can lead to air wasting when speaking and cause a sensation of running out of air.[69] In the case of bilateral cord paralysis, patients initially present with poor phonation, but the cords may move medially over time resulting in improved phonation but worsening of airway patency.[70]

Injuries to the nerves can result from damage anywhere along the course of the nerves. In the neck, the vagus nerves travel along the carotid sheath on their respective sides. On the left, the recurrent laryngeal nerve is given off at the level of the arch of the aorta at which time it wraps around the arch and travels back in a cephalad direction within the tracheoesophageal groove. While traveling between the cricoid and thyroid cartilage on its way to the larynx, the nerve is believed to be vulnerable to injury related to intubation.[69] On the right, the recurrent laryngeal nerve is given off at the level of the subclavian artery. The nerve then wraps around the subclavian and moves in a cephalad direction to reach the larynx. This long course leaves the nerves vulnerable to pathology of areas ranging from the brain to the mediastinum.

The superior laryngeal nerve innervates the cricothyroid muscle, which normally serves to pull the anterior ring of the cricoid cartilage toward the thyroid cartilage. This movement results in the arytenoids, attached to the lamina of the cricoid, being rotated posteriorly and therefore placing tension on the vocal cords. Loss of function on one side results in deviation of the arytenoid toward the side of the lesion.[7]

The recurrent laryngeal nerve innervates all intrinsic muscles of the larynx. As the thyroarytenoid muscle atrophies, it results in multiple changes that are visible on CT and MRI such as ventricular enlargement, anteromedial displacement of the ipsilateral arytenoid, and enlargement of the ipsilateral piriform sinus.[7]

CT or MRI imaging also plays an important role in diagnosing lesions along the course of the nerves that may affect nerve function. In the case of vocal cord paralysis, a workup should include imaging from the skull base to the clavicle if the paralysis is on the right, and skull base to the arch of the aorta if the paralysis is on the left.[69]

Treatment for unilateral vocal cord paralysis is generally surgical. Multiple methods are used but the underlying principle is medialization of the paralyzed cord, thereby restoring glottic competence[69] (**Fig. 5-16**). For bilateral paralysis, tracheostomy may be required in cases with severe airway impairment. If the airway is not severely compromised, more conservative treatment such as posterior cordotomy can be attempted.[70]

Radiation Changes

Treatment of laryngeal neoplasms with radiation therapy can lead to changes in the anatomy and physiology of the larynx that can significantly change the appearance on CT and MRI (**Fig. 5-17**). The most common side effect of radiation therapy is persistent laryngeal edema.[71] In general, CT will show diffuse thickening of the epiglottis and soft tissue prominence in the aryepiglottic folds, false vocal cords, and arytenoids. There is also increased attenuation of the pre-epiglottic and paraglottic spaces. The true cords and subglottis usually remain normal but can be edematous.[7,72] These imaging changes may persist for up to 2 years.[11]

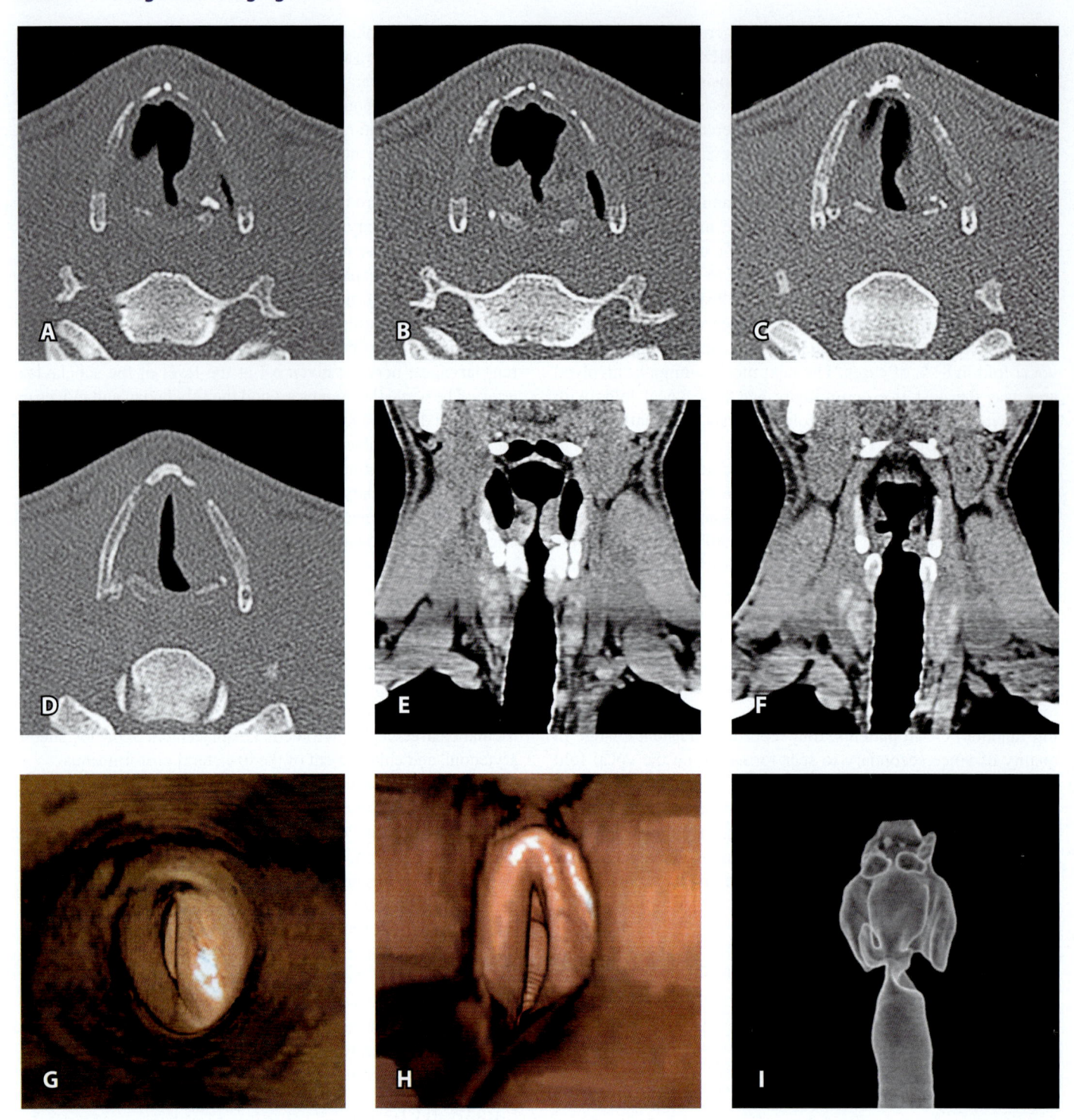

Figure 5-15 Vocal Cord Paralysis
Axial NECT images (**A–D**) show a left paralyzed vocal cord in an adducted position, obliterating the left ventricle of the glottis. The right normal vocal cord is fully abducted, facilitating breathing. Note the superior deflection of the left arytenoid cartilage (**A**), resulting from overcompensation of the left aryepiglottic. Coronal NECT images (**E–F**) show an anterior deflection left arytenoid cartilage with only slight asymmetry of the false cords (**E**). Note that dilitation of the vallecula, sometimes seen with vocal cord paralysis is not seen in this patient (**E**). Demonstrates a downward and medially displaced left vocal cord with an oblitterated left ventricle. Virtual endoscopic reformated images (**G–H**) show the paralytic adducted vocal cord at midline as seen from a cephalad view from below (**G**). Caudal view from above (**H**) show the paralytic left cord on the true left of the image with superior bulging of tissues into the venticular space. Coronal CT reconstruction representing the airway of the larynx (**I**) shows an inward deflection in airway contour at the level of the left vocal cord and ventricle, caused by the paralytic left cord and associated compensation of left accessory tissue.

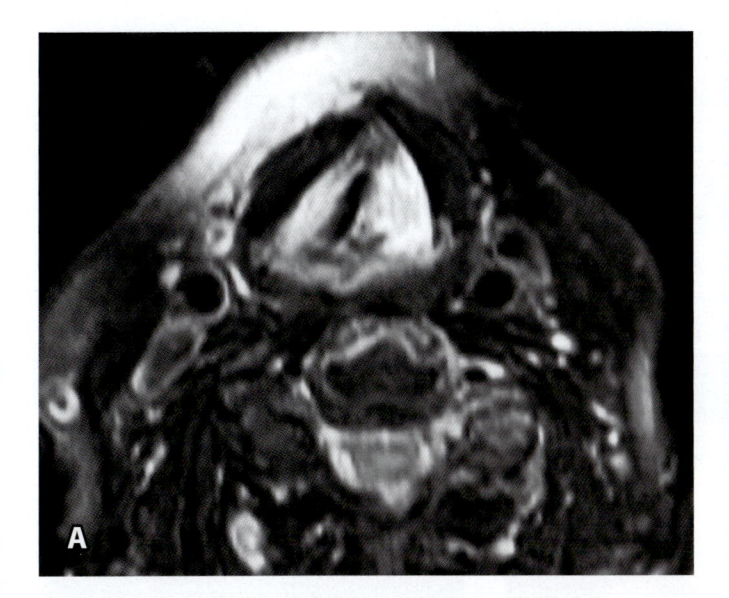

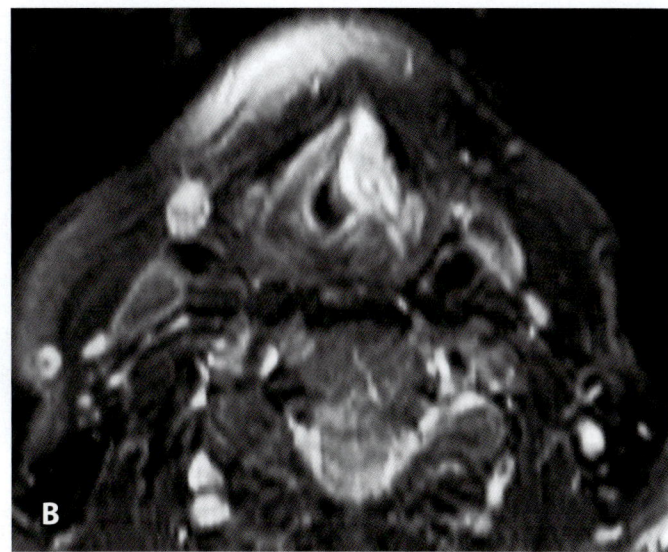

Figure 5-16 Teflon Vocal Cord Injection
Benign causes of glottic deformity. (**A, B**) Axial T2-weighted images show thickening and high signal in the left glottic region as a result of recent Teflon injections to approximate a paralyzed vocal cord.

The laryngeal cartilages generally remain unchanged, however when there is exposure to high doses radiation-induced chondronecrosis can occur. This is a devastating and at times fatal complication that is generally irreversible. Once developed, laryngectomy may be required due to associated laryngeal and therefore airway instability. Radiation associated chondronecrosis has been reported to occur with an incidence of 1% to 5%.[71]

Clinical correlation is important when evaluating possible chondronecrosis as changes on CT are nonspecific; however, there are some signs that can improve the physician's confidence of the presence of chondronecrosis such as gas bubbles in the soft tissue adjacent to the cartilage in question, collapse of thyroid cartilage, and sloughing of arytenoid cartilage.[10] Findings in MRI are similar, with increased intensity on T2-weighted images as a result of edema.[28] With both imaging modalities it can be difficult to distinguish chondronecrosis from recurrent tumor. In contrast, PET scanning has shown 80% accuracy in differentiating between the two.[71]

Postsurgical Changes

Total Laryngectomy

A total laryngectomy consists of complete removal of all laryngeal structures including the hyoid bone and the subglottic space.[28,72,73] A permanent tracheostome is required after surgery. Removal of the larynx allows the esophagus to assume a more anterior positioning and circular appearance.[72] A neopharynx is generally created during the procedure when the layers of the surgical site are closed. This structure is generally partially collapsed and shows variable enhancement of its lining mucosa.[28,74]

In general, complications after this procedure relate to the newly created stoma. A possibility exists however for the development of a carotid artery fistula, developed secondary to close contact with salivary drainage. Care must be taken during the surgery to avoid such a complication.[8] Late developing dysphagia is also a worrisome complication as it may be a sign of recurrence.

Supraglottic Laryngectomy

Supraglottic laryngectomy involves removal of all structures above the level of the ventricle including the epiglottis, aryepiglottic folds, and false vocal cords.[28,72,75] The overlying portion of the thyroid cartilage must also be removed. In general, the hyoid is preserved, though large tumors that extend to this area may require its removal, further worsening postoperative swallowing. The glottic and subglottic regions remain unchanged when viewed postoperatively; however, the removal of the epiglottis requires that the remaining larynx be elevated toward the base of the tongue so that the arytenoids may be opposed against the base of the tongue during swallowing in order to prevent aspiration. As a result, the distance of the remaining larynx to the hyoid bone will appear reduced on imaging.[28]

Complications of this procedure are generally related to swallowing, especially if the surgery is extended to include an arytenoid and/or the tongue base.[8] Generally, these problems can be overcome with therapy but a minority of patients may require total laryngectomy secondary to persistent aspiration.[8]

Vertical Hemilaryngectomy

This technique is used to treat glottic neoplasms, generally T2 or T3 tumors. The thyroid lamina overlying the area of the lesion is excised as is the true vocal cord and the anterior commissure. This procedure may also include the arytenoid and anterior third of the contralateral true vocal cord if necessary.[28,75]

This procedure is generally well tolerated with relatively few complications. Airway is generally well maintained and speech is still possible after this procedure; however, one tends to come at the cost of the other. In other words, a more stable airway often results in worse speech quality and vice versa.[8] If

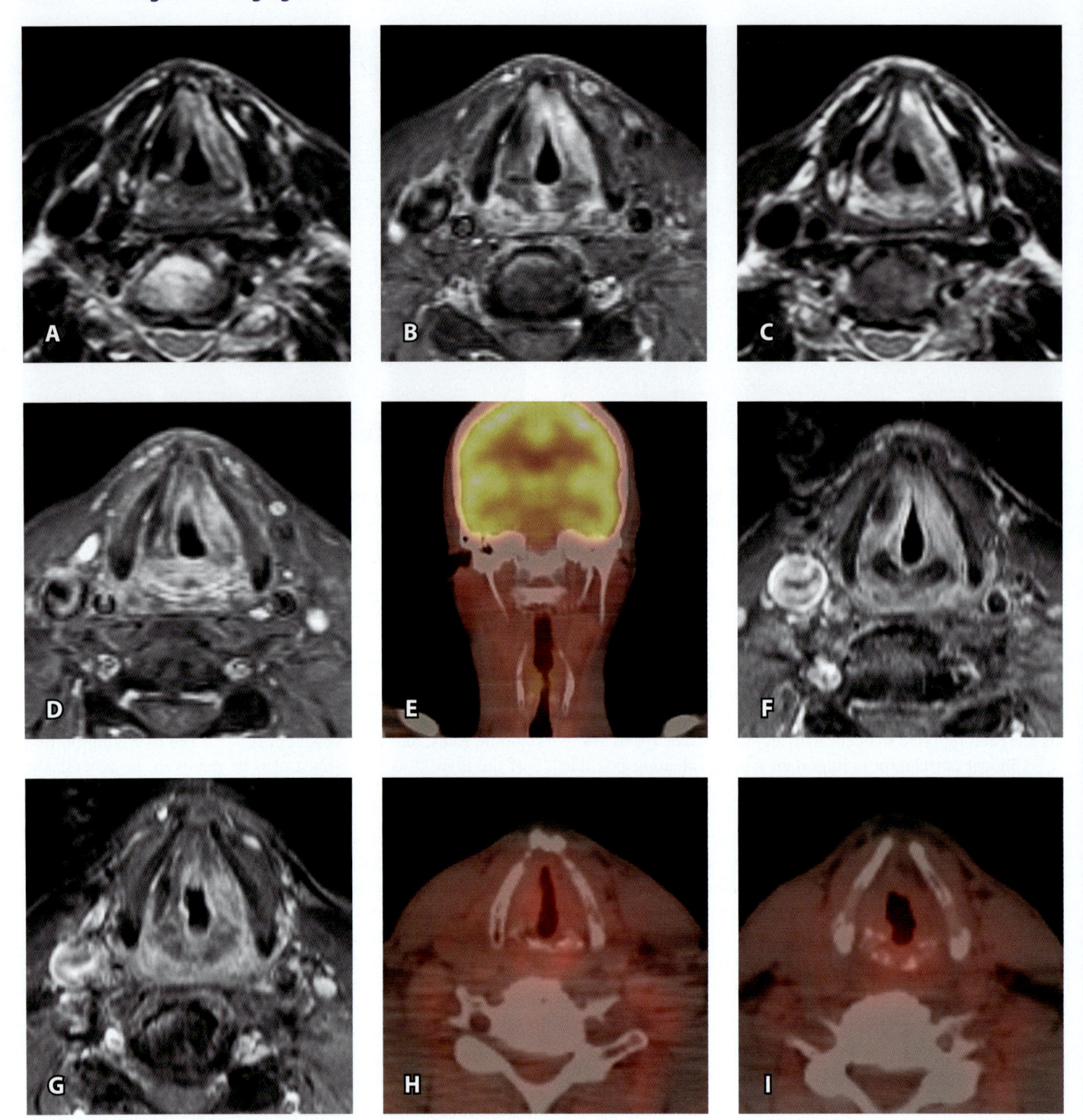

Figure 5-17 Early and Late Radiation Necrosis of the Larynx

This patient had chemoradiation for a T3 lesion four years prior and developed progressive pain and hoarseness. Early radiation necrosis: (**A–B**) Axial T2-weighted MRI shows increased signal in the left true and false cord regions extending in to the anterior commissure. (**C–D**) Axial postcontrast fat saturated T1-weighted images showing intense enhancement in these regions extending posteriorly into the cricoid cartilage. (**E**) Coregistered PET/CT shows a relatively "cold" lesion in the left side of the larynx without evidence of recurrent tumor. Images obtained nine months following previous scans. (**F–G**) Axial T2-weighted postcontrast fat saturation images showing thickening of the mucosa, deformity of the airway and both glottic and paraglottic enhancement. In the interval there is increased deformity and signal abnormality involving the left side of the glottis. (**H, I**) Two consecutive coregistered PET/CT images following injection of FDG18 which show no uptake in the regions of contrast enhancement consistent with radiation necrosis.

complications arise they tend to be with deglutition as removal of the arytenoid results in loss of the medial wall of the piriform sinus.[8]

REFERENCES

1. Sadler TW: Langman's medical embryology. 10th ed. Baltimore: Lippincott Williams & Wilkins; 2006.
2. Moore KL and Persaud TVN: The Developing human: clinically oriented embryology. 6th ed. Philadelphia: W.B. Saunders Company; 1998.
3. Gosling JA, Harris PF, Humpherson JR, Whitmore I, and Willan PLT: Human anatomy: text and color atlas. 2nd ed. New York: Gower Medical Publishing; 1990.
4. Tucker HM: The larynx. 2nd ed. New York: Thieme; 1993.
5. Schünke M, Schulte E, Schumacher U, Ross LM, and Lamperti ED: In: Ross LM and Lamperti ED, eds. Atlas of anatomy: neck and internal organs. New York: Thieme; 2006.
6. Ferlito A, ed.: Diseases of the larynx. New York: Oxford University Press; 2000.
7. Som PM and Curtin HD, eds.: Head and neck imaging, 4th ed. St Louis: Mosby; 2003.
8. Ossoff RH, Shapshay SM, Woodson GE, and Netterville JL, eds.: The larynx. Philadelphia: Lippincott Williams & Wilkins; 2003.
9. Hermans R: Staging of laryngeal and hypopharyngeal cancer: value of imaging studies. Head Neck 2006;16:2386–2400.
10. Joshi AS, et al.: CT scan, larynx. eMedicine. http://imedicine.com/DisplayTopic.asp?bookid=4&topic=390.2007.
11. Mafee MF, Valvassori GE, and Becker M: Valvassori's imaging of the head and neck. 2nd ed. New York: Thieme; 2005.
12. Becker M: Neoplastic invasion of laryngeal cartilage: radiologic diagnosis and therapeutic implications. Eur J Radiol 2000;33:216–229.
13. Becker M, Zbären P, Laeng H, et al.: Neoplastic invasion of the laryngeal cartilage: comparison of MR imaging and CT with histopathologic correlation. Head Neck Radiol 1995;194:661–669
14. Zimmer LA, Branstetter BF, Nayak JV, and Johnson JT: Current use of 18Fflurodeoxyglucose positron emission tomography and combined positron emission tomography and computed tomography in squamous cell carcinoma of the head and neck. Laryngoscope 2005;115:2029–2034.
15. Iqbal N, et al.: Laryngeal carcinoma. eMedicine. http://imedicine.com/DisplayTopic. asp?bookid=12&topic=384. 2007.
16. Kubota K, Yokoyama J, Yamaguchi K, et al.: FDG-PET delayed imaging for the detection of head and neck cancer recurrence after radiochemotherapy: comparison with MRI/CT. Eur J Nucl Med Mol Imaging 2004;31:590–595.
17. Fakhry N, Lussato D, Jacob T, Giorgi R, Giovanni A, and Zanaret M: Comparison between PET and PET/CT in recurrent head and neck cancer and clinical implications. Eur Arch Otorhinolaryngol 2007;264:531–538.
18. Connell CA, Corry J, Milner AD, et al.: Clinical Impact of, and Prognostic Stratification by, F-18 FDG PET/CT in Head and Neck Mucosal Squamous Cell Carcinoma. New York: Wiley Interscience; 2007.
19. Thompson LDR, ed.: Head and neck pathology. New York: Churchill Livingstone Elsevier; 2006.
20. Pilch BZ, ed.: Head and neck surgical pathology. Philadelphia: Lippincott Williams & Wilkins; 2001.
21. Zbären P, Becker M, and Lang H: Staging of laryngeal cancer: endoscopy, computed tomography and magnetic resonance versus histopathology. Eur Arch Otorhinolaryngol 1997;254:S117–S122.
22. Hornig JD, et al.: Supraglottic cancer. eMedicine. http://imedicine.com/DisplayTopic.asp?bookid=4&topic=687.2006.
23. Lydiatt WM, et al.: Glottic cancer. eMedicine. http://imedicine.com/DisplayTopic.asp?bookid=4&topic=688.2006.
24. Pfister DG, Laurie SA, Weinstein GS, et al.: American society of clinical oncology clinical practice guideline for the use of larynx-preservation strategies in the treatment of laryngeal cancer. J Clin Oncol 2006;24:3693–3704.
25. Grant DG, Salassa JR, Hinni ML, et al.: Transoral laser microsurgery for carcinoma of the supraglottic larynx. Otolaryngol Head Neck Surg 2007;136:900–906.
26. Motta G, et al.: CO2 Laser Treatment of Supraglottic Cancer. New York: Wiley Interscience; 2003.
27. Grant DG, Salassa JR, Hinni ML, et al.: Transoral laser microsurgery for untreated glottic carcinoma. Otolaryngol Head Neck Surg 2007;137:482–486.
28. Hermans R, ed.: Imaging of the larynx. New York: Springer 2003.
29. Lippert BM, Schlüter E, Claassen H, et al.: Leiomyosarcoma of the larynx. Eur Arch Otorhinolaryngol 1997;254:466–469.
30. Prince JS, Duhamel DR, Levin DL, et al.: Nonneoplastic lesions of the tracheobronchial wall. Radiologic findings with bronchoscopic correlation. Radiographics 2002;22:S215–S230.
31. Andrus JG and Shapshay SM: Contemporary management of laryngeal papilloma in adults and children. Otolaryngol Clin North Am 2006;39:135–158.
32. Rosen FS, Pou AM, and Quinn FB Jr.: Obstructive supraglottic schwannoma: a case report and review of the literature. Laryngoscope 2002;112:997–1002.
33. Newton JR, Ruckley RW, and Earl UM: Laryngeal neurilemmoma: a case report. Ear Nose Throat J 2006;85:448–449.
34. Kumar V, Abbas AK, and Fausto N, eds. Robbins and Cotran's Pathologic Basis of Disease. Philadelphia: Elsevier Saunders; 2005.
35. Malcolm PN, Saks AM, Howlett DC, and Ayers AB: Case report: magnetic resonance imaging (MRI) appearances of benign schwannoma of the larynx. Clin Radiol 1997;52:75–76.
36. Cohen S, Sincacori JT, and Courey MS: Laryngeal schwannoma: diagnosis and management. Otolaryngol Head Neck Surg 2004;130:363–365.
37. Baatenburg de Jong RJ, Van Lent S, and Hogendoorn PCW: Chondroma and chondrosarcoma of the larynx. Curr Opin Otolaryngol Head Neck Surg 2004;12:98–105.
38. Casiraghi O, Martinez-Madrigal F, Pineda-Daboin K, et al.: Chondroid tumors of the larynx: a clinicopathologic study of 19 cases, including two dedifferentiated chondrosarcomas. Ann Diagn Pathol 2004;8:189–197.
39. Wang SJ, Borges A, Lufkin RB, et al.: Chondroid tumors of the larynx: computed tomography findings. Am J Otolaryngol 1999;20:379–382.
40. Piazza C, Casirati C, Peretti G, et al.: Granular cell tumor of the hypopharynx treated by endoscopic CO(2) laser excision: report of two cases. Head Neck 2000;22(5)524–529.
41. Victoria LV, Hoffman HT, and Robinson RA: Granular cell tumour of the larynx. J Laryngol Otol 1998;112(4)373–376.
42. Sataloff RT, Ressue JC, Portell M, et al.: Granular cell tumors of the larynx. J Voice 2000;14(1):119–134.
43. Yoskovitch A, Cambronero E, Said S, et al.: Giant lipoma of the larynx: a case report and literature review. Ear Nose Throat J 1999;78(2)122–125.
44. El-Monem MHA, Gaafar AH, and Magdy EA: Lipomas of the head and neck: presentation variability and diagnostic work-up. J Laryngol Otol 2006;120:47–55.
45. Sesterhenn AM, Folz BJ, Lippert BM, et al.: Laser surgical treatment of laryngeal paraganglioma. J Laryngol Otol 2003;117:641–646.
46. Myssiorek D, Rinaldo A, Barnes L, and Ferlito A: Laryngeal paraganglioma: an updated critical review. Acta Otolaryngol 2004;124:995–999.
47. Brown SM and Myssiorek D: Lateral thyrotomy for excision of laryngeal paragangliomas. Laryngoscope 2006;116:157–159.
48. LaBagnara J, Hitchcock E, and Spitzer T: Rhabdomyoma of the true vocal fold. J Voice; 13:289–293.
49. Brys AK, Sakai O, DeRosa J, et al.: Rhabdomyoma of the larynx: case report and clinic and pathologic review. Ear Nose Throat J 2005;84:437–440.
50. Liess BD, Zitsch RP, Lane R, et al.: Multifocal adult rhabdomyoma: a case report and literature review. Am J of Otolaryngol-Head Neck Med Surg 2005;26:214–217.
51. Jensen K and Swartz K: A rare case of rhabdomyoma of the larynx causing airway obstruction. Ear Nose Throat J 2006;85:116–118.
52. Liang GS, Loevner LA, and Kumar P: Laryngeal rhabdomyoma involving the paraglottic space. Am J Roentgenol 2000;174:1285–1287.
53. Dedo HH and Izdebski K: Laryngeal amyloidosis in 10 patients. Laryngoscope 2004;114:1742–1746.
54. Alaani A, Warfield AT, and Pracy JP: Management of laryngeal amyloidosis. J Laryngol Oncol 2004;118:279–283.
55. Bartels H, Dikkers FG, van der Wal JE, et al.: Laryngeal amyloidosis: localized versus systemic disease and update on diagnosis and therapy. Ann Otol Rhinol Laryngol 2004;113:741–748.
56. Dursun G, Ozgursoy OB, Beton S, and Batikhan H: Current diagnosis and treatment of laryngocele in adults. Otolaryngol-Head Neck Surg 2007;136:211–215.

57. Alvi A, Weissman J, Myssiorek D, et al.: Computed tomographic and magnetic resonance imaging characteristics of laryngocele and its variants. Am J Otolaryngol 1998;19:251–256.
58. Pransky SM and Canto C: Management of subglottic hemangioma. Curr Opin Otolaryngol Head Neck Surg 2004;12:509–512.
59. Bitar MA, Moukarbel RV, and Zalzal GH: Management of congenital subglottic hemangioma: trends and success over the past 17 years. Otolaryngol Head Neck Surg 2005;132:226–231.
60. Rahbar R, Nicollas R, Roger G, et al.: The biology and management of subglottic hemangioma: past, present, future. Laryngoscope 2004;114:1880–1891.
61. Fitzsimons MG, Peralta R, and Hurford W: Cricoid fracture after physical assault. J Trauma 2005;59:1237–1238.
62. Chowdhury R, Crocco AG, and El-Hakim H: An isolated hyoid fracture secondary to sport injury: a case report and review of literature. Int J Pediatr Otorhinolaryngol 2005;69:411–414.
63. Hwang SY and Yeak SCL: Management dilemmas in laryngeal trauma. J Laryngol Otol 2004;118:325–328.
64. Mello-Filho FV and Carrau R: The management of laryngeal fractures using internal fixation. Laryngoscope 2000;110:2143–2146.
65. Cummings CW, et al.: Otolaryngology head and neck surgery. 4th ed. Philadelphia: Mosby; 2005.
66. Wang CC, Lin CC, Wang CP, et al.: Laryngeal tuberculosis: a review of 26 cases. Otolaryngol Head Neck Surg 2007;137:582–586.
67. Brazeau-Lamontagne L, Charlin B, Levesque RY, et al.: Cricoarytenoiditis: CT assessment in rheumatoid arthritis. Radiology 1986;158:463–466.
68. Chen JJ, Branstetter BF, and Myers EN: Cricoarytenoid rheumatoid arthritis: an important consideration in aggressive lesions of the larynx. Am J Neuroradiol 2005;26:970–972.
69. Rosen CA, et al.: Vocal fold paralysis, unilateral. eMedicine. http://imedicine.com/DisplayTopic.asp?bookid=4&topic=347.2006.
70. Ernster JA, et al.: Vocal fold paralysis, bilateral. eMedicine. http://imedicine.com/DisplayTopic.asp?bookid=4&topic=348.2006.
71. Dean R, et al.: Chondronecrosis of the larynx. eMedicine. http://imedicine.com/DisplayTopic.asp?bookid=4&topic=580.2006.
72. Mukherji SK and Weadock WJ: Imaging of the post-treatment larynx. Eur J Radiol 2002;44:108–119.
73. Maroldi R, Battaglia G, Nicolai P, et al.: CT appearance of the larynx after conservative and radical surgery for carcinomas. Eur Radiol 1997;7:418–431.
74. DiSantis DJ, Balfe DM, Hayden RE, et al.: The neck after total laryngectomy: CT study. Radiology 1984;153:713–717.
75. Keisch TA and Patel U: Partial laryngectomy imaging. Semin Ultrasound CT MRI 2003;24:147–156.

The Pharynx and Oral Cavity

Stephanie Channual, MD
Christopher R. Trimble, MD, MBA
Anton N. Hasso, MD, FACR

EMBRYOLOGY AND DEVELOPMENT

The dorsal end of the first pharyngeal arch forms the lateral wall of the nasopharynx. As the head of the embryo enlarges, the dorsal end of the first pharyngeal pouch deepens and eventually merges with the second pharyngeal pouch.[1] With the lateral wall of the nasopharynx, these contribute to the formation of the tubotympanic recess. The tubotympanic recess eventually forms the eustachian tube and tympanic cavity. The tonsillar fossa is also formed from the dorsal portion of the second pharyngeal pouch. The endodermal epithelium of the ventral second pouch proliferates to form the palatine tonsillar crypts. The lymphatic tissue of the palatine tonsil is formed by the mesenchyme of the second pharyngeal arch.

The mesoderm of the first pharyngeal arch gives rise to the muscles of mastication, the tensor veli palatini, and anterior belly of the digastrics muscles.[2] These muscles are all innervated by the mandibular division of the trigeminal nerve. Muscles arising from the second pharyngeal arch mesoderm include the posterior belly of the digastrics muscle, stylohyoid muscle, and muscles of facial expression, which are all innervated by the facial nerve. The third pharyngeal arch forms the stylopharyngeus, which is innervated by the glossopharyngeal nerve. The same arch also gives rise to the mucosa covering the base of the tongue. The palatopharyngeus muscle may also be a derivative of the third pharyngeal arch. The pharyngeal constrictor and levator veli palatini muscles are derived from the mesenchyme of the fourth to sixth pharyngeal arches and are innervated by the pharyngeal nervous plexus.

The formation of the structures of the oral cavity is based on the dynamics of the development of the first pharyngeal arch.[1] The first arch splits into two entities, which are the mandibular and maxillary portions. After the fourth week of development, these form into two maxillary, two mandibular, and a frontal nasal process. Neurocrest cells invade these tissues and are responsible for their growth. A small gap becomes the mouth. The philtrum or upper lip is formed where the nasomedial and maxillary processes meet during embryo development. Cleft palate can result when the processes fail to fuse fully. Mesoderm from the first arch will form the anterior two-thirds of the tongue, up to the foramen cecum. At four weeks, the oral tongue appears as two lateral lingual swellings and one medial swelling. Additional tissue from occipital somites contributes to the musculature of the tongue. Innervation to this tissue is supplied by the hypoglossal nerve.

ANATOMY

Nasopharynx

The nasopharynx is an epithelium-lined cavity located behind the nasal choanae in the upper part of the pharynx (**Fig. 6-1** and **Table 6-1**). The nasopharynx communicates with the oropharynx through the pharyngeal isthmus, which is bounded anteriorly by the soft palate and posteriorly by the ridge of Passavant, formed by the superior fibers of the superior pharyngeal constrictor muscle. The roof and posterior walls of the nasopharynx are formed by the inferior surface of the sphenoid body, basioccipital and anterior atlantooccipital membrane, anterior arch of the atlas, and body of the second cervical vertebra.[3]

The orifice of the eustachian tube lies on the lateral wall of the nasopharynx, about 1 to 1.25 cm behind and below the posterior end of the inferior turbinate.[3] The fibers of the superior pharyngeal constrictor muscle will curve below the eustachian tube and levator veli palatini. The eustachian tube and levator palatini muscle pierces the sinus of Morgagni to enter the pharynx. This sinus is a defect in the anterior portion of the pharyngobasilar fascia, and is located above the superior pharyngeal constrictor muscle and along the upper posterior border of the medial pterygoid plate. The close proximity of this sinus to the foramen lacerum and foramen ovale creates a potential pathway for cancer to spread to the cranial cavity.[4]

Superior and posterior to the eustachian tube orifice is the torus tubarius, a mucosal elevation marking the pharyngeal end

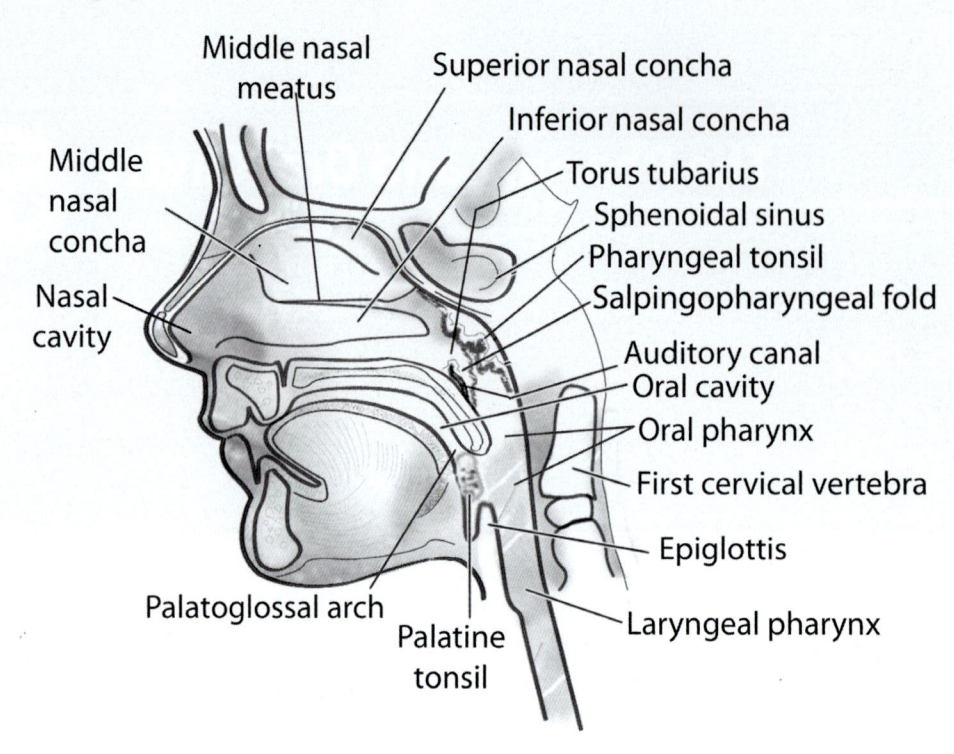

Figure 6-1 Pharynx
A midline sagittal view of the pharynx is shown. The posterior pharyngeal wall starts at the inferior aspect of the nasopharynx in the region of the soft palate and extends to the level of the epiglottis inferiorly. The fossa of Rosenmuller (not shown) is a deep recess posterior and superior to the torus tubarius and is a common site for origin of nasopharyngeal cancer.

Table 6-1 Nasopharynx Structures, Innervation, and Blood Supply

Structures Within the Nasopharynx
- Pharyngobasilar fascia
- Pharyngeal tonsil
- Torus tubarius
- Levator veli palatini muscle
- Tensor veli palatini muscle
- Fossa of Rosenmuller

Innervation
- Sensory: upper part (ciliated epithelia), CN V2; lower part (squamous epithilia), CN IX
- Motor: pharyngeal plexus, with the exception of the tensor veli palatini muscle (CN V3)

Blood Supply
- Branches of the external carotid artery, including the ascending pharyngeal artery, ascending and descending palatine arteries, pharyngeal branch of the sphenopalatine artery

CN = cranial nerve.

of the cartilaginous part of the tube. The fossa of Rosenmuller is a deep recess posterior and superior this tubal elevation and is a common site for origin of nasopharyngeal cancer.[5] The salpingopharyngeal fold descends from the posterior part of the torus tubarius and contains the salpingopharyngeus muscle (**Fig. 6-2**). The torus levatorius is an elevation between orifice of the eustachian tube and the soft palate, which contains the levator veli palatini muscles. The levator veli palatini and the tensor veli palatini muscles both originate lateral to the pharyngobasilar fascia but insert on the soft palate medial to the fascia.

Pharyngeal Tonsil and Pharyngeal Bursa

The pharyngeal tonsil is a collection of lymphoid tissue that is initially detectable at the midline roof and posterior wall of the nasopharynx. Hypertrophy of this tissue occurs in early childhood followed by gradual involution around the time of puberty. Large adenoid masses may extend laterally into the fossa of Rosenmuller. Asymmetry of hypertrophic adenoidal tissue may suggest cancer. Superior to the pharyngeal tonsil is the pharyngeal bursa, which is a depression of the mucous membrane that may extend up to the basilar process of the occipital bone.

Fascial Layers and Spaces

Three main coats, which are the mucosa, fibrous, and muscular layers, line the pharynx. The pharyngobasilar fascia is located between the mucosa and muscular layers and forms the connective tissue lining the lateral and posterior walls the nasopharynx.

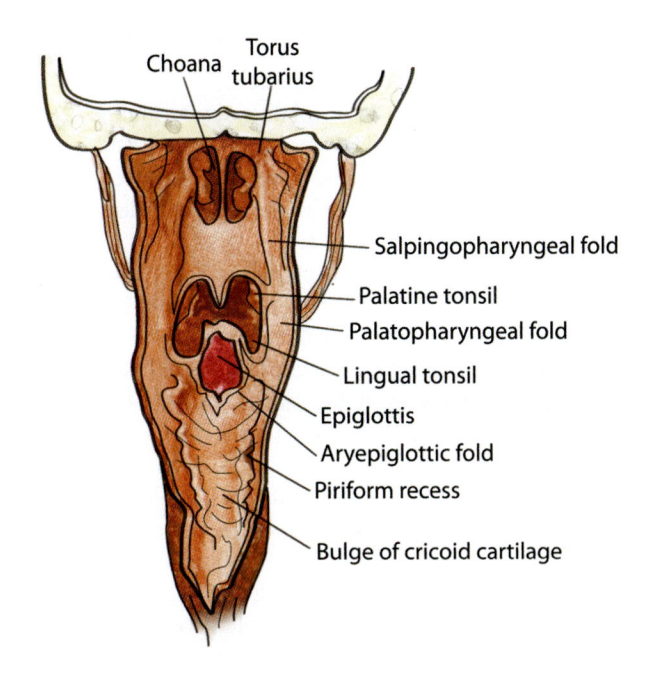

Figure 6-2 A View into the Pharynx from the Posterior Side
The wall of the pharynx has been opened with a longitudinal cut to show the connections of the nasal cavity, oral cavity, and larynx into the pharynx.

It is thick superiorly where it fuses to the basiocciput and petrous temporal bones. The fascia gradually diminishes in thickness as it descends. Midline posteriorly, the fascia condenses to form the median raphe, which provides the attachment for the pharyngeal constrictor muscles.

The buccopharyngeal fascia surrounds the nasopharyngeal mucosa and the outer surface of the pharyngeal constrictor muscles and extends anteriorly over the pterygomandibular ligament to the surface of the buccinator muscles. The fascia is attached to the carotid sheath laterally and the prevertebral fascia midline posteriorly. It unites with the pharyngobasilar fascia superiorly to form a single layer in the sinus of Morgagni. It may serve as a potential barrier to the spread of disease.[4]

The retropharyngeal space lies posterior to the nasopharynx and separates it from the prevertebral fascia. This space contains the retropharyngeal lymph nodes, including the node of Rouviere. The parapharyngeal space is predominantly fat filled, and is situated laterally to the pharynx and extends from the skull base to the superior mediastinum.[3] The masticator space is bounded by the superficial layer of deep cervical fascia and contains muscles of mastication and the ramus and posterior body of the mandible. Local spread of nasopharyngeal cancer can occur to these sites.

Blood Supply

Arterial supply to the nasopharynx all originate from the external carotid artery and its branches, which include the ascending pharyngeal, ascending and descending palatine, and pharyngeal branch of the sphenopalatine. The pharyngeal venous plexus drains superiorly into the pterygoid plexus or inferiorly into the facial or internal jugular veins.

Innervation

Branches of the maxillary division of the trigeminal nerve provide sensory innervation to the upper part of the nasopharynx, while the glossopharyngeal nerve provides sensory innervation to the lower part of the nasopharynx. The pharyngeal plexus, which comprised pharyngeal branches from the glossopharyngeal, vagus, spinal accessory cranial nerves, and cervical sympathetic plexus supply the motor innervation for the nasopharynx. The tensor veli palatini muscle receives its motor innervation from the mandibular division of the trigeminal nerve.

Lymphatic Drainage

The nasopharynx has a rich lymphatic plexus that primarily drains into the ipsilateral and contralateral upper deep cervical lymph nodes. Nasopharyngeal cancers often spread to the lateral retropharyngeal nodes of Rouviere, but can also spread to the jugulodigastric nodes (level II) and spinal accessory chain (level V) as well.

Oropharynx

The oropharynx is located in the mid portion of the pharynx and is bounded anteriorly by the oral cavity. The oropharynx is separated from the nasopharynx by the soft palate and from the hypopharynx by pharyngoepiglottic folds. The superior and middle pharyngeal constrictor muscles form the posterior and lateral boundaries of the oropharynx at the level of the second and third cervical vertebrae.[3] The oropharynx is divided into the posterior wall, soft palate, lateral walls or tonsillar regions, and tongue base (posterior third of the tongue).

The oropharyngeal isthmus connects the oropharynx to the oral cavity. The junction of the hard palate and the soft palate forms the superior part of this isthmus. The hard palate is considered a structure of the oral cavity while the lower surface of the soft palate is part of the oropharynx (the upper surface is considered as part of the nasopharynx). The soft palate is a fibromuscular structure that extends posteriorly and downward into the oropharynx. The levator veli palatini muscle, tensor veli palatini muscle, palatoglossus muscle, palatopharyngeus muscle, and musculus uvulae contribute to its structure. The anterior tonsillar pillar forms the lateral part of the oropharyngeal isthmus. The inferior part of the isthmus is formed by the circumvallate papillae, dome-shaped structures on the back of the tongue.[6]

The tonsillar fossa is defined by the anterior and posterior tonsillar pillar, which are mucosal folds produced by underlying muscles. The palatoglossus muscle is the anterior muscle and connects the soft palate with the base of the tongue. The palatopharyngeus muscle is the posterior muscle that contributes the formation of the pharyngeal wall. The palatine tonsil, which consists of irregular surface filled crypts, lies within the tonsillar fossa. The palatine tonsil forms part of Waldeyer ring, which also consists of the lingual tonsil in the base of the tongue and the pharyngeal tonsil in the roof of the nasopharynx.

The tongue base extends from the circumvallate papillae to the glossoepiglottic and pharyngoepiglottic fold. The glossoepiglottic fold runs from the tongue base to the epiglottis and divides the pit between the base of the tongue to separate both valleculae, which is also considered part of the oropharynx.

Blood Supply

The oropharynx is supplied by branches of the external carotid artery, which include the ascending pharyngeal, dorsal lingual, facial, and internal maxillary arteries. The peritonsillar veins are the main venous drainage system for the oropharynx. These veins pierce the superior pharyngeal constrictor muscle to drain into the common facial vein and the pharyngeal plexus.

Innervation

The glossopharyngeal and vagus cranial nerves provide motor and sensory innervation to the oropharynx. The base of the tongue receives its motor innervation from the hypoglossal nerve. The maxillary and mandibular divisions of the trigeminal nerve supply motor and most of the sensory innervation to the soft palate.

Lymphatic Drainage

The oropharynx has a rich lymphatic drainage. The primary lymphatic drainage is to the upper and mid-jugular nodes (levels II and III). Midline structures such as the posterior pharyngeal wall, soft palate, and tongue base drain to both sides of the neck, and can drain to the retropharyngeal node and parapharyngeal lymph nodes.

Oral Cavity

Oral Tongue

The oral tongue extends past the posterior border of the mouth and into the oropharynx (**Fig. 6-3**). The anterior two-thirds of the tongue lie mostly in the mouth while the posterior third faces the oropharynx. The terminal sulcus is a V-shaped groove that marks the separation of these two parts.

The tongue is divided in two halves by a midline septum, called the lingual septum. The lingual septum arises from the hyoglossus membrane and hyoid bone. Also referred to as the midline low-density plane, it can be seen as a hypodense midline structure on CT.

The tongue is composed of intrinsic and extrinsic muscles. Intrinsic muscles of the tongue include the inferior longitudinal, superior longitudinal, vertical, and transverse fibers, which are not connected to any structure besides the tongue. Extrinsic muscles include the hyoglossus, styloglossus, genioglossus, and palatoglossus fibers that are involved with the hyoid bone, styloid process, chin, and palate, respectively. The intrinsic muscles of the tongue are best visualized with MRI. On T1- and T2-weighted sequences, low signal intensity intrinsic muscle bundles are surrounded by high signal intensity fibrofatty supporting tissue. On MRI, intrinsic muscles of the tongue demonstrate greater signal intensity than the extrinsic muscles, but less than squamous cell carcinoma (SCCa).[7–9] Extrinsic muscles of the tongue may be well visualized on axial and coronal CT and MRI images. They are of low signal intensity on T1- and T2-weighted sequences.

Motor and sensory innervations to the intrinsic and extrinsic tongue muscles are provided by the hypoglossal nerve. The lingual nerve, which is a branch from the mandibular nerve, provides sensation to the anterior part of the tongue, while the chorda tympani supply its taste. The glossopharyngeal nerve provides touch, taste, and gag sensation to the posterior one-third of the tongue (**Fig. 6-4**).

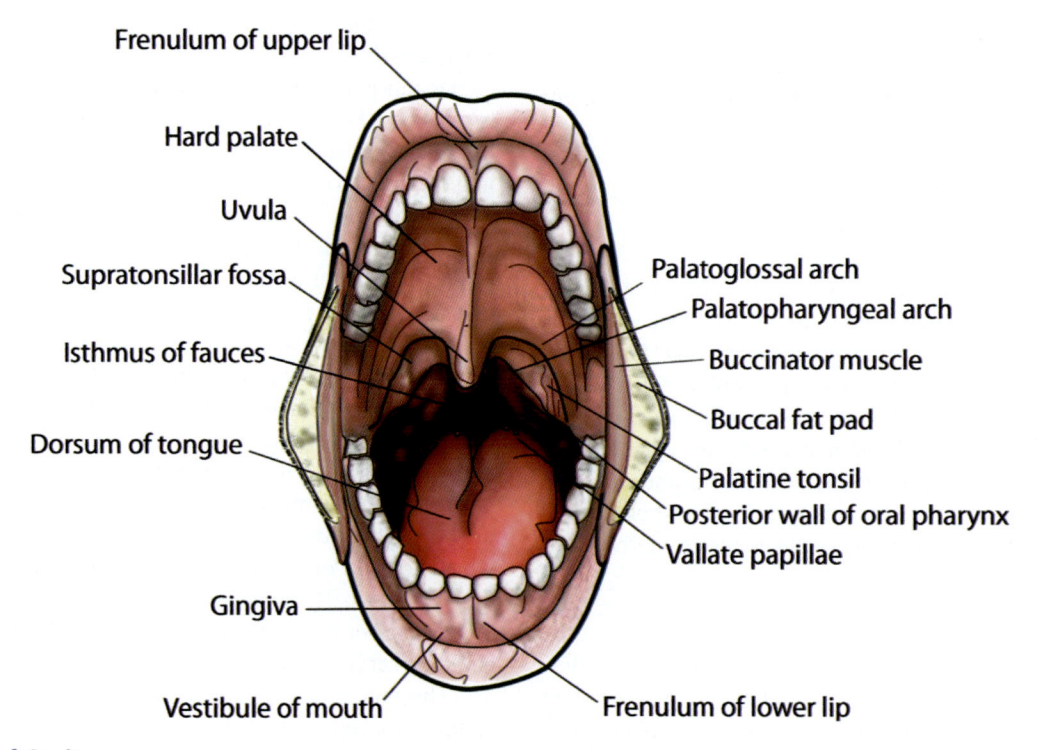

Figure 6-3 Oral Cavity
The pharyngeal arches are seen from anteriorly. The lip is the most common location for squamous cell carcinoma of the oral cavity.

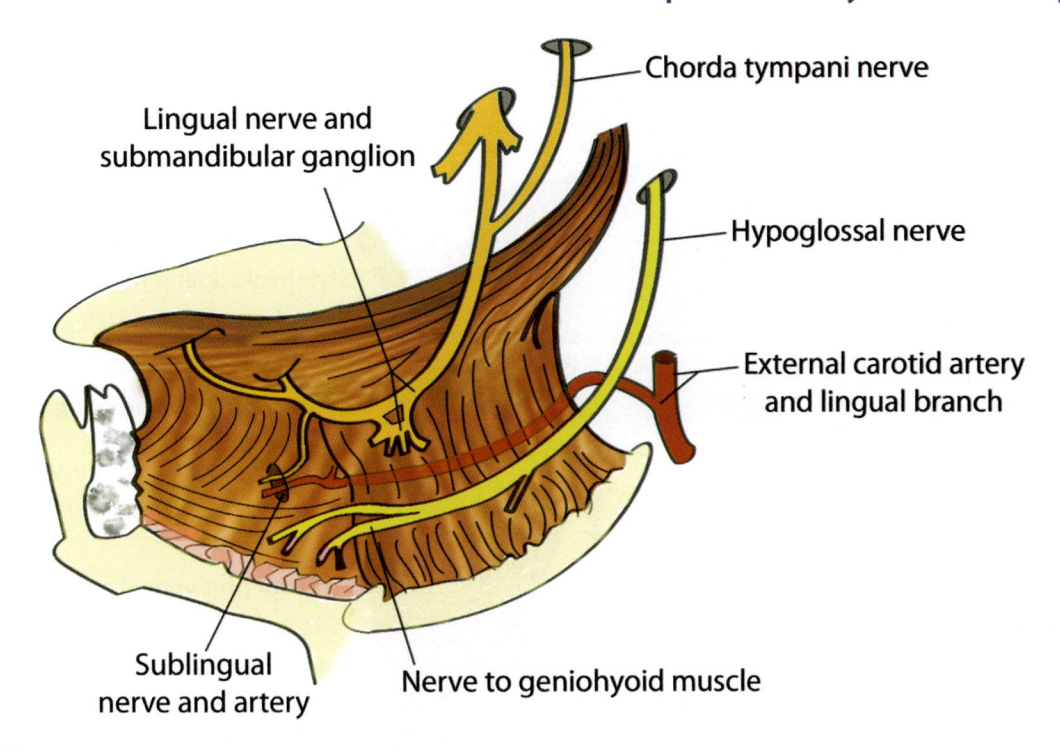

Figure 6-4 Oral Nerves
The nerves in the floor of the oral cavity on the left side is shown. Cancer of the base of the tongue may spread posteriorly to invade the styloid muscles or along the lingual vessels toward the external carotid artery.

Blood supply to the tongue includes the lingual artery and vein, which runs along the hypoglossal nerve and two separate lymphatic systems. The anterior tongue is drained by central and marginal system while the posterior tongue drains into ipsilateral and contralateral deep cervical nodes. The oral tongue may also drain into the submandibular and internal jugular nodes (levels I and II).

Floor of the Mouth

The floor of the mouth is a crescent-shaped area located between the undersurface of the tongue and the lower gingivae. The anterior floor of the mouth is the inferior to the mobile tongue. The lateral floor of the mouth is located laterally and inferiorly to the tongue.

Mylohyoid muscle is triangular in shape and is the main supporting structure of the floor of the mouth. It arises from mylohyoid ridge on the inner surface of the mandible. The muscle extends anteriorly to posteriorly from the mandibular symphysis to the last molar tooth. The anterior and middle fibers insert into the midline raphe, while the posterior fibers insert into the body of the hyoid bone. There is communication between the sublingual and submandibular spaces due to the free posterior border of the mylohyoid muscle.

The anterior belly of the digastric muscle lies superficially to the mylohyoid muscle. The anterior belly courses anteriorly and medially from the greater horn of the hyoid bone to the digastric fossa, which is located on the inferior border of the mandible.

The geniohyoid muscle lies on the superior surface of the mylohyoid muscle. It arises from the inferior genial tubercle on inner surface of mandible and passes dorsally to insert onto the anterior surface of the hyoid bone (**Fig. 6-5**).

The mylohyoid muscle separates the lower oral cavity into two spaces, which are the sublingual and submandibular spaces. Sublingual region is located superomedial to the mylohyoid muscle, lateral to genioglossus-geniohyoid muscle, and below the mucosa of the floor of the mouth. It contains the anterior extension if of the hyoglossus muscle, lingual nerve, artery and veins, cranial nerves IX and XII, sublingual glands and ducts, and the deep submandibular glands and ducts. The submandibular space is located inferior to mylohyoid muscle. It contains the anterior belly of the digastric muscle, inferior loop of cranial nerve XII, submandibular and submental nodes, superficial portion of the submandibular gland, and facial artery and vein.

Lymphatic drainage of the floor of the mouth is to the submental, submandibular, and/or internal jugular nodes (levels I and II).

Lips and Gingivobuccal Region

The lips are mainly composed of orbicularis oris muscle. The orbicularis oris comprised several muscles, which include the levator labii superioris alaeque nasi, levator labii superioris, levator anguli oris, zygomaticus major, depressor anguli oris, platysma, risorius, and buccinators muscles.

The gingival is composed of a mucosal covering that overlies both the lingual and buccal aspects of the alveolar process of the mandible and maxilla. Gingivobuccal sulcus is a term that describes the junction of the gingival with the buccal mucosa. This region is a common location for squamous cell carcinoma.

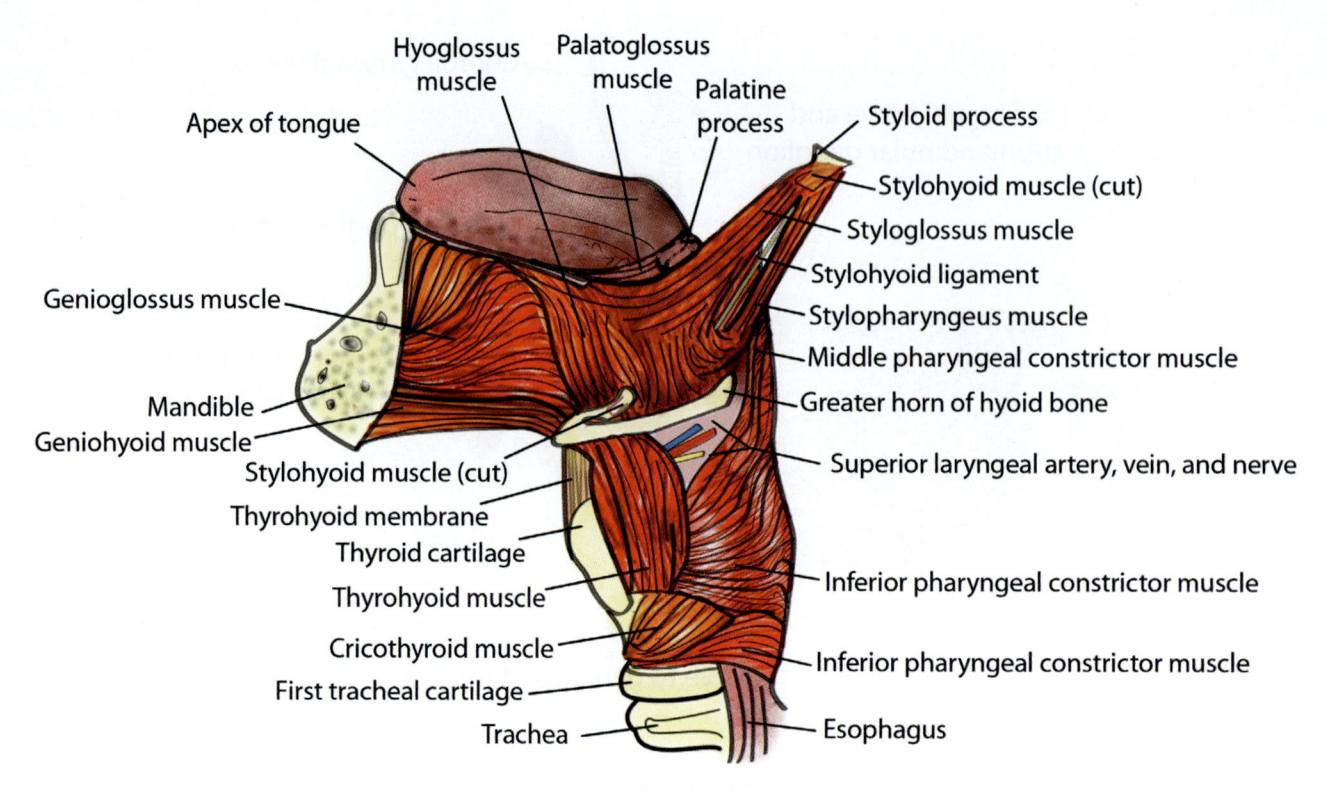

Figure 6-5 Pharynx Musculature
A view of the left side of the pharynx is shown. The pharyngeal constrictor muscles constitute the framework of the pharyngeal wall. Tonsil carcinoma can extend through the pharyngeal constrictor muscles into the parapharyngeal space.

To clearly view the gingivobuccal region on imaging, patients are generally instructed to puff their cheeks.

Motor innervation to the lips is via branches of the facial nerve. The lips drain to submental and/or submandibular (level I) lymph nodes.

Buccomasseteric Region

The buccomasseteric region includes masseter, buccinator muscles, buccal space, and the interior body of mandible. The masticator nerve innervates the masseter, which is a branch of the mandibular division of the trigeminal nerve. A branch of the facial nerve innervates the buccinator muscle. The buccal division of facial nerve and buccal branch of mandibular nerve are not normally identified on cross-sectional images.

Hard Palate and Retromolar Trigone

The hard palate is a thin horizontal bony plate of the skull that is located in the roof of the mouth. The palatine process of the maxilla and the horizontal plate of the palatine bone form the hard palate. The palatine nerve pierces the hard palate. The retromolar trigone is a portion of mucosa that covers the ascending ramus of the mandible from the third mandibular molar below the maxillary tubercle. It is situated between the buccal mucosa laterally and the anterior tonsillar pillar medially and posteriorly.

Hypopharynx

The hypopharynx is the most caudal portion of the pharynx that extends from the oropharynx to the esophageal verge. The hypopharynx continues inferiorly as the cervical esophagus to the level of the thoracic inlet. Anterior to the hypopharynx is the larynx. The retropharygeal space is located posteriorly to the hypopharynx.

Three distinct regions make up the hypopharynx, which include the posterior hypopharyngeal wall, postcricoid region, and pyriform sinus. The posterior boundary of the hypopharynx is formed by the posterior hypopharyngeal wall, which extends from the aryepiglottic folds superiorly to the esophageal verge inferiorly. The anterior boundary is formed by the postcricoid region that extends from the posterior surface of the arytenoids cartilage to the esophageal verge. The arygepiglottic folds separate the pyriform sinus from the larynx. The pyriform sinus resembles an inverted pyramid, and is formed by the anterior, medial, and lateral walls. The entrance to the pyriform sinus is at the base of the pyramid at the level of the pharyngoepiglottic folds. The apex is located at the inferior margin of the cricoid cartilage.

The boundary between the pyriform sinus and lateral neck compartment is formed by the thyrohyoid membrane. Because the superior laryngeal neurovascular bundle courses through the thyrohyoid membrane, tumors from the visceral compartment may also potentially spread into the extrapharyngeal soft tissue through this route.[7] The sensory axons of the superior laryngeal nerve continue superiorly to join the Arnold nerve within the jugular foramen.

Blood Supply

The lower pharynx is supplied by branches of the superior and inferior thyroid arteries. The veins drain superiorly into the pharyngeal plexus. Inferiorly, venous drainage is into the superior and inferior thyroid veins and into pharyngeal veins that drain into the internal jugular vein.

Innervation

The glossopharyngeal nerve and the internal laryngeal branch of the superior laryngeal nerve provide sensory innervation to the hypopharynx.

Lymphatic Drainage

The pyriform sinus is drained by a lymphatic network directed to level II and III nodes and secondarily to level V nodes. The posterior wall of the hyopharynx lymphatics drains to the retropharyngeal nodes and level II and III nodes. The lymphatics of the postcricoid drains into level III, IV, and VI nodes.

PHYSIOLOGY AND FUNCTION

Respiration

The nasopharynx warms and humidifies air breathed in through the nares before it travels down to the oropharynx. It also channels mucus produced by the membranes within the nasal cavity down the throat.

Deglutition

Deglutition is separated into three phases: the oral phase, the pharyngeal phase, and the esophageal phase. During the oral phase, the soft palate is pulled forward while the base of the tongue is elevated to prevent food bolus from entering into the pharynx too soon.[10] At the end of the oral phase, the bolus is propelled between the tongue and palate into the oropharynx. The styloglossus and palatoglossus muscles raise the tongue base, which elevates the uvula as well, and closes off the nasopharynx to prevent nasal aspiration. During the pharyngeal phase, through sequential contractions of the pharyngeal constrictor muscles, the bolus is propelled from the pharynx into the esophagus. The levator veli palatini muscle elevates the soft palate to the posterior nasopharyngeal wall. Contraction of the superior pharyngeal constrictor muscles brings the posterior tonsillar arches on each side closer to prevent large boluses from passing through.

IMAGING

Computed Tomography

Multidetector CT (MDCT) is the preferred CT imaging technique for evaluating the pharynx. MDCT requires a short imaging time compared to other conventional CT scanners. It also allows the entire scan to be performed in a single breath-hold with limited motion artifact. However, CT may be disadvantageous, as it requires radiation exposure and relatively high doses of iodinated contrast materials.

For evaluation of the pharynx and oral cavity with CT, axial images of the pharynx with the patient lying supine and head aligned in the cephalocaudad axis, is recommended (**Table 6-2**). The hard palate should lie perpendicular to the table top while the scan plane should be parallel to the inferior orbital meatal plane.[11] Coronal imaging allows the best detection for early erosion of the skull base or hard palate. Therefore, direct or reformatted coronal imaging is recommended for patients with suspicion of nasopharyngeal, palatal, or skull base carcinoma. Dental metal products may produce severe artifacts, requiring additional imaging to be performed with a gantry angulation along the mandible plane. The optimal field of view depends on patient size, but can vary between 14 and 18 cm. The slice thickness is preferentially between 4 and 5 mm for evaluation of nasopharyngeal and regional anatomy, while 2 and 3 mm is recommended for smaller lesions and subtle bone invasion by neoplasms. Soft tissue and bone reconstruction algorithms should be used on all studies.

Thin-section (3-mm) CT reconstructed with bone algorithm in coronal and axial planes is an accurate technique to detect mandibular and maxilla involvement by squamous cell carcinoma of the oral cavity and oropharynx.[12,13] Lymph node metastases in the neck are optimally evaluated by contrast CT with 5-mm axial sections.[13] CT is preferred in the evaluation of cervical node enlargement as it may be useful in detecting nodal necrosis and extracapsular involvement. However, differentiation between neoplastic tissue from muscle and lymphoid tissue on CT may be difficult.

Intravenous contrast is recommended for all neck studies, unless contraindicated. Contrast is important for evaluating cervical lymph nodes, the skull base, and can increase the conspicuity of pathology.

Magnetic Resonance Imaging

MRI is useful because of its multiplanar capabilities and superior depiction of soft tissue details.[14] Drawbacks to MRI as compared to CT are its relatively long examination time, cost, and limited availability.

MR imaging of the pharynx and oral cavity can be performed with a head volume coil. To obtain the best quality of scan, the patient must be instructed to minimize any movement, such as talking or swallowing. While dental artifacts can also occur as with CT imaging, these artifacts are less disruptive on MR studies.[15] Since a common diagnostic problem of CT is dental filling artifacts and MRI is motion artifacts due to swallowing, imaging of lesions located in the floor of the mouth and tongue base should be performed by CT, while MRI is recommended for lesions involving the palate and tongue. Axial T1W, axial fast spin-echo T2W, and sagittal T1W spin-echo images are obtained for routine MR examination (**Table 6-3**). Coronal T1W images can provide an additional view of the superior nasopharynx and skull base. While coronal images of the oropharynx are not essential, they can provide valuable assessment of the craniocaudal extent of pathology.[7] Sagittal sections should be added for paramidline lesions involving the tongue, lips, and anterior floor of the mouth.[13] Level V nodes are also best seen on coronal images.

Intravenous paramagnetic contrast is important for evaluating pharynx malignancies. Initial noncontrast T1W image will help distinguish areas of high signal intensity (i.e., high protein content, fat, etc.) from areas with contrast enhancement

Table 6-2 Nasopharynx, Oropharynx, Oral Cavity, and Tongue CT Protocol

		Nasopharynx	Soft and Hard Palate	Oropharynx, Oral Cavity, and Floor of Mouth
Indications:		Tumor, inflammatory disease, infection	Tumor, inflammatory disease, infection	Tumor, inflammatory disease, infection excluding involvement of the soft and hard palates
Scanner setting:		kV(p): 140; mA: 250–350 through nasopharynx and skull base; 220–260 through upper neck	kV(p): 140; mA: 250–350 through the maxillofacial area; 220–260 through upper neck	kV(p): 140; mA: 250–350 through the maxillofacial area; 220–260 through upper neck
Oral contrast:		None	None	None
Phase of respiration:		Quiet breathing	Quiet breathing	Quiet breathing
Rotation time:		0.5–0.8 s	0.5–0.8 s	0.5–0.8 s
Acquisition slice thickness:		1.0–1.25 mm through nasopharynx and skull base; 2.5–3 mm through rest of the neck	1.0–1.25 mm through nasal cavity, oral cavity, and oropharynx; 2.5–3 mm through rest of the neck	1.0–1.25 mm through oropharynx; 2.5–3 mm through rest of the neck
Pitch		• 0.75–1.0 (HQ = 3:1) through nasopharynx and skull base • 1.0–1.5 (HS = 6:1) through the rest of the neck • If the scanner is unable to perform the multislice helical imaging mode with the gantry in angled position, change for axial imaging plane, the gantry angle to 0 degrees, and reconstruct the images in the desired plane or use the multislice axial imaging mode. Also, obtain coronal images using the multislice axial imaging mode	• 0.75–1.0 (HQ = 3:1) through the nasal cavity, oral cavity, and oropharynx • 1.0–1.5 (HS = 6:1) through the rest of the neck • If the scanner is unable to perform the multislice helical imaging mode with the gantry in angled position, change for axial imaging plane, the gantry angle to 0 degrees, and reconstruct the images in the desired plane or use the multislice axial imaging mode. Also, obtain coronal images using the multislice axial imaging mode	• 0.75–1.0 (HQ = 3:1) through oropharynx • 1.0–1.5 (HS = 6:1) through the rest of the neck • If the scanner is unable to perform the multislice helical imaging mode with the gantry in angled position, change the gantry angle to 0 degrees, and reconstruct the images in the desired plane or use the multislice axial imaging mode
Multiplanar reconstruction slice thickness/interval for filming:		2.5–3.0 mm /2.5–3.0 mm	2.5–3.0 mm /2.5–3.0 mm	2.5–3.0 mm /2.5–3.0 mm
IV contrast	Concentration	LOCM 300–320 mg iodine/ml or HOCM 282 mg iodine/ml, 60% solution	LOCM 300–320 mg iodine/ml or HOCM 282 mg iodine/ml, 60% solution	LOCM 300–320 mg iodine/ml or HOCM 282 mg iodine/ml, 60% solution
	Rate	1 ml/s	1 ml/s	1 ml/s
	Scan delay	60 s	60 s	60 s
	Total volume	150 ml (minimum catheter size = 22 G)	150 ml (minimum catheter size = 22 G)	100 ml (minimum catheter size = 22 G)

Modified with permission from Silverman RM. Multislice Computed Tomography: A Practical Approach to Clinical Protocols. Philadelphia: Lippincott Williams & Wilkins, 2002: 78–79, 84–85, and 87–88.

Table 6-3 Nasopharynx, Oropharynx, Oral Cavity, and Tongue MRI Protocol	
Sagittal T1	Top of frontal sinus to top of manubrium
Coronal T1	Top of frontal sinus to top of manubrium
Axial T1	Top of frontal sinus to top of manubrium
Axial T2	Fast spin echo with fat-saturation
Slice thickness	4–5 mm sections
FOV	16–18 cm for T1-weighted images; 18–20 cm for T2-weighted images
Pixel size	<1 × 1 mm
Matrix	256 × 256–512 × 512
IV contrast	Obtain pre- and postcontrast T1-weighted images

on contrast enhanced T1W images. Fat suppression techniques after contrast administration are useful in delineating tumor extent and short tau inversion recovery images are sensitive in detecting marrow infiltration and small lesions.

While both CT and MRI are adequate techniques to assess nodal metastasis, MRI is superior to CT for detecting tumor recurrence. Nevertheless, MRI is limited in differentiating recurrence from postradiation fibrosis. MRI is superior to CT for detecting perineural spread of malignancy. CT is superior to MRI for identifying early cortical involvement and bone invasion, while MRI is more sensitive in detecting skull base marrow changes.

Positron Emission Tomography (PET)

Nuclear medicine studies are mainly used for the detection of metastatic disease to the bone. PET scanning may also be indicated in search of an unknown primary tumor in patients who have a neck mass or where CT is inconclusive for metastatic lymph nodes in the neck.[13] Studies have found that FDG-PET stages nodal and metastatic disease of NPC more accurately and sensitively than does the conventional workup.[16] Patients with distant metastases (advanced nodal stage, N3) would benefit the most from FDG-PET. FDG-PET may also be useful in detecting NPC recurrence following radiotherapy when MRI findings are indeterminate.[17]

A study by Goerres et al. examined the accuracy of conventional CT with that of PET/CT and SPECT/CT in the detection of bone invasion in 34 patients scheduled to undergo surgery for clinically suspected oral cavity carcinoma with possible bone invasion.[18] With histologic findings as the standard of reference, the accuracy of SPECT/CT (88%) was lower than that of PET/CT and contrast-enhanced CT (94% and 97%, respectively). Sensitivity (100%) was highest with PET/CT and specificity (100%) was highest with contrast-enhanced CT. FDG uptake seen on two sides of the same cortical bone was not a helpful imaging pattern for better identifying bone invasion in patients without evident cortical erosion on CT scans. The study concluded that while the assessment of cortical erosion with contrast-enhanced CT and the CT information from PET/CT are the most reliable methods for detecting bone invasion in patients with oral cavity carcinoma, FDG uptake seen on PET/CT images does not improve identification of bone infiltration.

However, a recent study performed by Babin et al. also examined the advantages of PET/CT when evaluating bone involvement in patients with squamous cell carcinoma of the oral cavity and/or of the oropharynx.[19] Their study specifically focused on mandibular involvement of the cancer. Each patient benefitted from PET, CT, and PET/CT fusion. Positron emission tomography/CT fusion shows sensitivity of 100% with specificity of 85%. Their study encourages the use of PET/CT when assessing mandibular invasion.

The combination of PET and CT may also be useful for patients with nasopharyngeal carcinoma. Gordin et al.'s assessment of FDG PET/CT in patients with nasopharyngeal carcinoma concluded that PET/CT is better than that of stand-alone PET or conventional imaging in providing anatomic localization of foci with abnormal FDG uptake in the assessment of locoregional disease.[20] Nevertheless, MRI appears to be superior to PET/CT for the assessment of locoregional invasion and retropharyngeal nodal metastasis.[21] Regardless, PET/CT is more accurate than MRI for determining cervical nodal metastasis.

Ultrasonography

Ultrasonography (US) can be used for evaluation of the floor of the mouth and tongue. Due to radiation exposure, US and MRI are the methods of first choice for children.[15] Significant drawbacks in the use of US is that it is operator dependent and does not allow complete sectional imaging of anatomical structures as with CT or MR imaging. Evaluation of the oral cavity with US is best performed using curved array or linear array broadband transducers with a frequency of 5 to 12 MHz. Color or power Doppler imaging is not necessary as most diagnoses are made with the standard gray scale technique. Minor salivary gland lesions in the mucosa of oral cavity and pharynx are not accessible by conventional ultrasound.[22]

PATHOLOGY

Malignant Neoplasms

Nasopharyngeal Carcinoma

Although nasopharyngeal carcinoma (NPC) is uncommon in the United States, it is endemic in East Asia and Africa.[23] NPC occurs more commonly in men. The incidence is highest in middle-aged persons in high-risk populations and declines thereafter. However, the incidence for low-risk population increases with age.[24]

Many factors have been recognized as a risk for developing the disease. In endemic populations, risk of NPC appears to be related to infection with Epstein-Barr virus (EBV). Specific serologic responses to various gene products of EBV are demonstrated in NPC patients. Studies have shown that genetic factors, such as HLA haplotypes, genetic polymorphisms, and chromosomal alterations may increase the risk of NPC susceptibility in certain ethnic groups.[25, 26] Intake of salted fish high in nitrosamine is also another important risk factor.[27] Common risk factors in the United States and Europe include consumption of alcohol and cigarette smoking.[28]

According to the World Health Organization (WHO, 2005), NPC is classified into three histologic types: keratinizing squamous cell carcinoma (WHO type I), nonkeratinizing carcinoma (WHO type II for differentiated and WHO type III for undifferentiated carcinoma), and basaloid squamous cell carcinoma.[24] The squamous cell type is similar to other squamous cell cancers of the head and neck. Lymphoepithelioma is a term used to describe nonkeratinizing nasopharyngeal carcinoma with abundant infiltration of lymphocytes. This infiltration may deter regional metastasis of undifferentiated NPC cancer cells to cervical nodes.[29] The endemic form of NPC is the most common and is commonly the undifferentiated, nonkeratinizing type. It has a more favorable prognosis than the sporadic form of NPC (more commonly, the keratinizing type) due to its higher radiosensitivity.

Many of the patients with NPC present with headache from cranial nerve involvement and neck mass from cervical node metastases. Cranial nerves III to VI are commonly affected by paracavernous sinus tumor invasion, resulting in neurologic symptoms. Nasal obstruction with epistaxis and serous otitis media can also occur (Fig. 6-6). Patients may remain asymptomatic for small lesions, resulting in the majority of patients presenting with advanced disease at initial presentation.[30]

Tumor Origin and Spread

Anterior Spread

Erosion of the maxillary sinus may occur if tumor spreads anteriorly into the nasal fossa. The tumor may then infiltrate the pterygopalatine fossa (PPF) through the sphenopalatine foramen (Fig. 6-7).[31,32] CT or MRI may reveal a replacement of normal fat content by the tumor.

From the PPF, the tumor can spread into many sites, including the foramen rotundum along the maxillary nerve to enter the cranium. Contrast-enhanced MRI can be used to detect perineural infiltration of the maxillary nerve. The tumor may also extend into the inferior orbital fissure and apex, and then through the superior orbital fissure. From the PPF, the tumor can also invade the infratemporal fossa, posing risk to the masticator muscles. In addition, the tumor can extend along the pterygoid nerve into the vidian canal.[33]

Lateral Spread

Lateral extension of tumor can be recognized by tumor infiltrating the parapharyngeal space (PPS). Infiltration of the PPS by a neoplasm indicates deep invasion of the tumor. The PPS is best defined on T1W MR images. Invasion of the space can occur directly through the pharyngobasilar fascia, or indirectly through the sinus of Morgagni. Tumor spread to the PPS is the most common direction of spread and can be recognized by effacement of fat from the PPS. An aggressive, enhancing mass infiltrating the deep fascial planes and spaces of the nasopharynx is a reliable indicator for malignancy. Further tumor extension may involve the masticator space (MS) and muscles of mastication.[34] The mandibular nerve lies within the MS and may be subject to perineural infiltration. Tumor infiltration of the mandibular nerve can be detected well with MR imaging. Extension along the mandibular nerve may lead to infiltration of the foramen ovale.

Posterior Spread

Posterior spread of tumor can infiltrate the prevertebral muscles and RPS. In advanced cases, vertebral body destruction and spinal canal involvement can occur. Infiltration of the carotid sheath can occur in posterolateral spread of tumor. Posterosuperior spread of tumor may infiltrate the jugular foramen and hypoglossal canal, and eventually spread into the posterior cranial fossa.[35]

Involvement of the tumor to the hypoglossal canal may affect the cranial nerves IX to XII. Patients with hypoglossal nerve involvement may present with tongue fasciculation or atrophy of the tongue musculature. The affected tongue may be displaced posteriorly on axial images, which is best detected on lower sections of the posterior tongue.[32] This displacement may give the impression of an increased tongue length. Contrast enhancement and high T2 intensity changes of the tongue can be seen as a result of perineural infiltration of the hypoglossal nerve.

Inferior Spread

Tumors may spread inferiorly along the pharyngeal wall into the oropharynx (Fig. 6-8). The spread often occurs along the submucosal plane. Submucosal spread of tumors is best detected on imaging studies rather than endoscopy. Gross wall thickening of the oropharyngeal wall may be detected on imaging, especially with MRI. Coronal and/or sagittal MRI is recommended to detect inferior extension of the nasopharyngeal tumor into the oropharynx, while axial images are best to evaluate tumors extending inferior to C1/2 vertebra.[36] Nasopharyngeal tumor may also extend inferiorly along the retropharyngeal space.

Superior Spread

Superior spread of tumor may erode the clivus, foramen lacerum, and sphenoid sinus floor. Nasopharyngeal tumors can extend intracranial through different pathways, such as via the

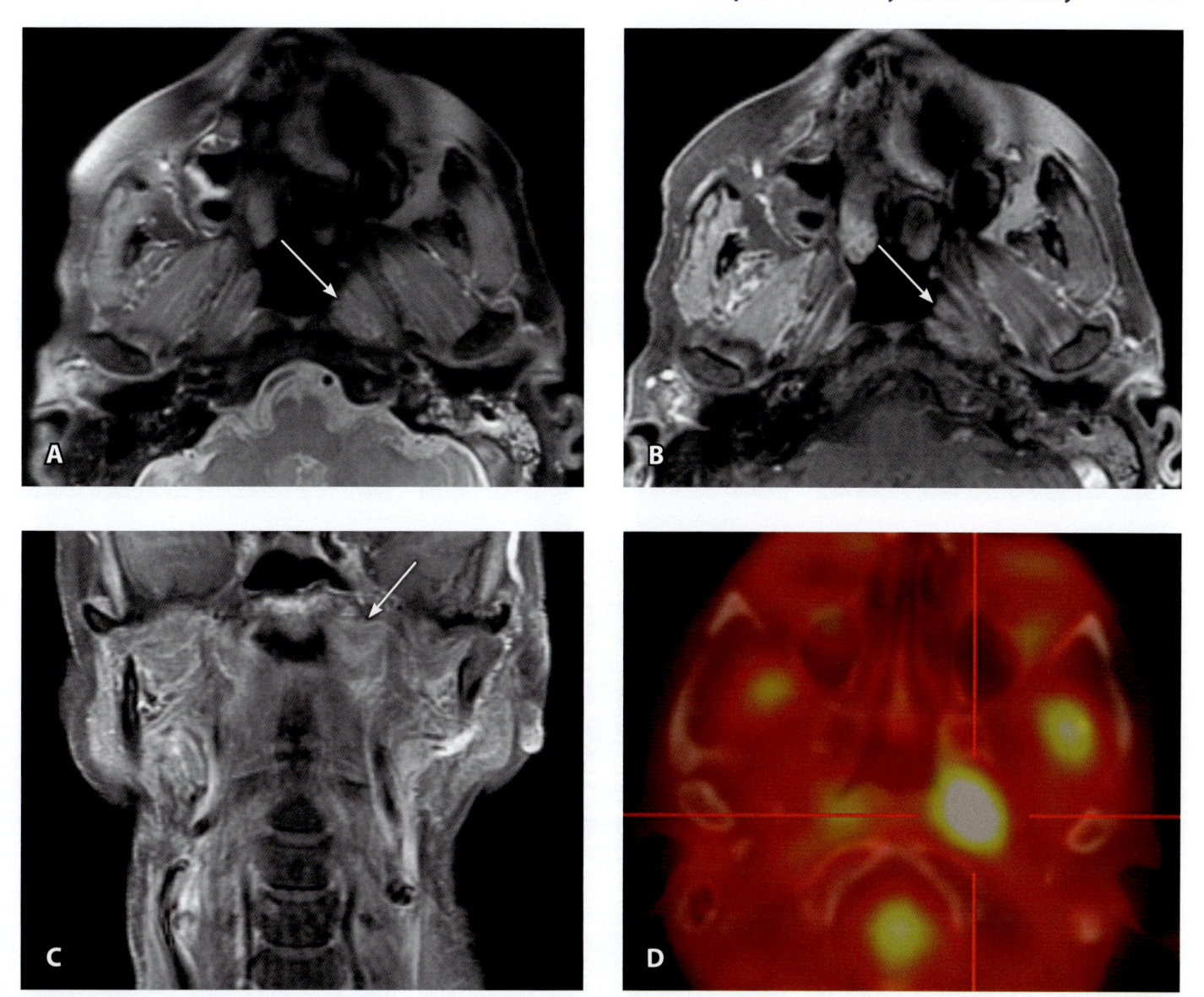

Figure 6-6 Nasopharyngeal Carcinoma
(**A**) Axial T2, (**B**) axial and (**C**) coronal postcontrast T1 with fat-saturated MR scans. (**D**) Axial fused PET/CT image. There is a focal, primarily submucosal mass filling the left fossa of Rosenmuller and extending into the adjacent pharyngeal muscles (*arrows*, **A–C**).

foramen lacerum, the foramen ovale, or skull base erosion. Skull base erosion is the most common route detected based on CT studies.[33] On MRI, the foramen ovale is the most common route detected. MRI is more sensitive than CT in detecting intracranial lesions. Intracranial spread of tumor is usually extracerebral. MRI can detect dural thickening along the middle cranial fossa floor, which many signify intracranial infiltration of tumor. However, reactive hyperplasia may also result in dural thickening. Nasopharyngeal tumor can invade the cavernous sinus, endangering cranial nerves III to VI.

Lymphatic Spread
NPC commonly metastasizes to cervical lymph nodes. About 75% to 95% of patients with NPC present with cervical lymphadenopathy. In addition, a majority of these cases are bilateral. Nodal metastasis tends to spread inferiorly. The first nodes involved are usually the retropharyngeal lymph nodes.

Compared with other head and neck tumors, NPC shows a higher frequency of distant metastasis. Patients with low cervical lymph node enlargement are at an increased risk for distant metastasis. The supraclavicular fossa is considered one of the last defensive barriers for malignant cell spread in lymphatic vessels.[33] From there, these cells may enter the subclavian vein and thoracic duct, resulting in the spread of cancer cells to the systemic circulation. Systemic dissemination of these cells can also occur via parapharyngeal venous plexus from tumor cells invading the PPS.

Distant metastasis may alter prognosis. The most frequent site of metastasis is the bone, following by lung and liver. Liver ultrasound and chest X-ray are performed during the staging

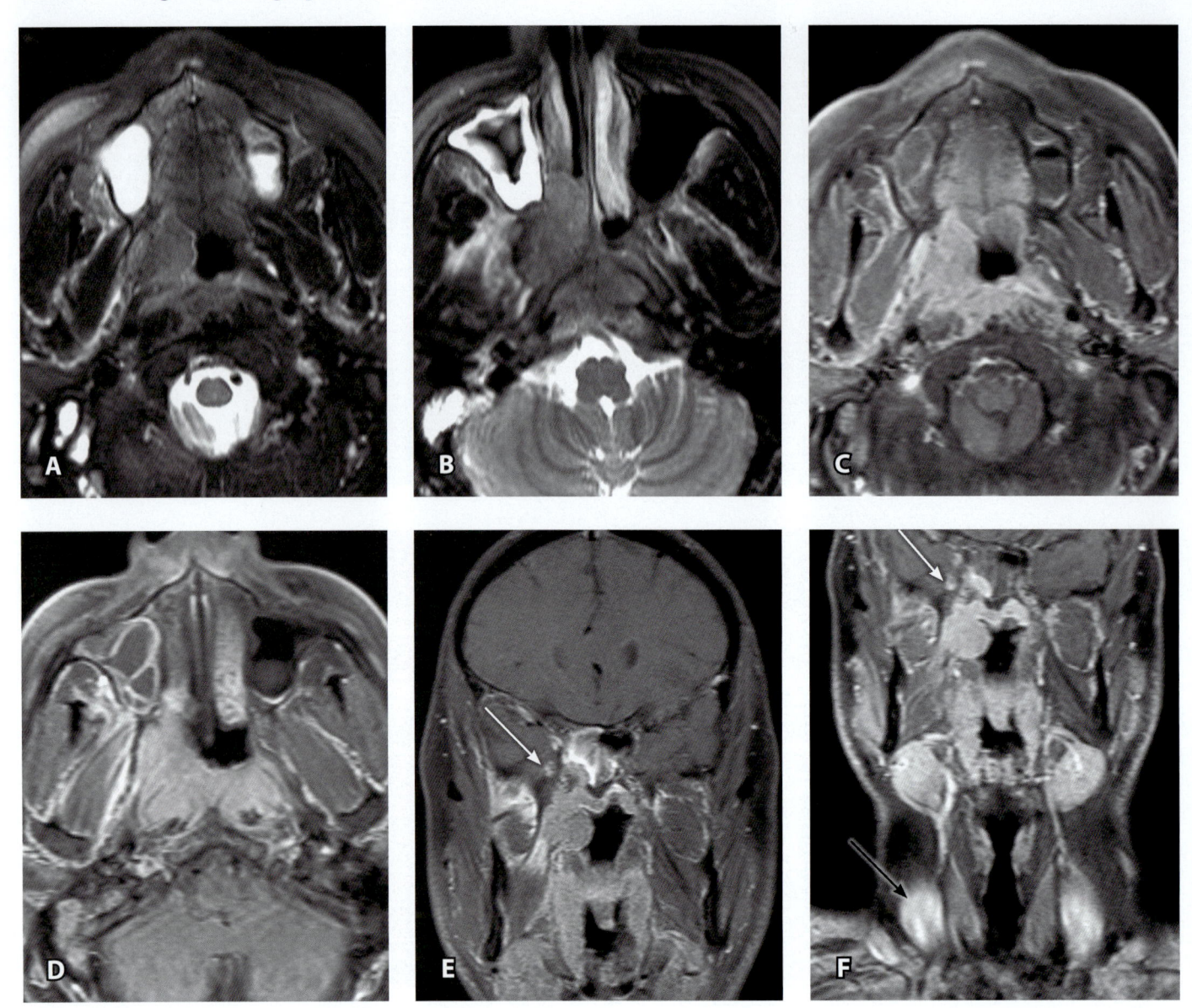

Figure 6-7 Undifferentiated Nasopharyngeal Carcinoma
Axial T2 (**A, B**) and postcontrast with fat-saturated axial (**C, D**) and coronal (**E, F**) MR scans. There is a bulky right nasopharyngeal tumor with growth into right nasal cavity and pterygopalatine fossa anteriorly, masticator space laterally, and retropharyngeal musculature posteriorly. There is subtle extension into the right foramen rotundum (*arrows*, **E, F**). There is bulky bilateral cervical nodal metastasis (*black arrow*, **F**) and opacification of the right mastoid air cells consistent with obstruction of the eustachian tube.

procedure. Abdominal or chest CT may be ordered if further evaluation is necessary. In the suspicion of bone metastases, bone scans can be performed. PET imaging can be used to evaluate occult neck adenopathies.

Tumor Classification and Staging

Imaging plays an important role in the staging of nasopharyngeal carcinoma (Table 6-4). Accurate staging is imperative as treatment is directly dependent on stage. Clinical examination may provide information on mucosal involvement but is unable to detect the deep extension or presence of skull base invasion or intracranial spread.[37]

CT currently remains one of the most commonly used imaging modality for staging NPC. While CT staging is adequate for most patients, MRI is the preferred imaging modality as it is superior to CT in demonstrating tumor extent, tumor recurrence, and postradiation complications.[38,39] Intensity-modulated radiation therapy and 3D comformal radiation therapy allow for accurate mapping of the tumor.

Because MRI is more sensitive in detecting skull base marrow changes, the significance of these marrow changes may be questionable and patients may be upstaged based on these findings. Clinically, marrow changes detected by MRI are included within the radiation treatment field. As the nasopharynx is a

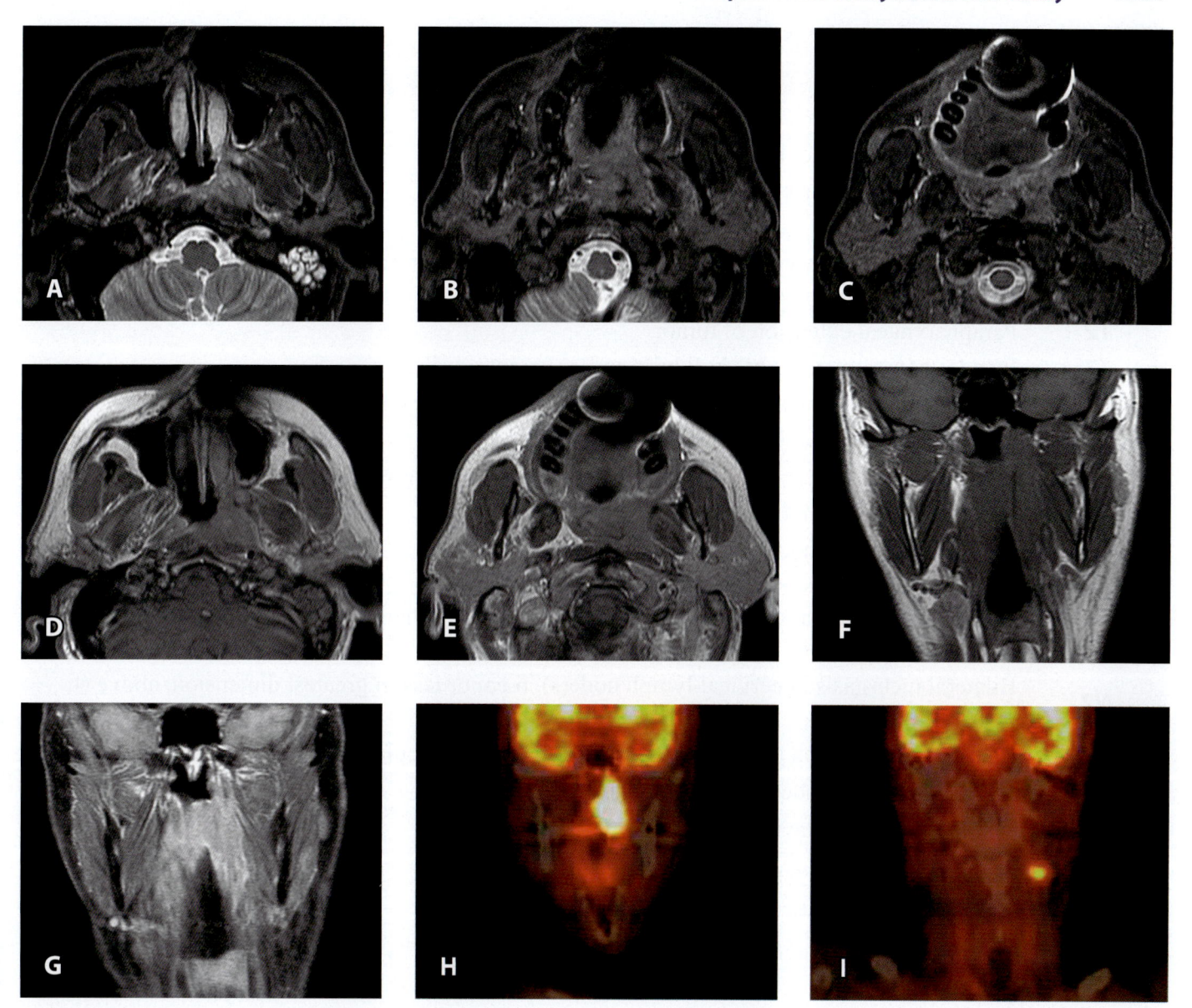

Figure 6-8 Invasive Nasopharyngeal Carcinoma
(**A–C**) Axial T2, (**D**) and (**E**) axial and (**F**) coronal T1, (**G**) Coronal postcontrast T1 with fat-saturated MR scans. (**H**) and (**I**) coronal fused PET/CT images. There is a longitudinally oriented tumor extending from the left fossa of Rosenmuller inferiorly along the pharyngeal submucosal space and invades the retropharyngeal musculature. In addition, there is a solitary 1 cm diameter left level II lymph node seen in (**I**).

relatively surgical inaccessible area, histopathologic confirmation of lesions in the skull base cannot be performed. Radiation therapy is thus the mainstay treatment for these lesions.

Studies have revealed that tumor volume is an independent prognostic indicator of NPC.[40,41] Tumor volume has shown to be more accurate than the TNM classification system in predicting treatment outcome. Further investigation is being done to determine whether tumor volume measurements could potentially be incorporated into the NPC TNM system.[42–44]

In a study conducted by Liao et al., MRI showed dramatic changes in the results of T stage and clinical staging and should be preferred to CT in staging NPC.[45] The study found that MRI demonstrated early primary tumor involvement more precisely and deep primary tumor infiltration more easily. They concluded that patients would benefit from changes in treatment strategies resulting from the use of MRI.

Oropharyngeal and Hypopharyngeal Carcinoma

The vast majority of encountered tumors of the oropharynx are squamous cell carcinoma. Cancer of the oropharynx is usually locally advanced at the time of clinical presentation. Typically, the cancer involves patients in the fifth through seventh decade of life. Men are affected more often than women. Overall survival rate is at approximately 50%. Risk factors for oropharyngeal carcinoma include cigarette smoking and alcohol abuse.

Table 6-4 Nasopharyngeal Carcinoma Tumor Staging

	Primary Tumor
TX	Primary tumor cannot be assessed
T0	No evidence of primary tumor
Tis	Carcinoma in situ
T1	Confined to nasopharynx, or extends to oropharynx and/or nasal cavity without parapharyngeal extension
T2	Parapharyngeal extension of tumor
T3	Invades bony structures of skull base and/or paranasal sinuses
T4	Intracranial extension and/or involvement of cranial nerves, infratemporal fossa/masticator space, hypopharynx, or orbit
	Nodal Staging
NX	Regional nodes cannot be assessed
N0	No regional lymph node metastasis
N1	Unilateral metastasis in cervical lymph node(s), 6 cm or less in greatest dimension, above supraclavicular fossa, and/or unilateral or bilateral, retropharyngeal lymph nodes, 6 cm or less in greatest dimension
N2	Bilateral metastasis in cervical lymph node(s), 6 cm or less in greatest dimension, above supraclavicular fossa
N3	Metastasis in a lymph node(s) >6 cm and/or to supraclavicular fossa
N3a	Metastasis in any node >6 cm in greatest dimension
N3b	Extension to supraclavicular fossa
	Distant Metastasis
M0	No distant metastasis
M1	Distant metastasis

Human papillomavirus (HPV), particularly with HPV-16, is a common risk factor in the United States and Europe.

Tumor Origin and Spread

Anterior Tonsillar Pillar

Most tonsillar cancers originate from the anterior tonsillar pillar (**Fig. 6-9**). These cancers commonly spread along the palatoglossal muscle and can extend superiorly and medially to invade the soft palate and hard palate. From there, the tumor can spread to the tensor and levator veli palatini muscles.

Anterior tonsillar pillar cancers can also extend interoinferiorly along the palatoglossus muscle to invade the base of the tongue. Anteromedial spread may involve the superior constrictor muscle and extend to the pterygomandibular raphe. Cancer may spread anteriorly and laterally along the pharyngeal constrictor muscle to the retromolar trigone and pterygomandibular raphe into the buccinator muscle. Advanced lesions may invade the mandible or infratemporal space. Primary lymphatic drainage of anterior tonsillar pillar tumors is to the submandibular and upper jugular lymph nodes.

Posterior Tonsillar Pillar

Posterior tonsillar pillar cancer is rare. When present, these cancers may spread superiorly to invade the soft palate. Tumor may also spread inferiorly along the palatopharyngeal muscle to invade the pharyngoepiglottic fold.[46] It may extend posteriorly into the posterior pharyngeal wall. Lymphatic drainage of these tumors is primarily to the upper jugular nodes.

Tonsillar Fossa

Tonsillar carcinomas usually involve the upper pole of the tonsil (**Figs. 6-10** and **6-11**). Tumors in this region are often occult, and a sore throat may be the only presenting symptom. The tumor may spread anteriorly or posteriorly to the tonsillar pillars. The cancer may also extend posteriorly and laterally to the lateral pharyngeal wall and parapharyngeal space. Tonsillar carcinomas can extend superiorly to invade the soft palate and

Chapter 6: The Pharynx and Oral Cavity   **239**

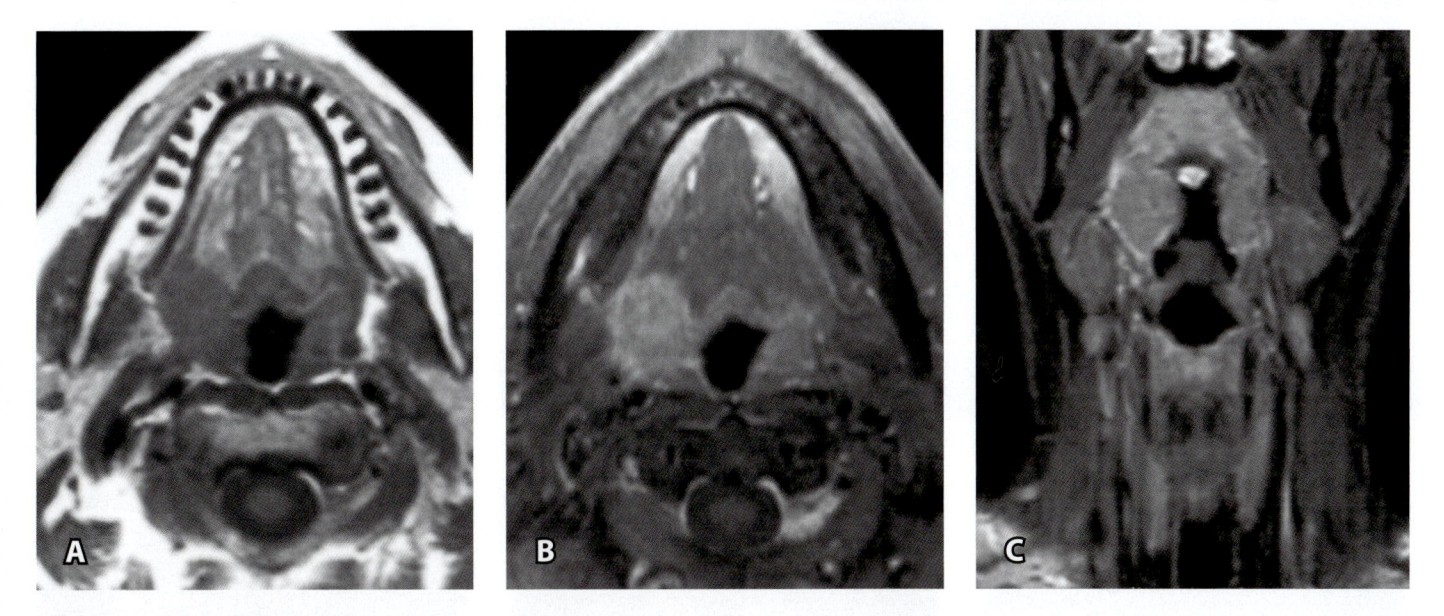

Figure 6-9 Tonsil Carcinoma
Axial plain T1 (**A**) and T2 (**B**) images of patient with a right-sided tonsillar cancer. The soft-tissue mass involves the palatine tonsil, grows through the pharyngeal constrictor muscles into the parapharyngeal space. Coronal image (**C**) demonstrates large right-sided tonsillar cancer.

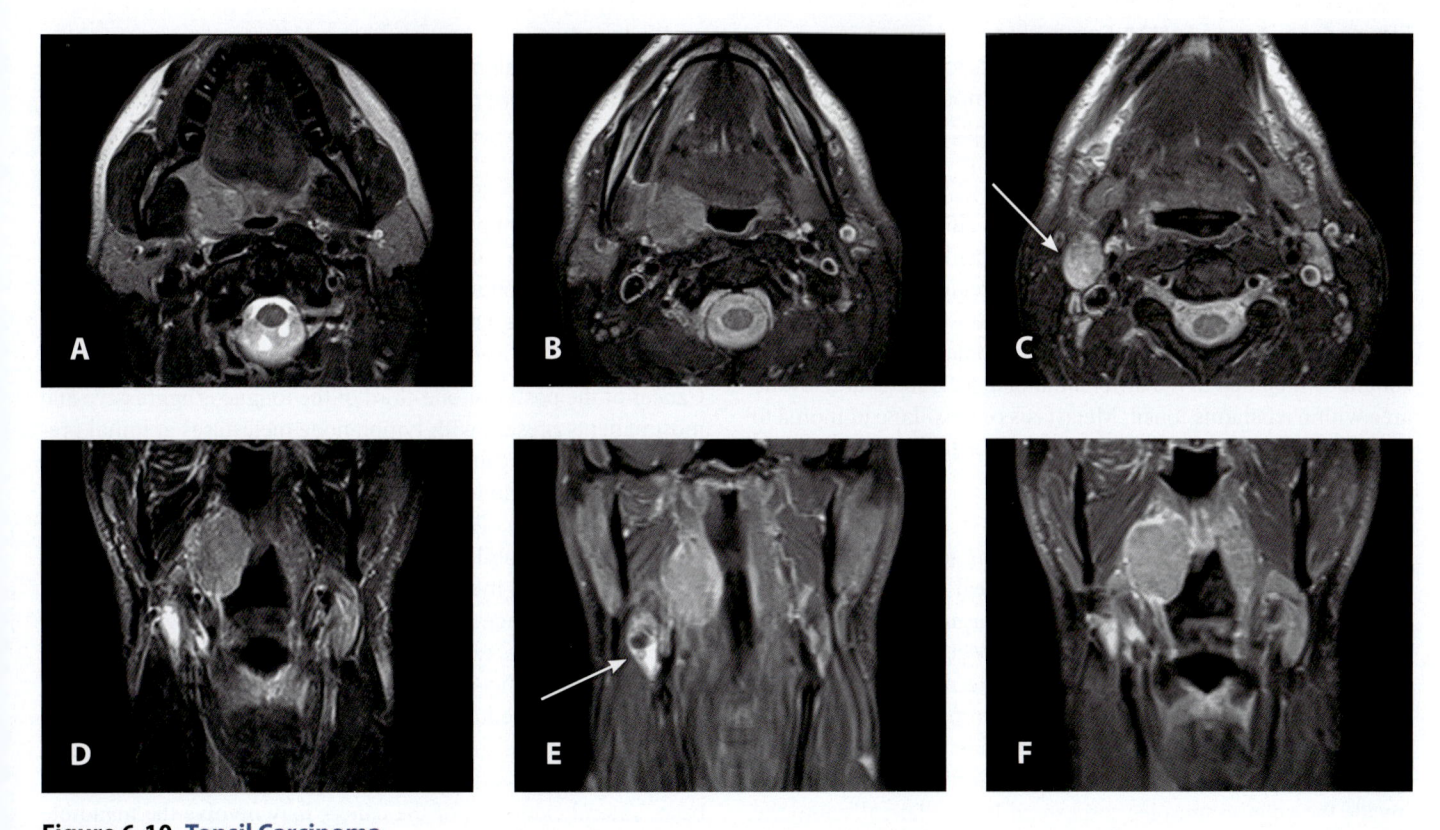

Figure 6-10 Tonsil Carcinoma
(**A–C**) Axial T2, (**D**) coronal T2, and (**E, F**) coronal postcontrast T1 with fat-saturated MR scans. There is a bulky mass centered in the right tonsillar fossa that shows intermediate T2 signal and moderate enhancement. Also noted is a large right level II nodal mass (*arrows*, **C, E**).

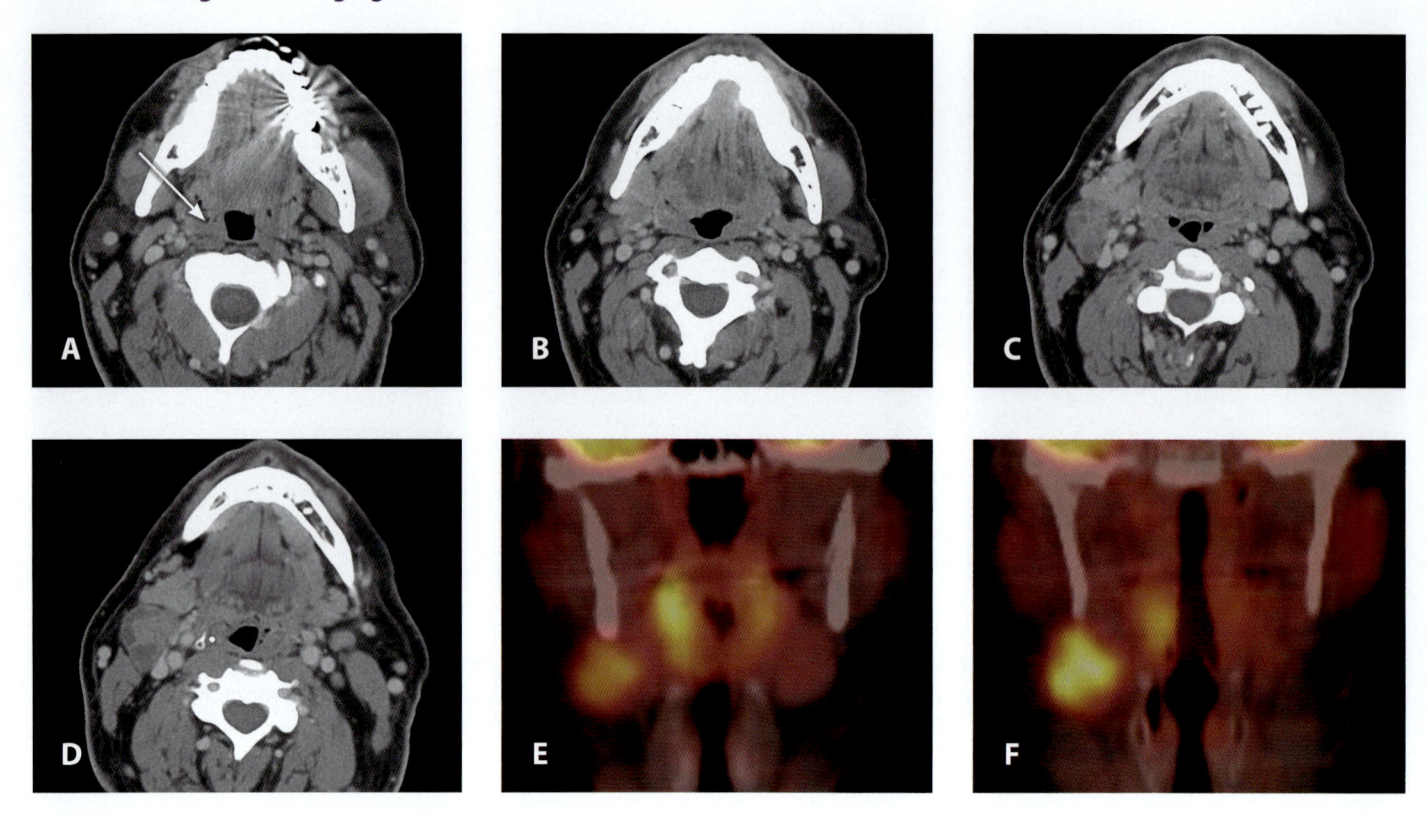

Figure 6-11 Tonsil T1N2A Carcinoma
(**A–D**) Axial postcontrast CT scans and coronal fused PET/CT images. There is a small mass centered in the right tonsillar fossa (*arrow*, **A**) and a much larger right level II nodal mass showing differential enhancement on CT. The fused PET/CT scans (**E–F**) show similar findings as well as additional uptake in the palatine tonsils bilaterally.

nasopharynx, or inferiorly to invade the glossotonsillar sulcus or base of the tongue.[7,8] Although the tonsillar fossa is usually asymmetric, asymmetry of the tonsillar region should be carefully evaluated when there is a metastatic lesion in the neck from an unknown primary tumor. Lymphoma, abscess, or tumor should be included in the differential diagnosis for a large cystic area within a palatine tonsil. Metastasis of tonsillar carcinoma to lymph nodes occurs primarily to the upper jugular or retropharyngeal lymph nodes.

Soft Palate
Soft palate carcinoma, most commonly the squamous cell type, has the best prognosis of all oropharyngeal cancers. However, minor salivary gland cancers can be seen in the posterior soft palate. Tumors usually occur on oral aspect of the soft palate. Though rare, carcinoma of the soft palate may spread superiorly to the nasopharynx in advanced, untreated cases. It may also extend inferiorly and laterally to invade the tonsillar pillars or anteriorly to invade the hard palate. Soft palate tumor may invade the palatini muscles and extend further laterally into the parapharyngeal space.[46] The palatine branches of the maxillary nerve may be at risk for tumor infiltration.[47] Lymphatic drainage of soft palate tumors is to level II nodes, and then to mid-jugular and retropharyngeal nodes.

Coronal images of the soft palate are recommended when evaluating the region since the soft palate lies in the axial plane (**Fig. 6-12**). Tumor and soft palate may be of similar density and display similar enhancement patterns CT. However, T1W MR images can clearly differentiate soft palate, filled with fat and mucous glands, from tumor based on its higher signal intensity. Tumor in the soft palate is detected as a region of lower signal intensity.

Tongue Base
Cancer of the posterior one-third of the tongue is aggressive and most patients present with lymph node metastases at initial presentation as these cancers are often clinically silent. However, symptoms may include pain, dysphagia, and otalgia from cranial nerve involvement. Tumor can spread anteriorly into the floor of the mouth or mobile tongue. From there, it may extend along the mylohyoid and hyoglossal muscles. Cancer may also spread posteriorly to invade the styloid muscles or along the lingual vessels toward the external carotid artery.[48] A tumor mass of 2 cm or more predicts perineural and vascular spread, which is associated with a reduced patient survival.[49] Perineural and vascular spread can be suspected in patients with tumor infiltrating the normal fatty tissue planes of the sublingual space or tongue base. Lateral extension of the cancer may involve the mandible and medial pterygoid muscles. Tumor can extend superiorly to invade the tonsillar fossa or soft palate. Tumor may also spread inferiorly to the valleculae, piriform sinuses into the preepiglottic space, and epiglottis (**Fig. 6-13**). Tongue base cancer that extends across the midline precludes surgical treatment, as one lingual neurovascular pedicle must be conserved to allow for safe swallowing postsurgical cure (**Fig. 6-14**).

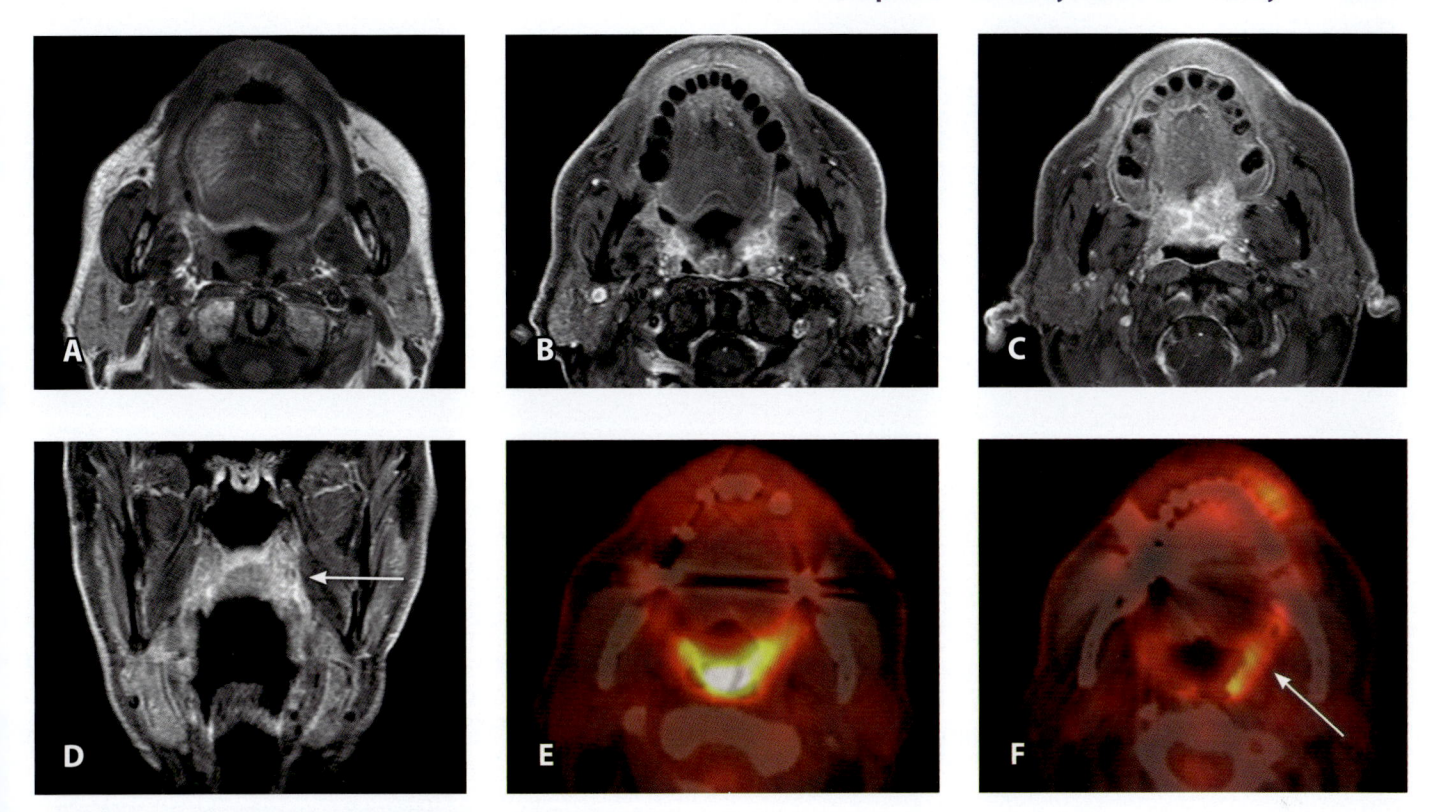

Figure 6-12 Soft Palate T3N2C Carcinoma
Plain axial T1 (**A**) and axial T2 (**B**), axial (**C**) and coronal (**D**) postcontrast with fat-saturated MR scans and axial fused PET/CT images (**E** and **F**). There is an irregular soft-tissue mass involving both sides of the soft palate, slightly greater on the left side where there is a small extension into the lateral pharyngeal wall (*arrows*, **D, F**).

It is difficult to differentiate tongue base neoplasm from lymphoid tissue based on imaging. Endoscopic biopsies are therefore recommended to accurately differentiate the two. However, imaging of cancer may reveal deep infiltration of soft-tissue structures. Noncontrast T1W MR imaging is helpful in revealing the extent of the lesion. It may be useful to detect tumor that has crossed the midline to determine potential partial glossectomy candidates. The tongue base has a rich lymphatic network, which primarily drains to upper and lower jugular nodes.

Posterior Oropharyngeal Wall

Cancer of the posterior oropharyngeal wall more commonly originates from cancer in the lateral oropharyngeal wall. Carcinoma of the posterior oropharyngeal wall has the worst prognosis of all oropharyngeal cancers. Symptoms may include pain, bleeding, and presence of a neck mass. Tumor may spread superiorly to the nasopharynx or inferiorly to the hypopharynx.[46]

These tumors commonly spread along the submucosa to invade the retropharyngeal fat but are limited by the prevertebral fascia, which acts as a barrier to tumor spread. Invasion of this fascia signifies a poor prognosis and also precludes surgical resection. CT and MR may reveal obliteration of the retropharyngeal fat plane with tumor invasion[50] (**Fig. 6-15**). However, cross-sectional imaging is poor in detecting the extent of involvement. Retropharyngeal fat plane obliteration, asymmetric enlargement of prevertebral muscles on CT imaging, and signal abnormalities on MRI imaging are generally poor diagnostic markers for tumor extension into the prevertebral space. Direct evaluation with open neck exploration is recommended for an accurate diagnosis. Nevertheless, a majority of posterior oropharyngeal wall cancer is treated by radiotherapy or combined chemotherapy and radiotherapy. In addition, cure rates are similar to that of surgery alone or combined surgery and radiotherapy.

Hypopharyngeal Carcinoma

More than 95% of hypopharyngeal malignancies arise from the epithelium of the mucosa, and are therefore SCCa.[7] Patients diagnosed with hypopharyngeal tumors are typically men aged 55 to 70 years with a history of tobacco abuse or alcohol ingestion. While the majority of patients remain asymptomatic, some patients may present with referred otalgia. This pain is referred to the ear via the Arnold nerve, a division of the vagus nerve, and suggests underlying malignancy.[7] Cervical lymph node metastases occur as the presenting symptom in approximately 75% of cases.

Superficial mucosal lesions in the pyriform sinus can be seen on barium studies. A nondistended pyriform sinus can mimic a tumor on CT and MR studies. CT and MR imaging can be used to detect submucosal spread when tumor is not apparent on direct clinical observation or barium studies (**Figs. 6-16 and 6-17**). In advanced cases, tumors of the pyriform sinus may spread to the larynx.

Pyriform sinus carcinomas may spread submucosally into the posterior wall of the hypopharynx, along the aryepiglottic

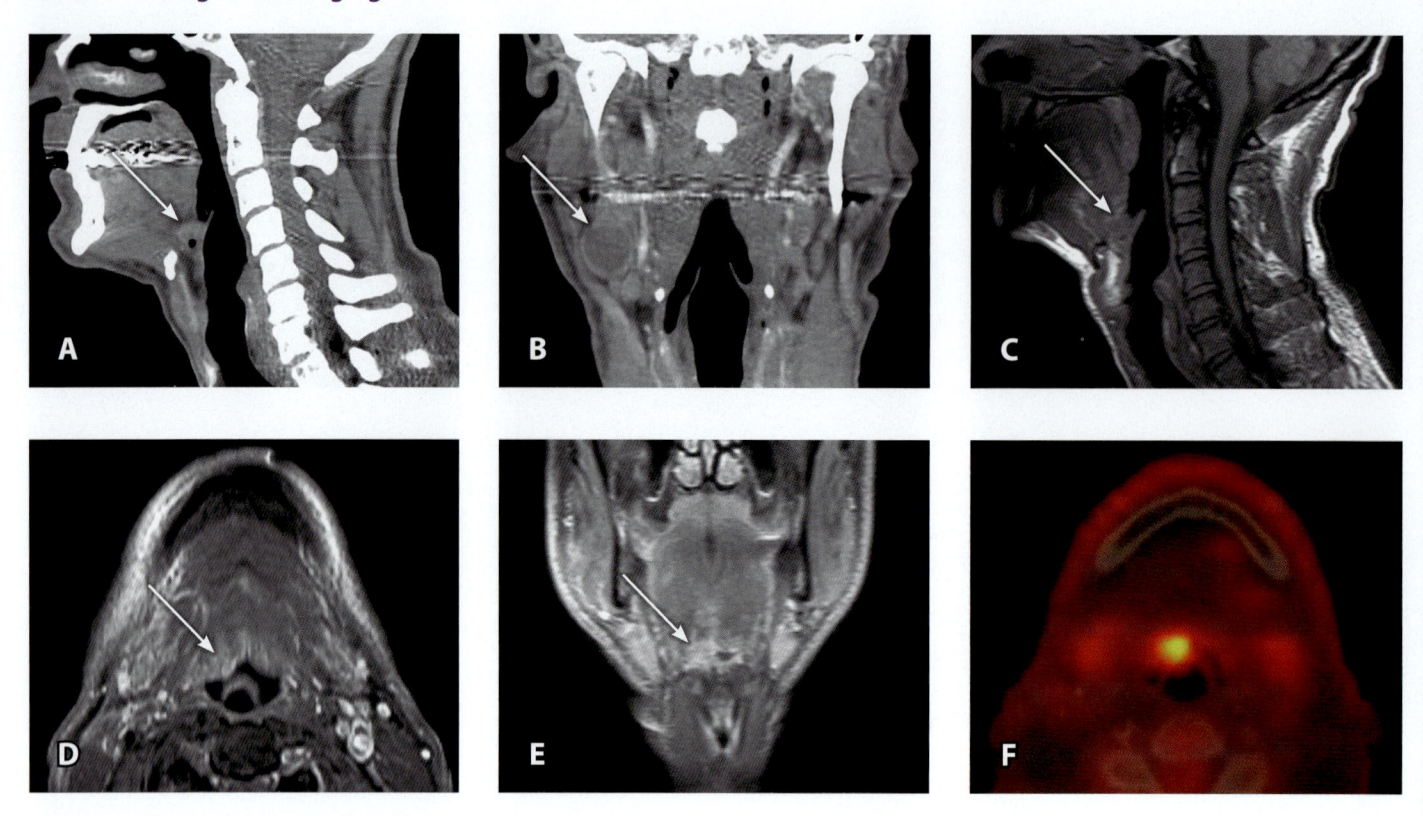

Figure 6-13 Base of Tongue T1N1 Carcinoma
Postcontrast reformatted sagittal (**A**) and coronal (**B**) CT scans prior to resection of the right neck node. The small primary tumor in the right base of tongue (*arrow*, **A**) was missed on initial clinical evaluation and CT imaging. The large right level II lymph node showing differential enhancement (*arrow*, **B**) was detected and surgically resected. Following surgery, plain sagittal MR scan (**C**), postcontrast with fat-saturated axial (**D**) and coronal (**E**) MR scans and axial fused PET/CT image (**F**) clearly show the small primary tumor in the base of tongue (*arrows*, **C, D, E**). Such multimodality imaging is essential in the accurate diagnosis and staging of head and neck cancers, particularly in the search for an unknown primary tumor when nodal metastasis is detected.

fold or the anterior wall in the postcricoid region. Tumors may invade the tongue base or extend into the paraglottic and preglottic fat. Cancer arising from the apex or lateral wall of the pyriform sinus often are found to invade the thyroid cartilage at the first diagnostic visit. Tumor involving the aryepiglottic fold may invade the arytenoids cartilage or false vocal cords.

Postcricoid tumors are usually not confined. These tumors can spread to the posterior larynx to cause vocal cord paralysis. Tumors may be large enough to narrow the lumen of the hypopharynx and spread through the cricopharyngeus to the esophageal verge (**Fig. 6-18**). Preoperative detection of esophageal verge involvement may alter surgical treatment.

Plummer-Vinson syndrome is a major risk factor for developing postcricoid hypopharyngeal cancer. More females than males have this syndrome. Patients may present with cervical esophageal and hyopharyngeal webs, dysphagia, iron deficiency anemia, and weight loss. Cancer development in the postcricoid region may be related to stasis about the webs.

Tumors of the posterior wall of the hypopharynx may extend cranially to the posterior wall of the oropharynx. Posterior wall tumors may invade the prevertebral muscles and even the vertebrae. Tumor fixation to the longus colli muscles can be detected by CT and MRI as obliteration of prevertebral fat planes by the tumor.[8] This invasion can best be seen on T2-weighted MR images where low signal intensity of muscle is replaced by intermediate signal intensity of the tumor. However, such findings may also be seen with inflammation of the muscles.

Lymphatic Spread

The upper parajugular lymph nodes are the first nodes to be involved in tumor spread. Retropharyngeal adenopathy is common, with or without involvement of other lymph nodes. Bilateral adenopathy is common in tongue base and soft palate cancer.

Tumor Classification and Staging

Oropharyngeal carcinoma is staged on size criteria (**Table 6-5**). MRI is the preferred method for staging squamous cell carcinoma of the oropharynx. MRI is more sensitive than CT in evaluating small tumors due to its superior soft-tissue contrast.

A study by Kim et al. assessed the utility of FDG PET in the preoperative staging of oropharyngeal SCCa by comparing it to MR and CT. FDG PET had higher sensitivities than CT/MRI for primary tumor detection and for identification of cervical metastases on neck side bases.[51] In contrast, the specificity of

Chapter 6: The Pharynx and Oral Cavity 243

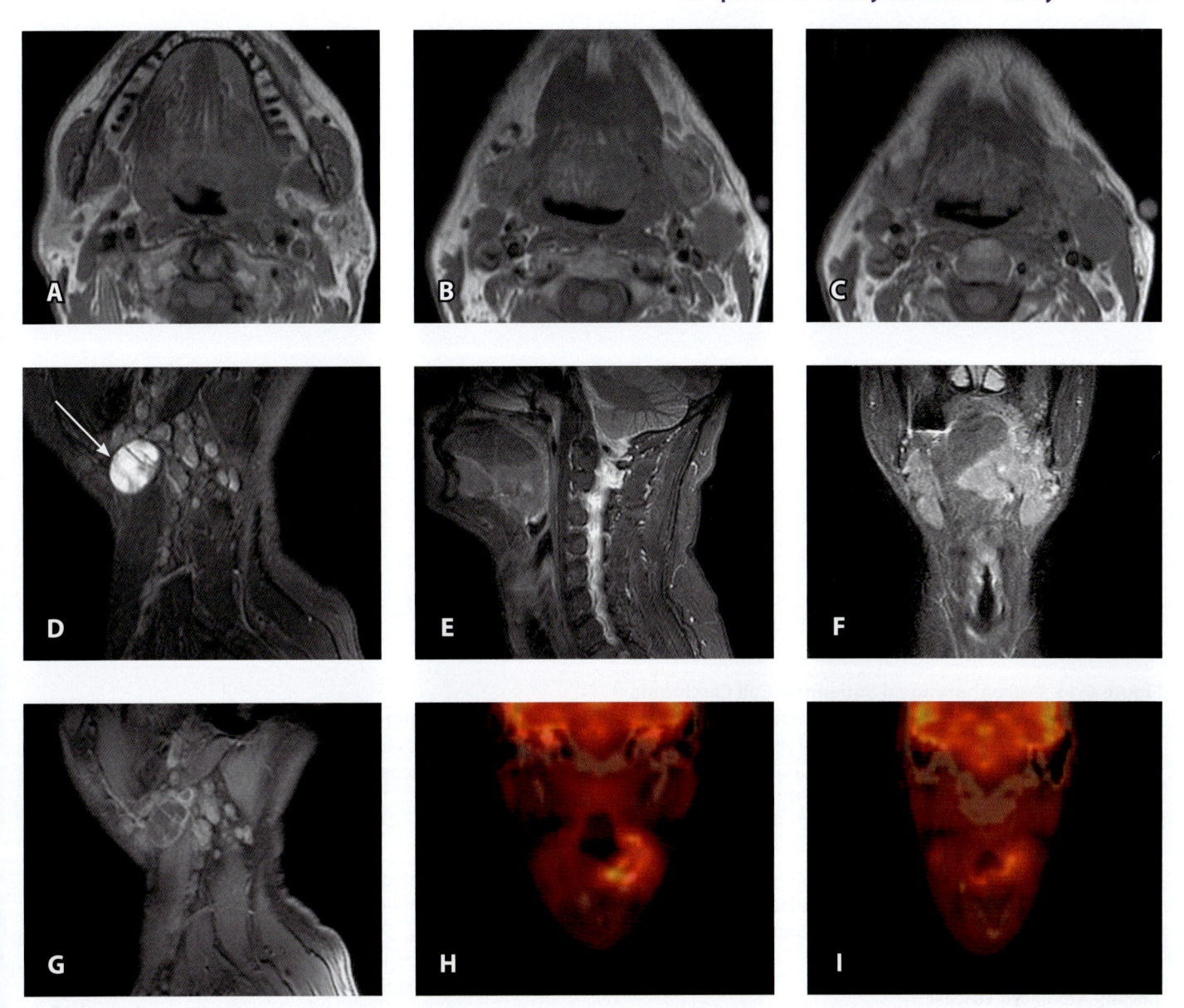

Figure 6-14 Base of Tongue T3N2C Carcinoma
Plain axial T1 (**A–C**) sagittal T2 (**D** and **E**) and postcontrast fat-saturated coronal (**F**) and sagittal (**G**) MR scans and coronal fused PET/CT (**H** and **I**) images. There is a large, widely infiltrating tumor in the left base of tongue extending downward into the vallecula showing deep invasion into both sides of the oral tongue. There are multiple bilateral levels II and III nodal metastasis, greater on the left side where there is a dominant cystic nodal mass (*arrow*, **D**). Such cystic cancer nodes must not be confused with a variety of cystic neck masses such as branchial cleft cysts or lymphangiomas (cystic hygromas).

---

the two methods did not differ significantly. They concluded that improved preoperative staging of FDG PET may help in planning treatment, but its accuracy is insufficient to replace pathologic staging based on neck dissection.

Treatment Based on Staging

Early Stage Disease
Patients are treated with surgery or radiation therapy. The advantage of radiation therapy over surgery is the ability to encompass areas at high risk, such as the cervical lymph nodes, without adding morbidity.

A few patients with nasopharyngeal carcinoma will present with early stage disease. These patients remain asymptomatic for prolonged periods. Due to the anatomical constraints of the nasopharynx, radiation therapy is recommended over surgical resection.

Most soft palate tumors are diagnosed at an early stage. Radiation therapy is the preferred treatment for these cancers. Elective neck treatment can be performed on patients with high risk of occult disease. Radiation therapy is also the modality of choice for treatment of early tonsillar cancers. While surgery provides similar survival rates, it is associated with significant

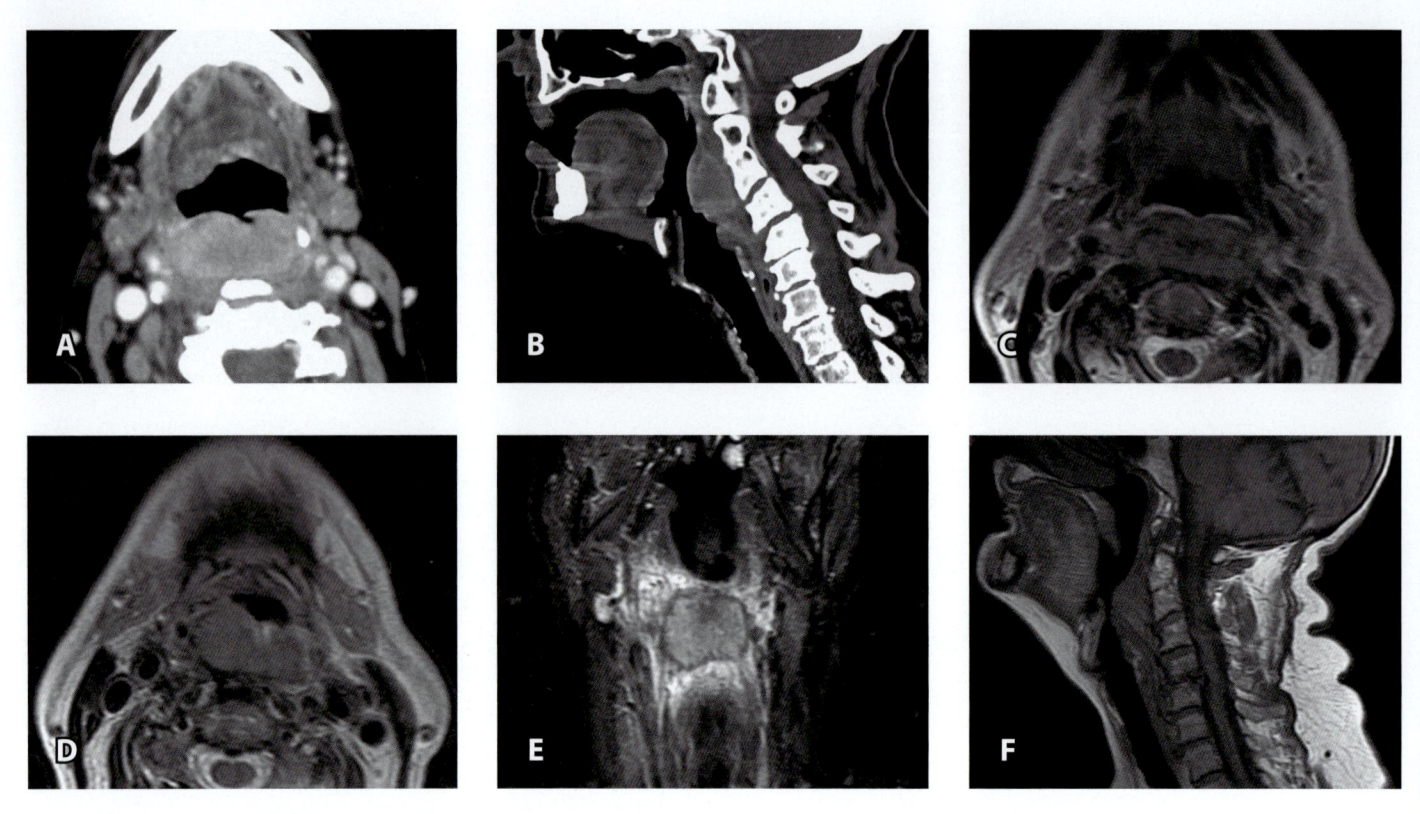

Figure 6-15 Retropharyngeal Squamous Cell Carcinoma
Postcontrast axial (**A**) and sagittal reformatted (**B**) CT scans. Plain axial (**C** and **D**) and coronal (**E**) T2 and plain sagittal T1 MR scans. There is a bulky bilateral retropharyngeal tumor with on biopsy proved to be a squamous cell carcinoma. Such bilateral retropharyngeal tumors are typically lymphomas or other sarcomas, but submucosal epithelial tumors of the postcricoid hypopharynx can be a close mimic, as in this case.

morbidity, such as those that affect swallowing. For patients with cancer on the tongue base and a clinically negative neck, bilateral prophylactic neck treatment is recommended due to the high risk of occult lymph node disease.

Locally Advanced Disease
Treatment for locoregional-advanced cancers may involve a combination of chemotherapy, surgery, and radiation therapy. A nonoperative approach is favored for patients with oropharyngeal carcinoma. Patients with oropharyngeal cancer may be treated with chemoradiotherapy and expect similar survival rates to those treated with surgery and radiation therapy. Surgery is therefore generally reserved for salvage therapy. Nasopharyngeal carcinoma in the majority of patients is not surgically resection. Patients are usually treated with chemoradiotherapy followed by adjuvant chemotherapy.

Distant Metastatic and Recurrent Disease
Chemotherapy provides palliative benefit in patients with symptomatic metastatic or incurable disease. However, it is uncertain whether this regimen prolongs survival.

Patients may present with locoregional recurrent disease, but no metastatic disease. Patients who were previously retreated with surgery should receive radiation therapy, while patients who were previously irradiated should undergo resection of the disease.[52] If surgery is not possible for previously irradiated patients, possible treatments include reirradiating the patient and adding chemotherapy or palliative chemotherapy.

Persistent asymmetry of tissue or increased enhancement after therapy may signify tumor recurrence. To evaluate recurrent disease, comparison with a baseline posttreatment CT or MRI study is recommended. Enlargement of node or mass along the margins of the surgical resection may indicate tumor recurrence. Differentiating tumor recurrence from fibrosis may be difficult on CT because of their similar density. Both immature scars and tumor display contrast enhancement on MRI and are hyperintense on T2W images. However, mature scars do not enhance with contrast and are of low signal intensity on T2W MR images. FDG, thallium-201, and MR spectroscopy can also be used to evaluate for recurrent disease.

Posttreatment

Radiation Changes
Radiation therapy has been used to treat pharyngeal carcinomas. Complete resolution of tumor usually occurs within 3 months following radiation therapy. Treatment of pharyngeal neoplasms with radiation can lead to changes in anatomy and physiology of the pharynx and can change their appearance on imaging. The posterior pharyngeal wall can thicken from a normal 2 to 3 mm to 6 to 7 mm after radiation therapy. In

Chapter 6: The Pharynx and Oral Cavity   **245**

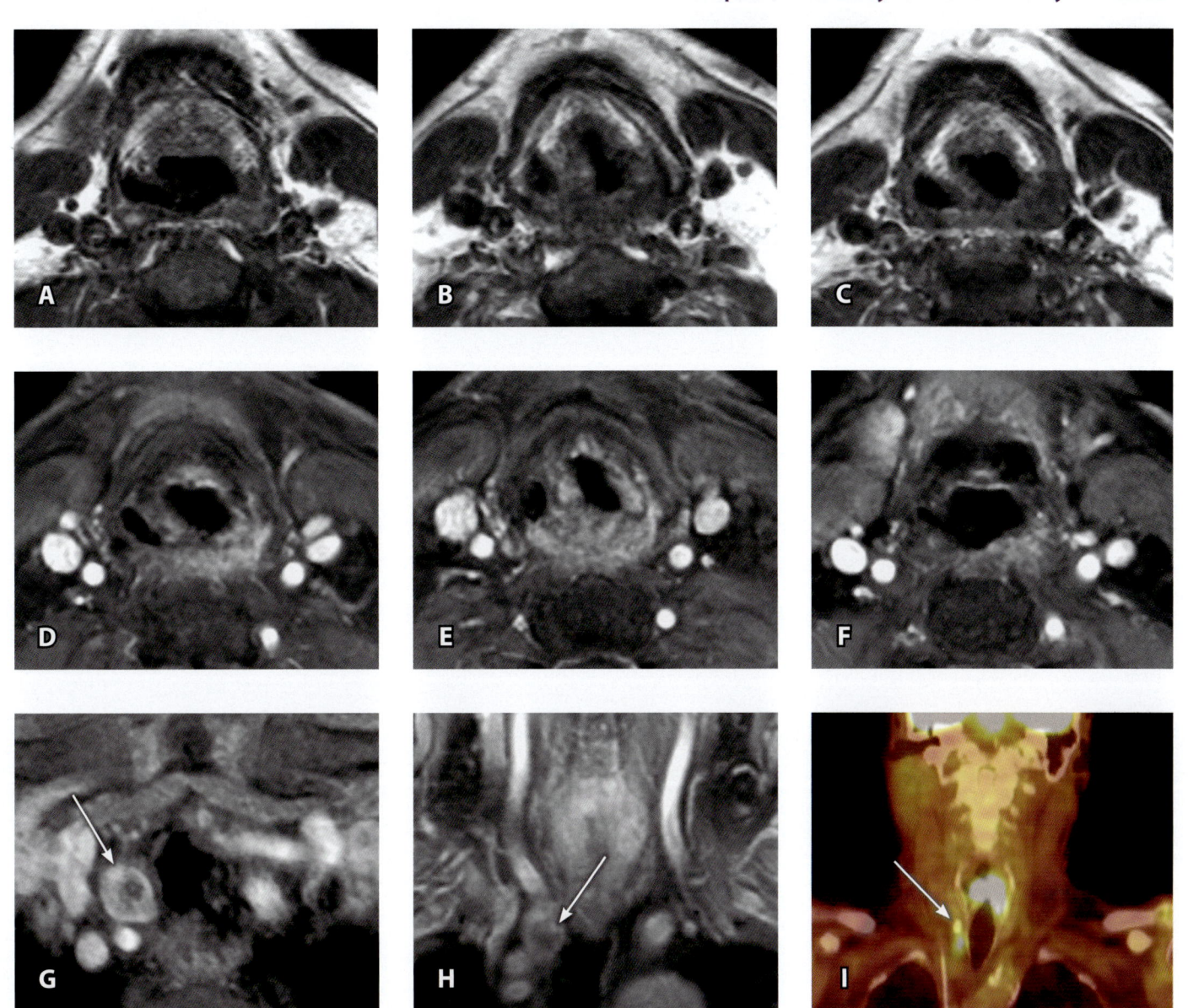

Figure 6-16 Hypopharyngeal Carcinoma with Level VI Nodal Metastasis
(**A–C**) Plain axial T1, (**D–H**) Postcontrast with fat-saturated axial T1 MR images and coronal fused PET/CT scan. There is a tumor in the left pyriform sinus showing extensive inferior and posterior growth into the postcricoid region bilaterally. A metastatic right-sided level VI nodal mass is evident (*arrows*, **G, H, I**). Such distal nodal metastasis is consistent with hypopharyngeal origin, but may also be detected in esophageal cancers that invade the postcricoid region. MR or CT imaging is superior to stand-alone PET imaging in making an accurate differential diagnosis.

addition, edema of the retropharyngeal space may be detected on imaging. The pharyngeal mucosa may be enhanced due to the formation of telangiectatic vessels that arise as a result of radiation-induced mucositis.

It is best to compare pretreatment imaging studies with post-treatment studies in order to differentiate residual changes from radiation from a residual tumor. Thickening of the soft tissue caused by radiation therapy will not progressively enlarge, as would a tumor. Tumor also has an imaging density similar to muscle, while edematous changes tend to be of lower density. Postradiation treatment complications include nerve paralysis and pharyngeal stenosis.

Cranial nerves are relatively resistant to radiation. The hypoglossal nerve is the most commonly affected nerve. The optic nerve, abducens nerve, and vagus nerve can also be affected. A study by Lin et al. suggested that patients with nasopharyngeal carcinoma radiotherapy may develop hypoglossal, vagus, or recurrent laryngeal nerve palsy from radiation-related fibrosis of the neck.[53] The pathway that these nerves travel is an important risk factor for the development of palsy.

After radiotherapy, the muscular pharyngeal walls may appear thickened and retropharyngeal edema may be detected on imaging. There may also be an increased attenuation of fatty tissue plane.

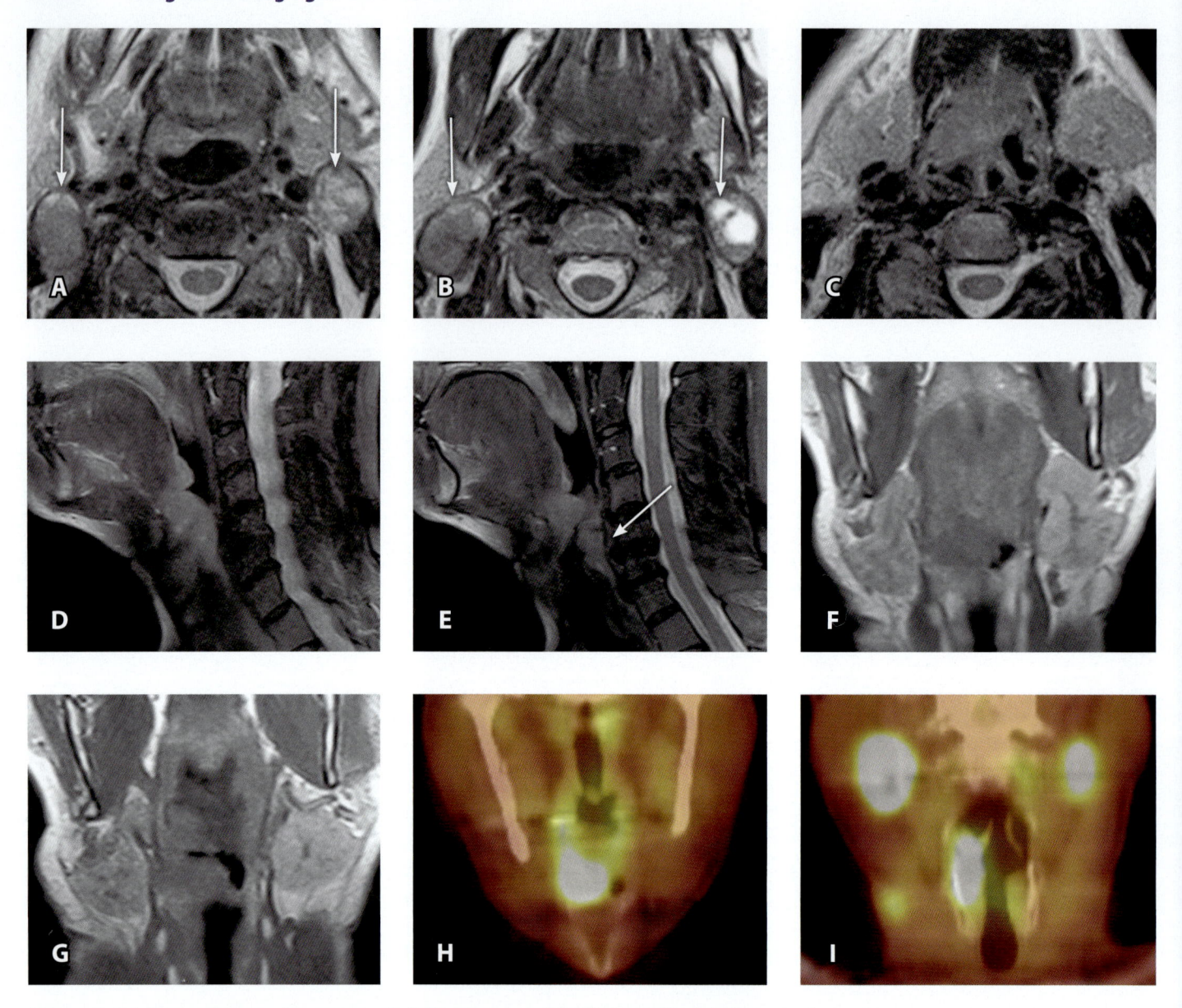

Figure 6-17 Hypopharynx Squamous Cell Carcinoma with Bilateral Nodal Metastasis
(**A–C**) Axial T2, (**D, E**) coronal T2, (**F, G**) coronal postcontrast T1 without fat-saturated MR scans and (**H** and **I**) coronal fused PET/CT images. There is a bulky tumor involving the right side of the superior hypopharynx with circumferential growth upward into the vallecula, tongue base and pre-epiglottic space. Involvement of the mid portion of the posterior pharyngeal wall (*arrow*, **E**), indicates bilateral spread, which is also detected in large bilateral level III nodal masses. The right nodal mass is primarily solid; the left nodal mass is primarily cystic (*arrows* **A, B**).

Postsurgical Changes

Resection of malignancies may result in distortion of the normal anatomy, making interpretation of postsurgical studies difficult. After surgical treatment, the pharyngeal wall is usually smooth and thin.

It is difficult to evaluate the postsurgical neck after extensive resection. After postsurgical treatment, contrast-enhanced CT or MRI cannot differentiate a tumor from granulation or scar tissue caused by the treatment as all of these enhance on imaging.

Oral Carcinoma

Although cancers of the head and neck account for only 5% of all cancers in the human body, 30% of these cancers occur in the oral cavity. Squamous cell carcinoma accounts for 90% of malignant oral cavity lesions. It typically affects men more than women and older individuals in the fifth to seventh decade of life.[54] Known risk factors include tobacco use, alcohol abuse, and infection with HPV. Clinical presentation may also include dysphagia, odynophagia, sore throat, and bleeding in the mouth. Early superficial mucosa lesions may be detected on visual

Chapter 6: The Pharynx and Oral Cavity

Table 6-5 Oropharyngeal/Hypopharyngeal Carcinoma Tumor Staging

	Primary Tumor
TX	Primary tumor cannot be assessed
T0	No evidence of primary tumor
Tis	Carcinoma in situ
T1	Tumor 2 cm or less in greatest dimension
T2	Tumor more than 2 cm but not more than 4 cm in greatest dimension
T3	Tumor more than 4 cm in greatest dimension or extension to lingual surface of epiglottis
T4a	Tumor invades the larynx, extrinsic muscle of tongue, medial pterygoid, hard palate, or mandible
T4b	Tumor invades lateral pterygoid muscle, pterygoid plates, lateral nasopharynx, or skull base, or encases the carotid artery
	Nodal Staging
NX	Regional lymph nodes cannot be assessed
N0	No regional lymph node metastasis
N1	Metastasis in a single ipsilateral lymph node, 3 cm or less in greatest dimension
N2	Metastasis in a single ipsilateral lymph node, more than 3 cm but not more than 6 cm in greatest dimension, or in multiple ipsilateral lymph nodes, none more than 6 cm in greatest dimension, or in bilateral or contralateral lymph nodes, none more than 6 cm in greatest dimension
N2a	Metastasis in a single ipsilateral lymph node more than 3 cm but not more than 6 cm in greatest dimension
N2b	Metastasis in multiple ipsilateral lymph nodes, none more than 6 cm in greatest dimension
N2c	Metastasis in bilateral or contralateral lymph nodes, none more than 6 cm in greatest dimension
N3	Metastasis in a lymph node more than 6 cm in greatest dimension
	Distant Metastasis
M0	No distant metastasis
M1	Distant metastasis

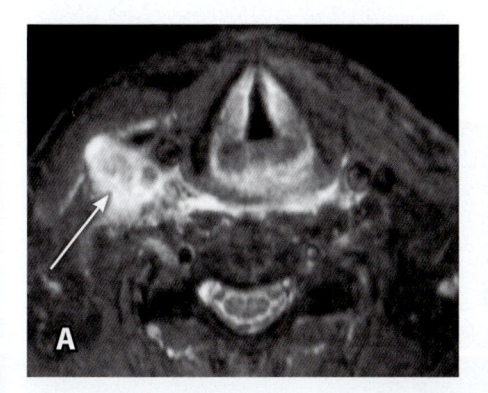

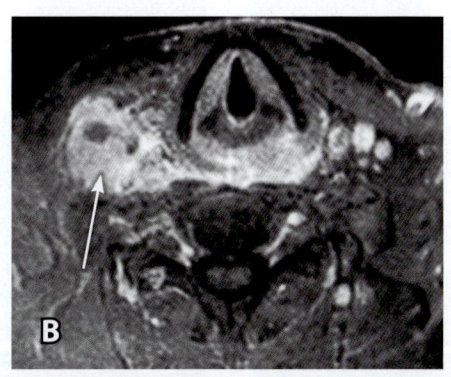

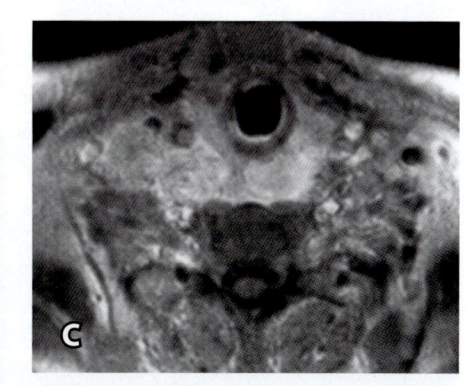

Figure 6-18 Hypopharyngeal Retrocricoid Carcinoma with Retrotracheal Extension
Axial T2 (**A**) and axial postcontrast with fat-saturated T1 (**B, C**) MR scans. The tumor with mucosal origin in the left postcricoid region of the hypopharynx has invaded the posterior musculature and extending inferiorly to the level of the trachea (**C**). There is also direct extension and/or metastasis to right cervical lymph nodes. The nodal mass is markedly irregular in outline consistent with extranodal spread into the adjacent soft tissues (*arrows*, **A, B**).

inspection as either patches of leukoplakia or erythroplakia. Because the oral tongue and the floor of the mouth are rich in lymphatics, they are at higher risk of nodal metastases compared with other locations, such as the gingival and hard palate.[55]

Tumor Origin and Spread

Lip

In the oral cavity, the lip is the most common location for SCCa. SCCa of the lip can involve the orbicularis oris muscle, while more advanced lesions can extend to involve the buccal mucosa. Deep extension of the tumor requires evaluation with CT or MRI. The mandibular cortex, mandibular marrow, inferior alveolar, and mental nerves should be assessed. Lymphatic drainage of these tumors is to submental, submandibular, and internal jugular nodes.

Floor of Mouth

Most tumors of the floor of the mouth are located anteriorly near the midline (Figs. 6-19 and 6-20). Cross-sectional imaging is needed to evaluate deep tumor infiltration. In ultrasound, the transducer should be tilted so that the anterior part of the floor of the mouth can be evaluated. Soft-tissue invasion occurs before mylohyoid muscle or mandible invasion.[56] The tumor can cross midline and invade the contralateral neurovascular bundle. Superior extension of the tumor can also involve the oral tongue. Involvement of the contralateral tongue and/or neurovascular bundle precludes radical surgical resection of the tumor. Inferior spread can occur along the hyoglossus muscle to the attachment of the hyoid bone. The tumor can extend posteriorly and laterally along the mylohyoid muscle and inner surface of the mandible. The submandibular gland or Wharton's duct may also

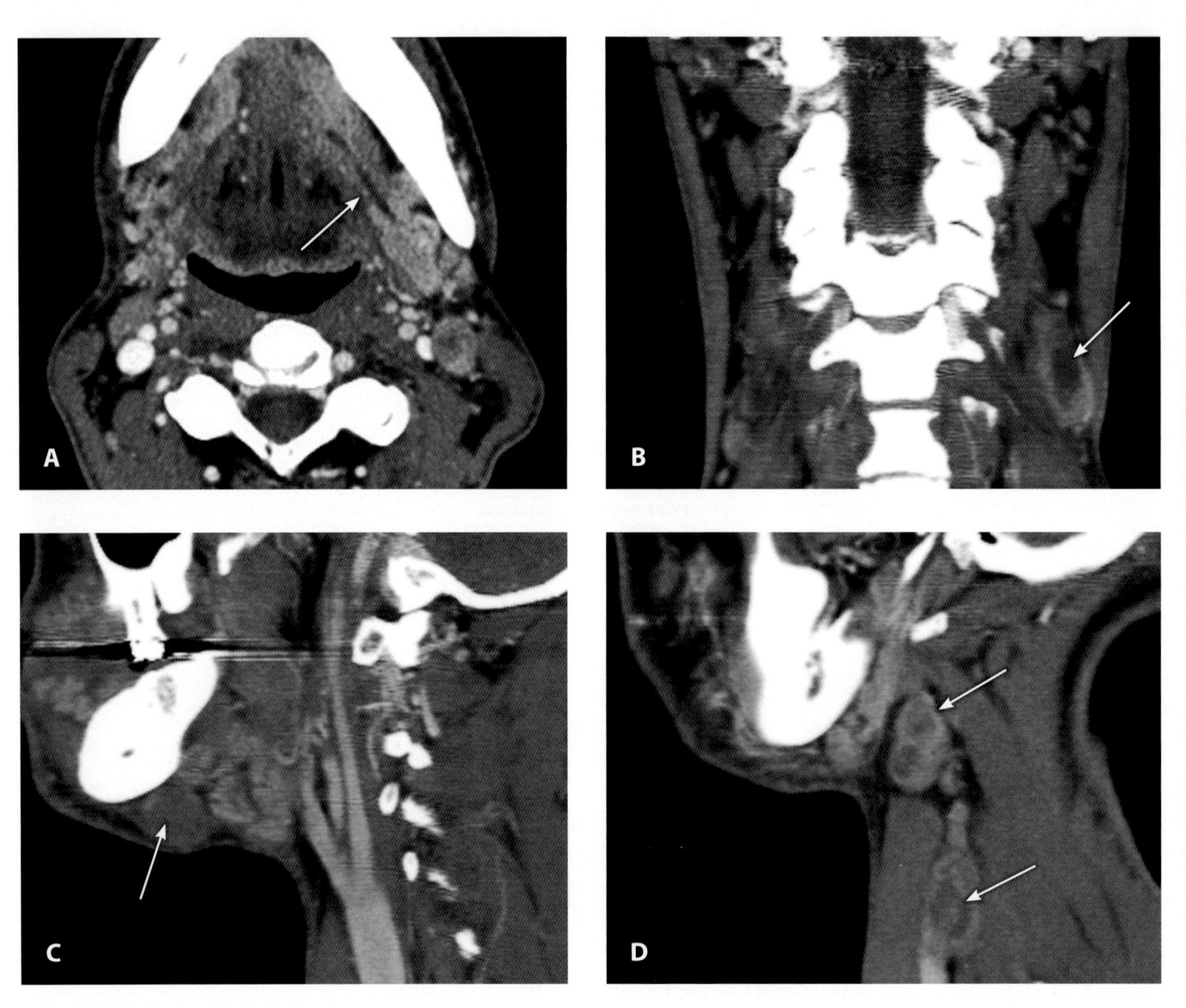

Figure 6-19 Floor of Mouth Carcinoma
(A) Axial, (B) coronal reformatted and (C, D) sagittal reformatted postcontrast CT scans. There is a mass in the left floor of mouth showing abnormal enhancement. The lesion obstructs the adjacent dilated Wharton submandibular duct (*arrow*, A). There are multiple bulky nodal metastasis in the left level I and level II cervical lymph nodes (*arrows*, B, C, D).

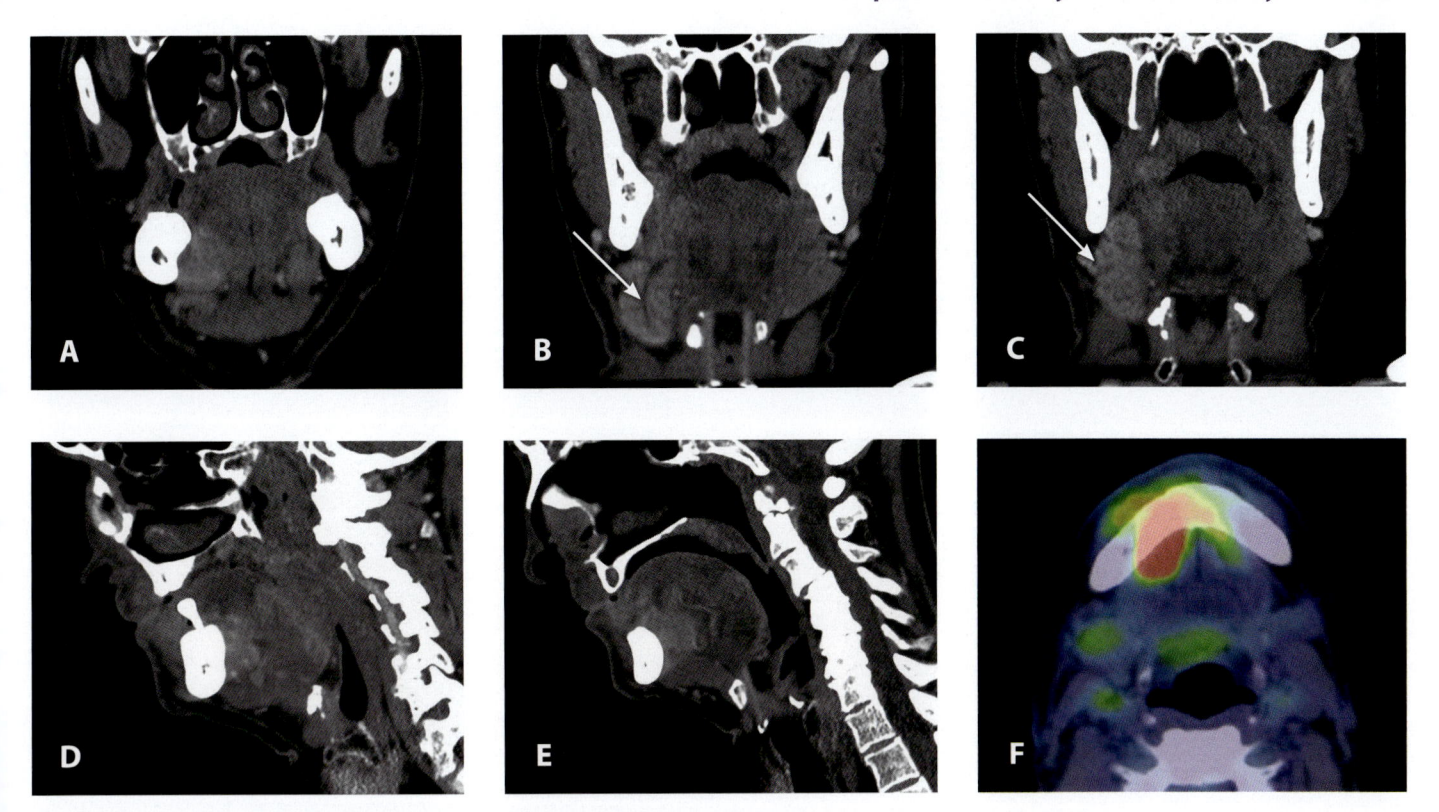

Figure 6-20 Floor of Mouth Squamous Cell Carcinoma
(**A–C**) Coronal reformatted, (**D, E**) sagittal reformatted contrast-enhanced CT scans and (**F**) axial fused PET/CT image. There is an enhancing tumor in the right anterior floor of mouth adjacent to the body of the mandible. The mass obstructs the intraglandular ducts in the right submandibular gland (*arrows*, **B**) and is associated with what appears to be pathologically enlarged right level IB metastatic nodes (*arrow*, **C**). However, the fused PET/CT (**F**) shows only modest uptake in this region indicating the "nodal mass" is an enlarged and obstructed submandibular gland with reactive adenopathy.

be infiltrated, and result in duct dilatation or obstructive inflammatory changes.

In tumors of the floor of the mouth, both MRI and CT should be performed in the initial work-up, especially for cases in which there is a clinical doubt about mandibular extension of disease.[14,57] Tumors of the anterior part of the floor of the mouth can spread via internal jugular (level I or II), submental, and/or submandibular lymph nodes. The greater depth of tumor invasion may increase the likelihood for cervical lymph node metastases.

Oral Tongue

Cancer of the oral tongue occurs most often on the ventrolateral surface (**Figs. 6-21** and **6-22**). Most of the lateral legions originate from the middle or posterior one-third of the lateral tongue. Tongue cancers can easily invade the intrinsic muscles or spread along extrinsic muscles to invade their sites of attachment, which include the hyoid bone, mandible, or styloid process.[56] Tumors of the tongue can invade the ipsilateral neurovascular bundle, tongue base, gingival mucosa. It is important to evaluate tumor extension with respect to the midline and to the contralateral sublingual space and neurovascular bundle.[49] Lymphatic drainage of oral tongue cancer is to the submandibular and internal jugular nodes (level I and II).

Gingival/Buccal Mucosa

Buccal mucosa is continuous with the gingival covering on the buccal surface of the maxillary and mandibular alveolar ridges and the retromolar trigone. SCCa of the gingival and buccal mucosa may eventually invade the maxillary or mandibular cortex, which may require extensive resection with segmental mandibulectomy or partial maxillectomy.[56] Invasion such as this is best detected on axial slices. SCCa of the buccal mucosa most commonly originates on the lateral walls. Lateral submucosal extension can occur along the buccinators muscle to the pterygomandibular raphe (**Fig. 6-23**).

Retromolar Trigone

Primary SCCa of the retromolar trigone is rare and characterized by early spread. SCCa of the retromolar trigone is located on the superoposterior part of the oral cavity and may involve the oropharyngeal regions (**Fig. 6-24**). The tumor many extend medially toward the hard palate and laterally to the buccinators space. Anteriorly, the tumor may infiltrate the gingival mucosa. Superior extension of the tumor can involve buccal mucosa and maxillary alveolar ridge. The tumors can spread posteriorly to affect the tonsillar pillar, soft palate, and pharyngeal tonsil. Deeply, infiltration can occur along the pterygomandibular space, mandible, and superior pharyngeal constrictor muscle.[58] Extension

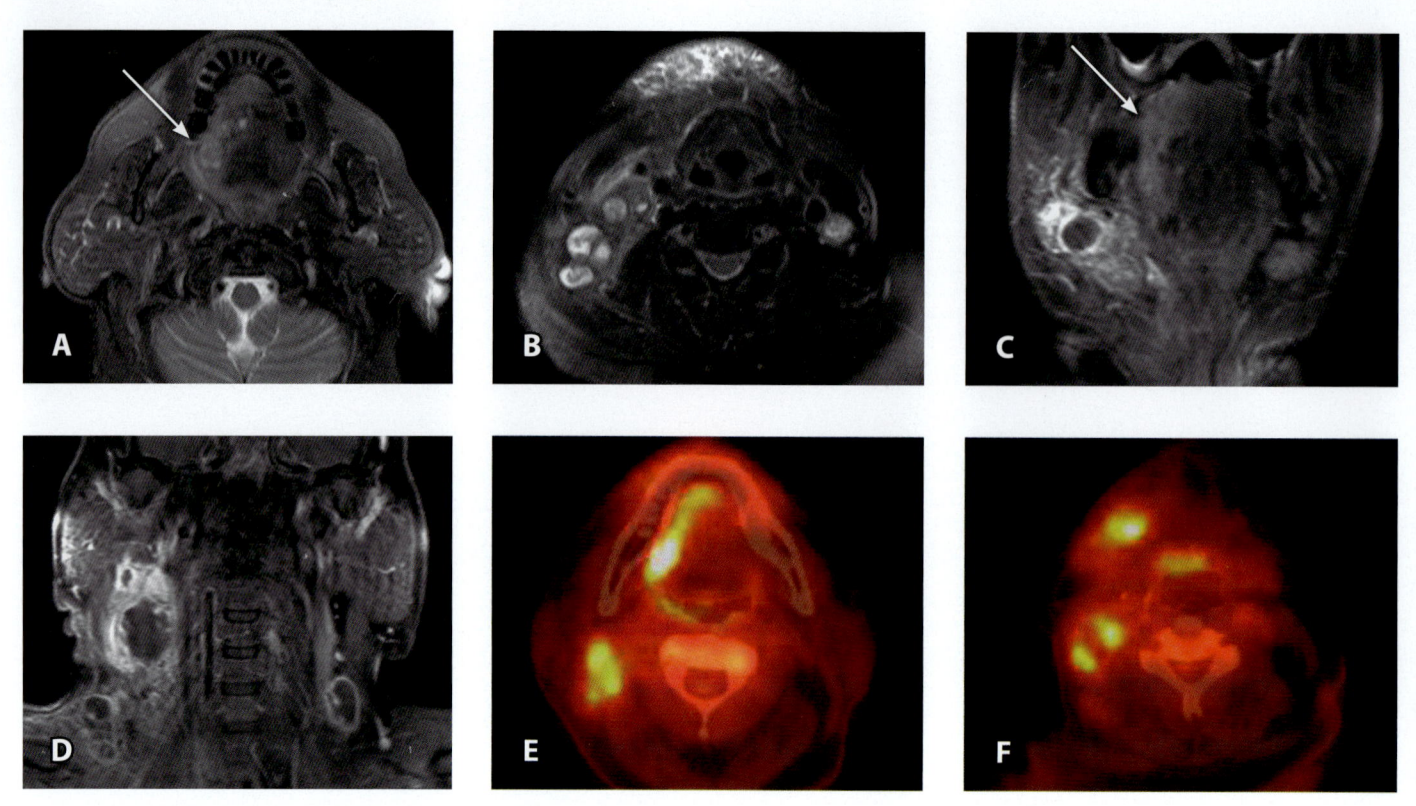

Figure 6-21 Oral Tongue T4N3 Squamous Cell Carcinoma
Axial (**A, B**) and coronal (**C, D**) T2 MR scans and axial fused PET/CT images (**E, F**). There is a large tumor mass extending along the length of the right oral tongue (*arrows*, **A, C**). Multiple foci of cervical nodal metastasis are evident, with a left level II necrotic mass and multiple solitary and confluent nodal masses throughout the right involving levels II, III, and V. There is direct extra-nodal extension of tumor into the soft tissues of the right neck. Such extranodal spread of cancer carries a poor prognosis and is better seen on MRI than on PET/CT (**E, F**).

of tumor into the pterygopalatine fossa may result in perineural spread of tumor.

Hard Palate

Close evaluation of the adjacent bone must be performed for tumors of the mucosal layer of the hard palate. Tumors can erode into the floor of the nasal cavity and the maxillary sinus. Tumor of the hard palate can best be seen on coronal CT or MR image using a bone window. The greater and lesser palatine canals and the incisive canals should be evaluated closely for perineural spread along the palatine nerves toward the pterygopalatine fossa. The maxillary division of the trigeminal nerve may also be involved. MRI may be used to detect perineural spread as thickening and contrast enhancement of the nerve. CT may reveal cortical erosions of the bony canals.

Inferior and Superior Alveolar Ridge Carcinoma

Alveolar ridge carcinoma accounts for approximately 10% of oral carcinomas. Inferior alveolar ridge carcinoma is much more common than superior alveolar ridge carcinoma. The majority of tumors arise in an edentulous area. Patients who chew tobacco are at greatest risk. Bone invasion may occur early due to close proximity, while cervical metastasis is rare. Superior alveolar ridge carcinoma can spread to the periosteum, buccal mucosa, and sinus[12] (**Fig. 6-25**). Inferior alveolar ridge carcinoma can spread to the periosteum, buccal mucosa, or floor of the mouth (**Figs. 6-26** and **6-27**). A perineural spread along the inferior alveolar nerve is also possible. Surgical therapy often involves partial maxillectomy or mandibulectomy.

Tumor Classification and Staging

The goal of diagnostic imaging is to establish the location, the size, and the extent of tumor. Important is the determination of tumor margins with respect to anatomic landmark structures as well as assessing for tumor spread across the midline (**Table 6-6**). These findings play an important role in therapeutic planning.[59]

Small superficial T1 tumors may not be visible on CT and MR images.[60] However, with increasing size, SCC can infiltrate deeper submucosal structures. CT and MRI can be used for an accurate evaluation of deep tumor infiltration.[61,62] In general, MRI is more sensitive and specific than CT in evaluating the oral cavity. Unenhanced T1-weighted sequences should be used as the basic pulse sequence for MR imaging of tumors of the oral cavity.[63] T2-weighted fast spin echo and contrast enhanced T1-weighted sequences can be added when tumor margins are not clearly defined by T1-weighted sequences. T2-weighted images can be helpful in assessing depth of invasion of the primary tumor of the oral tongue, as depth of invasion has been shown to correlate with the risk for nodal metastases and outcome.[64]

Chapter 6: The Pharynx and Oral Cavity   **251**

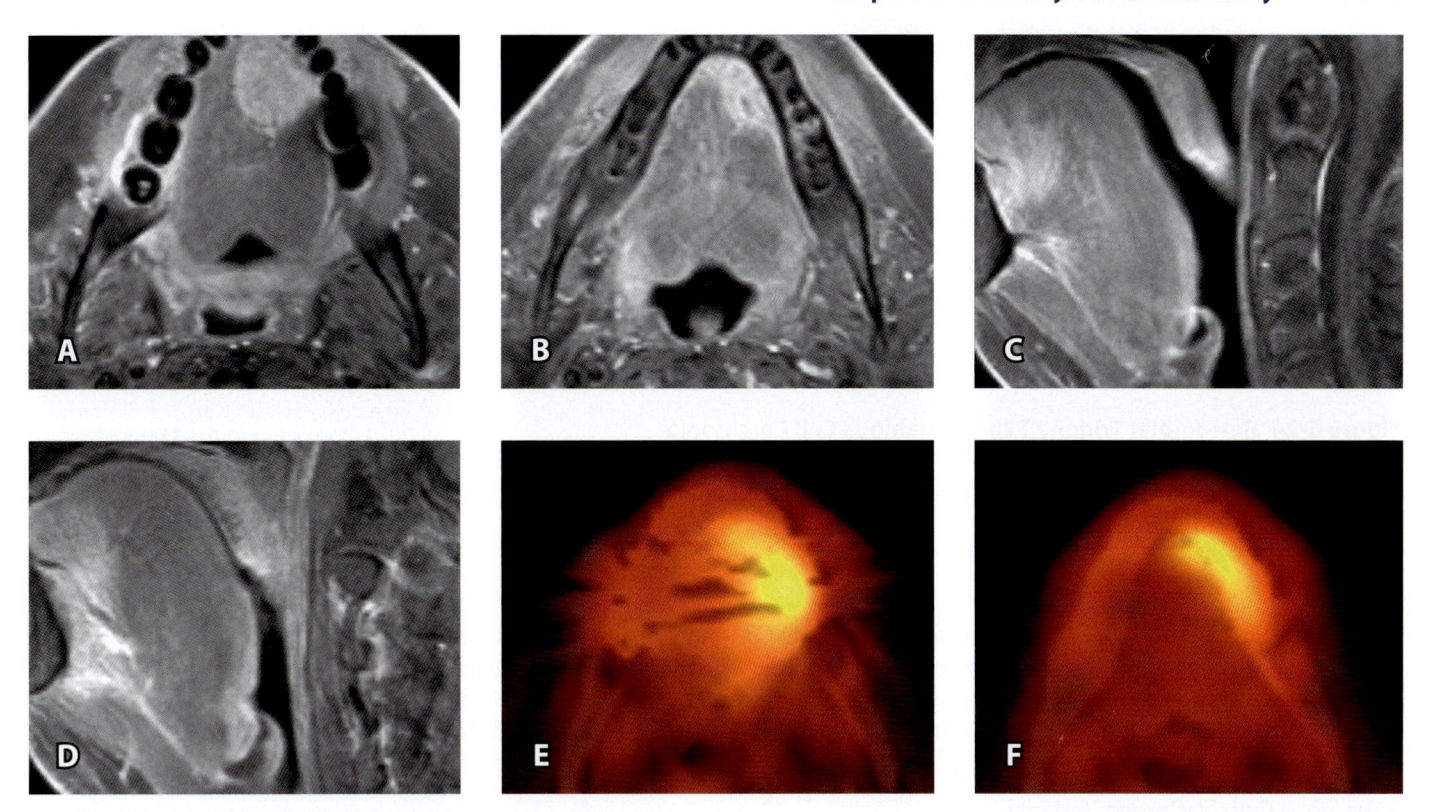

Figure 6-22 Oral Tongue Squamous Cell Carcinoma
Axial (**A, B**) and sagittal (**C, D**) contrast enhanced with fat-saturated T1 MR scans and axial fused PET/CT images. The enhancing tumor in the left anterior oral tongue adjacent to the lingual surface of the mandible is well seen on both examinations. However, the depth of invasion is an important prognostic sign and is difficult to determine by PET/CT (**E, F**).

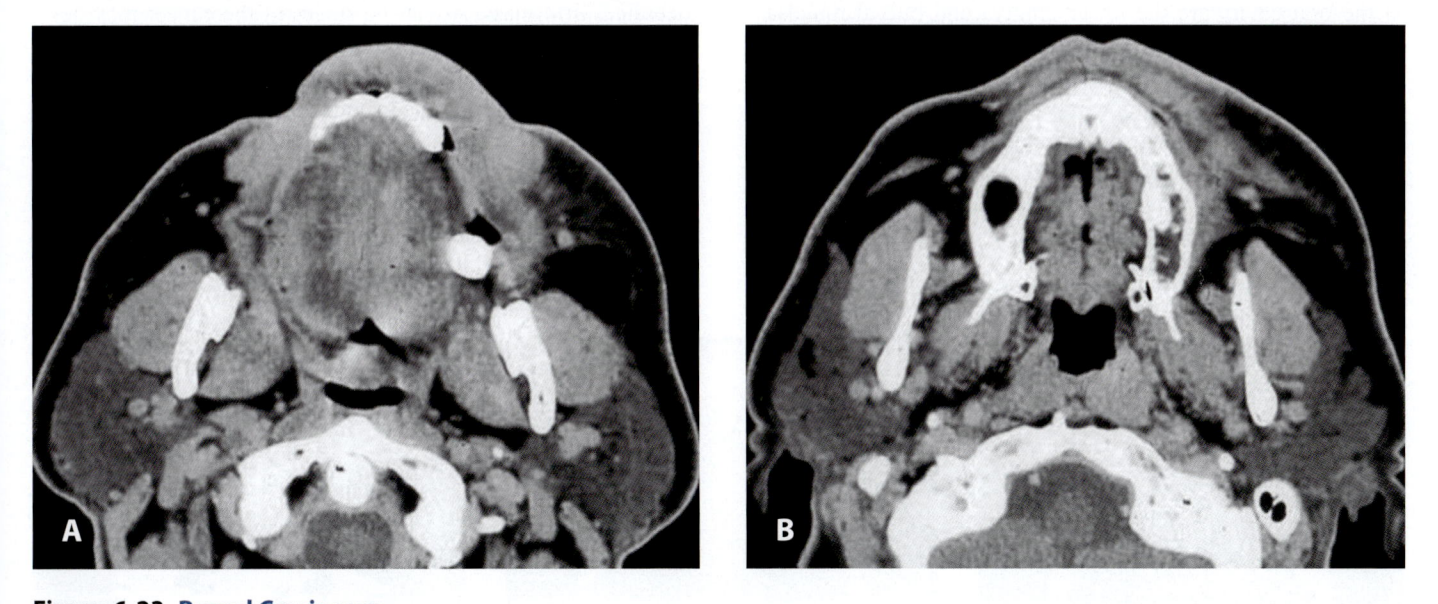

Figure 6-23 Buccal Carcinoma
(**A** and **B**) Axial contrast-enhanced CT scans. There is a bulky mass in the left side of the upper lip extending laterally underneath the skin surface of the left cheek and into the buccinator and platysma muscles.

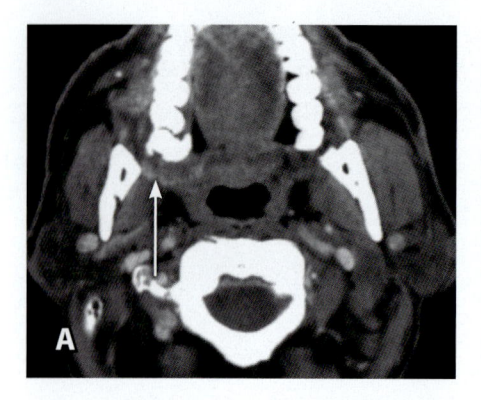

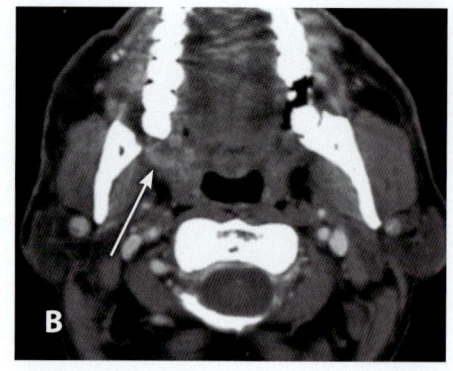

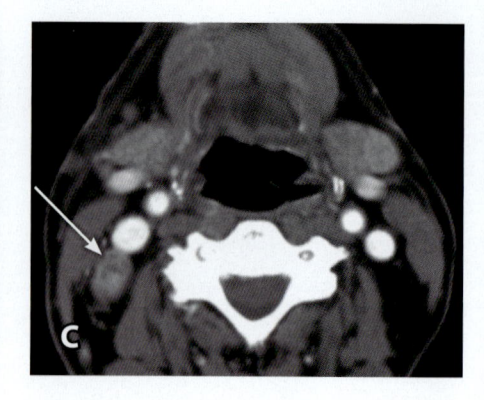

Figure 6-24 Retromolar Trigone T2N1 Squamous Cell Carcinoma
(**A–C**) Axial contrast-enhanced CT scans. There is a focal mass surrounding the right maxillary tuberosity (*arrows*, **A, B**). An enlarged right level II node showing differential enhancement characteristic of nodal metastasis is evident just posterior to the internal jugular vein (*arrow*, **C**).

Nevertheless, FDG PET has been found to be superior to CT and MRI for detecting occult neck metastasis of oral SCC.[65] Cervical lymph node metastases occur in approximately half of the patients with oral SCCa. Lymph node involvement is accepted to be the single most important prognostic parameter.[66]

Squamous Cell Carcinoma Variants

Verrucous Carcinoma

Verrucous carcinoma or Ackerman tumor is an uncommon variant of squamous cell carcinoma. Patients with oral verrucous carcinoma may be at greater risk for oral squamous cell carcinoma, which has a worse prognosis. Common sites affected in the oral cavity are the lower gingiva and buccal mucosa.[67] Reports of the cancer involving the alveolar mucosa, hard palate, and floor of the mouth have also been reported.[68] Verrucous carcinoma occurs more frequently in men older than 60 years. Risk factors for verrucous carcinoma include chewing tobacco or infection with HPV. Clinically, patients may present with a bulky, exophytic outgrowth. Verrucous carcinoma may be difficult to differentiate from other types of squamous cell carcinoma by imaging techniques.[69] There may be moderate enhancement of the tumor after contrast administration. However, no data on the radiological characteristics of the cancer in the oral cavity has been published. Metastasis to different parts of the body is rare.[69] The preferred treatment is with surgical excision.

Basaloid Squamous Cell Carcinoma

Basaloid squamous cell carcinoma has a predilection for the tonsils, tongue base, and floor of the mouth.[70–72] The cancer occurs more often in men than women. It usually presents in the sixth or seventh decade of life. Risk factors include smoking and alcohol abuse. On clinical exam, the tumor may appear as an ulcerated, firm mass. Advanced stages of the cancer may demonstrate perineural invasion and cervical lymph node metastases. On macroscopic histologic examination, tumor lobules are seen dispersed within and surrounded by fibrovascular stroma. A distinct lobulated enhancement pattern may thus be detected on enhanced T1-weighted MR images.[69] This pattern is not seen with squamous cell carcinoma. Treatment of basaloid squamous cell carcinoma is surgery followed by radiotherapy. Additional

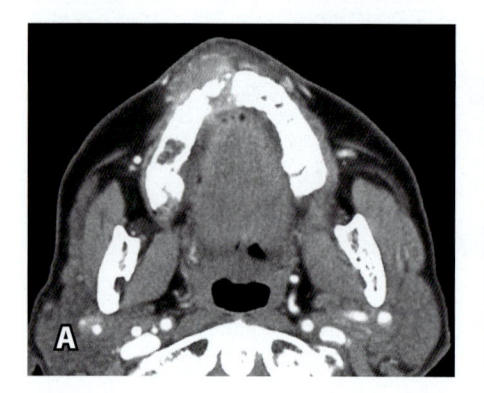

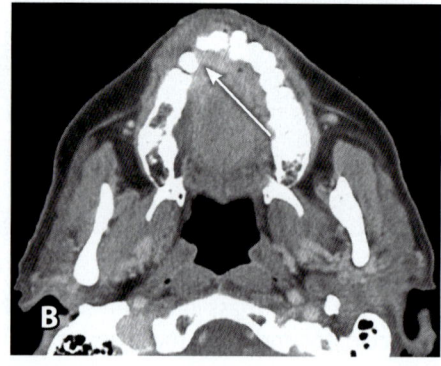

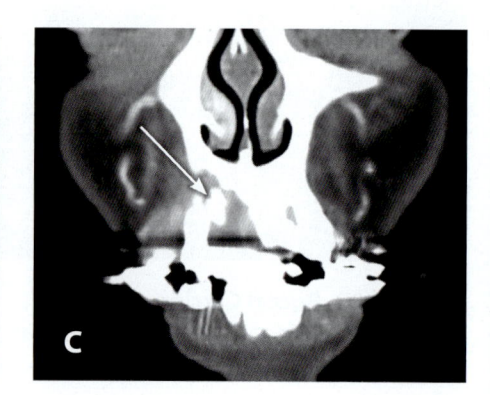

Figure 6-25 Upper Alveolar Ridge Squamous Cell Carcinoma
(**A, B**) Axial and (**C**) coronal reformatted contrast-enhanced CT scans. There is a destructive lesion in the right side of the maxillary alveolar ridge extending both anteriorly into the buccal and posteriorly into the lingual surface and causing disruption of the right canine tooth (*arrows*, **B, C**).

Chapter 6: The Pharynx and Oral Cavity **253**

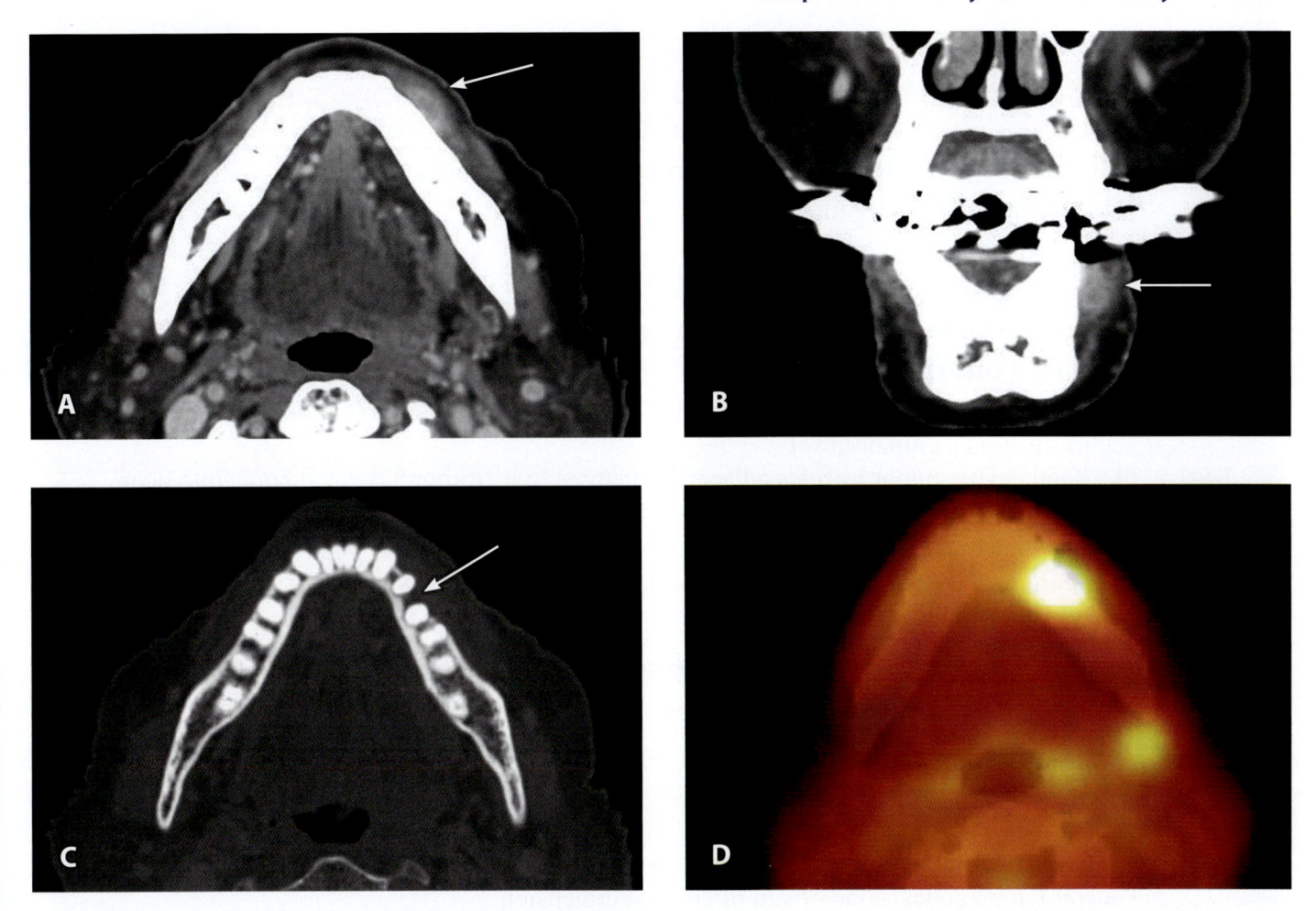

Figure 6-26 Inferior Alveolar Ridge Squamous Cell Carcinoma
Axial CT (**A**), reformatted coronal CT (**B**), axial bone windowed postcontrast CT (**C**) and axial fused PET/CT (**D**) images. There is an irregularly enhancing soft-tissue mass along the buccal surface of the left inferior alveolar ridge (*arrows*, **A, B**). Note the thinning of the cortex of the body of the mandible just beneath the tumor (*arrow*, **C**) consistent with bony invasion. The PET/CT confirms likely bone invasion by the tumor.

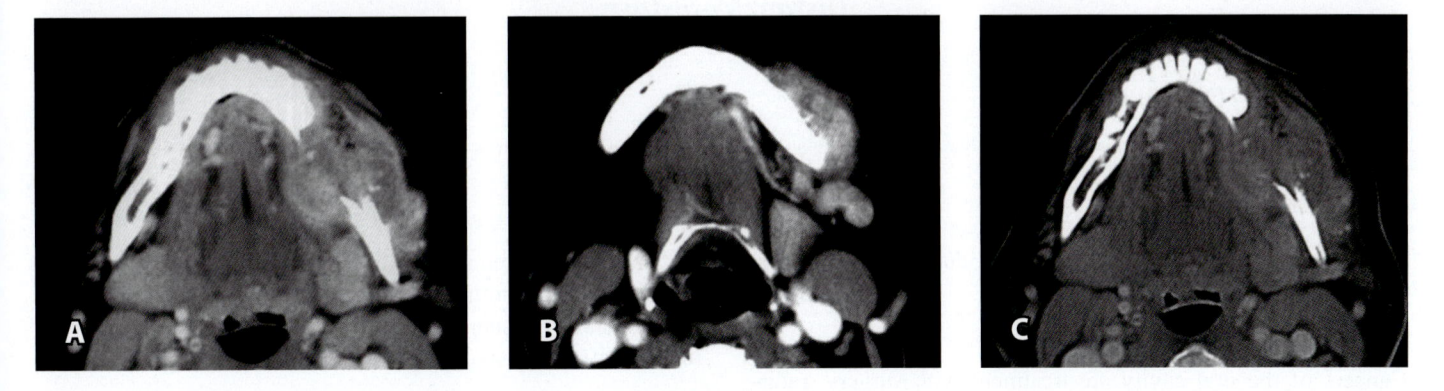

Figure 6-27 Inferior Alveolar Ridge Squamous Cell Carcinoma
(**A–C**) Axial contrast-enhanced CT scans. The soft-tissue images (**A** and **B**) show a bulky left lower alveolar ridge mass that encircles the body of the mandible with extension anteriorly into the buccal space and posteriorly into the floor of mouth. There are multiple enlarged left submandibular space nodal metastases. The bone image (**C**) shows destruction of the mid-body portion of the right mandible.

Table 6-6 Lip and Oral Cavity Tumor Staging

Primary Tumor*

TX	Minimum requirements to assess the primary tumor cannot be met
T0	No evidence of primary tumor
Tis	Carcinoma in situ
T1	Tumor 2 cm or less in greatest diameter
T2	Tumor >2 cm but not >4 cm in greatest dimension
T3	Tumor >4 cm in greatest dimension
T4a	• Lip: tumor invades through cortical bone, inferior alveolar nerve, floor of mouth, or skin of face (i.e., chin or nose) • Oral cavity: tumor invades adjacent structures [e.g., through cortical bone, into deep (extrinsic) muscles of tongue (genioglossus, hypoglossus, palatoglossus, and styloglossus), maxillary sinus, skin of face]
T4b	Tumor invades masticator space, pterygoid plates, or skull base and/or encases internal carotid artery

Nodal Staging

NX	Regional lymph nodes cannot be assessed
N0	No regional lymph node metastasis
N1	Metastasis in a single ipsilateral lymph node, 3 cm or less in greatest dimension
N2	Metastasis in a single ipsilateral lymph node, >3 cm but not >6 cm in greatest dimension, or in multiple ipsilateral lymph nodes, none >6 cm in greatest dimension, or in bilateral or contralateral lymph nodes, none >6 cm in greatest dimension
N2a	Metastasis in a single ipsilateral lymph node >3 cm but not >6 cm in greatest dimension
N2b	Metastasis in multiple ipsilateral lymph nodes, not >6 cm in greatest dimension
N2c	Metastasis in bilateral or contralateral lymph nodes, not >6 cm in greatest dimension
N3	Metastasis in a lymph node >6 cm in greatest dimension

Distant Metastasis

M0	No distant metastasis
M1	Distant metastasis

*Superficial erosion alone of bone/tooth socket by gingival primary is not sufficient to classify a tumor as T4.

adjuvant chemotherapy may be included due to the high incidence of distant metastases.[70]

Treatment Based on Staging

Cancers of the oral cavity are treatment with surgery, radiation therapy, and chemotherapy. Chemotherapy is often used to reduce the size of the tumor prior to surgery. In advanced cancers, reconstructive surgery may be needed. Invasion of the mandibular cortex requires marginal mandibulectomy, while invasion of the mandibular marrow requires segmental mandibulectomy with local reconstruction.

Stage I and stage II cancers require either surgery or radiation therapy for successful control of cancer. Stage III and stage IV cancers will often require combinations of surgery, radiation therapy, and chemotherapy. The 5-year survival rate is about 70% for stage I or stage II disease. The 5-year survival rate drops to about 50% for stage II cancers and 35% for stage IV cancers.

Other Malignant Neoplasms

Lymphomas

Lymphoma is the most common lymphoproliferative disorder in the extracranial head and neck. Hodgkin's lymphoma (HL) peaks during young adulthood and then over the age of 55 years. Males are more commonly affected than females. Patients may complain of constitutional symptoms such as night sweats, weight loss, and fever. The presence of Reed-Sternberg cells on nodal biopsy is characteristic of Hodgkin's disease. HL extends by means of contiguous nodal spread. Though rare, extranodal sites include the spleen and liver. Other sites include hematogenous spread to the bone marrow and direct extension to the lung.

Non-Hodgkins lymphoma (NHL) predominantly occurs in older patients. Males are also commonly more affected than females. Congenital and acquired immunodeficiency states are predisposing risk factors of the disease. Most patients have advanced disease at the time of initial presentation. NHL more frequently affects extranodal regions, especially areas within the head and neck, compared to HL.[73] Patients may have similar clinical symptoms in patients with SCCa. For example, patients can present with serous otitis media from an NHL located within the nasopharynx. From there, the tumor may invade the skull base. Waldeyer ring, which is particularly rich in lymphoid tissue, is a common extranodal site for NHL (**Fig. 6-28**). Other sites include the palate, gingival, eyelid, and lacrimal gland. The parotid gland can be affected in patients with a prior history of Sjogren syndrome.

Extranodal nasal type natural killer (NK)/T-cell lymphoma is an aggressive form of lymphoma that is usually associated with EBV. It is called NK/T because of the uncertainty regarding its cellular lineage, but an origin of immature NK cells is postulated. The frequency of NK/T-cell lymphoma is increased in Asia and in parts of Africa where Burkitt lymphoma is endemic.

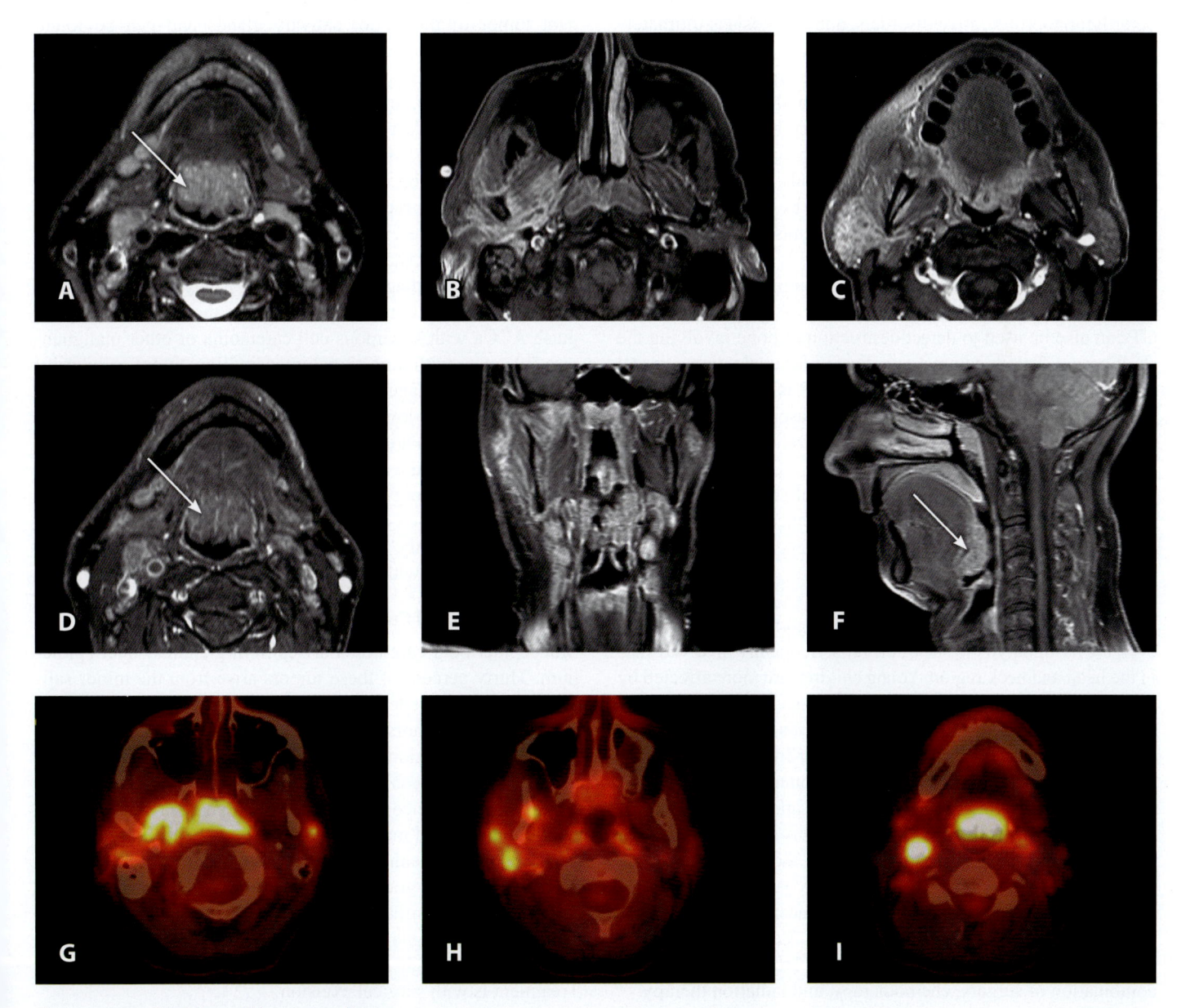

Figure 6-28 Waldeyer Ring Lymphoma
Axial T2 (**A**), axial contrast T1 enhanced with fat-saturated axial (**B–D**), coronal (**E**) and sagittal (**F**) MRI scans and axial fused PET/CT images (**G–I**). There is slight prominence of the lymphoid tissues in the nasopharynx and palatine tonsils, with marked hypertrophy of bilateral lingual tonsils (*arrows*, **A, D, F**). There are multiple bilateral cervical lymphadenopathies, particularly in the right level 1 and bilateral levels II and III documented on both the MRI and fused PET/CT images.

While it can affect patients of any age, it occurs more often in young adults. Men are more commonly affected than women. NK/T-cell lymphoma commonly present in the midfacial region but can occur in other extranodal sites, such as Waldeyer ring.[74] The tumor can present with nasal obstruction, and invade the sinuses and palate. Diagnosis is made based on specimen evaluation of involved areas. However, since the morphology of this tumor is variable, one should consider this disease in the diagnosis for all extranodal lymphoma demonstrating angioinvasion and necrosis.

On imaging studies, these tumors may appear large and homogenously enhanced. Similar findings can also be seen in poorly differentiated SCCa. Therefore, CT and MR imaging cannot clearly distinguish the different types of lymphoma and other lymphoproliferative disorders, and diagnosis is ultimately based on histologic examination of tissue. However, certain characteristics of the tumor may reveal its type on imaging. HL is most commonly located in the neck and the mediastinum, while NHL prefers extranodal regions such as the nasopharynx or Waldeyer ring. NHL manifests as a submucosal lesion accompanied by polypoid masses with a smooth mucosal surface.[75] NK/T cell lymphomas are characterized by destruction of the maxilla and bones around the paranasal sinuses, similar to bony destruction by other SCCa.

On CT, lymphomas have a density similar to that of muscle. Irregular margins and areas of necrosis may be detected. CT can also be used to detect destruction of bone involving the skull base. CT with contrast is indicated for evaluating cervical lymph nodes, chest, and mediastinum. MR is preferred to assess extension of the lymphoma to different fascial spaces.[75] MR is also performed for soft tissue detail in extranodal disease, especially when there is intracranial extension.[76] Lymphomas appear hypointense on T1W images and may be of variable intensity on T2W images. They have low contrast enhancement postcontrast administration.

Rhabdomyosarcoma

Rhabdomyosarcomas can be found throughout the body. However, the nasopharynx is one of the most frequently involved sites in the head and neck region. Young children are more affected by these tumors than adults. Symptoms for nasopharyngeal rhabdomyosarcoma include sore throat, serous otitis media, and rhinorrhea. Cavernous sinus syndrome can occur from tumor invasion of the skull base. Distant metastases are common.

On CT, the tumor may appear as an infiltrating soft-tissue mass invading the posterior maxillary sinus and skull base. On MRI, features of the tumor are similar to those of other SCCa. However, rhabdomyosarcomas are mainly submucosal tumors. There may be a variable amount of enhancement after IV contrast administration. Neuroblastoma and rhabdoid tumor may mimic rhabdomyosarcomas in children. Treatment involves a combination of surgery, chemotherapy, and radiation therapy.

Chordoma

Chordoma is a rare malignant neoplasm arising from cellular remnants of the primitive notochord. They frequently involve the nasopharynx, dorsum sella, skull base, and clivus. Those occurring in the nasopharynx appear as a bulky soft tissue mass, which can be confused with other nasopharyngeal tumors. When evaluating chordoma by imaging, both CT and MR imaging are used. CT is preferred to evaluate bony involvement, while MR is ideal for evaluating soft tissue and extension to nearby structures.[77] On CT, nasopharyngeal chordoma can appear as a lobular low-density soft-tissue mass with calcification and destruction of the sphenoid bone may be detected. However, MRI is recommended for both pretreatment and posttreatment evaluation. On T2W MR sequences, chordomas appear predominantly hyperintense compared with muscle.

Adenoid Cystic Carcinoma

Adenoid cystic carcinoma (ACCa) is the most common malignant tumor of the minor salivary glands and can be found throughout the oral cavity. Cases of involvement with minor salivary glands in the hard palate, buccal mucosa, floor of the mouth, tongue, lip, and retromolar trigone have been reported (**Fig. 6-29**).[78] ACCa typically occurs in patients in the fifth or sixth decade of life. Men and women are affected about equally. Clinical examination may reveal a submucosal bulge. Submucosal biopsies are required for an adequate diagnosis. While metastasis to the cervical nodes is rare, advanced stages of the carcinoma can metastasize to the lung, bone, and brain.[79]

At the time of diagnosis, MRI and CT may demonstrate submucosal spread of tumor. MRI and CT cannot be used to distinguish ACCa with squamous cell carcinoma or other malignancies.[80] Tumors with high signal intensity (low tumor cellularity) on T2-weighted images signify a better prognosis for the patient, while tumors with low signal intensity (high tumor cellularity) on T2-weighted images may predict a poorer prognosis.[81] ACCa may spread along the second and third divisions of the trigeminal nerve.[82] The ptergyopalatine fossa, foramen rotundum, pterygoid canal, foramen ovale, and cavernous sinus should thus be inspected thoroughly. Treatment involves surgery and radiation therapy combined with chemotherapy.

Mucoepidermoid Carcinoma

Mucoepidermoid carcinoma arises from glandular duct epithelium. Thirty percent of these tumors arise from the minor salivary glands that are located primarily in the buccal mucosa and palate.[83] These tumors can be classified as low-, intermediate-, and high-grade lesions. Women are more commonly affected than men with a mean age onset of 50 years.

Low-grade mucoepidermoid carcinoma may appear as a well-circumscribed mass with cystic components with the solid components being enhanced (**Fig. 6-30**). Calcifications may also be present.[84] High-grade tumors may have ill-defined margins, appear solid, and infiltrate locally. The tumor demonstrates low to intermediate signal intensity on T1-weighted images, and intermediate to high signal intensity on T2-weighted images. Treatment is with surgical excision.

Liposarcoma

Liposarcoma is very rare in the head and neck. Within the oral cavity, cases of involvement with the tongue, cheek, palate, floor of the mouth, and submental regions have been reported.[85] Middle-aged

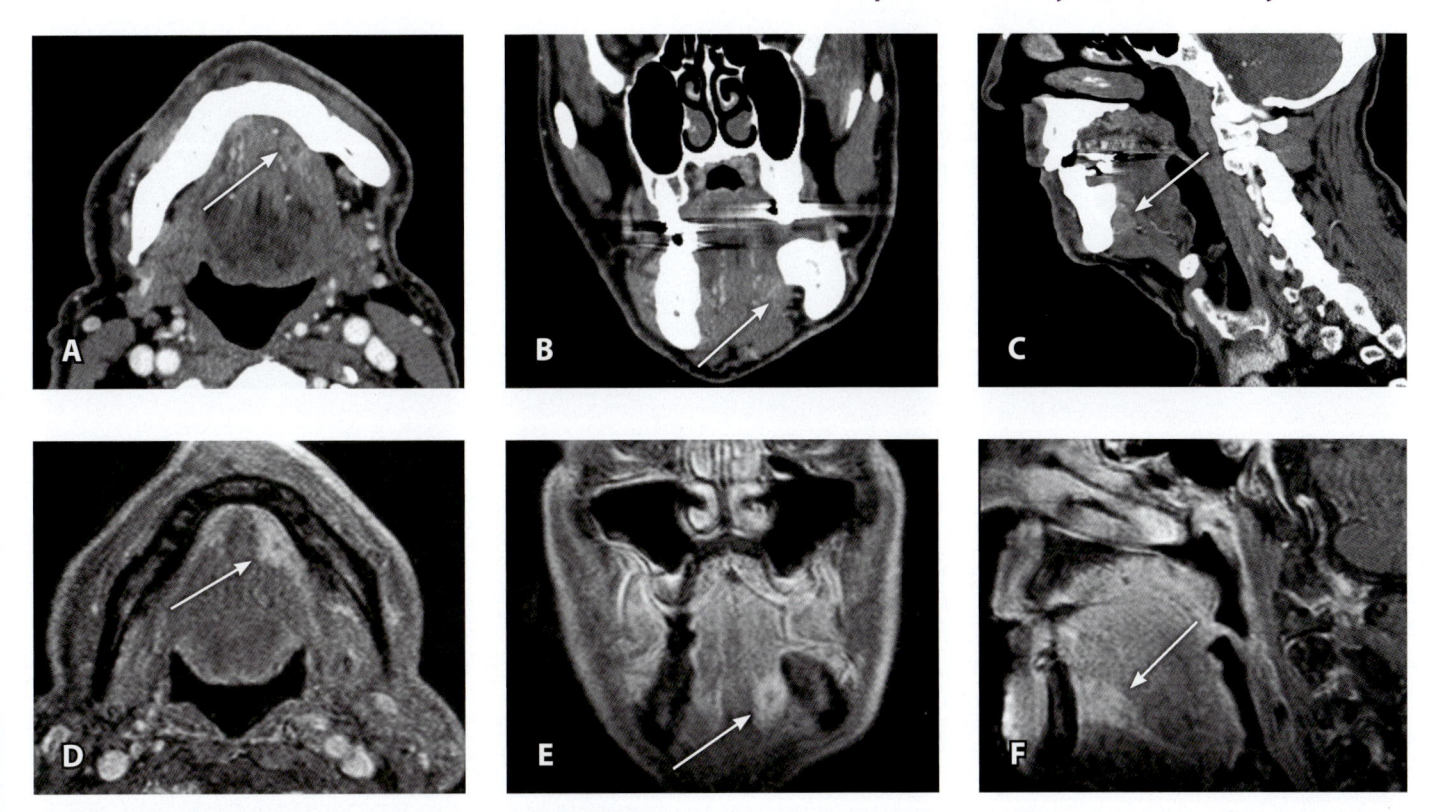

Figure 6-29 Floor of Mouth Adenoid Cystic Carcinoma
(**A**) Axial, (**B**) reformatted coronal, (**C**) reformatted sagittal enhanced CT scans and (**D**) axial, (**E**) coronal and (**F**) sagittal T1 enhanced with fat-saturated MRI scans. There is a small enhancing lesion in the left anterior floor of mouth abutting the lingual surface of the mandible (*arrows*, all images). The biopsy showed adenoid cystic carcinoma of the minor salivary glands, but the findings on imaging are nonspecific and would be consistent with squamous cell carcinoma. (Case courtesy of Wendy Smoker, MD.)

and older males are more often affected. However, they may occur in any age group and do not evolve from preexisting lipomas. The histologic tumor type correlates with the clinical behavior.

On CT, well-differentiated liposarcomas appear as heterogenous lesions with a density greater than subcutaneous fat.[86] They are usually composed of soft-tissue elements and fat. Infiltrating borders may be detected along with heterogenous contrast enhancement. Well-differentiated liposarcomas have signal intensities lower than fat on T1-weighted MR images (**Fig. 6-31**). Fat-suppressed contrast-enhanced T1-weighted images may reveal patchy, heterogenous enhancement of the lesion. Treatment is wide surgical excision.

Malignant Fibrous Histiocytoma

Ten percent of malignant fibrous histiocytoma (MFH) occur in the head and neck, and about 10% of these arise in the oral cavity.[87] It is usually seen in adults over 50 years of age with male predominance. Prior radiation therapy of the oral cavity is considered as a predisposing risk factor, and the prognosis for these patients is very poor. CT and MRI may reveal a large, homogenously enhancing soft-tissue mass without ulceration or necrosis. It may be associated with soft-tissue invasion and bone destruction on CT and MR images.[88] Surgery is the treatment of choice as MFH is resistant to radiation and chemotherapy.

Benign Neoplasms

Benign neoplasms rarely occur in the nasopharynx and oropharynx. Reports of these benign neoplasms include lipomas, polyps, teratomas, hamartomas, rhabdomyomas, dermoids, epidermoids, schwannomas, and neurofibromas. While 12% of fibromatoses involve the head and neck regions, these lesions rarely occur in the nasopharynx or oropharynx. In addition, CT findings of these lesions are generally nonspecific.

Rhabdomyomas are benign tumors of skeletal muscle that can involve regions of the oropharynx and nasopharynx, base of the tongue, and floor of the mouth. However, unlike cardiac rhabdomyomas, these rhabdomyomas are not associated with tuberous sclerosis. Rhabdomyomas have a density and intensity similar to muscle on CT and MR imaging, and are generally well circumscribed. Thirteen percent of schwannomas are located in the extracranial head and neck, but still rarely involve the pharynx or tongue. Schwannomas can occur in the submucosal space. While imaging is important to determine extent of spread, tissue sampling of the lesion is required for an accurate diagnosis. On CT, they appear as homogenous soft-tissue density masses with variable enhancement after contrast administration. They appear isointense to muscle on T1-weighted MR images and hyperintense to muscle on T2-weighted MR images. Neurofibromas involving pharynx or oral cavity are most likely

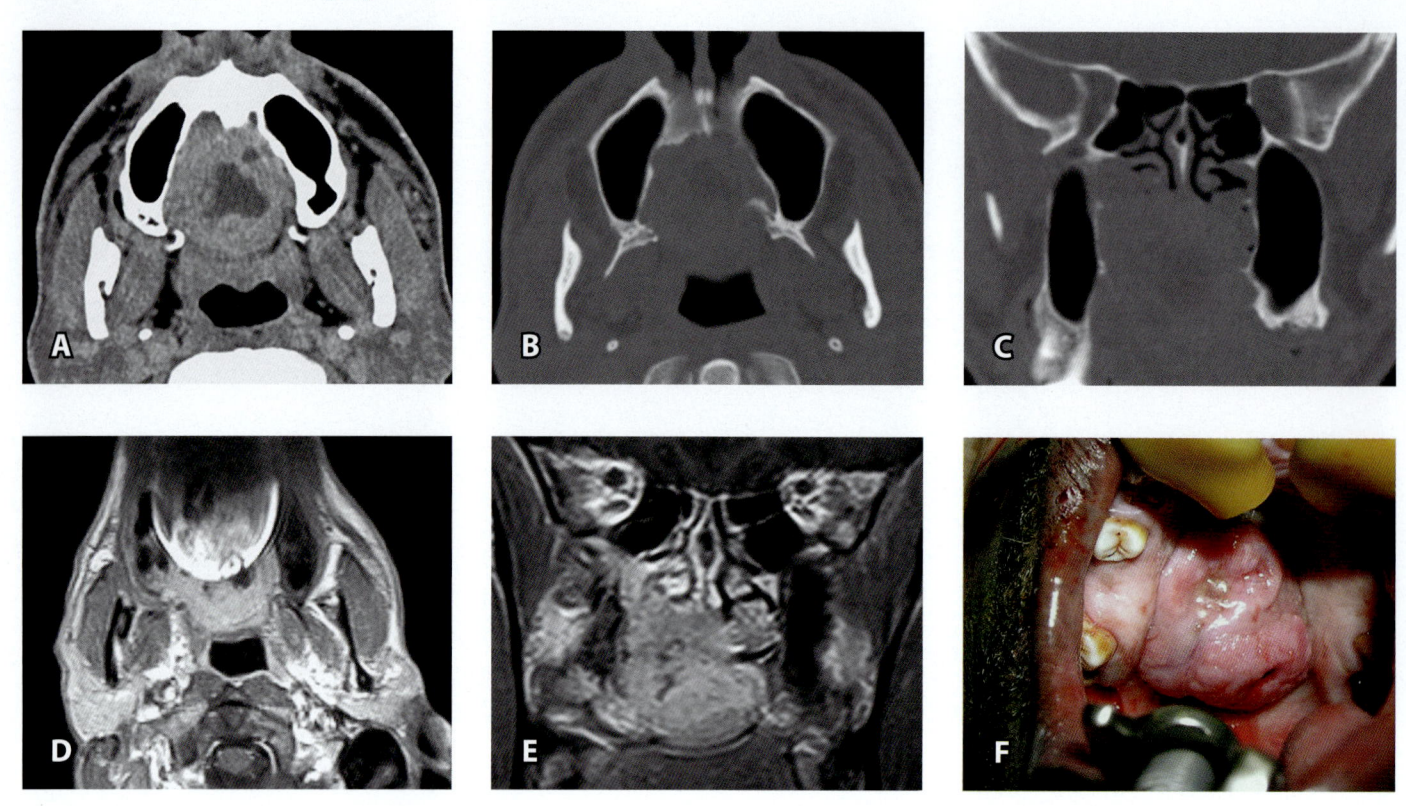

Figure 6-30 Hard Palate Mucoepidermoid
(**A**) Axial soft-tissue window, (**B**) axial and (**C**) coronal bone windowed unenhanced CT scans and (**D**) axial and (**E**) coronal enhanced T1 with fat-saturated MRI images. There is a bulky, markedly heterogenous tumor mass with complete destruction of the hard palate and extension into the bilateral nasal cavities, particularly on the right side. The intraoperative photo (**F**) shows the pinkish solid mass that fills the upper portion of the oral cavity. Pathological evaluation of the specimen documented a mucoepidermoid carcinoma of the minor salivary glands. (Case courtesy of Wendy Smoker, MD / Photo courtesy of DL Reede, MD.)

associated with neurofibromatosis and present as solitary or multiple ovoid masses on CT and MR scans.

Pleomorphic Adenomas

Pleomorphic adenoma (benign mixed tumor) is the most common benign-mixed salivary gland tumor comprising combination of epithelial and myothelial cells. It is usually seen in adults over 40 years of age and occurs more often in men than in women. While pleomorphic adenomas most commonly occur in the parotid gland, this tumor may occur in the submandibular, sublingual, and minor salivary glands as well. Most are asymptomatic and can present as a parotid mass on routine physical examination.

Although pleomorphic adenomas are typically smooth, well-marginated tumors, nodularity along the outer surface may be present. On CT, attenuation may be higher than the surrounding gland, but lower attenuation may also be detected. These adenomas are poorly enhanced in the early phase of contrast enhancement.[89] Large pleomorphic adenomas can develop a heterogenous appearance with areas of hemorrhage, calcification, and cysts (**Fig. 6-32**).[22] On MRI, pleomorphic adenomas may appear as a mixture of epithelial and fibromyxoid tissues with possible degenerative changes. This may result in heterogenous appearance of varying signals on T2-weighted images and variable contrast enhancement.[90,91] Pleomorphic adenomas are usually hypointense to muscle in T1-weighted images. The tumor has a slow growth pattern compared to malignant tumors. Treatment is generally with surgical resection, but can also include radiation therapy or chemotherapy.

Aggressive Fibromatosis

Tumors of fibrous origin can range from benign fibrous lesions such as keloid to fibrosarcoma. Aggressive fibromatosis, also called extraabdominal desmoids tumor, is in between these extremes. They occur most commonly in children and young adults. Recurrence rates are high. Although these tumors commonly infiltrate adjacent structures, they have no metastasizing potential. In the head and neck region, they typically affect the face and supraclavicular region, and rarely involve the oral cavity. There have been reports of tongue involvement.[92,93]

On CT, there is only slight enhancement of the lesion. The lesion may thus be inseparable from adjacent muscle. On MRI, there is variable signal intensity in T1- and T2-weighted images. On T1-weighted images, they are typically isointense or slightly hypointense. On T2-weighted images, they are hypointense to hyperintense. The lesion may be enhanced with contrast. Treatment is with surgical excision.

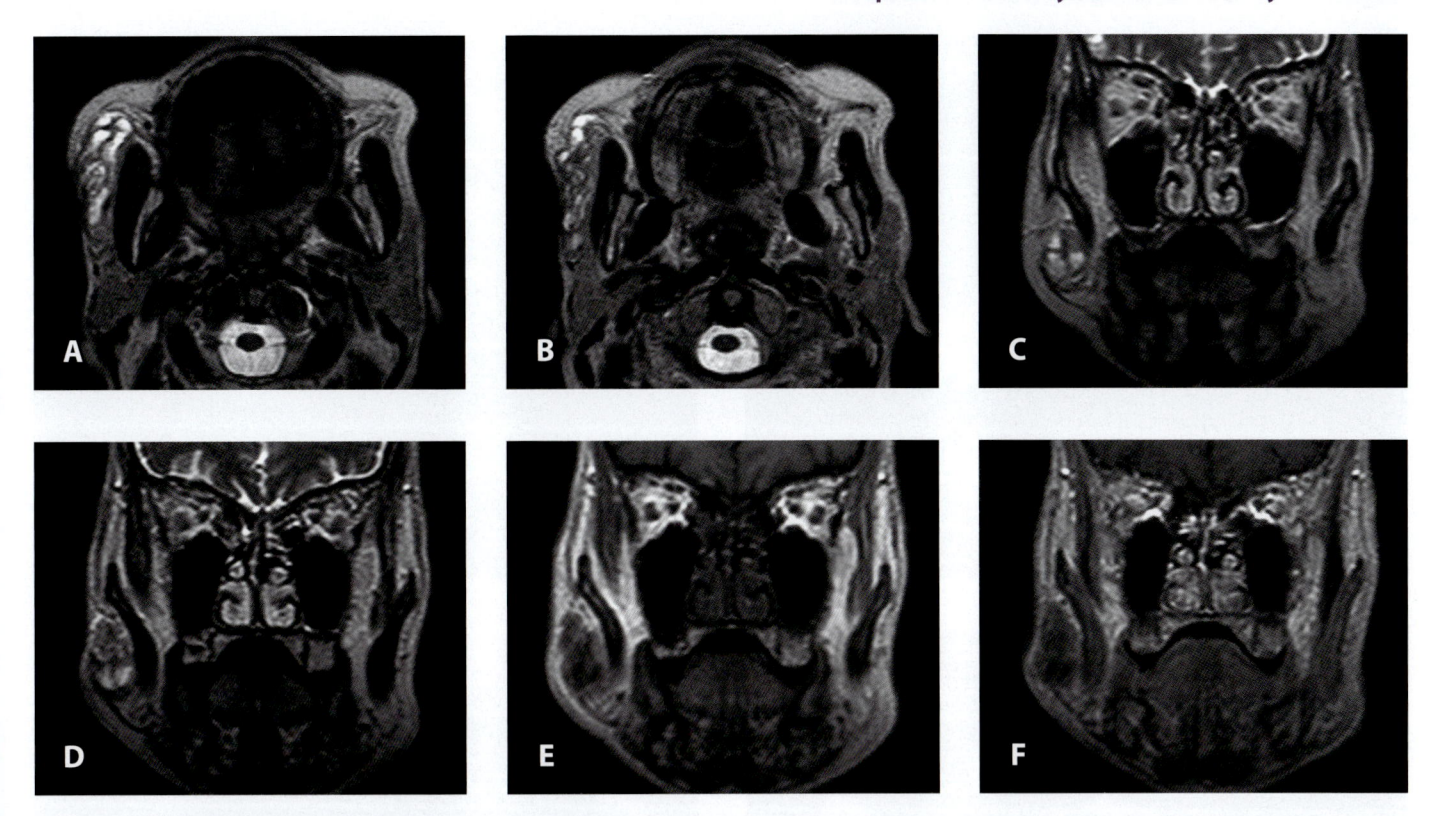

Figure 6-31 Buccal Space Spindle Cell Liposarcoma
(**A, B**) Axial and (**C, D**) coronal T2 and (**E, F**) coronal unenhanced T1 MR images. There is a heterogenous mass lesion in the right buccal space with foci of high T2 signal (**A–D**) and low T1 signal (**E, F**). The tumor is surrounded by typical fat intensity and the final pathologic diagnosis was of a spindle cell liposarcoma of buccal fat pad. (Case courtesy of Wendy Smoker, MD.)

Lipomas

Only 13% of lipomas arise in the extracranial head and neck.[94] Within the oral cavity, lipomas appear in order of decreasing frequency in the cheek, tongue, floor of the mouth, palate, and submental region.[95] The peak age of occurrence is 40 years and males are more commonly affected.

On CT, lipomas appear as a homogenous and nonenhancing lesion with attenuation values around −100 HU. On MRI, lipoma has similar signal intensity as subcutaneous fat on all pulse sequences. It appears hyperintense on T1-weighted images and hypointense on T2-weighted images and fat-suppressed T1-weighted images. Lipomas generally do not infiltrate nearby structures and are sometimes separated by thin septae. Liposarcoma should be suspected if portions of the lipoma have density or signal intensity characteristic of other soft tissues. Treatment of lipoma is with surgical excision.

Exostoses

Torus palatinus is benign thickening of cortical and medullary bone on the oral surface of the hard palate.[96] It is usually located midline. Most palatal tori have a diameter of less than 2 cm but can continue to grow throughout life. Palatal tori are more common in women. Their shape, including flat, spindle, nodular, and lobulated appearances, often categorizes the tori.

On CT, small lesions of palatal tori appear as dense cortical bone protruding inferiorly from oral aspect of hard palate. They are best evaluated on coronal planes. Large palatal tori appear as well-corticated cancellous bone on CT and may present with a midline fissure. Palatal tori are usually a clinical finding and treatment is unnecessary. If removal of the tori is needed, surgery can be performed to reduce the amount of bone present.

Developmental Lesions

Tornwaldt's Cyst

Tornwaldt's cyst is a remnant of the embryonic notochord usually located midline of the nasopharynx. The pharyngeal bursa, a cystic medial mass derived from a persisting remnant of the cranial end of the embryonic notochord, becomes obliterated following pharyngitis, thereby forming Tornwaldt's cyst. Persistent purulent discharge and eustachian tube obstruction may occur with infection. It often presents with sore throat, postnasal drip, and sinus congestion.

The cyst is detected more often on MRI. The cyst usually appears hyperintense on T1-weighted, T2-weighted, and fluid-attenuated inversion-recovery MR images.[97,98] No contrast enhancement can be seen on CT scans unless the cyst is infected.

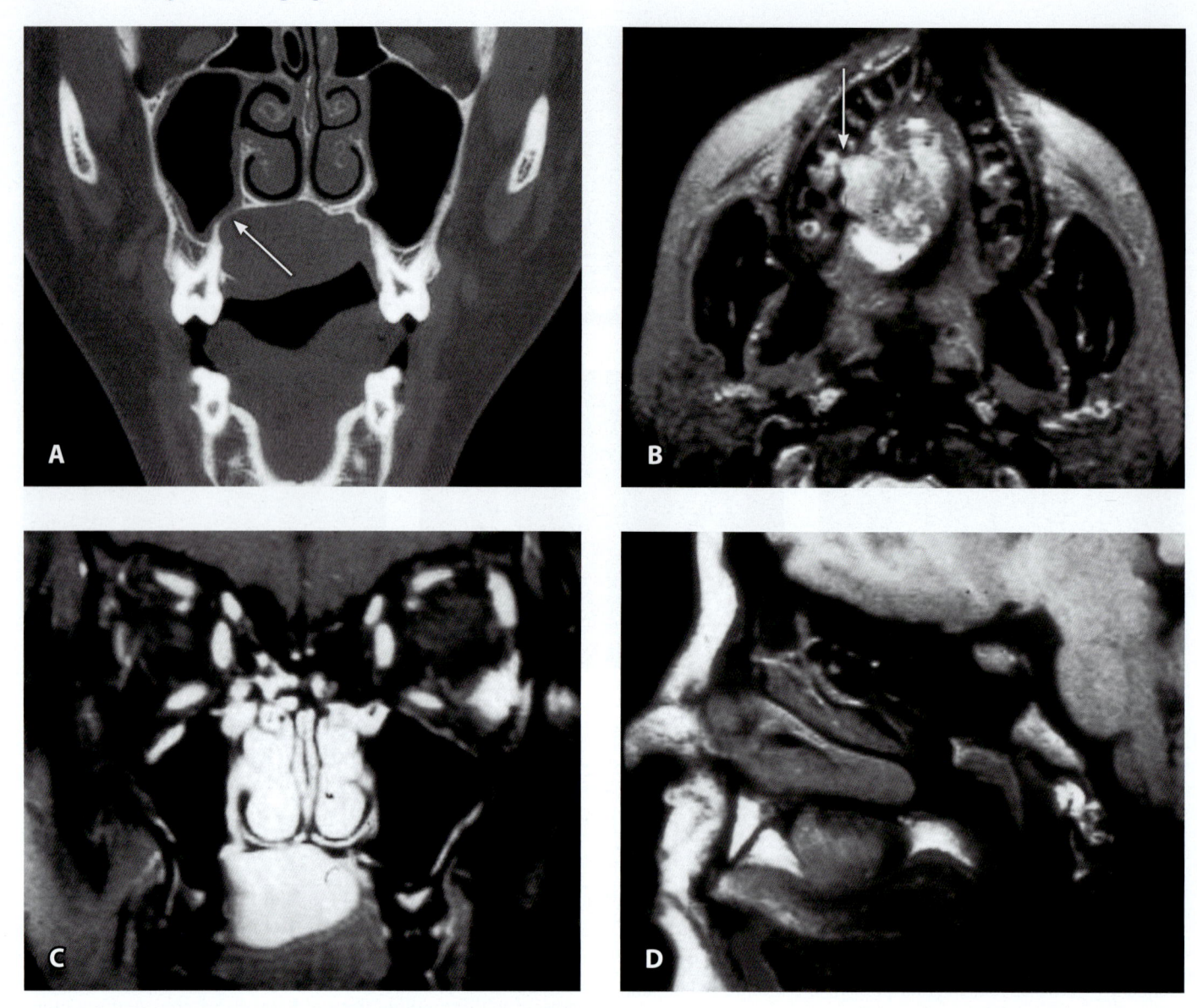

Figure 6-32 Soft Palate Pleomorphic Adenoma
(**A, B**) Axial and (**C, D**) coronal T2 and (**E, F**) coronal unenhanced T1 MR images. There is a heterogenous mass lesion in the right buccal space with foci of high T2 signal (**A–D**) and low T1 signal (**E, F**). The tumor is surrounded by typical fat intensity and the final pathologic diagnosis was of a spindle cell liposarcoma of buccal fat pad.

When infected, the cyst may blend in with surrounding nasopharyngeal soft tissue. Treatment consists of marsupialization or excision.

Extracranial Craniopharyngioma

During embryogenesis, Rathke's pouch courses through the mesenchyme of the sphenoid bone before it is ossified, allowing epithelial rests from the pouch to be entrapped within the sphenoid bone. Extracranial craniopharyngioma is thus formed from these residual epithelial elements. The mass is usually located midline and in close proximity to the sella turcica. Clinical presentation can include nasal obstruction or snoring.

Extracranial craniopharyngioma appears hyperintense on both T1-weighted and T2-weighted MR images and can extend into the infratemporal fossa.[99] MRI is the preferred imaging modality for this lesion, although CT may be helpful in defining bony anatomy, especially when planning surgical excision. The preferred management for extracranial craniopharyngioma is still a subject of debate, but could involve complete or partial resection or radiation of the mass.[100]

Nasopharyngeal Teratoma

Nasopharyngeal teratoma is a benign congenital neoplasm. It is a germ cell tumor comprising three germ layers, and contains foreign tissue. These lesions most commonly arise in the soft palate or the fossa of Rosenmuller. The teratoma may appear sessile or pedunculated and can protrude through the mouth. Most frequent symptoms include nasal obstruction, dyspnea, and dysphagia, though symptoms can vary depending on lesion size and location.

On CT and MRI, it can present as cystic and solid areas of fat density, and oftentimes include areas of bone and tooth formation. Nasopharyngeal teratomas are well encapsulated with no intracranial extension. Treatment is generally with surgical excision.

Accessory Parotid Tissue

Accessory parotid glands are true parotid tissue that is distinctly separate from parotid gland proper. They are found in 20% of the population. They are usually located anterior to the parotid gland hilum and superior to the parotid duct in the buccal space. The tissue overlies the anterior margin of the masseter muscle, and drain into Stensen's duct. There are no appreciable histopathologic differences between the accessory gland and the main gland. Accessory parotid tissues are more often detected on CT than MRI.[101]

Digastric Muscle Anomalies

Anomalies to the anterior digastric muscle are uncommon. Both unilateral and bilateral accessory digastric muscles have been described in the literature.[102,103] It is important to be familiar with these anomalies as they can be confused on CT and MR images as enlarged submental lymph nodes or masses in the floor of the mouth.[104] Hypoplasia or aplasia of the digastric muscle has also been reported and may be mistaken as denervation atrophy from mylohyoid nerve injury. However, identification of a normal ipsilateral mylohyoid muscle may suggest an intact mylohyoid nerve.

Dermoid Cysts

Dermoid cyst is an uncommon congenital neck lesion. The term "dermoid cyst" refers to all epidermoid, dermoid, and teratoid forms. Epithelial remnants become enclaved during early midline closure of the first and second pharyngeal arches, resulting in dermoid cysts. When the oral cavity is involved, the most common location of dermoid cyst is the floor of the mouth.[105] The sublingual region is the most common area involved, followed by the submental and submandibular regions. The cyst may present as a painless subcutaneous or submucosal lesion. When large, the cyst can displace the tongue and result in dysphagia, dysphonia, or dyspnea.[106]

Simple dermoid cyst appears as a well-circumscribed hypodense mass on CT. The wall may be enhanced after contrast administration. The cyst appears hypointense on T1-weighted images and hyperintense on T2-weighted images. When located in the sublingual space, a dermoid cyst may simulate a ranula. Compound dermoid cysts are more variable in appearance, which is dependent on their fat content. Multiple fat globules present within the cyst may give an appearance of a "sack of marbles," which is pathognomonic for dermoid cyst.[15,107] Compound dermoid cyst may appear hyperintense on T1-weighted images. Proton density and T2-weighted images also reveal a hyperintense mass surrounded by a thin rim of low signal intensity.

Treatment of dermoid cysts of the floor of the mouth involves extracapsular excision with an intraoral or external approach, depending on the size of the lesion and the position relative to the mylohyoid muscle.[108] Due to its malignant potential and to prevent recurrence, the entire cyst must be removed.

Thyroglossal Duct Cysts

Thyroglossal duct cysts are the most common nonodontogenic cysts that occur in the neck. They are fibrous cysts that form from a persistent thyroglossal duct, and can involve areas between the tongue base (foramen cecum) to the thyroid gland. The most common location for the cyst is the infrahyoid neck. It usually presents as a painless midline neck mass, unless infected. Clinical presentation in adults can include difficulty breathing, dysphagia, and/or dyspepsia. The thyroglossal cyst will move upward with protrusion of the tongue.

On CT or MRI, midline/paramedian cystic mass with or without rim enhancement is seen.[109] The cyst contents may have mucoid attenuation on CT. An uncomplicated cyst may appear hypointense on T1-weighted images and hyperintense on T2-weighted images. Ultrasound may reveal a hypoechoic mass with a thin outer line involving the floor of the mouth or tongue base.

Although rare, the persistent duct can become cancerous. Cancerous cells are ectopic thyroid tissue that has been deposited along the thyroglossal duct, usually following radiation exposure. Treatment for a thyroglossal cyst is surgical resection, often requiring removal of the midsection of the hyoid bone.

Lingual Thyroid

Lingual thyroid is thyroid tissue located at the lingual area due to failure of the thyroid gland to descend from the foramen cecum to the lower neck, resulting in residual thyroid tissue along the thyroglossal duct tract. It occurs more commonly in women than in men. The midline dorsum of tongue is the most common location for the ectopic thyroid gland.[110,111] While lingual thyroids are usually discovered incidentally, patients may present with complaints of dysphagia, dyspnea, and hoarseness. Malignancy transformation of lingual thyroid tissue is rare. Most patients with lingual thyroid have no other functioning tissue. Therefore, surgical excision of lingual thyroid tissue in the absence of other functioning thyroid tissue results in permanent hypothyroidism.

Iodine-123 radionuclide scanning is the best diagnostic modality for lingual thyroid. The tissue may appear hyperdense on pre- and postcontrast CT. It may appear only slightly hyperintense on both T1- and T2-weighted precontrast MRI images. In general, thyroid tissue displays strong contrast enhancement.

Infection

Infectious Mononucleosis

The Epstein-Barr virus causes infectious mononucleosis. It is a systemic and self-limiting lymphoproliferative disease that clinically presents with fever, tonsillar pharyngitis, hepatosplenomegaly, and lymphadenopathy.

Complications of IM include peritonsillar abscess and obstruction of airway by massive enlargement of lymphoid tissue. Cervical CT is recommended when such complications are suspected. CT with contrast may reveal enlargement and

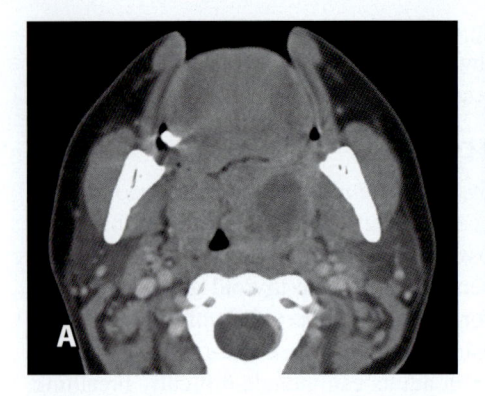

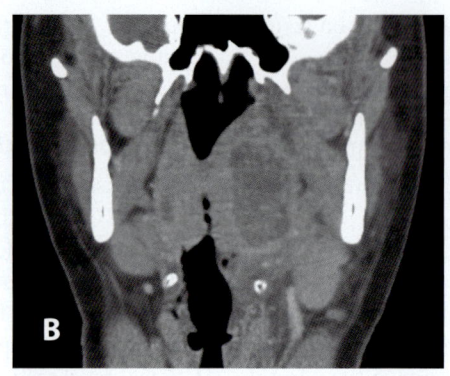

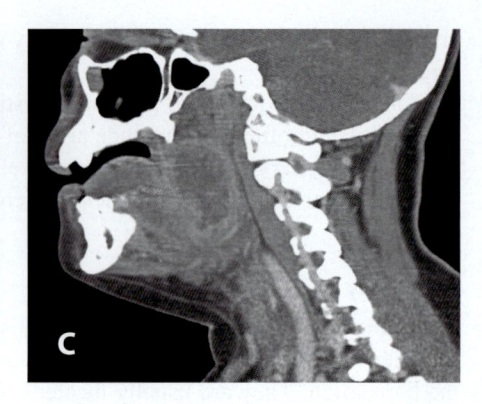

Figure 6-33 Tonsillitis with Abscess
(**A**) Axial contrast-enhanced CT scan shows diffuse thickening of tonsils consistent with inflammation with tonsillar abscesses. (**B–C**) Coronal and sagittal views show compression of oropharyngeal airway by bilateral tonsillar abscesses.

enhancement of tonsils. The lymphoid tissue may sometimes display streaky heterogenous enhancement with interspersed low attenuation, indicative of adenoidal edema.[112] Enlargement of posterior cervical lymph nodes, palatine tonsils, and adenoids may be detected on imaging.

Tonsillitis and Peritonsillar Abscess

Acute tonsillitis may result from viral and bacterial infection and is usually self-limiting. However, severe infection may result in peritonsillar abscess. Peritonsillar abscess is the most common deep infection of the head and neck, and may involve the lateral parapharyngeal or retropharyngeal space (**Figs. 6-33** and **6-34**). It may present with unilateral enlargement and medial displacement of the tonsil with contralateral deviation of the uvula. Patients will often complain of sore throat, odynophagia, or ipsilateral ear pain.

Tonsillar crypts may contain calcification due to prior infection. Contrast-enhanced CT scans can delineate the enhancing rim of the mature abscess and is the imaging of choice for diagnosing peritonsillar abscess. The inflammatory process appears hypodense to isodense on CT scans, and hypointense to isointense to surrounding muscles on T1-weighted and hyperintense on T2-weighted MR images. Treatment includes antibiotic administration, and surgical incision and drainage of the abscess.

Retropharyngeal Infections

Although retropharyngeal space infections are uncommon in adults, it is one of the most common causes of soft-tissue enlargement in children. In adults, these infections are most often a result of direct trauma to the pharyngeal wall. In children, infections from the nasal cavity, throat, middle ear, and paranasal sinuses generally drain into the retropharyngeal lymph node chains, causing enlargement of the lymph node tissue. Atrophy of the retropharyngeal lymph node chains following puberty may explain why retropharyngeal infections are more common in the pediatric population. Patients with these infections may present with fever, sore throat, neck stiffness, and swelling near the soft palate.

The infection begins at region of the lateral retropharyngeal lymph node but may extend to the retropharyngeal space. Abscesses may develop when the lymph node tissue becomes necrotic and suppurative.[10] A lateral neck radiograph may be used to identify the infection, which is generally localized at the level of the oropharynx or nasopharynx. Enlargement of the lymph nodes and edema of the retropharyngeal tissue can compromise the pharyngeal airway.

Radiographic imaging of thickened retropharyngeal tissue is nonspecific and cannot delineate between lymphadenopathy and abscess. However, air or an air-fluid level noted within the retropharyngeal tissue is a reliable indication of abscess formation. On CT, the abscess appears as a hypodense focal area with a rim of contrast enhancement within the retropharyngeal soft tissues. On MRI, the abscess appears hypointense on T1-weighted images and hyperintense on T2-weighted images.

Complications of retropharyngeal abscess include dissection of the abscess into the mediastinum and thrombophlebitis.[113,114] Because treatment of retropharyngeal abscess typically requires surgical drainage, it is important to distinguish these abscesses from other infections, such as cellulitis and suppurative lymphadenitis, both are managed by conservative treatment.

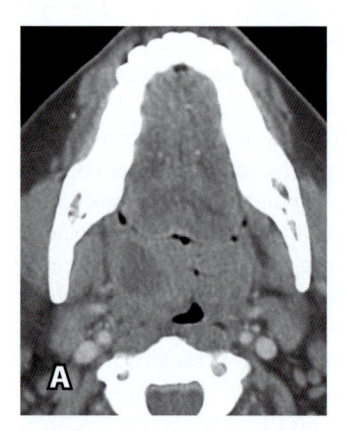

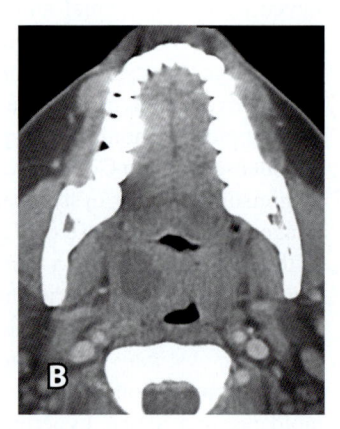

Figure 6-34 Tonsil Abscess
(**A, B**) Axial CT scans with contrast show bilateral tonsillar abscess within tonsillar fossa nearly obstructing oropharyngeal airway.

Adenoidal Hypertrophies

Hypertrophy of the lymphoid tissue in the adenoids generally occur in children, and regress around the age of puberty. Hypertrophic adenoids may appear as a homogenous, superficial soft tissue in the nasopharyngeal mucosal space and can potentially obliterate the fossa of Rosenmuller and obstruct the nasopharyngeal airway.

The adenoids have a density similar to muscle on CT images and may present with small cysts and calcifications. Adenoids are isointense on T1-weighted and hyperintense on T2-weighted MR images. Postcontrast studies reveal enhancement of the pharyngobasilar fascia as a thin continuous line outlining the adenoid surface. Interruption of this line may suggest cancer in the nasopharyngeal roof. An endoscopic biopsy is needed to distinguish nasopharyngeal lymphoma with hypertrophic adenoids, as delineating the two with MRI and CT may be difficult.

Acquired Immunodeficiency Syndrome

AIDS is caused by human T-cell lymphotropic virus type III (HTLV III). This disease progressively reduces the effectiveness of the immune system, leaving individuals susceptible to opportunistic infections and malignancies. Malignancies include Kaposi's sarcoma, Burkitt's lymphoma, non-Burkitt's lymphoma, and large B-cell NHL.

Kaposi's sarcoma may involve the oropharynx or any part of the aerodigestive tract. These tumors may present as small nodules or lobulated masses. Lymphoma can involve the tonsillar lymphoid tissues and can extend to the cavernous sinus. Early nasopharyngeal lesions may mimic diffuse adenoidal hypertrophy. If large, patients may present with airway obstruction. AIDS patients frequently present with hyperplasia of Waldeyer ring.[115] Studies have suspected an association of SCCa with HIV. Tumors are also more aggressive in patients with HIV, with a worse prognosis.

Odontogenic Abscesses

Inflammation of odontogenic origin may lead to abscess formation. Odontogenic abscesses spread in a variable fashion depending on their origin. Maxillary molar infection may produce abscesses in the buccal and masticator spaces.[116] From there, the abscess may spread into the retromolar trigone, parapharyngeal space, submandibular space, and floor of the mouth. The roots of the lower second and third molars reach below the attachments of the mylohyoid muscle, allowing infections to spread into the submandibular space. In contrast, roots of the mandibular first molar and premolar teeth do not reach below the attachments of the mylohyoid muscle. Infections of the mandibular first molar and premolar teeth instead involve the sublingual space.

On CT, abscesses may appear as single or multiloculated low-density areas with peripheral rim enhancement. They usually conform to fascial spaces. On MRI, they may appear hyperintense on T2-weighted images and hypointense on T1-weighted images. In addition to antibiotics, surgical opening and drainage of the abscess remain the treatment of choice.

Ludwig's Angina

Ludwig's angina is an infection of the floor of the mouth, usually occurring in adults with dental infections, especially from staphylococcal and streptococcal bacteria. Grodinsky developed strict criteria for the diagnosis of Ludwig's angina, which includes five characteristics.[117] Ludwig's angina is (i) a cellulitis of the submandibular space, and not an abscess; (ii) never involves only one space, but is frequently bilateral; (iii) can cause gangrene with serosanguineous infiltration but very little or no frank pus; (iv) attacks connective tissue, fascia, and muscles, but not glandular structures; (v) and is spread by continuity, not by the lymphatics. Presenting symptoms include swelling, pain and elevation of the tongue, dysphagia, and in severe cases, stridor and difficulty breathing.

Imaging can be used to evaluate the integrity of the airway. It is also useful in detecting any gas-forming organisms and neck abscesses.[118] On CT, cellulitis, edema, myositis of floor of mouth may be detected. Treatment involves appropriate antibiotic medication, airway management, and urgent surgery to incise and drain the collections.

Inflammation

Diffuse inflammatory changes may occur in the nasopharynx. Infection of the petrous apex of the temporal bone may be secondary to chronic infection of the ear due to malignant external otitis from *Pseudomonas*. Fungal infections from sinonasal cavities may spread to surrounding structures, such as the base of the skull and the nasopharynx. MRI can be used to detect for early marrow changes, while CT can be used to detect later bone destruction.[99]

Miscellaneous Pathology

Denervation Muscle Atrophy

The hypoglossal nerve, facial nerve, and mandibular division of the trigeminal nerve provide motor innervation to the oral cavity musculature and masticator space. Damage to these nerves may result in denervation and eventual muscle atrophy with fatty tissue replacement, which may be detected on CT during chronic stages. MRI may detect denervation earlier than CT. In general, image findings depend on the chronicity of the process.

During the acute/subacute phases of muscle denervation, there is a T2 prolongation of denervated muscle due to increase in extracellular water. This may be associated with an increase in muscle volume and may reveal abnormal enhancement and increased vascularity. During early chronic denervation changes, there is visible fatty muscle replacement but no increase in muscle mass. However, long-standing chronic denervation may reveal severe muscle volume loss with fatty replacement.[119] There is no abnormal enhancement on T2-weighted MR images for long-standing denervation.

Benign Masseteric Hypertrophy

Benign masseteric hypertrophy (BMH) should be included in the differential for masses in parotid area.[120] It is an enlargement of the masseter muscle and is generally idiopathic. It occurs more often in men than in women, and usually presents bilaterally. While etiology is currently unknown, there are familial and acquired forms of BMH.

CT and MRI may reveal muscle enlargement with preservation of surrounding fascial plains and margins. The muscles appear the same as normal muscle. Hyperostosis may be present at the mandibular insertion of the masseter muscle due to muscle hypertrophy.

Macroglossia and Acute Tongue Swelling

Macroglossia is an enlargement of the tongue. It is generally a clinical diagnosis. It can occur in multiple cases, including cretins and amyloidosis. In amyloidosis of the tongue, there may be symmetrical enlargement of both extrinsic and intrinsic tongue muscles without any focal masses. MRI may reveal normal signal intensities on T1- and T2-weighted MR images and no abnormal contrast enhancement.

Acute tongue swelling can result from compression of the tongue base, anaphylactic reactions, and spinal surgery complications.[121] Swelling occurs from massive edema and involve all tongue muscles. To prevent airway obstruction, corticosteroids should be administered.

Though macroglossia and acute tongue swelling are usually diagnosed clinically, imaging can be used to assist in the diagnosis and also exclude other pathologies.

REFERENCES

1. Sadler TW: Langman's medical embryology. Baltimore: Lippincott Williams & Wilkins; 2006.
2. Moore KL and Persaud TVN: The developing human: clinically oriented embryology. Philadelphia: W.B. Saunders Company; 1998.
3. Ross LM and Lamperti ED: Atlas of anatomy: neck and internal organs. New York: Thieme; 2006.
4. Thompson LDR, ed.: Head and neck pathology. New York: Churchill Livingstone Elsevier; 2006.
5. Pilch BZ, ed.: Head and neck surgical pathology. Philadelphia: Lippincott Williams & Wilkins; 2001.
6. Gosling JA and Harris PF: Anatomy: text and color atlas. New York: Gower Medical Publishing; 1990.
7. Becker M: Oral cavity, oropharynx, and hypopharynx. Semin Roentgenol 2000;35:21–30.
8. Becker M and Hasso M: Imaging of malignant neoplasms of the pharynx and larynx. In: Taveras JM and Ferruci JT, eds. Radiology: diagnosis-Imaging-Intervention. Philadelphia: JB Lippincott; 1996:1–16.
9. Lenz M and Hermans R: Imaging of the oropharynx and oral cavity. Part II: pathology. Eur Radiol 1996;6:536–549.
10. Bailey BJ, Johnson JT, and Newlands SD: Head and neck surgery otolaryngology. 4th ed. Philadelphia: Lippincott Williams & Wilkins; 2006.
11. Sigal R: Oral cavity, oropharynx, and salivary glands. Neuroimaging Clin N Am 1996;6:379–400.
12. Mukherji SK, Isaacs DL, Creager A, et al.: CT detection of mandibular invasion by squamous cell carcinoma of the oral cavity. Am J Roentgenol 2001;177:237–243.
13. Weber AL, Romo L, and Hashmi S: Malignant tumors of the oral cavity and oropharynx: clinical, pathologic, and radiologic evaluation. Neuroimaging Clin N Am 2003;13:443–464.
14. Sigal R, Zagdanski AM, Schwaab G, et al.: CT and MR imaging of squamous cell carcinoma of the tongue and floor of the mouth. Radiographics 1996;16:787–810.
15. Beil CM and Keberle M: Oral and oropharyngeal tumors. Eur J Radiol 2008;66:448–459.
16. Chang JT, Chan SC, Yen TC, et al.: Nasopharyngeal carcinoma staging by (18)F-fluorodeoxyglucose positron emission tomography. Int J Radiat Oncol Biol Phys 2005;62:501–507.
17. Tsai MH, Shiau YC, Kao CH, et al.: Detection of recurrent nasopharyngeal carcinomas with positron emission tomography using 18-fluoro-2-deoxyglucose in patients with indeterminate magnetic resonance imaging findings after radiotherapy. J Cancer Res Clin Oncol 2002;128:279–282.
18. Goerres GW, Schmid DT, Schuknecht B, et al.: Bone invasion in patients with oral cavity cancer: comparison of conventional CT with PET/CT and SPECT/CT. Radiology 2005;237:281–287.
19. Babin E, Desmonts C, Hamon M, et al.: PET/ CT for assessing mandibular invasion by intraoral squamous cell carcinomas. Clin Otolaryngol 2008;33:47–51.
20. Gordin A, Golz A, Daitzchman M, et al.: Fluorine-18 fluorodeoxyglucose positron emission tomography/computed tomography imaging in patients with carcinoma of the nasopharynx: diagnostic accuracy and impact on clinical management. Int J Radiat Oncol Biol Phys 2007;68:370–376.
21. Ng SH, Chan SC, Yen TC, et al.: Staging of untreated nasopharyngeal carcinoma with PET/CT: comparison with conventional imaging work-up. Eur J Nucl Med Mol Imaging 2009;36:12–22.
22. Lee YY, Wong KT, King AD, et al.: Imaging of salivary gland tumours. Eur J Radiol 2008;66:419–436.
23. Chang ET and Adami HO: The enigmatic epidemiology of nasopharyngeal carcinoma. Cancer Epidemiol Biomarkers Prev 2006;15:1766–1777.
24. Barnes L, Eveson JW, Reichart P, et al.: World health organization classification of tumors. Lyon: IARC Press; 2005.
25. Zou X, Cui J, Macias V, et al.: The progress on genetic analysis of nasopharyngeal carcinoma. Comp Funct Genomics 2007:57513.
26. Lo KW, To KF, and Huang DP: Focus on nasopharyngeal carcinoma. Cancer Cell 2004;5:423–428.
27. Yuan JM, Wang XL, Xiang YB, et al.: Preserved foods in relation to risk of nasopharyngeal carcinoma in Shanghai, China. Int J Cancer 2000;85:358–363.
28. Vaughan TL, Shapiro JA, Burt RD, et al.: Nasopharyngeal cancer in a low-risk population: defining risk factors by histological type. Cancer Epidemiol Biomarkers Prev 1996;5:587–593.
29. Jayasurya A, Bay BH, Yap WM, et al.: Lymphocytic infiltration in undifferentiated nasopharyngeal cancer. Arch Otolaryngol Head Neck Surg 2000;126:1329–1332.
30. Leong JL, Fong KW, and Low WK: Factors contributing to delayed diagnosis in nasopharyngeal carcinoma. J Laryngol Otol 1999;113:633–636.
31. Chong VF and Fan YF: Pterygopalatine fossa and maxillary nerve infiltration in nasopharyngeal carcinoma. Head Neck 1997;19:121–125.
32. Chong VFH: Neoplasms of the nasopharynx. In: Hermans R, ed. Head and neck cancer imaging. New York: Springer; 2006:143–159.
33. Dubrulle F, Souillard R, and Hermans R: Extension patterns of nasopharyngeal carcinoma. Eur Radiol 2007;17:2622–2630.
34. Chong VF: Masticator space in nasopharyngeal carcinoma. Ann Otol Rhinol Laryngol 1997;106:979.
35. Chong VF and Fan YF: Jugular foramen involvement in nasopharyngeal carcinoma. J Laryngol Otol 1996;110:987–990.
36. Chong VF and Ong CK: Nasopharyngeal carcinoma. Eur J Radiol 2008;66:437–447.
37. Chong VF, Mukherji SK, Ng SH, et al.: Nasopharyngeal carcinoma: review of how imaging affects staging. J Comput Assist Tomogr 1999;23:984–993.
38. Ng SH, Chong VF, Ko SF, et al.: Magnetic resonance imaging of nasopharyngeal carcinoma. Top Magn Reson Imaging 1999;10:290–303.
39. Ng SH, Chang JT, Ko SF, et al.: MRI in recurrent nasopharyngeal carcinoma. Neuroradiology 1999;411:855–862.
40. Chong VF, Zhou JY, Khoo JB, et al.: Nasopharyngeal cacinoma tumor volume measurement. Radiology 2004;231:914–921.
41. Mukherji SK, Schmalfuss IM, Castelijns J, et al.: Clinical applications of tumor volume measurements for predicting outcome in patients with squamous cell carcinoma of the upper aerodigestive tract. Am J Neuroradiol 2004;25:1425–1432.
42. Willner J, Baier K, Pfreundner L, et al.: Tumor volume and local control in primary radiotherapy of nasopharyngeal carcinoma. Acta Oncol 1999;38:1025–1030.
43. Sze WM, Lee AW, Yau TK, et al.: Primary tumor volume of nasopharyngeal carcinoma: prognostic significance for local control. Int J Radiat Oncol Biol Phys 2004;59:21–27.
44. Chen MK, Chen TH, Liu JP, et al.: Better prediction of prognosis for patients with nasopharyngeal carcinoma using primary tumor volume. Cancer 2004;100:2160–2166.
45. Liao XB, Mao YP, Liu LZ, et al.: How does magnetic resonance imaging influence staging according to AJCC staging system for nasopharyngeal

carcinoma compared with computed tomography? Int J Radiat Oncol Biol Phys 2008;72:1368–1377.
46. Mukherji SK, Pillsbury HR, and Castillo M: Imaging squamous cell carcinomas of the upper aerodigestive tract: what clinicians need to know. Radiology 1997;205:629–646.
47. Ginsberg LE and DeMonte F: Imaging of perineural tumor spread from palatal carcinoma. Am J Neuroradiol 1998;19:1417–1422.
48. Dubin MG, Ebert CS, Mukherji SK, et al.: Computed tomography's ability to predict sacrifice of hypoglossal nerve at resection. Laryngoscope 2002;112:2181–2185.
49. Mukherji SK, Weeks SM, Castillo M, et al.: Squamous cell carcinomas that arise in the oral cavity and tongue base: can CT help predict perineural or vascular invasion? Radiology 1996;198:157–162.
50. Hsu WC, Loevner LA, Karpati R, et al.: Accuracy of magnetic resonance imaging in predicting absence of fixation of head and neck cancer to the prevertebral space. Head Neck 2005;27:95–100.
51. Kim MR, Roh JL, Kim JS, et al.: Utility of 18F-fluorodeoxyglucose positron emission tomography in the preoperative staging of squamous cell carcinoma of the oropharynx. Eur J Surg Oncol 2007;33:633–638.
52. Hao SP, Tsang NM, and Chang CN: Salvage surgery for recurrent nasopharyngeal carcinoma. Arch Otolaryngol Head Neck Surg 2002;128:63–67.
53. Lin YS, Jen YM, and Lin JC: Radiation-related cranial nerve palsy in patients with nasopharyngeal carcinoma. Cancer 2002;95:404–409.
54. Martin-Granizo R, Rodriguez-Campo F, Naval L, et al.: Squamous cell carcinoma of the oral cavity in patients younger than 40 years. Otolaryngol Head Neck Surg 1997;117:268–275.
55. Stambuk HE, Karimi S, Lee N, et al.: Oral cavity and oropharynx tumors. Radiol Clin North Am 2007;45:1–20.
56. Brown JS, Lowe D, Kalavrezos N, et al.: Patterns of invasion and routes of tumor entry into the mandible by oral squamous cell carcinoma. Head Neck 2002;24:370–383.
57. Brown JS and Lewis-Jones H: Evidence for imaging the mandible in the management of oral squamous cell carcinoma: a review. Br J Oral Maxillofac Surg 2001;39:411–418.
58. Lane AP, Buckmire RA, Mukherji SK, et al.: Use of computed tomography in the assessment of mandibular invasion in carcinoma of the retromolar trigone. Otolaryngol Head Neck Surg 2000;122:673–677.
59. Lenz M, Greess H, Baum U, et al.: Oropharynx, oral cavity, floor of the mouth: CT and MRI. Eur J Radiol 2000;33:203–215.
60. Keberle M, Kenn W, Tschammler A, et al.: Current value of double-contrast pharyngography and of computed tomography for the detection and for staging of hypopharyngeal, oropharyngeal and supraglottic tumors. Eur Radiol 1999;9:1843–1850.
61. Kösling S, Schmidtke M, Vothel F, et al.: The value of spiral CT in the staging of carcinomas of the oral cavity and of the oro- and hypopharynx. Radiologe 2000;40:632–639.
62. Leslie A, Fyfe E, Guest P, et al.: Staging of squamous cell carcinoma of the oral cavity and oropharynx: a comparison of MRI and CT in T- and N-staging. J Comput Assist Tomogr 1999;23:43–49.
63. Yasumoto M, Shibuya H, Takeda M, et al.: Squamous cell carcinoma of the oral cavity: MR findings and value of T1-versus T2-weighted fast spin-echo images. AJR Am J Roentgenol 1995;164:981–987.
64. Spiro RH, Huvos AG, Wong GY, et al.: Predictive value of tumor thickness in squamous carcinoma confined to the tongue and floor of the mouth. Am J Surg 1986;152:345–350.
65. Ng SH, Yen TC, Chang JT, et al.: Prospective study of [^{18}F]fluorodeoxyglucose positron emission tomography and computed tomography and magnetic resonance imaging in oral cavity squamous cell carcinoma with palpably negative neck. J Clin Oncol 2006;24:4367–4368.
66. Magrin J and Kowalski L: Bilateral radical neck dissection: results in 193 cases. J Surg Oncol 2000;75:232–240.
67. Koch BB, Trask DK, Hoffman HT, et al.: Commission on Cancer, American College of Surgeons; American Cancer Society. National survey of head and neck verrucous carcinoma: patterns of presentation, care, and outcome. Cancer 2001;92:110–120.
68. Walvekar RR, Chaukar DA, Deshpande MS, et al.: Verrucous carcinoma of the oral cavity: a clinical and pathological study of 101 cases. Oral Oncol 2009;45:47–51.
69. Becker M, Moulin G, Kurt AM, et al.: Atypical squamous cell carcinoma of the larynx and hypopharynx: radiologic features and pathologic correlation. Eur Radiol 1998;8:1541–1551.
70. Ide F, Shimoyama T, Horie N, et al.: Basaloid squamous cell carcinoma of the oral mucosa: a new case and review of 45 cases in the literature. Oral Oncol 2002;38:120–124.
71. Paulino AF, Singh B, Shah JP, et al.: Basaloid squamous cell carcinoma of the head and neck. Laryngoscope 2000;110:1479–1482.
72. Altavilla G, Mannarà GM, Rinaldo A, et al.: Basaloid squamous cell carcinoma of oral cavity and oropharynx. J Otorhinolaryngol Relat Spec 1999;61:169–173.
73. Urquhart A and Berg R: Hodgkin's and non-Hodgkin's lymphoma of the head and neck. Laryngoscope 2001;111:1565–1569.
74. Li YX, Fang H, Liu QF, et al.: Clinical features and treatment outcome of nasal type NK/T-cell lymphoma of Waldeyer ring. Blood 2008;112:3057–3064.
75. Weber AL, Rahemtullah A, and Ferry JA: Hodgkin and non-Hodgkin lymphoma of the head and neck: clinical, pathologic, and imaging evaluation. Neuroimaging Clin N Am 2003;13:371–392.
76. Aiken AH and Glastonbury C: Imaging Hodgkin and non-Hodgkin lymphoma in the head and neck. Radiol Clin North Am 2008;46:363–378.
77. Nguyen RP, Salzman KL, Stambuk HE, et al.: Extraosseous chordoma of the nasopharynx. Am J Neuroradiol 2009;30:803–807.
78. Beckhardt RN, Weber RS, Zane R, et al.: Minor salivary gland tumors of the palate: clinical and pathologic correlates of outcome. Laryngoscope 1995;105:1155–1160.
79. Kim KH, Sung MW, Chung PS, et al.: Adenoid cystic carcinoma of the head and neck. Arch Otolaryngol Head Neck Surg 1994;120:721–726.
80. Becker M, Moulin G, Kurt AM, et al.: Non-squamous cell neoplasms of the larynx: radiologic-pathologic correlation. Radiographics 1998;18:1189–1209.
81. Sigal R, Monnet O, de Baere T, et al.: Adenoid cystic carcinoma of the head and neck: evaluation with MR imaging and clinicalpathologic correlation in 27 patients. Radiology 1992;184:95–101.
82. Parker GD and Harnsberger HR: Clinical-radiologic issues in perineural tumor spread of malignant diseases of the extracranial head and neck. Radiographics 1991;11:383–399.
83. Triantafillidou K, Dimitrakopoulos J, Iordanidis F, et al.: Mucoepidermoid carcinoma of minor salivary glands: a clinical study of 16 cases and review of the literature. Oral Dis 2006;12:364–370.
84. Yoon JH, Ahn SG, Kim SG, et al.: Calcifications in a clear cell mucoepidermoid carcinoma of the hard palate. Int J Oral Maxillofac Surg 2005;34:927–929.
85. Nascimento AF, McMenamin ME, and Fletcher CD: Liposarcomas/atypical lipomatous tumors of the oral cavity: a clinicopathologic study of 23 cases. Ann Diagn Pathol 2002;6:83–93.
86. Dooms GC, Hricak H, Sollitto RA, et al.: Lipomatous tumors and tumors with fatty component: MR imaging potential and comparison of MR and CT results. Radiology 1985;157:479–483.
87. Poli P, Floretti G, and Tessitori G: Malignant fibrous histiocytoma of the floor of the mouth: case report. J Laryngol Otol 1995;109:680–682.
88. Park SW, Kim HJ, Lee JH, et al.: Malignant fibrous histiocytoma of the head and neck: CT and MR imaging findings. Am J Neuroradiol 2009;30:71–76.
89. Lev MH, Khanduja K, Morris PP, et al.: Parotid pleomorphic adenomas: delayed CT enhancement. Am J Neuroradiol 1998;19:1835–1839.
90. Okahara M, Kiyosue H, Hori Y, et al.: Parotid tumors: MR imaging with pathological correlation. Eur Radiol 2003;(Suppl 4):L25–L33.
91. Keberle M, Ströbel P, and Relic A: Synchronous pleomorphic adenoma of the parotid and submandibular glands. Fortschr Röntgenstr 2005;177:436–438.
92. Suresh CS and Ali AA: Desmoid tumor of the tongue. Med Oral Patol Oral Cir Bucal 2008;13:E761–E764.
93. Roychoudhury A, Parkash H, Kumar S, and Chopra P: Infantile desmoid fibromatosis of the submandibular region. J Oral Maxillofac Surg 2002;60:1198–1202.
94. Som PM, Scherl MP, Rao VM, et al.: Rare presentations of ordinary lipomas of the head and neck: a review. Am J Neuroradiol 1986;7:657–664.
95. Epivatianos A, Markopoulos AK, and Papanayotou P: Benign tumors of adipose tissue of the oral cavity: a clinicopathologic study of 13 cases. J Oral Maxillofac Surg 2000;58:1113–1117.
96. Naidich TP, Valente M, Abrams K, et al.: Torus palatinus. Int J Neuroradiol 1997;3:229–243.
97. Ikushima I, Korogi Y, Makita O, et al.: MR imaging of Tornwaldt's cysts. Am J Roentgenol 1999;172:1663–1665.

98. Magliulo G, Fusconi M, D'Amico R, et al.: Tornwaldt's cyst and magnetic resonance imaging. Ann Otol Rhinol Laryngol 2001;110:895–866.
99. Mafee MF, Valvassori GE, and Becker M, eds.: Atlas of Head and Neck Imaging: the extracranial head and neck. New York: Thieme; 2004.
100. Stripp DC, Maity A, Janss AJ, et al.: Surgery with or without radiation therapy in the management of craniopharyngiomas in children and young adults. Int J Radiat Oncol Biol Phys 2004;58:714–720.
101. Tart RP, Kotzur IM, Mancuso AA, et al.: CT and MR imaging of the buccal space and buccal space masses. Radiographics 1995;15:531–550.
102. Aktekin M, Kurtoglu Z, and Oztürk AH: A bilateral and symmetrical variation of the anterior belly of the digastric muscle. Acta Med Okayama 2003;57:205–207.
103. Sehirli U and Cavdar S: An accessory mylohyoid muscle. Surg Radiol Anat 1996;18:57–59.
104. Uzun A, Aluclu A, and Kavakli A: Bilateral accessory anterior bellies of the digastric muscle and review of the literature. Auris Nasus Larynx 2001;28:181–183.
105. De Ponte FS, Brunelli A, Marchetti E, et al.: Sublingual epidermoid cyst. J Craniofac Surg 2002;13:308–310.
106. Fuchshuber S, Grevers G, and Issing WJ: Dermoid cyst of the floor of the mouth–A case report. Eur Arch Otorhinolaryngol 2002;259:60–62.
107. Koeller KK, Alamo L, Adair CF, et al.: Congenital cystic masses of the neck: radiologic-pathologic correlation. Radiographics 1999;19:121–146.
108. Vogl TJ, Steger W, Ihrler S, et al.: Cystic masses in the floor of the mouth: value of MR imaging in planning surgery. Am J Roentgenol 1993;161:183–186.
109. Reede DL, Bergeron RT, and Som PM: CT of thyroglossal duct cysts. Radiology 1985;157:121–125.
110. Douglas PS and Baker AW: Lingual thyroid. Br J Oral Maxillofac Surg 1994;32:123–124.
111. Takashima S, Ueda M, Shibata A, et al.: MR imaging of the lingual thyroid. Comparison to other submucosal lesions. Acta Radiol 2001;42:376–382.
112. Kutuya N, Kurosaki Y, Suzuki K, et al.: Pharyngitis of infectious mononucleosis: computed tomography findings. Radiat Med 2008;26:248–251.
113. Brochu B, Dubois J, Garel L, et al.: Complications of ENT infections: pseudoaneurysm of the internal carotid artery. Pediatr Radiol 2004;34:417–420.
114. De Sena S, Rosenfeld DL, Santos S, et al.: Jugular thrombophlebitis complicating bacterial pharyngitis (Lemierre's syndrome). Pediatr Radiol 1996;26:141–144.
115. Kirshenbaum KJ, Nadimpalli SR, Friedman M, et al.: Benign lymphoepithelial parotid tumors in AIDS patients: CT and MR findings in nine cases. Am J Neuroradiol 1991;12:271–274.
116. Yousem DM and Chalian AA: Oral cavity and pharynx. Radiol Clin North Am 1998;36:967–981.
117. Grodinsky MD: Ludwig's angina: an anatomical and clinical study with review of the literature. Surgery 1939;5:678–696.
118. Nguyen VD, Potter JL, and Hersh-Schick MR: Ludwig angina: an uncommon and potentially lethal neck infection. Am J Neuroradiol 1992;13:215–219.
119. Russo CP, Smoker WR, and Weissman JL: MR appearance of trigeminal and hypoglossal motor denervation. Am J Neuroradiol 1997;18:1375–1383.
120. Fyfe EC, Kabala J, and Guest PG: Magnetic resonance imaging in the diagnosis of asymmetrical bilateral masseteric hypertrophy. Dentomaxillofac Radiol 1999;28:52–54.
121. Krnacik MJ and Heggeness MH: Severe angioedema causing airway obstruction after anterior cervical surgery. Spine (Phila Pa 1976) 1997;22:2188–2190.

The Neck and Brachial Plexus

Wende N. Gibbs, MS, MD
Vincent Whelan, BS
Anton N. Hasso, MD, FACR

EMBRYOLOGY AND ANATOMY

Embryology of the Neck

The Branchial Apparatus

Structural development of the head and neck begins with the appearance of the branchial apparatus on the 24th day of gestation. Components of the branchial apparatus are transitory and undergo significant remodeling until the eighth week of development. Aberrant development of these structures into their adult forms results in a variety of congenital anomalies.

Early in the fourth week of development, neural crest cells migrate into the future head and neck regions. These cells differentiate into the mesenchyme, which along with lateral plate mesoderm, forms the tissues of the neck. Neural crest cells travel ventrally, around the developing brain, forming the trigeminal, facial, glossopharyngeal, and vagus nerve ganglia. In addition, these cells develop into the branchial arch cartilaginous components, which become the regional bones and ligaments. The lateral plate mesoderm forms the laryngeal cartilages and regional connective tissue, including skeletal musculature and vascular endothelia.

Once the neural crest cells have migrated, they differentiate into mesenchyme. The resultant thickening of mesoderm creates a series of six rounded arches. The dorsal aspects of these arches are attached to the sides of the head, and their ventral aspects meet at the midline of the neck. Only four of these arches are visible on the external surface of the embryo. The first, or mandibular arch, plays a major role in the development of face. The maxillary prominence of the mandibular arch forms the maxilla, zygomatic bone, and squamous temporal bone, while the mandibular prominence forms the mandible. The second, or hyoid arch, contributes to the formation of the hyoid bone. By the fourth week of development, the remaining arches have appeared. The fifth arch is rudimentary or absent, and the fourth and sixth arches partially fuse to form a combined fourth arch.

Each arch consists of an outer covering of ectoderm, an inner covering of endoderm, and a middle core of mesenchyme. In addition, each arch has its own cartilaginous, muscular, neural, and vascular component and derivatives. Arch cartilages either ossify to become bone, or their perichondrium thickens to form ligaments. Derivatives of branchial arch muscular components form the striated muscles of the head and neck. Each arch is supplied by its own cranial nerve. The special visceral efferent component of the nerve supplies the muscles derived from that arch, while special visceral afferents supply the skin and mucous membranes. Derivates of branchial aortic arch arteries become the arterial system of the head and neck. They arise from the primordial heart, travel around the pharynx, and enter the dorsal aorta **(Fig. 7-1)**.

The branchial arches are separated externally by ectoderm-lined clefts, and internally, within the primitive pharynx, by endoderm-lined pouches. Organs of the head and neck develop from the endodermal lining of the pouches. DiGeorge Syndrome results if the third and fourth pouches fail to differentiate.[1]

Four pairs of branchial clefts, or grooves separate the branchial arches externally. The first pair of grooves forms the external auditory meati. The remaining pairs do not develop into adult structures. If the first pair of branchial clefts do not fully develop, remnants can be seen in the adult as auricular sinuses or cysts in the skin anterior to the auricle of the ear, in or around the parotid gland, or at the angle of the mandible.[1,2,3] During the fifth week of development, the second arch grows caudally to cover the third and fourth arches. This area then sinks to form a surface depression called the cervical sinus, which is eventually obliterated in normal neck development. If the second branchial groove is not completely eliminated, a variety of congenital anomalies, including branchial cysts, sinuses, and fistulas may result.

A branchial cleft cyst is an enclosed epithelia-lined structure. If an opening to either the skin or foregut is present, the lesion is considered a sinus. Persistence of a branchial cleft will create a sinus opening externally in the skin, while a sinus

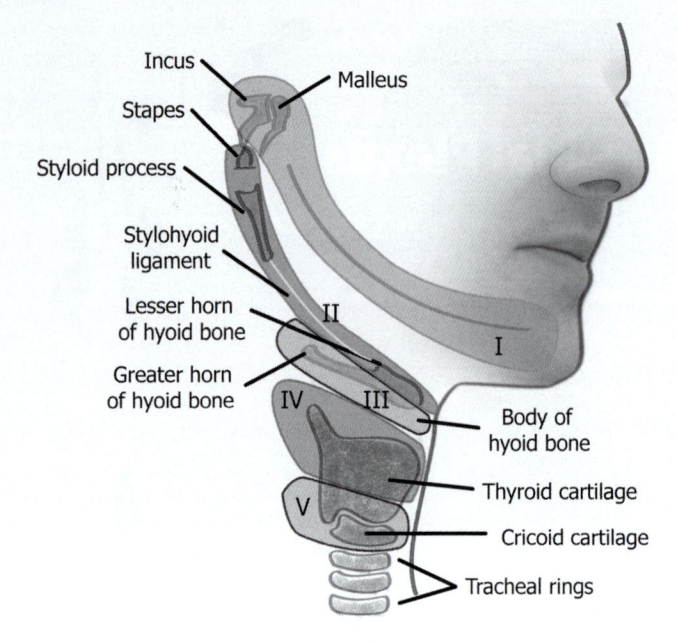

Figure 7-1 Derivatives of the Branchial Arches

opening internally results from the persistence of a branchial pouch. A fistula is a tract that communicates between the skin externally and the foregut internally.

Branchial membranes are formed by the intersection of endoderm from the branchial pouch with the ectoderm of the branchial cleft. Only the first pair of membranes persists in the adult, forming the tympanic membrane.

Thyroid Gland

The thyroid gland is the first endocrine gland to appear in embryonic development, starting on the 24th day. An endodermal thickening on the floor of the primordial pharynx forms an outpouching called the thyroid diverticulum. The diverticulum descends through the tongue and mylohyoid muscle, into the neck anterior to the developing hyoid. It then loops upward behind the hyoid, and descends anterior to the thyrohyoid membrane and strap muscles to reach its final position at the thyroid isthmus. This diverticulum, which connects the oral cavity to the thyroid gland, is called the thyroglossal duct. By the eighth week, the thyroglossal duct has degenerated and the thyroid gland has taken its adult shape and position. A pyramidal lobe of the thyroid, found in 50% of individuals, is the remnant of the distal end of the thyroglossal duct. A small blind pit, the foramen cecum of the tongue, is a remnant of the proximal opening of the duct.

The primordial thyroid consists of a solid mass of endodermal cells that become vascularized by the ingrowth of mesenchyme. The follicular structure of the gland develops by the 10th week, and by the 11th week, colloid has been formed and thyroid hormones are synthesized. A derivative of the fourth branchial pouch, the ultimobranchial body, is incorporated into the lateral lobes of the thyroid gland. The cells of the ultimobranchial body are thought to develop into the calcitonin-secreting parafollicular, or C cells.[4]

Abnormal development of the thyroid gland can result in several types of anomaly. Persistent epithelial elements of the thyroglossal duct can form thyroglossal duct cysts and sinuses anywhere along its descending developmental path. These cysts present as painless, progressively enlarging, mobile masses located in the cervical midline, anywhere between the foramen cecum of the tongue and the thyroid gland. If the cyst is below the hyoid bone, it may be found in a slightly paramedian location, usually on the left side.[5] If the persistent element of the duct is near the tongue, the duct can form a fistula that opens through the foramen cecum. These lingual fistulas may enlarge and produce symptoms of pharyngeal discomfort and dysphagia. Incomplete descent of the thyroid gland may result in solid nodules of ectopic thyroid tissue anywhere along the descending course of the gland. The most common location of ectopic thyroid tissue is at the base of the tongue. This lingual thyroid gland is found immediately inferior to the foramen cecum. If the descent of the thyroid was arrested at some point along the development path to the adult position, a sublingual thyroid gland is the result. Lingual and sublingual thyroid glands are often the only functional thyroid tissue of the body; therefore, these tissues must be identified and preserved in surgery.[6] Accessory ectopic thyroid tissue is functional glandular material found outside of the normal developmental path.

Salivary Glands

In the sixth and seventh weeks, the salivary glands begin to form as solid epithelial buds in the primordial oral cavity. These buds grow into the underlying mesenchyme. The connective tissue of the glands is derived from neural crest cells, while the secretory tissue is formed by oral epithelium.

The parotid glands are the first to appear, early in the sixth week. They form as buds from the proliferating oral ectoderm near the angles of the primordial mouth. The buds grow toward the ears and branch to form solid cords that later canalize and become ducts. Acini form from the rounded ends of the cords. Glandular secretion begins at 18 weeks.

Late in the sixth week, the submandibular glands emerge as endodermal buds on the floor of the primordial mouth. Solid cellular processes grow lateral to the tongue, then branch and differentiate. Acini form at 12 weeks and secretory activity begins at 16 weeks.

In the eighth week, the sublingual glands appear as multiple endodermal epithelial buds in the paralingual sulcus. They branch and canalize to form ten to twelve ducts that open into the floor of the mouth.

Thymus and Inferior Parathyroid Glands

During the sixth week of development, epithelium of the dorsal aspects of the third branchial pouches differentiates into the inferior parathyroid glands. Epithelium of the ventral aspects of the pouches comes together in the median plane of the neck to form the bilobed thymus. In the seventh week, the inferior parathyroid glands and thymus lose their connection with the pharynx and migrate into the neck. The inferior parathyroid glands then separate from the thymus and travel to the dorsal surface of the thyroid. The superior parathyroid glands develop from the fourth branchial pouches and migrate independently. Fragmentation of parathyroid tissue during migration can result in the formation of accessory parathyroid glands.[7]

The thymus migrates to the superior mediastinum, and continues to grow and develop after birth. The thymus is a large organ, and may extend into the root of the neck. At puberty, the thymus undergoes involution, and by adulthood, fat increasingly infiltrates the cortex of the gland. Thymic tissue remnants can form thymic cysts or accessory lobes that usually lie below the thyroid cartilage.[7]

Lymph Nodes

The lymphatic system begins to develop late in the sixth week of gestation in parallel with the vascular system. The exact developmental mechanism of the lymphatic system is still unknown due to a lack of specific lymphatic markers and growth factors.[8] Lymphatic vessels develop, join to form a lymphatic network, and make connections with the venous system.

There are six primary lymph sacs at the end of the embryonic period. The paired jugular lymphatic sacs appear in the lateral angle between the internal jugular veins and the subclavian veins. By the end of the ninth week, lymphatic vessels link the lymphatic sacs and travel along major veins from the jugular lymph sacs to the head, neck, and upper limbs. Two large channels, the right and left thoracic ducts, connect the jugular lymph sacs with the cisterna chyli. This linkage produces a bilateral system of lymphatic trunks, connected across the midline by numerous anastomoses.

The thoracic duct develops from the inferior part of the right thoracic duct, the superior part of the left thoracic duct, and the anastomosis between the thoracic ducts at the levels of the fourth, fifth, and sixth thoracic segments. The course and termination of the adult thoracic duct is highly variable.[9] The jugular sacs are the only primitive sacs to acquire permanent connections with the venous system. The jugular sac and the superior termination of the thoracic duct connect with the left subclavian vein. The right lymphatic duct is derived from the superior part of the right thoracic duct. The right lymphatic duct connects with the venous system at the angle between the right internal jugular and subclavian veins.

The lymph sacs are transformed into groups of lymph nodes during the early fetal period. Primordial lymph sinuses are created in the fifth fetal month when mesenchymal cells invade the lymph sac and break up its cavity into a network of lymphatic channels. Other mesenchymal cells give rise to the capsule and connective tissue framework of the lymph node. This process continues throughout fetal development, and true nodal cortex with germinal centers is not present until after birth.

Anatomy of the Neck

Thyroid Gland

The thyroid gland lies deep to the sternothyroid and sternohyoid muscles and anterolateral to the larynx and trachea. Normally, the gland lies within the thyroid bed, a region bounded superiorly by the oblique line of the tracheal cartilage and inferiorly by the fourth or fifth tracheal cartilage. The gland is variable in size, depending on gender, age, and weight. The average lobe is 5 cm long and weighs approximately 20 to 25 g in men, and is slightly larger in women.[10] The two elongated lateral lobes are connected by a median isthmus that overlies the second to fourth tracheal rings. Occasionally, the isthmus is absent and the gland exists as two distinct lobes. Fifty percent of individuals have a variably shaped pyramidal lobe.[6] The pyramidal lobe may ascend from the isthmus or from the adjacent part of either lobe toward the hyoid bone, to which it may be attached by a fibrous or muscular band.[11] The thyroid gland is encased in a thin fibrous capsule. The deep surface of the capsule adheres to the cricoid cartilage and superior tracheal rings by dense connective tissue. This surface is also in contact with the parathyroid glands and recurrent laryngeal nerves. The anterior surface of the gland faces the pretracheal layer of deep cervical fascia (DCF) that extends posteriorly to envelop the trachea, esophagus, and recurrent laryngeal nerves.

The vascular supply of the thyroid gland consists of two arteries and three veins associated with each lobe. The superior and inferior thyroid arteries lie between the capsule of the gland and the pretracheal layer of DCF. The vessels are large and form numerous anastomoses. Ten percent of individuals possess a small, unpaired thyroid ima artery. This is a single vessel that usually originates from the brachiocephalic trunk, but can also arise from the aortic arch, the right common carotid, the subclavian, or the internal thoracic arteries. It ascends on the anterior surface of the trachea and branches at the isthmus of the thyroid gland.[6]

The superior thyroid artery is the first anterior branch of the external carotid artery. In rare cases, it may arise from the common carotid artery just before its bifurcation. The artery runs anteroinferiorly deep to the infrahyoid muscles to the anterior border of the lateral lobe. There it sends a branch deep into the gland before curving toward the isthmus where it anastomoses with the contralateral artery.

The inferior thyroid artery arises from the thyrocervical trunk, a branch of the subclavian artery. It ascends vertically and then curves medially to enter the tracheoesophageal groove posterior to the carotid sheath. Most of its branches penetrate the posterior aspect of the lateral lobe. The inferior thyroid artery has a variable branching pattern and is associated closely with the recurrent laryngeal nerve.

Three pairs of veins provide venous drainage to the thyroid gland. The superior thyroid vein descends along the superior thyroid artery and drains into the internal jugular vein. The middle thyroid vein follows a direct course laterally to the internal jugular vein. The inferior thyroid veins empty into the innominate vein. Occasionally, both inferior veins form a common trunk called the thyroid ima vein, which empties into the left brachiocephalic vein.

Lymphatic vessels course through the interlobular connective tissue, surrounding the arteries, and communicate in the capsule of the gland. Lymphatic drainage of the thyroid gland is extensive and flows from the upper portion of the gland to the pretracheal and cervical lymph nodes, and from the lower portion of the gland to the paratracheal and lower deep cervical nodes. The lymphatic vessels terminate in the thoracic duct.

Principal innervation of the thyroid gland derives from the autonomic nervous system. Parasympathetic fibers come from the vagus nerves. Sympathetic fibers originate from the superior, middle, and inferior cervical sympathetic ganglia, and form plexuses that accompany the thyroid arteries.

Parathyroid Glands

The small, ovoid parathyroid glands lie on the posterior surface of each lobe of the thyroid gland, inside the sheath of the gland's fibrous capsule. Normally there are four parathyroid glands, but 5% of individuals have more than four.[6] Parathyroid glands are approximately 6 mm long, 4 mm wide, and 2 mm deep.[10]

Embryologically, the superior parathyroid glands are derived from the fourth branchial pouch and descend with the thyroid gland. Therefore, they are more constant in location, usually located near the middle of the posterior border of the lateral lobe of the thyroid. Ectopic superior glands may be located along or within the carotid sheath or deep to the esophageal or pharynx.[12]

The inferior parathyroid glands arise from the third branchial pouch along with the thymus; therefore their position is more variable. Normally, the inferior parathyroid glands lie on the posterior or lateral surface of the inferior poles of the thyroid gland. However, they may be found near or within the thymus in the superior mediastinum. Occasionally, ectopic inferior parathyroid glands may be located within the thyroid capsule or within the gland.[10] In addition, numerous small islands of parathyroid tissue may be found scattered in the cervical fat and connective tissue near the parathyroid glands.[11]

The parathyroid glands are supplied mainly by the inferior thyroid arteries, and drained by the parathyroid veins. The veins drain into a plexus on the anterior surface of the thyroid gland and trachea. Lymphatic drainage accompanies lymphatic vessels from the thyroid into the deep cervical and paratracheal lymph nodes. The parathyroid glands are innervated by thyroid branches from the cervical sympathetic ganglia.

Salivary Glands

There are three major groups of paired salivary glands: the parotid glands, the submandibular glands, and the sublingual glands. In addition, small accessory salivary glands can be found scattered over the palate, lips, tonsils, tongue, nasal sinuses, larynx, and pharynx.[13] The majority of minor salivary glands are found in the hard palate and lateral pharyngeal wall.[14]

The salivary glands serve numerous functions including lubrication, enzymatic degradation of food substances, production of hormones, antibodies, and other blood group–reactive substances, mediation of taste, and antimicrobial protection. The regulation of salivary flow is primarily through the parasympathetic division of the autonomic nervous system.

Saliva is produced in the glandular subunit. The fluid component of the saliva is derived from the perfusing blood vessels in proximity to the gland, while the macromolecular composition is derived from secretory granules within the acinar cells. The saliva is produced in the acinus. Myoepithelial cells are located along the periphery of the acinus. Upon contraction, the saliva is secreted into the ductal system.

The exact mechanism of salivary secretion is not completely understood but is believed to be under the influence of adenosine 3′, 5′-cyclic monophosphate (cAMP) and a calcium-activated phosphorylation mechanism. The salivary secretions are then modified by a variety of cell types along a series of ducts, including the striated, intercalated, and excretory ducts, before finally entering the oral cavity.

Parotid Gland

The irregularly shaped parotid gland is the largest salivary gland. It is wedged into a region called the parotid bed, bounded by the external acoustic meatus, the mandibular ramus, and the mastoid process. The gland is encased in a tough fascial capsule derived from the superficial layer of DCF that suspends it from the zygomatic arch. The main body of the gland overlies the masseter muscle. The deep portion of the gland lies in the stylomandibular tunnel, a region bounded anteriorly by the posterior edge of the mandibular ramus, dorsally by the anterior borders of the sternocleidomastoid and posterior belly of the digastric, and deeply by the stylomandibular ligament.

The parotid gland is unilobular, but for descriptive purposes is divided by the facial nerve into a deep and superficial lobe. Nearly 80% of the gland is considered superficial. The deep lobe is anterior to the styloid process and the carotid sheath. The average size of the gland in males is 5.8 cm craniocaudally and 3.4 cm ventrodorsally, but it is smaller in females.[15]

The parotid duct, or Stensen duct, exits the superficial lobe anteriorly, 1.5 cm below the zygomatic arch, and passes horizontally across the masseter to its anterior border. The duct then turns medially, pierces the buccinator, and enters the oral cavity opposite the second maxillary molar. The normal parotid duct is approximately 7 cm long.

The facial nerve and its branches, the external carotid artery, the retromandibular vein, and parotid lymph nodes are found within the body of the gland. The facial nerve exits the skull through the stylomastoid foramen and travels anterolaterally to enter the parotid gland. Immediately after entering the gland, it bifurcates into an upper and lower division, and subsequently divides into its five terminal branches. The retromandibular vein lies medial to the nerve and runs parallel with it. The parotid capsule is formed late in its development, resulting in lymph nodes located within the body and capsule of the gland. A superficial layer of draining lymph nodes lies beneath the capsule, and a deeper layer lies within the parotid parenchyma.

Branches of the external carotid and the superficial temporal arteries provide arterial supply to the gland and duct. The venous drainage flows into the retromandibular veins. The lymphatic vessels end in the superficial and deep cervical lymph nodes. The auriculotemporal nerve is closely related to the parotid gland and passes superior to it with the superficial temporal vessels. This nerve conveys secretory fibers from the glossopharyngeal nerve via the otic ganglion. Sympathetic fibers are derived from the cervical ganglia through the external carotid nerve plexus on the external carotid artery.

Submandibular Gland

The submandibular glands lie along the body of the mandible and wraps around the dorsal edge of the mylohyoid muscle. It is encapsulated with a fascial layer derived from the superficial layer of DCF like the parotid gland. For descriptive purposes, it is divided into superficial and deep portions. The superficial portion of the gland is located lateral to the mylohyoid and the deep portion lies between the mylohyoid and the hyoglossus. Posteriorly, the gland is separated from the parotid gland by the stylomandibular ligament. The marginal mandibular branch of the facial nerve and the anterior facial vein pass superficially over the gland. The facial artery crosses the deep portion of the gland and then runs anteriorly between the gland and the mandible.

The submandibular, or Wharton, duct emerges from the middle of the deep portion of the gland and travels anteriorly in the plane between the hyoglossus and the mylohyoid muscles, medial to the sublingual gland. The duct is approximately 5 cm long, and opens into the oral cavity lateral to the frenulum of the tongue. The inelasticity of the duct results in pain upon when it is obstructed.

The lingual nerve and submandibular ganglion are located superior and lateral to the submandibular gland and deep to the mylohyoid muscle. The hypoglossal nerve lies deep to the gland and inferior to the submandibular duct.

The arterial blood supply is from the facial artery that enters the gland superior to the posterior belly of the digastric muscle. The anterior facial vein provides venous drainage. The lymphatic drainage is to the submandibular lymph nodes, then to the deep cervical nodes. The chorda tympani nerve innervates the both the submandibular and the sublingual glands.

Sublingual Glands

The unencapsulated sublingual glands are the smallest of the major salivary glands. The sublingual gland is a flat, oblong structure that accompanies and occupies the same plane as the distal half of the submandibular duct. Each gland lies medial to the body of the mandible, superior to the mylohyoid muscle and deep to the mucosa of the mouth floor. The lingual nerve descends laterally to the anterior end of the sublingual gland and runs along its inferior border. Anteriorly, the lingual nerve and submandibular duct run parallel until the lingual nerve ascends into the tongue.

The sublingual glands have from 8 to 20 small ducts, the ducts of Rivinus, which penetrate the floor of mouth mucosa to enter the oral cavity laterally and posteriorly to the submandibular duct. A minority of the ducts join to form the ducts of Bartholin. These major ducts can drain into the submandibular duct. Arterial supply is from the sublingual and submental arteries. Lymphatic drainage is to the submental and submandibular lymph nodes, then to the deep cervical lymph nodes.

Minor Salivary Glands

Numerous minor salivary glands are located throughout the paranasal sinuses, nasal cavity, oral mucosa, hard and soft palate, pharynx, and larynx. The hard and soft palate contain the greatest number of minor salivary glands. Each gland is a discrete unit with its own duct opening into the oral cavity. The minor salivary glands are innervated by the trigeminal nerve via the pterygopalatine ganglion.

Cervical Fascia

The cervical fascia is composed of layers of dense connective tissue, which invests muscles and encloses anatomical spaces. Fascial planes function to both direct and limit the spread of disease processes in the neck. Spatial anatomical description of neck pathology and structures is well-suited to the axial views provided by MR and CT imaging, and provides a more useful basis for differential diagnosis than traditional descriptions based upon the triangles of the neck.

Layers of Cervical Fascia

The superficial cervical fascia (SCF) is a loose fat-filled layer of connective tissue that surrounds the head and neck just below the skin. This tissue allows the skin to move easily over the deeper neck structures. It contains the platysma and muscles of facial expression, as well as blood vessels, cutaneous nerves, and superficial lymph nodes.

The DCF forms sheets and corresponds to the fascial layers surrounding the musculature of the neck. It is subdivided into the superficial, middle, and deep layers of the DCF. While the three layers are not apparent on imaging, their location is inferred from other structures.

The superficial, or investing layer of DCF, lies immediately under the SCF, completely encircling the neck. It splits to invest the sternocleidomastoid and trapezius muscles, and encloses the muscles of mastication and the parotid gland. It forms a fascial sling around the inferior belly of the omohyoid and contributes to the carotid sheath.

The middle, or visceral layer of DCF, surrounds the viscera of the neck and splits to encapsulate the thyroid gland. This layer encircles the larynx, trachea, esophagus, thyroid and parathyroid glands, recurrent laryngeal nerves, and paraesophageal lymph nodes. It continues in the suprahyoid neck as the buccopharyngeal fascia.

The deep layer of DCF surrounds the prevertebral and paraspinous musculature. From its attachment at the skull base, it splits into an anterior alar and a posterior prevertebral component. The alar fascia is separated from the prevertebral fascia by the danger space, which is made of loose connective tissue, extending inferiorly to the diaphragm. Serious deep neck infections are common within this space. On imaging, the danger space cannot be distinguished from the retropharyngeal space (RPS).

The carotid sheath is a fascial layer that receives contributions from all three layers of DCF. It continues from the skull base through the neck, along the anterior surface of the prevertebral fascia, and enters the chest behind the clavicle. It contains the carotid arteries, internal jugular veins, and vagus nerves.

Spaces of the Neck

The three layers of DCF converge at the hyoid bone, dividing the neck into suprahyoid and infrahyoid compartments. The main spaces of the neck are grouped by their location in one of these compartments. The suprahyoid spaces include the masticator, parapharyngeal, retropharyngeal, carotid, parotid, and prevertebral spaces. The carotid, retropharyngeal, and prevertebral spaces span the entire neck, and are therefore also infrahyoid spaces. The submandibular and sublingual spaces lie within the oral cavity. Masses in the suprahyoid neck characteristically displace the parapharyngeal space, allowing for localization of the origin of the lesion to one of the surrounding spaces. Similarly, masses originating in the infrahyoid spaces displace the prevertebral muscles in a distinctive manner.

PAROTID SPACE

The Parotid space encloses the parotid gland, neurovascular structures which traverse the parenchyma, and intra and periparotid lymph nodes. Therefore, most lesions found in this space will involve inflammatory and neoplastic processes in the gland. Most lesions are easily seen and palpated on the cheek. However, lesions of the deep lobe of the parotid may be asymptomatic and go unrecognized on clinical examination. On imaging, lesions of the deep lobe of the parotid gland will characteristically displace the parapharyngeal space medially. Deeper lesions from adjacent spaces may push the parotid gland laterally, creating the false impression of a parotid gland mass. Accessory parotid tissue is a normal and common anatomical variant that may appear as an asymmetric mass on the masseter muscle. Similarly, the parotid tail may extend below the angle of the mandible, mimicking a mass in this region.

Malignancies from the parotid space (PS) can extend into the temporal bone via the facial nerve. Sixty percent of adenoid cystic carcinoma, the second most common parotid malignancy, will demonstrate perineural spread. The facial nerve should be evaluated carefully and completely, from parotid to cerebellopontine angle, for tumor invasion.

Anatomy of the Parotid Space

The PS is located posterior to the ramus of the mandible, where the superficial layer of DCF splits to enclose the parotid gland. The gland is located anterior to mastoid tip and external auditory canal, inferior to zygomatic arch, and superior to the lower border of the angle of the mandible. Anteriorly, it overlaps the masseter muscle. Stenson's duct enters oral cavity through the buccal mucosa opposite upper second molar. The medial border of the PS abuts the parapharyngeal space. The masticator space is anterior to the PS, and the posterior border relates to the carotid sheath vessels, the styloid process, and the posterior belly of the digastric muscle.

The parotid gland and the structures it contains are the main components of this space. The PS is transected by the facial nerve, artificially separating the gland into a superficial lobe and deep lobe. The facial nerve fibers originate at the pontomedullary junction, leave the posterior cranial fossa through the internal acoustic meatus, and enter the facial canal in the petrous temporal bone. The motor root traverses the facial canal and innervates the stapedius muscle. From there, it descends and emerges from the stylomastoid foramen to enter the parotid gland. Parasympathetic secretory afferents to the parotid leave the inferior salivary nucleus with the glossopharyngeal nerve and travel via Jacobson's plexus in the middle ear to synapse in the otic ganglion, just below foramen ovale. Postsynaptic fibers are distributed to the parotid by the auriculotemporal nerve.

The major vessels of the PS are the external carotid artery and the retromandibular vein. The external carotid artery (ECA) terminates in the parotid, where is gives off two terminal branches, the superficial termportal, and the maxillary artery. The superficial temporal and maxillary veins unite in the parotid to form the retromandibular vein. The vein lies lateral to the artery, and the facial nerve lies lateral to the vein. In addition, the PS contains numerous parotid lymph nodes within the glandular parenchyma.

Congenital Anomalies of the Parotid Space

First Branchial Cleft Cyst

Patients with a first branchial cleft cyst present with a compressible neck mass in or around the parotid gland. An external sinus may be seen opening at the angle of the mandible. The differential diagnosis includes cystic hygroma, neck abscess, and suppurative lymph node. Imaging demonstrates a cystic mass within or around the parotid gland. The cyst is usually hypointense on T1-weighted images and hyperintense on T2-weighted images. The signal intensity on T1-weighted images increases with the protein content of the cyst. The thickness of the cyst's wall will vary according to the degree of inflammation, and enhances with contrast (**Fig. 7-2**).

Vasoformative Anomalies of the Parotid Space

Hemangiomas in the PS usually involve the entire parotid gland. Nearly all hemangiomas involute by the age of 10 years, therefore intervention is usually unnecessary. However, parotid hemangiomas may obstruct the external auditory canal. Surgery in this region is difficult because of the location of the facial nerve.

The tumor is soft and compressible with an overlying bluish skin discoloration. On imaging, the lobulated mass is poorly marginated, with low signal intensity on T1-weighted images and high intensity on T2. Contrast enhancement is intense.

Lymphatic malformations and cystic hygromas are also discovered at an early age, but may spontaneously appear in adulthood, usually following trauma. Unlike hemangiomas, they do not involute. The facial nerve, cranial nerve VII, passes through the parotid gland, and can be injured in surgery. These cystic lesions are multiloculated, with low signal intensity on T1-weighted images and high intensity on T2-weighted images. There is little contrast enhancement of the cyst walls, unless they are thickened by inflammation (**Fig. 7-3**).

Inflammatory Lesions of the Parotid Space

Sialadenitis is a painful infection that usually is caused by staphylococcus, streptococcus, or anaerobic bacteria. Although it is very common among elderly adults with salivary gland stones, sialadenitis can also occur in children. Risk factors include dehydration, recent surgery, prematurity, malnutrition, eating disorders, chronic illness, and cancer. Medications, such as antihistamines, diuretics, psychiatric medications, beta-blockers, and barbiturates also contribute. Without proper treatment, sialadenitis can develop into a severe infection, especially in people who are debilitated or elderly.

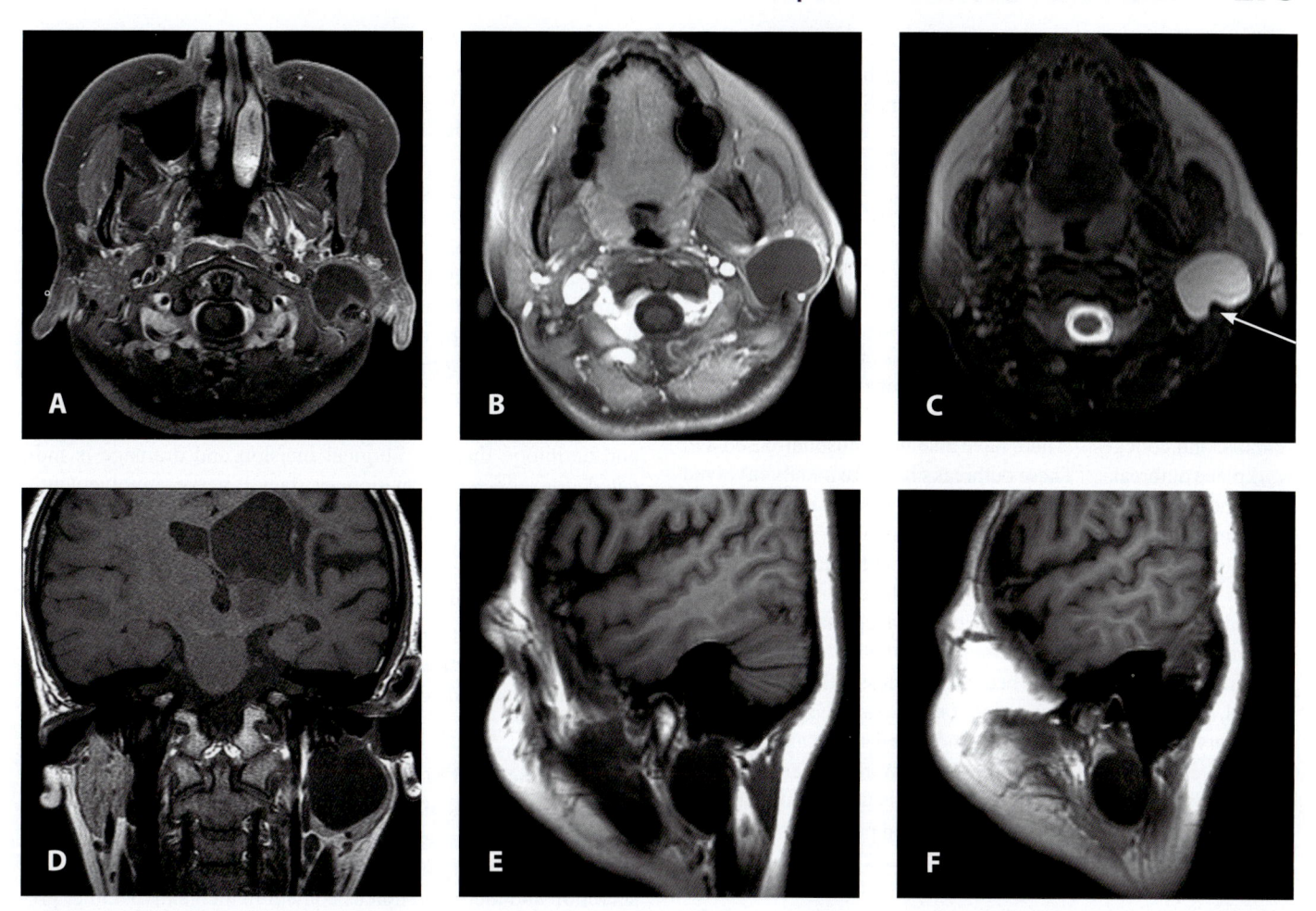

Figure 7-2 First Branchial Cleft Cyst
(**A, B**) Axial enhanced T1 with fat-saturated, (**C**) T2 axial, (**D**) coronal and (**E, F**) sagittal T1 MRI scans. There is a smoothly marginated, purely cystic lesion within the left parotid gland showing no postcontrast enhancement (**A, B**). The lesion abuts the left mastoid process that forms a focal indentation posteriorly (*arrow*, **C**). The coronal view shows left hemispheric infarction with encephalomalacia (**D**). The sagittal images clearly show the location behind the ramus of the mandible (**E, F**).

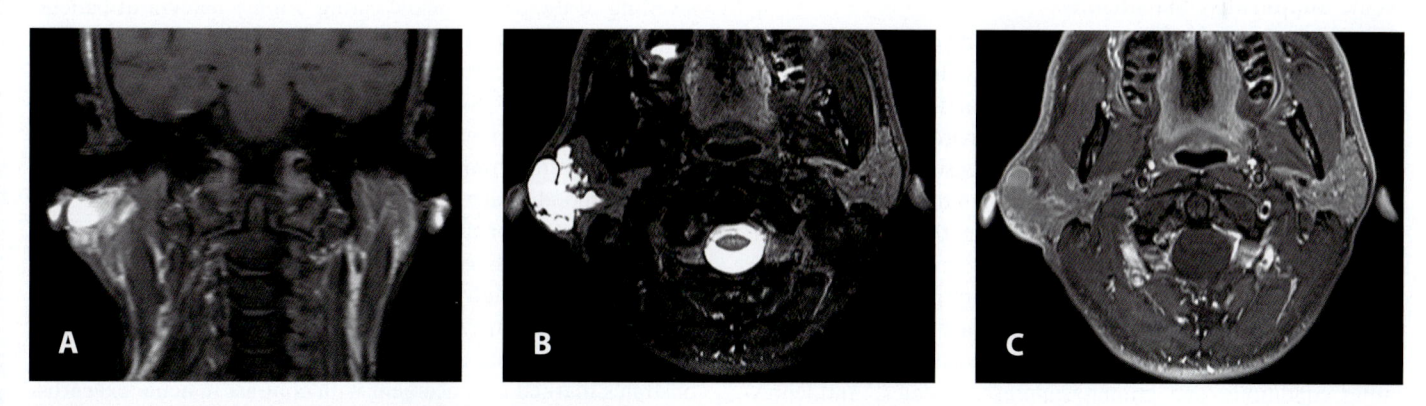

Figure 7-3 Parotid Lymphangioma with Hemorrhage
(**A**) Coronal T1WI, (**B**) axial T2WI, and (**C**) axial contrast-enhanced fat-saturated T1WI MR scans. There is a multicystic lesion in the right parotid gland, which shows high signal blood products on T1 (**A**) and intense T2 increased signal (**B**). There is no postcontrast enhancement, characteristic of a lymphangioma (**C**). These lesions have a propensity for hemorrhage despite lack of enhancement.

Acute sialadenitis

Acute sialadenitis can result from viral or bacterial infections. The identification of abscess is of primary importance, as this requires immediate surgical treatment.

Acute Viral Sialadenitis

Paramyxovirus is the most common viral cause of parotitis. Acute bilateral swelling of the parotid glands is accompanied by pain, erythema, tenderness, malaise, fever, and occasionally trismus. Peak incidence is in children 4 to 6 years old. The development of an effective the U.S. vaccine strategy has led to a significant decline in the incidence of mumps cases since 1967. However, there have been a number of sporadic mumps outbreaks reported in cohorts of susceptible individuals from military barracks, high schools, and colleges.[16] There have also been hospital-based and workplace outbreaks.[17] These outbreaks have frequently involved older individuals who are at risk for more serious morbidity and for complications requiring hospital admission.

Mumps infection frequently presents with a nonspecific prodrome, followed within 48 hours by the development of parotitis, which is due to direct infection of ductal epithelium and local inflammation. All but 10% of cases present with bilateral parotid swelling. The parotid glands become progressively enlarged and painful, and on physical examination the orifice of the Stensen duct is erythematous and swollen. Increased serum amylase supports the clinical diagnosis. The parotid swelling can last up to 10 days. Symptomatic infection in adults is usually more severe than in children. In the presence of bilateral parotitis, the clinical diagnosis is usually straightforward. Other causes of unilateral or bilateral parotitis include other viral infections, such as parainfluenza, coxsackievirus, influenza A, Epstein-Barr virus, adenovirus, and bacterial infections such as *Staphylococcus aureus*. Noninfectious etiologies include salivary calculi, tumors, sarcoidosis, Sjorgren's syndrome, and thiazide diuretics.

On T1-weighted images, the high signal of the fatty parotid is replaced by intermediate signal intensity. T2-weighted images have high signal intensity, and the glands enhance with contrast.

Acute Suppurative Sialadenitis

Acute suppurative parotitis is a bacterial infection of the parotid gland that occurs when decreased salivary flow allows bacteria to travel up the Stenson's duct into the gland parenchyma. Bacterial infection is more common in the parotid than the other salivary glands. The opening of the Stenson's duct is larger and more prone to injury than the Wharton duct, and the serous parotid secretions are less bacteriostatic than the mucinous secretions of the submandibular gland.

Most cases of acute suppurative parotitis occur in the elderly, although neonatal and premature infants are also at risk.[18] Factors that increase risk include postoperative dehydration, debilitating conditions, and immunosuppressive states. Antidepressants, anticholinergics, and diuretics can cause dehydration.[19] Ductal obstruction from sialolithiasis, tumor, or foreign bodies may also lead to bacterial infection.

Patients present with fever, pain, and an erythematous, swollen, indurated cheek. In 15% to 25% of cases, swelling will be bilateral.[20] The Stenson's duct may exude purulent discharge. In 80% of cases *Staphylococcus aureus* is the causal organism. *Streptococcus viridans, Streptococcus pneumonia, Haemophilus influenzae, Streptococcus pyogenes,* and *Escherichia coli* may also be the cause of the infection. The incidence of infection from strict anaerobes, such as *Peptostreptococcus* and *Bacteroides*, is rising.[21]

On imaging, the gland is enlarged and the normal architecture is obscured. The infection is normally limited to the gland, but there have been reports of spread into contiguous neck spaces.[22] T2-weighted images will show diffuse high signal from edema, but signal will be decreased with significant cellular infiltration. The enlarged gland will have moderate diffuse enhancement with contrast. An abscess will have a low signal intensity center surrounded by rim enhancement.

Treatment includes rehydration to increase salivary flow, and antibiotic therapy. Surgical incision and drainage is indicated for abscess formation or facial nerve involvement.[21] Superficial parotidectomy may be efficacious when conservative management fails.[23]

Chronic Sialadenitis

Common causes of chronic parotid inflammation include recurrent bacterial infection, granulomatous disease, such as sarcoidosis, autoimmune disorders, most commonly Sjögren's disease, or irradiation.

Chronic Bacterial Sialadenitis

Chronic bacterial sialadenitis is a low-grade chronic infection that can eventually lead to destruction of the salivary gland. It may occur more commonly in patients with decreased salivary secretion and increased mucus content in their saliva. Other predisposing factors include stones, strictures, and trauma.

Patients with chronic bacterial sialadenitis generally have intermittent exacerbations of acute sialadenitis. The onset of the chronic inflammatory process induces alterations in salivary chemistry and enzyme and immunoglobulin content. Sialectasis, ductal ectasia, and acinar atrophy occur, accompanied by a lymphocytic infiltrate. Patients present with recurrent painful swelling of the parotid while eating. Eighty percent of patients experience permanent xerostomia.

In children, recurrent parotitis usually affects males between 3 and 6 years old.[20] Swelling may be unilateral or bilateral, and lasts from days to weeks. Patients may have accompanying pain and fever. Symptoms may resolve at puberty or continue into adulthood. Bacterial cultures from saliva generally produce *S. viridans* or another low-virulence bacteria considered normal oral flora. Even between attacks, bacteria are present in the saliva. Sialography reveal punctate sialectasis as in Sjögren disease. Even when symptoms are unilateral, sialectasis is commonly demonstrated in the opposite gland. MR imaging demonstrates marked enhancement with contrast in acute exacerbations, and can show extensive cystic malformed acini in chronic disease.[24] MR signal intensity reflects the relative amounts of edema versus inflammatory cellular infiltrate.

Treatment is initially conservative with a search for predisposing factors such as a calculus or stricture. If unsuccessful, ductal dilatation, ligation, tympanic neurectomy, irradiation of the gland, or excision of the gland may be performed.[25]

Granulomatous Disease of the Parotid Space

Granulomatous disease may affect the parotid lymph nodes or the gland parenchyma as part of the systemic disease process. Sarcoidosis, tuberculosis, atypical mycobacterial infection, syphilis, toxoplasmosis, cat-scratch disease, and actinomycosis are granulomatous diseases that may involve the salivary glands.

Sarcoidosis

Sarcoidosis is a multisystem granulomatous disorder of unknown etiology that is characterized pathologically by the accumulation of T lymphocytes and mononuclear phagocytes, and the presence of noncaseating granulomas in involved organs. The immune granuloma cells are organized spatially resulting from an immunological response to an antigenic trigger.[26] Genetic predisposition is determined by the varying effects of several genes, with both linkage and functional relevance.

The lungs are affected in approximately 90% of patients, and pulmonary disease accounts for the majority of the morbidity and mortality associated with this disease. It typically affects young adults, and generally presents with bilateral hilar adenopathy, pulmonary infiltrates, skin lesion, eye lesions, or any combination of these features.

Sarcoidosis most frequently involves the lung, and patients present with cough, dyspnea, and chest pain. Other symptoms include fatigue, malaise, fever, and weight loss. Painless swelling of the salivary glands occurs in approximately 4% of patients with sarcoidosis. The constellation of lacrimal gland enlargement, xerostomia, and xerophthalmia is referred to as keratoconjunctivitis sicca. Facial palsy has also been reported. Heerfordt's syndrome is characterized by mild fever, painless parotid enlargement, uveitis, and cranial nerve involvement, usually seen as a transient seventh nerve paralysis.[27] Asymptomatic swelling of the parotid gland accompanied by reduced salivary flow or enlarged cervical nodes may suggest an apparently silent systemic sarcoidosis.[28]

MR images demonstrate one or more benign, noncavitating masses with cystic and solid features. There is often associated reactive cervical adenopathy. Treatment is symptomatic. Corticosteroids are used in severe cases.

Sjogren Syndrome

Sjogren syndrome (SS) is a chronic inflammatory disorder characterized by lymphocytic infiltration of exocrine glands, especially the lacrimal and salivary glands. The population prevalence is approximately 0.5%, and the female to male ratio is 9:1.[29] There are two age peaks; one in the second and third decades, and one after menopause in the fifth decade.[29]

SS can exist as a primary autoimmune disorder or as a condition in association with another autoimmune process such as rheumatoid arthritis, systemic lupus erythematosus, or scleroderma. A new international consensus for diagnosis requires objective signs and symptoms of dryness, including a characteristic biopsy appearance from a minor salivary gland, or autoantibody such as anti-SS-A. Exclusions to the diagnosis include infections with HIV, human T-lymphotropic virus type I, or hepatitis C virus, and previous radiotherapy to the head and neck, lymphoma, sarcoidosis, graft-versus-host disease.[29] Although the processes that underlie autoimmunity in SS are not known, disturbances of T and B lymphocytes as well as of glandular cells, such as the ductal epithelial cells, are important.[30]

The disease involves chronic lymphocytic inflammation, impaired function, and finally destruction of the lacrimal and salivary glands. Salivary gland involvement is confirmed by sialography or labial gland biopsy (**Fig. 7-4**). Salivary gland

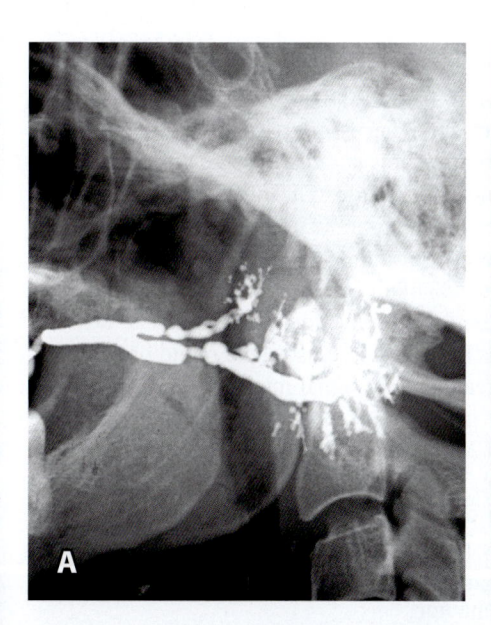

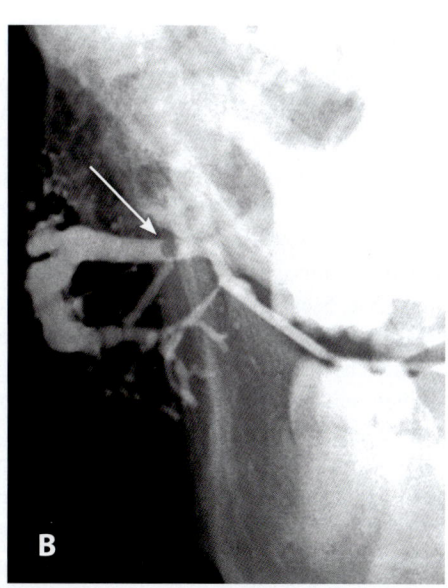

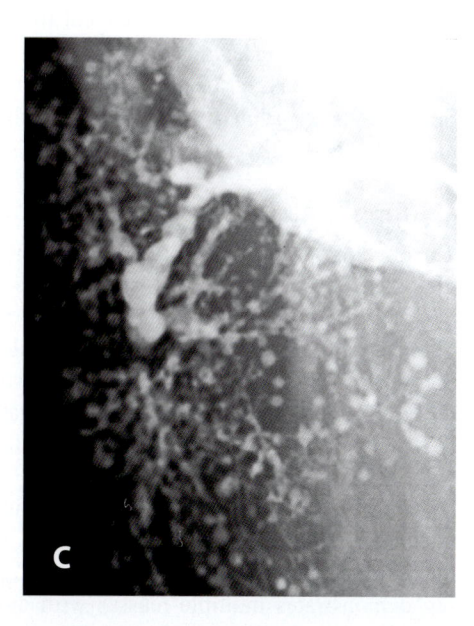

Figure 7-4 Sjörgen Syndrome Sialectasis
Images following right parotid duct cannulation for sialography. On sagittal view (**A**), the dilated primary trunk bifurcates into two portions of the parotid gland. On coronal view (**B**), a small air bubble is seen intermixed with the water-soluble contrast agent (*arrow*). The intraductal sialectasis is well-shown. In coronal view (**C**), the marked dilatation of the secondary ducts and glandular structures.

enlargement occurs in 30% to 50% of patients with SS at some point in the course of the disease. The glands are usually firm, diffuse, and nontender. These changes are most obvious in the parotid glands, but the submandibular glands may be equally affected. Salivary gland enlargement may be chronic, or episodic, with swelling and reduction over a few weeks. A particularly hard or nodular gland may suggest a neoplasm.

Non-invasive MR sialography is the best method for evaluating salivary glands in suspected SS.[31–33] Contrast-enhanced MRI with heavily T2-weighted sequences and digital subtraction methods for suppression of fat signal can be used to distinguish ductal pathology. The Stensen duct and primary branching ducts can be reliably depicted. Globular or cavitary changes appear as areas of high T2 signal. In the early stages of SS, the salivary glands will appear normal. As the disease progresses, and the parotid gland enlarges, globular collections of watery saliva can be seen on T1-weighted images as discrete low signal foci. Contrast-enhanced T1-weighted images show mild heterogeneous enhancement of the nodular, fibrous parenchyma. Cystic change will appear as nonenhancing foci. Cystic change is a rare development, and may resemble HIV-associated lymphoepithelial cysts. The entities can be distinguished clinically, and on imaging, by the presence of cervical adenopathy in the latter condition.

Postirradiation Sialadenitis

Post-irradiation sialadenitis has both acute and chronic presentations. The acute form can occur within 24 hours following a single radiation dose of more than 1,000 cGy. Symptoms, which include pain, tenderness, and xerostomia, resolve in several days. Edema in the gland will have increased signal on T2-weighted images.

Chronic postirradiation sialadenitis may result from radiotherapy for oral cavity or pharyngeal tumors. Both major and minor salivary glands are affected. The parenchyma is replaced by dense fibrous tissue containing numerous lymphocytes. Serous cells are primarily affected.[34] MR shows diminished signal on T1- and T2-weighted images.

Lymphoepithelial Cysts of the Parotid Space

The development of benign lymphoepithelial cysts in the parotid gland is well described in patients with human immunodeficiency virus. The size of the cysts vary from 0.5 to 5 cm in diameter, and they may be unilateral or bilateral. They develop secondary to lymphatic infiltration of salivary parenchyma that provokes a lymphoepithelial lesion of striated ducts with basal cell hyperplasia.[35] Their diagnosis is based on the characteristic clear brown fluid aspirated from the cysts.

These lesions may be difficult to distinguish from Sjogren syndrome and sarcoidosis if no clinical history is provided, but with known HIV, the diagnosis is straightforward. Imaging demonstrates multiple masses with cystic areas and solid components representing lymphoid aggregates in enlarged parotid glands.[36] Associated reactive cervical lymphadenopathy and tonsillar hyperplasia is common. T1-weighted images will show low signal cysts, and variable signal in solid areas. On T2-weighted images, the rounded, well-defined cysts will have high signal. Contrast will demonstrate rim-enhancement of the cysts, and heterogenous enhancement of solid lymphoid areas.

Treatment includes repeat percutaneous aspiration, superficial parotidectomy, radiation, azidothymidine, and use of tetracycline and doxycycline sclerotherapy.[37] These patients are susceptible to the development of B-cell lymphoma, so continued monitoring is important.

Benign Tumors of the Parotid Space

In the PS, smooth, well-defined masses, which enhance homogeneously, are usually benign tumors. Eighty percent to 90% of these will be benign mixed tumors, also called pleomorphic adenomas. Another 10% will be Warthin's tumors. These are tumors, derived from salivary gland tissue in the parotid lymph nodes, are unique to this space. The final 10% comprise lipomas, oncocytomas, and schwannomas of the facial nerve.

Preoperatively, it is important for the radiologist to determine the relationship of tumor to surrounding structures, and if possible, determine whether the tumor is benign or malignant. Benign tumors are treated with local excision or superficial parotidectomy, while malignant tumors are removed with total parotidectomy with or without facial nerve resection.

Benign Mixed Tumor (Pleomorphic Adenoma)

Benign mixed tumors (BMT) are epithelium-derived benign tumors that show both epithelial and mesenchymal differentiation. They are the most common benign tumor of the parotid gland.

The tumor is believed to arise from myoepithelial or ductal reserve cell origin.[38] BMT comprise a mixture of epithelial elements in a matrix with variable amounts of myxoid, hyaline, chondroid, and osseous elements. The tumor is ovoid and well-defined, with a partially developed capsule. Most are smaller than 6 cm.

The typical patient is in their fifth decade presenting with a painless, slow-growing mass in the cheek. Surgical resection is the mainstay of treatment of accessory parotid gland neoplasms. The recommended treatment is surgical resection of tumor with wide margins around the capsule. The prognosis is excellent; only 4% recur. Recurrent tumors are frequently multinodular.[39] Twenty-five percent of untreated BMT undergo malignant change. Nearly 2% to 5% of all BMT, treated or not, will degenerate to carcinoma ex pleomorphic adenoma.

Small adenomas are well-circumscribed, ovoid or spherical masses with homogeneous low signal intensity on T1-weighted images and low to intermediate contrast enhancement. There is high signal on T2-weighted images, reflecting the myxoid content of the tumor. Larger tumors demonstrate mixed T1 and T2 signal, with foci of necrosis and hemorrhage (**Figs. 7-5** and **7-6**). Carcinoma ex pleomorphic adenoma can appear identical to BMT on imaging. Necrosis and invasive margins suggest aggressive tumor behavior.

Twenty percent of individuals have accessory parotid gland tissue. While the parotid gland has primarily serous cells, accessory parotid tissue resembles submandibular gland tissue, with mucinous and serous composition. One percent to 8% of parotid tumors arise in this accessory gland. The rate of malignancy

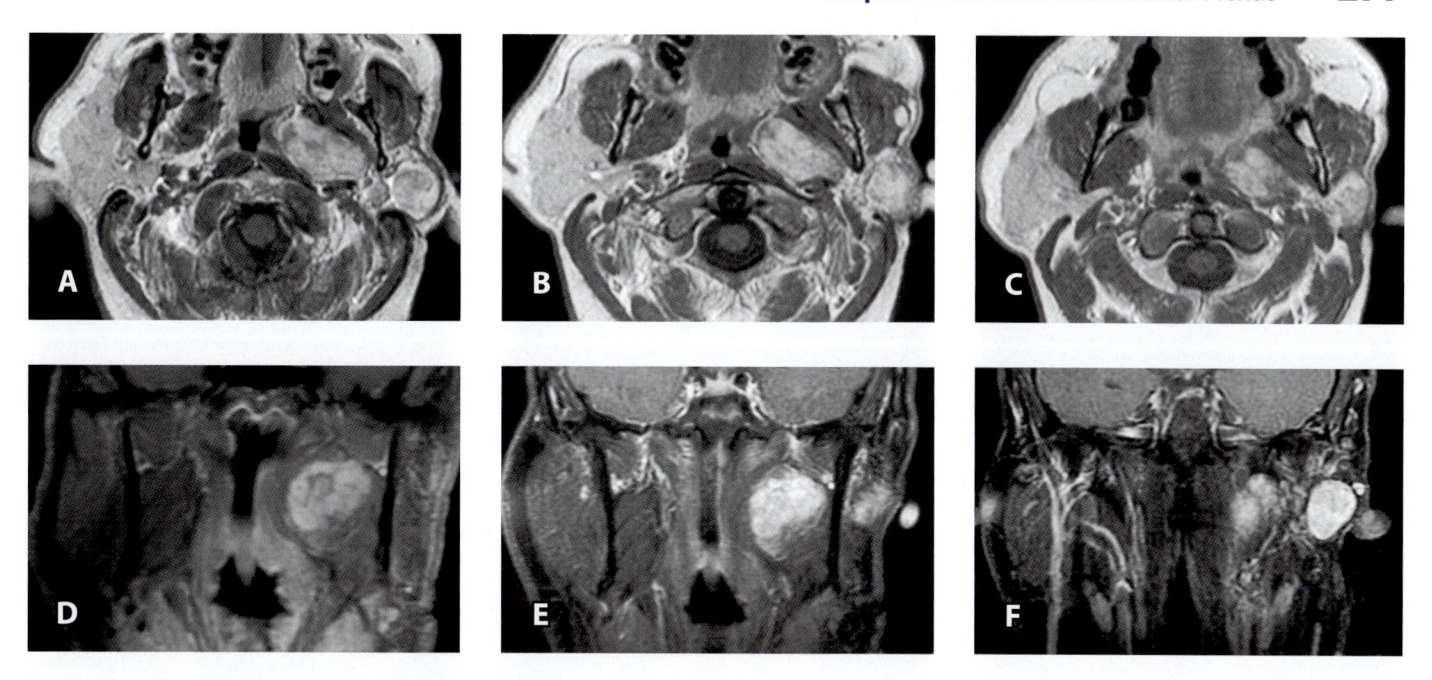

Figure 7-5 Benign Mixed Tumor of the Parotid
Axial T1WI (**A–C**) and coronal postcontrast T1WI with fat-saturated (**D–F**) MR images. There is a heterogeneous signal mass in both the superficial and deep lobes of the left parotid gland. The deep component extends toward the parapharyngeal space, which is displaced medially. The inferior row of enhanced images shows the complex nature of the tumor.

has been reported to be from 26% to 50%.[40,41] The majority of benign tumors are BMT.

Warthin's Tumor

Warthin's tumor, or papillary cystadenoma lymphomatosum, is the second most common benign lesion of the parotid gland comprising 2% to 10% of all parotid tumors. They are believed to arise from small salivary gland tissue rests in the parotid lymphoid tissue. These tumors are found almost exclusively in the parotid gland, as no other salivary glands contain lymph nodes.

Ten percent are bilateral. It is the most common lesion to present in a multifocal unilateral or bilateral presentation. The tumors are small, encapsulated masses, which most often develop in the superficial aspect of the parotid. Cyst formation is common in large tumors, and nodules may be seen along the cysts, which distinguishes them from lymphoepithelial cysts. The papillary cystic spaces are filled with a mucinous or serous secretion.[39] On microscopic examination, the spaces are lined by a double layer of epithelial cells resting on a dense lymphoid stroma, with occasional germinal centers.[38]

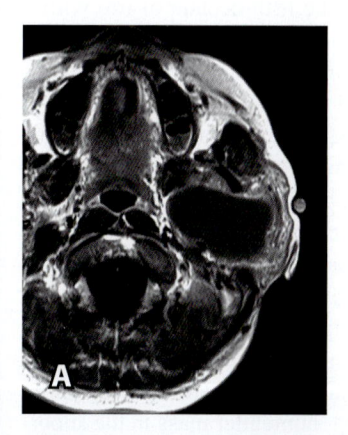

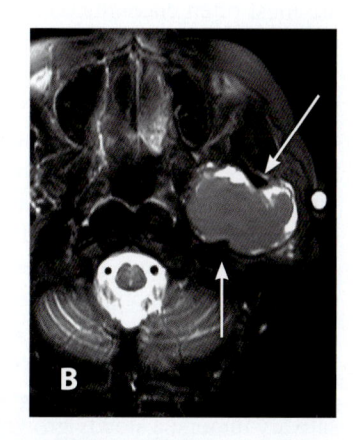

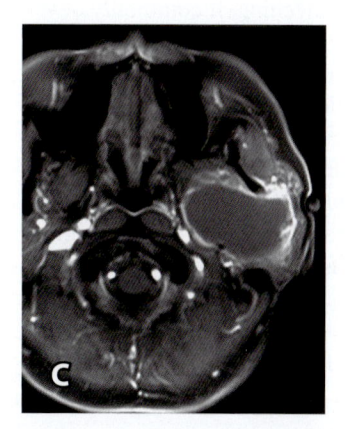

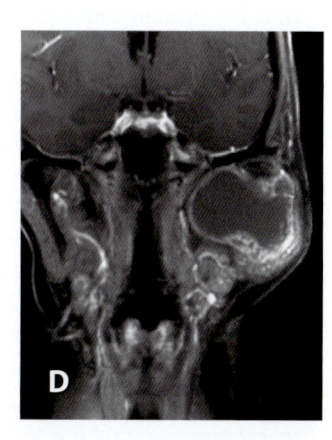

Figure 7-6 Benign Mixed Tumor of the Parotid
(**A**) Axial T1WI, (**B**) axial T2WI, and contrast-enhanced with fat-saturated (axial, **C** and coronal, **D**) MR images. A large cystic mass is evident in the left parotid gland with extension into the deep lobe through the stylomandibular notch, best visualized in **B** (*arrows*). Most of the content within the cystic portion of the tumor is devoid of signal on all sequences, commonly seen in highly proteinaceous materials. There is enhancement of the surrounding solid portions of the tumor (**C, D**).

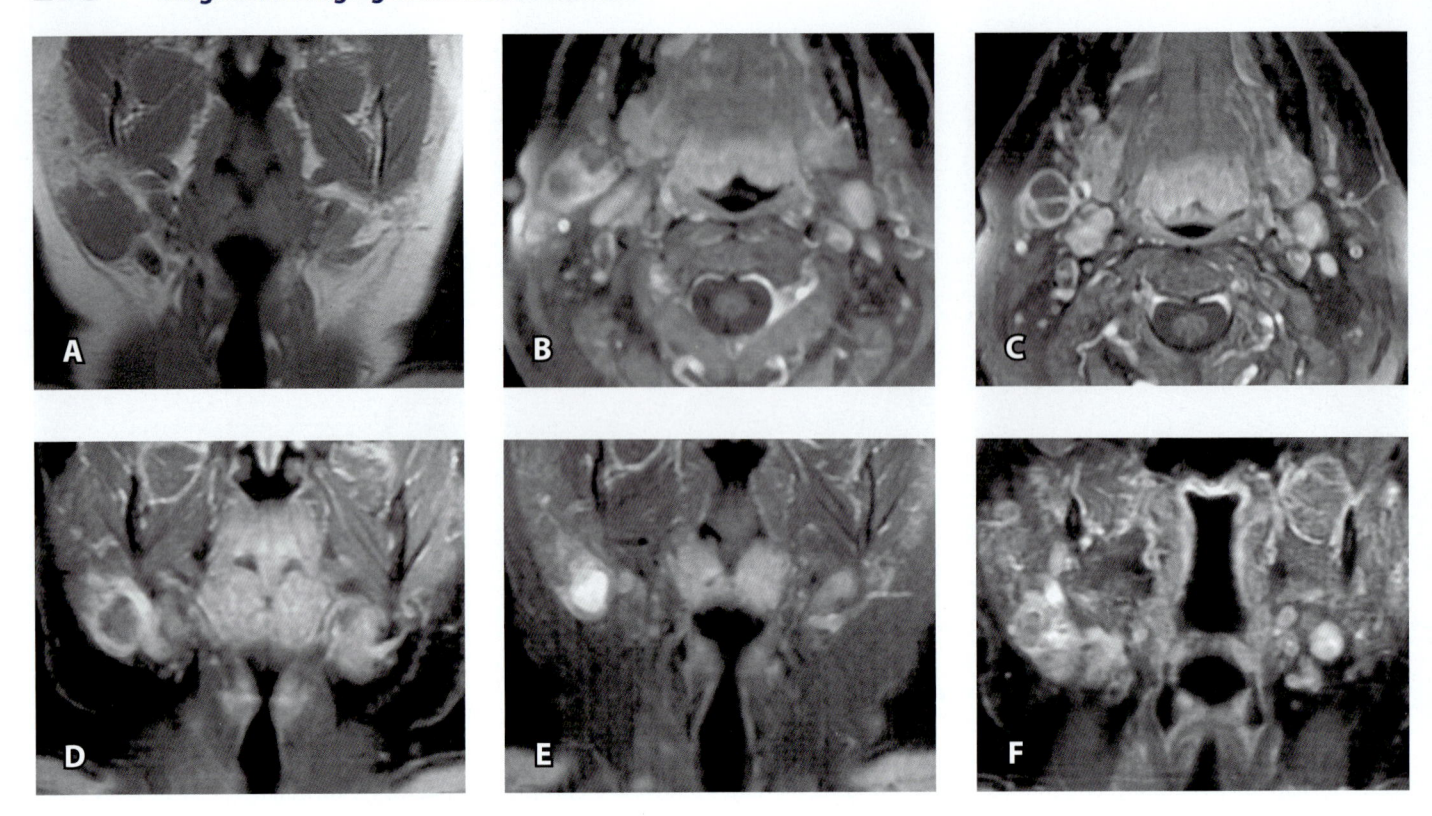

Figure 7-7 Parotid Warthin Tumor and Mucoepidermoid
(**A**) Coronal T1, and contrast-enhanced fat-saturated axial (**A, B**) and coronal (**D–F**) MR scans. Multiple submandibular nodal masses are evident (**A–C**), some of which show differential enhancement, consistent with malignancy. The tail of the right parotid gland contains an enhancing tumor mass, which histologically proved to be a mucoepidermoid tumor. In addition, multiple bilateral parotid tumors were detected and were proven to be multicentric papillary cystadenoma lymphomatosum (Warthin tumor).

Patients are most often 40 to 70 years old, though the range extends from 2 to 92 years of age. Almost all patients with this tumor are white. Males are more commonly affected, but the number of females has increased in the last few decades, perhaps due to the increase in women smokers. Smokers have an eight-fold increase in risk for development of these tumors.[42] Patients commonly present with a painless swelling. It commonly develops in the inferior pole of the superficial lobe of the parotid. The masses are usually 2 to 5 cm in diameter, and easily palpable. Treatment is limited partial parotidectomy.[34] Recurrence occurs in 2% of patients after complete resection, most likely due to multicentric disease with tumor development in a new site.

Warthin's tumors are difficult to distinguish from benign mixed tumors on imaging. They have low signal on T1-weighted images and high signal on T2 (**Fig. 7-7**). The presence of cysts may help in differentiation. Large tumor cysts may resemble second branchial cleft cysts or necrotic lymph nodes. The presence of multiple intrinsic parotid masses, unilaterally or bilaterally, also suggests Warthin's tumor (**Fig. 7-8**).

Oncocytoma

Oncocytomas are rare tumors that comprise less than 1% of salivary gland tumors, and occur most commonly in the parotid. Oncocytes are epithelial cells filled with mitochondria, which impart a granular appearance to the cytoplasm. The abundance of mitochondria may reflect a metabolic defect, in which mitochondrial hyperplasia develops to compensate for decreased adenosine triphosphate production.[43] By the age of 70 years, the majority of individuals will have oncocytes in their parotid glands.[44] They develop from acinar and ductal epithelial cells that have undergone an inexplicable cytoplasmic change.[39] They are most often encountered after the fifth decade of life with a nearly equal male-to-female ratio. While the majority of these tumors affect the parotid gland, up to 10% affect the submandibular gland and minor salivary glands in the palate, buccal mucosa, or tongue. In 7% of cases, the tumors are bilateral. Multicentricity has been reported as well, so with suspicion of this tumor, both parotid glands should be carefully evaluated. Rarely, oncocytosis will occur as a diffuse hyperplastic process.[35]

In the parotid, oncocytomas are encapsulated, well-circumscribed tumors with a smooth surface that may be divided into lobules by fibrous tissue septae. Microscopically, there are sheets, nests, or cords of uniform oncocytes. The clinical presentation of oncocytomas is essentially identical to other benign salivary tumors; a slowly growing, nontender mass in the superficial lobe of the parotid. They are painless, firm, and mobile. Pain or facial nerve paralysis suggests malignant transformation. Malignant oncocytoma may arise from a benign tumor, or de novo. Malignancy is judged by evidence of vascular invasion, infiltrative growth, and perineural extension. Treatment

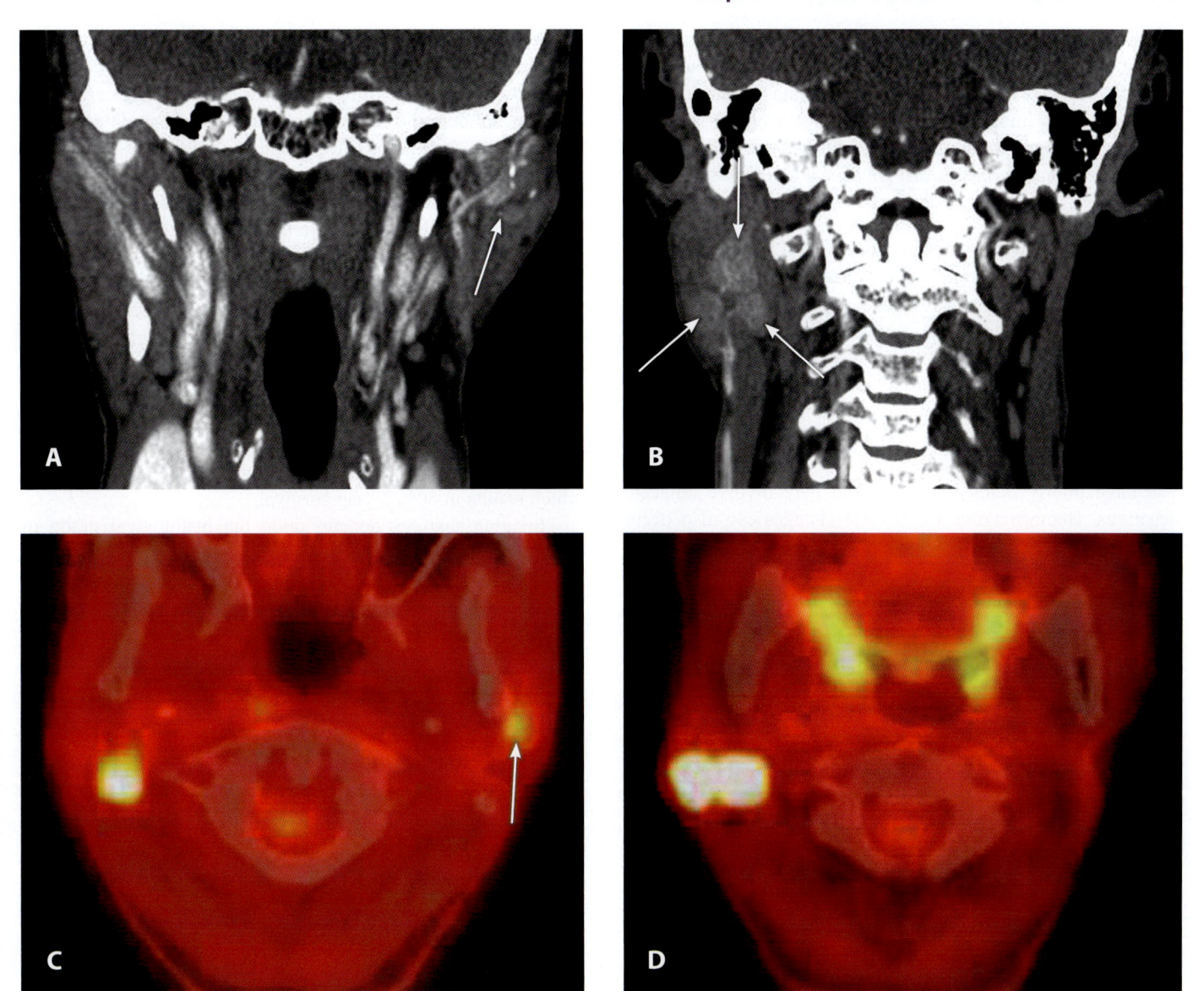

Figure 7-8 Multicentric Warthin Tumor
(**A, B**) Reformatted coronal contrast-enhanced CT scans and (**C, D**) fused PET/CT images. There are at least two separate minimally enhancing nodules in an enlarged right parotid gland (*arrows*, **B**). A smaller lesion is seen on the left side (*arrow*, **A**). The multiple bilateral lesions are highly FDG avid on PET/CT, including the small lesion in the left gland (*arrow*, **C**).

is surgical excision with wide margins. There is a low rate of recurrence with complete removal.

On imaging, these masses are sharply marginated, and may be singular, bilateral, and multicentric. T1-weighted images show an intermediate signal mass, which will enhance diffusely with contrast. T2-weighted images are variable, normally with intermediate to low signal. Pleomorphic adenomas demonstrate increased signal T2-weighted, differentiating these two tumors. Oncocytomas and Warthin's tumors demonstrate increased uptake of pertechnetate anion due to their high mitochondrial content, and therefore can be distinguished from other primary or metastatic neoplasms on technetium-99m pertechnetate scintigraphy.

Schwannoma

Primary tumors of the facial nerve are uncommon. Schwannomas are benign encapsulated tumors that arise from Schwann cells. They are composed of compact, Antoni A cells, and loosely packed, Antoni B cell areas. These tumors most commonly occur at the geniculate ganglion, but can arise anywhere from the cerebellopontine angle to the parotid gland (**See Fig. 9-42**). Patients with extratemporal facial nerve schwannoma may present with a facial twitch, followed by a facial palsy. They may be diagnosed with idiopathic Bell's palsy, but the condition does not resolve. Symptoms of sensorineural hearing loss, tinnitus, vestibular dysfunction imply that lesion is at the cerebellopontine angle or internal auditory canal.

In the PS, a schwannoma will appear as a sharply defined tubular mass following the expected course of the facial nerve through the parotid. They have intermediate signal intensity on T1-weighted images, high signal intensity on T2, and they enhance with contrast. On CT, these tumors are well-defined, intermediate density masses that enhance with contrast.

Lipoma

Lipomas develop within or adjacent to the parotid, and represent up to 10% of parotid tumors. Ten percent of these are actually diffuse fatty infiltration of the parotid gland, or lipomatosis.[39] Patients are typically in their fifth or sixth decade, and men are 5 to 10 times more likely than women to develop these tumors. The mass is soft, mobile, and nontender. They enlarge slowly, reaching 1 to 8 cm in diameter. Treatment is complete excision.

MR imaging shows increased T1-weighted signal and low T2 signal, without contrast enhancement. The infiltrating lipomas have poorly defined margins and may involve adjacent structures. Hemorrhaging and fibrotic changes can also occur within these.

Malignant Tumors of the Parotid Space

The malignant nature of salivary gland carcinomas is not always clinically apparent. Benign and malignant parotid tumors both tend to present as asymptomatic swellings. Facial nerve paralysis or fixation of the overlying skin are fairly reliable indicators of malignancy, but are not always evident. The prognosis for malignant parotid cancer is strongly influenced by tumor stage, particularly if the lesion is metastatic (**Figs. 7-9–7-12**). True measures of clinical outcome require extended patient follow-up, sometimes up to 20 years.

Mucoepidermoid Carcinoma

Mucoepidermoid carcinoma is the most common malignant salivary gland tumor, both in children and adults, accounting for 30% of parotid malignancies.[45] Patients are most often female in their fifth decade. These carcinomas may demonstrate any combination of solid and cystic growth. Their cellular composition is often a mixture of mucous cells, intermediate cells, clear cells, and epidermoid cells. Tumors are graded based upon clinical behavior and tumor differentiation. Low-grade lesions are well-circumscribed masses with cystic areas of mucinous material and mature cellular elements. High-grade lesions are solid with an infiltrative growth pattern. They are hypercellular, with noticeable cellular atypia and frequent mitotic figures. Differentiation between these tumors and squamous cell carcinoma can be difficult. Positive immunohistochemical staining for mucin confirms a high-grade mucoepidermoid carcinoma.

These tumors tend to present as slow growing, painless, masses that are "rock hard". One quarter of patients with high-grade lesions have facial nerve dysfunction. Treatment for low-grade lesions is wide excision, which results in a 5-year survival rate of 75%. High-grade lesions require surgery and radiation, which results in 50% 5-year survival.[45]

Imaging features depend upon the histological grade of the tumor. Low grade lesions are well-defined and resemble a benign mixed tumor. Cysts containing mucin will appear as hyperintense areas within the tumor on both T1 and T2-weighted images. The surrounding tumor will have low signal intensity on T2, representing fibrous tissue (**Fig. 7-13**). High-grade lesions are aggressive, with poorly defined, heterogeneous internal architecture.

Adenoid Cystic Carcinoma

Adenoid cystic carcinomas (ACC)[46] represent malignant transformation of terminal duct reserve cells. They comprise 10% to 20% of all salivary gland tumors, and 2% to 6% of parotid tumors. The tumor grows relentlessly, with poor long-term survival. The cancer usually arises in the fifth through seventh decades, affecting women more slightly more often than men.

ACC arises from major and minor salivary gland tissue. Three histologic patterns have been identified: tubular, cribriform, and solid. Most tumors contain varying amounts of all three types. The solid type has the worst prognosis due to advanced stage and development of distant metastases.[47] The tumor is slow-growing, and metastasizes to lungs and bones rather than to lymph nodes. Perineural spread occurs in 40% to 60% of cases. Invasion into gland parenchyma and soft tissue is also common. Patients may present with only a mass, or may have pain and paresthesias indicating neural involvement. Treatment is surgical excision, with postoperative radiation therapy.[48] Despite treatment, multiple recurrences are common.[47] Survival is 75% at 5 years, but drops to 20% at 20 years.[39]

On imaging, adenoid cystic carcinoma in the parotid may resemble a benign tumor, with well-demarcated borders. Perineural spread along the facial or mandibular nerve to the skull base enhances with contrast on MR images. On T1 and T2-weighted images, the tumor will have low to intermediate signal intensity (**Figs. 7-14** and **7-15**).

Acinic Cell Carcinoma

Acinic cell carcinomas are low-grade adenocarcinomas that demonstrate serous acinar differentiation. These tumors represent 10%

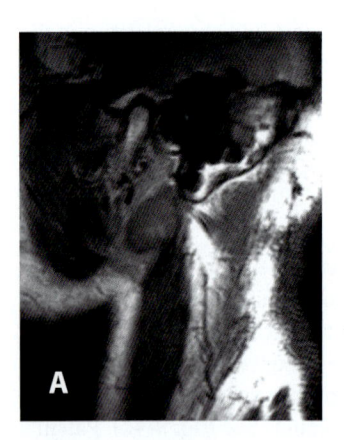

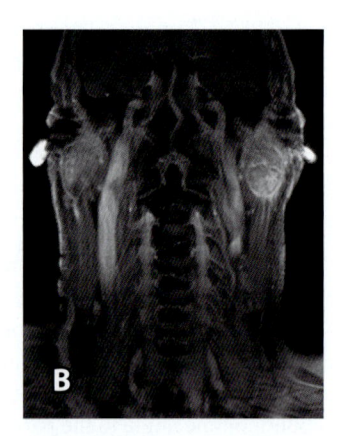

Figure 7-9 Parotid Metastatic Melanoma
(**A**) Sagittal T1WI and (**B**) contrast-enhanced fat-saturated coronal images show a solitary enhancing tumor in the left lobe of the parotid gland. The findings are nonspecific and could represent either primary or metastatic tumor as in this case.

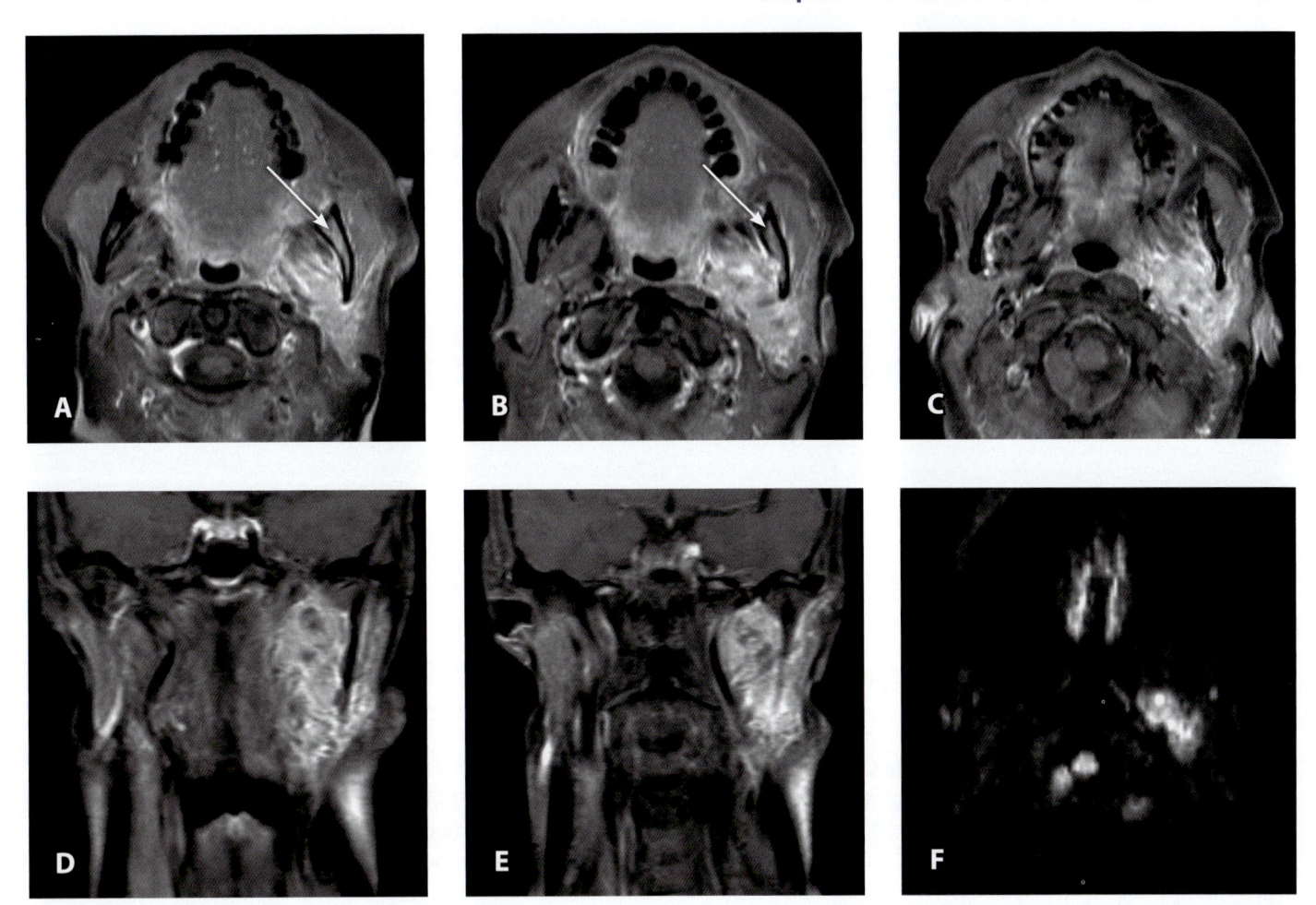

Figure 7-10 Metastasis to Parotid Region
(**A–C**) Axial and (**D, E**) coronal contrast-enhanced fat-saturated images and (**F**) axial DWI scans. A highly invasive, heterogeneously enhancing tumor incorporates portions of the parotid gland, the masticator space, and encircles the ramus of the mandible up to the skull base. There is likely invasion of the marrow within the left ramus, which shows increased signal (*arrows,* **A, B**) on the left, unlike the uninvolved right ramus showing dark signal. The DWI image shows restricted diffusion, a feature more commonly seen in malignant tumors having a high nuclear to cytoplasm ratio.

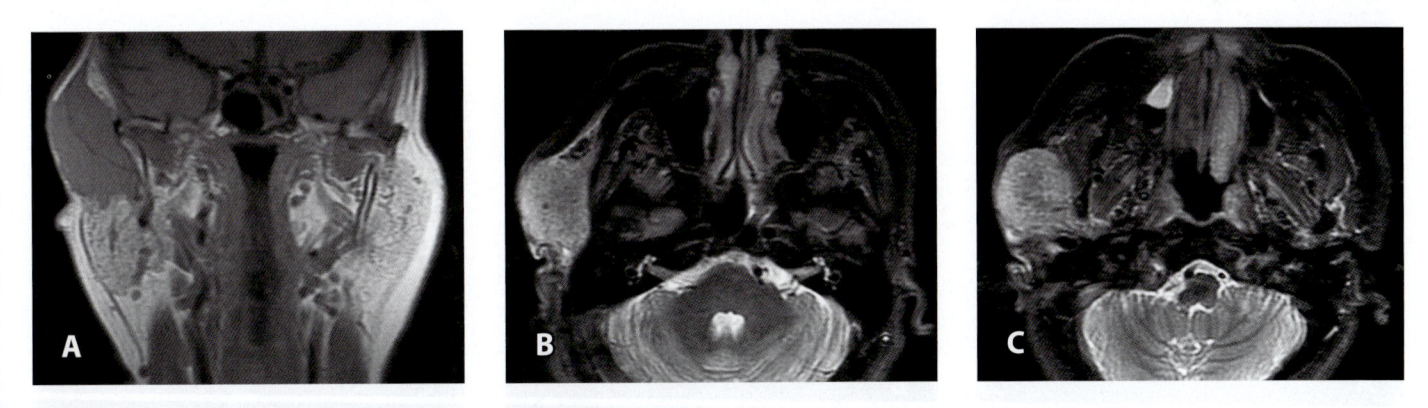

Figure 7-11 Eccrine Tumor Metastasis to Parotid
(**A**) Coronal T1WI and (**B, C**) axial T2 unenhanced images. There is a fairly homogeneous mass that extends into the skin overlying the superior portion of the right parotid gland. Such tumors of the skin or adnexal structures may directly invade the parotid gland as in this case.

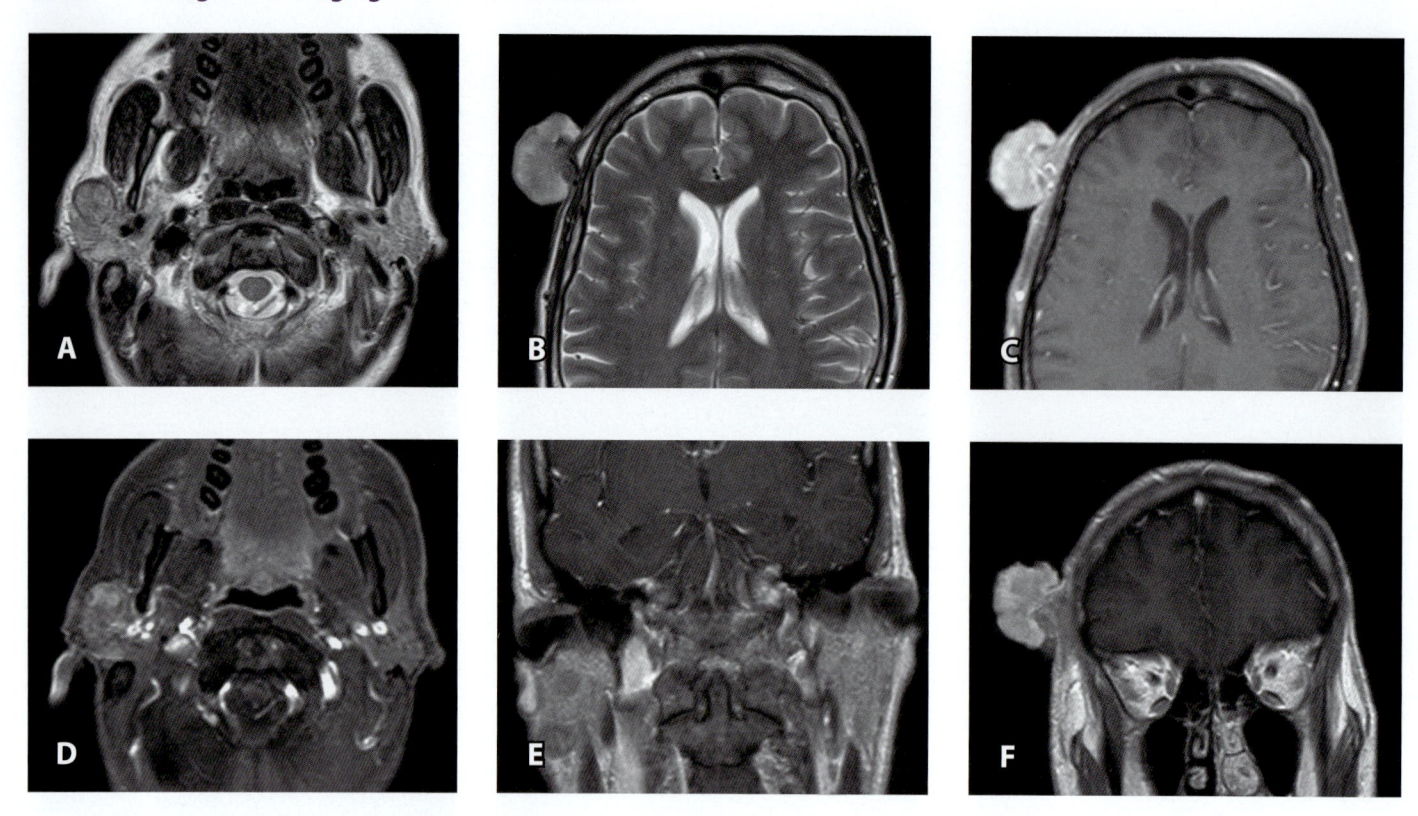

Figure 7-12 Metastatic Parotid Spindle Cell Tumor
(**A, B**) Axial T2WI and contrast-enhanced fat-saturated axial (**C, D**) and coronal (**E, F**) MR images. The primary tumor is located in the right parotid gland, showing heterogeneous T2 signal and modest enhancement (**D, E**). Also noted is a horn-like lesion emitting from the right anterior scalp, which proved to be a focus of metastasis from the primary parotid spindle cell carcinoma.

to 15% of malignant salivary gland tumors, and occur mainly in the parotid gland.[45] Women are more frequently affected than men, and the age distribution is fairly uniform from the third to the eighth decades of life.[44] Acinic cell adenocarcinoma is the second most common malignant salivary gland tumor in children.

The tumor is composed of round circumscribed nodules. The cut surface is solid but may show cystic degeneration and hemorrhage. The microscopic features of acinic cell adenocarcinoma are extremely variable. The pattern of growth may be solid, microcystic, papillary-cystic, or follicular.[49] According to their malignant potential, acinic cell carcinomas are divided into three grades. Grade I, or low-grade malignancy, includes completely encapsulated tumors without local infiltration; grade II, moderate malignancy, tumors show signs of capsular invasion; and grade III, high-grade malignancy, have papillary-cystic zones and infiltrate the surrounding tissues.

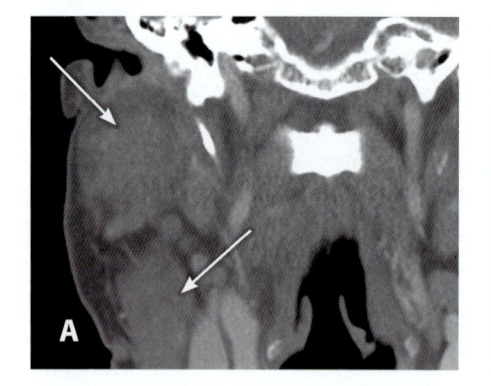

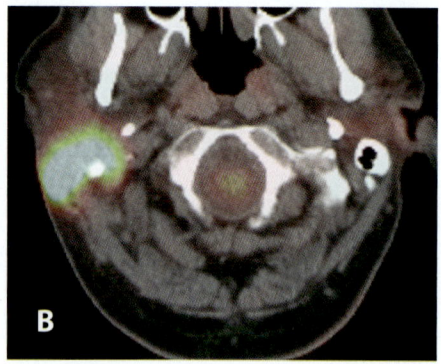

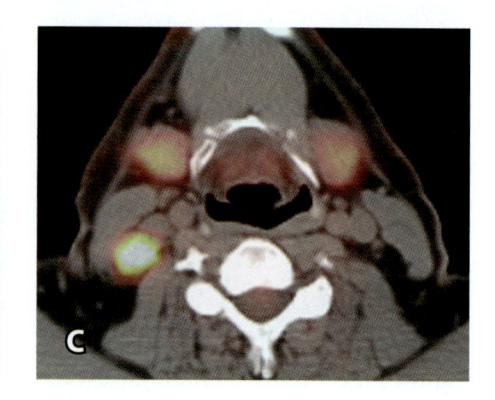

Figure 7-13 Parotid Mucoepidermoid with Nodal Metastasis
(**A**) Coronal reformatted CT scan with contrast and (**B, C**) axial fused PET/CT images. There are two masses seen in the right neck, one in the parotid gland and one large nodal mass inferior to the gland (*arrows*, **A**). There is intense avid FDG uptake in both lesions (*arrows*, **B, C**). Less intense activity is noted incidentally in both submandibular glands, indicating normal physiologic secretion.

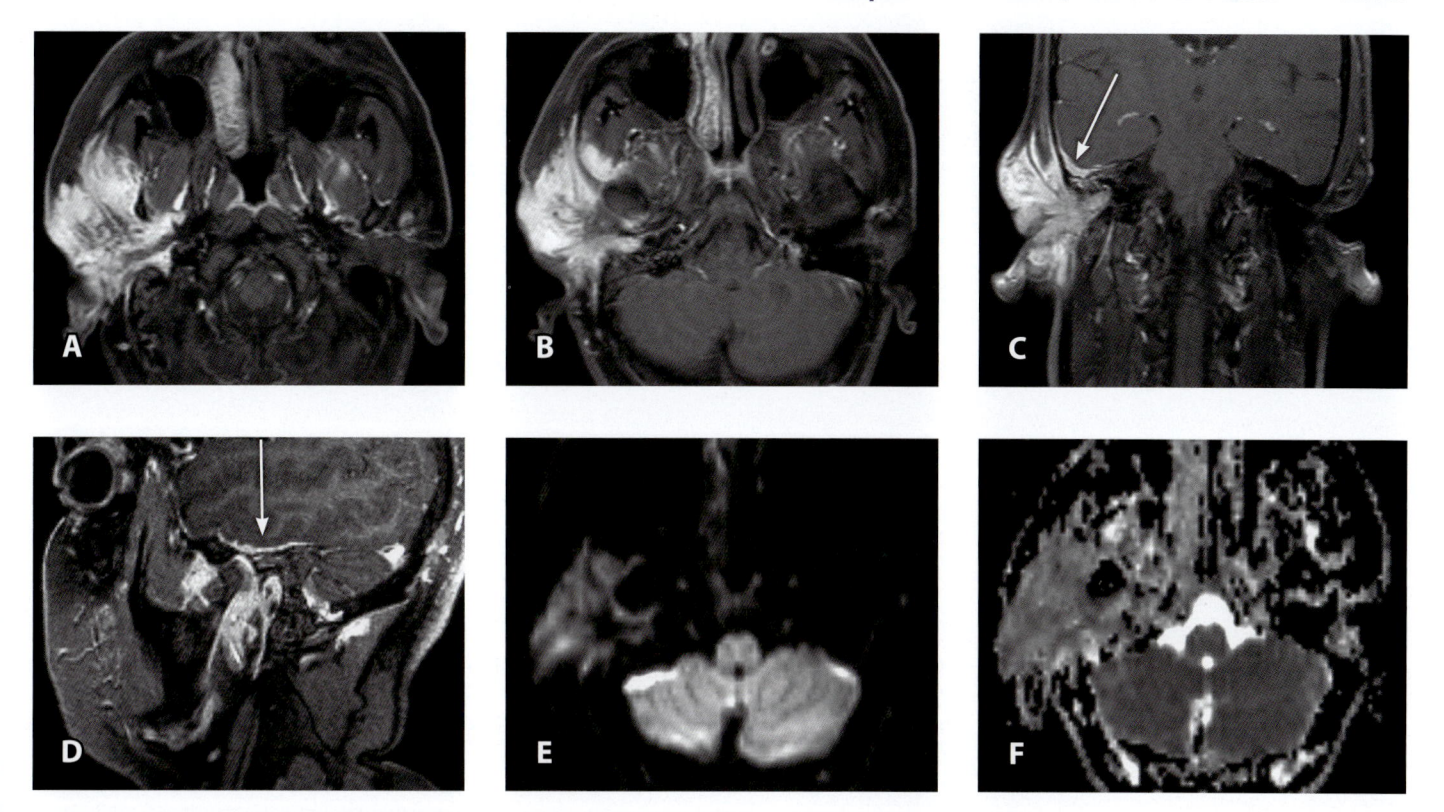

Figure 7-14 Parotid Adenoid Cystic Carcinoma with Perineural and Meningeal Spread
Contrast-enhanced fat-saturated axial (**A, B**), coronal (**C**) and sagittal (**D**) MR scans and axial DWI (**E**) and ADC (**F**) MR sequences. The widely infiltrating, markedly enhancing tumor mass extends beyond the parotid gland into the surrounding architecture of the neck and skull base. The tumor has invaded the floor of the middle fossa with perineural extension to the meninges along the branches of the fifth nerve (*arrows*, **C, D**). Such perineural spread is common with adenoid cystic carcinoma is mildly restricted diffusion, as shown in **E** and **F**.

Patients present most commonly with a slow-growing, painless mass. Pain and facial nerve involvement are rare.[45] Acinic cell carcinoma occurs bilaterally 3% of the time, making it the second most common bilateral tumor after Warthin's tumor.[39] Treatment is surgical excision with negative margins. Superficial lobectomy is sufficient for most tumors, but those involving the deep lobe require total parotidectomy. The recurrence rate after adequate resection is approximately 30%.[50]

Imaging findings are nonspecific, and acinic cell carcinoma can resemble a benign mixed tumor. Cystic areas and central hemorrhage and necrosis are more common in acinic cell carcinoma.[51] The tumor demonstrates low signal on T1, high signal on T2, and mild contrast enhancement.[52]

Lymphoma

Nearly 1% to 2% of parotid malignancies are primary or disseminated lymphoma. Men and women are equally affected and are usually in their fifth decade at the time of presentation. Most are non Hodgkin's lymphoma. Patients with SS have a 40 times greater risk of developing parotid lymphoma.[45] On imaging, lymphoma will appear as multiple, well-defined lesions within the parotid gland. T1- and T2-weighted images will have homogeneously intermediate signal intensity and mild enhancement with contrast. Prognosis is good with chemotherapy and radiation therapy.

Squamous Cell Carcinoma

Primary squamous cell carcinoma (SCCa), which develops from metaplasia of parotid duct epithelium, is rare, comprising 0.1% to 0.5% of parotid tumors.[39] These tumors are aggressive and widely infiltrating. Sixty percent of patients will present with cervical lymph node metastases and facial nerve involvement.[45] Primary SCCas tend to be moderately to well-differentiated tumors with glassy pink cytoplasm, intracellular bridges, and squamous pearls. In regions of tumor, infiltrated areas will show extensive replacement of salivary gland parenchyma by a prominent desmoplastic reaction.[49]

More commonly, SCCa involving the parotid gland take the form of metastases or direct extension from overlying facial skin. The finding of a SCC in the parotid should prompt an examination of the scalp and facial skin with careful attention to the preauricular area, ear, and cheek. Mucoepidermoid carcinoma must be ruled out with a mucin stain, which will be negative for SCCa.

Patients present with a rapidly enlarging mass, which may be fixed to adjacent structures. In some cases, the patient may have pain or facial nerve involvement. Imaging demonstrates low to

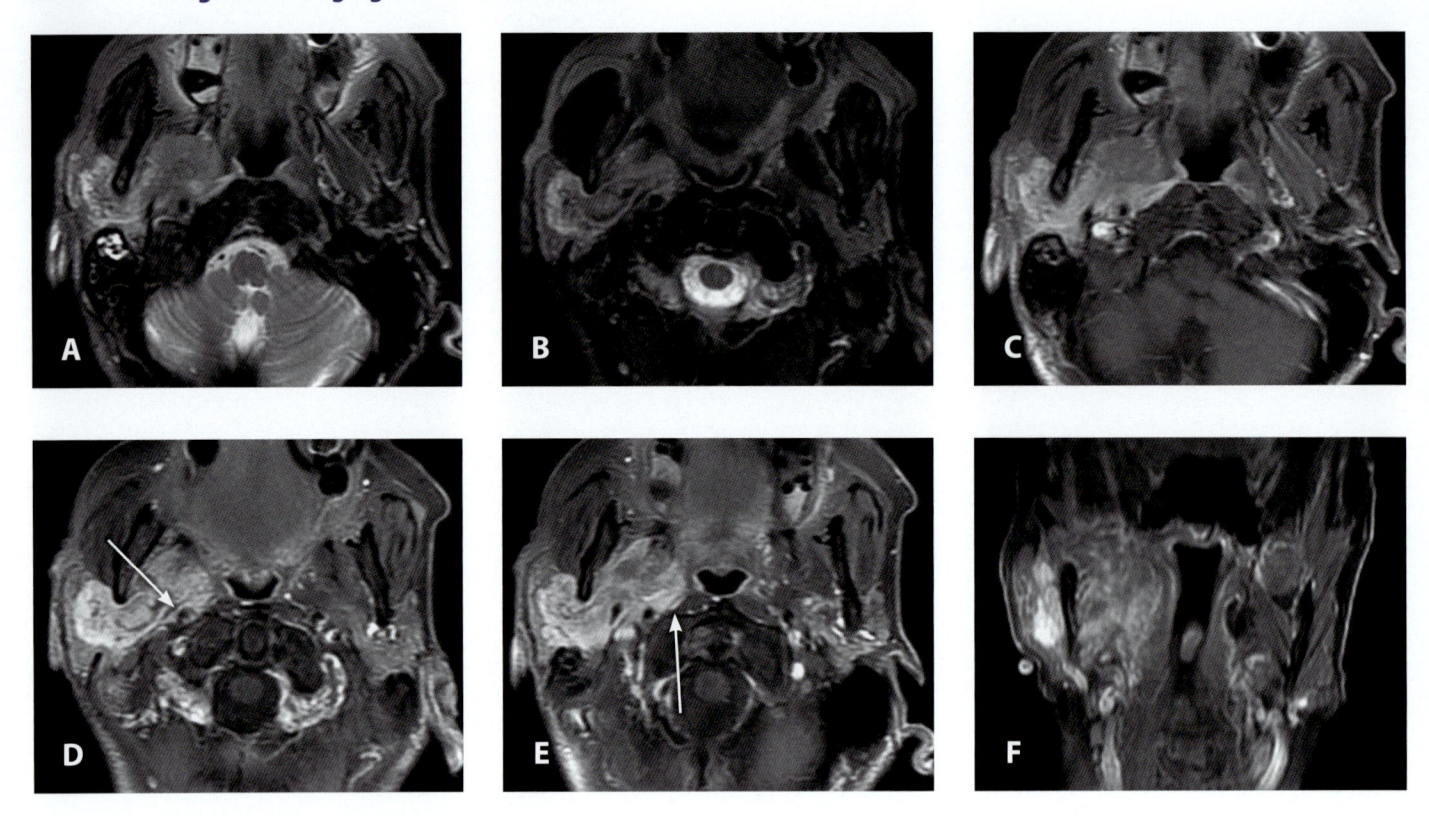

Figure 7-15 Parotid Adenoid Cystic Carcinoma
(**A, B**) Axial T2WI and contrast-enhanced with fat-saturation axial (**C–E**) and coronal (**F**) MR scans. There is a heterogenous mass in both the superficial and deep lobes of the parotid with extension into the right prevertebral muscles just beneath the mucosa of the nasopharynx (*arrow*, **E**). There is probable tumor surrounding the right carotid artery (*arrow*, **D**), making surgical resection difficult.

intermediate signal on T1 and T2 images (**Fig. 7-16**). Central necrosis will increase T2 signal within the mass. Treatment of primary or metastatic SCCa is resection and neck dissection, with postoperative radiation therapy. Most patients are older men, presenting with advanced disease, and thus, prognosis is poor.

SUBMANDIBULAR AND SUBLINGUAL SPACES

The submandibular space (SMS) and the sublingual space (SLS) are the two major spaces of the oral cavity. The salivary glands dominate these spaces, and are subject to a variety of inflammatory and neoplastic lesions. In adults, the most common lesion in this space is nodal metastases from squamous cell carcinoma. The submandibular lymph nodes are the most common site for metastases in squamous cell carcinoma of the floor of mouth. The majority of involved nodes are less than 1cm, necessitating careful imaging evaluation. The main SMS/SLS lesions in the pediatric population are second branchial cleft cysts.

Anatomy

The SMS is located between the floor of the mouth and the hyoid bone. It is enclosed within the superficial layer of deep cervical fascia, except for the posterior border, where it has free communication with the inferior parapharyngeal space and posterior sublingual space. There is also free communication between the two sides of the SMS, allowing disease processes to spread throughout the horseshoe-shaped space. Specifically, the superficial layer of the deep cervical fascia (SLDCF), which encloses the paired, contiguous submandibular spaces, runs along the mylohyoid muscle and the deep aspect of the platysma.

Contents of the SMS include the anterior belly of the digastric muscle, the superficial portion of the submandibular gland, submandibular and submental lymph nodes, the facial vein and artery, and the inferior loop of hypoglossal nerve. Diseases of this space primarily originate in the submandibular gland or the lymph nodes.

The mylohyoid muscle separates the SMS from the paired, contiguous sublingual spaces. These lie superomedial to the SMS, on each side of the genioglossus muscles and are not lined by fascia. The posterior free edge of the mylohyoid provides open communication between these two spaces. The SLS is a potential space with no true fascial lining. The SLS lies within the mandibular arch, and is bounded anteriorly by the mandible, medially by the genioglossus and geniohyoid muscles, inferiorly by the mylohyoid muscle, and superiorly by the mucosa in the floor of the mouth.

Numerous neurovascular structures are located within the SLS, including the sensory branch of cranial nerve V3, the chorda

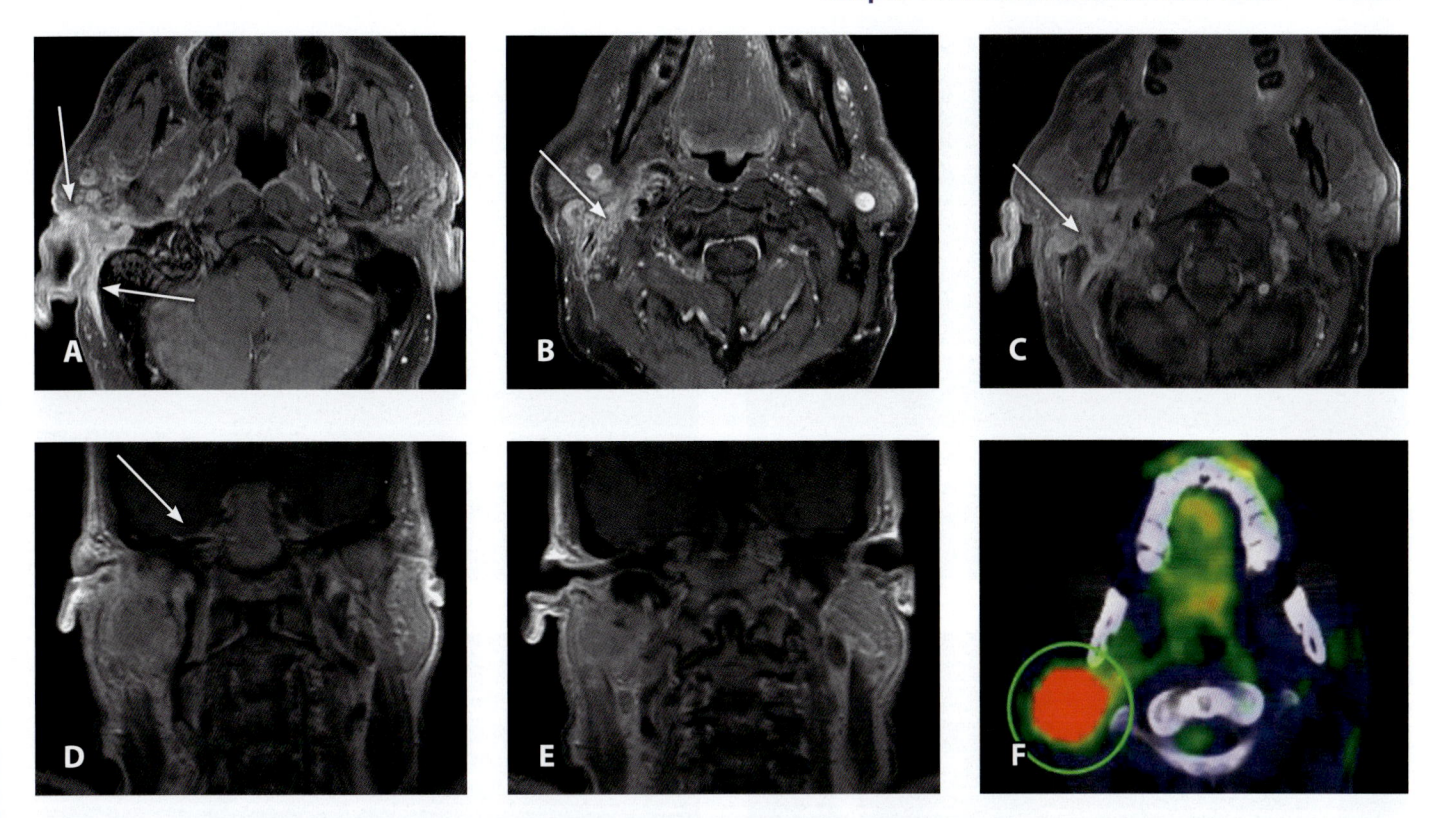

Figure 7-16 Extension of Squamous Cell Carcinoma from the External Auditory Canal
Axial contrast-enhanced with fat saturation **A–C**, coronal contrast-enhanced without fat saturation (**D, E**) MR images and axial fused PET/CT scan. There is a mass originating in the skin surrounding the right ear and external auditory canal (*arrows*, **A**). There is tumor invasion of the superior portion of the parotid gland, surrounding the styloid process and the adjacent skull base at the location of the stylo-mastoid foramen (*arrows*, **B, C**). The lack of fat suppression in **D** and **E**, limits detection of bony and soft tissue involvement, but improves subtle intracranial extension into the dura of right middle cranial fossa (*arrow*, **D**). Detection of such subtle skull base invasion may be difficult with PET/CT (**F**).

tympani branch of cranial nerve VII, cranial nerves IX and XII, and the lingual artery and vein. The submandibular gland wraps around the back of the mylohyoid, with the superficial aspect in the lying in the submandibular space, and the deep aspect, along with the submandibular duct, in the SLS. In addition, this space contains the sublingual glands and ducts. The submandibular duct runs with the lingual nerve laterally to the hyoglossus muscle, while the lingual artery and vein lie deep to the hyoglossus.

Congenital Anomalies of the Submandibular and Sublingual Spaces

Thyroglossal Duct Cyst

Thyroglossal duct cysts are the most common congenital neck masses in childhood. Twenty percent of these anomalies are located in the suprahyoid neck. Suprahyoid thyroglossal duct cysts in the SMS are midline masses that cause a fullness in the floor of the mouth. Thyroglossal duct cysts are low signal on T1-weighted images, hyperintense on T2-weighted images, and they do not enhance unless infected. A sagittal MR image is useful in the case of suprahyoid cysts, as it demonstrates the full course of the lesion through the complicated anatomy of the mouth floor (**Fig. 7-17**).

Second Branchial Cleft Cyst

Second branchial cleft cysts are the most common anomalies of the branchial apparatus. They are most often located in the posterior aspect of the SMS (**Fig. 7-18**). Therefore, as these lesions enlarge, the submandibular gland is pushed anteromedially, the sternocleidomastoid muscle is displaced posterolaterally, and the carotid space moves medially.

MR imaging is useful in defining the total extent of the lesion for complete surgical resection. The lesion appears as a unilocular cystic mass in the posterior SMS at the angle of the mandible.

Vasoformative Malformations

Hemangioma

Hemangiomas are most often seen in infants and children under the age of seven years. They are present at or soon after birth, and enter a proliferative phase which lasts until nine or ten months of age. This is followed by a slower involuting phase that lasts five to ten years. These tumors are nontender, soft, mobile masses with a bright red hue in the overlying skin if the lesion is superficial, or bluish hue if the lesion is deep. Imaging characteristics depend upon the growth phase of the tumor. Proliferating hemangiomas appear as low signal masses on T1-weighted images and high signal masses on T2-weighted images, with intense T1

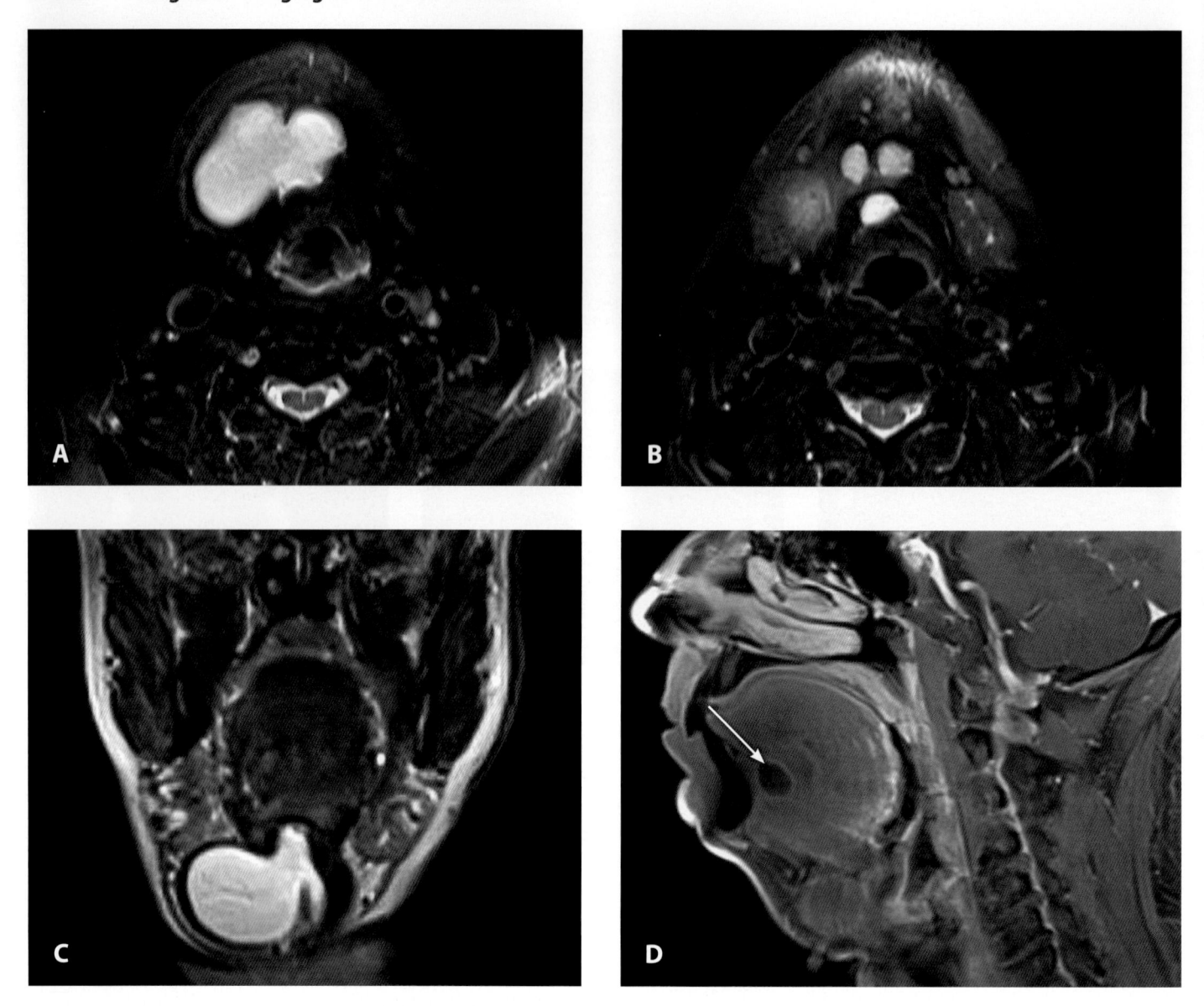

Figure 7-17 Atypical Thyroglossal Duct Cyst
Axial T2 (**A, B**), coronal FSE T2, and sagittal contrast-enhanced with fat-saturated MR images. There is a cystic mass that is located primarily in the submandibular space (**A, C**) with only small components extending down to the level of the hyoid bone (**B**). The tiny cystic component in the base of the tongue (*arrow*, **D**) shows no enhancement which rules out any thyroid remnants in this location.

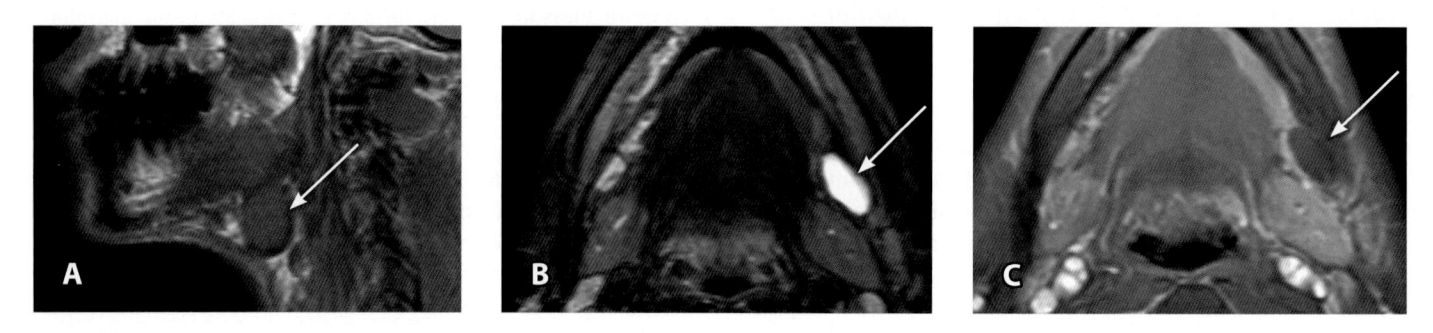

Figure 7-18 Second Branchial Cleft Cyst
Sagittal T1 (**A**), axial T2 (**B**) and contrast-enhanced T1 with fat-saturated (**C**) MR images. There is a purely cystic mass beneath the left angle of the mandible (*arrows*, **A–C**) showing no contrast enhancement.

postgadolinium enhancement and flow voids. In the involuting phase, vascularity decreases, and fibroadipose tissue characterizes the lesion. T1-weighted images appear as high signal masses and T2-weighted images appear as low signal masses. There are no longer flow voids and there is no postcontrast enhancement.

Lymphatic Malformation

In children, large lymphatic malformations, or cystic hygromas, are most often found in the posterior cervical space, but in adults, they are often seen in the SMS, sublingual space, and PS.[5] These lesions present as slowly growing, asymptomatic, soft cervical masses of variable size. The differential diagnosis for cystic hygromas includes a Second Branchial Cleft cyst, a Thyroglossal duct cyst, and a neck abscess. On MR imaging, the cystic hygroma is an insinuating, multilocular fluid intensity mass, with low signal on T1-weighted images, high signal on T2-weighted images, and little to no rim enhancement with contrast.

Inflammatory Lesions of the Submandibular and Sublingual Spaces

Cellulitis (Ludwig's Angina)

Ludwig's angina is a potentially life-threatening, rapidly expanding, diffuse inflammation of the submandibular and sublingual spaces that occurs most often in young adults with odontogenic infections. The anterior teeth are responsible for the initial SLS infection, while the second and third molars, whose apical abscesses tend to perforate the lingual cortex of the mandible below the mylohyoid insertion, cause an initial submaxillary space infection (**Fig. 7-19**). The inflammation is typically caused by cellulitis but can have a component of gangrenous myositis. Causative bacteria include streptococci, staphylococci, gram-negative and anaerobic organisms. Symptoms include severe neck pain and swelling, fever, malaise, and dysphagia. Examination may reveal carious molar teeth, neck rigidity, or drooling. The presence of stridor, dyspnea, decreased air movement, or cyanosis suggests impending airway compromise. Once established, infection evolves rapidly. The tongue may enlarge to two or three times its normal size and distend posteriorly into the hypopharynx, superiorly against the palate, and anteriorly out of the mouth. Immediate posterior extension of the process will directly involve the epiglottis. As the styloglossus muscle leaves the tongue and passes between the middle and superior constrictor muscles to attach on the styloid process, a space called the buccopharyngeal gap is formed. Through this gap, infection can spread to the submandibular and parapharyngeal spaces (**Fig. 7-20**). From the parapharyngeal space (PPS), cellulitis can spread directly into the superior mediastinum.

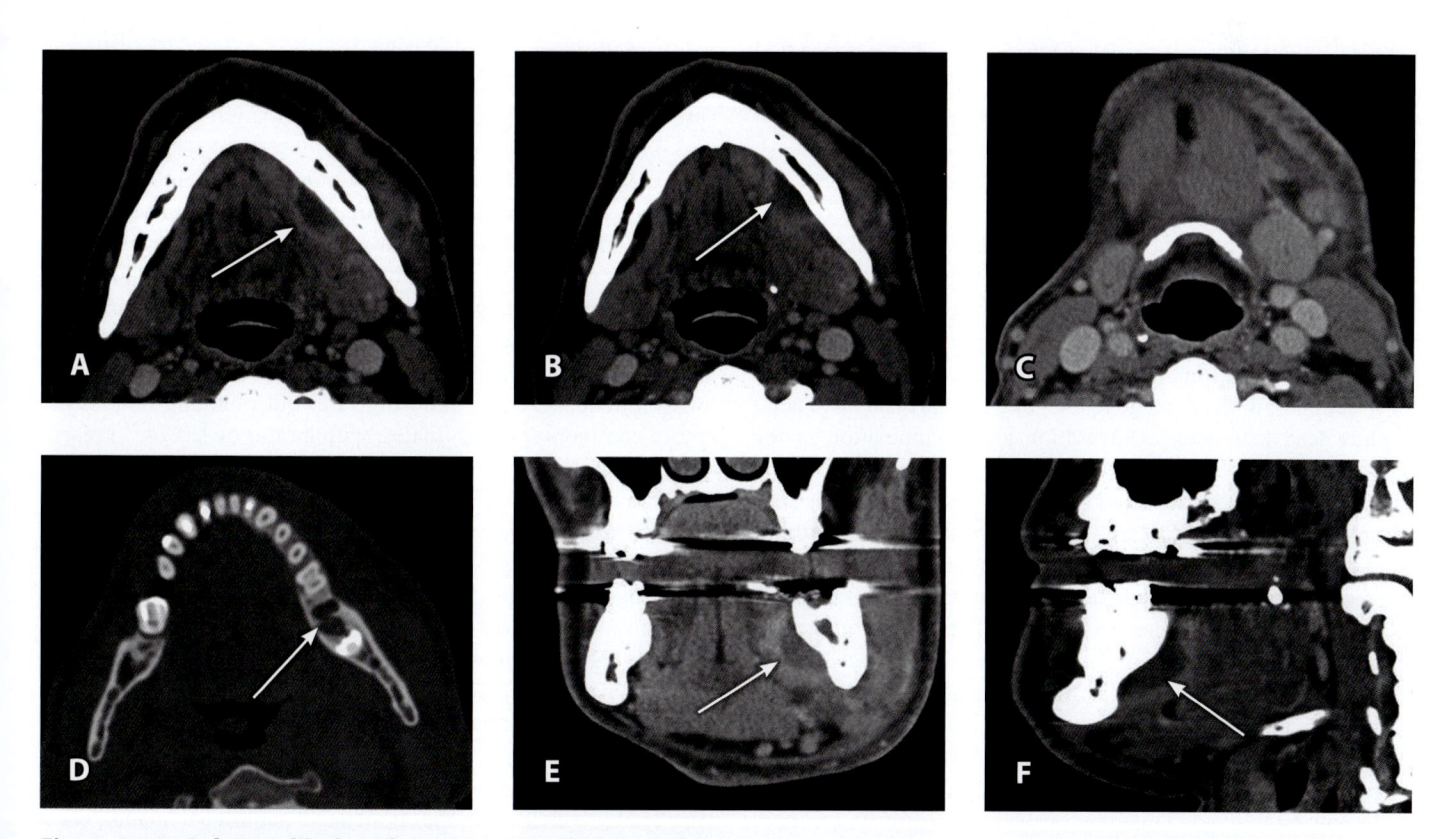

Figure 7-19 Submandibular Abscess Post Tooth Extraction
Axial soft tissue (**A–C**), axial bone algorithm (**D**) reformatted coronal (**E**) and sagittal (**F**) contrast-enhanced CT scans. There is a peripherally enhancing, lucent mass along the lingual surface of the left mandible adjacent to the bony margin (*arrows*, **A, B**). There is extensive left submandibular adenopathy and thickening of the skin and platysma muscle with interstitial lymphatic engorgement, all of which are consistent with cellulitis and myositis. The surgical bed of the extracted molar tooth no. 31 is well-seen (*arrow*, **D**). An abscess of the submandibular space is well-seen in **E** and **F** (*arrows*).

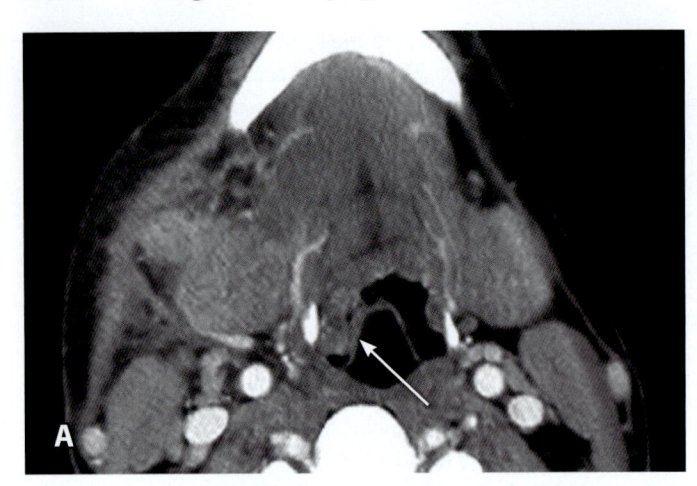

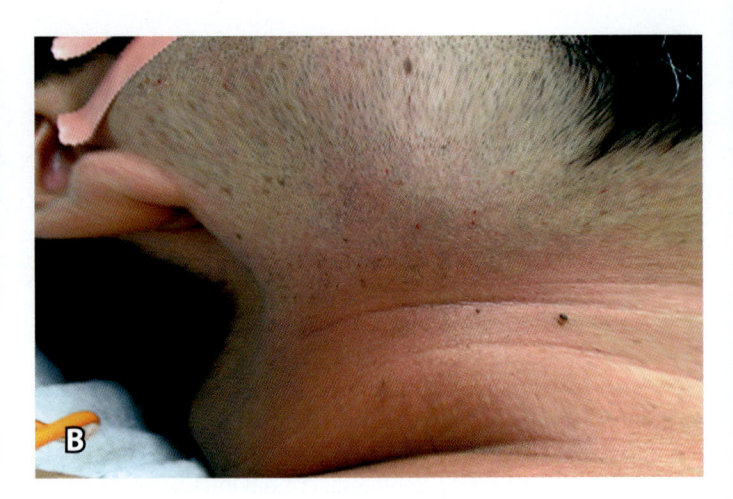

Figure 7-20 Odontogenic Submandibular Cellulitis
Axial contrast-enhanced CT scan (**A**) and photo of the right side of the neck (**B**). The extensive myositic changes in the right neck muscles with submandibular inflammatory changes, including fat stranding and nodal hypertrophy is well seen. Note that the infectious process has extended medially into the vallecula along the right side of the airway (*arrow*, **A**). It is essential that these infectious are identified early by recognizing skin erythema and swelling in the cervical soft tissues (**B**).

Treatment includes protection of the airway, parenteral antibiotics, immediate surgical consultation and possible operative drainage.

SMS infection has high signal intensity on T2-weighted images and strongly enhances with contrast. CT is a better tool to evaluate this region, as it can identify calculi, bone erosion, and gas pockets.

Ranula

Ranulas, also called mucoceles, are mucous retention cysts associated with obstruction or trauma to the sublingual or minor salivary glands. Congenital ranulas can arise secondary to an imperforate salivary duct or ostial adhesion. These are very rare and have been known to spontaneously resolve. Posttraumatic ranulas arise from trauma to the sublingual gland, which causes obstruction or direct damage to the duct. Backpressure and acini rupture lead to mucus extravasation and accumulation in the surrounding tissues. An intense inflammatory reaction to the protein and amylase-rich fluid collection is believed to mediate pseudocyst formation.[53] Rarely, partial obstruction of a sublingual duct will lead to formation of a retention cyst. Oral ranulas are more common on the left side, with a left to ratio of 1:0.62.[54] Simple ranulas are confined to the floor of the mouth, above the mylohyoid muscle.

Large, "plunging" ranulas develop when the wall of the simple ranula ruptures. They extend to other spaces and can present as a unilateral neck mass. Plunging ranulas can develop via several pathways. A retention cyst may penetrate through a dehiscent mylohyoid. This may occur spontaneously, or, more commonly, after surgery for a simple ranula has left scar tissue on the ranula's superior surface. In the latter case, recurrence of the ranula will create a plunging ranula, as the lesion follows the path of least resistance through the mylohyoid. Alternatively, a sublingual gland may penetrate the mylohyoid or an ectopic gland on the cervical aspect of the mylohyoid may develop into a ranula. A third path involves the merging of the submandibular gland or duct with a sublingual duct, which may produce a ranula posterior to the mylohyoid muscle. Rarely, they can arise independently of the oral component. These are pseudocysts, with loose vascularized connective tissue, rather than an epithelial capsule, surrounding a mucinous mass. These lesions are more common on the right side, with a left to right ratio of 1:1.16.[54]

On examination, a ranula will most often present as a painless bluish cyst on the underside of the tongue. They do not change size with chewing or swallowing. Plunging ranulas will appear as neck masses, with or without associated pathology in the oral cavity. Plunging ranulas can expand to an impressive size, with reports of extension to the nasopharynx, skull base, and mediastinum. Simple ranulas are more common in females, with a male to female ratio of 1:1.2, but plunging ranulas are more commonly seen in males, with a ratio of 1:0.74.[54] Presentation is most frequently in the second and third decades of life, with an age range of 2 to 61 years.[55]

Ranulas are sharply marginated, homogenous masses with low signal intensity on T1-weighted images and high signal on T2-weighted images. On CT, these thin-walled cystic lesions have low attenuation (**Fig. 7-21**). Simple ranulas will be found in the SLS, while plunging ranulas have their bulk in the SMS, with a smaller "tail" in the SLS. Ranulas must be differentiated from second branchial cleft cysts, cystic hygromas, and other cystic neck masses.[56]

Ranulas are commonly treated with complete excision of the lesion, often with the associated sublingual gland, via a transoral approach. Recurrence after removal of the gland and lesion is 1.20%.[54] If complete excision is not possible, marsupialization and suturing of the pseudocyst wall to the oral mucosa may be effective, but in this case, the recurrence rate is 66.7%.[54] Plunging ranulas may require both an intraoral and transcervical approach for complete excision. Surgical complications are

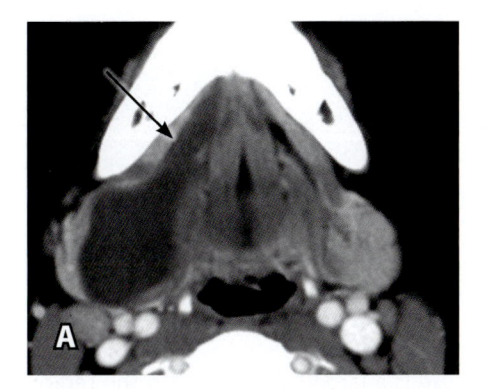

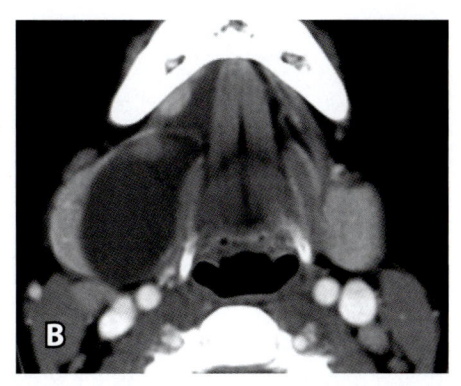

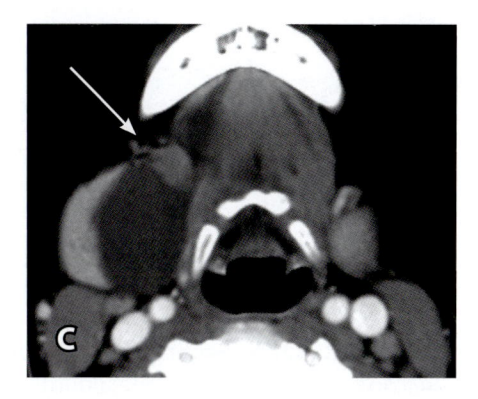

Figure 7-21 Plunging Ranula from the Sublingual into the Submandibular Space
(**A–C**) Axial CT contrast-enhanced CT scans. There is a lucency in the righ side of the floor of the mouth extending longitudinally from anterior to posterior (*arrow*, **A**). The largest component of the cyst extends posteriorly and inferiorly into the adjacent submandibular space. The right submandibular gland is compressed and displaced anteriorly (*arrow*, **C**). (Case courtesy of Wendy Smoker, MD.)

minor and self-limited.[57] Carbon dioxide laser and intracystic injection therapy with OK-432 appear to be safe and effective alternatives to surgery.[58] In pediatric patients, a 5-month period of observation in anticipation of spontaneous resolution is recommended.[53]

Sialoadenitis

Acute submandibular sialadenitis is an inflammation of a submandibular gland resulting from obstruction, stricture, infection, or trauma. Patients present with pain, tenderness, erythema, and swelling. There may be cellulitis, induration of adjacent soft tissues, and expression of purulent material from the submandibular duct (**Fig. 7-22**). The majority of patients are between 31 and 55 years old.[59] Although less common in children, sialadenitis may present with addition symptoms of irritablility and failure to thrive.

In most cases, the inflammation is caused by a calculus in the gland or duct (**Fig. 7-23**). Inflammation of the duct, sialodochitis, usually presents with dilation proximal to the obstruction, or multiple areas of dilation interspersed with stenosis. In cases of bacterial infection, the causative organism is most commonly Staphylococcus aureus. *S. viridans*, *Haemophilus influenzae*, *S. pyogenes*, and *E. coli* are also found. Commonly, the infection results from dehydration, with overgrowth of the oral flora. The major causes are postoperative dehydration, radiation therapy, and immunosuppression from diabetes mellitus, chemotherapy, human immunodeficiency virus, and organ transplant. In addition, mumps, HIV, coxsackievirus, parainfluenza, influenza A, and herpes viruses have been implicated in the development of infectious sialadenitis.

In acute sialoadenitis, edema in the gland will have high signal on T2-weighted images. If sialadenitis is secondary to a calculus, contrast-enhanced, fat-suppressed T1-weighted images will show a unilateral, enhancing gland, and possibly cellulitis and myositis. Calculi may or may not be visualized depending on their size.

Chronic sialadenitis is a slowly progressive inflammatory process, also more commonly seen in adults. It is associated

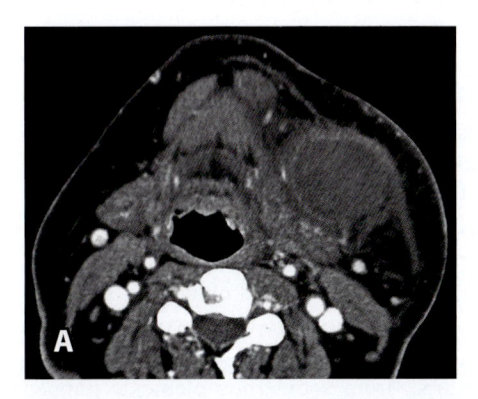

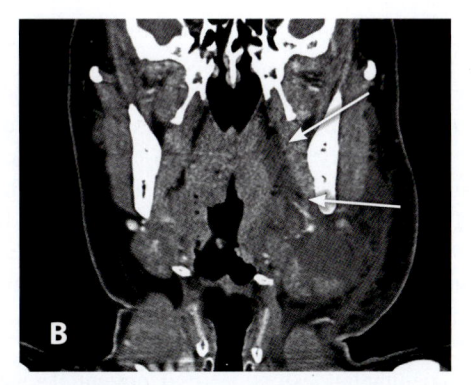

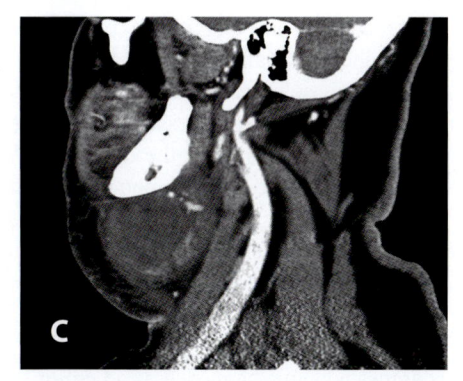

Figure 7-22 Submandibular Sialoadenitis with Parapharyngeal Abscess
Axial (**A**), reformatted coronal (**B**), and reformatted sagittal (**C**) contrast-enhanced CT scans. A large lucent mass is seen beneath the angle of the left mandible with contiguity superiorly and posteriorly with the parapharyngeal space (*arrows*, **B**). Such extensions of submandibular infections into the parapharyngeal space relate to the lack of a natural fascial boundary between these two structures.

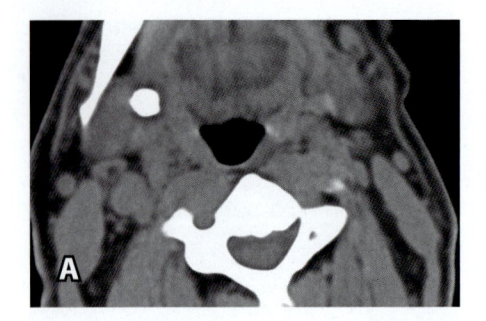

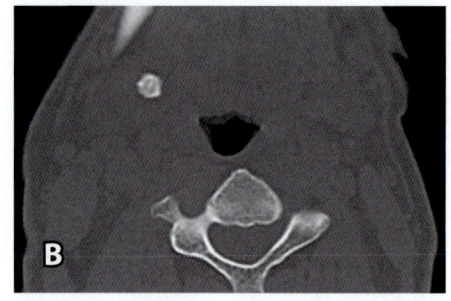

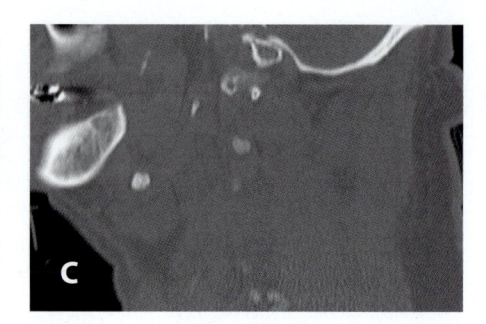

Figure 7-23 Submandibular Gland Duct Calculus
Axial soft tissue (**A**), axial bone algorithm (**B**), and reformatted sagittal (**C**) CT scans. There is a large calcification in the region of the right Wharton duct. Such calculi are difficult to detect with MR and require conventional Panorex images or CT scans for optimal detection.

with conditions linked to decreased salivary flow, including calculi, salivary stasis, repeated acute infections, trauma, radiation, and immunocompromise. Retrograde infection from normal oral flora and recurring acute infections cause inflammatory change in the ductal epithelium. Secretions have increased mucin content, which can lead to slow flow and obstruction. Squamous, oncocytic, or mucous cell metaplasia may develop in the ductal epithelium. Radiation-induced disease is characterized by targeted destruction of serous cells, and replacement with fibrosis and lymphocytic infiltrate consisting primarily of CD4+ subsets.[34]

Patients present with intermittent, painful, bilateral swelling of the glands after eating. The gland is enlarged, with chronic inflammatory infiltrate. T1-weighted MR images will have low signal intensity and T2-weighted images will have intermediate to high signal. There will still be enhancement with contrast. CECT will demonstrate enhancement and possibly scattered, small calcifications. The differential diagnosis includes sarcoidosis, sialotithiasis, granulomatous disease, inflammatory pseudotumor, SS, and Mikulicz syndrome.

Sialadenosis is the noninflammatory, nonneoplastic swelling of a salivary gland in association with acinar hypertrophy and ductal atrophy. Nutritional deficiencies, endocrine disease, metabolic derangements, autoimmune conditions, and certain drugs are causative. Patients present with painless bilateral swelling of the glands.

Chronic sclerosing sialadenitis (CSS), or Kuttner tumor, is a relatively uncommon disease in which the submandibular gland swells and hardens, with the development of progressive periductal sclerosis, dense lymphocytic infiltrate with a predominance of CD8+ cytotoxic T cells, lymphoid follicle formation, fibrosis, and obliterative phlebitis.[60] Chronic sclerosing inflammatory lesions are found diffusely in periductal or interlobular connective tissue and also within lobules, with variable destruction or atrophy of the salivary glandular lobules or acini. CSS is sometimes misdiagnosed as a benign lymphoepithelial lesion or tumor.[61] The exact immunologic etiology is still unknown. CSS is occasionally reported to be associated with sclerosing pancreatitis, an IgG4-related disease,[62] sclerosing cholangitis, and retroperitoneal fibrosis. Imaging findings are non-specific, resembling those in chronic sialadenitis. The submandibular gland is enlarged, with low to intermediate T1 signal, intermediate to high T2 signal, and avid contrast enhancement.

Reactive Adenopathy

The submandibular and submental lymph nodes are found between the hyoid bone and mylohyoid muscle, anterior to a line drawn through the posterior edge of the submandibular gland. The submental nodes, or Level IA, lie between the medial margins of the anterior bellies of the digastric muscles. The submandibular nodes, Level IB, are found posterolateral to the medial edge of the anterior belly of the digastric muscle, anterior to the posterior edge of the submandibular gland.

Level I nodes can be larger than other groups because they are chronically challenged through life, as the primary draining nodes for oropharyngeal, sinus, and facial infection. The differential of an inflammatory process includes bacterial, viral, fungal, and mycobacterial infections, as well as granulomatous diseases. The majority of patients will present with fever and tender lymph nodes.

Benign Tumors of the Submandibular and Sublingual Spaces

Dermoid, Epidermoid, and Teratoid Cysts

Dermoid and epidermoid cysts are developmental or acquired lesions that occur in the head and neck with an incidence of approximately 7%.[63] Twenty-five percent of these are found on the anterior aspect of the floor of the mouth. Other commonly involved areas include the lips, tongue, and buccal mucosa. Epidermoid cysts consist of simple squamous cell epithelium with a fibrous wall. Dermoid, or compound, cysts have various skin appendages, such as hair follicles and sebaceous glands, in addition the epidermoid elements. Teratoid, or complex, cysts contain diverse tissues derived from all three germ layers.

Congenital cysts arise from ectodermic elements trapped during the midline fusion of the first and second branchial arches between the third and fourth weeks of intrauterine life.[64] Alternatively, they may arise from the tuberculum impar of His. This structure, along with the mandibular arches, forms the floor of the mouth and the body of the tongue. Acquired cysts arise from traumatic or iatrogenic implantation of epithelial cells or from the occlusion of a sebaceous gland duct.

Most lesions occur as slowly enlarging masses in the second or third decade of life. On palpation, they are soft and usually smaller than 2 cm. They are painless, but can displace the tongue. Patients may present with dysphagia, dysphonia, and dyspnea.

Epidermoid and dermoid cysts are usually unilocular midline masses, which are well-circumscribed with thin walls. Epidermoids are filled with desquamated keratin, which forms a thick, "cheese-like" paste. They have low signal intensity on T1-weighted images and high signal on T2. Dermoids have a fatty contents, and therefore have high signal on T1-weighted images. On CT, dermoids and epidermoids have a similar appearance, unless the dermoid contains fat. The wall of the cyst usually enhances with contrast. The differential diagnosis of a midline cyst includes thyroglossal duct cyst, ranula, lymphoepithelial cyst, lymphangioma, and cystic hygroma.

Treatment is surgical, with an intraoral or transcutaneous cervical approach depending upon the location and size of the mass. Prognosis is good, with a low incidence of relapse.[65] Epidermoids and dermoids are most often benign, but malignant transformation of a long-standing dermoid cyst to squamous cell carcinoma has been reported.[66]

Benign Mixed Tumor (Pleomorphic Adenoma)

BMT are the most common salivary gland neoplasms. Approximately half of submandibular tumors are benign, and pleomorphic adenomas make up 90% of these lesions.[67] Grossly, the tumors are smooth and encapsulated. The capsule, however, is incomplete microscopically, and tumor pseudopodia may extend beyond the margin of the apparent capsule. The contents of the tumor appear varied depending on the cellularity and the myxoid content. The characteristic feature of the tumor is morphologic diversity, with presence of both epithelial and mesenchymal elements. Epithelial cells make up the majority of the cellular regions, and myoepithelial cells make up stromal areas. The ratio of cellular elements to stromal elements can vary widely. The stromal component may have a myxoid, fibroid, or chondroid appearance. In the submandibular gland, these tumors present as a painless, isolated mass. Malignant transformation occurs in 2% to 5% of all salivary gland BMT.[68] Treatment is complete surgical excision of the tumor with wide margins to capture microscopic pseudopodia and tumor budding, and thereby reduce the chances of recurrence.

Small BMT are solitary, well-circumscribed, spherical masses with low signal intensity on T1-weighted images, and high signal on T2. Contrast enhancement is low to intermediate. Larger adenomas may have foci of necrosis and hemorrhage and mixed T1 and T2 signal. On CT, focal calcification or ossification may be seen in larger tumors.

Lipoma

Lipomas are the most common soft tissue mesenchymal tumors. However, they comprise only 1% to 1.4% of all benign oral lesions.[69] In the oral cavity, they may occur in the major salivary glands, buccal mucosa, lip, tongue, palate, vestibule, and floor of mouth. The most common location in the maxillofacial region is the buccal mucosa.[70]

Lipomas will have high signal intensity on T1-weighted images and no contrast enhancement. Fat suppression will cause a concomitant decrease in signal for both the lesion and the subcutaneous fat.

Malignant Tumors of the Submandibular and Sublingual Spaces

Submandibular Gland Tumor

Submandibular and sublingual gland tumors are more aggressive than parotid tumors, with a worse prognosis. Approximately half of submandibular gland tumors are malignant. Tumor fixation to the mandible or infiltration of the skin suggest extraglandular malignant extension. Weakness of the tongue suggests hypoglossal or lingual nerve involvement.[45]

Treatment is wide local excision with adjuvant postoperative radiotherapy in the cases of perineural invasion, positive margins, or lymph node metastases. Positive cervical lymph nodes is an indication for modified radical neck dissection. Regional recurrence occurs in approximately half of patients.[71]

On imaging, carcinomas of the submandibular gland appear as invasive masses arising from the gland, often with adjacent malignant lymphadenopathy. The routine use of MRI evaluation in the postoperative period may identify changes indicative of recurrent disease months to years before it is clinically evident.[47]

Adenoid Cystic Carcinoma

Adenoid cystic carcinomas (ACC) comprise 10% of all salivary gland tumors, but are the most common malignant tumor of the submandibular gland.[71] The tumor grows slowly, but relentlessly, with good short-term survival, but poor survival at 10 to 20 years.[49] ACC metastasizes to distant sites, such as lungs and bones, rather than to lymph nodes. Women are more commonly affected than men, and the cancer usually arises in the fifth through seventh decades.

Grossly, adenoid cystic carcinomas are usually monolobular and nonencapsulated. They have a gray-pink color and infiltrate the surrounding normal tissue (**Fig. 7-24**). Microscopically, the tumors consist of basaloid epithelial elements that form cylindrical structures. Tumors are classified by the general architecture into three types. The cribriform pattern has a basophilic mucinous substance filling cystic spaces, resembling Swiss cheese. In the tubular pattern, the cells are arranged in smaller ducts and tubules with less prominent cystic spaces. This variety has the best prognosis. The solid type is characterized by sheets of neoplastic cells with few cystic spaces.[49] This subtype has a reported 10-year survival rate of 0%.[45] Any given tumor may contain all three patterns. All types have a propensity for perineural spread and aggressive behavior. Successful disease control is related to size of the original tumor, presence of perineural invasion, and positive tumor margins, which demonstrates the importance of preoperative imaging evaluation.[48]

Mucoepidermoid Carcinoma

Mucoepidermoid carcinoma is by far the most common malignant salivary gland tumor, in both adults and children. It occurs

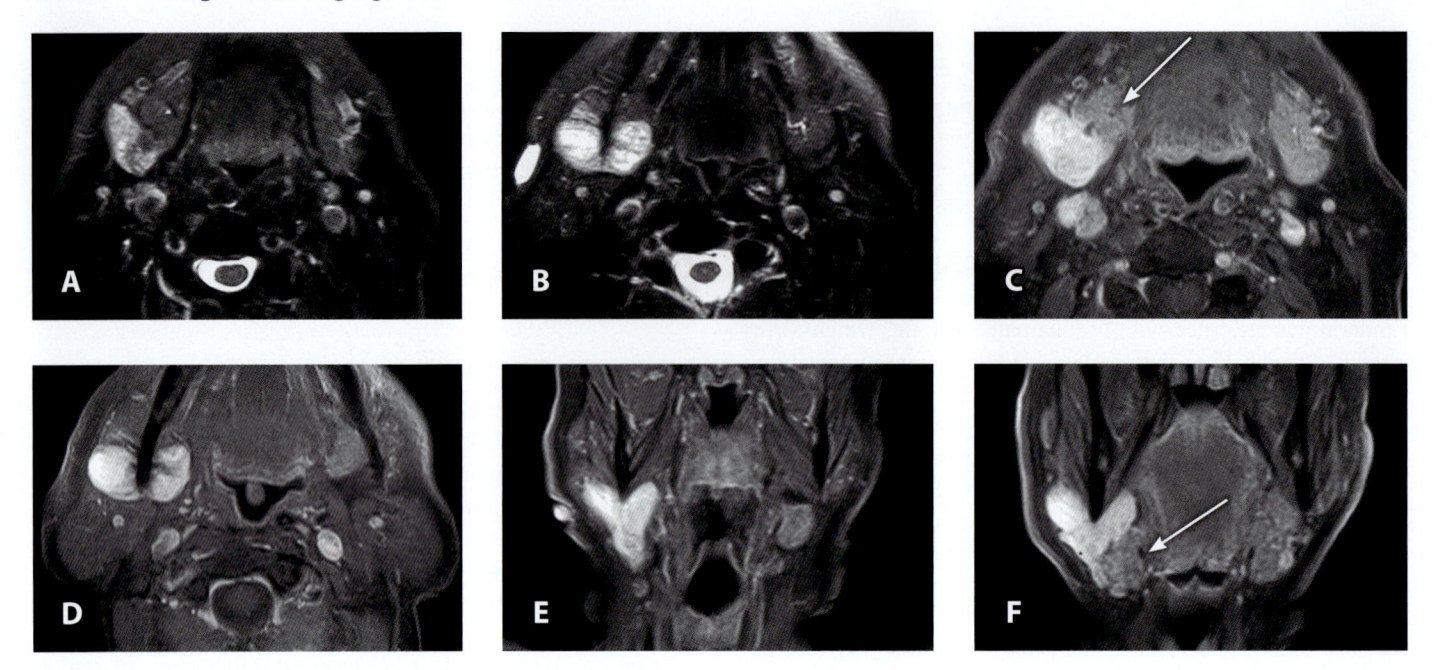

Figure 7-24 Submandibular Adenoid Cystic Carcinoma
Axial T2W (**A–B**) and contrast-enhanced T1W (axial, **D** and coronal **E–F**) MR images. The submandibular gland tumor straddles the inferior border of the angle of the right mandible with multiple adjacent foci of lymphadenopathy. There is exophytic growth along the posterior and lateral borders with preservation of a portion of the submandibular gland (*arrows*, **C, F**).

in the major and minor salivary glands, and is more common in women. These tumors normally present as painless, slow growing, cystic masses.

Mucoepidermoid carcinomas comprise a variable mixture of mucous cells, intermediate cells, clear cells, and epidermoid cells. Most tumors have a combination of solid and cystic growth. Submandibular gland mucoepidermoid carcinoma metastasizes more frequently than the same cancer in other salivary glands.[72] High-grade mucoepidermoid carcinomas with a predominance of anaplastic epidermoid cells must be differentiated from primary and metastatic squamous cell carcinoma. The distinction relies on the histochemical demonstration of mucin within tumor cells.[49]

Squamous Cell Carcinoma and Lymphoma

Primary SCCa does not normally occur in the submandibular and sublingual glands. It readily extends from the mucosal surface of the oral cavity, or due to anterior extension from the tongue base to invade the submandibular space. Level 1 and 2 nodes must be carefully assessed, as bilateral nodal spread is common. In one study, 88% of metastatic lymph nodes were less than or equal to 10 mm in diameter, making detection difficult.[73] Obstruction of the submandibular or sublingual glands is often a presenting symptom of carcinoma of the floor of the mouth. Nodal metastases from squamous cell carcinoma may demonstrate necrosis and excapsular spread. On T1-weighted images, nodes will be isointense with muscle. Necrosis will have low signal on T1, and will enhance with contrast. Necrosis has high signal intensity on T2-weighted images.

Primary lymphoma of the salivary glands is rare. Multiple, enlarged, nonnecrotic lymph nodes suggest non-Hodgkin's lymphoma. Patients will have many small, painless, rubbery masses in the submandibular space. Systemic symptoms may include fever, weight loss, fatigue, and night sweats. Lymphomas have low signal intensity on T1-weighted images and low to high in signal intensity on T2-weighted images, with variable contrast enhancement (**Fig. 7-25**).

THE MASTICATOR SPACE

The masticator space (MS) encloses the muscles of mastication, the temporalis, masseter, medial and lateral pterygoids, the ramus and posterior body of the mandible, the motor and sensory branches of the mandibular division of the trigeminal nerve (CN V3), and the inferior alveolar artery and vein. Lesions in this space are primarily infectious, most often from odontogenic sources, and neoplastic. In all cases of neoplastic disease, complete assessment of CN V3 for perineural spread is vital. The second and third molars abut the anterior aspect of the space, and are frequently the source of MS lesions. The buccal space, which includes the buccinator muscle, the distal portion of the parotid duct, the facial artery and vein, and the buccal fat pad, is also anterior to the MS, and is often involved by extension of inflammatory of neoplastic processes. The posteromedial border of the MS is shared with the fatty parapharyngeal space, which is displaced posteriorly or medially by expanding MS lesions. The parotid space lies posterior to mandibular ramus.

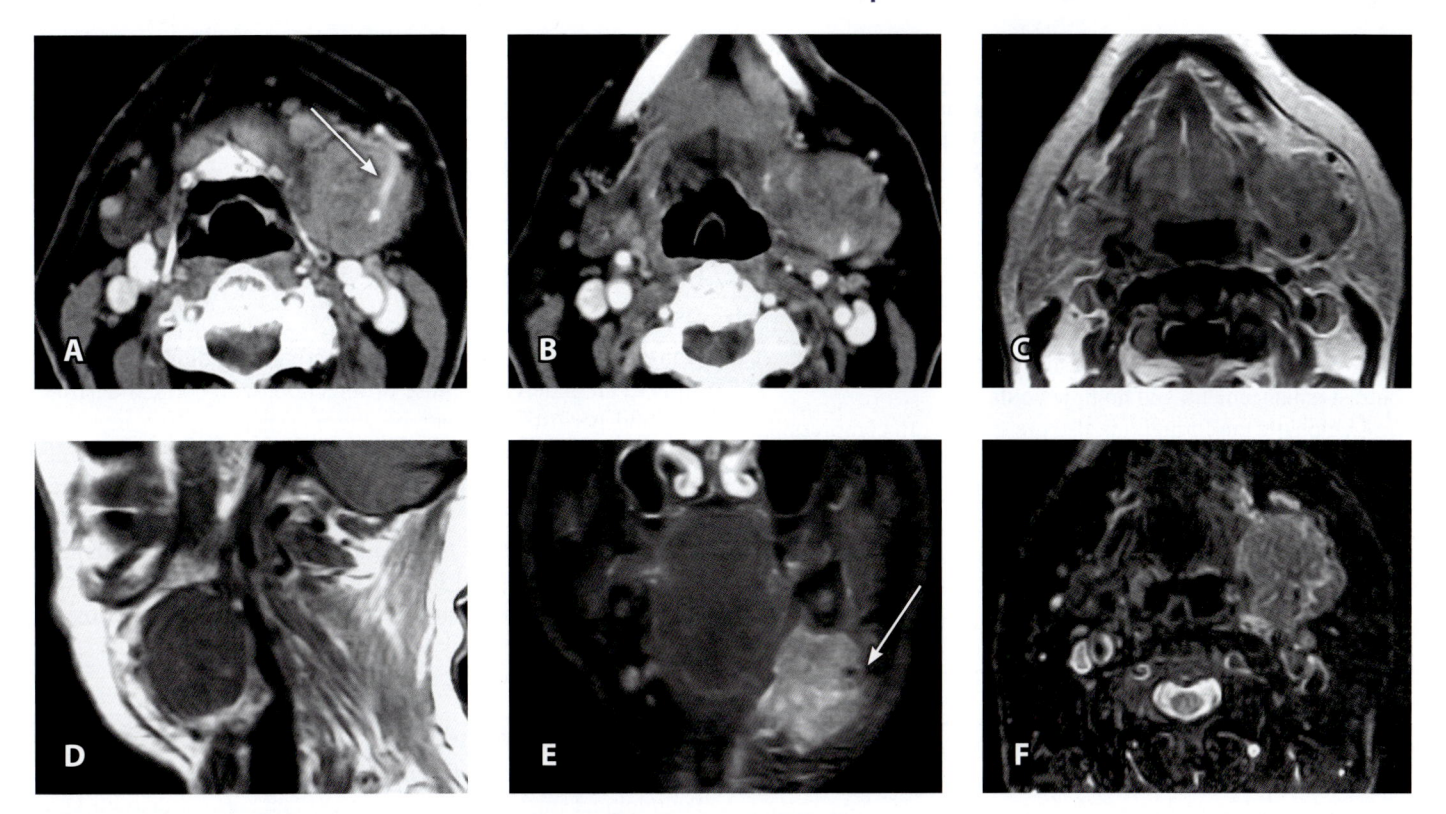

Figure 7-25 Submandibular Undifferentiated Squamous Cell Carcinoma
Axial contrast-enhanced CT scans (**A–B**), axial T1W (**C**), sagittal T1W (**D**), coronal T2W (**E**), and axial T2W (**F**) MR images. There is a bulky mass encompassing the entire left submandibular gland and surrounding its vascular supply (*arrows*, **A, E**).

Anatomy of the Masticator Space

The superficial layer of DCF extends from the clavicle, inferiorly, to the skull base superiorly. At the mandible, the DCF splits to enclose the MS. On the lateral aspect, the fascia extends over the masseter muscle, attaches to the zygomatic arch, covers the temporalis, and attaches to the cranial ridge. The medial or deep layer of DCF, which extends to the skull base, is attached from the medial pterygoid plate to the sphenoid spine. The deep fascial layer attaches to the skull base medial to the foramen ovale, allowing direct disease spread between the MS and intracranial compartment.

The mandibular branch of the fifth cranial nerve (V3), provides motor innervation to the muscular derivatives of the first pharyngeal arch: the masseter, temporalis, medial pterygoid, lateral pterygoid, mylohyoid, anterior belly of the digastric, tensor veli palatini, and tensor tympani. It also provides sensation to the face, teeth, mouth, nasal cavity, and dura. The small motor root and large sensory root of the trigeminal nerve extend from the lateral pons and course through the prepontine cistern to the petrous apex. From the trigeminal cistern in Meckels' cave, V3 emerges from the trigeminal ganglion and leaves the intracranial compartment through foramen ovale. Extracranially, V3 descends between the tensor veli palatini and lateral pterygoid muscles before dividing into muscular branches.

Perineural tumor spread can involve any portion of the nerve, transmitting disease from the MS intracranially, or from the brain to the MS. In addition, connections between branches of the trigeminal nerve and the cranial nerve VII via the auriculotemporal nerve, the vidian nerve, and the greater petrosal nerve permit further perineural spread.

Surgical procedures, lesion drainage, and radiotherapy planning require complete delineation of tumor or inflammation. Radiologic assessment of the MS should include its entire span, from the superolateral border on the cranial ridge, to the inferior extent at the submandibular space. Disease processes can extend a significant vertical distance because the superficial fascial layer covering the temporalis muscle attaches high on the scalp. The entire course of the trigeminal nerve should be evaluated, including foramen ovale and the mandibular foramen, because perineural spread allows for intracranial invasion and extension into the cavernous sinus. Similarly, fungi, such as Mucor, can enter the cranium through the vasculature. The pterygopalatine fossa is another vulnerable entry point for disease, allowing spread to the inferior orbital fissure and orbital apex. Several benign anatomic variations in this region can be mistaken for pathology. In 20% of patients, accessory parotid tissue surrounds the parotid duct, and should not be mistaken for a mass. Unilateral or bilateral hypertrophy of the masseter, often seen in patients with bruxism, can resemble pathologic change. Similarly, unilateral denervation atrophy can make the normal masseter appear pathologically enlarged.

Vasoformative Anomalies of the Masticator Space

Vascular malformations are common congenital anomalies found in the masticator space. Hemangiomas are soft, compressible, benign tumors that appear at birth or shortly thereafter. They proliferate in the first year of life, and then spontaneously regress. On MR imaging, hemangiomas appear as poorly marginated, lobulated masses. Signal intensity depends on the age of the lesion, with those in the proliferative stage appearing as high flow lesions and those in the involuting stage appearing as low flow lesions. In the proliferative phase, signal intensity is low on T1-weighted images, high on T2-weighted images, and contrast enhancement is intense. Focal flow voids and phleboliths may be present. The involuting phase produces high signal intensity on T1 images, low signal intensity on T2 images, no contrast enhancement, and no flow voids.

Lymphatic malformations also present as soft, compressible masses at birth, or within two years of birth. Unlike hemangiomas, they do not spontaneously involute. These lesions are most often cystic, with multiple dilated spaces and stromal septations. They are infiltrative and often invade multiple anatomic spaces. Skin, soft tissues, and bone can all be involved in the lesion. T1-weighted images have low signal, while T2-weighted images have high signal and fluid/fluid levels. There is usually no contrast enhancement, although there may be subtle enhancement of the rim or septations, especially if the lesion is infected. These are low flow lesions, and therefore no flow voids are present. Spontaneous intralesional hemorrhage alters the signal characteristics of the cystic content, increasing the signal on T1-weighted images, and variably changing T2-weighted images.

Inflammatory Lesions of the Masticator Space

Infection is a primary reason for focused evaluation of the masticator space, and odontogenic abscess is the most common lesion in this site. Infections commonly arise from extraction of a molar tooth, and less commonly can result from chronic dental caries, severe gingivitis, and traumatic osteomyelitis. It is vital to identify abscesses, which require antibiotic treatment and surgical drainage.

Cellulitis

Cellulitis appears as "dirty" fat, which represents dilated lymphatics and venules within the tissue. The fat will appear brighter than normal on CT, and similarly, will demonstrate increased T2 signal, and decreased T1 signal. Myositis appears as diffuse swelling of the muscles, with decreased attenuation on CT, and increased signal on T2-weighted MR images.

Odontogenic Abscess

Odontogenic abscesses in the MS result primarily from molar infections or dental procedures. Less often, osteomyelitis or malignant otitis externa in diabetic and immunocompromised patients can produce these lesions. Odontogenic abscesses are common in areas where dental care and antibiotics are not readily available, and in individuals with poor dental hygiene.

Trismus in often the presenting symptom, necessitating an imaging, rather than clinical evaluation. Fever, leukocytosis, and pain and swelling of the cheek are addition symptoms. Treatment includes aggressive intravenous antibiotics and surgical drainage. Untreated abscess can spread to the floor of the mouth and sublingual and submandibular spaces, or superiorly in the suprazygomatic MS and to the skull base. Antibiotic treatment of odontogenic infection may ameliorate systemic signs of infection, leaving a persistent local infection that can evolve into an abscess. CT has traditionally been the preferred imaging method for MS and mandibular lesions, but in some cases, MR imaging has provided improved visualization of inflammatory changes and differentiation of lesions in this space.[74]

Osteomyelitis

Non-enhanced CT is useful in detecting mandibular osteomyelitis as an underlying cause of infection, with cortical destruction and periosteal elevation, sclerotic changes, and myositis. Contrast enhancement will demonstrate the abscess, showing fluid density with a thick, enhancing rim. On MR, T1-weighted images will have low signal intensity around the mandible, loss of normal cortical bone signal void, and loss of medullary fat signal. T2-weighted images will highlight the abscess with high signal, and may show increased signal or subperiosteal fluid within the medullary cavity. On contrast-enhanced T1, the abscess will have low signal with an enhancing wall.

Osteoradionecrosis

Osteoradionecrosis of the mandible can mimic osteomyelitis. Pathological fractures, fragmentation, and cortical disruption of the bone can be visualized on CT. The overlying soft tissues will enhance and appear thickened. On MR, the bone marrow will have abnormal low intensity signal on T1, high signal intensity on T2, and intense contrast enhancement. Adjacent muscles will show thickening, appear hyperintense on T2-weighted images, and diffusely enhance.[75]

Benign Tumors of the Masticator Space

Nerve sheath tumors, schwannomas and neurofibromas, are the most common benign tumors of the masticator space. Rapid growth and pain may indicate malignant transformation.

Schwannoma

Schwannomas are slow-growing benign tumors of the peripheral nervous system that arise from Schwann cells and displace, rather than invade nerve fascicles.[76] Macroscopically, they are firm, rubber-like, encapsulated masses. Histologically, they are composed of compact, hypercellular Antoni A , and looser, cystic Antoni B tissue. Internal cystic change, associated with mucinous degeneration, hemorrhage, necrosis, and the formation of microcysts, becomes more prominent as the tumor increases in size.

Clinically, schwannomas present as slow-growing, painless masses. They are the most common asymptomatic mass in the deep facial soft tissues. Symptomatic cases present with masticator muscle weakness, facial pain or paresthesia, decreased sensation in the chin and mandible, and rarely, trismus.[77] Schwannomas may arise sporadically or may be associated with neurofibromatosis type 2. Typically, these tumors appear in the third or fourth decade, affecting both genders equally.

Fifty percent of trigeminal nerve schwannomas are found in Meckel's cave, 20% in the cisternal segment of the nerve, and

5% arise in the distal intracranial branches and extend extracranially.[78] In the masticator space, they appear as well-circumscribed fusiform or ovoid masses following the course of V3, which lies along the medial border of the lateral pterygoid muscle.

T1-weighted images demonstrate a mass that is iso- or hypointense to muscle. On T2, the tumors are isointense to muscle if they are very cellular or hyperintense if they contain cystic areas. Contrast-enhanced images show homogeneous enhancement. On non-enhanced CT, the tumors appear iso- to hypointense to muscle. Contrast enhancement is mild to moderate. CT nicely demonstrates the characteristic smooth enlargement of foramen ovale, the mandibular foramen, and the mental foramen where tumor remodels bone. Masticator muscle atrophy shows reduced volume and fatty infiltration with high signal.

Intraosseous schwannomas are rare, but well described.[79] The significant size and length of the trigeminal nerve in the inferior alveolar canal makes the mandible a common site for these lesions. They can cause bone destruction and expansion of the cortical plates of the mandible, displacement of teeth, and erosion of the root surface. The tumor can involve the bone by eroding it from the outside, or by arising within a nutrient canal or centrally within the bone. Differential diagnosis of an intraosseous schwannoma in the oral region includes desmoplastic fibroma, well-differentiated fibrosarcoma, odontogenic fibroma, benign fibrous histiocytoma, and neurofibroma. Strong, diffuse staining with antibodies for S-100 protein supports the diagnosis.

Traditionally, schwannomas are treated with surgical resection. Complete resection can be difficult, and may result in new neurological deficits. Subtotal resection commonly results in tumor recurrence.[80]

Neurofibroma

Neurofibromas are benign, well-circumscribed, nonencapsulated nerve sheath tumors composed of uniform fibroblasts and neuronal elements in a collagen matrix. They express S-100 protein, but less diffusely and strongly than schwannomas.[81] Neurofibromas exhibit different morphologies, grow at highly variable rates, and occur in multiple locations. One classification system stratifies these tumors into five types: localized cutaneous, diffuse cutaneous, localized intraneural, plexiform, and massive soft tissue neurofibromas. Only plexiform neurofibromas have malignant potential.

Solitary neurofibromas of the trigeminal nerve are very rare, but auriculotemporal nerve involvement has been reported.[82] The presence of neurofibroma in a young person, multiple fibromas, or plexiform neurofibromas, strongly suggests Neurofibromatosis Type 1. Symptoms result from tumor mass, functional disorder, or paresthesias resulting from nerve atrophy as the tumor replaces nerve tissue.

Management depends on the location and growth pattern of the neurofibroma. The majority are treated surgically when they produce functional or cosmetic deficits. Medical therapies have been investigated to arrest neurofibroma development by targeting environmental, cellular, and molecular targets.[83]

On contrast-enhanced CT, the tumor demonstrates homogenous enhancement, with significant fatty replacement and multiple cystic areas. These tumors remodel, but do not destroy bone unless there has been malignant transformation. They have intermediate signal intensity on T1-weighted images, and are hyperintense on T2.

Malignant Tumors of the Masticator Space

Muscle and bone are the main components of the masticator space, so it follows that sarcoma is the most common primary malignant tumor found in this compartment. Osteosarcoma, chondrosarcoma, synovial sarcoma, and rhabdomyosarcoma are the most commonly seen varieties. In children, a solid mass arising in the MS is considered a rhabdomyosarcoma until proven otherwise. Rarely, previous radiation therapy for head and neck tumors can cause the development of sarcomas after a latency of several years. Aggressive fibromatosis is an unusual tumor that is characterized by local invasion, but bland histology and no metastasis. Squamous cell carcinoma, the most common head and neck malignancy, can invade via direct extension from the aerodigestive tract, or by perineural spread on V3. Systemic non-Hodgkin's lymphoma and metastatic disease from lung, breast, colon, and prostate cancers may also be found in this space.

Sarcoma

One percent of all neoplasms are sarcomas. Of these, 5% to 15% occur in the adult head and neck, and 35% are found in the pediatric head and neck.[84] Fibrosarcomas are the most common soft tissue sarcomas in the adult, while rhabdomyosarcomas are the most common in children. In 80% of patients, sarcomas present as painless masses.[84] However, depending upon the location of the tumor, impingement by the tumor may cause compressive symptoms. Clinical examination will reveal a submucosal mass, differentiating these tumors from squamous cell carcinoma. Imaging studies can help with diagnosis of the non-specific mass, revealing size and location, bone destruction, intracranial involvement, and regional nodal disease. MRI has superior soft-tissue resolution and is best able to evaluate the primary lesion, perineural extension, dural involvement, bone marrow replacement, and orbital invasion. CT has increased sensitivity for bony abnormalities. For surgical planning, both modalities can be used in a complementary fashion. Contemporary management of sarcomas includes a multidisciplinary approach using a combination of surgery, radiotherapy, and chemotherapy specific for tumor type, histologic grade, and stage of disease. Radiotherapy can be employed as neoadjuvant, adjuvant, or primary local therapy depending on the site and type of tumor, the availability and acceptability of the surgical option, and the efficacy of the chemotherapy.

Fibrosarcoma

Fibrosarcoma is a tumor of mesenchymal cell origin that is composed of malignant fibroblasts in a collagen background. It can occur as a soft tissue mass or as a primary or secondary bone tumor. Primary fibrosarcoma develops within the medullary canal, or peripherally, from the periosteum. The more aggressive, secondary fibrosarcoma, arises from a pre-existing lesion or after radiotherapy to an area of bone or soft tissue.

Five percent of fibrosarcomas occur in the head and neck.[84] Patients are typically in their fourth to fifth decade, and present with a painless mass in the face, neck, or scalp. There is a slight male preponderance. The slow growing lesion will usually reach a substantial size before causing symptoms. Metastasis occurs in at least 60% of cases, and the 5-year disease-free survival rate is between 32% to 57%.[85] Treatment is wide surgical excision. High-grade tumors may require adjuvant radiation or chemotherapy.

In the head and neck it can be difficult to differentiate fibrosarcoma and aggressive fibromatosis. Both lesions destroy bone and aggressively invade surrounding structures. On T2-weighted MR images, these tumors have relatively low signal, reflecting high cellularity, increased nuclear-to-cytoplasm ratio, and the presence of fibrous tissue.[86] The tumor will show moderate enhancement with contrast. On CT, the homogeneous soft tissue mass may demonstrate areas of calcification, and will enhance with contrast.[87]

Rhabdomyosarcoma

Rhabdomyosarcomas are the most common soft tissue tumor of childhood, and the third most common extracranial solid tumor after neuroblastoma and Wilms tumor. They represent 3% to 4% of all malignancies in children. Most cases are appear to be sporadic, but the tumor has been associated with familial syndromes, such as neurofibromatosis and Li-Fraumeni syndrome.[88] Thirty-five percent of these tumors are found in the head and neck. In the MS, they typically present in children less than ten years old as a painless, rapidly enlarging mass which medially displaces the pharyngeal mucosa. Rhabdomyosarcomas in the head and neck may arise in the orbit, middle ear, nasopharynx, intratemporal fossa, paranasal sinuses, parotid gland, oral cavity, pharynx, thyroid, scalp, or neck. Tumors of these areas are most often of the embryonal subtype, with round and spindle cells.[89] This subtype is known to have loss of heterozygosity at the 11p15 locus, the site of the insulin-like growth factor (IGF-II) gene, and a loss of imprinting, leading to overexpression of IGF-II.[90]

Symptoms include trismus, resulting from masticator muscle or temporomandibular joint involvement, and sometimes pain from bone destruction and nerve involvement. The tumors can destroy the mandible and spread to the skull base and intracranial compartment.

Rhabdomyosarcomas fall under the category of small, round, blue-cell tumors of childhood. The four histological types include: embryonal, consisting of round and spindle cells; alveolar, with non-cohesive cells surrounding a central lightly populated area; pleomorphic, with pleomorphic and spindle-shaped cells, and mixed, which includes two or more cell types.

MR is the best imaging modality for assessment of these tumors because of its superior ability to characterize soft tissues. Diagnostic imaging describing tumor origin, size, local extent, invasiveness, and nodal spread is important for assigning risk-based therapy. In addition, MR is useful for postsurgical identification of residual or recurrent tumor.[91] Rhabdomyosarcomas are aggressive, but well-circumscribed. They are isointense to muscle on T1-weighted images and intermediate on T2. They enhance homogeneously with contrast, unless areas of necrosis are present (**Fig. 7-26**). MRI or CT of draining lymph nodes is also performed to identify regional nodal spread. PET/CT has also proven useful in this role, identifying unusual sites of soft tissue and bony metastases not appreciated on exam or by other imaging modalities. PET/CT is also useful in evaluating surgical margins.[91]

Prognosis is based upon ability to control local disease. Multimodality treatment protocols have significantly improved outcomes in recent decades.[92]

Osteosarcoma

After Multiple Myeloma, osteosarcoma is the most common primary malignant tumor of bone, accounting for approximately 20% of primary bone cancers. In children, osteosarcoma is the most common malignant bone tumor. Approximately 8% of osteosarcomas arise in the head and neck, with the majority of these found in the adult mandible and maxilla.[93] Seventy-five percent of all osteosarcomas occur in patients younger than 20 years of age. A second peak occurs in the fifth and sixth decades,

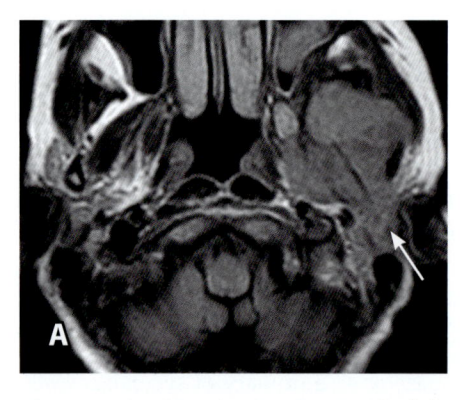

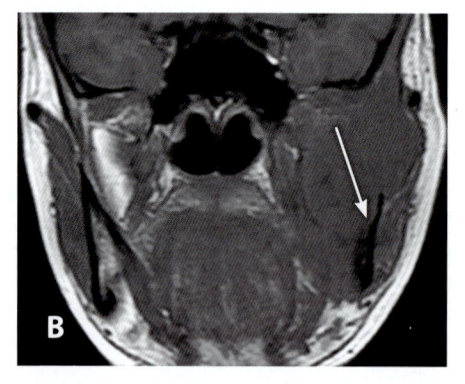

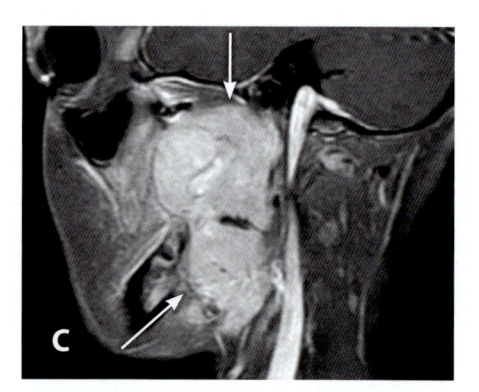

Figure 7-26 Masticator Space Rhabdomyosarcoma
Axial T1WI (**A**), coronal T1WI (**B**), and sagittal contrast-enhanced T1WI with fat saturation (**C**). There is a large, homogenously-enhancing circumscribed mass arising from the left masticator space with extension superiorly to the skull base (*arrows*, **C**), inferiorly into the submandibular space (*arrows*, **C**) and laterally into the parotid space (*arrow*, **A**). The mass has invaded the marrow and obliterated the inner cortical margin of the mandibular ramus (*arrow*, **B**). Postoperative pathology confirmed embryonal rhabdomyosarcoma.

when osteosarcoma represents a complication of Paget disease, irradiation, or bone infarcts. In patients with head and neck osteosarcoma, the tumor normally presents in the third or fourth decade.[85] Individuals with hereditary retinoblastoma are several hundred times more likely to develop osteosarcoma due to mutations in the Rb gene. Most tumors have some type of combined inactivation of the Rb and p53 tumor suppressor pathways.[94]

Grossly, osteosarcomas are gritty, gray-white tumors with hemorrhage and cystic degeneration.[38] They spread into the medullary canal, infiltrating and replacing marrow. The tumor cells create bone, and may additionally create cartilage and fibrous tissue.

Osteosarcomas typically present as painful, progressively enlarging masses. These lesions are highly malignant and metastasize aggressively. Head and neck osteosarcoma metastasizes less often than the same tumor at other sites, with 7% to 17% of individuals developing distant disease, usually in the lungs and brain.[85]

Treatment is amputation, or if possible, limb-sparing surgery, combined with chemotherapy. Adjuvant radiotherapy is important for disease control in high-grade soft-tissue sarcomas. Prognosis is clearly related to tumor grade and margin status.[93] Five-year survival is approximately 55% (Ha), and 5-year disease-free survival from 23% to 37%.[93] In some studies, disease of the mandible and maxilla have an better prognosis than other head and neck sites due to straightforward surgical access.[95]

Imaging demonstrates a large, destructive, mixed lytic and blastic mass with permeative margins. The tumor frequently breaks through the cortex and lifts the periosteum, resulting in reactive periosteal bone formation. Features on imaging studies reflect the most abundant histologic elements. Highly malignant lesions exhibit considerable similarity to one another on imaging studies. The degree of calcification and ossification will determine the appearance of osteosarcoma on both CT and MR images. CT images demonstrate tumor comprise dense bone or a soft tissue mass with associate bone destruction. A spiculated periosteal reaction in a "sunray" pattern is characteristic of this tumor. On MR images, dense mineralization appears as signal void. The soft tissue component of the tumor will have high T2-weighted signal and enhance. Infiltration of the marrow will appear as intermediate signal characteristic of tumor replacing the normally high signal marrow.

Chondrosarcoma

Chondrosarcoma is the second most common primary malignant bone tumor after osteosarcoma. The malignant cells of this tumor form from cartilage rather than osteoid. These tumors can arise in cartilaginous structures, bone derived from chondroid precursors, or areas where cartilage isn't found from cartilaginous differentiation of primitive mesenchymal cells.[96] Five to 10% of head and neck sarcomas are of this variety. Half are found in the sinonasal cavity and the other half in the mandible and larynx. Primary chondrosarcomas arise from normal tissues. Secondary chondrosarcomas, which make up 10% of the total, develop from pre-existing benign cartilaginous lesions such as enchondromas and osteochondromas, or from fibrous dysplasia or Paget's disease.[38]

The tumor is composed of malignant hyaline and myxoid cartilage. Nodules of grayish tissue comprise this bulky tumor. Calcifications and central necrosis are often present. The tumor pushes into surrounding tissue, differentiating it from the invasive action of aggressive fibromatosis. Adjacent cortex is thickened and eroded.[38]

MR images demonstrate the intramedullary and soft tissue extent of the tumor. CT images demonstrate the presence of cortical destruction and the character of matrix mineralization patterns. Chondrosarcomas typically have low signal intensity on T1-weighted images and intermediate to high signal on T2-weighted images. Heterogeneity on T1, T2, and postcontrast images correspond pathologic tumor composition. On T2-weighted images, mineralization will appear as low signal, while focal areas of high signal correspond to hyaline cartilage, focal cystic changes, or hemorrhage.[97] Patients present with a painful, enlarging mass. Treatment is surgical excision. The role of chemotherapy and radiotherapy has not been well-established. Five-year survival is 87.2%.[96]

Radiation-Induced Sarcoma

Radiation-induced sarcoma (RIS) is a complication of radiation treatment for head and neck cancer, seen in up to 0.8% of cases.[98] These cases are very rare, but could rise as increasingly effective therapies extend the lives of cancer patients, and as the number of patients in our aging population proliferates. The prognosis for patients with these tumors is poor, more so when the tumor in the head and neck, with one studying reporting a five-year disease-free survival rate of only 8%.[99] In a study of 15 patients treated for nasopharyngeal carcinoma, radiation-induced osteosarcoma developed in the maxilla of 5 patients and the mandible in 7 patients. The latent period ranged from 4 to 27 years.[100] RIS has a bimodal pattern of age distribution with the highest incidence at ages 10 to 19 years and a second peak after age 50.[101]

CT images of RIS demonstrate a soft tissue mass which destroys bone, as well as new tumor bone formation. The treatment for RIS includes surgery, radiotherapy, chemotherapy, or a combination of these.

Aggressive Fibromatosis (Desmoid Tumor)

Aggressive fibromatosis (AF) is a neoplastic process with unusually characteristics. These tumors present as large invasive lesions that often recur after excision, but histologically, they have a bland appearance, consisting of well-differentiated fibroblasts. They have infrequent mitoses and do not metastasize. The pathogenesis is most likely multifactorial, with genetic, environmental, and endocrine factors contributing to tumor development.[102] Up to 30% of cases are related to trauma.[103] Risk of developing AF is significantly increased in patients with the familial form of AF, familial adenomatous polyposis, and Gardener's syndrome, as all are due to mutations of the APC gene on chromosome 5q22.[104] The APC gene regulates the cellular level of beta-catenin, which when increased, leads to tumor proliferation. All desmoid tumors, even those without an APC mutation, overproduce beta-catenin.

These tumors can arise anywhere in the body. They are most often confined to the musculature and overlying aponeurosis or fascia. Occasional lesions may involve the periosteum and lead to bone erosion.[105] Twelve percent to 15% of all desmoids arise in the head and neck, most commonly in supraclavicular fossa, but also in the orbit, mandible, scalp, and palate.[106] In the head and neck, invasion of vascular structures and compression of the airway cause more severe symptoms and increased mortality. Morphologically, the tumors are gray or white, firm, poorly demarcated masses that are rubbery and infiltrate surrounding structures. The central part of the tumor is densely collagenous, and the younger periphery is occupied by plump fibroblasts.

Patients present between puberty and 40-years old, with a peak between 25 to 35 years old. In most cases, AF is a painless enlarging mass, although pain and neurologic symptoms have been reported.[105] AF in the pediatric population is rare. The age distribution of cases peaks at 8 years of age, and there is a slight male predominance.[102] Children with AF in the head and neck present at a slightly younger age. Treatment is surgical, unless there is a significant risk of mutilation or functional impairment. In these cases, varying combinations of external beam radiation, nonsteroidal anti-inflammatory drug (NSAIDs), tamoxifen, cytotoxic chemotherapy, or observation proved efficacious.[107] The recurrence rate is approximately 50%.[102] Spontaneous regression in sporadic cases has been reported.[108]

Imaging studies are essential in planning therapy and in posttreatment monitoring. Signal intensity can be variable on both T1 and T2-weighted images due to the inconsistent distribution of collagen, fibroblasts, and fibrosis in the tumor. In most cases, the tumor will be isointense on T1-weighted images, heterogeneously hyperintense on T2-weighted images, and will enhance avidly with contrast (**Fig. 7-27**). The mass may be

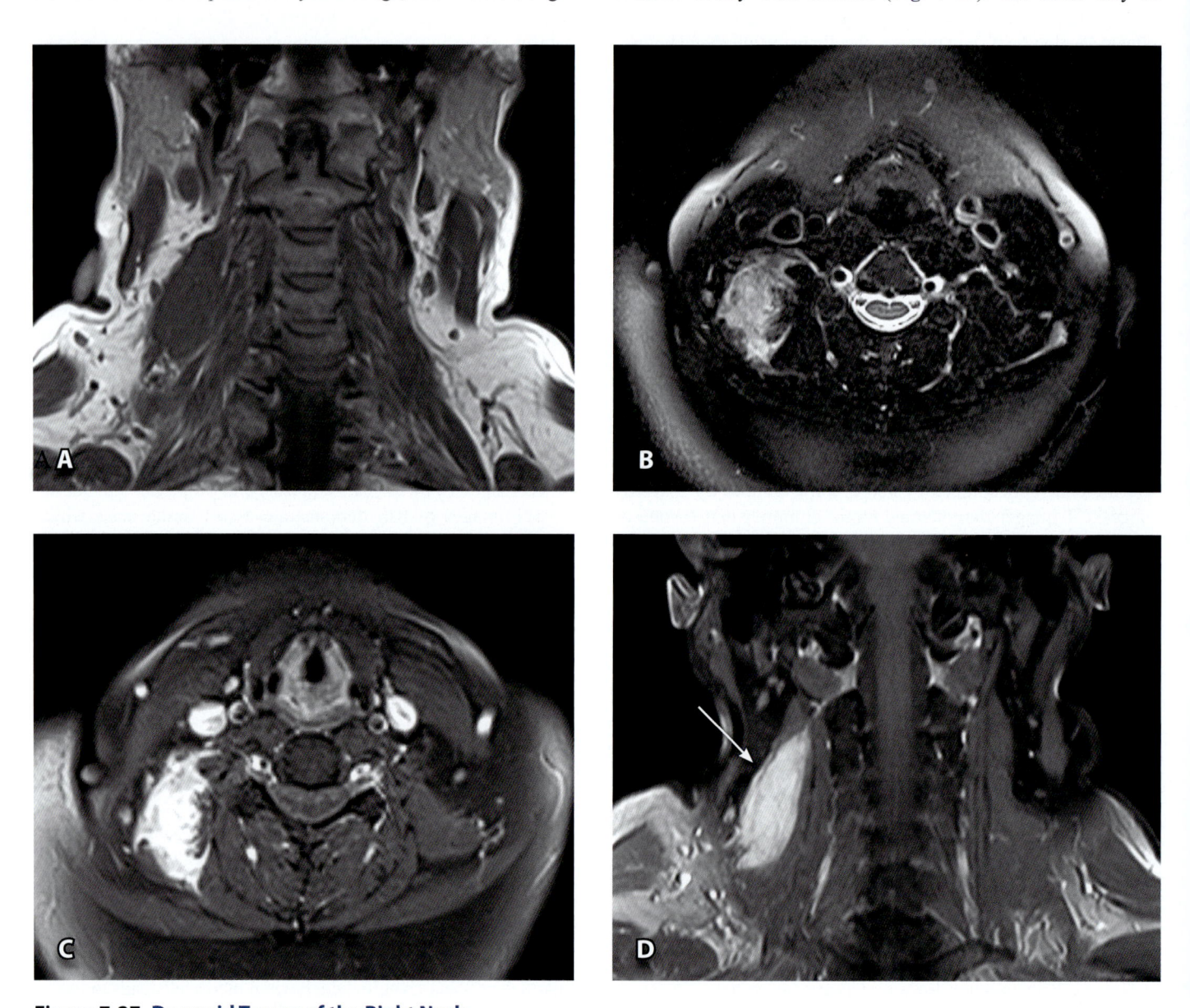

Figure 7-27 Desmoid Tumor of the Right Neck
Coronal T1W (**A**) axial T2W (**B**), axial contrast-enhanced (**C**) and coronal contrast-enhanced coronal (**D**) MR images. There is a nonspecific mass in the right posterior neck that appears to extend across natural fascial planes. Such tumors are typically highly-invasive and often recurr following surgical resection.

ovoid or irregular and may show low signal intensity bands on all images. Unlike soft-tissue sarcomas, they do not demonstrate central necrosis.[109]

Extension of Primary Malignancies

Squamous cell carcinoma is the most common malignancy to invade the MS. Tumor from the retromolar trigone and anterior tonsillar pillars are most commonly seen. Fascial planes, muscle, and bone can be invaded. Muscle invasion has intermediate signal intensity on T1-weighted images and intermediate to high signal on T2, differentiating the tumor from the surrounding low T2 signal of muscle. Contrast enhancement is moderate. Tumor replacement of bone marrow has the same imaging characteristics. Colon, prostate, breast, lung, or thyroid cancer can metastasize to the mandible, or less commonly, the maxilla. Lymphoma can infiltrate the MS muscles, bones, or lymph nodes. Patients with non-Hodgkin Lymphoma (NHL) in the MS may present with pain or trismus, with or without lymphadenopathy. On MR, lymphoma is isointense to muscle on T1, hyperintense on T2, and enhances diffusely. Nodes are not necrotic or calcified unless the patient has been treated.

THE CAROTID SPACE

Neurovascular structures dominate the carotid space (CS),[110] therefore most lesions of this area are vascular and neoplastic. Schwannomas and paragangliomas are the primary tumors of this space. Invasion from nearby sites of SCC and nodal metastases are also common. Vascular lesions such as internal jugular vein and carotid artery thrombosis and carotid aneurysm are additional lesions often found in the CS.

Tumors in this space will displace the internal carotid artery (ICA) anteriorly, in contrast to parotid gland pathology, which will displace the ICA posteriorly. In addition, lesions of the CS characteristically displace the parapharyngeal space anteriorly and the styloid process anterolaterally. Disease processes can spread from the CS to the intracranial compartment through the jugular foramen.

Anatomy of the Carotid Space

The CS extends from the skull base to the aortic arch. All three layers of deep cervical fascia contribute to its fascial boundary. Some consider the CS to be the retrostyloid compartment of the parapharyngeal space, as it is separated only by thin fascia of the styloid musculature. The suprahyoid portion of the CS stretches from the jugular foramen to the hyoid bone, and the infrahyoid portion extends from the hyoid to the aortic arch. The CS is bordered by the PPS anteriorly, the PS laterally, the RPS medially, and the vertebral bodies posteriorly.

The vascular contents of this space include the common carotid artery (CCA), ICA, and the internal jugular vein (IJV). The ICA branches from the CCA at the level of the hyoid bone. The IJV is the continuation of the sigmoid sinus as it emerges from the skull base, terminating where it joins the subclavian vein. The IJV lies posterolateral to the ICA and CCA near its origin, but becomes anterolateral to the lower CCA.

Cranial nerves IX–XII and the sympathetic plexus are the nervous structures of the CS. The sympathetic plexus lies within the medial fascial wall of the CS, between the CS and RPS. The Vagus nerve (CN X), travels with the CCA and IJV in the CS throughout the suprahyoid and infrahyoid neck, while cranial nerves IX, XI, and XII travel in the CS in the suprahyoid neck, through the level of the nasopharynx, and then exit at the level of the soft palate.

The internal jugular lymph nodes are closely related to the CS. The upper jugular, level 2 nodes originate at the intersection of the IJV and posterior belly of the digastric muscle and extend to the hyoid bone. The mid-jugular, level 3 nodes run from the hyoid to the cricoid cartilages. The lower jugular, level 4 nodes extend from the cricoid cartilage to the clavicle.

Anatomic features of the CS which can facilitate the identification and localization of lesions include its direct connection to the jugular foramen, and its proximity to other easily visualized spaces and structures.

Vascular Lesions of the Carotid Space

Carotid Artery Dissection and Pseudoaneurysm

Internal carotid artery pseudoaneurysm is a contained rupture of the artery resulting from loss of integrity of the arterial wall's three layers. It can arise as a rare complication of infection from the PPS or RPS,[111] or more commonly from blunt or penetrating trauma. Neoplastic blow-out, surgery, and radiation therapy also can produce pseudoaneurysms (**Figs. 7-28** and **7-29**).[112] Bacteria implicated in pseudoaneurysm formation, including *Staphylococcus*, *Streptococcus*, and *Bacteroides*, may provide a septic focus resulting in arteritis.[111] Salmonella and Klebsiella, which produce elastase, are commonly found in lesions in intravenous drug abusers. Other, less common causes of pseudoaneurysm include fibromuscular dysplasia, Ehlers-Danlos syndrome, Behcet's disease, and syphilis.

Patients may present with pain, fever, dysphonia, or dysphagia. Neurological symptoms, such as Horner's syndrome and lower cranial neuropathy may be evident. On exam, the pseudoaneurysm is an expanding pulsatile mass at the lateral aspect of the neck. Imaging will demonstrate an outpouching in the ICA wall. Contrast-enhanced CT demonstrates abnormal contrast accumulation contiguous with the vessel lumen.[113] On MR images, the ICA wall is enlarged, with variable signal due to a variety of blood products in the wall thrombus. Contrast-enhancement will demonstrate an enhancing lumen and wall, with low signal intensity thrombus. Angiography is the gold standard for evaluation of ICA pseudoaneurysm, but CTA and contrast-enhanced MRA are useful alternatives.[114,115]

Bacterial pseudoaneurysms are treated with endovascular occlusion with or without surgical ligation, and antimicrobial therapy.[111,116] To date, there have been no randomized controlled trials to establish optimum management of blunt carotid artery injury. Currently available treatment modalities are anticoagulation, antiplatelet therapy and open surgery. More recently, reports of endovascular treatment of these injuries have appeared and this may in time provide a viable alternative to the more invasive surgical options.

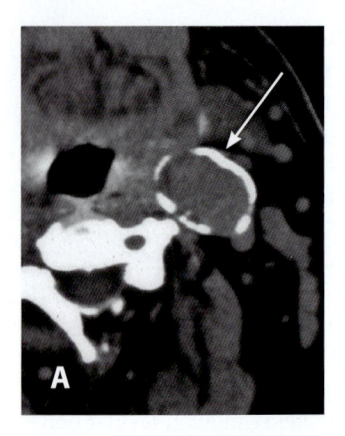

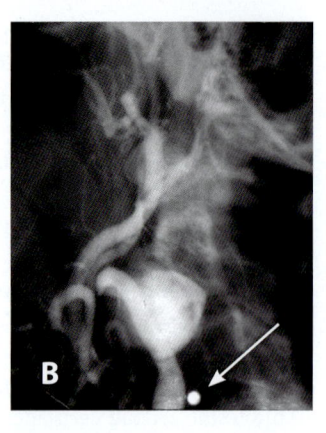

Figure 7-28 Traumatic Carotid Artery Pseudoaneurysm
(**A**) Axial unenhanced CT scan and (**B**) lateral angiographic view of the left common carotid artery. There are curvilinear calcifications within the left carotid space (*arrow*, **A**). A large pseudo-aneurysm of the left carotid artery is well seen on the angiogram. The patient had sustained a gunshot from a "B-B" gun with a metallic remnant in the neck (*arrow*, **B**).

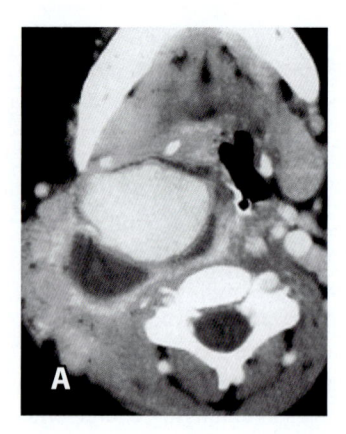

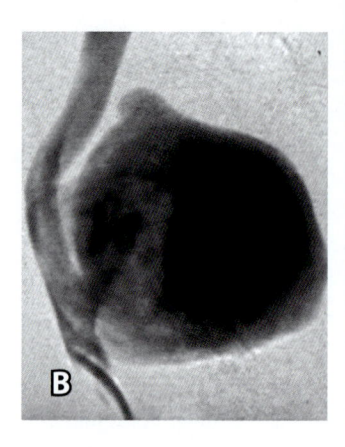

Figure 7-29 Internal Carotid Artery Pseudoaneurysm
(**A**) Axial CT scan with contrast. There is partial contrast filling of a large right neck mass. The unenhanced portion represents partial thrombosis of the internal carotid artery. (**B**) Selective right internal carotid angiogram showing the large pseudoaneurysm. (Case courtesy of Wende Smoker, MD and Susan Blaser, MD.)

ICA dissection results from an intimal tear, which allows blood to enter the potential space between the intima and media of the vessel wall. A subintimal dissection tends to result in stenosis of the arterial lumen, whereas a subadventitial dissection may cause aneurysmal dilatation of the artery. The hematoma can track from carotid bifurcation to skull base. Dissection is related to trauma, connective tissue disorders, neck manipulation, recent infection, and the presence of underlying vasculopathy.[117-119] Spontaneous carotid artery dissections occur in the United States at a rate of 2.5 to 3 per 100,000 annually.[119] These occur in all age groups, but are an important cause of stroke in young and middle age patients. The cause of spontaneous dissection is thought to be related to an underlying structural defect of the extracellular matrix, resulting from a combination of genetic and environmental factors. Individuals with Ehlers-Danlos syndrome type 4, Marfan's syndrome, and osteogenesis imperfecta type 1 are at increased risk.[120] Hypertension has also been implicated in the development of spontaneous dissection.[121] Patients present with a classic triad of severe neck pain, face pain, or headache, oculosympathetic palsy, and cerebral or retinal ischemia in one-third of cases. The presence of two of these symptoms strongly suggest the diagnosis.[119] Neurological symptoms most often occur within 24 hours, but can take as long as 2 months to manifest.[122] Treatment is anticoagulation, antiplatelet agents, or both.

An intimal flap or double lumen are pathognomonic findings, but occur in less than 10% of cases. In one-third of cases, an aneurysmal dilation will be seen. Normally, the vessel lumen will be narrowed compared to the normal vessel on the opposite side. On axial T1-weighted fat saturated MR images, a hyperintense crescent, representing intramural hematoma, will be visualized next to the ICA lumen (**Fig. 7-30**). T2-weighted images will also demonstrate the bright cresent. There is no enhancement with contrast. The radiological differential diagnosis includes infection or neoplasm adjacent to the vessel. These entities can be differentiated from dissection by clinical presentation and contrast enhancement.[123]

Jugular Vein Thrombosis

IJV thrombosis is most commonly the result of intravenous drug injection into the IJV or from an iatrogenic source, such as central venous catheter placement. Other causes include a history of neck surgery, trauma, infection, nodal disease, hypercoagulable state, and systemic malignancy (Trousseau's syndrome). Thrombophlebitis may lead to thrombosis, or the thrombosis may become secondarily infected, producing septic thrombophlebitis. Lemierre syndrome – thrombus precipitated by an oropharyngeal infection – is characterized by sepsis, IJV thrombophlebitis, and pulmonary or distant metastatic abscesses. It is rare since the widespread use of antibiotics, but may be found in underprivileged populations. Treatment is antibiotics and abscess drainage if necessary.

Spontaneous IJV thrombosis is rare, and is most commonly associated with central venous catheters.[124] It has been reported to result in pulmonary embolism in 16% of patients.[125] Gram positive organisms are found in this setting, while septic thrombophlebitis found in IV drug users is more commonly due to methicillin-resistant *S. aureus*.[126] IJV thrombosis complicates neck dissection in up to 30% of cases, most often due to wound infection, fistula, or radiation treatment.[127-130] Free flap reconstruction has a similar thrombosis rate, but patency is regained in greater than 90% of cases.[131]

Thrombophlebitis occurs when infections of the oropharynx, pharynx, sinuses, middle ear, or parotid glands spread to the CS. The infection spreads via local tissue planes, venules, or lymphatics. Sepsis may occur 7 to 10 days after onset.

Patients present with fever, leukocytosis, and neck pain and swelling. Important complications of IJV thrombosis and thrombophlebitis include pulmonary embolism, thrombosis of the

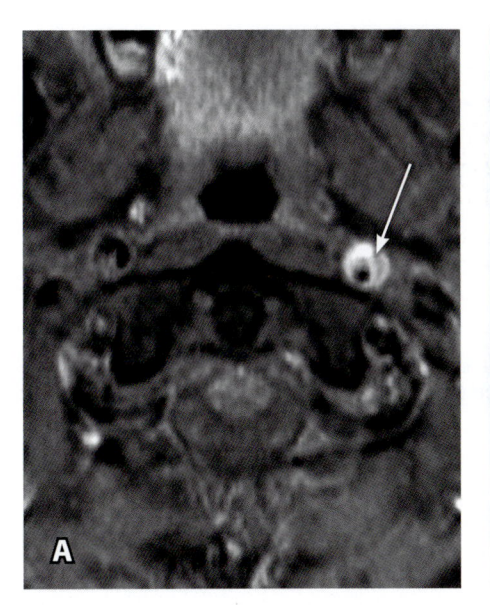

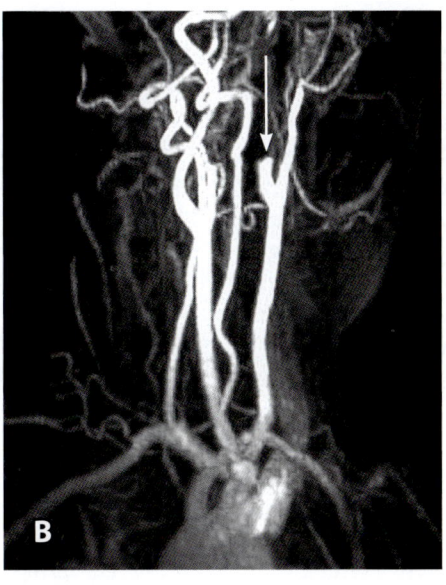

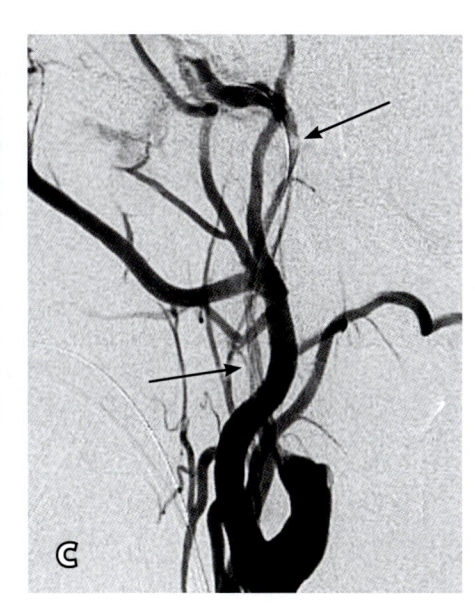

Figure 7-30 Traumatic Carotid Artery Dissection

(**A**) Axial T-1 unenhanced with fat-saturated MR image (**B**) time of flight MRA with contrast of neck vessels and lateral angiographic view of the left common carotid artery. There is a circumferential band of high signal surrounding a flow void (*arrow*, **A**) of the left internal carotid artery. This hemorrhage is located within the walls of the dissection. An abrupt cutoff of the left internal carotid artery is seen on the time of flight images (*arrow*, **B**). The nearly occluded internal carotid artery shows minimal flow on the angiogram done in conjunction with endovascular treatment (note micro-catheter within the lumen (*arrows*, **C**).

subclavian vein and superior sagittal sinus, superior vena cava syndrome, and airway edema. In addition, systemic sepsis and septic emboli may cause empyema, septic arthritis, renal failure, hepatic dysfunction, and cerebral edema.

On imaging, thrombophlebitis is characterized by a distended vessel surrounded by soft tissue inflammation. After a week, the inflammation will subside, and the thrombosis is considered chronic. On MR, signal intensity depends upon the age of the clot. On T2-weighted images, thrombosis will be bright in the acute phase, diminishing to low signal intensity in the subacute phase. With contrast, the thrombus will have low intensity with an enhancing wall. On contrast-enhanced CT, the thrombus will have low attenuation, and will be surrounded by a thickened, enhancing vasa vasorum (**Fig. 7-31**).

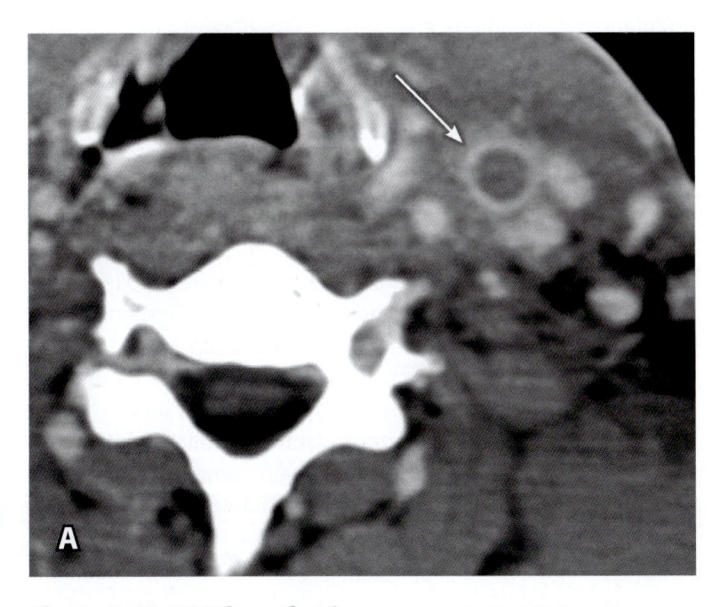

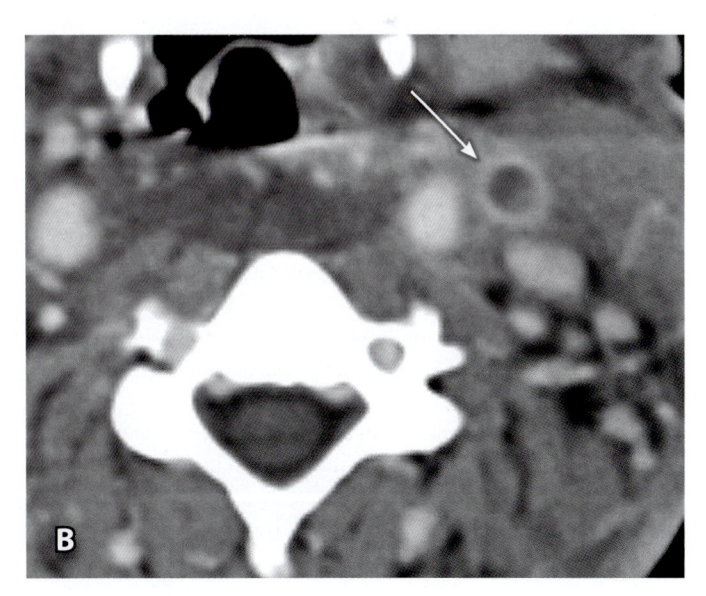

Figure 7-31 IJV Thrombosis

(**A, B**) Axial CT contrast-enhanced CT scans. There is a filling defect (*arrows*) in the left internal jugular vein with surrounding inflammatory changes in the soft tissues of the neck.

Benign Tumors of the Carotid Space

Paraganglioma

Paragangliomas are rare tumors that arise from widely dispersed, specialized neural crest cells that are associated with autonomic ganglia, and have the ability to secrete neuropeptides and catecholamines. The paraganglia of the head and neck migrate along the branchial mesoderm. Subtypes include carotid paraganglioma or carotid body tumor, found at the common carotid artery bifurcation; vagal paraganglioma or glomus vagale, arising from the nodose ganglion of the vagus nerve; jugular paraganglioma or glomus jugulare, arising from the jugular ganglion; and tympanic paraganglioma or glomus tympanicum, arising in association with the nerve of Jacobsen along the cochlear promontory. Rarely paragangliomas may be found in the larynx, orbit, and paranasal sinuses.[132]

Clinical presentation is typically associated with the site of tumor origin. Carotid body tumors typically present with a neck mass, whereas middle ear and jugular foramen tumors present with pulsatile tinnitus. In addition, jugular foramen tumors often present with symptoms referable to lower cranial neuropathies. MR imaging has greatly simplified the preoperative diagnosis of paragangliomas. These tumors are smooth, oval-shaped masses in the CS, which displace the ICA. A "salt and pepper" pattern of intense contrast enhancement studded with multiple flow voids on T2-weighted MR images is characteristic. The carotid paraganglioma, the most common paraganglioma of the head and neck, will characteristically splay the internal and external carotid arteries.

Ten percent to 50% of paragangliomas are inherited in an autosomal dominant manner by germline heterozygous inactivating mutations in mitochondrial complex II succinate dehydrogenase genes SDHB, SDHC, and SDHD.[133] The SDHD mutation plays a role in both hereditary and sporadic cases.[134] This mutation appears to be responsible for a chronic hypoxic signal, leading to chief cell proliferation and tumor formation. Spontaneous paragangliomas are seen more frequently in patients who live at high altitudes, are smokers, or who have COPD.[135] Hypoxia, as either an exogenous or endogenous factor seems to be important to the development of these tumors.

Multicentricity occurs in approximately 10% of sporadic, and in 30% to 40% of familial paragangliomas.[132] Familial paragangliomas typically occur in the second or third decade, while spontaneous tumors do not typically appear until the fourth decade or beyond. Genetic counseling and radiological screening are available for members of families with the hereditary forms.[136] On average, 5% to 10% are malignant: 2% to 4% of jugulotympanic tumors, 6% of carotid body tumors, and 16% to 19% of vagal tumors.[137] All paragangliomas contain neurosecretory granules, but very few reach levels of clinical significance. One percent of paragangliomas are considered functional. Those rare head and neck paragangliomas that do become functional produce vasoactive catecholamines, which can cause hypertension, headaches, palpitations, sweating, nervousness, and weight loss.

Carotid Paragangliomas

In the head and neck, 60% of paragangliomas are tumors of the carotid body, located at the bifurcation of the common carotid artery, or along the internal or external carotid arteries. Clinically, they present as a painless, slowly enlarging mass located anterior to the sternocleidomastoid muscle at the level of the hyoid bone. The tumor may transmit a carotid pulse or bruit. Enlargement and compression of the pharynx, carotid vessels, and cranial nerves 10 to 12 may cause cranial nerve deficits, dysphagia, odynophagia, or hoarseness. Tumor growth will encase the arteries, but will not narrow their lumens.[138]

Carotid paragangliomas tumors splay the carotid bifurcation with posterolateral displacement of the internal carotid artery. On MR imaging, T1-weighted images demonstrate a smooth, oval-shaped tumor with an intermediate signal intensity background matrix and scattered areas of signal void. Contrast administration produces intense homogeneous enhancement. On T2-weighted images, the classic "salt and pepper" appearance, reflecting areas of high and low flow, is present in most lesions larger than 2 cm.

Paragangliomas have a high density of somatostatin type 2 receptors on their cell surface and can be imaged using Indium-111 octreotide. Digital subtraction angiography is the gold standard of paraganglioma imaging, but is often not necessary with a classic appearance on MR. It can be a valuable tool in evaluation for surgery demonstrating displacement of blood vessels, tumor invasion in vessels, and the adequacy of intracranial circulation to determine the feasibility of ICA sacrifice. The tumor appears as a hypervascular mass with enlarged feeding arteries, and intense blush, and early draining veins.

Treatment is primarily surgical. Preoperative embolization may be used to minimize blood loss. The vagus, hypoglossal, and spinal accessory nerves must be identified for preservation. Patients with large or recurrent tumors often require vascular reconstruction, which requires through preoperative planning. Elderly patients and other poor surgical candidates may be treated with radiation therapy.

Jugulotympanic Paraganglioma

Jugular paragangliomas, arising from the superior vagal (jugular) ganglion are located in the region of the jugular foramen, where they commonly traverse the skull base to be located both intra and extracranially. Growth of the dumbbell-shaped tumor may extend superiorly into the posterior fossa or inferiorly into the intratemporal space. Lateral extension may involve the middle ear structures. Clinically, patients with these tumors present with pulsatile tinnitus, dizziness, blurred vision, Horner's syndrome, and neck masses. In most cases, large jugular and tympanic paragangliomas cannot be differentiated, and thus the combined term. Treatment is surgery, radiation, or a combination of the two.

On T1-weighted MR images, tumors larger than 2 cm will display the characteristic salt and pepper appearance. There is avid enhancement with contrast. Contrast-enhanced CT also demonstrates intense enhancement. Non-contrast CT will display destruction of bone in the jugular foramen. The tumor will appear as a hypervascular mass with intense tumor blush and early draining veins on angiography (See **Fig. 9-47**).

Vagal Paraganglioma

Vagal paragangliomas, which typically occur in association with the nodose ganglion, account for less than 5% of head and neck paragangliomas. The paraganglia from which these tumors arise are dispersed within the perineurium or between the nerve fiber fascicles. These tumors are found above the carotid bifurcation, with blood supply most commonly from the ascending pharyngeal and occipital arteries. The most common presenting sign is the presence of a painless neck mass accompanied occasionally by dysphagia and hoarseness. There may be medial deviation of the oropharynx indicating parapharyngeal space involvement. Cranial nerve dysfunction occurs more frequently than with carotid paragangliomas, but less than jugulotympanic paragangliomas. Surgical resection of vagal paragangliomas is typically by a cervical approach, unless there is intracranial extension. The facial, hypoglossal, and spinal accessory nerves, and the carotid artery and the jugular vein must be identified for preservation. Surgical treatment may be complicated by cranial nerve dysfunction.[139]

T1-weighted images demonstrate the classic salt and pepper appearance, and contrast enhancement is intense. T2-weighted images have high signal with hypointense flow voids seen within the tumor. Vagal paragangliomas will displace both the internal and external carotid arteries anteriorly, and is associated with erosion and widening of the jugular foramen (see **Fig. 9-49**).

Schwannoma

Schwannomas are benign neoplasms of the nerve sheath that can originate from almost any peripheral nerve. They are slow-growing tumors that cause symptoms by compressing the nerve or surrounding structures. Schwannomas are encapsulated, and stretch the nerve, but do not invade. Two distinct areas are usually observed in these tumors: Antoni A regions with tightly packed, spindle-shaped cells, and Antoni B areas, which are loosely packed. They are usually solitary, but may be multiple in patients with Neurofibromatosis Type 1.

These tumors present in patients between the second and fifth decades with equal gender prevalence. Twenty-five to 45% of these tumors are found in the head and neck, and most of these are found in the combined parapharyngeal/CS.[39] Patients may present with lower cranial neuropathy or with no symptoms except a neck mass. These tumors are almost always benign, although malignant degeneration has been reported. Treatment consists of tumor resection via a transcervical approach. The tumor is normally separated from the nerve by a fibrous capsule, enabling the surgeon to excise or enucleate the tumor without damage to the nerve. If the nerve cannot be preserved, a nerve graft or end-to-end anastomosis may preserve function.[140] The recurrence rate for these tumors after gross total resection is low.

On MR, these are normally round or ovoid, well-circumscribed lesions. MR signal intensity may be homogeneous or heterogeneous due to cyst formation and hemorrhage. T1-weighted images can show any level of signal intensity, while T2-weighted images have intermediate to high signal. With contrast, they demonstrate intense, homogeneous enhancement. Occasionally, flow voids may be seen, in which case these tumors may be difficult to distinguish from paragangliomas. Adjacent bony structures may be remodeled, but will not show infiltration. Schwannomas of the vagus nerve will separate the carotid artery from the jugular vein, differentiating them from schwannomas of the cervical sympathetic chain, which is located posterior to the carotid sheath[141] (**Fig. 7-32**) (see **Fig. 9-51**). In the infrahyoid neck, a large tumor will displace the thyroid and trachea to the opposite side.[142]

Malignant Tumors of the Carotid Space

Extension of Regional Malignancies

Squamous cell carcinoma may invade the CS via direct invasion from the primary site or by nodal metastases. Primaries are usually located in the mucosa of the nasopharynx, oropharynx, or hypopharynx. The fascia of the lower CS is not easily penetrated, but above the hyoid bone, the fascia is incomplete, allowing tumor spread from carotid bifurcation to skull base. Extracapsular extension of level 2 to 4 lymph node metastases can traverse the CS to reach the skull base.

A primary of the upper aerodigestive tract may be deeply infiltrative at the time of diagnosis, extending to involve the carotid artery. Circumferential involvement of greater than 270 degrees renders the tumor unresectable without carotid sacrifice. Treatment options include carotid artery resection, with or without reconstruction, shaving tumor from the artery for cure or palliation, or nonsurgical management with radiation and chemotherapy. Previously untreated patients with advanced cervical squamous cell carcinoma metastasis are usually treated with aggressive radiation and chemotherapy in attempt to eradicate both the primary and the cervical metastasis. Six to 8 weeks after radiation treatment, the patient receives a radical neck dissection. Cancers that are less radiosensitive, such as adenocarcinoma, adenoid cystic carcinoma, and melanoma, may be best treated initially with surgical resection and intraoperative radiation, followed by postoperative radiation. The prognosis for patients with recurrent or residual disease involving the carotid artery is very poor.[143]

On MR images, tumor will enhance with contrast and T2-weighted images will show high signal intensity. When evaluating for carotid artery involvement, obliteration of the fascial plane between the artery and the mass suggest involvement of the adventitia.

Lymphoma

Lymphoid cancers are a diverse, but closely related group of neoplasms, which include NHL, Hodgkin's lymphoma (HL), multiple myeloma, and acute and chronic lymphocytic leukemia. The etiology of lymphoid neoplasms remains largely unknown, but risk factors include certain infections, such as Epstein-Barr virus and HIV, and diseases and treatments which cause immunosuppression, including autoimmune disease, organ transplant, and primary or acquired immunodeficiency.[144]

The staging of lymphoid neoplasms involves a careful history and physical examination; imaging with chest X-ray, CT, gallium scan, bone scan, ultrasound, or MRI of the chest, abdomen, pelvis; biopsy of the bone marrow; and blood tests, including lactate dehydrogenase, albumin, or beta2-microglobulin levels. 18F-FDG PET has emerged as a promising tool for staging and monitoring early therapeutic responses.[145]

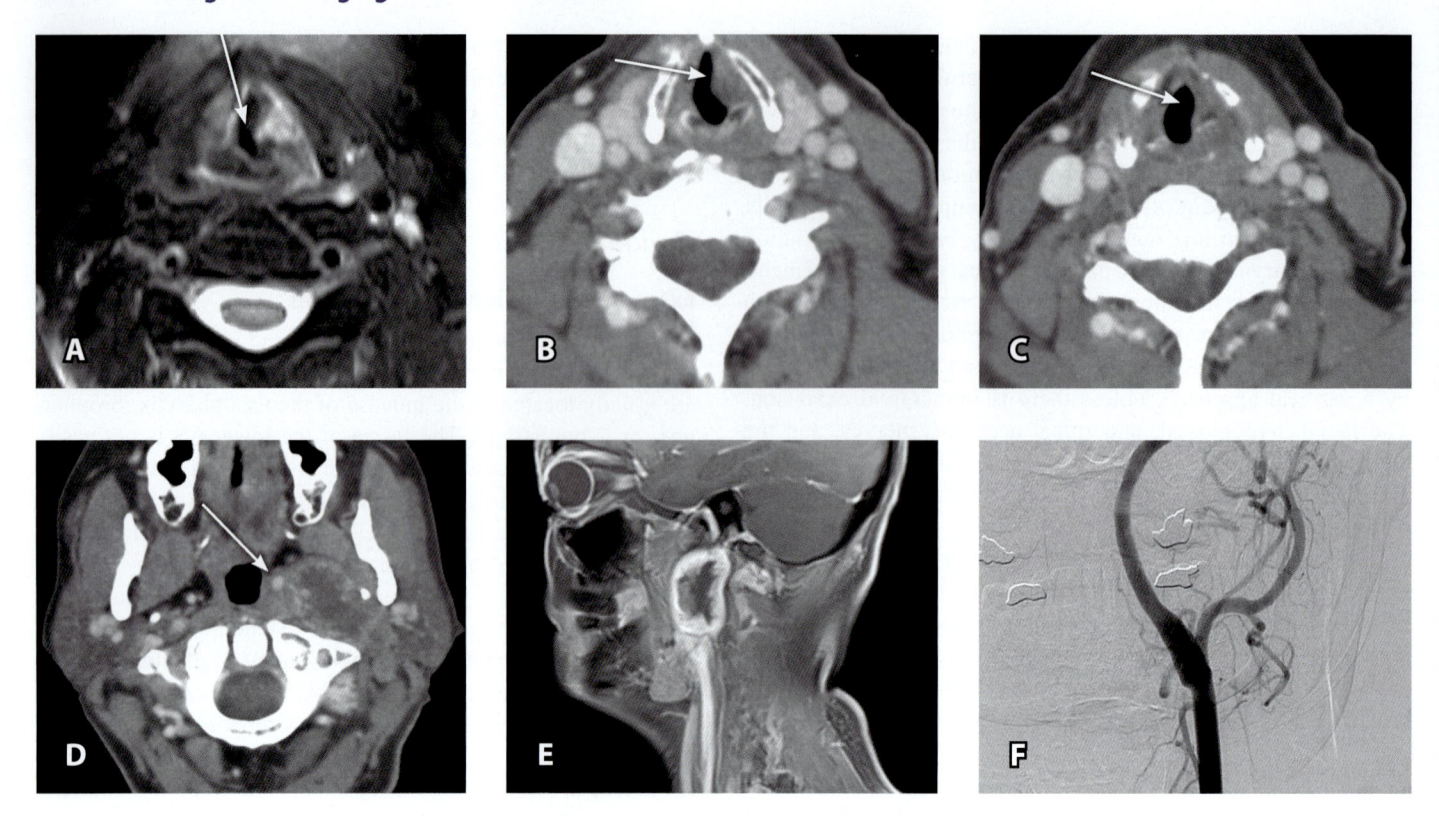

Figure 7-32 Schwannoma of the Xth Nerve (Patient with Vocal Cord Paralysis)
(**A**) Axial T-2 MR image (**B–D**) axial contrast-enhanced CT scans (**E**) sagittal T-1 contrast-enhanced MR image and (**F**). AP angiographic view of the left common carotid artery. Scans through the vocal cords and supraglottic region show medialization of the left false and aryepiglottic folds (*arrows*, **A–C**) consistent with vocal cord paralysis. There is a large peripherally enhancing tumor within the left carotid space showing marked anterior displacement of the internal carotid artery (*arrow*, **D**). There are only a few branches within the tumor on the angiogram (**E**). This rules out a vagal paraganglioma, a lesion that typically shows many rapidly filling vascular pedicles.

Lymphoma is the second most common neoplasm of the head and neck and should be considered in the differential diagnosis of any lesion in this region, especially if the typical factors for squamous cell carcinoma are not present. NHL can involve any region, most commonly Waldeyer's ring, followed by orbit, paranasal sinuses, salivary glands, and thyroid.[146] Two-thirds of NHL, and nearly all cases of HL present with nontender nodal enlargement.[38]

Non-Hodgkin's Lymphoma

Lymphoma encompasses a diverse group of neoplasms. In most cases, the phenotype of the lymphoid neoplastic cell resembles a stage of normal lymphocyte differentiation. HL is clinically and histologically unique, and is treated in a different manner than other lymphomas. NHL accounts for 4% of new cancer cases in the United States, and 3% of cancer deaths.[147] 85% of all lymphomas. The most common types of NHL include lymphoblastic, small non-cleaved or Burkitt lymphoma (**Fig. 7-33**), large cell or diffuse histocytic, and follicular. The lymphoblastic type most often involves T-cells, but can involve B-cells. It usually occurs with a mass in the chest and enlarged lymph nodes with or without the involvement of bone marrow and the central nervous system. Small non-cleaved cell lymphoma originating in Africa is most commonly associated with the Epstein-Barr virus and involves a jaw mass and central nervous system disease. In North America, small non-cleaved cell lymphoma is not associated with Epstein-Barr virus. It arises in the abdomen and often spreads to bone marrow. Large cell or diffuse histiocytic NHL involves B or T-cells and accounts for about 30% of lymphoma cases.[148] It is more common in adults, but affects all ages. Large cell B cell lymphoma often originates in the abdomen and can spread to the bone marrow and central nervous system. Thirty percent of cases are extra-nodal.[38] The follicular type comprises 22% of NHL.[148] It is common in the elderly, advanced at presentation, and has an indolent clinical course.

Staging for NHL is less useful in guiding treatment than in Hodgkin's lymphoma, because disease spread is less predictable. Patients are assumed to have systemic disease at presentation.

The primary treatment for non-Hodgkin's lymphoma is chemotherapy. Radiation and bone marrow transplant are also used. Radioimmunotherapy, which uses monoclonal antibodies with a radionuclide to deliver radiation to the tumor site, has shown great promise in treating NHL.[149]

Hodgkin's Lymphoma

HL is a group of cancers characterized by Reed-Sternberg cells in an appropriate reactive cellular background. The disease arises within lymph nodes and spreads in an orderly fashion to

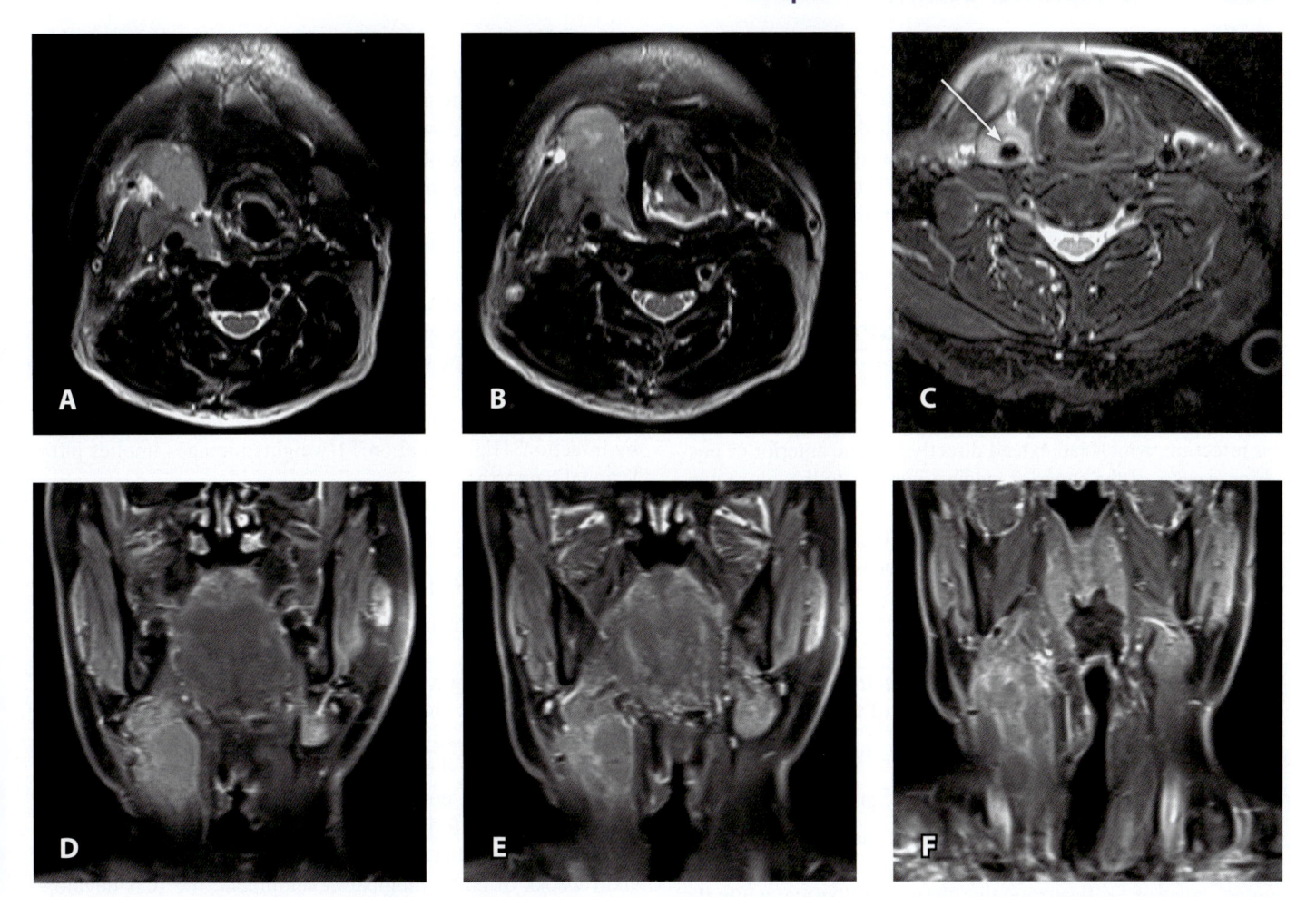

Figure 7-33 Burkitt Lymphoma of the Carotid Space
Axial T2W (**A–C**) and coronal contrast-enhanced with fat-saturated T1W (**D–F**) MR images. These scans demonstrate a nodular-appearing mass extending across the length of the right carotid space and completely surrounding the flow void of the common carotid artery (*arrow*, **C**). This tumor appears to originate from multiple nodal masses within the carotid space.

contiguous nodes. Late in the course of the disease, vascular invasion leads to widespread hematogenous dissemination.

HL peaks in young adults and again in those 50 years and older. It is slightly more common in males than females, and is more common in Caucasians. This disease is very rare in children younger than 5 years and tends to cluster in families. The four types of Hodgkin's disease include nodular sclerosing, mixed cellularity, lymphocyte predominance, and lymphocyte depleted. Nodular sclerosing accounts for 40 % of all HL and 70% of HL in adolescents. This is the only form of HL that is more prevalent in women. Thirty percent of HL is the mixed cellularity type, which is an advanced disease that usually affects children under 10 years of age. Lymphocyte predominance type accounts for 10% to 15% of HS. It is usually is localized and has the best likelihood of a good outcome. It is mainly found in males and younger patients. The widespread, lymphocyte depleted type is more common in HIV-positive adults.

The majority of patients present with overt disease, most often as an asymptomatic enlarged lymph node or a mass on chest X-ray. However, the presenting symptoms and signs may be relatively nonspecific and more compatible with infection than malignant disease. HL presents as a painless mass in approximately 70% of cases. The involved lymph node is usually nontender with a rubbery consistency. The most common involved site is in the neck, with 60% to 80% of patients having enlarged cervical or supraclavicular nodes. The spread of disease is predictable, from nodes, to spleen, to liver, to bone marrow and extranodal disease.[38]

The most common treatments for Hodgkin's disease are radiation and/or chemotherapy, or bone marrow transplant. Treatments vary depending on the stage of the cancer and age of the patient.

A diagnosis of lymphoma should be considered when multiple, large, nonnecrotic lymph nodes are present or multiple sites of disease are identified in extranodal tissue. Imaging cannot differentiate HL and NHL; however, based upon the predilection of the different types for certain areas of the body, and clinical findings, a diagnosis can usually be suggested. The enlarged lymph nodes of both HL and NHL will range from 2 to 10 cm in diameter. Most lymph nodes will not be necrotic unless there has been chemotherapy or radiation treatment. An exception is found in HL and Burkitt's lymphoma, which may show necrosis before treatment. Likewise, calcification is not normally present in pretreatment nodes, but may appear after treatment.[146] Extranodal spread is bulky and lobulated, covered by intact mucosa. Aggressive tumors will destroy bone. Lymphomas have low signal intensity on T1-weighted images, with variable contrast enhancement. They have variable signal intensity on T2-weighted images depending on the degree of extracellular water and fibrosis.

THE RETROPHARYNGEAL SPACE

Lymph nodes and fat are the only structures native to the retropharyngeal space (RPS). Yet it is an extremely important conduit for infection, which can extend directly into the anterior or posterior aspects of the superior mediastinum, or to the entire posterior mediastinum via the danger space. Infectious processes, including cellulitis, suppurative adenopathy, and abscess, and nodal metastases, most often from squamous cell carcinoma, are the most common lesions found in the RPS. On imaging, disease processes of the infrahyoid RPS will appear as flattened masses anterior to the prevertebral musculature, displacing these muscles posteriorly. In the suprahyoid neck, retropharyngeal nodal masses will displace the posterior aspect of the parapharyngeal space anterolaterally.

Anatomy of the Retropharyngeal Space

The RPS is a potential space located in the midline, directly behind the pharynx. The anterior boundary of the RPS is the middle layer of DCF surrounding the visceral space, while the posterior and lateral boundaries are composed of the deep, or alar layer of DCF. This space extends from the skull base to the upper mediastinum between the levels of C6 and T4. A slip of DCF separates the RPS from the potential space which lies behind it: the danger space. The danger space extends caudally into the mediastinum and provides a conduit for disease.

In the suprahyoid neck, the RPS contains the retropharyngeal lymph nodes, which drain the paranasal sinuses, auditory tube, and nasopharynx. In the infrahyoid neck, the RPS contains only adipose tissue. Imaging of this space is especially important because of its proximity to the airway and the difficulty in clinically evaluating nodal disease in this area. The lateral retropharyngeal nodes are located anterior to the alar fascia, medial to the ICA, at the level of the transverse process of the atlas. These are well seen on MRI. The upper and lower medial retropharyngeal nodes, when present, are located medial to the lateral nodes. No nodes are found below the level of the hyoid bone. Retropharyngeal nodes are normally prominent in children and gradually decrease in size. By adulthood, these nodes should normally be less than 8 mm in short axis dimension.

Vasoformative Anomalies of the Retropharyngeal Space

Hemangiomas and lymphatic malformations can be found anywhere in the nasopharynx and oropharynx. MR imaging of hemangiomas is characteristic, but depends upon the growth phase of the lesion. In the proliferating phase, hemangiomas are well-defined, lobulated soft tissue masses that are isointense or slightly hyperintense to muscle on T1-weighted images and hyperintense on T2-weighted images. Hemangiomas are high-flow lesions, and exhibit multiple flow voids. Contrast enhancement of the tumor is intense and relatively uniform. As the tumor involutes, vascularity decreases, and fibrous and adipose tissue replaces the tumor. The adipose tissue appears as high intensity foci within the lesion on T1-weighted imaging.

Characteristic imaging findings of lymphatic malformations include low signal T1-weighted images and high signal T2-weighted images with fluid/fluid levels. There is no central enhancement with contrast, but there may be an enhancing tumor rim and septations, especially if the walls have been thickened by infection. High signal on T1-weighted images implies intralesional hemorrhage.

Vascular Anomalies of the Retropharyngeal Space

Anomalous Internal Carotid Artery

Carotid artery anomalies are common, occurring in 10% to 40% of the population.[150]

Excessive length of the ICA is seen in 10% to 43% of angiograms, taking the form of a coil, bends, or kinking.[151] The cervical ICA normally ascends straight from the carotid bifurcation, anterior to the transverse processes of the upper three cervical vertebrae, posterolateral to the PPS, lateral to the tonsillar fossa, and inferior to the superior pharyngeal constrictor, to the carotid canal in the petrous temporal bone. In the fifth and sixth weeks of embryological development, the ICA develops from the third branchial arch arteries and the cranial aspect of the dorsal aorta. A loop forms at the junction of the two arteries, which is usually straightened by descent of the vessels and heart into the mediastinum. If this process is disrupted in some way, by incomplete development or accelerated growth, the loop may persist. Vascular transposition is bilateral in 31% of cases and unilateral in 67%.[152]

Paulsen, et al described the four most common variations of the ICA: straight to the skull base, medial, lateral, ventral, or dorsal displacement with an S or C shape; kinking of one or more segments, and coiling.[150] Coiling is most likely due to developmental factors, curving may be related to aging, and kinking is thought to be associated with atherosclerosis, hypertension, and fibromuscular dysplasia.[151]

Medial dislocation of the ICA into the RPS at the level of the pharynx is a common anomaly. It will often appear as an asymptomatic, pulsating submucosal mass on the posterior pharyngeal wall. Symptomatic cases present with dysphagia, globus sensation, or obstructive sleep apnea.[153] More serious complications of ICA anomalies include cerebral hypoxia, TIA, and stroke. These cases require medical or surgical treatment.[46]

Routine pharyngeal surgeries, such as adenoidectomy, tonsillectomy, uvulopalatopharyngoplasty, or incision and drainage of peritonsillar abscesses, in a patient with undiagnosed RPS ICA is extremely dangerous, making an imaging diagnosis very important. The radiologist should consider this diagnosis and alert the otolaryngologist/head and neck surgeon when observing an asymmetry of the posterior pharyngeal wall on a preoperative CT or MRI. Three-dimensional TOF MRA and Doppler ultrasound have been useful in evaluating these anomalies.[154]

Inflammatory Lesions of the Retropharyngeal Space

Imaging a vital tool in effective diagnosis and treatment of infection in the RPS. The anatomy of the deep neck is highly complex and imaging is necessary to accurately localize the extent and, if unknown, the origin of the infection. In addition, lesions within this space are covered by unaffected superficial soft tissue, and are therefore difficult to palpate and visualize externally. Preoperative imaging is important, because surgical access to this space can place intervening neurovascular and soft tissue structures at risk. Imaging can also identify surrounding structures which may have become involved in the infectious process, which can lead to thrombosis, osteomyelitis, and neural dysfunction.

Cellulitis and Abscess

The RPS and SMS are the spaces most commonly infiltrated by direct extension of infection. Infections from lingual and faucial tonsils, adenoids, salivary glands, and mandible often spread to the RPS lymph nodes. The nodes become enlarged and suppurative, and the surrounding retropharyngeal fat becomes edematous due to cellulitis. Symptoms may be vague, and include fever, irritability, and dysphonia. More acute symptoms include dysphagia and dyspnea due to local mass effect resulting from laryngeal edema. Abscess formation follows rupture of the nodal capsule. Abscesses require antibiotics and surgical drainage.

In children, infections in the pharynx or sinuses commonly involve the retropharyngeal nodes. In adults, distant spread from peritonsillar abscess or odontogenic infection is seen in the RPS. Deep neck abscesses often contain multiple organisms; the most common are *S. viridans* and *S. aureus*. Tuberculous retropharyngeal abscess is usually due to spinal tuberculosis. It is rare, and is most common in children. Symptoms include fever, weight loss, dysphagia, respiratory distress, spinal deformation, and neurological symptoms. Treatment is transoral drainage and anti-tuberculosis therapy. Other causes of an edematous RPS include jugular venous or lymphatic obstruction, a history of radiation therapy, trauma, or a non-infectious inflammatory process. Four to six weeks after radiation therapy, fluid may fill the RPS. It is of no clinical significance, and will normally disappear within 12 weeks.[155]

Complications are secondary to mass effect, rupture of the abscess, or spread of infection. The most acute complication involves an abscess expanding against the pharynx or trachea, causing airway compression. Rupture of the abscess can cause aspiration of pus, resulting in asphyxiation or pneumonia. Spread of the infection to the mediastinum can result in mediastinitis, purulent pericarditis and tamponade, pyopneumothorax, pleuritis, empyema, or bronchial erosion. Spread of the infection laterally can involve the carotid sheath and cause jugular vein thrombosis or carotid artery rupture. Posterior spread of infection can result in osteomyelitis and erosion of the spinal column, causing vertebral subluxation and spinal cord injury. Neurologic symptoms may indicate spinal epidural abscess.[156] Mediastinitis has a high mortality rate secondary to sepsis. The mediastinum is drained via a cervicomediastinal or a transthoracic approach. If the infection is in the danger space, a thoracotomy is indicated.

T1-weighted MR images show intermediate signal intensity in enlarged retropharyngeal lymph nodes that are involved in infection. Suppuration is indicated by rim enhancement. On T2-weighted images, inflamed nodes have high signal intensity, as does cellulitis in the surrounding soft tissues. Inflamed lymph nodes and cellulitis strongly enhance with contrast. On CT, suppurative lymph nodes will be enlarged, with central hypodensity, and can be surrounded by phlegmon. Abscesses will also appear hypodense, developing rim enhancement as they mature. Cellulitis is also hyperdense on CT images. In early stages of RPS involvement, inflamed lymph nodes and cellulitis may be unilateral, with asymmetric deformation of the PMS. In later stages, fluid can fill the width of the RPS, and expand anteriorly to compress the pharyngeal wall, posteriorly to flatten the prevertebral muscles, and laterally, displacing the carotid sheaths.

Foreign Bodies and Penetrating Injury of the Retropharyngeal Space

Children swallow a variety of foreign objects, and can also lacerate the esophagus after falling with objects in their mouths. Adults often swallow chicken or fish bones, and senile, stuporous, or psychiatric patients can inhale objects, such as dentures. Iatrogenic causes of penetrating injury include instrumentation with laryngoscopy, endotracheal intubation, surgery, endoscopy, feeding tube placement, and dental procedures. Objects that perforate the esophagus or pharynx can migrate to the RPS, and are a common source of infection.

Symptoms of a swallowed foreign body include respiratory distress, drooling, pain, dysphagia, and if infection has developed, fever and sepsis. Patients with no symptoms may develop infection and abscess insidiously. In this setting of a swallowed object and respiratory distress, CT is more commonly used than MRI to localize the object. Rapid treatment may be undertaken endoscopically, while more complicated cases require surgical removal of the object and antibiotic treatment.

Reactive Lymphadenopathy of the Retropharyngeal Space

Reactive nodes can be difficult to differentiate from malignant nodes without clinical information. The former condition is assumed in young adults and children, while malignancy should be suspected in adult patients. Patients may have systemic illness, or localized neck infection, such as pharyngitis. Retropharyngeal effusion may also be present (**Fig. 7-34**). Reactive RPS nodes will generally be smaller than 10 mm in diameter and oval in shape. On MR, T1-weighted images will have homogeneous low to intermediate signal intensity with minimal contrast enhancement. T2-weighted images will have

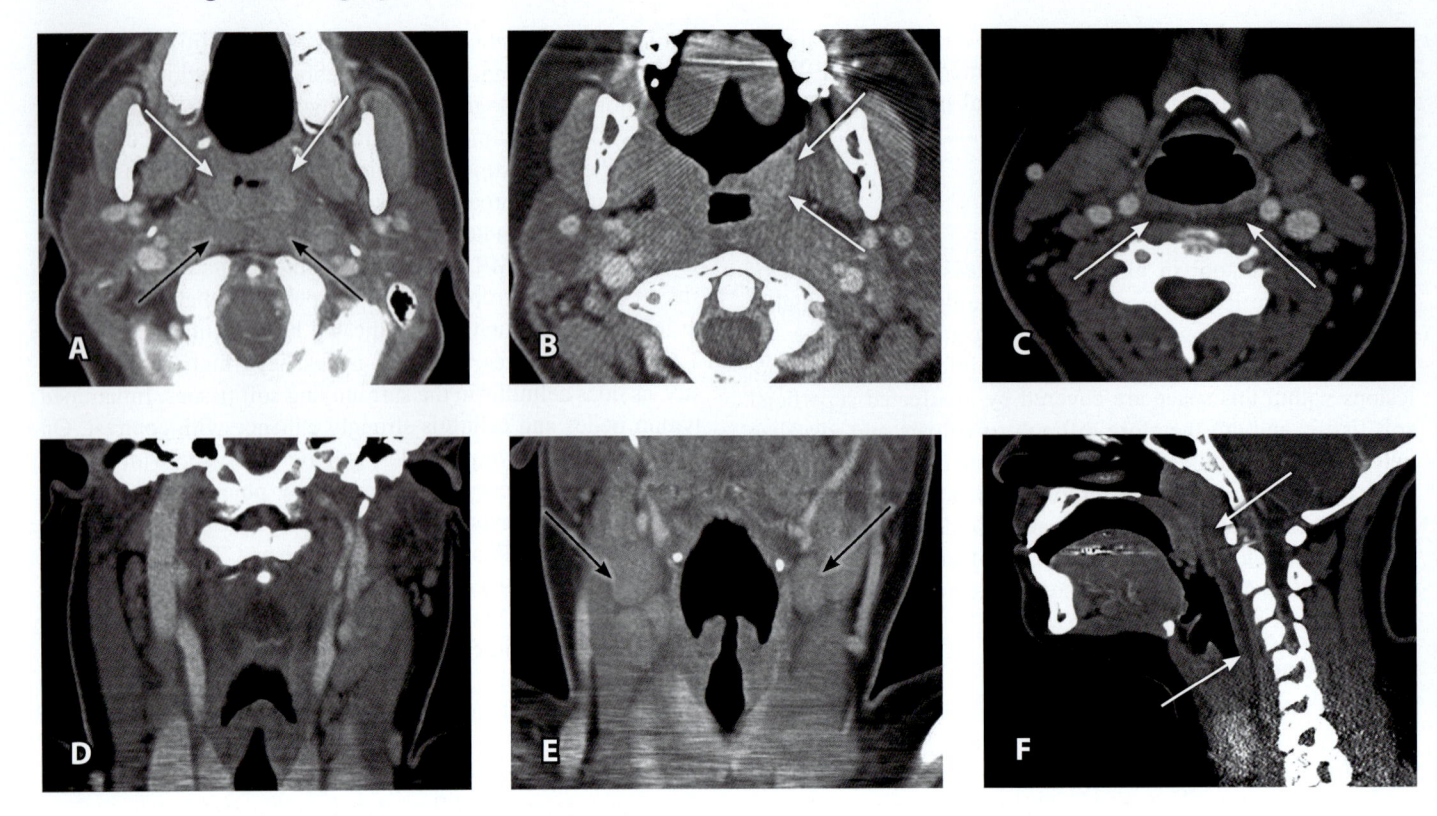

Figure 7-34 Retropharyngeal Lymphadenopathy and Effusion
Axial (**A–C**), coronal (**D, E**), and sagittal (**F**) CECT images. There are enlarged adenoids (*white arrows*, **A**) and heterogenous enhancement within an enlarged left palatine tonsil (*arrows*, **B**), consistent with an early infectious process. There are also enlarged retropharyngeal (*black arrows*, **A**) and cervical (*arrows*, **E**) lymph nodes. The low density retropharyngeal fluid has dissected from the level of C1 to C7, but does not enhance or demonstrate significant mass effect, suggesting reactive rather than infectious etiology.

intermediate signal intensity. Suppuration can lead to RPS abscess.

Benign Tumors of the Retropharyngeal Space

Lipoma

Thirteen percent of lipomas occur in the head and neck, and they are the most common lesions of mesenchymal origin in the neck.[76] They are soft and freely mobile, usually arising in the submucosa of the RPS, PPS, or PS. They are slow-growing, and often asymptomatic until they reach a large size. In the RPS, compressive symptoms include a globus sensation, respiratory difficulty, and dysphagia.

Lipomas are discrete, encapsulated, homogeneous fatty masses, which have high signal intensity on T1-weighted MR images and diminished intensity on T2. Lipomas do not enhance with contrast. On CT, they have low attenuation and are hypodense. Areas of high T2 signal, nodular or globular nonadipose areas within the tumor, thickened septa, or associated nonadipose masses suggest the diagnosis of liposarcoma. However, necrosis or infarction can produce heterogeneity within a lipoma. Well-differentiated liposarcomas tend to be larger than lipomas, are often traversed by dense bands of collagen, have gelatinous areas, and have adipocytes that show greater variation in size.[157,158]

Malignant Tumors of the Retropharyngeal Space

Malignancy in the RPS can take the form of direct extension from a contiguous primary, or nodal metastases. Direct extension will most likely come from the PMS, CS, perivertebral space, or vertebral column. Nodal metastases to the RPS arise from nasopharyngeal carcinoma in the majority of cases, as well as thyroid cancer and melanoma. Non-Hodgkin's lymphoma can involve lymph nodes, or appear as extralymphatic tumor in the RPS. Synovial sarcoma can involve the head and neck; most commonly the RPS. One-third of these tumors resemble benign masses, making diagnosis difficult.

Direct Extension of Carcinoma and Nodal Metastases

Due to their remote location, the retropharyngeal lymph nodes are often not evaluated in the standard head and neck examination, therefore imaging assessment is of key importance. The medial retropharyngeal lymph nodes, located anterior to the prevertebral muscles on each side of the midline, are normally small and not well-visualized on CT or MRI unless they are pathologically enlarged. The lateral retropharyngeal nodes are normally 3 to 7 mm in adults. They are found between the internal carotid artery and the longus colli muscle. Lymph nodes are only found in the suprahyoid RPS.

Medial retropharyngeal lymph nodes are rarely visualized on imaging, therefore malignancy is suspected when they are apparent. Other criteria for malignancy include size larger than 8 mm and nodal necrosis. Intranodal tumor necrosis has a heterogeneous signal intensity on both T1- and T2-weighted images representing keratin pooling, fibrous tissue, edema, and tumor cells. With contrast, necrotic nodes have low signal intensity centrally with a peripheral zone of enhancement. Contrast-enhanced fat-suppressed T1-weighted MR imaging sequences improve this differentiation and increase visualization of extracapsular tumor spread.

The lateral retropharyngeal lymph nodes, and level 2 and 5 lymph nodes drain the nasopharynx. RPS nodes associated with squamous cell carcinoma most commonly arise from nasopharyngeal carcinoma, but can also be associated with primaries in the posterior wall of the oropharynx or the hypopharynx. Nodes associated with thyroid cancer may have calcium or prominent cystic change,[159] and are hyperintense on T1-weighted images due to thyroglobulin content. They are usually seen with extensive cervical lymphadenopathy. Lymph node metastasis from differentiated thyroid cancer has little influence on long-term survival or recurrence in patients less than 45-years-old. Above this age, lymphadenopathy is associated with increased rates of recurrence.[160]

Lymphoma

Lymphoma of Waldeyer's ring is especially likely to spread to the RPS. Nodal lymphomas may present as a single, homogeneous, well-marginated, lobulated round mass. Aggressive lesions may invade surrounding soft tissue structures. Extranodal lymphoma appears as a bulky submucosal mass. Lymphoma rarely demonstrates ulceration or calcification unless there has been chemotherapy or radiation. High grade, aggressive lymphomas may have these characteristics, in addition to lytic bone destruction. T1-weighted MR images have low signal intensity. The signal of T2-weighted lesions varies depending upon the cellular composition of the tumor.

Synovial Sarcoma

Synovial sarcomas account for 10% of soft tissue sarcomas. The majority arise in the lower limbs of young adults, but 3% of primary lesions are found within the head and neck, especially in the RS. SS at this location have a significantly better prognosis than tumors located elsewhere, with 5-year survival rates ranging from 47% to 82%.[161] The cellular and molecular mechanisms of synovial sarcoma are poorly understood. The characteristic translocation t(X;18) (p11.2;q11.2) and its resulting SYT/SSX1 or SYT/SSX2 fusion transcript are the only well-described findings.[162] This diagnostic translocation creates a unique promise for targeted immunotherapy.[163]

Patients with head and neck SS can present with a painful, slow-growing mass. This tumor has a tendency to lie latent for long periods of time before exerting a burst of aggressive behavior.[164] If the tumor is near the pharynx, patients may have hoarseness, dysphagia, or dyspnea. On MR, T1-weighted images show a mass which is iso- or hyperintense to muscle. T2-weighted images demonstrate heterogeneous hyperintensity. Most tumors heterogeneously enhance with contrast. Imaging may also demonstrate hemorrhage, necrosis, cystic areas, and calcification, but these are not consistent findings.[165] One-third of tumors are septated, well-circumscribed masses which resemble benign tumors on MR imaging.[166]

Recommended treatment includes wide excision with negative margins, postoperative radiotherapy to improve local control rates, and adjuvant chemotherapy to prevent or delay the occurrence of distant metastases.[165]

THE PARAPHARYNGEAL SPACE

The centrally located PPS contains few structures, and produces few intrinsic lesions. However, lesions in surrounding compartments compress or displace the PPS in a predictable manner, allowing radiologists to identify their origin by observing the deformation of this key space. Lesions in the CS, posterior to the PPS, will displace it anteriorly, while lesions in the MS will displace the PPS posteriorly. Masses in the parotid gland will displace the PPS from lateral to midline, while lesions arising in the pharyngeal mucosal space will impinge upon the medial aspect of the PPS and push it laterally. Those rare intrinsic lesions of the PPS will displace the carotid artery posteriorly, the parotid laterally, the pharynx medially, and the pterygoid muscles anteriolaterally. Lesions must be surrounded by fat on all sides to be considered intrinsic to the PPS. Fortunately, fat is easily visualized on both CT and MR, making this a valuable tool in localizing lesions in this area.

The PPS is primarily fat-filled, with scant rests of minor salivary gland tissue and lymph nodes. Most mass lesions of the space arise from these components, while infection extends into the space from contiguous regions. The space also contains branches of CN V3, the internal maxillary artery, the ascending pharyngeal artery, the pharyngeal venous plexus, and the tensor veli palatini and pharyngeal constrictor muscles.

Anatomy of the Parapharyngeal Space

The PPS is a centrally located fatty triangle, which extends from the skull base to the hyoid bone. It is not enclosed in fascia, but is bounded by surrounding spaces, and continuous with the SMS inferiorly. The exact definition of the space is controversial, and many surgeons consider the PPS to include the CS as its poststyloid compartment. The two spaces are separated by the fascia of the stylopharyngeus, styloglossus, and tensor veli palatini muscles.

Superiorly, the PPS attaches to the skull base medial to the foramen ovale and foramen spinosum. The medial border is composed of the middle layer of DCF that covers the pharyngeal mucosal space. The superficial layer of deep cervical fascia enclosing the masticator and parotid spaces forms the lateral border, with the deep aspect of the parotid gland extending into the space. The pterygomandibular raphe forms the narrow anterior boundary of the space. The PPS extends to the hyoid bone, but some consider the styloglossus muscle the inferior extent of the PPS.

Congenital Anomalies of the Parapharyngeal Space

Atypical Second Branchial Cleft Cyst

Branchial cleft cysts in the PPS are atypical, rare lesions, arising from remnants of the first, or more commonly, the second branchial arch.[167] They are usually found in the medial aspect of the space, deep to the tonsillar fossa, from which they project cephalad toward the skull base. Second branchial cleft cysts are the most common branchial apparatus anomalies, but they are usually found in high in the lateral neck, deep to the anterior border of the sternocleidomastoid muscle. In the PPS, a second branchial cleft cyst may present as a bulge in the parotid gland or in the posterolateral pharyngeal wall. These lesions may rapidly increase in size after an upper respiratory tract infection.

On MR imaging, these cystic lesions have a low signal on T1-weighted images and high signal on T2-weighted images. Infection increases the T1-weighted signal and decreases signal on T2-weighted images. Infection also results in changes in the thickness and enhancement of the cyst wall (**Fig. 7-35**).

Vasoformative Anomalies

Vasoformative anomalies, such as hemangiomas, may occur anywhere in the nasopharynx and oropharynx. These lesions are isointense to muscle on T1-weighted images and hyperintense on T2-weighted images. High flow lesions will demonstrate flow voids. Venous malformations in this space may compress the airway.

Aneurysm and Pseudoaneurysm of the Parapharyngeal Space

Trauma and surgery can produce pseudoaneurysms of head and neck vessels, with large-diameter vessels more commonly involved. Pseudoaneurysms typically develop over weeks to months. Injury to the arterial wall produces a hematoma which develops central liquefaction and an outer wall of fibrous connective tissue as an inflammatory response. The hematoma will pulsate and enlarge, and may eventually rupture, causing severe hemorrhage. In deep locations, such as the PPS, there may be no symptoms prior to rupture. The internal maxillary artery is rarely involved because of its small caliber.[168] The large vascular anomaly is easily seen on CT and MR, and is best evaluated with angiography. Embolization is the preferred treatment.[169,170]

Inflammatory Lesions of the Parapharyngeal Space

PPS infections usually result from spread from contiguous spaces. In all cases, the source of the infection must be found for effective treatment. CT is the imaging modality of choice to assess osteomyelitis and calculus disease.

Abscesses in the PPS commonly develop after pharyngitis or tonsillitis via the pharyngeal mucosal space. In children, infections are most often due to multiple aerobic bacterial species, with Group A beta-hemolytic *Streptococcus* the most common pathogen.[171] Patients present with sore throat, dysphagia, trismus, and systemic symptoms including fever, malaise, and leukocytosis. An abscess in the tonsil can usually be differentiated from a parapharyngeal abscess by the presence of neck swelling, induration, and limited or painful neck movement in the later. Both will impinge upon the pharyngeal mucosal space, obstructing the airway. Surgical drainage has traditionally been performed via an external neck approach at the level of the carotid bifurcation, with visualization and protection of the neurovascular bundle, but recent pediatric studies have shown success with a transoral approach.[172,173] Contrast-enhanced CT can identify both the abscess and the relative position of the great

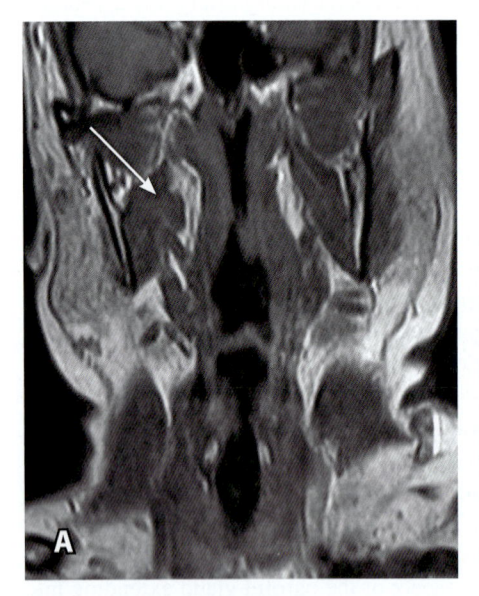

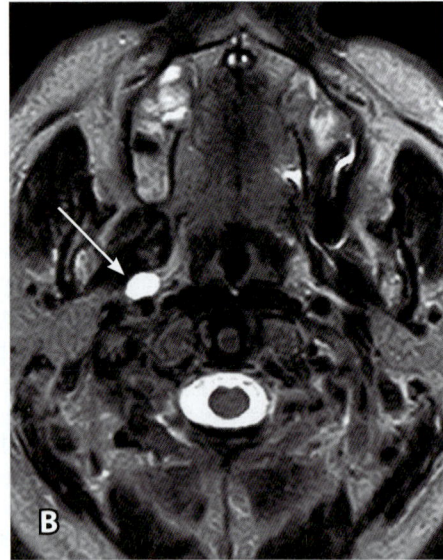

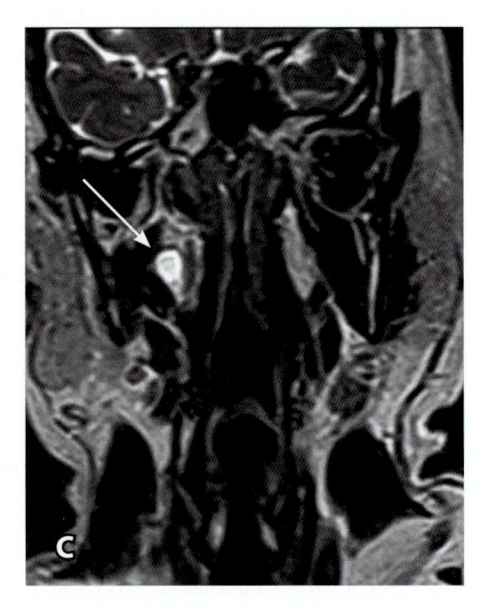

Figure 7-35 Atypical Parapharyngeal Branchial Cleft Cyst
Coronal T1W (**A**) and T2W (axial, **B** and coronal, **C**) MR images. There is a purely cystic mass entirely located within the parapharyngeal space (*arrows*, **A–C**). Such remnants of second branchial cleft cysts may simulate more aggressive entities, such as minor salivary gland or deep lobe of parotid tumors.

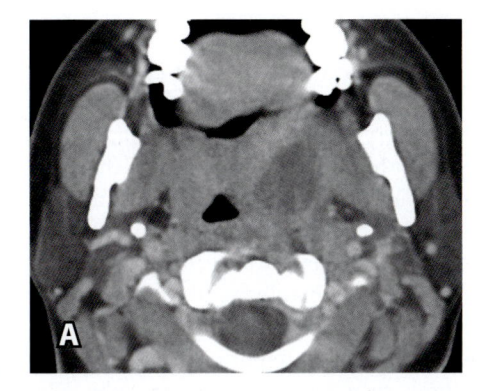

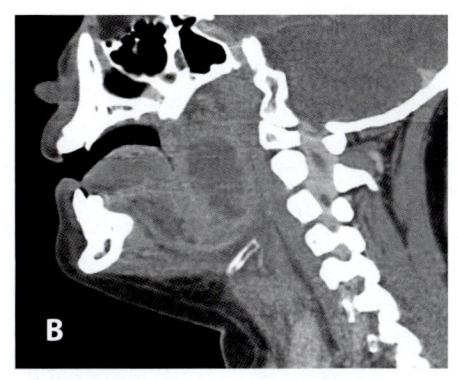

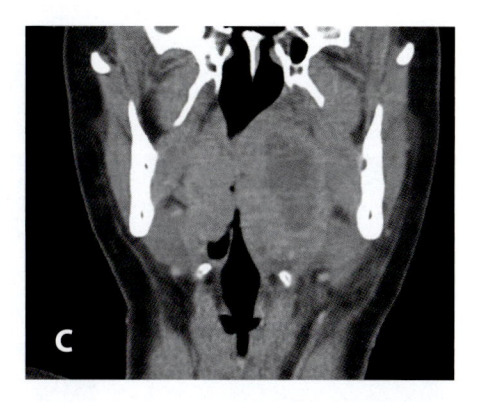

Figure 7-36 Oropharyngeal Abscess with Tonsillitis
Axial (**A**), sagittal reformatted (**B**), and coronal reformatted (**C**) contrast-enhanced CT images. The differentiation of phlegmon vs a well-defined abscess is less important than recognizing the potential of airway compromise that requires emergent treatment. Endoscopic drainage is helpful in reducing the morbidity of such infections.

vessels; information which is important for both medical and surgical treatment. Abscess will be seen as an area of central hypodensity, with or without ring enhancement (**Fig. 7-36**).

Benign Tumors of the Parapharyngeal Space

Pleomorphic Adenoma

The PPS contains only fat and rests of minor salivary gland tissue. Therefore, intrinsic neoplasms of this space are few. The most common is the extraparotid pleomorphic adenoma arising from the rests of glandular tissue.

Pleomorphic adenoma is the most common salivary gland tumor. They are rounded, well-circumscribed masses with a capsule which is not always fully developed. The dominant histologic feature of these tumors is significant heterogeneity. Epithelial and mesenchymal components are present, with an inner epithelial layer representing the former, and an outer layer of myoepithelial cells representing the latter. The stroma may contain variable amounts of mucoid, fibroid, cartilaginous, vascular, or myxochondroid elements. Most tumors show areas of cartilaginous differentiation.[89] It is believed that all neoplastic elements are either myoepithelial or ductal reserve cell origin. Infarction may occur, but tumor necrosis suggests malignant transformation.[89]

Clinically, extraparotid pleomorphic adenomas in the PPS present as painless, slow-growing, mobile, discrete masses. The deep location of this space makes it difficult to examine clinically, so masses smaller than 2 cm are often discovered incidentally. Neoplasms in this space will begin to displace the lateral wall of the pharyngeal mucosal space when they grow larger than 2 cm, and must achieve a significant size to displace the parotid gland.

On CT, these tumors appear as low attenuation masses, with areas of high attenuation representing hemorrhage or calcification in the stroma. More detail can be appreciated on MR imaging. On T1-weighted images, the tumors are low to intermediate signal intensity, while on T2, they have high signal due to areas of mucoid stroma or cystic degeneration. They enhance mildly with contrast.

It is important to distinguish extraparotid masses from those in the deep lobe, as this will alter the surgical approach. Treatment is complete resection via a transcervical approach. The rate of recurrence with adequate resection is 4%, but incomplete resection leads to recurrence in 25%.[38]

Incidence of malignant transformation increases with the age of the tumor, from 2% for tumors present less than 5 years, to 10% for those in place for more than 15 years. These cancers are typically adenocarcinoma or undifferentiated carcinoma, and are among the most aggressive salivary gland neoplasms, with a 30% to 50% mortality in 5 years.[38]

Schwannoma

Schwannomas are benign encapsulated tumors which arise from Schwann cells. In the PPS, the most common sites of origin are the vagus nerve and the sympathetic chain. On T1-weighted MR images, these lesions have intermediate signal intensity and enhance with contrast. On T2-weighted images, they demonstrate high signal intensity. On CT, these tumors are well-defined, intermediate density masses that enhance with contrast.

Neurofibroma

Neurofibromas are unencapsulated and intimately involved with the nerve of origin. Neurofibromas are often multiple. They may occur as a manifestation of the neurofibromatosis type 1, and in these patients, the incidence of malignant transformation is increased. The nerve of origin usually has to be sacrificed during excision to ensure complete removal of the neoplasm.

Lipoma

Lipomas are the most common mesenchymal tumors of soft tissue. They are painless benign masses, which most commonly grow subcutaneously. Deep neck lipomas grow insidiously and cause few symptoms other than those of a localized mass or mechanical displacement of adjacent structures. In these cases, patient may present with airway obstruction or dysphagia.[174,175]

Radiological imaging is critical for an accurate preoperative evaluation and planning the surgical approach. MR images demonstrate signal intensity of fat, with high signal on T1-weighted

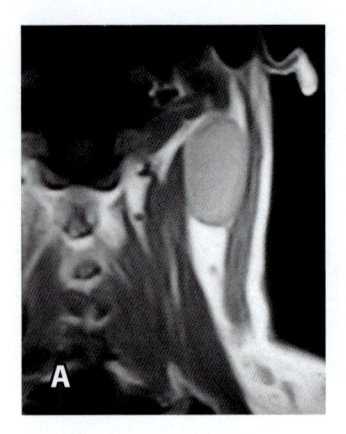

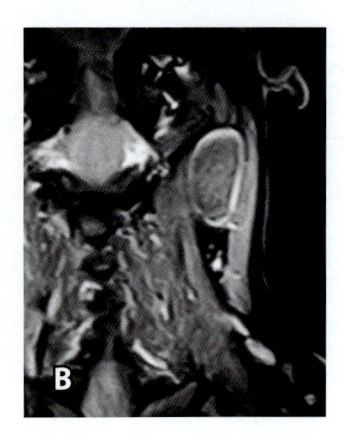

Figure 7-37 Encapsulated Lipoma
Coronal T1W and coronal contrast-enhanced T1W with fat-saturated MR images. The mildly hyperintense tumor (**A**) completely fades on the fat saturation image (**B**) with a smoothly enhancing capsule.

images and low signal on T2 (**Fig. 7-37**). Fat suppression will produce a low signal intensity. Lipomas do not enhance with contrast.

Management is surgical excision if the tumor produces symptoms. Lipomas are known to recur in 5% cases. Liposarcomas mostly arise de novo but a few cases of malignant change has been described[176] (**Fig. 7-38**).

Malignant Tumors of the Parapharyngeal Space

Extension of Regional Malignancies

The most common malignancy in the PPS is extension from surrounding regions. The vast majority of these are squamous cell carcinoma, but lymphoma is also seen. Oropharyngeal cancers from the anterior tonsillar pillar and soft palate are common. Nasopharyngeal carcinoma spreads to the parapharyngeal space in almost half of cases. Nasopharyngeal carcinoma is treated with combinded modality chemotherapy and radiotherapy.

T1-weighted images demonstrate a tumor with intermediate signal intensity amidst high signal fat of the PPS.

Malignant Salivary Gland Tumors

Half of primary PPS neoplasms are of salivary gland origin. These may arise from the deep lobe of the parotid gland, ectopic salivary rests, or minor salivary glands of the lateral pharyngeal wall. The prevalence of neoplasms that arise within the deep lobe of the parotid gland is identical to that of those that arise in the superficial lobe. The most common PPS lesion is the pleomorphic adenoma, which represents 80% to 90% of salivary neoplasms in this space. Other benign salivary lesions, including Warthin tumors and oncocytomas are also found. Mucoepidermoid carcinoma is the most common tumor of the parapharyngeal space, followed closely by carcinoma ex pleomorphic adenoma and adenoid cystic carcinoma (**Fig. 7-39**). Approximately 20% of all salivary lesions in the PPS are malignant.

LYMPH NODES OF THE NECK

The lymphatic system is composed of a vascular network of thin-walled capillaries that drain lymph from the extracellular spaces within most organs. The capillaries extend into larger vessels that pass into lymph nodes. All lymph is filtered through at least one, but usually several nodes. Efferent lymphatic collecting vessels return the lymph to the venous circulation via the thoracic and right lymphatic ducts. The lymphatic system also includes lymphoid organs such as the lymph nodes, tonsils, Peyer's patches, spleen, and thymus, all of which play an important role in the immune response.

Lymph nodes are ovoid, round, or bean-shaped nodular structures, composed of dense lymphoid tissue. Cervical nodes vary in size, with the largest nodes belonging to the internal jugular group, which are situated around the jugular vein. The average neck node is less than 10 mm in diameter. The nodes are partially or fully embedded in the fibrous adipose tissue, which facilitates smooth motion of the muscles, vessels and nerves.

Normal lymph flow enters the lymph nodes via afferent vessels and traverses the reticular meshwork of the marginal sinuses. It then flows to the cortical, and finally the medullary sinuses. Lymph leaves the nodes through efferent channels in the hilum.

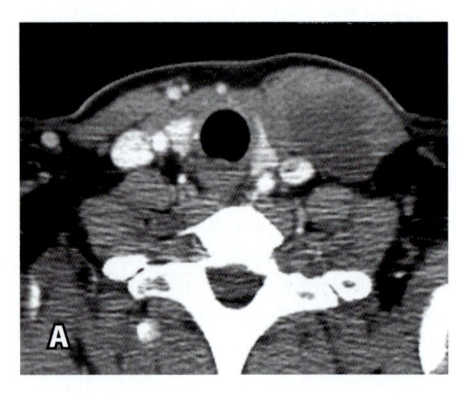

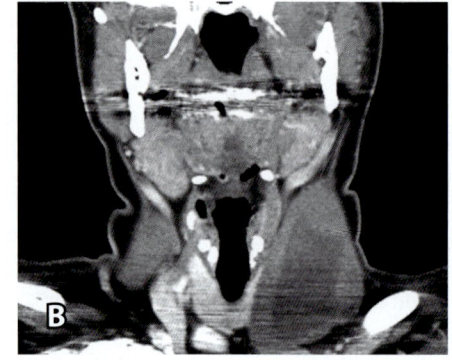

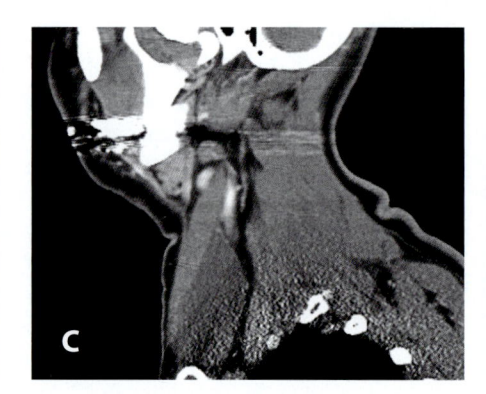

Figure 7-38 Liposarcoma of the Neck
Axial (**A**), coronal reformatted (**B**), and sagittal reformatted (**C**) contrast-enhanced CT images. There is a relatively lucent mass with irregular borders that is encompassed within the left sternocleidomastoid muscle. Pathologic diagnosis was that of a liposarcoma. Note that CT is less specific than MRI (Fig. 7-37).

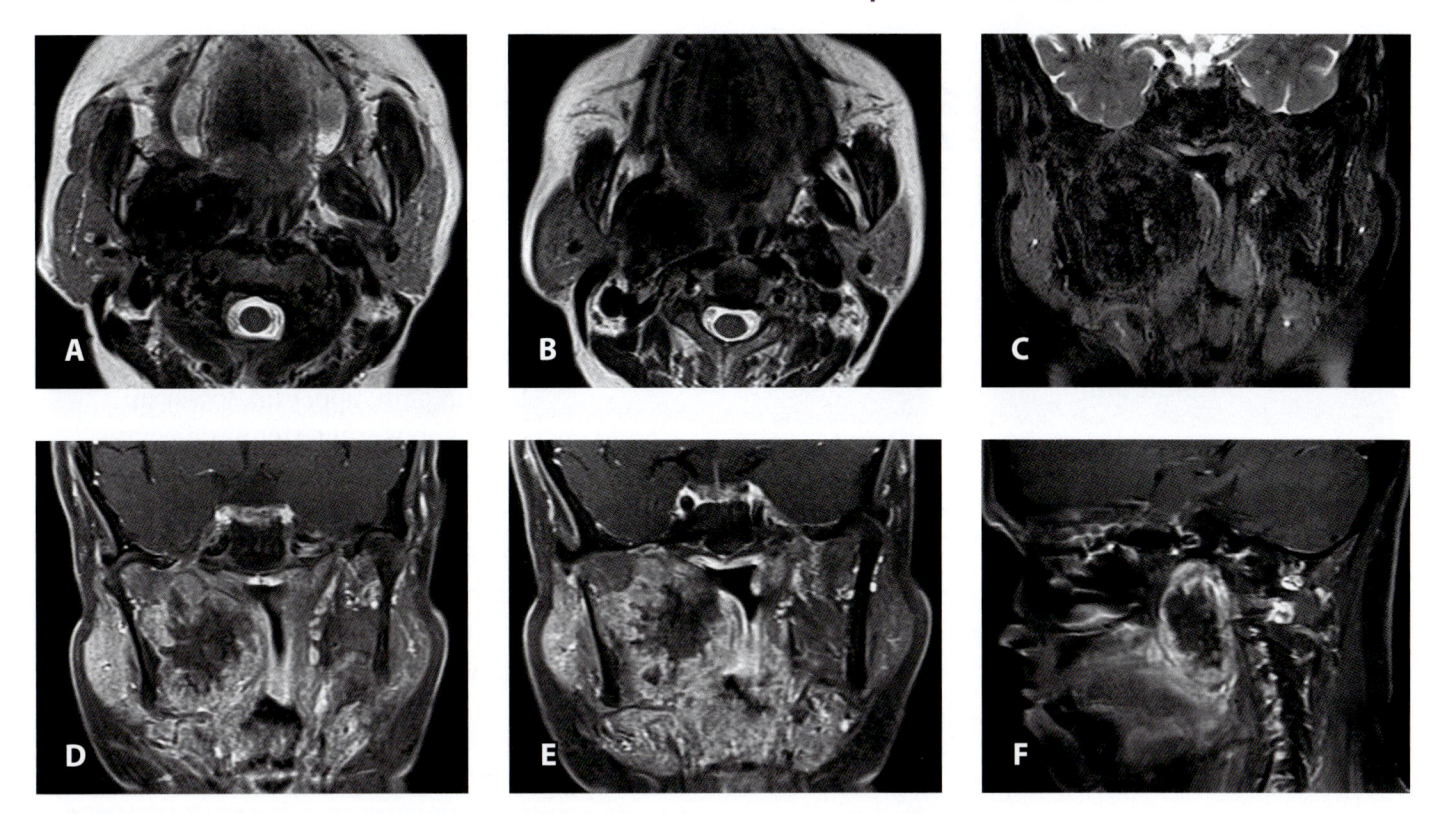

Figure 7-39 Parapharyngeal Mucoepidermoid Carcinoma with Central Calcifications
Axial FSE T2W (**A, B**), coronal T2W (**C**), and contrast-enhanced T1W with fat-saturated (coronal, **D, E**, and sagittal, **F**) MR scans. On all images the central portion of the right parapharyngeal space tumor remains devoid of signal, consistent with a dense calcified matrix. The surrounding regions of enhancement extend beyond the parapharyngeal space into the adjacent masticator space and deep lobe of the parotid gland.

More than one-third of the body's lymph nodes are in the neck. In the head and neck, only the orbit and the muscles lack direct lymphatics. The cervical lymphatics are arranged in clusters and chains which each have a characteristic drainage pattern. An understanding of the location and drainage of the nodes is important to identify which regions are the most likely to be affected by metastatic disease or infection **(Fig. 7-40)**. Drainage patterns and disease spread can be more easily understood by examining the embryologic origins of cervical structures.

The classification and terminology of the 300 cervical lymph nodes is complex and still developing. Classification systems based upon Rouviere's "lymphoid collar" have largely been replaced by the standardized nomenclature of the American Joint Committee on Cancer (AJCC) classification, which separates nodal regions into anatomical levels **(Table 7-1)**.

Imaging of Neck Lymph Nodes

One of the main indications for performing CT and MR imaging of the neck is the evaluation of cervical lymph nodes. Imaging studies are utilized both in cases of unknown neck mass and to investigate potential metastasis from known mucosal malignancies.

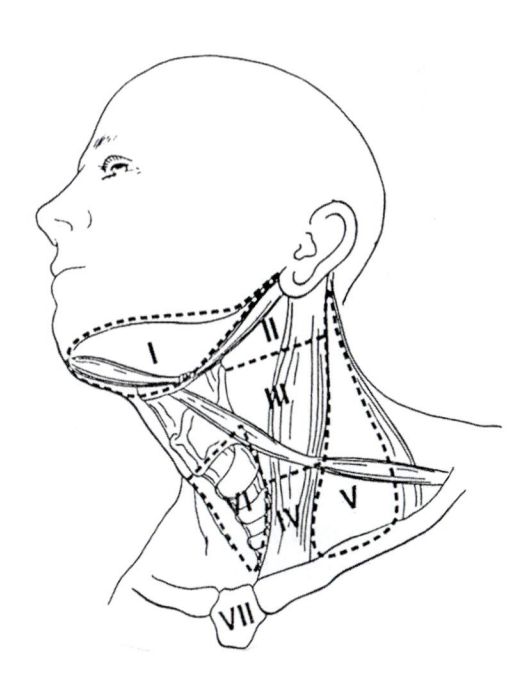

Figure 7-40 Anatomic Subsites of Nodes

Table 7-1 Nodal Anatomic Subsites – American Joint Committee on Cancer 2002

Level	Nodal Group	Location and Boundaries	Drainage
I	Submental mandibular	Contains the submental and submandibular triangles. Bounded by the anterior and posterior bellies of the digastric muscle, the hyoid bone inferiorly, and the mandibular body superiorly	**Submental** Chin, mid-lower lip, cheeks, anterior gingiva, floor of mouth, lower incisors, tip of tongue **Submandibular** Lateral chin, upper lip, lower lip, cheeks, nose, anterior nasal cavity, gums, teeth (except lower incisors, palate, medial eyelids, floor of mouth, submandibular and sublingual glands)
II	Upper jugular	Borders include the skull base superiorly to hyoid bone inferiorly	Submandibular, parotid, and retropharyngeal nodes; tonsil, pharynx, larynx, esophagus, thyroid glands
III	Mid-jugular	Bounded by the hyoid bone superiorly and the cricoid cartilage inferiorly	
IV	Lower jugular	Extends from the cricoid cartilage superiorly to the clavicle interiorly	
V	Posterior triangle	**Posterior Triangle** Includes the posterior triangle, with boundaries formed by the anterior aspect of the trapezius posteriorly, the posterior border of the sternocleidomastoid anteriorly, and the clavicle inferiorly	Occipital region at the apex of the posterior triangle
		Spinal Accessory Along the course of the spinal accessory nerve and in the posterior triangle of the neck	parotid region, occipital region, lateral neck, shoulder
		Transverse Cervical Above the clavicle and along the course of the transverse cervical vessels	Internal jugular and posterior triangle nodes, infraclavicular regions, skin of anterolateral neck
VI	Prelaryngeal (Delphian) pretracheal paratracheal	Includes the anterior central compartment. Extends from the hyoid bone superiorly to the suprasternal notch inferiorly. The lateral borders are formed by the medial aspects of the carotid sheaths.	**Prelaryngeal** Larynx **Pretracheal** Skin and muscles of the anterior neck **Paratracheal** Supraglottic and subglottic larynx, pyriform sinus, thyroid, trachea, and esophagus

Table 7-1 Nodal Anatomic Subsites – American Joint Committee on Cancer 2002 (*Continued*)			
Level	Nodal Group	Location and Boundaries	Drainage
VI	Upper mediastinal	Includes the upper mediastinum, inferior to the suprasternal notch	
Others	Suboccipital		
	Retropharyngeal		Nasopharynx, oropharynx
	Buccinator		Eyelids, cheek, mid-face
	Preauricular		Skin of head and neck
	Periparotid		Skin of head and neck
	Intraparotid		Parotid glands, forehead and temporal region, middle and lateral face, auricle, external auditory canal, Eustachian tube, posterior cheek, buccal mucous membrane, gums

Cor = best assessed in coronal CT sections; Axi = best assessed in axial CT sections.

Important aspects of the assessment include the presence, location, extent, and spread of metastases to critical adjacent structures, such as the carotid artery, internal jugular veins, and skull base. Worldwide, palpation is the most common method of staging the neck. Palpation of cervical lymph nodes is inexpensive and easy to perform, but is generally considered to be inaccurate. The sensitivity and specificity of this staging method are in the range of 60% to 70% depending on the tumor studied.[177] The low sensitivity of this method increases the risk for unrecognized occult metastasis. The sensitivity of CT and MR for accurately detecting nodal metastases has been reported as 84% and 92%, respectively.[178] Imaging can help detect occult metastases, determine operability in patients with palpable lymph nodes, and can be both prognostically and therapeutically relevant if vital structures have been invaded.

MR has replaced CT in the majority of extracranial lesions of the head and neck. There are proponents for each modality, and numerous investigators have assessed their relative accuracy and sensitivity in neck node evaluation. MR is generally considered superior to CT in the evaluation of the nasopharynx, paranasal sinuses, salivary glands, oropharynx, and the retropharyngeal and prevertebral spaces. CT has greater accuracy in the evaluation of regions subject to motion artifact, such as the larynx. In addition, it is faster, less expensive, and useful for patients with contraindications for MR.[179]

Normal lymph nodes have the same density as muscle on unenhanced CT. Intravenous contrast increases nodal enhancement. Similarly, on unenhanced T1-weighted MR, lymph nodes have the same signal intensity as muscle, while contrast produces a slight increase in signal. Comparison of pre- and postcontrast sequences is useful in identifying skull base invasion and perineural tumor spread. T1 images without contrast show fine anatomic detail and distortion of fat planes, while T2-weighted images more clearly demonstrate lesions and abnormalities.[179] A normal lymph node is oblong or oval-shaped with a well-defined border. The lucent hilum of the node is composed of fat, and can be mistaken for a necrotic node on CT.[180]

Evaluation of Neck Lymph Nodes

Imaging is especially useful to patient management if a metastatic node or nodes are found in a clinically negative neck. The main imaging criteria for assessing nodal metastases include the size and shape of the node, the presence of necrosis, and the presence of a localized group of nodes in an expected nodal draining area for a specific primary tumor.

There is disagreement about the best way to measure nodes, but in the simplest case, nodes are considered abnormal if they are larger than 10 mm in diameter. Exceptions include the larger level II nodes and the smaller retropharyngeal nodes, which are considered abnormal if their diameter exceeds 15 mm and 8 mm, respectively.[181] Microscopic tumor foci cannot yet be identified by imaging.[182] Normal nodes are oval or oblong, while metastatic nodes are round or spherical.[159]

Central nodal necrosis is considered a more specific sign of metastasis. Evaluation sensitivity is enhanced significantly when both necrosis and nodal size are used as criteria. On CT, necrosis appears as a rim of irregular enhancement surrounding a hypoattenuated central region. On postcontrast, fat-suppressed, T1-weighted MR images, peripheral enhancement surrounds a central hypointensity.[159]

Extra-nodal tumor spread decreases survival by 50% compared to confined tumors.[183] Extranodal extension is seen on CT images as a poorly defined nodal border with variable enhancement. In addition, there may be obliterated fat planes adjacent to the node. It should be noted that infection, prior surgery, or irradiation can produce similar findings.[159]

Staging of Neck Lymph Nodes

Accurate staging is the most important factor in assessment, treatment planning, and prognosis in patients with head and neck cancer. The AJCC TNM staging system incorporates three aspects of tumor growth: the extent of primary tumor (T), the involvement of regional lymph nodes (N), and distant metastasis (M).

THYROID GLAND

Anatomy of the Thyroid Gland

The normal thyroid gland is located between the thyroid cartilage and the fifth or sixth tracheal ring. It is firm and rubbery, surrounded by a fibrous capsule, and enclosed in a fascial compartment formed by the pretracheal fascia. The normal gland surrounds the anterior and lateral circumference of the trachea. Each lobe is approximately 5 cm long, 3 cm wide, and 2 cm thick, but the size varies with sex and nutritional status. The isthmus of the gland is firmly adhered to the second or third tracheal cartilage. In half of all individuals a pyramidal lobe extends from the gland. The prevertebral fascia covering the long muscles of the neck lies behind the gland, while the carotid sheath lies laterally. At the lower pole, fat separates the gland from the longus colli muscles.

The thyroid is composed of a supporting stoma with blood vessels and nerves, and the gland parenchyma, which is divided into lobules composed of 20 to 40 thyroid follicles. The normal weight of the tissue is between 15 and 20 g. Physiological stress causes the gland to increase in size and activity. Transient hyperplasia is marked by the growth of follicular cells, which become tall and columnar and form buds or papillae. When the stress is removed, involution and colloid accumulation occurs, and the follicular cells return to their normal size and shape.

MR Imaging of the Thyroid Gland

Normal thyroid tissue is hypointense relative to muscle on T1-weighted images and intermediate between the intensities of fat and muscle on T2-weighted images. The strap muscles can be distinguished from the subcutaneous fat and the immediately abutting thyroid gland because of their relatively low signal intensity. Portions of the inferior thyroid veins can be seen between the lobes anteriorly. The esophagus can be seen posterior to the trachea, with its mucosal layers showing higher intensity than the muscular wall on T2-weighted images.[184,185]

Thyroid abnormalities are evaluated primarily by nuclear medicine scans and ultrasonography. Functional status of the gland is determined by radionucleotide scintigraphy, histological diagnosis is made by percutaneous needle biopsy, and sonography is used to distinguish cystic from solid lesions and to monitor the size of nodules. MR imaging is indicated in the assessment of large tumors, the mediastinal extension of large goiters, and identifying sites of recurrence of thyroid carcinoma. T1-weighted images distinguish tumor from fat, while T2-weighted images differentiate tumor and muscle. Tumor invasion will change the signal characteristics of the muscle, causing it to be hyperintense to the contralateral muscle on T2-weighted images. In addition, MR imaging can demonstrate the involvement of the trachea and esophagus, as well as lymphadenopathy. In the investigation of large goiters, coronal images can show cervical and thoracic components, and are useful for preoperative planning. Postoperatively, characteristic imaging findings can differentiate between recurrent carcinoma and fibrosis.[186]

MR imaging has the advantage of excellent tissue contrast, allowing for discrimination of various tissues and the numerous tissue planes of the neck. Surface coils designed especially for the neck allow for thin sections and small fields of view. In visualizing the vasculature, no contrast media is required. On spin-echo images, flowing blood is represented by a flow void. Contrast is used to differentiate normal and pathological tissues. MR imaging with contrast is superior to CT because the contrast does not interfere with iodide uptake or organification by the thyroid gland.

Inflammatory and Metabolic Lesions of the Thyroid Gland

Thyroiditis

Inflammation of the thyroid gland, thyroiditis, encompasses a diverse group of disorders with a range of consequences. Acute conditions, such as infectious (suppurative) thyroiditis and subacute granulomatous (De Quervain's) thyroiditis, usually present with significant pain but little dysfunction of the gland. On the other end of the spectrum, subacute lymphocytic thyroiditis and Reidel (fibrous) thyroiditis, produce relatively little inflammation or pain, but substantial thyroid dysfunction. Hashimoto thyroiditis, an autoimmune disease, is chronic and painless, but demonstrates inflammation and gradual thyroid dysfunction, and has systemic consequences. There are no specific MR imaging findings that allow for the differentiation of the inflammatory disease processes involving the thyroid, with the exception of the hypointensity on all sequences found in Riedel thyroiditis.

Hashimoto Thyroiditis

Hashimoto thyroiditis is a chronic lymphocytic autoimmune disease characterized by gradual destruction of the thyroid gland with resultant hypothyroidism. It is the most common cause of hypothyroidism in the United States and in areas of the world with sufficient dietary iodine levels. This disease occurs predominantly in women between the ages of 40 and 60 years. It has a significant genetic component, clustering in families. Cases have been associated with the presence of major histocompatibility haplotypes HLA-DR5 and HLA-DR3, implying different pathologic mechanisms leading to its development.[187] Hashimoto thyroiditis is associated with an increased incidence of other autoimmune diseases, such as systemic lupus erythematosus and rheumatoid arthritis, as well as B cell lymphomas.

Clinically, Hashimoto thyroiditis presents as a painless unilateral or bilateral enlargement of the thyroid and with some degree of hypothyroidism. On palpation, the gland is moderately enlarged, firm, and occasionally multinodular, without necrosis or calcification. In approximately 12% of patients

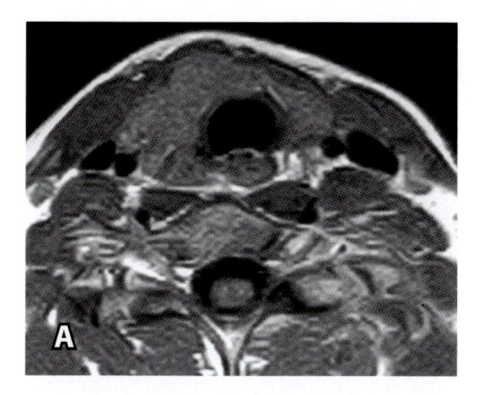

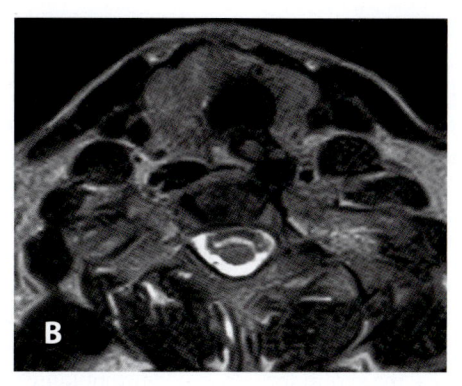

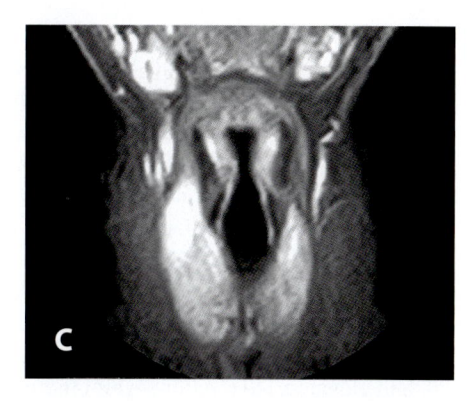

Figure 7-41 Hashimoto Thyroiditis with Lymphoma
Axial T1 (**A**), axial T2 (**B**) and coronal contrast-enhanced with fat-saturated (**C**) MR scans. There is heterogenous signal and nodularity throughout both lobes of the thyroid gland and thyroid isthmus, greater on the right side. Following contrast infusion, there is intense enhancement without a focal mass (**C**). The findings are nonspecific; however, sudden increases in the size of the thyroid gland in patients with known Hashimoto thyroiditis should raise suspicion of an associated autoimmune neoplasm such as lymphoma.

there is extensive fibrosis and a large symptomatic goiter which can cause symptoms of dyspnea and dysphagia. These cases most often occur in men.[188]

Morphologically, the gland is diffusely enlarged with an intact capsule. Histologically, there is a lymphocytic infiltration with plasma cells and well-developed germinal centers. In addition, there is oncocytic cellular change of follicular cells and atrophy of follicles with scant colloid. Laboratory tests demonstrate autoantibodies against thyroglobulin, thyroid peroxidase, and thyroid stimulating hormone (TSH) receptor.

MR imaging shows a diffusely enlarged gland with a heterogenous and sometimes nodular appearance. T2-weighted images of the gland demonstrate increased signal intensity. In some cases, lower intensity bands are present, indicating fibrosis (**Fig. 7-41**).

Hormone deficiency is treated with replacement therapy. Prognosis for the disease is good with proper treatment.

Riedel (Fibrous) Thyroiditis

Reidel thyroiditis (RT) is a rare disorder marked by extensive fibrosis of the thyroid gland and surrounding structures. The disease may be associated with other fibrogenic disorders, including retroperitoneal and mediastinal fibrosis, sclerosing cholangitis, and orbital pseudotumor. The etiology of this disease is still unknown. Women are affected more often than men.

Patients present with a rapidly enlarging thyroid mass which may cause local pressure symptoms of dyspnea, dysphagia, and hoarseness. The gland is often asymmetrical and non-tender, with a "stony hard" goiter. Symptoms of hypothyroidism are usually present.

Morphologically, the gland is diffusely enlarged. Fibrosis extends beyond the capsule, infiltrating adjacent musculature. Vasculitis is also present, with small arteries and veins showing fibro-inflammatory involvement. Histologically, RT demonstrates atrophic thyroid follicles surrounded by an inflammatory infiltrate of lymphocytes, plasma cells, and eosinophils, and dense bands of fibrosis.

The characteristic finding on MR imaging is hypointensity on T1- and T2-weighted images with homogenous enhancement or decreased enhancement.[188] It is believed that fibrotic replacement of normal thyroid parenchyma and vasculature explain the lack of enhancement following iodinated contrast on CT and gadolinium administration on MR imaging.[189] The gland is irregularly enlarged with obliteration of adjacent soft tissue planes, indicating an infiltrative mass. RT is the only thyroid disorder that is easily distinguishable on the basis of MR signal intensity. While other thyroid diseases show homogeneous or heterogeneous hyperintensity, especially on T2-weighted images, RT appears homogeneously hypointense on all sequences due to the extensive fibrosis.[190] Airway deviation and stenosis are common findings. In addition, adjacent structures including the strap muscles, CS, tracheoesophageal groove and retropharyngeal regions are often invaded.[191]

In general, RT is self-limiting disease with a good prognosis. Limited surgical intervention may be required to treat compressive symptoms. RT resembles thyroid malignancy, but because of the significant differences in treatment, staging, and prognosis, it is important to differentiate these diseases before surgery. Potential surgical complications include injury to vital surrounding structures, such as the carotid arteries, recurrent laryngeal nerves, and parathyroid glands. Corticosteroids have been used successfully to slow progression of the disease. Tamoxifen has also show success, possibly due to its ability to stimulate the release of transforming growth factor-beta, which inhibits fibroblast proliferation.[192]

Granulomatous Subacute (De Quervain's) Thyroiditis

Granulomatous subacute thyroiditis (GST) is another inflammatory thyroid disorder of uncertain etiology. It is believed that GST is caused by a viral infection or postviral inflammatory response, as the majority of patients develop the disease after an acute upper respiratory infection. Cytotoxic T lymphocytes damage thyroid follicles causing an excessive release of thyroid hormones and transient hyperthyroidism. Unlike autoimmune diseases, the process is limited rather than chronic. Women between the ages of 30 and 50 years old are predominantly affected. There is a strong association with HLA-B35.

Patients present with pain in the neck, especially when swallowing. In addition, there are constitutional symptoms of fever, fatigue, anorexia, and myalgia. Onset may be gradual or sudden. The thyroid gland is enlarged and painful. Initially, serum levels of T3 and T4 are high, while TSH levels are low. Unlike most cases of hyperthyroidism, radioactive iodine uptake is diminished, due to low TSH levels. As the disease progresses, a hypothyroid state develops, with decreased levels of T3 and T4, and elevated TSH. After several more weeks, the serum levels return to normal.

The gland is firm and unilaterally or bilaterally enlarged. The capsule is intact, and may be slightly adherent to the adjacent structures. Histologically, damaged thyroid follicles are surrounded by inflammatory aggregates of lymphocytes and plasma cells. Multinucleate giant cells surround pools of colloid. As the disease progresses, inflammatory infiltrate and fibrosis fill the site of injury.

MR imaging shows a diffusely enlarged gland with high signal intensity on T1- and T2-weighted images.[191] Diagnosis is made on clinical grounds.

The disease is self-limiting, with a good prognosis. Patients are typically hyperthyroid for several weeks, followed by a brief hypothyroid phase. Thyroid function returns to normal after one to two months. The painless variant of this disease may resemble a tumor, necessitating a core needle biopsy for diagnosis.[188]

Acute Infectious (Suppurative) Thyroiditis

Acute infective thyroiditis is a rare, self-limited infectious process which does not significantly impair thyroid function. Infections reach the thyroid by direct seeding of the gland via a fistula from the piriform sinus, or by hematogenous spread. Causative pathogens include *Streptococcus hemolyticus*, *Staphylococcus*, *Pneumococcus*, *Mycobacterium tuberculosis*, and several species of fungi. Glandular enlargement is secondary to edema. Liquification necrosis and abscess formation may occur.

Symptoms of acute thyroiditis include neck pain and tenderness, fever, and dysphagia. Patients present with a swollen, tender thyroid gland. MR imaging is utilized to exclude fistulas from the piriform sinus or thyroglossal duct as causes of the infection. Images demonstrate neck swelling, within and around the gland, and abscess formation.[193]

Fine-needle thyroid aspiration is utilized to obtain material for culture. Immediate parenteral antibiotic therapy is used to prevent abscess formation. Surgery may be indicated if a developmental abnormality is the cause of the infectious process.

Graves Disease

Graves disease is another autoimmune disorder, with thyroid dysfunction resulting from autoantibodies against the TSH receptor. It is the most common cause of endogenous hyperthyroidism. This disease is very common, predominantly affecting women between the ages of 20 and 40 years. Genetic factors are important in this disease, with family clustering and high concordance (60%) in monozygotic twins. HLA-B8 and HLA-DR3 are commonly associated with the disease.[187] Patients with Graves disease have an increased probability of developing other autoimmune diseases, including systemic lupus erythematosus, pernicious anemia, type 1 diabetes, and Addison disease.

Patients with Grave's disease present with diffuse enlargement of the thyroid gland and hyperthyroidism. In addition, exophthalmos is a common finding, and pretibial myxedema occurs in a minority of patients. Hyperactivity of the thyroid gland causes symptoms such as heat intolerance, weight loss, fatigue, insomnia, tremors, palpitations, and agitation.

Morphologically, there is diffuse hypertrophy and hyperplasia of the thyroid follicular epithelial cells. Histologically, there is prominent vascular congestion and follicular hyperplasia, but lobular architecture is retained. Colloid is scant and pale, with scalloping at the periphery. Laboratory findings demonstrate elevated free T4 and T3 levels and depressed TSH levels.

On MR imaging, the gland is enlarged with diffusely increased signal intensity on T1- and T2-weighted images and avid enhancement. In addition, there are numerous coarse bands within the gland representing fibrous tissue around thyroid lobules, as well as dilated vessels representing venous structures.[184,185] Iodine uptake is markedly increased on radioiodine scans, within the enlarged, nonfocal, hot gland.

The goal of treatment is to decrease the aspects of hyperthyroidism caused by increased beta-adrenergic tone. Administration of thioamides, such as propylthiouracil, radioactive iodine obliteration of the gland, or surgical thyroidectomy are common. None of these options removes the underlying immune disorder. Graves disease is a chronic illness with no true cure.

Simple and Multinodular Goiter

The most common manifestation of thyroid disease is enlargement of the thyroid gland, or goiter. Impaired synthesis of thyroid hormone results in diffuse or multinodular goiter. Endemic goiter, the most common cause of goiter worldwide, is caused by iodine deficiency, while sporadic goiter, the most common form in the developed countries, results from other causes, including autoimmune disorders, hyper- or hypothyroidism, and thyroid carcinoma. Puberty and pregnancy are common, benign causes of goiter in which estrogen causes diffuse enlargement of the thyroid. When the size of the gland is doubled, it becomes palpable, and when it reaches three times the normal mass, the goiter becomes visible.[10] Large goiters often mimic or hide neoplastic disease.

A goiter which is diffusely enlarged without nodularity is called a simple goiter. In the hyperplastic stage, the gland is diffusely and symmetrically enlarged. In the resolving phase, the follicular epithelium involutes to form an enlarged, colloid-rich gland.

Over time, repeated cycles of enlargement and involution produce a multinodular goiter. These lesions can produce dramatic enlargement of the gland, with goiters reaching up to 2,000 g.[187] Uneven follicular hyperplasia and colloid accumulation leads to scarring, hemorrhages, and calcification. Nodularity arises from the expanded parenchyma within the restraints of the gland's stromal framework.

Patients are usually older women with an asymptomatic unilateral or bilateral mass in the lower neck. The enlarged gland may compress the airway, causing dysphagia, or may compress the large vessels of the neck and upper thorax. A minority of patients may have symptoms indicative of hyperthyroidism or hypothyroidism.

Morphologically, the gland is asymmetrically enlarged and multilobulated. The gland can compress adjacent structures laterally, or it can extend behind the sternum or into the mediastinum. Histologically, there are areas of follicular epithelial hypertrophy mixed with regions of flattened, inactive epithelium filled with colloid. Hemorrhage, fibrosis, and calcification represent regressive change.

MR imaging is utilized to assess the volume and morphology of the gland, visualize the status of the airway and evaluate compression of adjacent structures, detect features of malignant degeneration, and direct fine needle aspiration.[191] Determining the extent of the goiter is vital for preoperative planning.

These lesions are composed of solid matrix, colloid cysts, blood degradation products, fibrosis, and calcification, therefore imaging findings vary. Commonly, the lesion appears heterogeneous with nodularity and isointense signal on T1-weighted images.[184,185] Hemorrhagic foci are present in the majority of cases and the lesions are heterogenous on T2-weighted images.[193] Multinodular goiters demonstrate well-defined borders and lobules, differentiating them from neoplastic processes. Tracheal deviation or stenosis are often present.[188]

Treatment may involve surgery if there are compressive symptoms or for cosmetic reasons. The recurrence rate following nontotal bilateral thyroidectomy is 21%.[10] Antithyroid medications and radioiodine are nonsurgical alternatives for decreasing the gland's volume.

Benign Lesions of the Thyroid

Thyroid Adenoma

Adenomas are the most common benign thyroid tumors. The majority are discrete, solitary masses derived from follicular epithelium. Increases in intracellular levels of cAMP activate genes that control the production of thyroid hormone and proliferation of thyroid epithelial cells. Fifty percent to 75% of autonomously functioning thyroid adenomas are caused by somatic mutations that lead to the constitutive activation of cAMP.[187]

The discovery of thyroid adenoma is often an incidental finding. These masses are painless, but large tumors may cause local pressure symptoms, such as dysphagia. Follicular adenomas appear in all age groups and are slightly more common in women. The size of these tumors is variable, but most are smaller than 3 cm.[193]

On gross inspection, these lesions are solitary masses with complete fibrous capsules. They may have foci of necrosis, hemorrhage, or cystic degeneration. There is clear distinction from surrounding structures, and compression of adjacent thyroid tissue. Microscopically, there are uniform colloid-filled follicles. Different subtypes are categorized by colloid content and the degree of follicle formation. Most adenomas appear as cold nodules on radioiodine scans, although rare hyperfunctional adenomas that cause hyperthyroidism (Plummer's disease) appear as hot nodules. Cold nodules have a significantly higher rate of malignancy.

Adenomas, like multinodular goiters, are hypo- to isointense compared to normal thyroid tissue on T1-weighted images and are hyperintense on T2-weighted images. Foci of increased signal on T1 may represent hemorrhage and areas of low signal may represent hyaline degeneration or calcification.[186] Significant contrast enhancement is due to the vascularity and increased extracellular space of the adenoma compared to normal thyroid tissue.[184,185]

Adenomas are removed surgically for definitive diagnosis. Inspection of the capsule is vital, as follicular carcinomas are differentiated from adenomas by extracapsular spread and invasion of blood vessels.

Benign Cyst

Benign thyroid cysts constitute approximately 20% of solitary nodules.[188] The majority result from degeneration of thyroid adenomas, and a minority arise in multinodular goiters. They are filled with blood, hemosiderin, and cell debris.

Cysts demonstrate high or low signal intensity on T1-weighted images, and uniformly high signal on T2-weighted images. Colloid cysts are homogenous and hyperintense on both T1- and T2 images (**Fig. 7-42**). Noncolloid cysts are hypointense on T1. Hemorrhagic cysts are

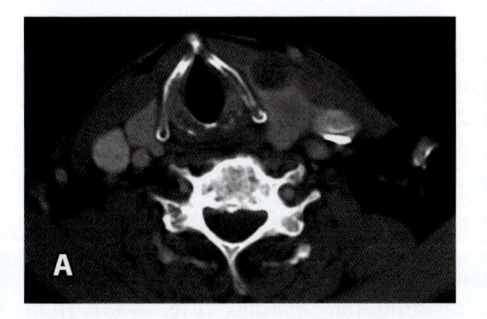

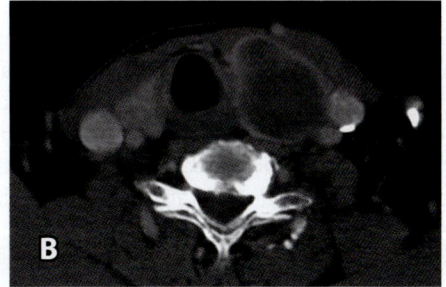

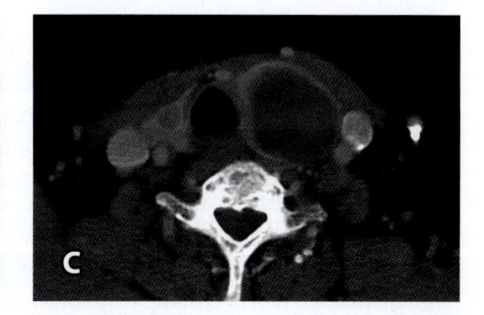

Figure 7-42 Thyroid Gland Colloid Cysts
(**A–C**) Axial contrast-enhanced CT scans. The left lobe of the thyroid is markedly enlarged and contains at least two smoothly marginated, nonenhancing cysts. Cystic thyroid neoplasms can have an identical appearance and cannot be ruled out without biopsy or PET/CT scans.

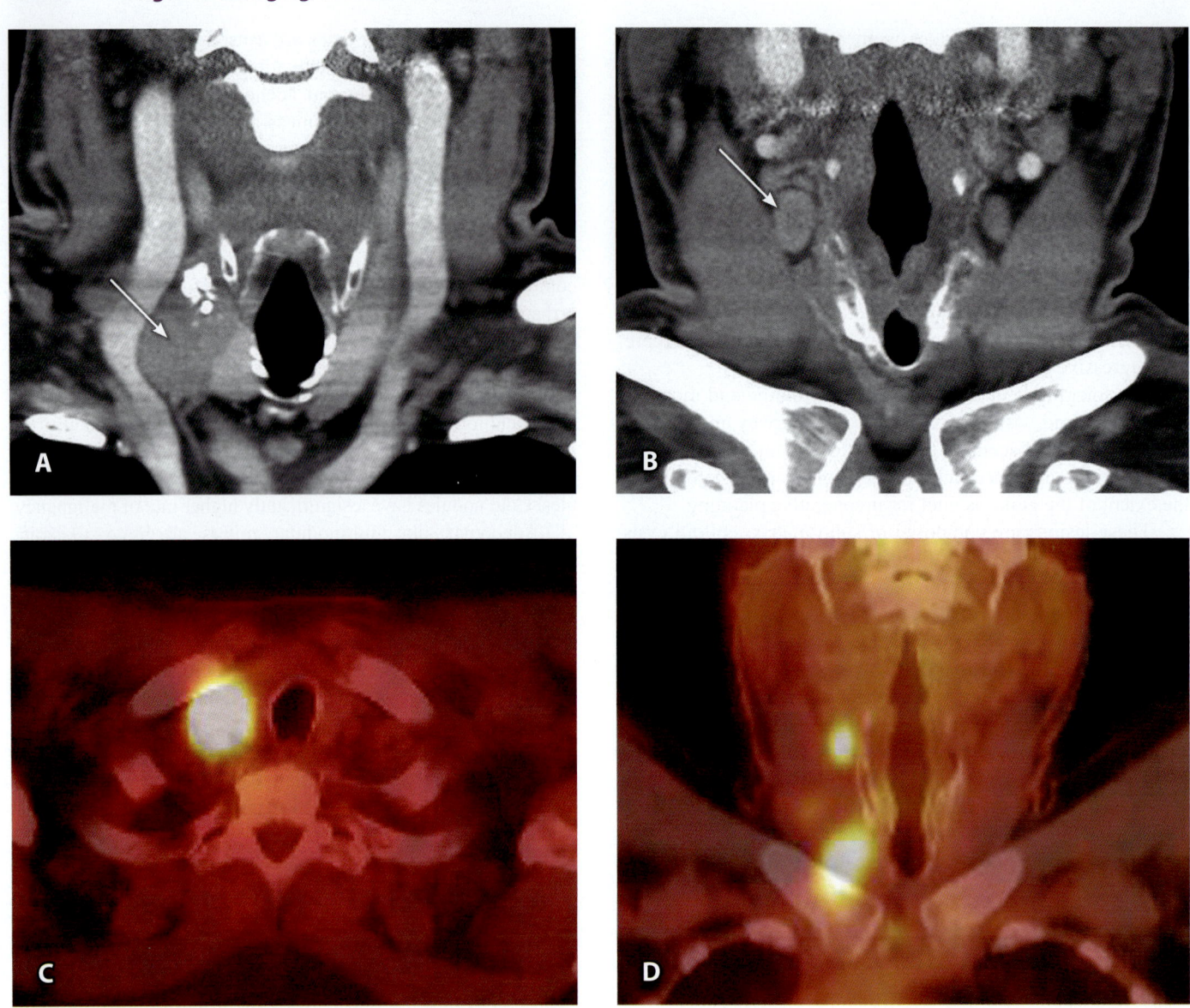

Figure 7-43 Metastasis to the Thyroid and Neck
(**A, B**) Reformatted coronal contrast-enhanced CT scans and (**C**). axial and (**D**). coronal PET/CT images. There is a mass with the right lobe of the thyroid (*arrow*, **A**) lying caudal to some irregular calcifications, likely in a colloid cyst. There is at least one pathologically enlarged lymph node in the adjacent soft tissues of the neck (*arrow*, **B**). The mass in the right thyroid and the neck node show avid FDG uptake (**C** and **D**), both were proven to be metastatic lesions from squamous cell carcinoma.

relatively hyperintense on both T1 and T2, and after 14 to 21 days, may demonstrate a "rim sign" of hypointensity on T2 which corresponds to a ring of hemosiderin-laden macrophages. Cystic degeneration within multinodular goiters or tumors may be hyper- or hypointense to normal thyroid tissue and other parts of the tumor on T2-weighted images. Hypointensity signifies hyaline degeneration.[186]

Malignant Lesions of the Thyroid

Thyroid carcinoma accounts for 1.5% of all cancers in the United States. Most cases occur in adults, with a female predominance that has been attributed to estrogen receptors on neoplastic thyroid epithelium. Most of these tumors are well-differentiated. Exposure to ionizing radiation, especially in youth, is a major risk factor. Other risk factors include thyroid diseases such as Hashimoto thyroiditis and nodular goiter. The activation or mutation of certain oncogenes is an important factor in the development of these lesions. The thyroid can also be the site of non-Hodgkin's lymphoma, which has a strong relationship with Hashimoto thyroiditis.

Thyroid malignancy commonly appears as a unilateral intrathyroid mass with infiltrating margins (**Fig. 7-43**). Both benign and malignant tumors generally have low signal intensity on T1-weighted images and high intensity on T2-weighted images. MR imaging can aid in the diagnosis of thyroid cancers by detecting malignant lymphadenopathy.

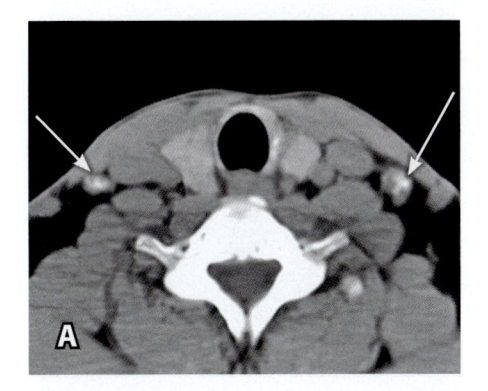

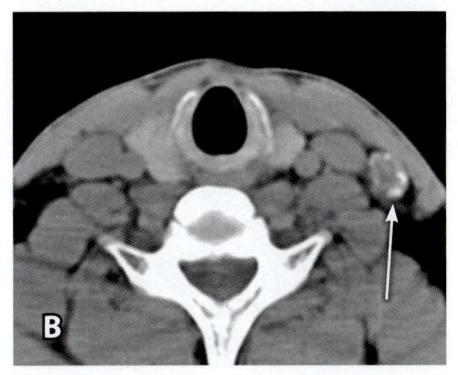

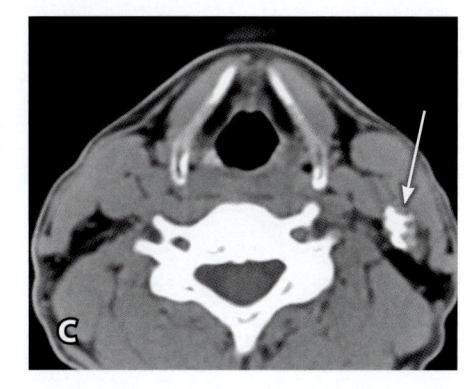

Figure 7-44 Thyroid Papillary Carcinoma with Calcified Nodal Metastasis
Axial CT scans (**A–C**) without contrast. A portion of the left lobe of the thyroid gland has been surgically resected. There are multiple calcified nodal masses in both sides of the neck (*arrows*). Such lesions are characteristic of metastasis from thyroid papillary carcinoma.

Papillary Carcinoma

Papillary carcinoma is the most common thyroid malignancy, constituting 75% to 85% of all thyroid malignancies. They occur most often in women between 20 and 40 years, and are strongly associated with previous exposure to ionizing radiation. Most of these tumors are well-differentiated and indolent, but an aggressive variant can invade the trachea, larynx, and esophagus. Rearrangements in chromosome 10 result in a mutated gene called the papillary thyroid carcinoma oncogene (RET/PTC), which is constitutively active and provides unregulated growth signals to thyroid cells.

Patients may present with asymptomatic thyroid nodules or with a mass in a cervical lymph node (**Fig. 7-44**). In advanced disease, symptoms of dysphagia, dyspnea, hoarseness, or cough may be present. Papillary masses are cold nodules on radioiodine scans. Fine needle aspiration is necessary to differentiate benign from malignant lesions.

Papillary carcinomas can be uni- or multifocal lesions within the gland. Some are well circumscribed, while others are infiltrative, with ill-defined margins. The lesions are often cystic, and contain areas of fibrosis and calcification (**Fig. 7-45**). Definitive diagnosis is made upon microscopic exam, which shows psammoma bodies, ground glass nuclei, and branching papillae with dense fibrovascular cores.[187]

On MR imaging, the tumor is isointense with muscle on T1-weighted images and intermediate to high intensity on T2-weighted images, with a heterogeneous enhancement pattern. Cystic and hemorrhagic components have high intensity on both T1- and T2-weighted images.

Surgery is the therapy of choice for all primary lesions. The prognosis for papillary carcinoma is good, with a 10-year survival rate of 98%.[187] Patients with extrathyroid invasion and distant metastasis have a poorer prognosis, as do male patients, elderly patients, and those with tumors larger than 5 cm.[188]

Follicular Carcinoma

Follicular carcinoma is the second most common type of thyroid carcinoma, accounting for 10% to 20% of cases. This disease is more prevalent in women between the ages of 40 and 50 years. Iodine deficiency and nodular goiter may predispose individuals to the development of this disease.

The majority of these tumors are well-circumscribed and slow growing, resembling an adenoma. Invasiveness is evident on microscopic inspection, and is diagnostic. The aggressive form of follicular carcinoma is invasive, penetrating the surrounding tissue and airway. Histologically, the colloid-filled follicles are uniform, resembling normal thyroid tissue. Psammoma bodies and nuclear features of papillary carcinoma are not present.

Imaging findings are the same as those for other papillary carcinoma and other malignant tumors. The lesion may be confined to the gland or it may invade surrounding structures, and show necrosis and calcification (**Fig. 7-46**).

Capsular and vascular invasion indicates distant metastases in 50% to 75% of cases. Lymph node metastases are rare, but vascular invasion, with metastases to lungs, liver, brain, and bone, are common.[188] Treatment is lobectomy or thyroidectomy followed by treatment with thyroid hormone to suppress endogenous TSH.

Medullary Carcinoma

Medullary carcinoma comprises approximately 5% of thyroid carcinomas. This neuroendocrine tumor arises from the parafollicular, or C cells of the thyroid. Like normal C cells, this tumor secretes calcitonin, which can be used as a tumor marker. Eighty percent of cases are sporadic, while 20% are familial forms, with and without associated multiple endocrine neoplasia (MEN). The sporadic cases usually arise in individuals older than 50 years, and have a poorer prognosis than the familial form. The familial form is inherited as an autosomal dominant trait, and is more likely to appear in younger individuals. Tumors are generally unilateral in sporadic cases and bilateral in familial cases. Germline mutations in the RET protooncogene play an important role in the development of the familial form of the disease, and have been associated with some cases of the sporadic form.[187] Lymphatic spread is the primary mode of metastasis, but hematological spread is also common. Amyloid deposits appear in 90% of these tumors and are pathognomonic.

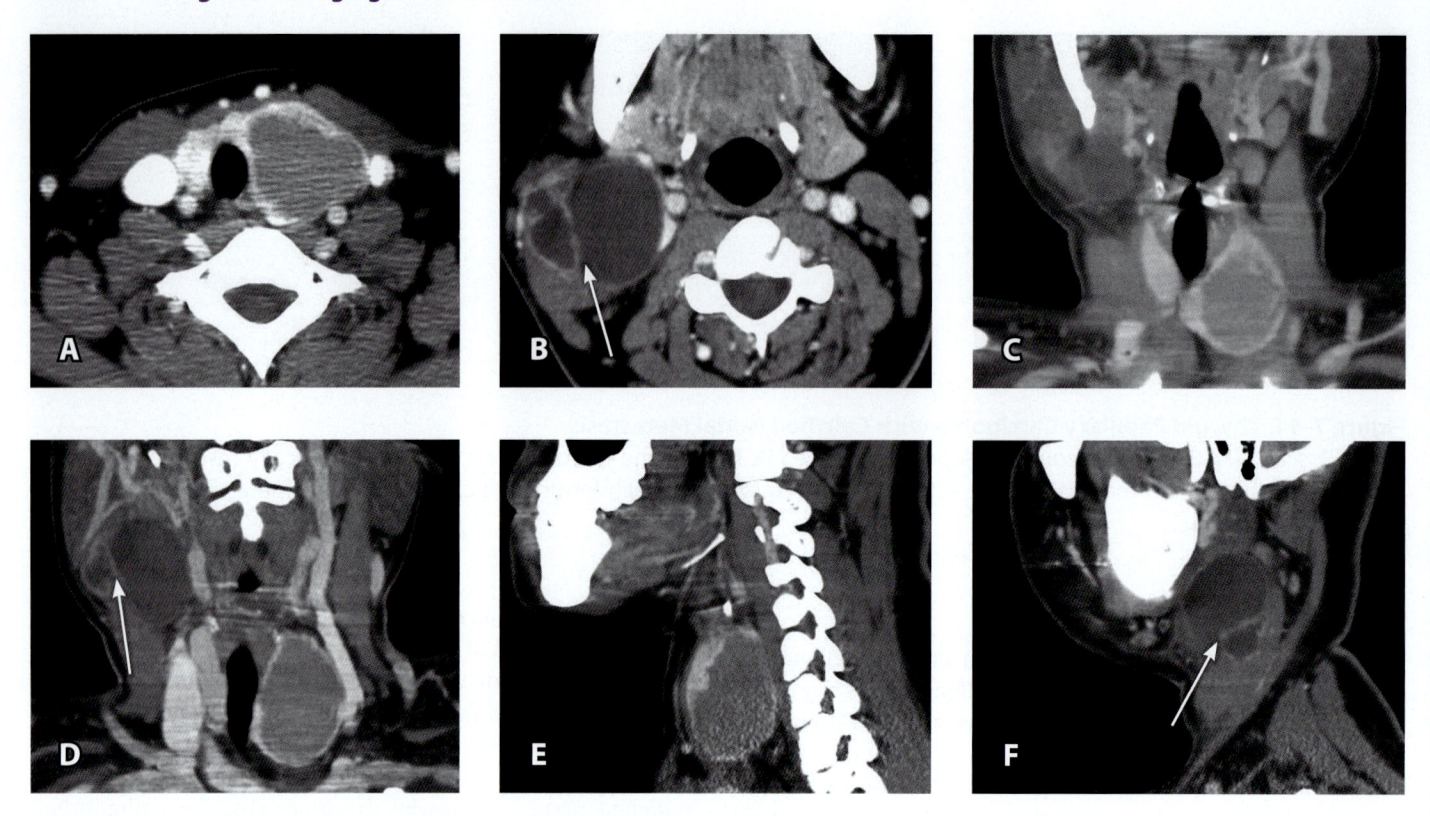

Figure 7-45 Cystic Thyroid Papillary Carcinoma with Cystic Nodal Metastasis
Axial (**A, B**), reformatted coronal (**C, D**) and reformatted sagittal (**E, F**) contrast-enhanced CT scans. A large cystic mass is noted in the left lobe of the thyroid gland. A separate multilocular cystic nodal mass is evident in the right level II nodes (*arrows*, **B, D,** and **F**). Such cystic neck masses should not be misdiagnosed as congenital lesions such as branchial cleft or thyroglossal cysts.

Patients present with a solid nodule, which grossly is well-circumscribed, firm, and nonencapsulated. In sporadic cases, medullary carcinoma may cause compressive symptoms, or may manifest as a paraneoplastic syndrome. In familial cases, the tumor is often asymptomatic.

The tumor is infiltrative and grows in nests of spindle- or polygonal-shaped cells. Hyalinized collagen, amyloid, and vascular stroma comprise the lesion. Foci of hemorrhage are often present.

On MR imaging, the tumor is solid, and may contain coarse calcifications and local invasion. In 50% of cases there is spread to the mediastinal and cervical lymph nodes. In 15% to 25% of cases, there is metastatic spread to lungs, liver, and bone[188] (**Fig. 7-47**).

Anaplastic Carcinoma

Anaplastic carcinoma is an undifferentiated tumor of the thyroid follicular epithelial cells. This aggressive cancer accounts for less than 5% of thyroid carcinomas, and has a poor prognosis, with mortality of 100%. Women above the age of 65 years are predominantly affected, and there is an association between this tumor and pre-existing goiter. This tumor is characterized by rapid growth and obliteration of adjacent tissue planes.

Patients commonly present with a rapidly enlarging neck mass that causes compressive symptoms and vocal cord paralysis. In most cases, the disease has already invaded adjacent neck structures and metastasized to the lungs at the time of presentation.

On gross examination, the tumor is firm with areas of necrosis and hemorrhage. Microscopically, a variety of patterns are seen within the same tumor. Spindle cell regions resembling sarcomas, and large, pleomorphic giant cells are common. There is invasive growth beyond the gland and vascular invasion.

Seventy-five percent to 80% of cases have metastatic spread to the lymph nodes. The internal carotid arteries and adjacent aerodigestive structures are invaded 34% to 55% of the time. There is no effective treatment, as the tumors are resistant to both radiation and chemotherapy, and death occurs in less than one year.[193]

Other sarcomas of the head and neck that have to be considered are malignant tumors of muscle origin (i.e., rhabdomyosarcoma), neurogenic origin (i.e., malignant schwannomas), cartilaginous origin (i.e., chondrosarcomas), or osseous origins (i.e., osteosarcomas). These lesion need to also be differentiated from rare benign entities such as nephrogenic calcinosis or benign vasoformative anomalies.

Lymphoma

Approximately 5% of thyroid malignancies are thyroid lymphomas. These tumors involve the thyroid primarily, or in a minority of cases, as part of a systemic lymphoma. Eighty percent of these cases are found in patients with Hashimoto thyroiditis. The majority of these lymphomas are non-Hodgkin's B-cell lymphomas.

Patients are usually women over the age of 60 years. They present with a rapidly enlarging, compressive, infiltrative mass. Eighty percent of cases involve solitary nodules, while 20% have multiple nodules.

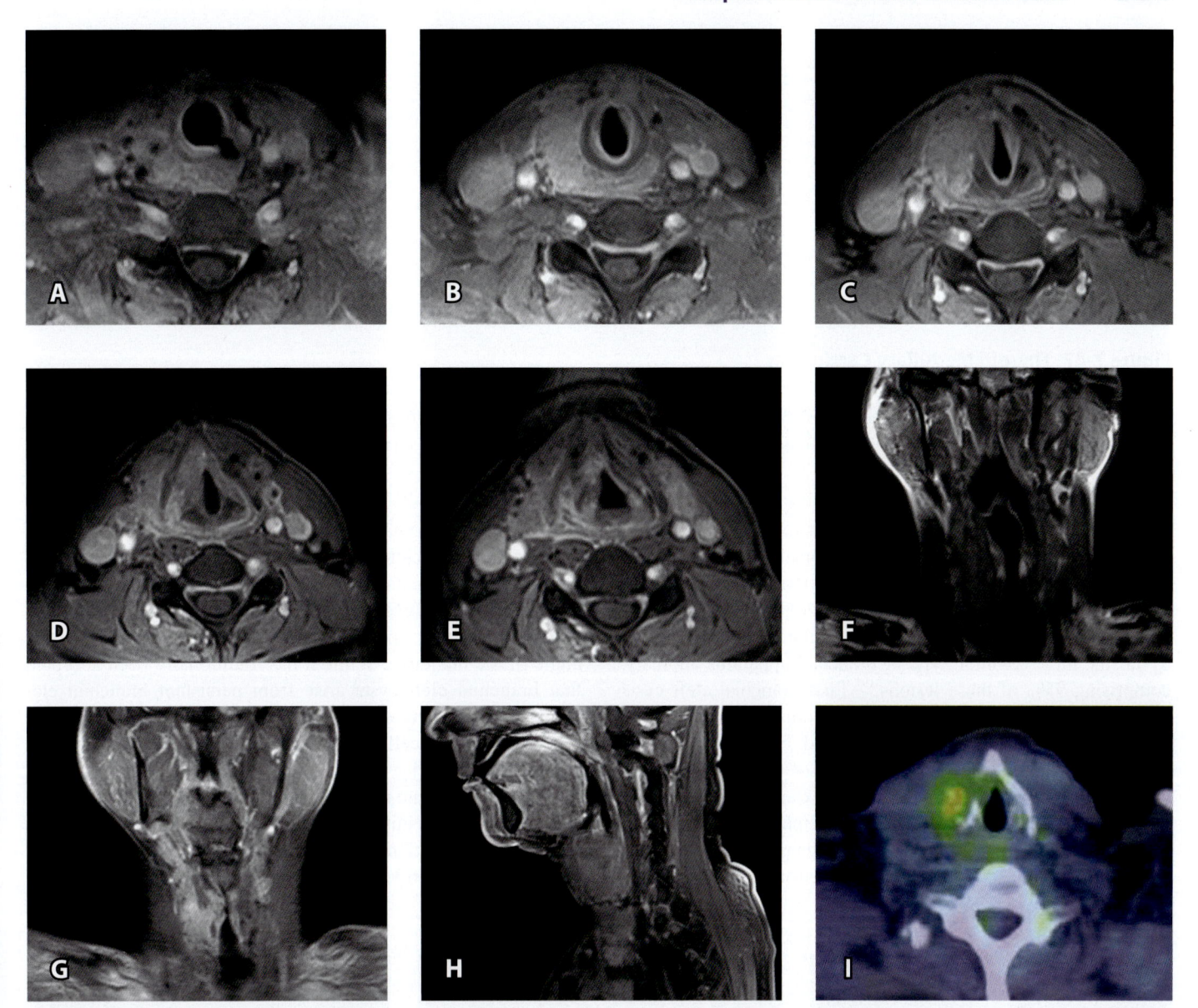

Figure 7-46 Radiation-induced Follicular Thyroid Carcinoma with Glottic Invasion
Serial axial (**A–E**) and coronal (**F–H**) contrast-enhanced T1 MR scans with fat-saturated and axial fused PET/CT image (**I**). The patient has a history of neck irradiation for thyroid gland carcinoma. There are multiple ferromagnetic artifacts in both sides of the thyroid bed that represent surgical clips placed at the time of prior thyroidectomy. There is an invasive tumor that invades the right side of the glottic structures and extends into the airway. The PET/CT image shows clear destruction of the right thyroid cartilage (**I**). Such radiation-induced neoplasms are highly aggressive and difficult to eradicate.

The gross pathology demonstrates a homogeneous solid mass with ill-defined margins and no capsule. Microscopically, the cells are monomorphic, noncohesive, atypical lymphoid cells.

Imaging studies do not differentiate between lymphoma and carcinoma. Both demonstrate an infiltrating mass with indistinct margins. Thyroid lymphoma has a lower frequency of calcification and necrosis. These tumors are generally homogenously hyperintense on T2-weighted images (**Fig. 7-41**).[193]

Treatment is based upon lymphoma subtype and extent of disease. Intermediate to high-grade lymphoma is treated with chemotherapy and radiation. Prognosis is good and there is a high cure rate.

THE PEDIATRIC NECK

Congenital Anomalies

First Branchial Cleft Cyst

The branchial apparatus begins to develop during the fourth week of gestation. The four ectodermal branchial clefts remain

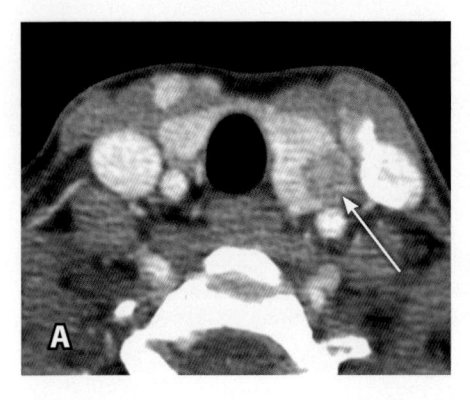

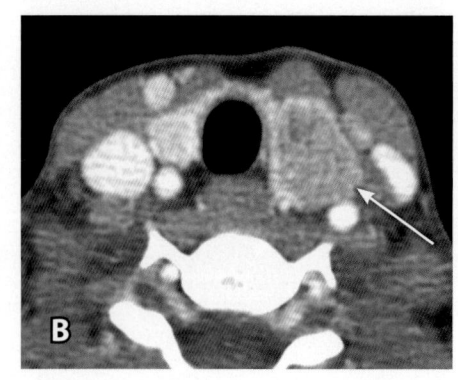

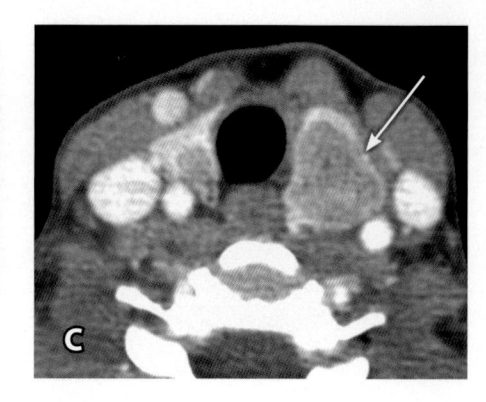

Figure 7-47 Thyroid Medullary Carcinoma
Axial contrast-enhanced CT scans. There are bilateral primarily low-density lesions in both lobes of the thyroid gland, much more evident on the left side (*arrows*). Biopsy showed medullary thyroid carcinoma. CT is often nonspecific in the evaluation of thyroid masses, particularly the differentiation of neoplasms from benign colloid cysts.

on the surface of the embryo through the sixth week, and then they are obliterated. Normally, only the dorsal portion of the first branchial cleft remains, becoming the external auditory canal. If the clefts fail to obliterate, branchial cleft cysts, sinuses, or fistulas may result (**Figs. 7-48**). Second branchial cleft cysts are by far the most common type of branchial apparatus anomaly, comprising 95% of these lesions.[194] First branchial cleft cysts account for only 1% to 8% of these anomalies.[195] Two types of first branchial cleft cyst are recognized, based upon distinct developmental processes. The first type of cyst arises from a duplication anomaly of the membranous external auditory canal. It is comprised of purely ectodermal elements. The cyst runs parallel to the normal external auditory canal, from a location medial to the concha, extending to the retroauricular region. A second type of anomaly is derived from persistent portions of the first branchial cleft and arch, along with portions of the second branchial arch, and contains both ectodermal and mesodermal elements. This cystic lesion is found in or around the parotid gland.[196] If a sinus opens to the skin, it is usually found at the angle of the mandible. While it has traditionally been accepted that branchial cleft cysts arise from persistent branchial elements, there is new evidence that some of these lesions may arise from buried cell rests or salivary gland inclusions within cervical lymph nodes.[187]

These lesions are most common in children below the age of ten years, but may initially appear well into adulthood. There is no gender predilection for this developmental anomaly. Acute or subacute infection often precipitates the spontaneous appearance

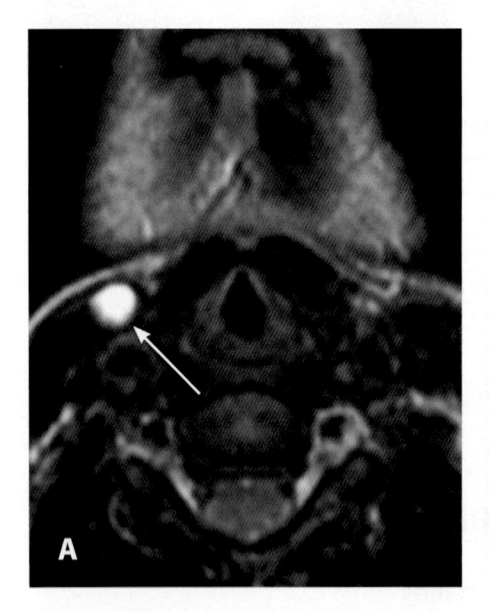

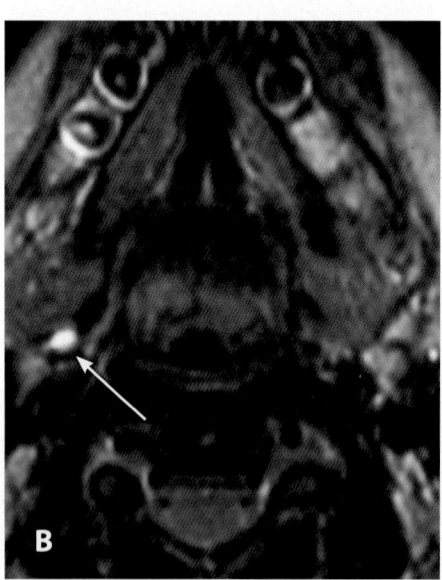

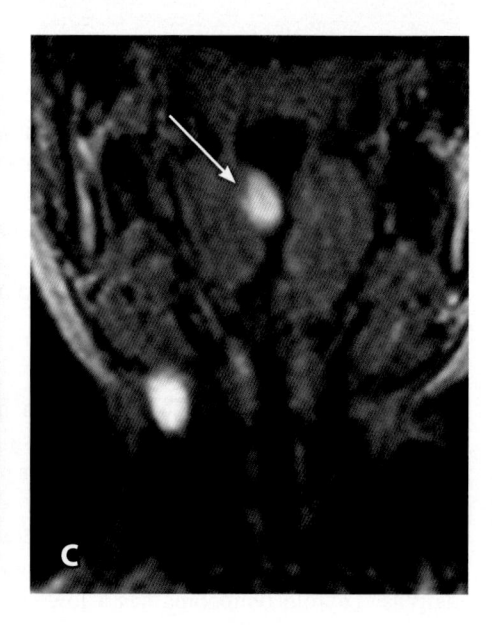

Figure 7-48 Remnant of a Second Branchial Cleft Fistula
Axial (**A, B**) and coronal (**C**) T2 MR scans. This child had previous resection of a cystic neck mass, but continues to have recurrent neck swelling. There are two cystic lesions relating to remnants of a second branchial cleft cyst. One cyst extends from the right neck into the parapharyngeal space (*arrows*, **A** and **B**) and another in the region of the right palatine tonsil (*arrow*, **C**).

of the cysts.[110] The differential diagnosis for a branchial cleft cyst includes metastatic malignant neoplasm, tuberculous cervical adenitis, cystic hygroma, hemangioma, dermoid cyst, primary lymphoma, neurofibroma, lipoma, thyroglossal duct cysts, cystic tumors in the tail of the parotid gland, accessory thymic remnants, and branchiogenic carcinoma.[197] The only successful treatment for branchial cleft cysts is complete surgical excision.[198]

Branchial cleft cysts are well-circumscribed, spherical or ovoid lesions, 2 to 5 cm in diameter. The thin, fibrous walls are lined by stratified squamous or pseudostratified columnar epithelium. Lymphoid tissue with reactive follicles often lies deep to the lining membrane. The cyst is filled with a clear or yellowish fluid.[187]

On MR imaging, these cystic lesions appear as homogenous masses with variable signal, depending upon the protein content of the cyst fluid. Usually, there is a low signal on T1-weighted images and high signal on T2-weighted images. However, a higher protein content, resulting from infection, can increase the T1 signal and cause dephasing and loss of signal on T2-weighted images. Infection also results in changes in the thickness and enhancement of the cyst wall.[194]

Second Branchial Cleft Cyst

In the fifth week of embryonic development, the second branchial arch overgrows the third and fourth arches, and subsequently forms a depression called the cervical sinus. In normal neck development, the sinus and arches are obliterated. If portions of the second arch remain, a second branchial cleft cyst, sinus, or fistula may form.

Second branchial cleft cysts are the most common branchial apparatus anomalies. They are normally found high in the lateral neck, deep to the anterior border of the sternocleidomastoid muscle, anywhere from the external auditory canal to the clavicle. The cysts may appear at any point along the developmental pathway of the second branchial arch, but are most commonly found at the level of the carotid artery bifurcation, lateral to the jugular vein.[194] Rarely, a second branchial cleft cyst may present as a bulge in the parotid gland or in the posterolateral pharyngeal wall.[199]

Patients of all ages may present with a second branchial cleft cyst, but they are usually identified by the age of 30 years.[198] These lesions are typically painless, fluctuant masses, which appear spontaneously following infection. Without treatment, the masses can slowly enlarge, and become painful due to secondary infection. Imaging characteristics of second branchial cleft cysts are identical to those of first branchial cleft cysts.

Thyroglossal Duct Cyst

The primordial thyroid develops between the third and fourth weeks of fetal development. It descends along the thyroglossal duct from the base of the tongue to the thyroid bed in the anterior visceral space of the neck. Normally, the thyroglossal duct involutes by the eighth week of gestation. If portions of the duct remain, a thyroglossal duct cyst can form in that location.

Thyroglossal duct cysts are the most common congenital neck masses in childhood.[63] Fifteen percent of these lesions are found at the hyoid bone, 65% are found just below the hyoid, and 20% are located in the suprahyoid neck.[200] Nearly 75% of these lesions are found in the midline.[201] Cysts which form more inferiorly may deviate from the midline due to the paramedian position of the bilobed thyroid gland. Suprahyoid thyroglossal duct cysts can be found as high as the tongue base, with lingual fistulas opening through the foramen cecum (**Fig. 7-49**).

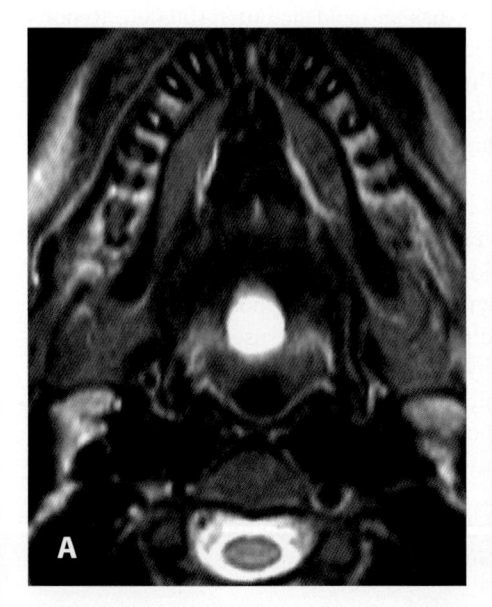

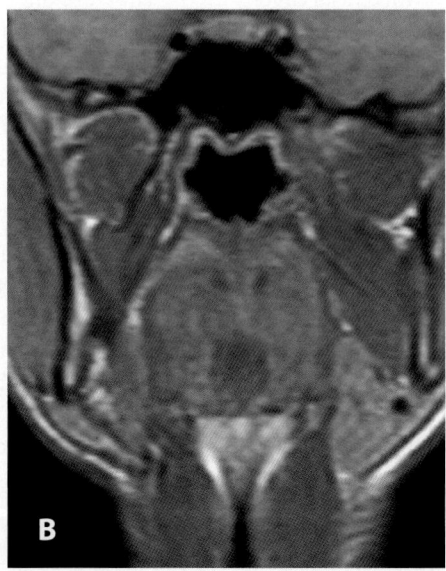

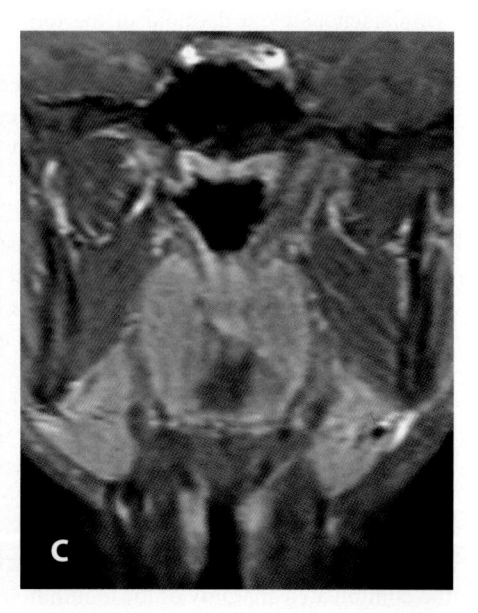

Figure 7-49 Foramen Cecum Thyroglossal Duct Cyst
(**A**) Axial T2, (**B**) coronal unenhanced T1 and (**C**) coronal contrast-enhanced T1 MR. scans. A purely cystic mass is located in the midline of the base of the tongue within the foramen cecum. A pure thyroglossal duct remnant, as in this case, shows no contrast enhancement (**C**), whereas an ectopic thyroid gland would demonstrate intense enhancement.

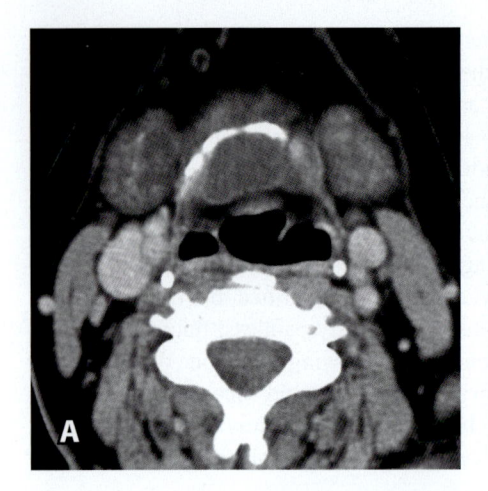

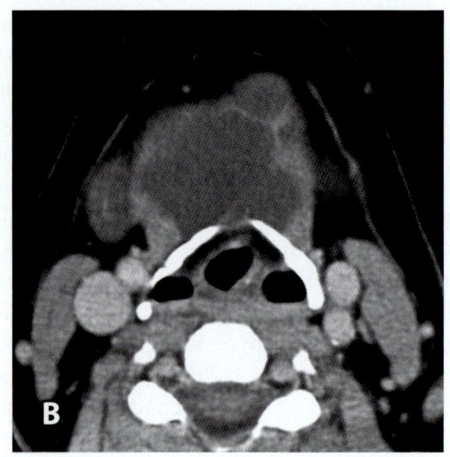

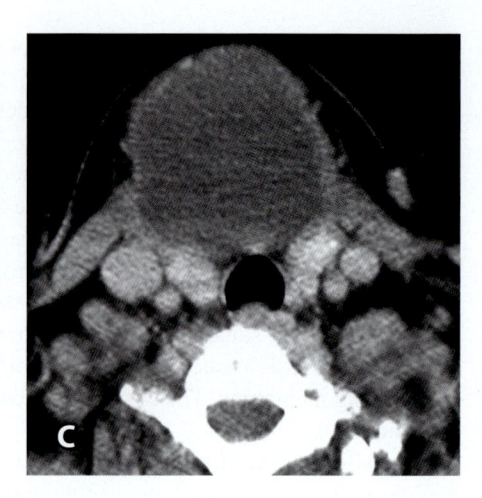

Figure 7-50 Large Thyroglossal Duct Cyst
Axial contrast-enhanced CT scans. There is a large nonenhancing multicystic mass in the anterior neck. The mass surrounds the hyoid bone (**A**) and extends downward past the thyroid cartilage (**B**) to the level of the midline pyramidal lobe of the thyroid gland (**C**). The use of contrast enhancement is essential in such cases to rule out an associated thyroid neoplasm within the contents of the thyroglossal cyst, which is not present in this case.

Infrahyoid thyroglossal duct cysts may appear slightly below the hyoid bone, or embedded in the infrahyoid strap muscles.

Thyroglossal duct cysts appear primarily in children, with 70% diagnosed by the age of 20 years.[63]

Patients present with an enlarging, asymptomatic, midline cervical mass which moves upward with tongue protrusion. Although the majority of these lesions are found below the hyoid bone, they can be found anywhere from the foramen cecum of the tongue to the thyroid gland. Recurrent infections are common, and the patient history may be positive for a previous abscess in the area. The differential diagnosis for a thyroglossal duct cyst includes a lingual or sublingual thyroid, lymphadenopathy, a dermoid of the tongue, a mixed laryngocele, or a malignant necrotic node. The treatment of choice for a thyroglossal duct cyst is the Sistrunk procedure, which involves complete surgical removal of the cyst, a central section of the hyoid bone, and a portion of the tongue musculature.[196,202] Failure to remove the entire squamous epithelial lining of the cyst results in recurrence.

Thyroglossal duct cysts are smooth, spherical or fusiform swellings approximately 2 to 3 cm in diameter (**Fig. 7-50**). They are filled with mucinous, clear secretions.[187] The walls of the cysts are lined with stratified squamous or ciliated pseudostratified columnar epithelium.[5]

Radiologically, the thyroglossal duct cyst is a unilocular cystic mass in the midline of the neck, or in a slightly paramedian position if the lesion is below the hyoid bone. "Beaking" of the infrahyoid strap muscles around the lesion is characteristic.[77] A sagittal MR image is useful in the case of suprahyoid cysts, as it demonstrates the full course of the lesion through the complicated anatomy of the mouth floor. Thyroglossal duct cysts are low signal on T1-weighted images and hyperintense on T2-weighted images. Normally, there is no enhancement with contrast, but the rim may enhance if it has been thickened by infection or inflammation. The presence of proteinaceous debris from infection or hemorrhage results in variable signal intensity.

Lingual and Sublingual Thyroid

The primordial thyroid gland descends from the foramen cecum of the tongue to its adult position in the neck. If the thyroid gland develops correctly, but fails to descend to the normal adult position, it is called an ectopic thyroid gland. The term lingual thyroid refers to a thyroid gland which has not descended due to failure of thyroglossal duct formation in the third week of development. It is found near its site of origin at the foramen cecum of the tongue, below the mucosa.

This rare anomaly has an incidence of 1:100,000. Reports of gender predominance range from a 3:1 to 4:1 female to male ratio.[203,204] Lingual thyroid is commonly asymptomatic, and the finding is incidental. The onset of symptoms often coincides with puberty, pregnancy, or the menopause, when raised levels of TSH cause hypertrophy of the gland. Upon examination, a raised, pink mass is found at the base of tongue. If the mass is large, patients may present with symptoms including dyspnea, dysphonia, a sensation of fullness in the floor of the mouth, and choking. Lingual thyroid often causes hypothyroidism.[203]

Radioactive iodine scintigraphy is used to determine the presence of other thyroid tissue in the neck. CT and MRI are useful but not definitive for thyroid malignancy. MRI findings will be identical to normal thyroid tissue.

Treatment involves hormonal therapy with levothyroxine to shrink the lesion. Surgery is utilized when there is airway obstruction or malignancy.[203] Lingual thyroid is very often the only thyroid tissue in the body, and must be preserved during neck surgery.

Rarely, the developing thyroid glands starts its descent, but its progress is arrested. This "sublingual thyroid gland" can be found anywhere in the normal course of descent, but is usually found at, or slightly below the hyoid bone. This anomaly presents as a rounded midline protuberance of the neck, and resembles a thyroglossal duct cyst. While a sublingual thyroid gland is much less common than a lingual thyroid gland, it is important because it may be inadvertently removed if it is misdiagnosed as a thyroglossal duct cyst. A sublingual thyroid gland is also often the only thyroid tissue of the body. Positive iodine scintigraphy is the only certain method of differentiating these lesions. Treatment involves the same hormonal regimen used for lingual thyroid.[203]

THE BRACHIAL PLEXUS

Sensory and motor function of the upper extremity is provided by the brachial plexus, which is a composite of the ventral roots of C5-T1, and occasionally C4 and T2.[205] These roots coalesce to form trunks, divisions, cords, and branches. The brachial plexus is difficult to clinically evaluate because palpation is not possible, making the localization of lesions difficult.[206] However, the brachial plexus is readily identifiable by CT and MR imaging, with MR being the preferred imaging method due to greater soft tissue contrast and the ability for multiplanar imaging.[207] Because the brachial plexus nerves are not routinely identified during imaging, it is important to be knowledgeable about pertinent imaging studies in evaluating brachial plexopathies. Such plexopathies can result from trauma, congenital anomalies, tumors, bony lesions, inflammatory conditions, and infections.

Anatomy

The lordotic curvature of the spine causes the superior nerve roots to be located anteriorly to the inferior nerve roots. The superior nerve roots run inferiorly, laterally, and anteriorly, passing between the anterior and middle scalene muscles.[205] Nerve roots C5 and C6 unite to form the superior trunk near the lateral border of the anterior scalene muscle (**Fig. 7-51**). The C7 nerve root forms the middle trunk, with no contributions from the other nerve roots. C8 and T1 unite to form the inferior trunk posterior to the anterior scalene muscle. The roots and trunks of the brachial plexus are found in the region known as the supraclavicular plexus.[208]

Each trunk divides to form an anterior and a posterior division. The superior and middle trunk divide at, or after passing laterally to, the anterior scalene muscle. The divisions of the inferior trunk are formed at or after the nerves cross the first rib. The divisions of the superior and middle trunks can be found superior to the subclavian artery, whereas the divisions of the inferior trunk can be found directly posterior to the subclavian artery.[205] Three divisions are found in the region known as the retroclavicular plexus in the costoclavicular space.[208] In all, six divisions are formed, which unite to form three cords named according to their relationship to the subclavian artery (**Table 7-2**). The lateral cord is formed by the anterior divisions of the upper and middle trunks, the posterior cord is formed by the posterior divisions of all three trunks, and the medial cord is formed by the anterior division of the inferior trunk.[206]

The Divisions form Three Cords

- *Lateral – from the anterior divisions of the upper and middle trunks*
- *Medial – from the anterior division of the lower trunk*
- *Posterior – from the posterior divisions of all three trunks*

The lateral and medial cords form in the lower neck, while the posterior cord forms in the axilla. They enter the

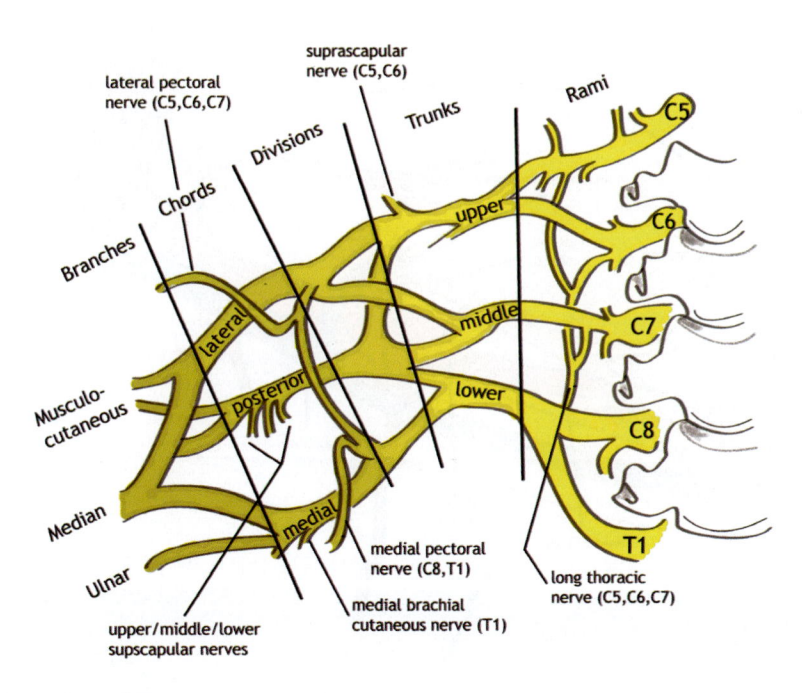

Figure 7-51 Brachial Plexus Schematic
Note the segments of the brachial plexus showing its typical origin from the ventral rami (roots) of C5–T1 and its distal arrangement into trunks, divisions, cords, and branches.

Table 7-2 Arteries of the Brachial Plexus

Artery	Course	Relationship to Brachial Plexus
Vertebral Artery	Cephalocaudad direction through transverse foramina	Roots of BP emerge from transverse processes of cervical vertebrae posterior to artery
Subclavian Artery	R. Subclavian A. is a branch of the Brachiocephalic A; L. Subclavian A. is a branch of the Aorta; both become Axillary A. Distally	Superior and Middle BP Trunks pass superior to Subclavian A.; Inferior Trunk passes posterior to Subclavian A.
Axillary Artery	R. Subclavian A. is a branch of the Brachiocephalic A; L. Subclavian A. is a branch of the Aorta; both become Axillary A. Distally	BP cords are named lateral, posterior, and medial based on relationship to artery

Demondion X, Boutry N, Drizenko A, et al.: Thoracic outlet: anatomic correlation with MR imaging. Am J Roentgenol 2000;175:417–422.

axilla between the clavicle and first rib, inside the axillary sheath, adjacent to the axillary vein and artery (**Fig. 7-52**). The three cords end in terminal branches in the retropectoralis minor space in the region known as the infraclavicular plexus.[208] These terminal branches supply the motor and sensory innervations to the upper extremity. The five terminal branches of the brachial plexus are the musculocutaneous nerve, axillary nerve, median nerve, radial nerve, and ulnar nerve (**Table 7-3**).[206]

Imaging

MR imaging of the brachial plexus is preferred to CT imaging due to the ability of imaging multiplanar views, which allows for easier mapping and more reliable differentiation between

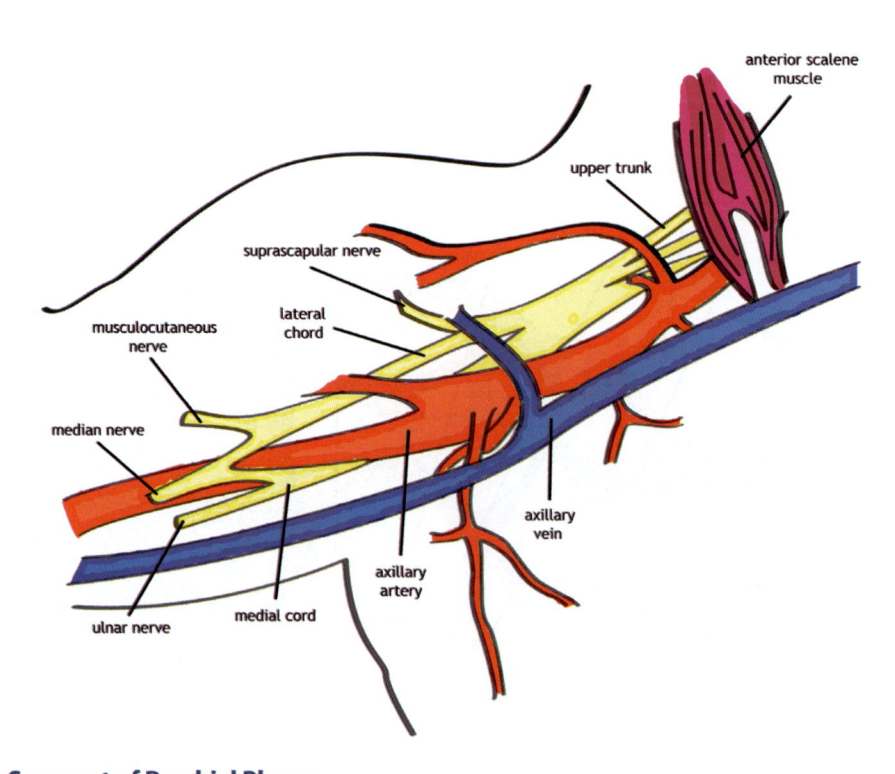

Figure 7-52 Axillary Segment of Brachial Plexus
The relationship of the trunks, cords, and branches of the brachial plexus to the axillary artery and subclavian vein in the axilla is intimate. Careless puncture of the axillary artery for endovascular access can lead to a brachial plexopathy.

Table 7-3 Brachial Plexus

Roots	Trunks	Divisions	Cords	Branches
C4* C5 C6	Superior trunk	Anterior/Posterior	Lateral (from the anterior divisions of superior and middle trunks)	Musculocutaneous Nerve (C5,6,7)
				Axillary Nerve (C5,6)
C7	Middle trunk	Anterior/Posterior	Medial (from anterior division of the inferior trunk)	Median Nerve (C5*,6,7,8,T1)
C8 T1 T2*	Inferior trunk	Anterior/Posterior	Posterior (from the posterior divisions of all trunks)	Radial Nerve (C5,6,7,8,T1*)
				Ulnar Nerve (C7*,8,T1)

*Denotes Inconstant Contribution.
Netter FH. Brachial Plexus: Schema. In: Atlas of Human Anatomy. 4th ed. Philadelphia, PA: Saunders/Elsevier, 2006, Plate 430.

vascular and nonvascular tissue without iodinated contrast. Furthermore, a major disadvantage of CT imaging of the lower neck region is that the only obtainable images are direct axial images, which are obscured by beam-hardening artifacts at the thoracic outlet. Even though the benefits of MR imaging allow for easier visualization, the form of imaging chosen should be determined on a case-by-case basis.[205]

Imaging studies of the brachial plexus are important for determining whether the lesion is postganglionic or preganglionic, which is of crucial importance when determining the course of treatment. In the case of preganglionic lesions, nerve transfers can be used to restore function to certain denervated muscles. Postganglionic lesions can be repaired with nerve grafting or are carefully monitored.[209]

For imaging of the brachial plexus, high-resolution unilateral imaging in two to three planes is preferred, although bilateral imaging can also be utilized (**Table 7-4**).[205] Axial and coronal planes allow for comparison between left and right sides. The sagittal plane consistently demonstrates the nerves of the brachial plexus and related vessels in cross section. The axial plane is very useful for visualizing the nerve roots exiting the foramina, because the imaging plane and the orientation of the nerve roots are parallel.[210]

Phased array-surface coils allow for optimal MR imaging of the brachial plexus, although this type of imaging may result in artifacts due to respiration. Alternatively, a body-coil on a 1.0 or 1.5 Tesla magnet can also be used. Several imaging protocols can be used: coronal localizer scout; sagittal T1-weighted images from the spinal canal to the lateral aspect of the clavicle on the affected side; axial T1-weighted images from the C4 vertebra to the carina, perpendicular to the axis of the trachea; oblique coronal T1-weighted images along the distal subclavian and proximal axillary arteries; and a T2-weighted sequence in the axial plane. Ideal slice thickness is no more than 5 mm.[205]

T1-weighted images are best used for displaying regional anatomy. T2-weighted images are used to display pathological conditions. Fat suppression is often used to prevent obstruction of abnormal intraneural signal intensity by the fat signal intensity.[205]

Table 7-4 MR Protocols for Plexopathies

- Coronal Short T1 Inversion Recovery Sequence (STIR) with fast spin-echo inversion recovery technique with TR of 3,000 ms, TE of 34 ms, and imaging time of 3.25 min with double acquisitions.
- Sagittal fat-saturated fast spin-echo proton-density with TR of 5,000 ms, TE of 40 ms, and imaging time of 4.40 min with double acquisitions.
- Axial three-dimensional FIESTA with 4 acquisitions and imaging time of 4.36 min.
- Axial T1 spin-echo with TR of 700 ms and imaging time of 4.40 min with single acquisition.
- Coronal T1 spin-echo with TR of 700 ms and imaging time of 4.40 min with single acquisition.
- Coronal postgadolinium T1 coronal spin-echo with TR of 700 ms and imaging time of 4.40 min with single acquisition.
- Axial postgadolinium T1 spin-echo with TR of 700 ms and imaging time of 4.36 min with double acquisitions.

Todd M, Shah GV, Mukherji SK. MR imaging of brachial plexus. Top Magn Reson Imaging 2004;15:113–125.

Magnetic resonance neurography, can be helpful in evaluating peripheral nerve disorders localized in small areas, especially if improved surface coils are used. This technique, which uses fat suppression and a heavily T2-weighted sequence, is also known as T2-weighted short tau inversion recovery (STIR) imaging.[210] This technique can cause nerves to become slightly hyperintense.[211]

If a torso coil is used, all three planes can be imaged at the same time. The involved side can also be compared to the contralateral side to help define the difference between normal anatomical variation and subtle pathological changes.[205]

The use of CT for brachial plexus imaging is largely reserved for cases in which patients that are unable to undergo standard MR imaging, or when a mass needs to be removed using CT guidance.[205]

Clinical Application
Trauma

Trauma accounts for approximately 50% of all brachial plexopathy cases.[205] Males form the highest percentage of traumatic plexopathy cases–almost 90% of cases in one study.[212] Concerns with trauma-induced plexopathies include cervical or clavicular fracture, or an avulsed, stretched, or compressed nerve root. Soft tissue swelling and/or hematomas in the brachial plexus region can cause similar symptoms.[205] A lesion affecting the upper brachial plexus involving nerves C5 and C6 may result in paralysis of the biceps and shoulder muscles (**Fig. 7-53**). If C7 is also affected, some wrist muscles may also be affected. A lesion affecting C8 and T1 may result in paralysis of the forearm flexor and intrinsic hand muscles. If the stellate ganglion or cervical sympathetic trunk is affected, it can result in Horner's syndrome, which is characterized by ipsilateral ptosis, miosis, and anhydrosis.[205,207,209]

Brachial Plexus injuries are classified as preganglionic, postganglionic, or a combination of both. Preganglionic lesions are characterized by avulsed nerve roots, whereas postganglionic lesions involve the nerve structure that is distal to the sensory ganglion. The subgroups of postganglionic lesions include nerve ruptures and nerve lesions in continuity.[209]

Cross-sectional imaging of the brachial plexus is usually done four to six weeks posttrauma to the brachial plexus region to differentiate between intraforaminal and extraforaminal cases. Intraforaminal injuries are characterized by traumatic pseudomeningoceles, nerve root avulsions, and spinal cord contusion. Extraforaminal injuries account for approximately 25% of traumatic brachial plexopathies. Extraforaminal injuries include: lesions immediately deep or inferior to the clavicle, and lesions distal to the plexus.[205]

In MR evaluation of patients with posttraumatic brachial plexopathy, analysis should focus on the integrity of the nerve roots in the central spinal axis rather than identification of pseudomeningoceles.[205]

In cases of nontraumatic brachial plexopathy, it should be determined if the plexopathy is idiopathic, since this benign condition usually resolves within three years. Unlike traumatic brachial plexus injuries, which present with motor deficiencies, nontraumatic brachial plexopathies more often present with sensory deficits in a patchy distribution (**Fig. 7-54**).[207] The most common cause of nontraumatic brachial plexopathy, however, is metastatic disease. In such cases, the mass is the suspected cause of the plexopathy if Horner's syndrome, lower plexus symptoms, and/or a history of neoplasm are present.[205]

Congenital Anomalies

Obstetric brachial plexus palsy occurs as a result of extreme lateral traction of the head during the final phase of delivery, stretching the brachial plexus. If the delivery is a breech delivery, the traction is exerted via the shoulder. If the delivery is a cephalic delivery, the traction is exerted via the head. In both cases, the upper roots are most vulnerable. Erb's palsy, often confused with obstetric brachial plexus palsy, characteristically involves the fifth and sixth cervical roots. Erb's palsy is characterized by weakness during shoulder abduction, external rotation, flexion, and supination of the elbow, and extension of the wrists and fingers.[205]

In many cases of obstetric brachial plexus injuries, infants recover with little or no residual functional impairment. In a study by Greenwald et al,[213] 61 cases in 30,000 live births in the United States had obstetric brachial plexus injuries, with "full" recovery in 96% of those cases. In a study of deliveries in an Eastern province of Saudi Arabia,[214] the most common causes of obstetric brachial plexus injuries were difficult deliveries (56%), large babies (35%), and the use of forceps or vacuum extraction during delivery (35%). Of the presentations in this study, most of them were vertex, although there were some breech and some shoulder presentations, as well.

Currently, MR Neurography (MRN) is the most useful means for evaluating birth-related brachial plexus injuries. This technique involves using axial and coronal STIR and T1-weighted imaging with and without gadolinium, and it provides better detail than standard imaging techniques.[215]

Abnormalities detected by MRN of patients with birth-related brachial plexus injuries include: pseudomeningocele; enhancement and/or thickening of nerve roots, which are suggestive of nerve scarring or neuroma; and a loss of the normal oblique rotation of the nerve root, suggestive of root avulsion without pseudomeningocele.[215] In a study of 11 infants,[215] MRN findings also included denervation changes consistent with muscle atrophy and abnormal muscle signal. Several of the infants also had T2 prolongation along the brachial plexus on the affected side.

Tumors and Mass Lesions

Lesions along the course of or adjacent to the brachial plexus cause brachial plexopathies. Cases of plexopathies typically present with pain and motor and sensory deficits of the upper extremities. If pain is present, it usually increases with neck traction, shoulder movement, or deep inspiration. There is often tenderness of the supraclavicular fossa. Long-term complications of brachial plexopathies include edema, muscle wasting, joint contractures, osteoporosis, and degenerative joint disease.[205]

The most common cause of lesions to the brachial plexus is motor vehicle accidents, with motorcycle accidents accounting for 84% of these lesions.[209,216] Because of traction forces, motorcycle accidents most commonly cause nerve root avulsions, whereas car accident injuries are more commonly crush-type injuries.[216] To detect a nerve root avulsion, T1-weighted imaging should be

Chapter 7: The Neck and Brachial Plexus   **331**

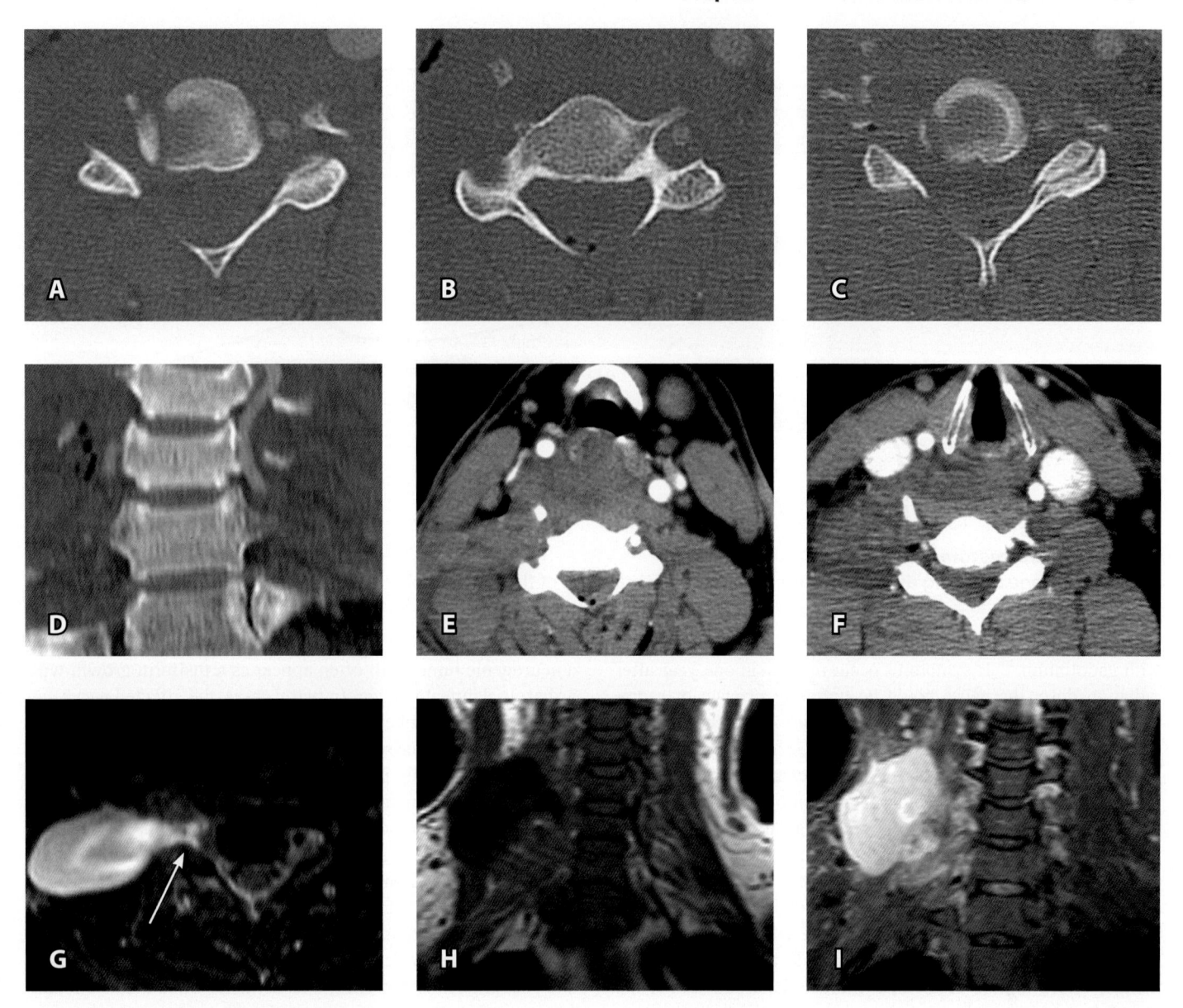

Figure 7-53 Penetrating C6 Injury
Axial (**A–C**), reformatted coronal (**D**) with bone windows, axial (**E, F**) with soft tissue windows contrast-enhanced CT scans and axial T2 (**G**), coronal T1 (**H**) and coronal T2 (**I**) MR images. The subject sustained a deep penetrating injury resulting in dual vascular and neural injuries. There is fracturing with distraction of the anterior and posterior horns of the right C6 transverse process and occlusion of the V2 segment of the right vertebral artery. There is marked swelling in the prevertebral and right paravertebral spaces and a soft tissue mass adjacent to the right scalene muscles (*arrows*, **E, F**). The MRI documents that the soft tissue mass is a large pseudomeningocele resulting from avulsion of the C6 nerve root (*arrow*, **G**).

used. Findings that are consistent with nerve root avulsion include absence of low intensity nerve root in the fat of the neural foramen. To detect crush-type injuries, T2-weighted imaging should be used. Findings consistent with crush-type injuries include a thickening of the brachial plexus with or without increased signal intensity. This occurs because of edema and fibrosis in the region.[206]

During neurologic evaluation, presence of Horner's syndrome typically correlates with involvement of the inferior trunk. In addition, a combination of brachial plexopathy and phrenic nerve dysfunction could be a result of a lesion in the superior trunk of the brachial plexus.[205]

Radiation-induced plexopathies result from radiation therapy to the axillary region. In such cases, it can be difficult to differentiate between recurrent or residual disease and radiation-induced neuropathy. Neurologic damage from radiation therapy typically occurs 5 to 30 months after radiotherapy is started. Damage is dose-dependent, with higher radiation doses resulting in greater neurological damage. If symptoms occur less than one year after a radiation dose of 60Gy or greater, the cause is most likely radiation damage.[205] Radiation-induced plexopathies typically present with low signal intensity on T1-weighted and T2-weighted images, but can have high signal intensity on T2-weighted

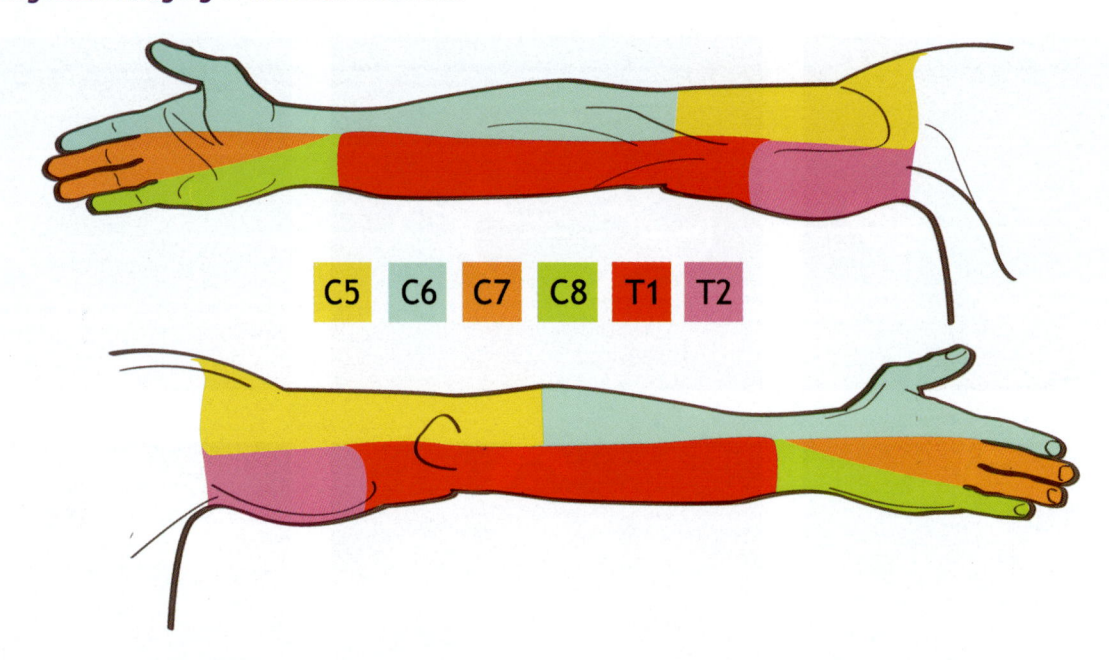

Figure 7-54 Dermatomes of the Arm
Schematic image outlining the distribution of the sensory branches of the brachial plexus.

sequences. Radiation-induced plexopathies can also enhance with gadolinium.[210] If symptoms occur more than one year after radiation dose, the cause could be tumor recurrence or radiation damage.[205] The most reliable distinction between radiation-induced plexopathies and tumors is the presence of a mass.[210]

Metastatic disease involving the brachial plexus region is often secondary to extrascapular extension of nodal metastases in the axilla, supraclavicular fossa, or scalene nodes. Melanomas and carcinomas of the breast, lung, gastrointestinal, thyroid, and head and neck may metastasize to these nodes (**Fig. 7-55**). Metastases from the breast into the brachial plexus are common because of the lymphatic drainage into the axillary region. Lung metastases from apical tumors can invade the lower brachial plexus. These tumors result in a characteristic pain down the arm, followed by numbness and weakness, particularly in distributions from C8 and T1.[205]

Superior sulcus tumors, also known as thoracic inlet tumors, are associated with lung tumors, namely, adenocarcinoma, squamous cell, and large cell and small cell carcinomas. MR imaging has markedly improved visualization of these tumors, with images taken in the coronal and sagittal planes allowing for determination of superior, inferior, anterior, and posterior extent of the tumor. Both planes also allow for the relationship between the brachial plexus and tumor to be easily shown.[210]

Primary neural tumors in the brachial plexus are rare, consisting of neurofibromas (**Fig. 7-56**), schwannomas (**Figs. 7-57 and 7-58**) and malignant peripheral nerve sheath tumors. Neurofibromas are the most common neural tumor that invade the brachial plexus.[205,210] One-third of these cases result from patients with Neurofibromatosis Type I, with the other two-thirds of the cases being sporadic.[205] Characteristically, if a neurogenic tumor is present, it will present with a low signal intensity T1-weighted imaging, an increased signal intensity on proton-density images, a high signal intensity on T2-weighted images,

and enhancement after gadolinium administration. Additionally, a neurogenic tumor will often appear as a fusiform growth with a sharply delineated edge. In many cases, the affected nerve can be seen entering and exiting the tumor.[210]

Pancoast's syndrome is associated with tumors of the lung apex; most commonly, nonsmall cell bronchiogenic carcinoma, with squamous cell carcinoma the most common, followed by adenocarcinoma and large cell carcinoma. Its signs and symptoms include shoulder and arm pain in the distribution of the C8, T1, and T2 nerve roots, Horner's syndrome, and atrophy of the hand muscles.[205]

Lesions involving the trunks and divisions of the brachial plexus typically occur in the posterior triangle of the neck, lateral to the anterior scalene muscle, and in the supraclavicular and retroclavicular regions. Pancoast tumors and metastatic disease are primarily found in this region.[205]

Bony Lesions

Cervical disk disease should be ruled out before expensive radiological evaluation is performed. Nearly 80% to 90% of cervical radiculopathy secondary to disk disease occurs at C6 and C7 root levels, mimicking symptoms seen in cases of brachial plexopathy.[205]

Bones in the cervical spine, shoulder, and thoracic outlet should be evaluated in brachial plexopathy cases. Cervical ribs, lesions of the first rib and clavicle, and primary bony lesions of the shoulder may mimic brachial plexopathy symptoms (**Fig. 7-59**).[205]

Inflammation and Infection

Chronic inflammatory demyelinating polyneuropathy is likely an immune-mediated neuropathy characterized by symmetric weakness and sensory loss in the arms and legs, and can also affect the brachial plexus. The process of demyelination, remyelination, and inflammation results in thickening of the peripheral nerves. Soft tissue inflammation, as a result of bacterial or viral

Chapter 7: The Neck and Brachial Plexus **333**

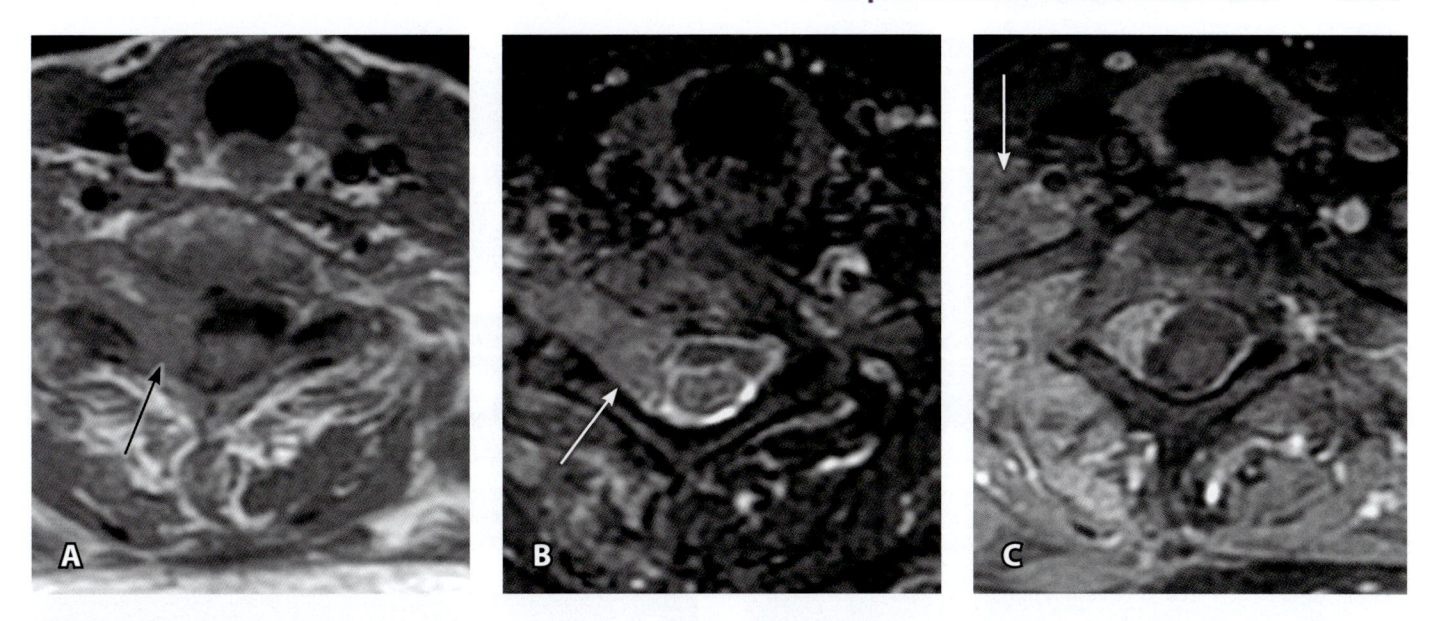

Figure 7-55 Melanoma with Neck Metastasis Cuasing Brachial Plexopathy
(**A**) Axial, T-1 (**B**) axial T-2 and (**C**) axial T1 contrast-enhanced with fat-saturated MR images. There is an irregular enhancing mass extending from the right C7 neural foramen (*arrows*, **A, B**) into the soft tissues of the lower neck including the scalene muscles (*arrows*, **C**).

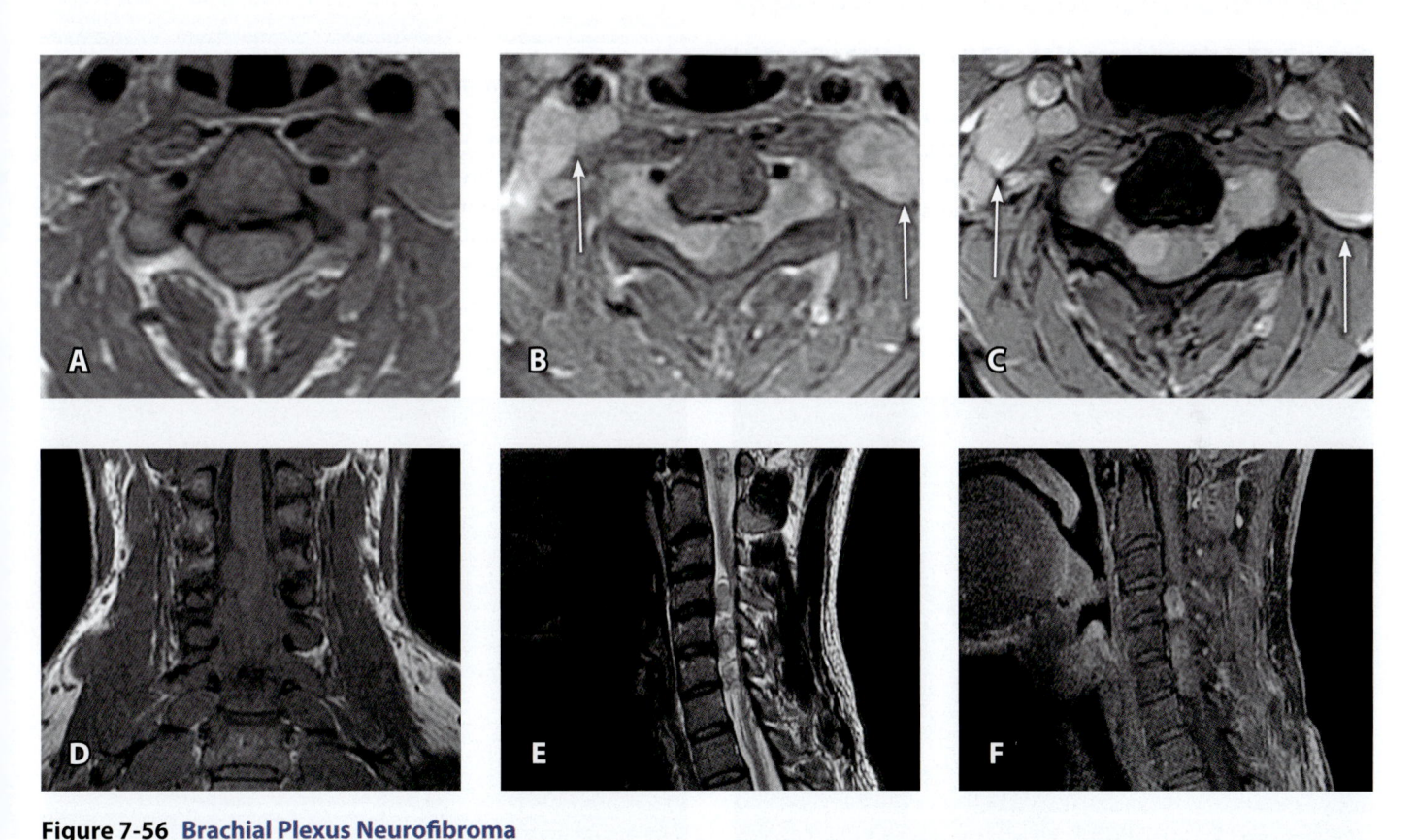

Figure 7-56 Brachial Plexus Neurofibroma
(**A**) Axial T-1, (**B**) axial T-1 and (**C**) axial T-2 contrast-enhanced, (**D**) coronal T-1, (**E**) sagittal T-2 and (**F**) sagittal T-1 contrast-enhanced with fat-saturated MR images. Multiple bilateral neurofibromas are evident at multiple levels through the cervical spine, both in the neural foramina and inside the spinal canal. Also seen are bilateral carotid space neurofibromas (*arrows*, **B, C**) in this patient with neurofibromatosis type I.

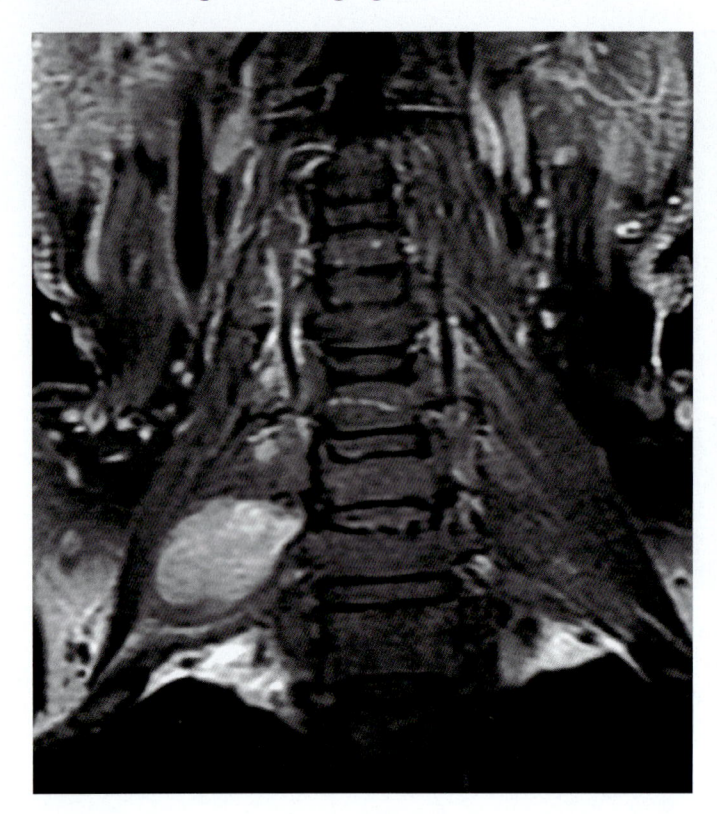

Figure 7-57 Schwannoma of the C7 Ramus of the Brachial Plexus
Coronal T-1 contrast-enhanced with fat-saturated MR image. There is an oval-shaped mass located within the right scalene muscles with a small medial protrusion into the adjacent neural foramen. Solitary neurogenic tumors may be randomly seen, whereas plexiform neurofibromas as only seen in cases of neurofibromatosis.

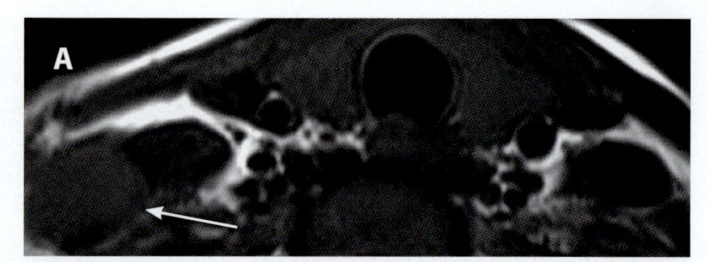

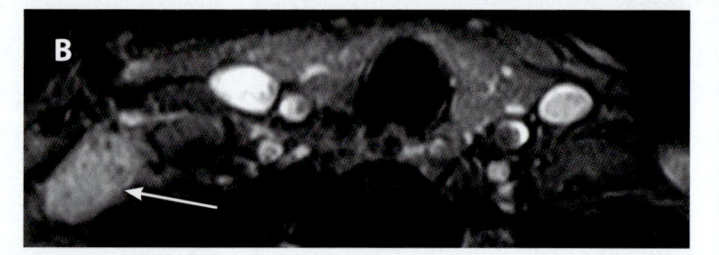

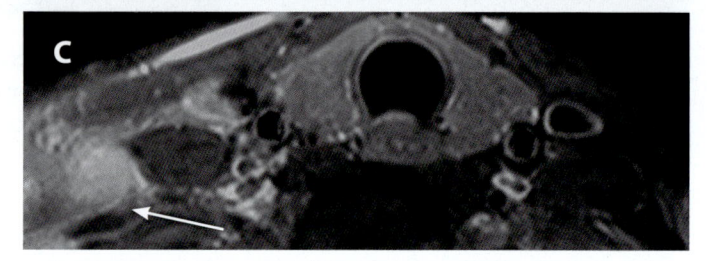

Figure 7-58 Schwannoma of the Superior Trunk of the Brachial Plexus
Axial T1 (**A**), T-2 (**B**) and contrast-enhanced with fat-saturated (**C**) MR images. There is a rounded enhancing mass located underneath the right clavicle lateral to the scalene muscles (*arrows*, **A–C**). At this point, the brachial plexus divides into superior, middle and inferior trunks, all in close proximity to each other.

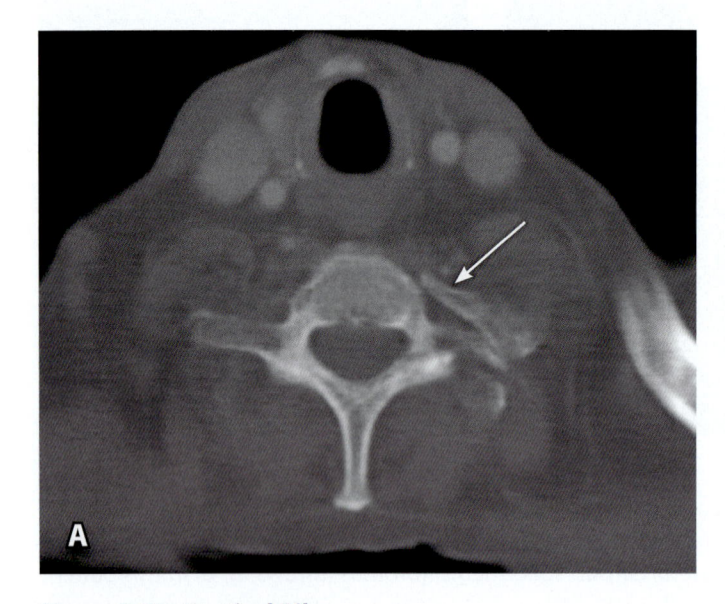

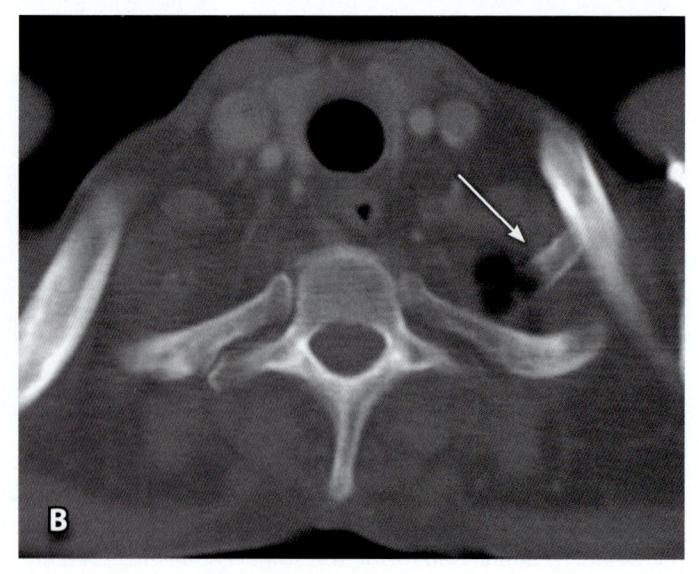

Figure 7-59 Cervical Rib
(**A, B**) Axial bone windowed CT scans. There is a bony protuberance (*arrows*) located adjacent to the left transverse process of C7 extending toward the clavicle above the left first rib.

infection, and thrombophlebitis in the subclavian and jugular veins can also affect the brachial plexus.[205]

Brachial neuritis is characterized by an acute onset of pain, which is followed by weakness and atrophy of the shoulder girdle muscles. The cause is currently unknown, but it is often preceded by viral infection or immunization.[205] MR imaging is often more helpful in excluding other possible diagnoses. However, T1- and T2-weighted axial and coronal series can show a thickened, abnormal high signal that is consistent with inflammation and possible brachial neuritis.[217]

REFERENCES

1. Moore KL and Persaud TVN: Study guide and review manual of human embryology. Philadelphia: WB Saunders; 1998.
2. Moore KL and Persaud TVN: Before we are born: essentials of embryology and birth defects. Philadelphia: WB Saunders; 1998.
3. Cummings CW: Otolaryngology—head and neck surgery. St. Louis: Mosby Year Book; 1993.
4. Gray H, Williams PL, and Bannister LH: Gray's anatomy: the anatomical basis of medicine and surgery. New York: Churchill Livingstone; 1995.
5. Koeller KK, Alamo L, Adair CF, and Smirniotopoulos JG: Congenital cystic masses of the neck: radiologic-pathologic correlation. Radiographics 1999;19:121–146; quiz 152–123.
6. Moore KL, Dalley AF, Donohoe LS, and Moore MF: Clinically oriented anatomy. Philadelphia: Lippincott Williams & Wilkins; 1999.
7. Richardson M and Sie K: The neck: embryoloogy and anatomy. In: Bluestone CD, ed. Pediatric otolaryngology. 4th ed. Philadelphia: Saunders;2003:1605–1620.
8. Oliver G and Detmar M: The rediscovery of the lymphatic system: old and new insights into the development and biological function of the lymphatic vasculature. Genes Dev 2002;16:773–783.
9. Skandalakis JE, Gray S, and Ricketts R: The lymphatic system. In: Skandalakis JE and Gray SW, eds.: Embryology for surgeons: the embryological basis for the treatment of congenital anomalies. 2nd ed. Baltimore: Williams & Wilkins; 1993:877–897.
10. Hendrix R: Diseases of the thyroid and parathyroid glands. In: Ballenger JJ and Snow JB, eds. Ballenger's otorhinolaryngology: head and neck surgery. 16th ed. Baltimore: Williams & Wilkins; 2003:1455–1483.
11. Williams P: Thyroid gland. In: Gray H, Williams PL, and Bannister LH, eds. Gray's Anatomy: the anatomical basis of medicine and surgery. 38th ed. New York: Churchill Livingstone; 1995:1891–1896.
12. Akerstrom G, Malmaeus J, and Bergstrom R: Surgical anatomy of human parathyroid glands. Surgery 1984;95:14–21.
13. Carol W and Morgan C: Disease of the salivary glands. In: Snow JB and Ballenger JJ, eds., Ballenger's otorhinolaryngology: head and neck surgery. 16th ed. Hamilton, Ont.: BC Decker; 2003:1441–1454.
14. Phelps P: The pharynx and larynx: the neck. In: Sutton D, ed., Textbook of radiology and imaging. 7th ed. Edinburgh: Churchill Livingstone; 2003:1489–1518.
15. Sinha UK and Ng M: Surgery of the salivary glands. Otolaryngol Clin North Am 1999;32:887–906.
16. Briss PA, Fehrs LJ, Parker RA, et al.: Sustained transmission of mumps in a highly vaccinated population: assessment of primary vaccine failure and waning vaccine-induced immunity. J Infect Dis 1994;169:77–82.
17. Wharton M, Cochi SL, Hutcheson RH, and Schaffner W: Mumps transmission in hospitals. Arch Intern Med 1990;150:47–49.
18. Spiegel R, Miron D, Sakran W, and Horovitz Y: Acute neonatal suppurative parotitis: case reports and review. Pediatr Infect Dis J 2004;23:76–78.
19. Fattahi TT, Lyu PE, and Van Sickels JE: Management of acute suppurative parotitis. J Oral Maxillofac Surg 2002;60:446–448.
20. Mandel L and Surattanont F: Bilateral parotid swelling: a review. Oral Surg Oral Med Oral Pathol Oral Radiol Endod 2002;93:221–237.
21. Brook I: Acute bacterial suppurative parotitis: microbiology and management. J Craniofac Surg 2003;14:37–40.
22. Cohen MA and Docktor JW: Acute suppurative parotitis with spread to the deep neck spaces. Am J Emerg Med 1999;17:46–49.
23. Sadeghi N, Black MJ, and Frenkiel S: Parotidectomy for the treatment of chronic recurrent parotitis. J Otolaryngol 1996;25:305–307.
24. Huisman TA, Holzmann D, and Nadal D: MRI of chronic recurrent parotitis in childhood. J Comput Assist Tomogr 2001;25:269–273.
25. Baurmash HD: Chronic recurrent parotitis: a closer look at its origin, diagnosis, and management. J Oral Maxillofac Surg 2004;62:1010–1018.
26. Baughman RP, Lower EE, and du Bois RM: Sarcoidosis. Lancet 2003;361:1111–1118.
27. Fischer T, Filimonow S, Petersein J, Zimmer C, Beyersdorff D, and Guski H: Diagnosis of Heerfordt's syndrome by state-of-the-art ultrasound in combination with parotid biopsy: a case report. Eur Radiol 2002;12:134–137.
28. Vairaktaris E, Vassiliou S, Yapijakis C, et al.: Salivary gland manifestations of sarcoidosis: report of three cases. J Oral Maxillofac Surg 2005;63:1016–1021.
29. Fox RI: Sjogren's syndrome. Lancet 2005;366:321–331.
30. Hansen A, Lipsky PE, and Dorner T: Immunopathogenesis of primary Sjogren's syndrome: Implications for disease management and therapy. Curr Opin Rheumatol 2005;17:558–565.
31. Jungehulsing M, Fischbach R, Schroder U, Kugel H, Damm M, and Eckel HE: Magnetic resonance sialography. Otolaryngol Head Neck Surg 1999;121:488–494.
32. Tonami H, Ogawa Y, Matoba M, et al.: MR sialography in patients with Sjogren syndrome. Am J Neuroradiol 1998;19:1199–1203.
33. Kalinowski M, Heverhagen JT, Rehberg E, Klose KJ, and Wagner HJ: Comparative study of MR sialography and digital subtraction sialography for benign salivary gland disorders. Am J Neuroradiol 2002;23:1485–1492.
34. Teymoortash A, Simolka N, Schrader C, Tiemann M, and Werner JA: Lymphocyte subsets in irradiation-induced sialadenitis of the submandibular gland. Histopathology 2005;47:493–500.
35. Mandel L and Carrao V: Bilateral parotid diffuse hyperplastic oncocytosis: Case report. J Oral Maxillofac Surg 2005;63:560–562.
36. Lowe LH, Stokes LS, Johnson JE, et al.: Swelling at the angle of the mandible: imaging of the pediatric parotid gland and periparotid region. Radiographics 2001;21:1211–1227.
37. Marcus A and Moore CE: Sodium morrhuate sclerotherapy for the treatment of benign lymphoepithelial cysts of the parotid gland in the HIV patient. Laryngoscope 2005;115:746–749.
38. Cotran RS, Kumar V, Collins T, and Robbins SL: Robbins pathologic basis of disease. Philadelphia: Saunders; 1999.
39. Barnes L: Surgical pathology of the head and neck. New York: Informa Healthcare; 2009.
40. Johnson FE and Spiro RH: Tumors arising in accessory parotid tissue. Am J Surg 1979;138:576–578.
41. Perzik SL and White IL: Surgical management of preauricular tumors of the accessory parotid apparatus. Am J Surg 1966;112:498–503.
42. Yu GY, Liu XB, Li ZL, and Peng X: Smoking and the development of Warthin's tumour of the parotid gland. Br J Oral Maxillofac Surg 1998;36:183–185.
43. Chang A and Harawi SJ: Oncocytes, oncocytosis, and oncocytic tumors. Pathol Annu 1992;27 Pt 1:263–304.
44. Ellis G and Auclair P: Atlas of tumor pathology, tumors of the salivary glands, Washington DC: Armed Forces Institute of Pathology; 1996:103.
45. Witt RL: Major salivary gland cancer. Surg Oncol Clin N Am 2004;13:113–127.
46. Ballotta E, Thiene G, Baracchini C, et al.: Surgical vs medical treatment for isolated internal carotid artery elongation with coiling or kinking in symptomatic patients: A prospective randomized clinical study. J Vasc Surg 2005;42:838–846.
47. Bradley PJ: Adenoid cystic carcinoma of the head and neck: a review. Curr Opin Otolaryngol Head Neck Surg 2004;12:127–132.
48. Gurney TA, Eisele DW, Weinberg V, Shin E, and Lee N: Adenoid cystic carcinoma of the major salivary glands treated with surgery and radiation. Laryngoscope 2005;115:1278–1282.
49. Westra WH: The surgical pathology of salivary gland neoplasms. Otolaryngol Clin North Am 1999;32:919–943.
50. Lewis JE, Olsen KD, and Weiland LH: Acinic cell carcinoma. Clinicopathologic review. Cancer 1991;67:172–179.
51. Suh SI, Seol HY, Kim TK, et al.: Acinic cell carcinoma of the head and neck: Radiologic-pathologic correlation. J Comput Assist Tomogr 2005;29:121–126.
52. Sakai O, Nakashima N, Takata Y, and Furuse M: Acinic cell carcinoma of the parotid gland: CT and MRI. Neuroradiology 1996;38:675–679.

53. Pandit RT and Park AH: Management of pediatric ranula. Otolaryngol Head Neck Surg 2002;127:115–118.
54. Zhao YF, Jia Y, Chen XM, and Zhang WF: Clinical review of 580 ranulas. Oral Surg Oral Med Oral Pathol Oral Radiol Endod 2004;98:281–287.
55. Davison MJ, Morton RP, and McIvor NP: Plunging ranula: clinical observations. Head Neck 1998;20:63–68.
56. Macdonald AJ, Salzman KL, and Harnsberger HR: Giant ranula of the neck: differentiation from cystic hygroma. Am J Neuroradiol 2003;24:757–761.
57. Zhao YF, Jia J, and Jia Y: Complications associated with surgical management of ranulas. J Oral Maxillofac Surg 2005;63:51–54.
58. Mintz S, Barak S, and Horowitz I: Carbon dioxide laser excision and vaporization of nonplunging ranulas: a comparison of two treatment protocols. J Oral Maxillofac Surg 1994;52:370–372.
59. Laskawi R, Schaffranietz F, Arglebe C, and Ellies M: Inflammatory diseases of the salivary glands in infants and adolescents. Int J Pediatr Otorhinolaryngol 2006;70:129–136.
60. Tiemann M, Teymoortash A, Schrader C, et al.: Chronic sclerosing sialadenitis of the submandibular gland is mainly due to a T lymphocyte immune reaction. Mod Pathol 2002;15:845–852.
61. Roh JL and Kim JM: Kuttner's tumor: Unusual presentation with bilateral involvement of the lacrimal and submandibular glands. Acta Otolaryngol 2005;125:792–796.
62. Kitagawa S, Zen Y, Harada K, et al.: Abundant IgG4-positive plasma cell infiltration characterizes chronic sclerosing sialadenitis (Kuttner's tumor). Am J Surg Pathol 2005;29:783–791.
63. Woodruff WW and Kennedy TL: Non-nodal neck masses. Semin Ultrasound CT MR 1997;18:182–204.
64. Smirniotopoulos JG and Chiechi MV: Teratomas, dermoids, and epidermoids of the head and neck. Radiographics 1995;15:1437–1455.
65. Longo F, Maremonti P, Mangone GM, De Maria G, and Califano L: Midline (dermoid) cysts of the floor of the mouth: report of 16 cases and review of surgical techniques. Plast Reconstr Surg 2003;112:1560–1565.
66. Devine JC and Jones DC: Carcinomatous transformation of a sublingual dermoid cyst. A case report. Int J Oral Maxillofac Surg 2000;29:126–127.
67. Weber RS, Byers RM, Petit B, Wolf P, Ang K, and Luna M: Submandibular gland tumors. Adverse histologic factors and therapeutic implications. Arch Otolaryngol Head Neck Surg 1990;116:1055–1060.
68. Silvers AR and Som PM: Salivary glands. Radiol Clin North Am 1998;36:941–966,vi.
69. Furlong MA, Fanburg-Smith JC, and Childers EL: Lipoma of the oral and maxillofacial region: site and subclassification of 125 cases. Oral Surg Oral Med Oral Pathol Oral Radiol Endod 2004;98:441–450.
70. Fregnani ER, Pires FR, Falzoni R, Lopes MA, and Vargas PA: Lipomas of the oral cavity: clinical findings, histological classification and proliferative activity of 46 cases. Int J Oral Maxillofac Surg 2003;32:49–53.
71. Camilleri IG, Malata CM, McLean NR, and Kelly CG: Malignant tumours of the submandibular salivary gland: a 15-year review. Br J Plast Surg 1998;51:181–185.
72. Goode RK, Auclair PL, and Ellis GL: Mucoepidermoid carcinoma of the major salivary glands: clinical and histopathologic analysis of 234 cases with evaluation of grading criteria. Cancer 1998;82:1217–1224.
73. DiNardo LJ: Lymphatics of the submandibular space: an anatomic, clinical, and pathologic study with applications to floor-of-mouth carcinoma. Laryngoscope 1998;108:206–214.
74. Jones KC, Silver J, Millar WS, and Mandel L: Chronic submasseteric abscess: anatomic, radiologic, and pathologic features. Am J Neuroradiol 2003;24:1159–1163.
75. Chong J, Hinckley LK, and Ginsberg LE: Masticator space abnormalities associated with mandibular osteoradionecrosis: MR and CT findings in five patients. Am J Neuroradiol 2000;21:175–178.
76. Hasso AN and Nickmeyer CA: Magnetic resonance imaging of soft tissues of the neck. Top Magn Reson Imaging 1994;6:254–274.
77. Harnsberger HR: Cystic masses of the head and neck. In: Handbook of head and neck imaging. 2nd ed. St. Louis: Mosby; 1995:199–223.
78. Majoie CB, Hulsmans FJ, Castelijns JA, et al.: Primary nerve-sheath tumours of the trigeminal nerve: clinical and MRI findings. Neuroradiology 1999;41:100–108.
79. Chi AC, Carey J, and Muller S: Intraosseous schwannoma of the mandible: a case report and review of the literature. Oral Surg Oral Med Oral Pathol Oral Radiol Endod 2003;96:54–65.
80. Zabel A, Debus J, Thilmann C, Schlegel W, and Wannenmacher M: Management of benign cranial nonacoustic schwannomas by fractionated stereotactic radiotherapy. Int J Cancer 2001;96:356–362.
81. Woodruff J: Pathology of major peripheral nerve sheath neoplasms. In: Weiss SW and Brooks JSJ, eds. United States and Canadian academy of pathology. Soft tissue tumors. Baltimore: Williams & Wilkins; 1996:129–161.
82. Cartellieri M and Swoboda H: Neurofibroma of the auriculotemporal nerve. Eur Arch Otorhinolaryngol 2000;257:396–398.
83. Gottfried ON, Viskochil DH, Fults DW, and Couldwell WT: Molecular, genetic, and cellular pathogenesis of neurofibromas and surgical implications. Neurosurgery 2006;58:1–16.
84. Potter BO and Sturgis EM: Sarcomas of the head and neck. Surg Oncol Clin N Am 2003;12:379–417.
85. Sturgis EM and Potter BO: Sarcomas of the head and neck region. Curr Opin Oncol 2003;15:239–252.
86. O'Connell TE, Castillo M, and Mukherji SK: Fibrosarcoma arising in the maxillary sinus: CT and MR features. J Comput Assist Tomogr 1996;20:736–738.
87. Eskey CJ, Robson CD, and Weber AL: Imaging of benign and malignant soft tissue tumors of the neck. Radiol Clin North Am 2000;38:1091–1104,xi.
88. Dagher R and Helman L: Rhabdomyosarcoma: an overview. Oncologist 1999;4:34–44.
89. Rice DH and Batsakis JG: Surgical pathology of the head and neck. Philadelphia: Lippincott Williams & Wilkins; 2000.
90. Zhan S, Shapiro DN, and Helman LJ: Activation of an imprinted allele of the insulin-like growth factor II gene implicated in rhabdomyosarcoma. J Clin Invest 1994;94:445–448.
91. McCarville MB, Spunt SL, and Pappo AS: Rhabdomyosarcoma in pediatric patients: the good, the bad, and the unusual. Am J Roentgenol 2001;176:1563–1569.
92. Gillespie MB, Marshall DT, Day TA, Mitchell AO, White DR, and Barredo JC: Pediatric rhabdomyosarcoma of the head and neck. Curr Treat Options Oncol 2006;7:13–22.
93. Smith RB, Apostolakis LW, Karnell LH, et al.: National Cancer Data Base report on osteosarcoma of the head and neck. Cancer 2003;98:1670–1680.
94. Gorlick R, Anderson P, Andrulis I, et al.: Biology of childhood osteogenic sarcoma and potential targets for therapeutic development: meeting summary. Clin Cancer Res 2003;9:5442–5453.
95. Kassir RR, Rassekh CH, Kinsella JB, Segas J, Carrau RL, and Hokanson JA: Osteosarcoma of the head and neck: meta-analysis of nonrandomized studies. Laryngoscope 1997;107:56–61.
96. Koch BB, Karnell LH, Hoffman HT, et al.: National cancer database report on chondrosarcoma of the head and neck. Head Neck 2000;22:408–425.
97. Collins MS, Koyama T, Swee RG, and Inwards CY: Clear cell chondrosarcoma: radiographic, computed tomographic, and magnetic resonance findings in 34 patients with pathologic correlation. Skeletal Radiol 2003;32:687–694.
98. Mark RJ, Poen J, Tran LM, Fu YS, Selch MT, and Parker RG: Postirradiation sarcomas. A single-institution study and review of the literature. Cancer 1994;73:2653–2662.
99. Mark RJ, Bailet JW, Poen J, et al.: Postirradiation sarcoma of the head and neck. Cancer 1993;72:887–893.
100. Wei-wei L, Qiu-liang W, Guo-hao W, Zhi-hua C, and Zong-yuan Z: Clinicopathologic features, treatment, and prognosis of postirradiation osteosarcoma in patients with nasopharyngeal cancer. Laryngoscope 2005;115:1574–1579.
101. Maghami EG, St-John M, Bhuta S, and Abemayor E: Postirradiation sarcoma: A case report and current review. Am J Otolaryngol 2005;26:71–74.
102. Buitendijk S, van de Ven CP, Dumans TG, et al.: Pediatric aggressive fibromatosis: a retrospective analysis of 13 patients and review of literature. Cancer 2005;104:1090–1099.
103. Schlemmer M: Desmoid tumors and deep fibromatoses. Hematol Oncol Clin North Am 2005;19:565–571,vii–viii.
104. Tejpar S, Nollet F, Li C, et al.: Predominance of beta-catenin mutations and beta-catenin dysregulation in sporadic aggressive fibromatosis (desmoid tumor). Oncogene 1999;18:6615–6620.
105. Hosalkar HS, Fox EJ, Delaney T, Torbert JT, Ogilvie CM, and Lackman RD: Desmoid tumors and current status of management. Orthop Clin North Am 2006;37:53–63.
106. Collins BJ, Fischer AC, and Tufaro AP: Desmoid tumors of the head and neck: a review. Ann Plast Surg 2005;54:103–108.

107. Lewis JJ, Boland PJ, Leung DH, Woodruff JM, and Brennan MF: The enigma of desmoid tumors. Ann Surg 1999; 229:866–872;discussion 872–863.
108. Dormans JP, Spiegel D, Meyer J, et al.: Fibromatoses in childhood: the desmoid/fibromatosis complex. Med Pediatr Oncol 2001;37:126–131.
109. Lee JC, Thomas JM, Phillips S, Fisher C, and Moskovic E: Aggressive fibromatosis: MRI features with pathologic correlation. AJR Am J Roentgenol 2006;186:247–254.
110. Karmody C: Developmental anomalies of the neck. In: Bluestone CD, ed. Pediatric otolaryngology. 4th ed. Philadelphia: Saunders; 2003: 1648–1663.
111. Reisner A, Marshall GS, Bryant K, Postel GC, and Eberly SM: Endovascular occlusion of a carotid pseudoaneurysm complicating deep neck space infection in a child. Case report. J Neurosurg 1999;91:510–514.
112. Levy EI, Horowitz MB, Koebbe C, and Jungreis CC: Target-specific multimodality endovascular management of carotid artery blow-out syndrome. Ear Nose Throat J 2002;81:115–118.
113. Nunez DB Jr., Torres-Leon M, Munera F: Vascular injuries of the neck and thoracic inlet: helical CT-angiographic correlation. Radiographics 2004;24:1087–1098;1099–1100.
114. Kraus RR, Bergstein JM, and DeBord JR: Diagnosis, treatment, and outcome of blunt carotid arterial injuries. Am J Surg 1999;178:190–193.
115. Phan T, Huston J, IIIrd, Bernstein MA, Riederer SJ, Brown RD Jr.: Contrast-enhanced magnetic resonance angiography of the cervical vessels: experience with 422 patients. Stroke 2001;32:2282–2286.
116. Kou B, Davidson J, Gilbert R, and Cheung G: Coil embolization of pseudoaneurysms of the external carotid artery: Case series. J Otolaryngol 2000;29:315–318.
117. Mazighi M, Saint Maurice JP, Rogopoulos A, and Houdart E: Extracranial vertebral and carotid dissection occurring in the course of subarachnoid hemorrhage. Neurology 2005;65:1471–1473.
118. Grau AJ, Brandt T, Buggle F, et al.: Association of cervical artery dissection with recent infection. Arch Neurol 1999;56.
119. Schievink WI: Spontaneous dissection of the carotid and vertebral arteries. N Engl J Med 2001;344:898–906.
120. Schievink WI, Wijdicks EF, Michels VV, Vockley J, and Godfrey M: Heritable connective tissue disorders in cervical artery dissections: a prospective study. Neurology 1998;50:1166–1169.
121. Pezzini A, Caso V, Zanferrari C, et al.: Arterial hypertension as risk factor for spontaneous cervical artery dissection. A case-control study. J Neurol Neurosurg Psychiatry 2006;77:95–97.
122. Beletsky V, Nadareishvili Z, Lynch J, Shuaib A, Woolfenden A, and Norris JW: Cervical arterial dissection: Time for a therapeutic trial? Stroke 2003;34:2856–2860.
123. Lasak JM, Kryzer TC, Walker M, and Berger R: Imaging case of the month. Extracranial internal carotid artery dissection. Otol Neurotol 2005;26:131–132.
124. Unsal EE, Karaca C, and Ensari S: Spontaneous internal jugular vein thrombosis associated with distant malignancies. Eur Arch Otorhinolaryngol 2003;260:39–41.
125. Monreal M, Raventos A, Lerma R, et al.: Pulmonary embolism in patients with upper extremity DVT associated to venous central lines—A prospective study. Thromb Haemost 1994;72:548–550.
126. Maki DG, Crnich CJ: Line sepsis in the ICU: Prevention, diagnosis, and management. Semin Respir Crit Care Med 2003;24:23–36.
127. Leontsinis TG, Currie AR, and Mannell A: Internal jugular vein thrombosis following functional neck dissection. Laryngoscope 1995;105:169–174.
128. Hudgins PA, Kingdom TT, Weissler MC, and Mukherji SK: Selective neck dissection: CT and MR imaging findings. AJNR Am J Neuroradiol 2005;26:1174–1177.
129. Prim MP, de Diego JI, Fernandez-Zubillaga A, Garcia-Raya P, Madero R, and Gavilan J: Patency and flow of the internal jugular vein after functional neck dissection. Laryngoscope 2000;110:47–50.
130. Quraishi HA, Wax MK, Granke K, and Rodman SM: Internal jugular vein thrombosis after functional and selective neck dissection. Arch Otolaryngol Head Neck Surg 1997;123:969–973.
131. Wax MK, Quraishi H, Rodman S, and Granke K: Internal jugular vein patency in patients undergoing microvascular reconstruction. Laryngoscope 1997;107:1245–1248.
132. Myssiorek D: Head and neck paragangliomas: an overview. Otolaryngol Clin North Am 2001;34:829–836,5.
133. Schiavi F, Boedeker CC, Bausch B, et al.: Predictors and prevalence of paraganglioma syndrome associated with mutations of the SDHC gene. JAMA 2005;294:2057–2063.
134. Baysal BE, Willett-Brozick JE, Filho PA, Lawrence EC, Myers EN, and Ferrell RE: An Alu-mediated partial SDHC deletion causes familial and sporadic paraganglioma. J Med Genet 2004;41:703–709.
135. van den Berg R: Imaging and management of head and neck paragangliomas. Eur Radiol 2005;15:1310–1318.
136. Dundee P, Clancy B, Wagstaff S, and Briggs R: Paraganglioma: the role of genetic counselling and radiological screening. J Clin Neurosci 2005;12:464–466.
137. Lee JH, Barich F, Karnell LH, et al.: National cancer data base report on malignant paragangliomas of the head and neck. Cancer 2002;94:730–737.
138. Rao AB, Koeller KK, and Adair CF: From the archives of the AFIP. Paragangliomas of the head and neck: radiologic-pathologic correlation. Armed Forces Institute of Pathology. Radiographics 1999;19:1605–1632.
139. Sharma PK and Massey BL: Avoiding pitfalls in surgery of the neck, parapharyngeal space, and infratemporal fossa. Otolaryngol Clin North Am 2005;38:795–808.
140. Colreavy MP, Lacy PD, Hughes J, et al.: Head and neck schwannomas—A 10 year review. J Laryngol Otol 2000;114:119–124.
141. Furukawa M, Furukawa MK, Katoh K, and Tsukuda M: Differentiation between schwannoma of the vagus nerve and schwannoma of the cervical sympathetic chain by imaging diagnosis. Laryngoscope 1996;106:1548–1552.
142. Harnsberger HR: The Carotid Space. In: Handbook of head and neck imaging. 2nd ed. St. Louis: Mosby; 1995:75–88.
143. Freeman SB, Hamaker RC, Borrowdale RB, and Huntley TC: Management of neck metastasis with carotid artery involvement. Laryngoscope 2004;114:20–24.
144. Fisher SG and Fisher RI: The epidemiology of non-Hodgkin's lymphoma. Oncogene 2004;23:6524–6534
145. Jerusalem G, Hustinx R, Beguin Y, and Fillet G: Evaluation of therapy for lymphoma. Semin Nucl Med 2005;35:186–196.
146. Weber AL, Rahemtullah A, and Ferry JA: Hodgkin and non-Hodgkin lymphoma of the head and neck: clinical, pathologic, and imaging evaluation. Neuroimaging Clin N Am 2003;13:371–392.
147. Jemal A, Murray T, Ward E, et al.: Cancer statistics, 2005. CA Cancer J Clin 2005;55:10–30.
148. Lu P: Staging and classification of lymphoma. Semin Nucl Med 2005;35:160–164.
149. Rao AV, Akabani G, and Rizzieri DA: Radioimmunotherapy for Non-Hodgkin's lymphoma. Clin Med Res 2005;3:157–165.
150. Paulsen F, Tillmann B, Christofides C, Richter W, and Koebke J: Curving and looping of the internal carotid artery in relation to the pharynx: Frequency, embryology and clinical implications. J Anat 2000;197 Pt 3:373–381.
151. Koskas F, Bahnini A, Walden R, and Kieffer E: Stenotic coiling and kinking of the internal carotid artery. Ann Vasc Surg 1993;7:530–540.
152. Vega J, Gervas C, Vega-Hazas G, Barrera C, and Biurrun C: Internal carotid artery transposition: another cause of widening of the retropharyngeal space. Eur Radiol 1999;9:347–348.
153. Smith D, Neal J, Rumboldt Z, and Gillespie MB: Radiology quiz case 3. Retropharyngeal carotid artery. Arch Otolaryngol Head Neck Surg 2005;131:75,78–79.
154. Galletti B, Bucolo S, Abbate G, et al.: Internal carotid artery transposition as risk factor in pharyngeal surgery. Laryngoscope 2002;112:1845–1848.
155. Chong VF and Fan YF: Radiology of the retropharyngeal space. Clin Radiol 2000;55:740–748.
156. Tsai YS and Lui CC: Retropharyngeal and epidural abscess from a swallowed fish bone. Am J Emerg Med 1997;15:381–382.
157. Kransdorf MJ, Bancroft LW, Peterson JJ, Murphey MD, Foster WC, and Temple HT: Imaging of fatty tumors: Distinction of lipoma and well-differentiated liposarcoma. Radiology 2002;224:99–104.
158. Gaskin CM and Helms CA: Lipomas, lipoma variants, and well-differentiated liposarcomas (atypical lipomas): Results of MRI evaluations of 126 consecutive fatty masses. Am J Roentgenol 2004;182:733–739.
159. Sakai O, Curtin HD, Romo LV, and Som PM: Lymph node pathology. Benign proliferative, lymphoma, and metastatic disease. Radiol Clin North Am 2000;38:979–998,10.
160. Shaha AR: Management of the neck in thyroid cancer. Otolaryngol Clin North Am 1998;31:823–831.

161. Roth JA, Enzinger FM, and Tannenbaum M: Synovial sarcoma of the neck: A followup study of 24 cases. Cancer 1975;35:1243–1253.
162. Olsen RJ, Lydiatt WM, Koepsell SA, et al.: C-erb-B2 (HER2/neu) expression in synovial sarcoma of the head and neck. Head Neck 2005;27:883–892.
163. Albritton KH and Randall RL: Prospects for targeted therapy of synovial sarcoma. J Pediatr Hematol Oncol 2005;27:219–222.
164. Mankin HJ and Hornicek FJ: Diagnosis, classification, and management of soft tissue sarcomas. Cancer Control 2005;12:5–21.
165. Rangheard AS, Vanel D, Viala J, Schwaab G, Casiraghi O, and Sigal R: Synovial sarcomas of the head and neck: CT and MR imaging findings of eight patients. Am J Neuroradiol 2001;22:851–857.
166. Blacksin MF, Siegel JR, Benevenia J, and Aisner SC: Synovial sarcoma: frequency of nonaggressive MR characteristics. J Comput Assist Tomogr 1997;21:785–789.
167. Shin JH, Lee HK, Kim SY, et al.: Parapharyngeal second branchial cyst manifesting as cranial nerve palsies: MR findings. Am J Neuroradiol 2001;22:510–512.
168. Bradley JP, Elahi M, and Kawamoto HK: Delayed presentation of pseudoaneurysm after Le Fort I osteotomy. J Craniofac Surg 2002;13:746–750.
169. Jay J, Shapiro BM, Komisar A, and Lawson W: Posttraumatic pseudoaneurysm of the extracranial middle meningeal artery. Arch Otolaryngol 1985;111:264–266.
170. Krishnan DG, Marashi A, and Malik A: Pseudoaneurysm of internal maxillary artery secondary to gunshot wound managed by endovascular technique. J Oral Maxillofac Surg 2004;62:500–502.
171. Nagy M, Pizzuto M, Backstrom J, and Brodsky L: Deep neck infections in children: a new approach to diagnosis and treatment. Laryngoscope 1997;107:1627–1634.
172. Cable BB, Brenner P, Bauman NM, and Mair EA: Image-guided surgical drainage of medial parapharyngeal abscesses in children: a novel adjuvant to a difficult approach. Ann Otol Rhinol Laryngol 2004;113:115–120.
173. Choi SS, Vezina LG, and Grundfast KM: Relative incidence and alternative approaches for surgical drainage of different types of deep neck abscesses in children. Arch Otolaryngol Head Neck Surg 1997;123:1271–1275.
174. Abdullah BJ, Liam CK, Kaur H, and Mathew KM: Parapharyngeal space lipoma causing sleep apnoea. Br J Radiol 1997;70:1063–1065.
175. Scott RF, Collins MM, and Wilson JA: Parapharyngeal lipoma. J Laryngol Otol 1999;113:935–937.
176. Kakani RS, Bahadur S, Kumar S, and Tandon DA: Parapharyngeal lipoma. J Laryngol Otol 1992;106:279–281.
177. van den Brekel MW: Lymph node metastases: CT and MRI. Eur J Radiol 2000;33:230–238.
178. Hillsamer PJ, Schuller DE, McGhee RB Jr., Chakeres D, Young DC: Improving diagnostic accuracy of cervical metastases with computed tomography and magnetic resonance imaging. Arch Otolaryngol Head Neck Surg 1990;116:1297–1301.
179. Lowe V, Stack JB, and Watson JR: Head and neck cancer imaging. In: Ensley JF, ed. Head and neck cancer: emerging perspectives. San Diego, Calif. London: Academic; 2002:23–32.
180. Branstetter BF, IVth and Weissman JL: Normal anatomy of the neck with CT and MR imaging correlation. Radiol Clin North Am 2000;38:925–940,9.
181. Mancuso AA, Harnsberger HR, Muraki AS, and Stevens MH: Computed tomography of cervical and retropharyngeal lymph nodes: normal anatomy, variants of normal, and applications in staging head and neck cancer. Part II: pathology. Radiology 1983;148:715–723.
182. Greene FL: American Joint Committee on Cancer, American Cancer Society. AJCC Cancer Staging Manual. New York: Springer;2002.
183. Collins S: Controversies in management of cancer of the neck. In: Thawley SE, Panje WR, Batsakis JG, and Lindberg RD, eds. Comprehensive management of head and neck tumors. Philadelphia: Saunders 1987; 1386–1443.
184. Higgins CB and Auffermann W: Endocrine Imaging : Textbook and Atlas. New York: Georg Thieme Verlag; Thieme Medical Publishers;1993.
185. Higgins CB and Auffermann W: Thyroid gland. In: Higgins CB and Auffermann W, eds. Endocrine imaging: textbook and atlas. Stuttgart; New York, NY: Georg Thieme Verlag; Thieme Medical Publishers;1993:43–84.
186. Gotway MB and Higgins CB: MR imaging of the thyroid and parathyroid glands. Magn Reson Imaging Clin N Am 2000;8:163–182,9.
187. Cotran RS, Kumar V, and Collins T: Head and neck. In: Cotran RS, Kumar V, Collins T, and Robbins SL, eds. Robbins pathologic basis of disease. 6th ed. Philadelphia: Saunders; 1999:756–774.
188. Weber AL, Randolph G, and Aksoy FG: The thyroid and parathyroid glands. CT and MR imaging and correlation with pathology and clinical findings. Radiol Clin North Am 2000;38:1105–1129.
189. Ozgen A and Cila A: Riedel's thyroiditis in multifocal fibrosclerosis: CT and MR imaging findings. AJNR Am J Neuroradiol 2000;21:320–321.
190. Papi G, Corrado S, Cesinaro AM, Novelli L, Smerieri A, and Carapezzi C: Riedel's thyroiditis: Clinical, pathological and imaging features. Int J Clin Pract 2002;56:65–67.
191. Lufkin RB, Borges A, and Villablanca P: Neck. In: Lufkin RB, Borges A, and Villablanca P, eds. Teaching atlas of head and neck imaging. New York: Thieme; 2000:107–184.
192. Few J, Thompson NW, Angelos P, Simeone D, Giordano T, and Reeve T: Riedel's Thyroiditis: treatment with tamoxifen. Surgery 1996;120: 993–999.
193. Yousem DM: Parathyroid and thyroid imaging. Neuroimaging Clin N Am 1996;6:435–459.
194. Mukherji SK, Fatterpekar G, Castillo M, Stone JA, and Chung CJ: Imaging of congenital anomalies of the branchial apparatus. Neuroimaging Clin N Am 2000;10:75–93,viii.
195. Donegan J: Congenital Neck Masses. In: Cummings CW, Fredrickson J, Harker L, Krause C, and Schuller D, eds. Otolaryngology—head and neck surgery. 2nd ed. St. Louis: Mosby Year Book;1993:1554–1565.
196. Cunningham MJ: The management of congenital neck masses. Am J Otolaryngol 1992;13:78–92.
197. Mandell DL: Head and neck anomalies related to the branchial apparatus. Otolaryngol Clin North Am 2000;33:1309–1332.
198. Rowe L: Congenital anomalies of the head and neck. In: Ballenger HC and Snow JB, eds. Ballenger's manual of otorhinolaryngology head and neck surgery. Hamilton: BC Decker; 2003:1073–1089.
199. Harnsberger HR: The parapharyngeal space and the pharyngeal mucosal space. In: Handbook of head and neck imaging. 2nd ed. St. Louis: Mosby; 1995:29–45.
200. Grossman RI and Yousem DM: Extramucosal disease of the head and neck. In: Neuroradiology: The requisites. St. Louis: Mosby; 1994:413–446.
201. Lev S and Lev MH: Imaging of cystic lesions. Radiol Clin North Am 2000;38:1013–1027.
202. Bauer P and Lusk R: Neck masses. In: Bluestone CD, ed. Pediatric otolaryngology. 4th ed. Philadelphia: Saunders; 2003:335–339.
203. Skandalakis JE, Gray S, and Todd N: Pharynx and its derivatives. In: Skandalakis JE and Gray SW, eds. Embryology for surgeons: the embryological basis for the treatment of congenital anomalies. 2nd ed. Baltimore: Williams & Wilkins; 1993:17–64.
204. Williams JD, Sclafani AP, Slupchinskij O, and Douge C: Evaluation and management of the lingual thyroid gland. Ann Otol Rhinol Laryngol 1996;105:312–316.
205. Reede D and Holliday R: Brachial Plexus. In: Som PM and Curtin HD, eds. Head and Neck Imaging. 4th ed. St. Louis, MO: Mosby; 2003:2216–2238.
206. Hyodoh K, Hyodoh H, Akiba H, et al.: Brachial plexus: Normal anatomy and pathological conditions. Curr Probl Diagn Radiol 2002;31:179–188.
207. Todd M, Shah GV, and Mukherji SK: MR imaging of brachial plexus. Top Magn Reson Imaging 2004;15:113–125.
208. Sureka J, Cherian RA, Alexander M, and Thomas BP: MRI of brachial plexopathies. Clin Radiol 2009;64:208–218.
209. Yoshikawa T, Hayashi N, Yamamoto S, et al.: Brachial plexus injury: Clinical manifestations, conventional imaging findings, and the latest imaging techniques. Radiographics 2006;26 Suppl 1:S133–S143.
210. van Es HW: MRI of the brachial plexus. Eur Radiol 2001;11:325–336.
211. Aagaard BD, Maravilla KR, and Kliot M: MR neurography. MR imaging of peripheral nerves. Magn Reson Imaging Clin N Am 1998;6:179–194.
212. Millesi H: Brachial plexus injuries in adults. Orthopade 1997;26:590–598.
213. Greenwald AG, Schute PC, Shiveley JL: Brachial plexus birth palsy: a 10-year report on the incidence and prognosis. J Pediatr Orthop 1984;4:689–692.
214. al-Rajeh S, Corea JR, al-Sibai MH, al-Umran K, and Sankarankutty M: Congenital brachial palsy in the eastern province of Saudi Arabia. J Child Neurol1990;5:35–38.
215. Smith AB, Gupta N, Strober J, and Chin C: Magnetic resonance neurography in children with birth-related brachial plexus injury. Pediatr Radiol 2008;38:159–163.
216. Lanaras TI, Schaller HE, and Sinis N: Brachial plexus lesions: 10 years of experience in a center for microsurgery in Germany. Microsurgery 2009;29:87–94.
217. Ayoub T, Raman V, and Chowdhury M: Brachial neuritis caused by varicella-zoster diagnosed by changes in brachial plexus on MRI. J Neurol 2009.

Vascular Anomalies and Vascular Tumors of the Head and Neck

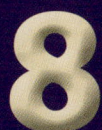

Jose A. Ospina, MD, PhD
Wende N. Gibbs, MS, MD
Anton N. Hasso, MD, FACR

Vasoformative malformations are common congenital anomalies, most often seen in infants and children. Diagnosis and treatment of these lesions has been aided by the biologic classification system of Mulliken and Glowacki, which distinguishes disorders using clinical, histochemical, and cellular criteria.[1] The vasoformative malformations are divided into two groups, hemangiomas and vascular malformations. Hemangiomas are characterized by rapid cellular proliferation shortly after birth, typically followed by spontaneous involution within several years. In contrast, vascular malformations are pure congenital anomalies, containing mature, orderly, nonproliferating endothelial cells. These lesions are usually present, though not necessarily visibly detectable, at birth, grow in parallel with the child, and do not typically regress in the absence of therapeutic intervention. The vascular malformations are further subdivided according to vessel type into lymphatic, capillary, venous, arteriovenous, and mixed subtypes (Fig. 8-1). Lesions are also categorized based on hemodynamic characteristics. Proliferative-phase hemangiomas, arterial malformations, and arteriovenous malformations and fistulas are considered high-flow lesions, while involuting hemangiomas, and capillary, venous, and lymphatic malformations are low-flow lesions.

HEMANGIOMAS

Hemangiomas are benign vascular neoplasms composed of proliferating endothelial cells that are most commonly seen as small, solitary lesions in the head and neck. They are characterized by a predictable evolution and duration, generally appearing within weeks after birth, proliferating rapidly during the first year, and then spontaneously involuting over a period of several years. Hemangiomas may be located superficially in the skin and mucous membranes, or may infiltrate the deeper structures of the head and neck. Superficial hemangiomas, historically termed "strawberry" hemangiomas, appear as well-defined, bright scarlet nodules or plaques on the skin. If the tumor lies deep within the subcutaneous tissue or muscle, the overlying skin may display a bruise-like faint bluish cast, or may even appear normal depending on the depth of the lesion. Though most hemangiomas tend to be small, up to 10% may grow rapidly and become problematic, particularly if they compromise the visual axis or airway.[2,3]

The nature and cellular location of the primary defect responsible for triggering, maintaining, and arresting this abnormal endothelial proliferation is still under investigation. Most begin as relatively inconspicuous macules that quickly enter a proliferative phase and expand into masses in the oral cavity, pharynx, parotid gland, or neck. This proliferative period is characterized by rapid cycling of the endothelial cells between multiplication, migration, and death, creating a multilaminar basement membrane. Approximately 2 to 5 years after birth, the proliferation slows and the hemangioma enters an involuting phase, in which endothelium is replaced by infiltrative fibrous and adipose tissue. Late in this phase, only a few thin-walled vascular channels remain. These channels resemble normal vasculature, with the exception they still possess a multilaminated basement membrane.[4] The proliferative and involuting phases are not distinct, as both processes occur simultaneously. However, at predictable intervals, one process is dominant. At the end of the cycle, the fully involuted hemangioma has a cavernous appearance, and may be mistaken for a venous malformation.

Hemangiomas are the most common tumors of the head and neck in infancy and childhood, accounting for approximately 7% of all benign soft-tissue tumors.[5] Almost all of these lesions become clinically evident by 6 months of age. Eighty percent of hemangiomas present as single lesions, while 20% appear as bilateral or multiple lesions.[6] The female to male prevalence ranges from 3:1 to 4:1, and Caucasians account for a significantly higher proportion of cases. Half of these tumors involute and resolve by the age of 5 years, and 70% have resolved by the age of 7 years.[7] Most hemangiomas do not require treatment, but some, such as those located in the subglottic region, can be problematic and even life threatening. In these cases, MR imaging is

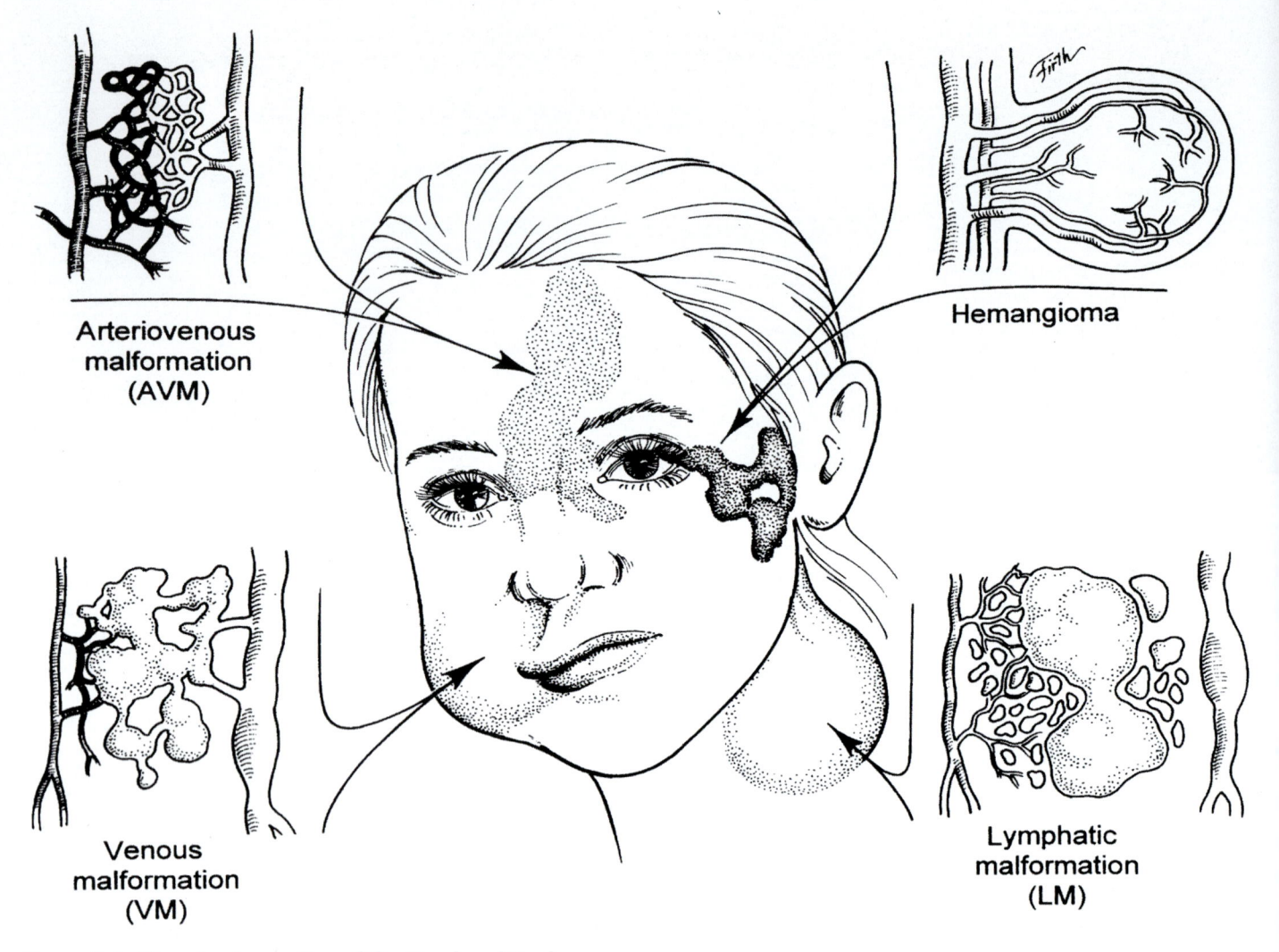

Figure 8-1 Vascular Anomalies of the Head and Neck
Schematic diagram depicting the morphologic appearance and gross histology of the most common vascular anomalies of the head and neck. Insets depict the aberrant angioarchitecture manifest by the various lesions.

indicated to evaluate the number and extent of the lesions. Disseminated neonatal hemangiomatosis is a rare life-threatening disease characterized by hemangiomas in more than three organ systems. Hemangiomas can also be associated with a variety of other intracranial arterial vascular anomalies and neurological abnormalities, or disease syndromes, such as PHACES and Kasabach-Merritt syndrome.[8]

Superficial, cutaneous hemangiomas are easily diagnosed by appearance. Early-phase subcutaneous hemangiomas, which have extended through the skin and have infiltrated underlying muscle, may be more subtle, resembling a scratch, bruise, or patch of hypopigmentation. In some cases, hemangiomas change in size during straining or crying. The tumors may deform skeletal structures, such as the mandible, skull, and orbit, secondary to mass displacement, but they rarely invade bone.[8] The differential diagnosis for hemangiomas includes fibrosarcoma, rhabdomyosarcoma, and neurofibroma (**Table 8-1**).

Grossly, hemangiomas are bright red tumors, which vary in size from a few millimeters to several centimeters in diameter. Histologically, they are unencapsulated, lobulated masses of vessels separated by minimal connective tissue stroma.

MR imaging of hemangiomas is characteristic, but depends upon the growth phase of the lesion (**Table 8-2**). In the proliferating phase, hemangiomas are well-defined, lobulated soft-tissue masses that are isointense or slightly hyperintense to muscle on T1-weighted images and hyperintense on T2-weighted images (**Fig. 8-2**). During the proliferative phase hemangiomas are characterized by high-flow physiology and thereby exhibit multiple flow voids on MRI (**Fig. 8-3**). Contrast enhancement of the tumor is intense and relatively uniform. As the tumor involutes, vascularity decreases, and fibrous and adipose tissue replaces the tumor. The adipose tissue appears as high intensity foci within the lesion on T1-weighted imaging (**Figs. 8-4** to **8-6**). In addition to characterizing the intrinsic imaging properties of hemangiomas, MR is invaluable in defining the extent of these lesions as well as any associated mass effect on adjacent structures.

Chapter 8: Vascular Anomalies and Vascular Tumors of the Head and Neck 341

Table 8-1 Hemangioma Differential Diagnosis

DDx	Description
Fibrosarcoma	• Rare infantile form appears shortly after birth • Rapidly growing • Locally aggressive • Imaging: low to intermediate signal intensity mass on T1 and T2, with moderate contrast enhancement.
Rhabdomyosarcoma	• Rapidly growing • Commonly invades bone • Spreads through neural foramina. • Imaging: heterogenous mass with diffuse enhancement and local bone destruction • Intratumoral hemorrhage may be present
Neurofibroma	• Slow growing • Painless soft-tissue tumor • Arises in ages 20 to 40 years • Imaging: low signal T1 and high signal T2 with variable contrast enhancement

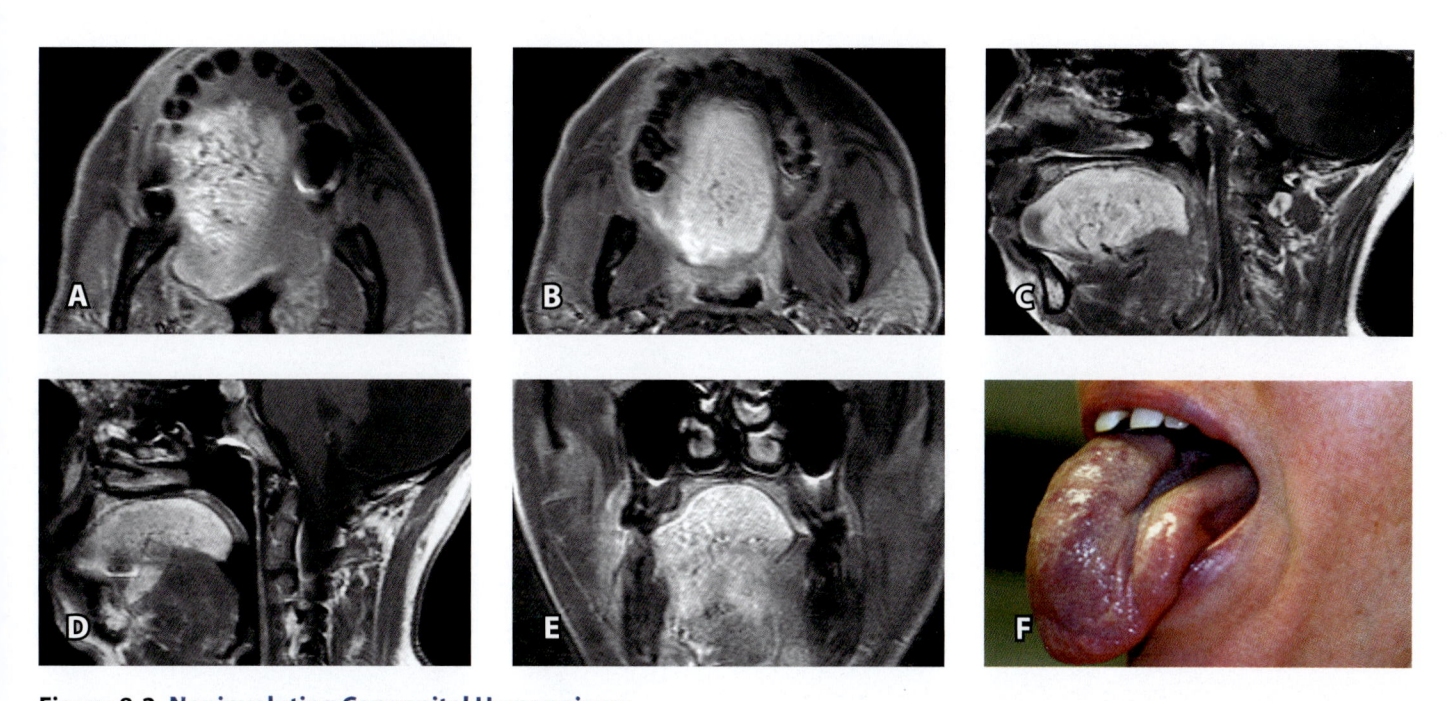

Figure 8-2 Noninvoluting Congenital Hemangioma
(**A–E**) T1 contrast-enhanced fat-saturated MR images. (**A, B**) Axial, (**C, D**) sagittal, and (**E**) coronal images showing an intensely enhancing lesion on the right side of the oral tongue with multiple small flow voids. This lesion was present since birth, grew rapidly, and has remained stable as the patient matured into adulthood. (**F**) Photo of patient's tongue.

Table 8-2 MR Imaging of Hemangiomas

Phase	Description	T1W MR Findings	Postcontrast T1W MR Findings	T2W MR Findings
Proliferative	• High-flow lesions	• Low signal • Flow voids	• Intense enhancement	• High signal • Flow voids
Involuting	• Lesions become low flow • Hypercellularity replaced by fibrous and adipose tissue	• High signal	• No enhancement	• Low signal

In addition, in deep or dangerous hemangiomas, MR imaging is utilized to assess the degree of airway impingement, and MR angiography or venography can be used to evaluate vascular compromise.

A variety of treatment options for disfiguring or dangerous hemangiomas exist, including surgical excision, pharmacotherapy, the use of sclerosing agents, and laser treatments. Surgical excision may be utilized to remove the fibrofatty tissue that remains after a hemangioma has involuted. Complications from this treatment include significant blood loss, tissue loss, and disfiguring cutaneous scarring. Sclerosing agents and continuous wave and pulsed dye lasers can arrest the proliferative phase and accelerate the involuting phase of the hemangioma, but can also result in cutaneous scarring. The newer Nd:YAG laser can also efficiently treat hemangiomas, and when utilized intralesionally, it minimizes cutaneous damage by transmitting energy directly to the lesion via a bare fiber delivery system. The potassium titanyl phosphate laser

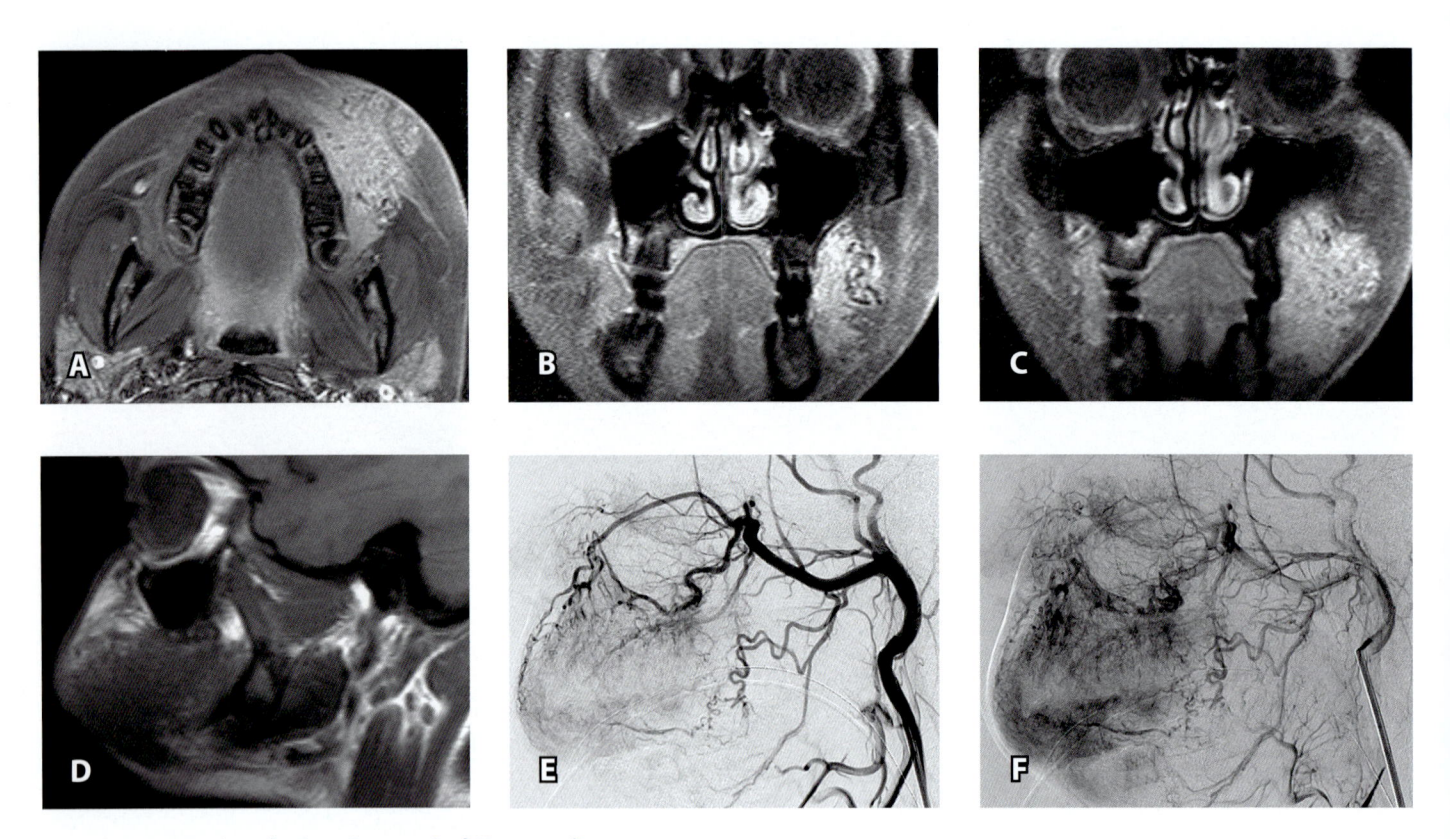

Figure 8-3 Noninvoluting Congenital Hemangioma
(**A**) Axial and (**B, C**) coronal T1 contrast-enhanced fat-saturated MR scans demonstrate a subcutaneous lesion in the left buccal space extending from the surface of the maxillary alveolar ridge to the surface. (**D**) Sagittal T1 unenhanced MR image showing no flow voids, as the vessels are too small to detect. (**E, F**) Lateral selective left maxillary artery angiograms in two phases. (**E**) The early phase shows a fine tangle of vessels throughout the mass lesion but no early draining veins. (**F**) The later phase shows an intense stain without any large feeders, but with a fine network of small vessels.

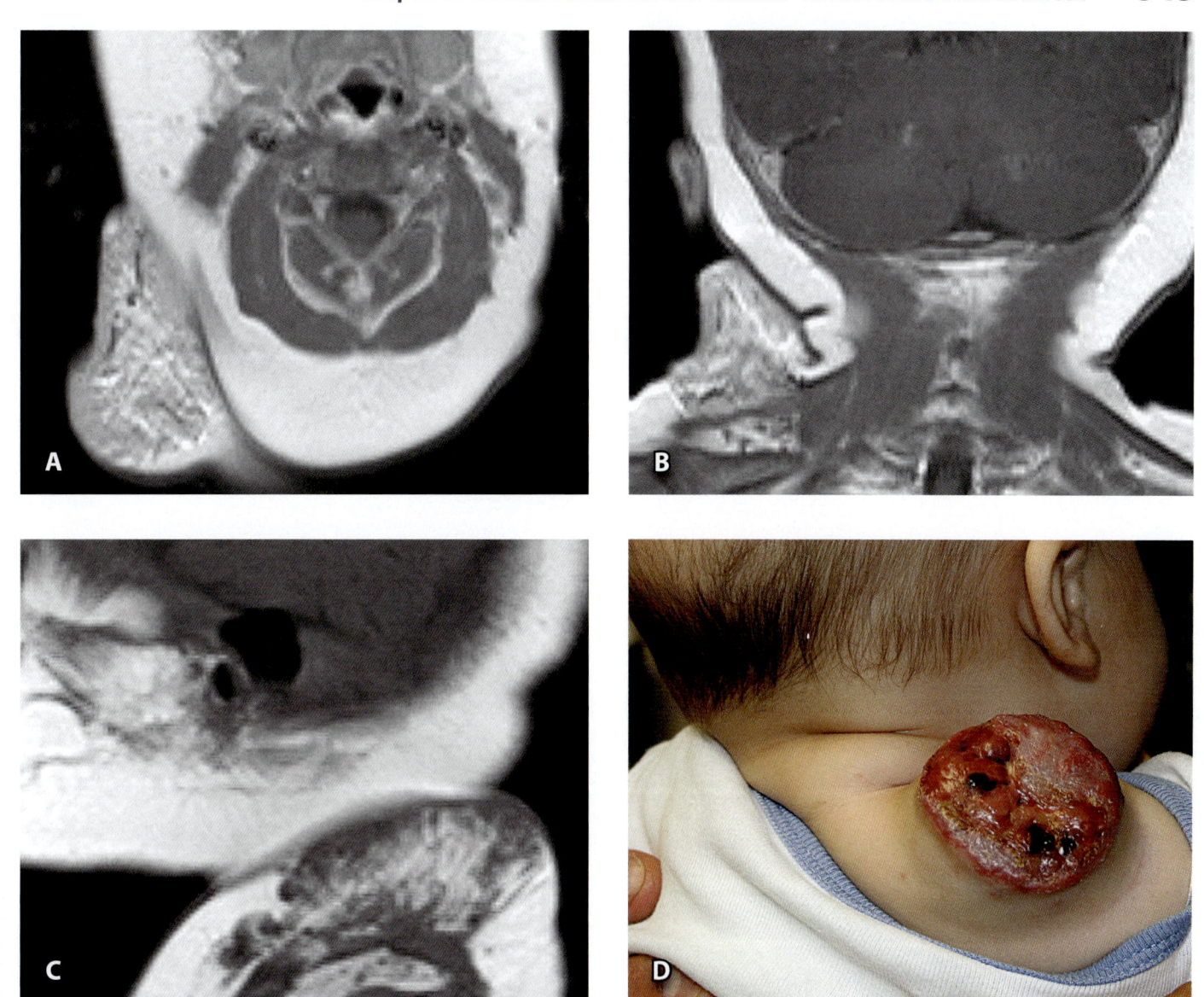

Figure 8-4 Rapidly Involuting Congenital Hemangioma
(**A**) Axial, (**B**) coronal T1 contrast-enhanced and (**C**) sagittal T1 unenhanced MR images demonstrate a large protruding mass in the right shoulder showing a heterogeneous appearance and some enhancement and a few flow voids. (**D**) Photo of the neck mass in a young child showing a lesion that has been present since birth, grew rapidly and has started to involute with increased coarseness and thickening of its skin surface.

(KTP) is a modified version of the Nd:YAG, which is more effective than the traditional Nd:YAG as it specifically targets hemoglobin.[9] These intralesional photocoagulation therapies show great promise in the treatment of both hemangiomas and venous malformations.[10]

Patients with rapidly proliferating hemangiomas that are cosmetically or functionally threatening may require aggressive pharmacological intervention. Corticosteroids have long been recognized to effectively treat up to 90% of proliferating hemangiomas,[11–13] putatively by inhibiting angiogenesis[14] and promoting vasoconstriction.[12] At present, steroids are typically reserved for growing tumors that are disfiguring or obstruct the visual axis, airways, digestive passageways, or auditory canal; for lesions causing congestive heart failure or consumptive coagulopathy; or for ulcerated, bleeding, or infected hemangiomas. Periocular hemangiomas, especially those involving the eyelid, are particularly responsive to intralesional steroid injections.[15] Alternatively, interferon-alpha-2 has been used successfully[16] when steroid therapy has failed, produced complications, or was contraindicated. Unfortunately, a high incidence of spastic diplegia, and other neurologic complications, limits the use of this agent.[17]

VASCULAR MALFORMATIONS

Vascular malformations result from errors in the morphogenesis of the embryonic vascular system between the fourth and eighth weeks of development. They are present at birth, but may not be

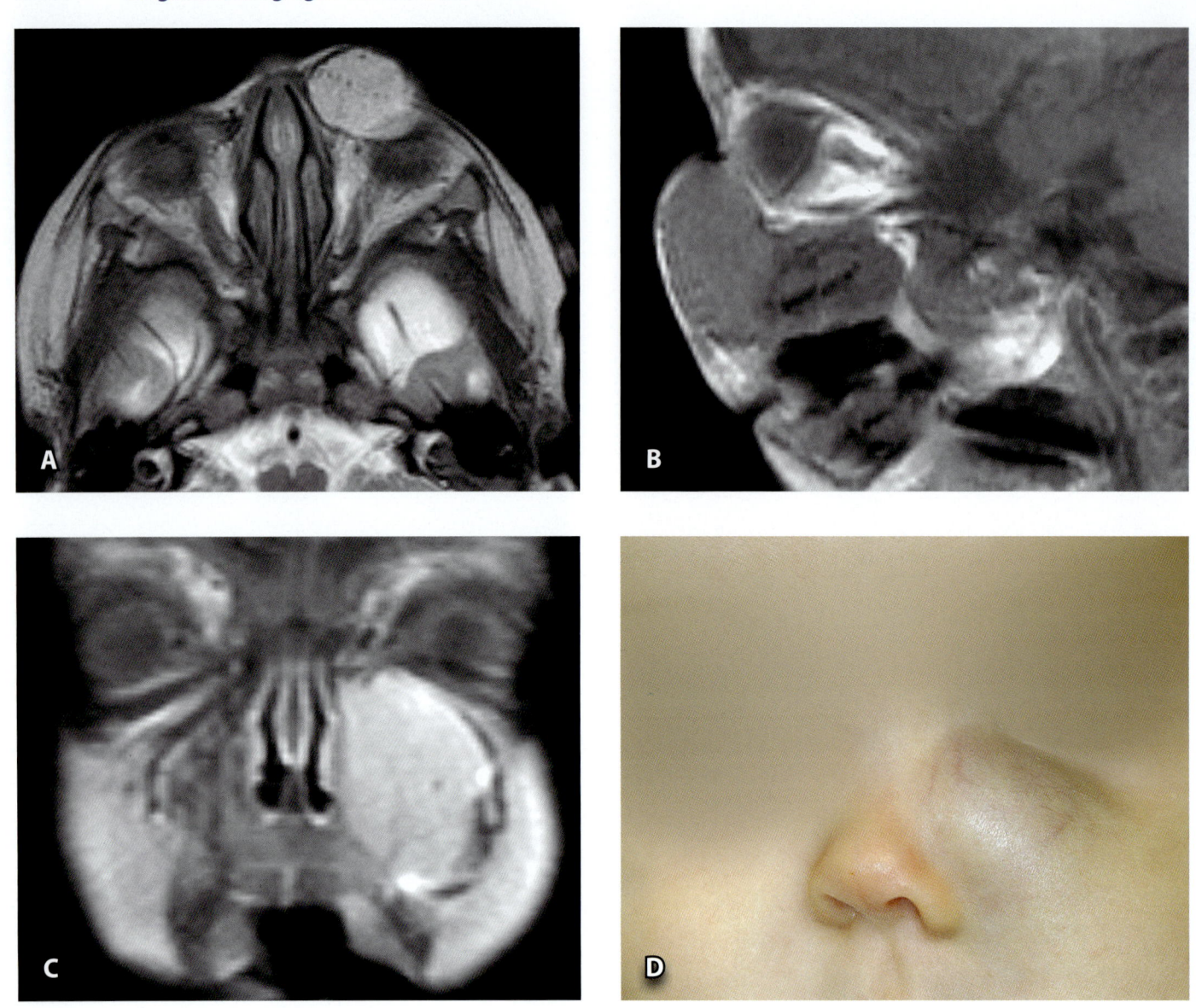

Figure 8-5 Involuting Hemangioma
(**A**) Axial T2, (**B**) sagittal T1, and (**C**) coronal T1 contrast-enhanced fat-saturated MR scans. An enhancing vascular lesion with a fine reticulated appearance is noted between the left eye and the nose within the nasolabial fold. (**D**) Photo of the lesion during the involuting phase of a hemangioma. This lesion was clinically evident soon after birth in this infant girl, expanded rapidly and then spontaneously involuted.

detected until adolescence or adulthood. Spontaneous enlargement may be induced by trauma, thrombosis, infection, or hormonal fluctuations. Cosmetic deformity and clinical difficulty are more common with vascular malformations than with hemangiomas. The low-flow vascular malformations often cause skeletal deformity, while the high-flow lesions cause destructive interosseous changes.[6] Unlike hemangiomas, these lesions show no gender predilection.

Lymphatic Malformations

Lymphatic malformations, commonly known as lymphangiomas or cystic hygromas, are low-flow anomalous lymphatic channels that result from aberrant morphogenis. These lesions comprise sequestered cystic spaces of various sizes that may be interconnected or isolated and filled with serous fluid or hyaline material,[18] and may be found on the skin or within deeper regions of the neck, axilla, mediastinum, and elsewhere. While lymphatic malformations are histologically benign, they increase in size after birth by filling with transudate and by budding from pre-existing channels.

Lymphatic malformations are often categorized according to size; however, they all share the same pathologic process and different types may be seen in the same lesion. The smaller, simple (capillary) lymphangiomas, are slightly elevated masses which are usually found subcutaneously in the head, neck, and axilla. They average 1 to 2 cm in diameter, and resemble capillary channels. At the opposite end of the spectrum, cavernous lymphangiomas (cystic hygromas), are larger lesions, which can

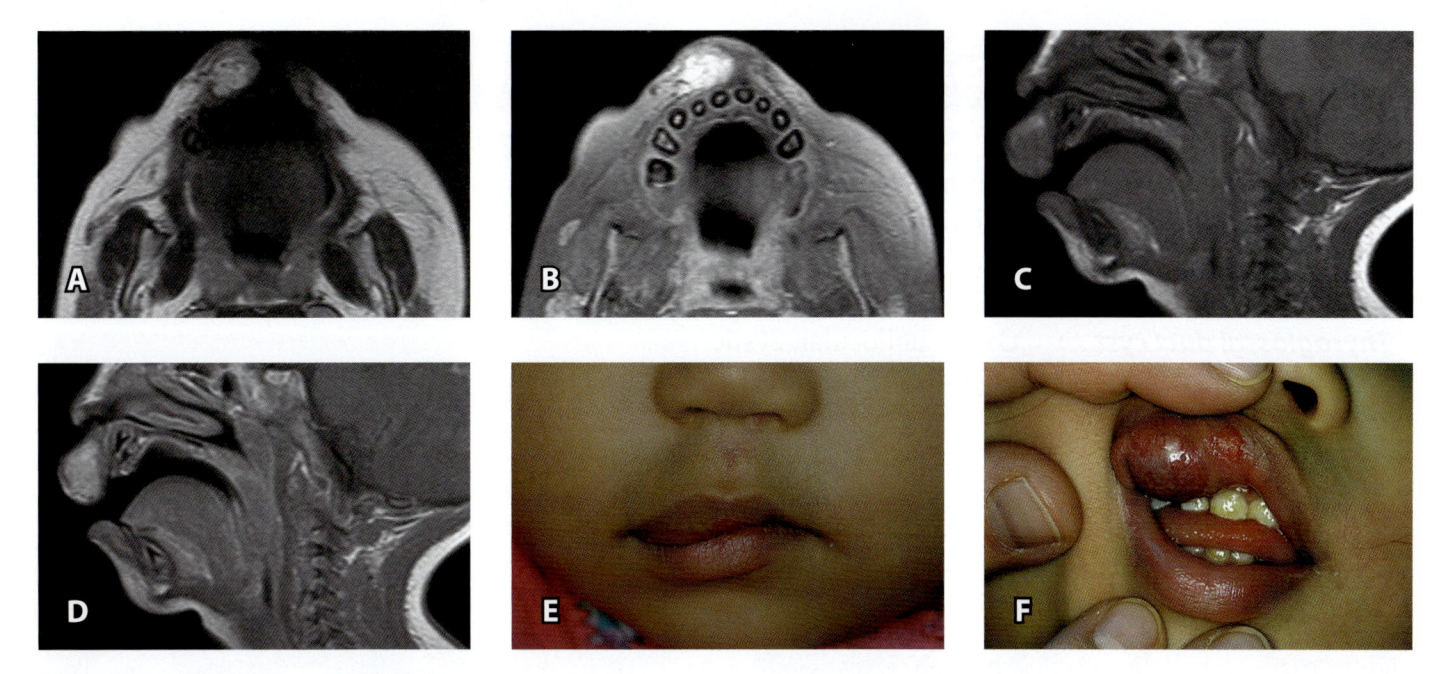

Figure 8-6 Involuting Hemangioma
T1 unenhanced (**A**) axial and (**C**) sagittal and T1 contrast-enhanced fat-saturated MR images showing an enhancing lesion with small-flow voids involving the upper right side lip. The lesion extends from the vermillion border to the underlying mucosal surface as depicted in this young child's photos (**E** and **F**).

grow up to 15 cm in diameter. The majority of these lesions occur in the neck or axilla, and commonly produce gross deformities. They are composed of massively dilated cystic spaces separated by minimal connective tissue stroma. These unencapsulated lesions have indistinct margins, making surgical removal difficult.[5] In recent years, it has been suggested that categorization of lymphatic malformations as microcystic versus macrocystic is perhaps more appropriate given the distinct morphologic, radiologic, and treatment differences between these two types of lesions.

Etiologically, it is believed that lymphatic malformations result from the failure of some lymphatic sacs to fuse with the central venous system during development, or from the obstruction of lymph flow between the developing channels and the venous system. The sequestration of the embryonic remnants in the former case my result in the smaller, peripheral lesions, while the obstruction in the later case would lead to larger, central lesions. Seventy-five percent of the larger cystic hygromas occur in the lower neck and upper mediastinum.[19] This tendency is most likely due to fusion failure in the jugular pair of lymphatic sacs. The tendency for lymphangiomas to bud and branch makes them infiltrative, and they can often involve multiple anatomic spaces.

As many as two-thirds of lymphatic malformations are noticed at birth, and approximately 90% of these lesions become obvious by the age of two.[20] Only a small percentage will be identified in young adults. These lesions can appear sporadically, with an otherwise normal lymphatic system, or as part of a syndrome, such as Turner's, Noonan's, or fetal alcohol syndrome. Most lymphatic malformations present as a slow-growing, painless, soft, compressible mass in the posterior triangle of the neck. Rapid expansion may occur with intralesional infection or hemorrhage and result in compression of structures that precipitate stridor, dyspnea, and dysphagia. Less commonly, these lesions involve the mucosal surface of the oral cavity and tongue impairing eating, and when large can compromise the airway thus necessitating emergency treatment.[20] When microcystic components infiltrate the skin and musculature, the presentation may be in the form of numerous cutaneous or mucosal vesicles.

Histologically, lymphatic malformations are composed of dilated lymphatic channels, which by their nature are thin walled. They also contain septations of variable thickness, which are characteristic of these lesions that can be seen on contrast-enhanced MR images. Pathologically, these lesions appear as smooth, nonencapsulated masses.

MR imaging is used to differentiate lymphatic malformations from other fluid-filled masses, as well as defining depth and extent of involvement (**Table 8-3**). Characteristic MR findings will reveal a mass with septations and multiple cystic spaces that extends through multiple fascial planes (**Table 8-4**). Typically, macrocystic lesions demonstrate low signal on T1-weighted images, high signal on T2-weighted images, and a lack of central enhancement following gadolinium administration (**Fig. 8-7**). However, septal or rim enhancement may be seen, particularly if the walls have been thickened by infection. Fluid–fluid levels may be seen with a recent history of sudden rapid enlargement. Findings with microcystic malformations are nonspecific and may simply appear as soft-tissue thickening.[21]

Complete surgical excision has long been touted as the choice therapeutic modality for permanent treatment of symptomatic lymphatic anomalies even though disappointing results are not unusual. Microcystic lesions can be especially challenging to resect because

346 Diagnostic Imaging of the Head and Neck

Table 8-3 Lymphatic Malformation Differential Diagnosis

DDx	Description
Second branchial cleft cyst	• Located at angle of mandible • Ovoid, unilocular • Characteristic displacement pattern
Thyroglossal duct cyst	• Located at midline near the hyoid bone • Ovoid, unilocular, cystic • Engulfed by infrahyoid strap muscles
Neck abscess	• Thick, enhancing wall surrounding fluid collection • Cellulitis, myositis and fasciitis in adjacent soft tissues

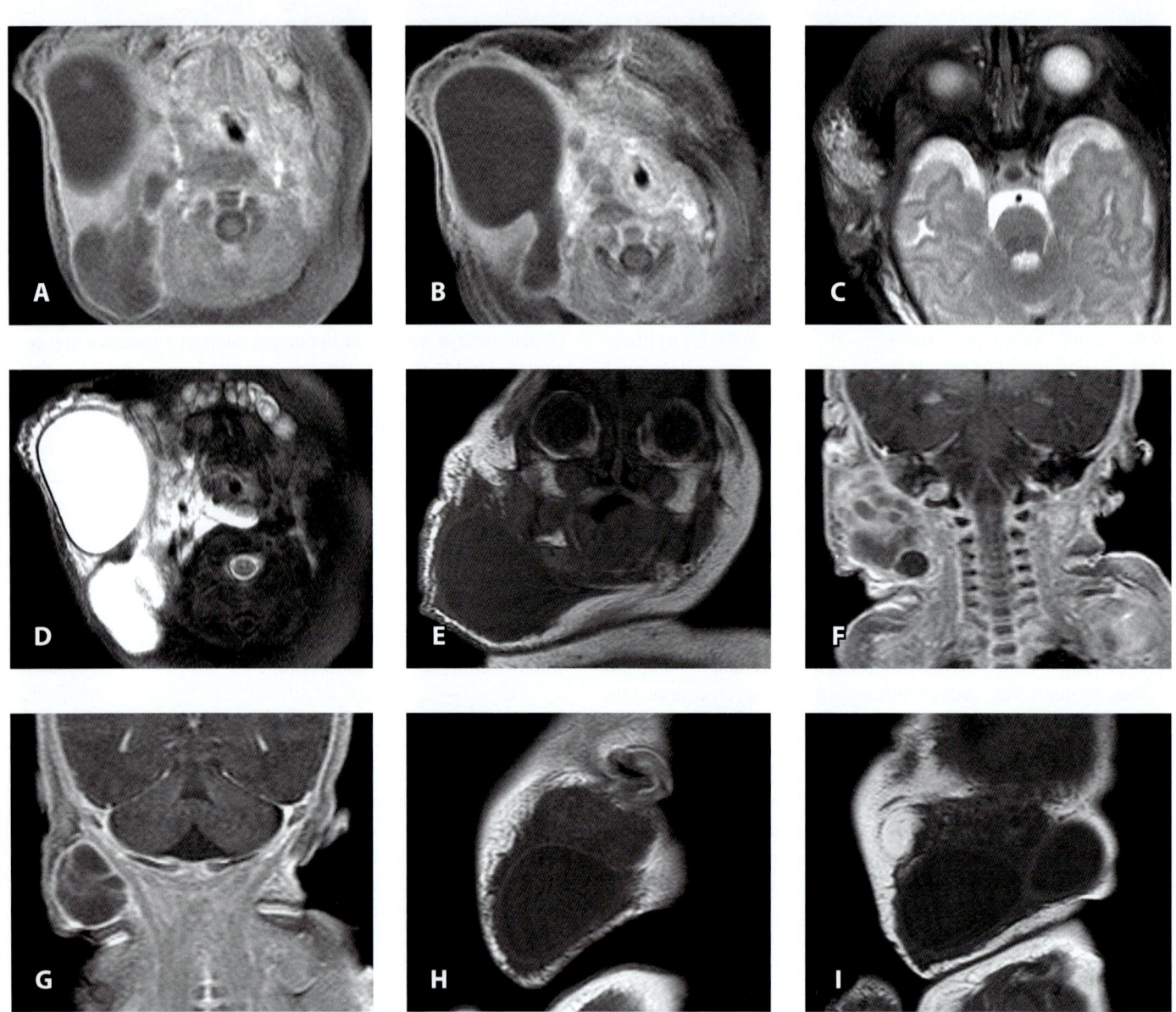

Figure 8-7 Lymphangioma
(**A, B**) Axial and (**F, G**) coronal T1 contrast-enhanced fat-saturated, (**C, D**) axial T2, and (**E**) coronal and (**H, I**) sagittal T1 MR images. There is a trans-spatial, cystic mass centered in the posterior triangle of the right neck that contains several large locules. Few delicate internal septations are noted within some of the locules and there is minimal rim enhancement.

Table 8-4 MR Imaging of Lymphatic Malformations

Description	T1W MR Findings	Postcontrast T1W MR Findings	T2W MR Findings
• Cystic • Multiloculated • Insinuating • Cross-spatial boundaries	• Low signal	• None • Possible slight enhancement of rim and/or septations, especially if infected.	• High signal • Fluid–fluid levels

they frequently infiltrate surrounding tissue and, in the neck, may encompass important neurovascular structures. Under these circumstances nerve injury is likely even with meticulous dissection. Furthermore, microscopic extension is often difficult to see during surgery making the incidence of recurrence high secondary to subtotal resection.[22] However, in those cases where infiltration can be visualized intraoperatively, or the lesion appears to be encapsulated, recurrence is less likely to occur following surgery.[18] Nevertheless, surgical extirpation with clean margins is indicated for the successful eradication of head and neck lymphatic malformations, particularly those that are microcystic in nature.

Percutaneous sclerotherapy is an important option with proven efficacy in the treatment of macrocystic lymphatic malformations, especially those that are challenging to resect due to location or insinuation around vital structures. Intralesional injection of agents like bleomycin, Ethibloc®, and ethyl alcohol have been used to sclerose cystic spaces;[22,23] however, significant local and systemic toxicities warrants extreme caution in their use. Picibanil (OK-432), a streptococcal derivative, is a sclerosing agent that has also been used very successfully in the treatment of macrocystic lymphatic malformations,[24] presumably by inducing the elaboration of pro-inflammatory cytokines and stimulating apoptosis.[20,25,26] This compound is almost universally effective in the treatment of macrocystic lesions,[25,27,28] although fair to excellent have also been achieved in microcystic malformations.[29] The efficacy of Picibanil appears to be limited to craniofacial lymphatic malformations as limited responsiveness has been seen in lesions outside the head and neck.[30] Unlike other agents that can cause marked scarring, Picibanil does not appear to hinder subsequent surgical excision.[20,31] Despite the lack of FDA approval for the management of lymphatic malformations, numerous studies in the scientific medical literature have documented a favorable safety profile for Picibanil.

Capillary Malformations

Capillary malformations, also erroneously called capillary hemangiomas, include port-wine stains and telangiectasias. These common lesions are composed of narrow, thin-walled vessels lined by a thin endothelium. At birth, these are flat cutaneous lesions, but they enlarge and thicken as the child grows. Soft-tissue hypertrophy and overgrowth of the affected area may lead to facial asymmetry.[32]

Capillary malformations are usually isolated lesions, but may be associated with other vascular malformations. The incidence of these lesions is approximately 0.3%. A small number of patients with port-wine stains have Sturge-Weber syndrome, in which a facial capillary lesion overlies an encephalo-trigeminal angiomatosis. In addition, capillary malformations are often the predominant cutaneous element in Wyburn-Mason syndrome and Cobb syndrome, which have capillary malformations overlying optic or spinal cord arteriovenous malformations, respectively.[21] MR imaging performed in patient's with capillary malformations is not directed at evaluating the lesion per se, but rather to assess syndromic abnormalities (**Fig. 8-8**).

Treatment of capillary malformations is primarily driven by the desire to improve the cosmetic appearance of patients. The treatment of choice for these lesions is photothermolysis using pulsed dye lasers with wavelengths in the range of 585 to 600 nm and pulses ranging from 0.45 to 10 ms. In cases refractory to pulsed dye laser, the uses of deeper penetrating lasers such Nd-YAG (1064 nm) or KTP (532 nm) may be used, albeit with a greater likelihood of adverse effects.[33] The clinical endpoint during treatment is to achieve a light purpura within minutes after treatment.

Venous Malformations

Venous malformations are the second most common vascular anomaly of the head and neck region. These lesions have historically been referred to as cavernous hemangiomas, varicose hemangiomas, or lymphangiohemangiomas. They may either consist of spongy masses of sinusoidal space with variable communications with adjacent veins, or they may be composed of varicosities or dysplasias of venous channels.

Like all vascular malformations, venous lesions are present at birth, and grow in a linear fashion with the child, tending to become nodular and thickened with age. They have a variable clinical presentation, depending upon the depth and extent of the lesion. These malformations may occur anywhere in the body, but are most common in the head and neck region which account for 40% of lesions.[34,35] Although most typically found on the lips, tongue (**Fig. 8-9**), buccal fat space (**Fig. 8-10**), and buccal mucosa, venous malformations may also present intramuscularly, periorbitally (**Figs. 8-11** and **8-12**), or in the parapharyngeal spaces.[36] They are typically soft, compressible masses, which may contain palpable phleboliths. The skin overlying the

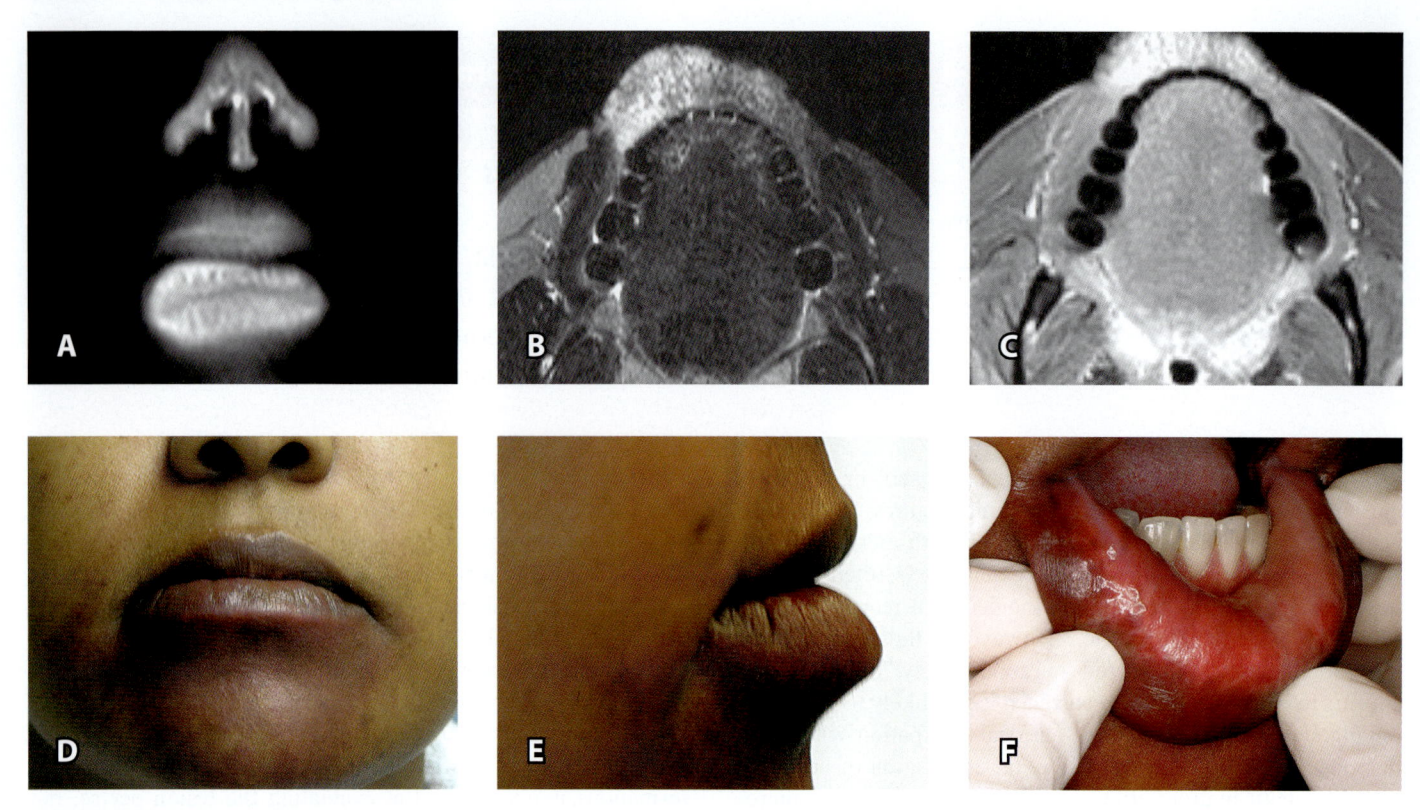

Figure 8-8 Port-wine Stain
(**A**) Coronal and (**B**) axial T2, and (**C**) axial T1 contrast-enhanced fat-saturated MR scans. There is a finely reticulated lesion expanding the right lower lip without flow voids, or calcifications, but with intense enhancement of the skin and underlying soft tissues. (**D–F**) Photographs of the lower lip and chin lesion in this adult woman. Over time, this lesion did not enlarge nor involute; however, it became thicker and more deforming of the lower lip. Earlier, the patient was able to hide the lesion with make-up, but ultimately laser treatment was a viable option.

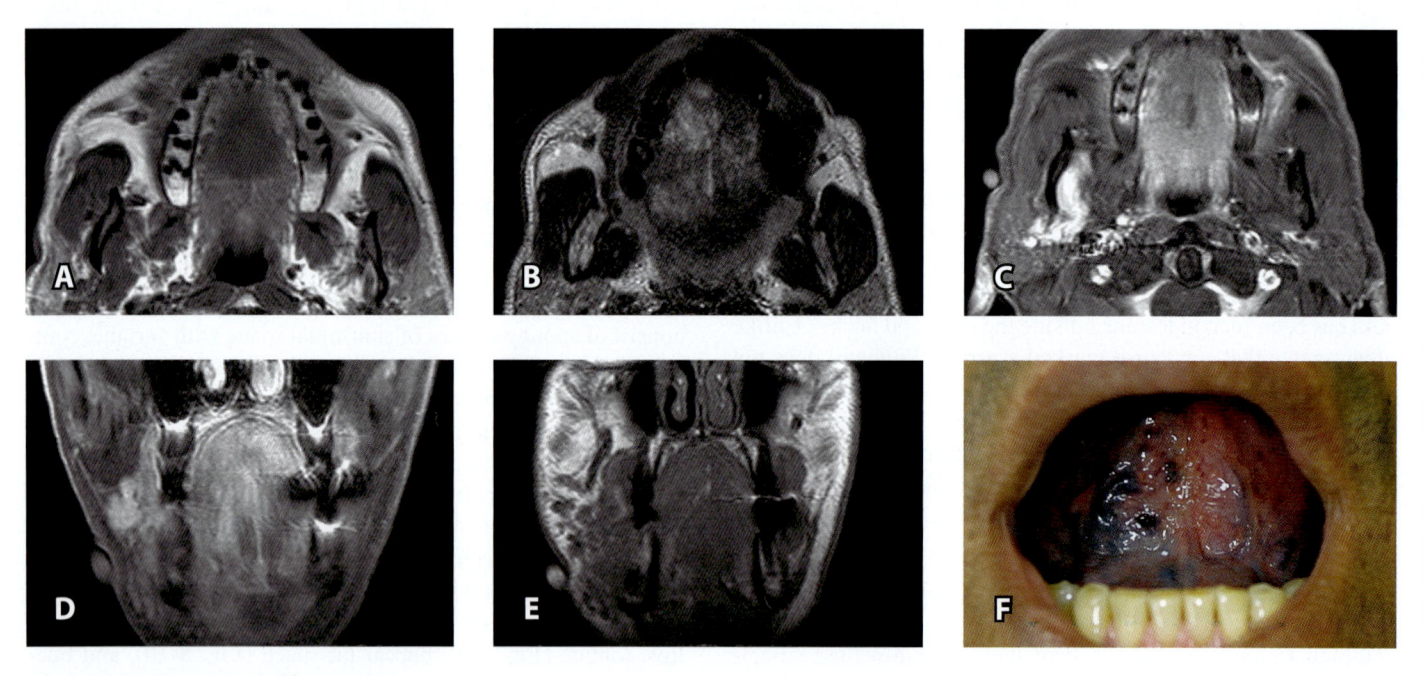

Figure 8-9 Venous Malformation
(**A**) Axial and (**E**) coronal T1, (**B**) axial T2, and (**C**) axial, and (**D**) coronal T1 contrast-enhanced fat-saturated MR images. There is an ill-defined enhancing lesion in the oral tongue that crosses fascial planes and extends into the right buccal space. No flow voids were identified. (**F**) Photo of the tongue shows a violaceous lesion along the undersurface mucosa.

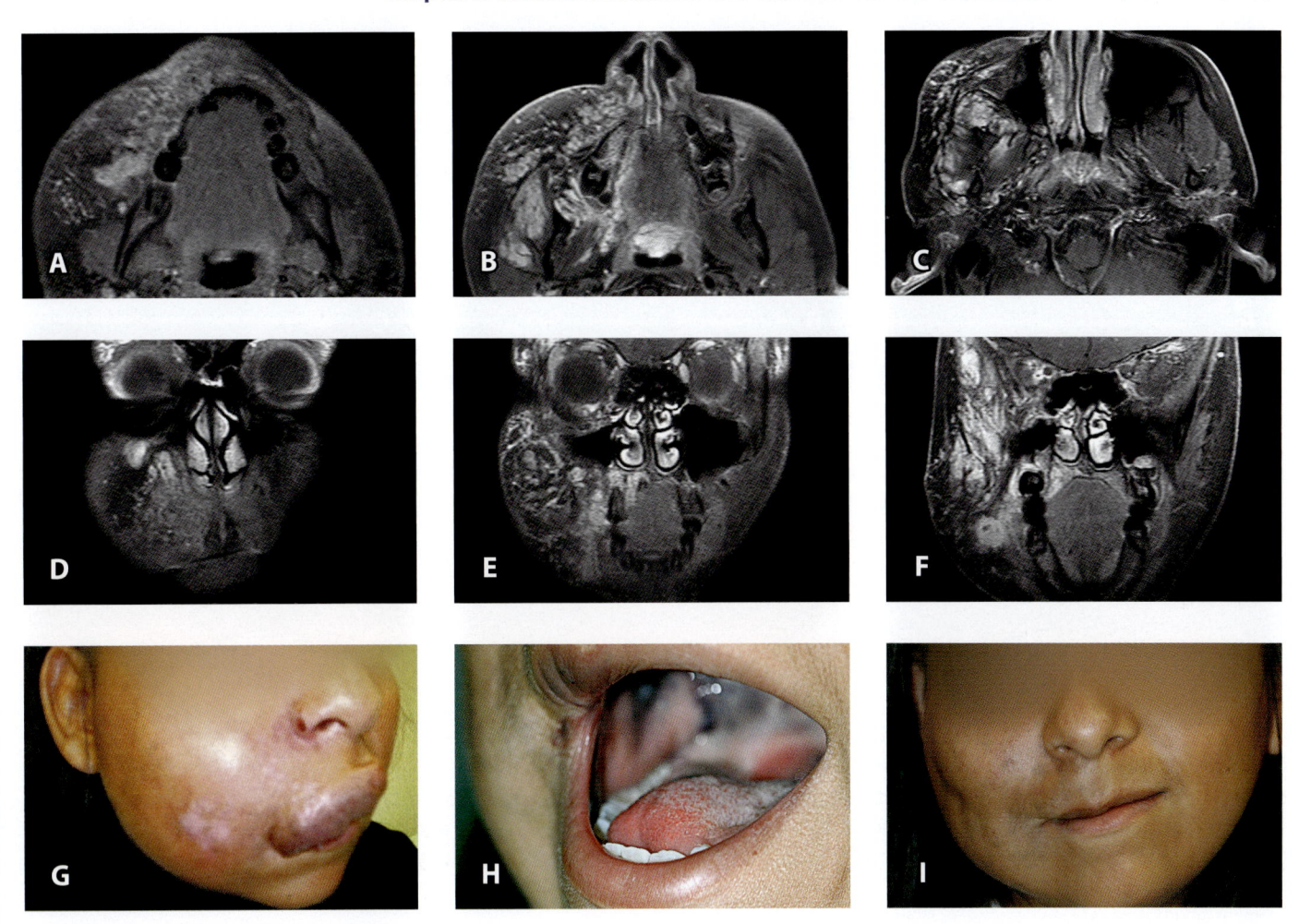

Figure 8-10 Venous Malformation
(**A–C**) Axial and (**D–F**) coronal T1 contrast-enhanced fat-saturated MR images reveal a poorly defined enhancing mass in the right cheek that extends to the right nasolabial fold and significantly involves the right upper lip in this young girl. No significant flow voids in this trans-spatial lesion was consistent with a low-flow venous malformation. (**G, H**) Photos of the face and tongue of this patient reveal marked facial deformity with purplish discoloration of the overlying skin and buccal mucosa. (**I**) Photograph of the patient posttreatment shows normal skin coloration and significantly improved cosmesis.

lesion appears blue or purple in color, and be cool to touch. Pulsations, bruits, or thrills should not be present. These venous lesions may become more pronounced with increased physical activity and during a Valsalva maneuver, and may abruptly enlarge after hemorrhage (**Fig. 8-12**). Deep venous malformations may present with pain, and those located in the parapharyngeal or retropharyngeal spaces may cause speech or airway complications.

MRI will reveal collections of serpentine structures separated by septations, with intermediate signal intensity on T1-weighted images and high signal intensity on T2-weighted images. Gadolinium administration will almost universally demonstrate diffuse enhancement throughout the lesion. Phleboliths are commonly present within venous malformations and are seen as round low signal intensity structures on MRI.[10] Venous malformations often involve more than one anatomic space, and may extend deeply through multiple tissue planes, including cutaneous tissue, muscle, and bone. Intraosseous involvement, however, is not a typical feature.[37] Unfortunately, imaging features such as location and morphology of the lesion fail to predict successful treatment outcomes.[38]

The preferred therapy for venous malformations is sclerotherapy or surgical excision, although laser treatments are becoming more effective and more widely used. These lesions resemble hemangiomas, and occasionally this results in improper treatment with radiotherapy. Various treatment options are currently recommended for head and neck venous malformations depending on depth, location, and extent. Laser therapy is increasingly being used for management of small, uncomplicated venous malformations. Pulsed dye, KTP,[39] and Nd:YAG laser therapy[40] can be used to photocoagulate small superficial cutaneous lesions with good results. Interstitial Nd:YAG or KTP laser therapy under image guidance is

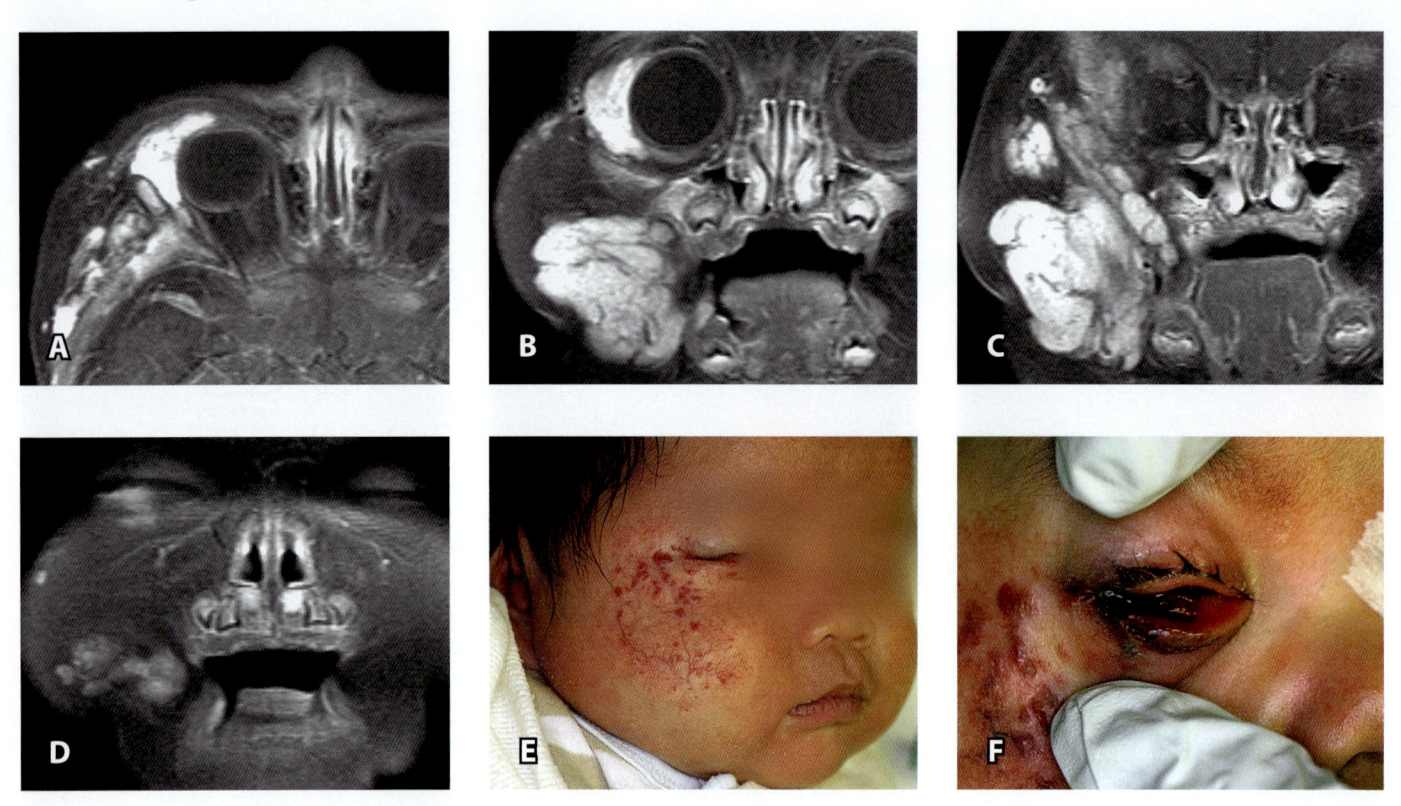

Figure 8-11 Venous Malformation
(**A**) Axial and (**B–D**) coronal T1 contrast-enhanced fat-saturated MR scans show an intensely enhancing trans-spatial mass centered in the right cheek, with extension into the right sphenotemporal buttress, and anterolateral orbit. No flow voids were seen. (**E, F**) Photos of the right face of this infant show crimson discoloration of the overlying skin with purple discoloration along the lateral canthus of the orbit.

preferred for deep cutaneous or subcutaneous lesions, or mixed lesions with a deep component.[41] Multiple treatments with imaging at follow-up are recommended to ensure the entire lesion is effectively treated otherwise to minimize the risk of recurrence.

Percutaneous, image-guided intralesional injection of a sclerosing agent alone or in combination with surgical excision is the preferred treatment for venous malformation that are extensive, deforming, or present with complications. Although a number of sclerosing substances are available for treatment of head and neck venous malformations, their selection depends on the size and site of the lesion.[42] Pure ethanol is a highly destructive agent that can cause significant complications, including tissue necrosis, ulceration, neurolysis, and pain, and should be used only in lesions not encompassing major nerves. When venous malformations are in close proximity to important nerves or in delicate cutaneous areas, especially in the vermillion, less toxic agents such as Sotradecol (sodium tetradecyl sulfate) or Polidocanol should be considered.[42,43] If the lesion is large, disfiguring, or compromises vital functioning surgical excision may follow sclerotherapy. Surgical resection alone is typically limited to treatment of intramuscular lesions confined to expendable muscles or muscle groups.[44]

Arteriovenous Malformations

Arteriovenous malformations (AVM) are rare vascular anomalies in which arteries and veins are connected without intervening arteriolar resistance vessels or capillary beds. This direct connection between the arterial and venous systems consists of a network of small vascular channels with feeding arteries and draining veins. AVMs are rarely discrete, but instead appear as field defects, involving multiple tissue types and anatomical spaces. In contrast, congenital arteriovenous fistulas are localized lesions that are often supplied by branches of the superficial temporal, vertebral, or subclavian artery.[45]

AVMs do not usually appear at birth, and may remain asymptomatic for many years. Like other vascular malformations, AVMs grow proportionally during childhood. However, they have been observed to expand rapidly after local trauma, infection, attempted excision, or hormonal changes such as puberty or pregnancy. These lesions enlarge by forming collateral vessels and recruiting adjacent normal vessels by connecting across low-resistance arteriovenous channels.[46] Although quite rare, extracranial arteriovenous malformations are most commonly found in the head and neck. Cervicofacial AVMs are most commonly seen in the cheek and ear (**Fig. 8-13**), while intraosseous AVMs often involve the mandible and maxilla.[45] The clinical examination reveals a warm, pulsatile,

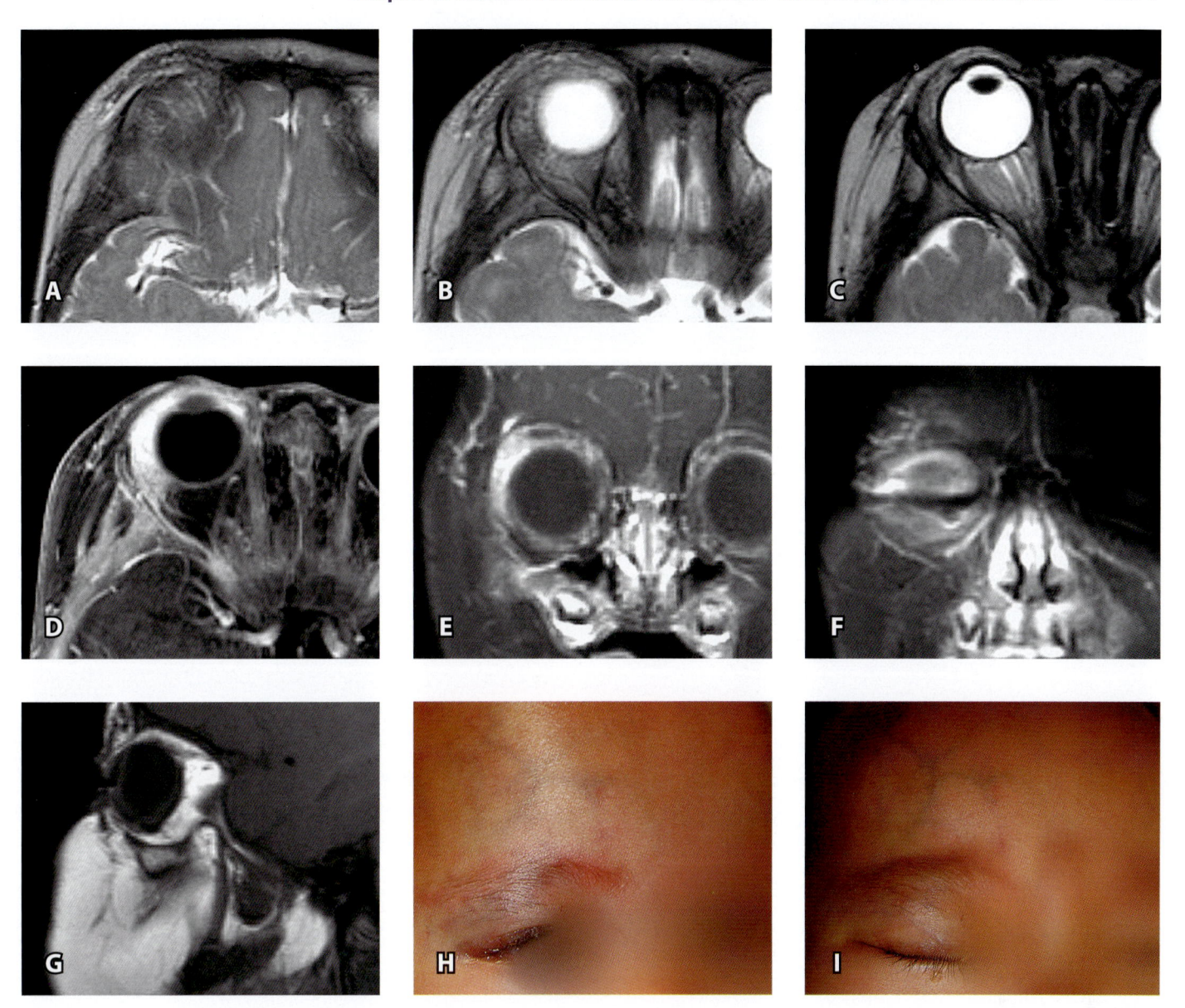

Figure 8-12 Venous Malformation of the Orbit
(**A–C**) Axial T2, and (**D**) axial, (**E, F**) coronal, and (**G**) sagittal T1 contrast-enhanced fat-saturated MR images demonstrate a right pre- and postseptal enhancing lesion in the right orbit without flow voids. (**H, I**) Photos of the right forehead show faint bluish skin discoloration. This perceived "bruise" had been present since birth and had remained stable in size, apart from intensifying during bouts of crying.

bluish mass with a palpable thrill and bruit secondary to the increase in blood flow. Patients may present with pain, bleeding and ulcerations, or even with a rapidly enlarging, disfiguring mass.

MR imaging of arteriovenous malformations yields information that differentiates them from other vascular anomalies, defines the extent of the disease, and demonstrates the high-flow characteristic of the lesion. MRI may reveal a heterogenous lesion with soft-tissue thickening that lacks a parenchymatous component. This feature distinguishes arteriovenous malformations from proliferating hemangiomas. Arteriovenous malformations display diffuse gadolinium enhancement, and serpentine flow voids will be evident on T1- and T2-weighted images. Bony involvement may be suspected if marrow signal intensity is decreased on T1-weighted images.[37] Confirmation, as well as mapping of the lesion, by digital subtraction angiography is invariably performed in anticipation of treatment. Angiography will typically demonstrate dilated tortuous arteries and veins, absence of parenchymal staining with contrast, and arteriovenous shunting.

AVMs are unpredictable lesions which are dangerous and very difficult to treat. Unlike other vascular malformations, irradiation, steroids, and laser therapy have not been effective and

352 Diagnostic Imaging of the Head and Neck

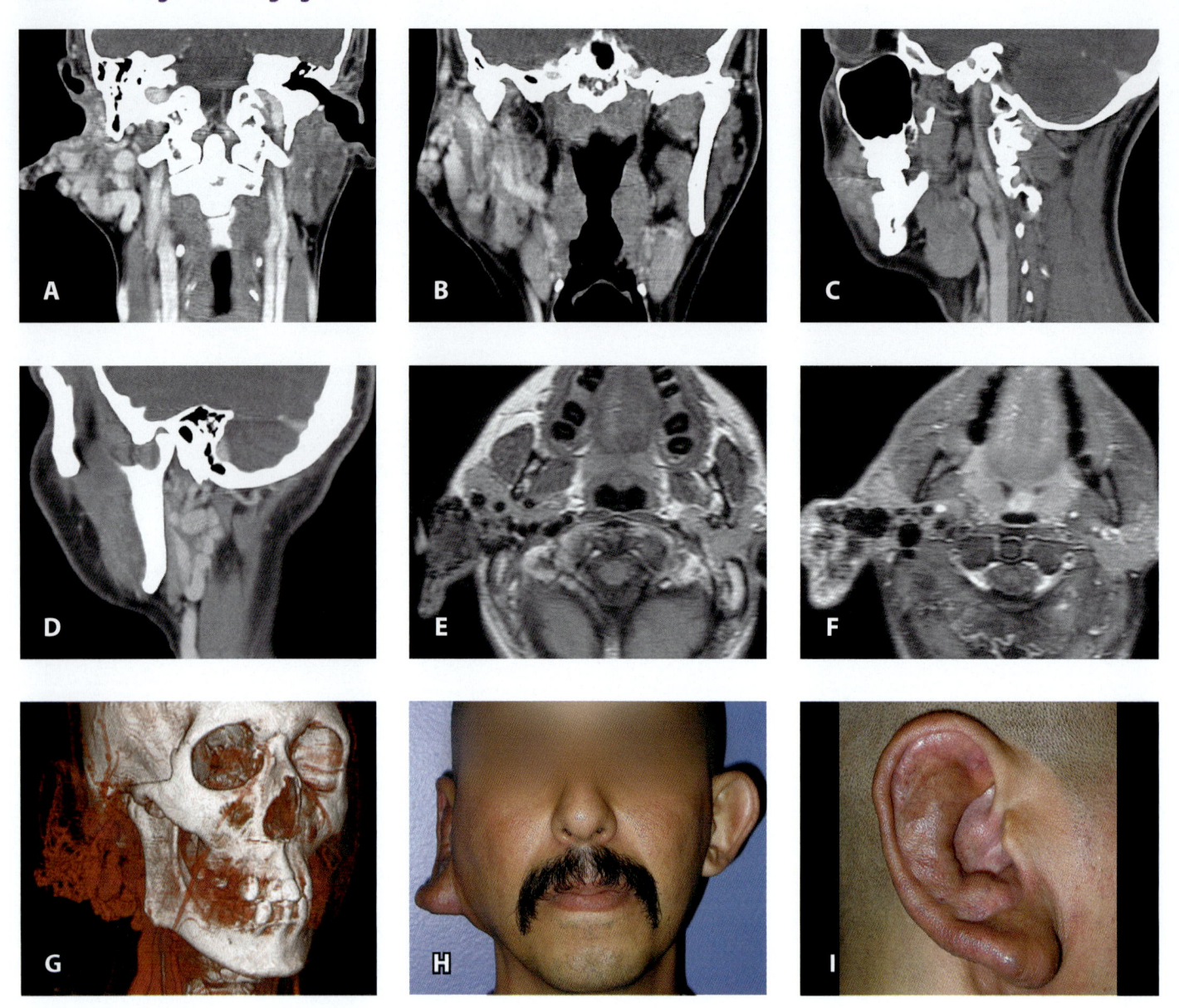

Figure 8-13 AV Fistula of the Maxillary Artery
Selected reformatted coronal (**A, B**) and sagittal (**C, D**) images from a CT angiogram. (**E**) Axial T1 unenhanced and (**F**) axial T1 contrast-enhanced fat-saturated MR images. (**G**) Color-coded reformatted 3D CT angiogram with surface rendering. Multiple large flow voids are noted within the right parotid gland and external ear. The vascular structures extend laterally from the region of the second portion of the maxillary artery, lying within the deep lobe of the parotid gland. There is rapid shunting of blood from arteries to veins as depicted in (**G**) consistent with an AV fistula. Photos of the patient who had sustained trauma to the right face, showing the discoloration and marked swelling of the pinna and adjacent parotid gland. Clinical palpation demonstrated a thrill and auscultation demonstrated a loud bruit.

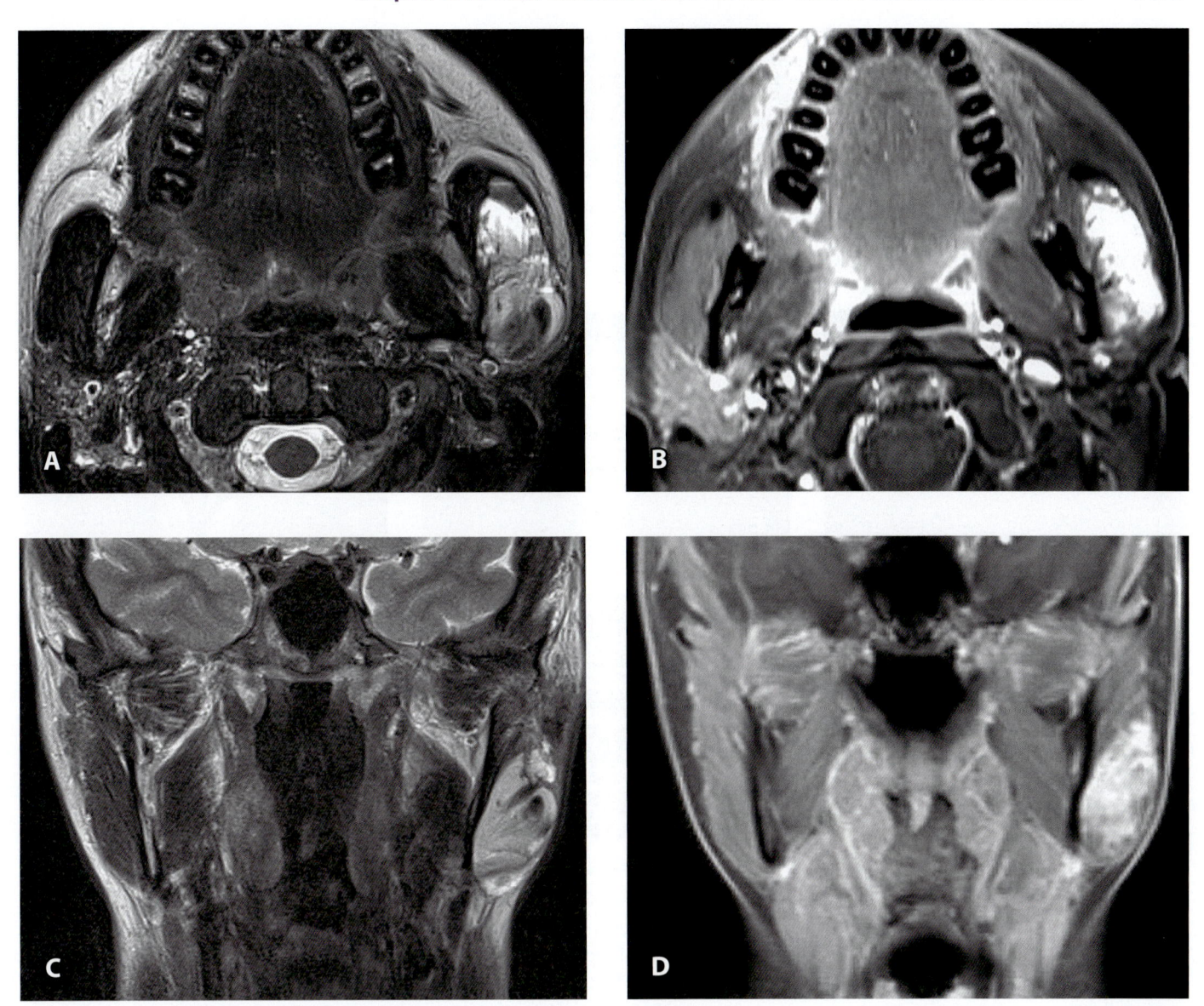

Figure 8-14 Venolymphatic Malformation of the Masticator Space
(**A**) Axial and (**B**) coronal T2, and (**C**) axial and (**D**) coronal T1 contrast-enhanced fat-saturated MR images. A heterogeneous, mixed intensity lesion is located within the left masseter muscle. The vascular channels are nonserpentine, primarily linear, with an occasional phlebolith (*arrow*, **C**). Only a portion of the lesion within the masseter muscle shows enhancement surrounding the phlebolith.

thus have no place in the management of arteriovenous malformations. Consequently, therapeutic management options are limited to aggressive embolotheraphy with or without complete surgical resection in order to achieve cure.

Combined Malformations

Arteries, veins, and lymphatics may all be involved in developmental vascular anomalies. Combined malformations may involve any number and type of vascular channel. They may or may not involve bone and soft tissues. Cutaneous capillary malformations are most often associated with deep AVMs, venous malformations, lymphatic malformations, or combined malformations (**Figs. 8-14** and **8-15**).[21] These lesions are often present in syndromes, such as Sturge-Weber syndrome. Sturge-Weber syndrome involves capillary malformations in the distribution of the trigeminal nerve, ocular and cerebrovascular anomalies, and facial overgrowth. Parkes-Weber syndrome is another example, consisting of a combined capillary-lymphatic-venous malformation.

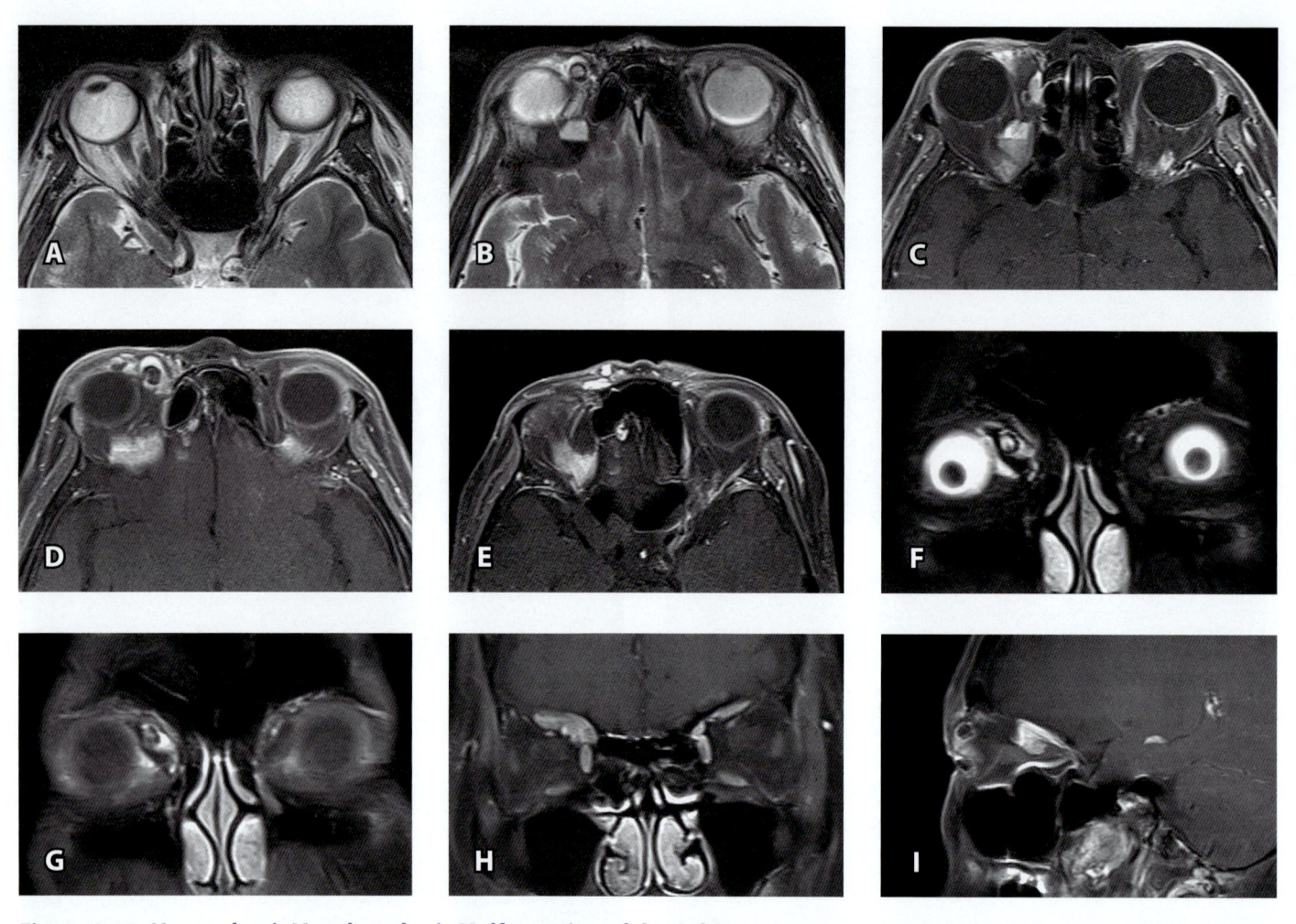

Figure 8-15 Hemorrhagic Venolymphatic Malformation of the Orbit
(**A, B**) Axial T2, (**C–E**) axial T1 contrast-enhanced fat-saturated, (**F, G**) coronal T2, (**H**) coronal and (**I**) sagittal T1 contrast-enhanced fat-saturated MR images. There is a complex partially enhancing intra- and extraconal lesion in the right orbit with fluid–fluid levels (*arrows*, **B, C**). Note that the lighter superior supernatant fluid has MR characteristics of serum, while the heavier infranatant fluid has MR characteristics of hematocrit in this supine patient, consistent with acute hemorrhage.

REFERENCES

1. Mulliken J: Classification of vascular birthmarks, in vascular birthmarks: hemangiomas and malformations, Mulliken J and Young A, eds. Philadelphia: W.B. Saunders Company; 1988:24–38.
2. Wegner G: Uber lymphangiome. Arch Klin Chir 1877;20:641.
3. Mulliken JB and Glowacki J: Hemangiomas and vascular malformations in infants and children: a classification based on endothelial characteristics. Plast Reconstr Surg 1982;69(3):412–422.
4. Mulliken J: Pathogenesis of hemangiomas, in vascular birthmarks: hemangiomas and malformations, Mulliken J, and Young A, eds. Philadelphia: W.B. Saunders Company; 1988:63–76.
5. Schoen F and Cotran R: Blood Vessels, in robbins pathologic basis of disease, Cotran RS, et al., eds.: Philadelphia: Saunders; 1999:493–542.
6. Mulliken J: The classification of vascular birthmarks, in management and treatment of benign cutaneous vascular lesions. Tan O, ed. Philadelphia: Lea & Febiger;1992:1–23.
7. Bauer P and Lusk R: Neck masses, in pediatric otolaryngology. Bluestone CD, ed. Philadelphia: Saunders;2003:1629–1647.
8. Metry DW and Hebert AA: Benign cutaneous vascular tumors of infancy: when to worry, what to do. Arch Dermatol 2000;136(7):905–914.
9. Achauer BM, Celikoz B, and VanderKam VM: Intralesional bare fiber laser treatment of hemangioma of infancy. Plast Reconstr Surg 1998:101(5); 1212–1217.
10. Hubbell RN and Ihm PS: Current surgical management of vascular anomalies. Curr Opin Otolaryngol Head Neck Surg 2000;8(6): 441–447.
11. Edgerton MT: The treatment of hemangiomas: with special reference to the role of steroid therapy. Ann Surg 1976;183(5):517–532.
12. Sasaki GH, Pang CY, and Wittliff JL: Pathogenesis and treatment of infant skin strawberry hemangiomas: clinical and in vitro studies of hormonal effects. Plast Reconstr Surg 1984;73(3):359–370.
13. Zarem HA and Edgerton MT: Induced resolution of cavernous hemangiomas following prednisolone therapy. Plast Reconstr Surg 1967;39(1):76–83.
14. Folkman J, Langer R, Linhardt RJ, et al.: Angiogenesis inhibition and tumor regression caused by heparin or a heparin fragment in the presence of cortisone. Science 1983;221(4612):719–725.
15. Kushner BJ: Intralesional corticosteroid injection for infantile adnexal hemangioma. Am J Ophthalmol 1982;93(4):496–506.
16. Ohlms LA, Jones DT, McGill TJ, et al.: Interferon alfa-2a therapy for airway hemangiomas. Ann Otol Rhinol Laryngol 1994;103(1):1–8.
17. Garza G, Fay A, and Rubin PA: Treatment of pediatric vascular lesions of the eyelid and orbit. Int Ophthalmol Clin 2001;41(4):43–55.

18. Fliegelman LJ, Friedland D, Brandwein M, et al.: Lymphatic malformation: predictive factors for recurrence. Otolaryngol Head Neck Surg 2000;123(6):706–710.
19. Zadvinskis DP, Benson MT, Kerr HH, et al.: Congenital malformations of the cervicothoracic lymphatic system: embryology and pathogenesis. Radiographics 1992;12(6):1175–1189.
20. Rowley H, Perez-Atayde AR, Burrows PE, et al.: Management of a giant lymphatic malformation of the tongue. Arch Otolaryngol Head Neck Surg 2002;128(2):190–194.
21. Burrows PE, Laor T, Paltiel H, et al.: Diagnostic imaging in the evaluation of vascular birthmarks. Dermatol Clin 1998;16(3):455–488.
22. Dubois J, Garel L, Abela A, et al.: Lymphangiomas in children: percutaneous sclerotherapy with an alcoholic solution of zein. Radiology 1997;204(3):651–654.
23. Sung MW, Chang SO, Choi JH, et al.: Bleomycin sclerotherapy in patients with congenital lymphatic malformation in the head and neck. Am J Otolaryngol 1995;16(4):236–241.
24. Karmody C: Developmental anomalies of the neck, in Pediatric Otolaryngology, Bluestone CD, ed. Philadelphia: Saunders;2003:1648–1663.
25. Ogita S, Tsuto T, Nakamura K, et al.: OK-432 therapy for lymphangioma in children: why and how does it work? J Pediatr Surg 1996;31(4):477–480.
26. Sung MW, Lee DW, Kim DY, et al.: Sclerotherapy with picibanil (OK-432) for congenital lymphatic malformation in the head and neck. Laryngoscope 2001;111(8):1430–1433.
27. Banieghbal B and Davies MR: Guidelines for the successful treatment of lymphangioma with OK-432. Eur J Pediatr Surg 2003;13(2):103–107.
28. Giguere CM, Bauman NM, Sato Y, et al.: Treatment of lymphangiomas with OK-432 (Picibanil) sclerotherapy: a prospective multi-institutional trial. Arch Otolaryngol Head Neck Surg 2002;128(10):1137–1144.
29. Claesson G and Kuylenstierna R: OK-432 therapy for lymphatic malformation in 32 patients (28 children). Int J Pediatr Otorhinolaryngol 2002;65(1):1–6.
30. Hall N, Ade-Ajayi N, Brewis C, et al.: Is intralesional injection of OK-432 effective in the treatment of lymphangioma in children? Surgery 2003;133(3):238–242.
31. Greinwald JH, Burke DK, Bonthius DJ, et al.: An update on the treatment of hemangiomas in children with interferon alfa-2a. Arch Otolaryngol Head Neck Surg 1999;125(1):21–27.
32. Morelli J and Weston W: Pulsed dye laser treatment of port-wine stains in children, in Management and treatment of benign cutaneous Vascular Lesions, Tan O, ed. Philadelphia: Lea & Febiger;1992:100–106.
33. Wall TL: Current concepts: laser treatment of adult vascular lesions. Semin Plast Surg 2007;21(3):147–158.
34. Dubois J and Garel L: Imaging and therapeutic approach of hemangiomas and vascular malformations in the pediatric age group. Pediatr Radiol 1999;29(12):879–893.
35. Very M, Nagy M, Carr M, et al.: Hemangiomas and vascular malformations: analysis of diagnostic accuracy. Laryngoscope 2002;112(4):612–615.
36. Enjolras O and Mulliken JB: The current management of vascular birthmarks. Pediatr Dermatol 1993;10(4):311–313.
37. Baker LL, Dillon WP, Hieshima GB, et al.: Hemangiomas and vascular malformations of the head and neck: MR characterization. Am J Neuroradiol 1993;14(2):307–314.
38. Berenguer B, Burrows PE, Zurakowski D, et al.: Sclerotherapy of craniofacial venous malformations: complications and results. Plast Reconstr Surg 1999;104(1):1–11; discussion 12–15.
39. Low DW: Management of adult facial vascular anomalies. Facial Plast Surg 2003;19(1):113–130.
40. Hochman M, Emre V, James S, et al.: Contemporary management of vascular lesions of the head and neck. Curr Opin Otolaryngol Head Neck Surg 1999;(7):161–166.
41. Werner JA, Lippert BM, Gottschlich, et al.: Ultrasound-guided interstitial Nd: YAG laser treatment of voluminous hemangiomas and vascular malformations in 92 patients. Laryngoscope 1998;108(4 Pt 1):463–470.
42. Gelbert F, Enjolras O, Deffrenne D, et al.: Percutaneous sclerotherapy for venous malformation of the lips: a retrospective study of 23 patients. Neuroradiology 2000;42(9):692–696.
43. Lewin JS, Merkle EM, Duerk JL, et al.: Low-flow vascular malformations in the head and neck: safety and feasibility of MR imaging-guided percutaneous sclerotherapy—preliminary experience with 14 procedures in three patients. Radiology 1999;211(2):566–570.
44. Hein KD, Mulliken JB, Kozakewich HP, et al.: Venous malformations of skeletal muscle. Plast Reconstr Surg 2002;110(7):1625–1635.
45. Robertson RL, Robson CD, Barnes PD, et al.: Head and neck vascular anomalies of childhood. Neuroimaging Clin N Am 1999;9(1):115–132.
46. Kohout MP, Hansen M, Pribaz JJ, et al.: Arteriovenous malformations of the head and neck: Natural history and management. Plast Reconstr Surg 1998;102(3):643–654.

The Cranial Nerves

Christopher R. Trimble, MD, MBA
Anton N. Hasso, MD, FACR

CRANIAL NERVE EMBRYOLOGY

Each of the 12 cranial nerves is present by the fourth week of development and consists of either a motor nucleus, a sensory ganglion, or both motor and sensory components. Similar to the organization of the spinal nerves, motor nuclei are contained within the brainstem and sensory ganglia are located peripherally.

Sensory ganglia originate from a combination of both ectodermal neuroepithelial swellings on the exterior surface of the embryo and also from neural crest cells.[1] Surface placodes induce the formation of sensory ganglia of CN I (nasal placode), CN II (lens placode), and CN XIII (otic placode). Additionally, four epibranchial placodes are located dorsal to pharyngeal arches and give rise to sensory ganglia for the nerves of the pharyngeal arches (CN V, VII, IX, and X). Neural crest cells also give rise to parasympathetic visceral efferent ganglia, whose fibers traverse along the course of CN III, VII, IX and X.[2] Finally, the motor nuclei of cranial nerves IV, V, VI, VII, IX, X, XI, and XII arise from eight segmental neuroepithelial proliferations of the neural tube known as rhombomeres.

Pharyngeal Arches

CN V, VII, IX, and X have embryologic origins as nerves of pharyngeal arches. The six segmental tissue proliferations that constitute the pharyngeal arches are discernable by gestational week 3 as rounded ridges on the sides of the head and will eventually form the face, nasal cavities, mouth, larynx, pharynx, and neck. Each arch consists of three histologic components, including 1) ectoderm lining the arches exteriorly, 2) endoderm bordering the primordial gut interiorly, and 3) a mesenchyme layer that is located between the endoderm and ectoderm.

Mesoderm proliferation in the mesenchyme layer forms the distinct body of each arch and is composed of a combination of both native arch mesenchyme, contributing to the muscular components, and neural crest cell migration, which contribute to the cartilaginous components of each arch. In addition to having discrete cartilaginous and muscle structures, each pharyngeal arch also develops a unique vascular (aortic arch) and a unique nervous (cranial nerve) supply. Of all the pharyngeal arches, arch 1 has two distinct mesenchyme swellings which form the maxillary and the mandibular prominences derive. Pharyngeal arch 5 forms incompletely and thus does not contribute significantly to anatomic development.[2] The structures of the pharyngeal arches are summarized in **Table 9-1**.

Pharyngeal Pouches, Grooves, and Membranes

Spatial relationships between each arch also create three distinct functional embryologic structures known as pharyngeal pouches, grooves, and membranes. Between each arch, pharyngeal grooves are formed by ectodermal depressions exteriorly and pharyngeal pouches are formed by endodermal indentations interiorly. Pharyngeal membranes are formed by the areas of thinly apposed ectoderm and endoderm between the pharyngeal pouches and grooves.

Of the pharyngeal grooves, only the first persists as the external auditory meatus. Other pharyngeal grooves contribute to the cervical sinuses, but are normally later overgrown by neck tissues. The first pharyngeal membrane is the only one to persist and forms the tympanic membrane. Pharyngeal pouches are responsible for the formation of several essential anatomic entities which are summarized in **Table 9-2**.

Pharyngeal Arch Abnormalities

Neural crest cells are essential to the structural formation of the pharyngeal arches. Any interference with their migration or function is liable to produce severe and disfiguring malformation of the arches and their structures. Abnormalities in pharyngeal arch development include Treacher Collins syndrome, Robin sequence, DiGeorge anomaly, and hemifacial microsomia. Neural crest cell abnormalities are generally inherited, though are also particularly affected by environmental teratogens, including retinoic acids and alcohol. Because neural crest cells also play a key role in endocardial cushion and aorticopulmonary vascular development, individuals with pharyngeal arch

Table 9-1 Pharyngeal Arch Contents

Pharyngeal Arch	Nerve Supply	Muscles	Vascular Supply	Cartilage & Bone
Arch 1 "Mandibular"	CN V, V2, V3	• Muscles of mastication • Mylohyoid • Anterior belly of digastric • Tensor palatine • Tensor tympani	• Maxillary artery	• Meckel cartilage • Malleus • Anterior ligament of malleus • Incus • Sphenomandibular ligament
Arch 2 "Hyoid"	CN VII	• Stapedius • Stylohyoid • Posterior belly of the digastric • Auricular • Muscles of facial expression	• Stapedial artery	• Reichert's cartilage • Lesser horn of hyoid • Upper part of hyoid body
Arch 3	CN IX	• Stylopharyngeus	• Common & internal carotid arteries	• Greater horn of hyoid • Lower part of hyoid body

Arch 4	CN X – superior laryngeal branch	• Cricothyroid
		• Levator palatini
		• Pharyngeal constrictors
			• Parts of aortic arch and right subclavian	• Laryngeal cartilage
				  • Thyroid
				  • Cricoid
				  • Arytenoid
				  • Corniculate
				  • Cuneiform

Arch 6	CN X – recurrent laryngeal branch	• Intrinsic laryngeal muscles	• Proximal pulmonary arteries	

Table 9-2 Pharyngeal Pouch Structures

Pharyngeal Pouch	Structures
Pouch 1	• Tympanic recess • Mastoid antrum • Auditory tube
Pouch 2	• Tonsillar sinus or fossa • Lymphatic tissue of crypts
Pouch 3	• Thymus • Inferior parathyroid gland
Pouch 4	• Superior parathyroid gland • Ultimopharyngeal (ultimobranchial body) • Parafollicular C cells

structural abnormalities are at a higher likelihood of certain cardiac defects, including tetralogy of Fallot, persistent truncus arteriosus, and transposition of the great vessels.[3,4]

GENERAL CRANIAL NERVE FUNCTION AND PATHOLOGY

The cranial nerves in the fully developed individual all exit the inferior brain or brainstem and, with the exception of CN VIII, extend outside the skull to provide sensory, motor, and autonomic innervation to the structures of the head and neck (**Fig. 9-1**). **Table 9-3** provides an overview of the cranial nerves and their functions. Several general pathologic processes may affect any single cranial nerve, regardless of anatomic location or course. However, cranial nerve pathology often affects specific clusters of nerves, dictated by their close anatomic relationships. Though there is much anatomic overlap between said regional clusters of nerves, the cranial nerves may be grouped regionally into the olfactory nerve (CN I), the optic nerve (CN II), the

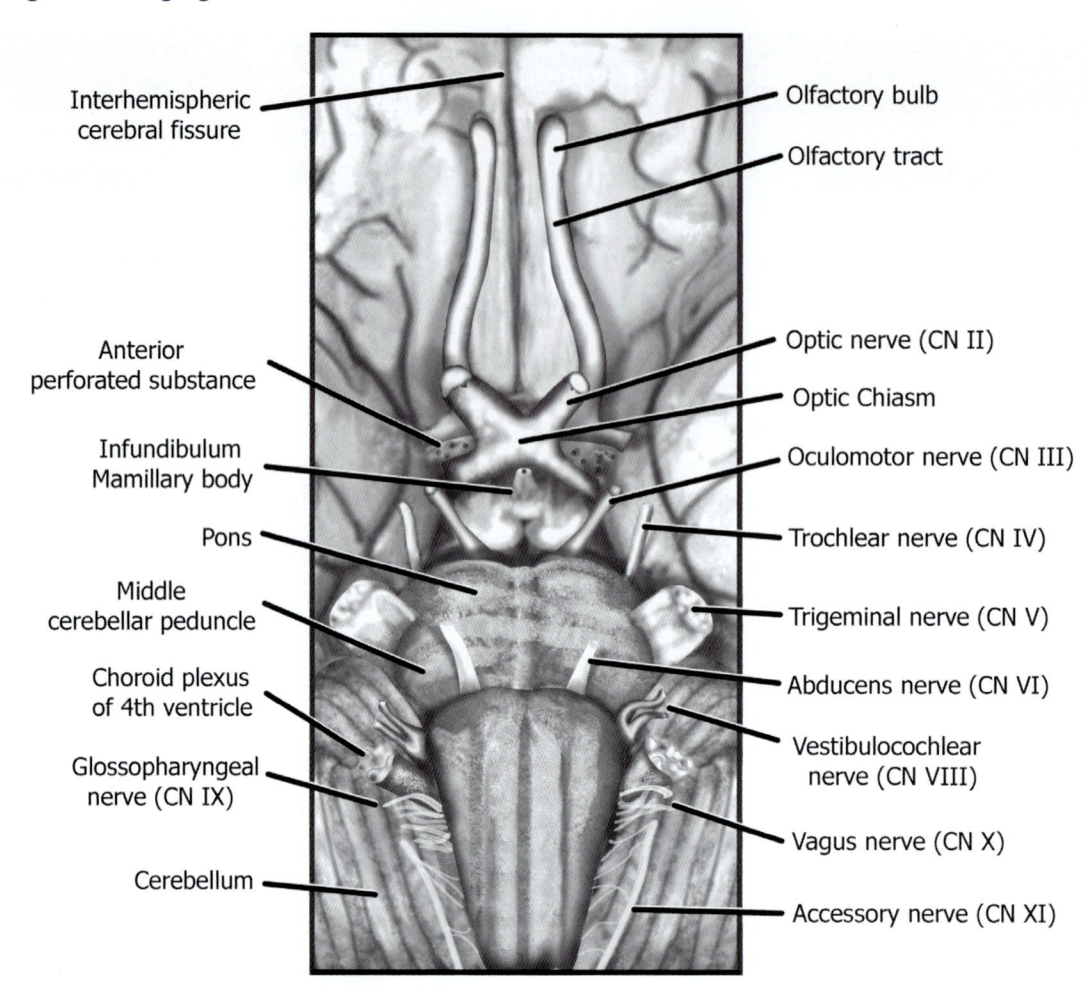

Figure 9-1 Anatomy Overview of the Cranial Nerves
Anterior brainstem as viewed from an inferior perspective, showing the root exit and entry zones of the 12 cranial nerves. Note that CN IV is the only nerve that exits the posterior brainstem.

extraocular muscle nerves (CN III, IV, and VI), the cerebellopontine angle nerves (CN V, VII, and VIII), the jugular foramen nerves (CN IX, X, and XI), and the hypoglossal nerve (CN XII).

Vascularization of the Cranial Nerves

Vascularization of the cranial nerves derives from the vertebrobasilar system, the internal carotid artery, and the external carotid artery. Cranial nerves are often supplied by more than one system through either multiple vascular tributaries or through complex anastomotic connections. Of note, the middle meningeal and accessory meningeal arteries from the external carotid system anastomose with branches of the inferolateral trunk of the internal carotid system to supply CN III, IV, V, VI, and VII in the region of the temporal bone and cavernous sinus; ischemic pathology in either of these systems may cause neuropathies to these nerves. Vascularization of CN VII is particularly diverse and includes tributaries from the middle meningeal, ascending pharyngeal, and posterior auricular branches of the external carotid artery. Other major vascular tributaries to cranial nerves include the ophthalmic artery, the meningohypophyseal trunk of the internal carotid, the anterior inferior cerebellar artery (AICA), and the posterior inferior cerebellar artery (PICA). **Table 9-4** highlights important vascular tributaries of the cranial nerves.[5–10]

Common Cranial Nerve Pathologies

Peripheral Nerve Sheath Tumors

Neurofibromatoses

Neurofibromatoses are autosomal dominant disorders that commonly cause disorders of the nervous system and skin pigmentation, for which they are also known as neurocutaneous syndromes. Neurofibromatosis 1 (NF-1) is associated with a defect in a suppressor protein involved in the RAS signalling pathway and results in neurofibromas, café-au-lait spots, skin fold freckling, optic gliomas, Lisch nodules (iris hamartomas), and bony dysplasia. Incidence of NF-1 is approximately 1 in 4,000 individuals. Neurofibromas are the classic features of NF-1 and consist of proliferating nerve sheath cells. Neurofibromas may be either solitary or plexiform and though benign, often can cause severe disfigurement. Plexiform neurofibromas affect nearly

Table 9-3 Overview of the Cranial Nerves

CN Group	CN	Major Functions	Transmitting Foramen
Olfactory Nerve	CN I olfactory	• Olfaction	cribriform plate
Optic Nerve	CN II optic	• Vision	optic canal
Oculomotor Muscle Nerves	CN III oculomotor	• Extraocular muscle movement	superior orbital fissure
	CN IV trochlear		
	CN VI abducens		
Cerebellopontine Angle Nerves	CN V trigeminal		
	CN V1 ophthalmic	• Sensory to superior face	
	CN V2 maxillary	• Sensory to mid face	foramen rotundum
	CN V3 mandibular	• Sensory to lower face • Motor to muscles of mastication	foramen ovale
	CN VII facial	• Motor to muscles of facial expression • Sensory to anterior tongue	stylomastoid foramen
	CN VIII vestibulocochlear	• Sensory to acoustic and vestibular organs	internal auditory canal
Jugular Foramen Nerves	CN IX glossopharyngeal	• Sensory to pharynx • Sensory to posterior tongue	jugular foramen
	CN X vagus	• Motor to vocal cords • Motor to pharyngeal constrictors • Sensory to epiglottis, glottis, esophagus	
	CN XI accessory	• Motor to trapezius • Motor to sternocleidomastoid	
Hypoglossal Nerve	CN XII hypoglossal	• Motor to intrinsic and extrinsic muscles of the tongue	hypoglossal canal

25% of individuals with NF-1 more commonly affect cranial nerves than do solitary neurofibromas. These lesions grow longitudinally along the nerve fascicles in the orbit, scalp, or parotid gland, or rarely in the neck, resembling a "bag of worms" on MR imaging (**Figs. 9-2–9-4**). The lesions are hyperintense on T2 imaging and strongly enhance with contrast administration. Surgery is the treatment of choice.[11–14]

Neurofibromatosis 2 (NF-2) is more rare than NF-1, having an incidence of 1 in 25,000. NF-2 arises because of the loss of a tumor suppressor protein involved in cytoskeletal signaling. The hallmark feature of NF-2 is schwannomas in motor fibers of cranial nerves. Particularly, it is associated bilateral vestibular schwannomas in 95% of cases and increases the incidence of nonvestibular schwannomas, especially in CN III and V. Other features of NF-2 may include meningioma, spinal tumors, foot drop due to amyotrophy, and facial mononeuropathy.[14,15] MR screening is recommended in all populations with NF-1 and NF-2.[16]

Table 9-4 Vascularization of the Cranial Nerves

	Arteries and Arterial Branches			CN Supplied
Internal Carotid Artery	ophthalmic C6 segment	ophthalmic artery		CN II, V1
	cavernous C4 segment	inferolateral trunk	superior branch	CN III, IV
			anteromedial branch	CN II, IV, VI, V1, V2, V3
			anterolateral branch	V2
			posterior branch	V3
		meningohypophyseal trunk	dorsal clival artery	CN VI in Dorello's canal
			tentorial artery	CN III, IV, trigeminal ganglion
External Carotid Artery	internal maxillary artery	middle meningeal artery; accessory meningeal artery		V2, V3
		middle meningeal artery	petrous artery	CN VII
	ascending pharyngeal artery	neuromeningeal trunk	jugular branch	CN IX, X, XI
			hypoglossal branch	CN XII
			musculospinal branch	CN XI
		inferior tympanic artery		CN VII
	posterior auricular artery	stylomastoid artery		CN VII
Basilar Artery	AICA	internal auditory artery		CN VIII
	PICA			CN IX, X

AICA = anterior inferior cerebellar artery; PICA = posterior inferior cerebellar artery.

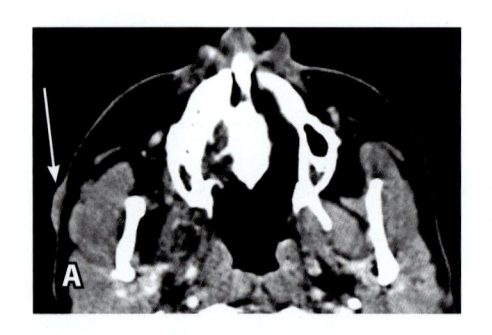

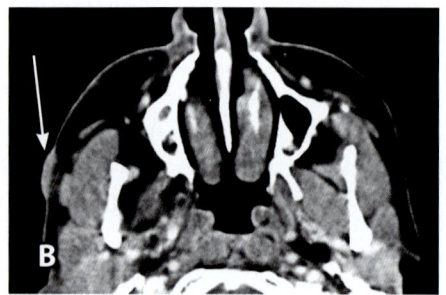

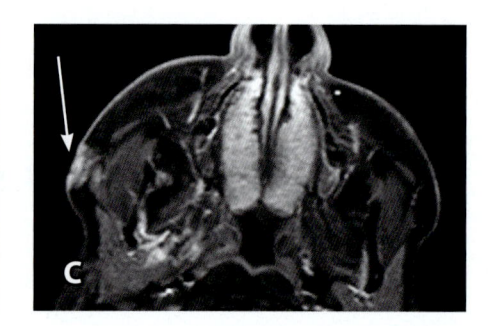

Figure 9-2 Cheek Neurofibroma
Neurofibroma of the right cheek in a patient with known NF-1. Axial CECT scans (**A–B**) demonstrate a soft tissue density lesion (*arrows*) over the zygomatic arch of the right cheek. Axial T1W postcontrast MR image (**C**) shows a superficial enhancing lesion (*arrow*), consistent with a single neurofibroma in the trigeminal nerve distribution.

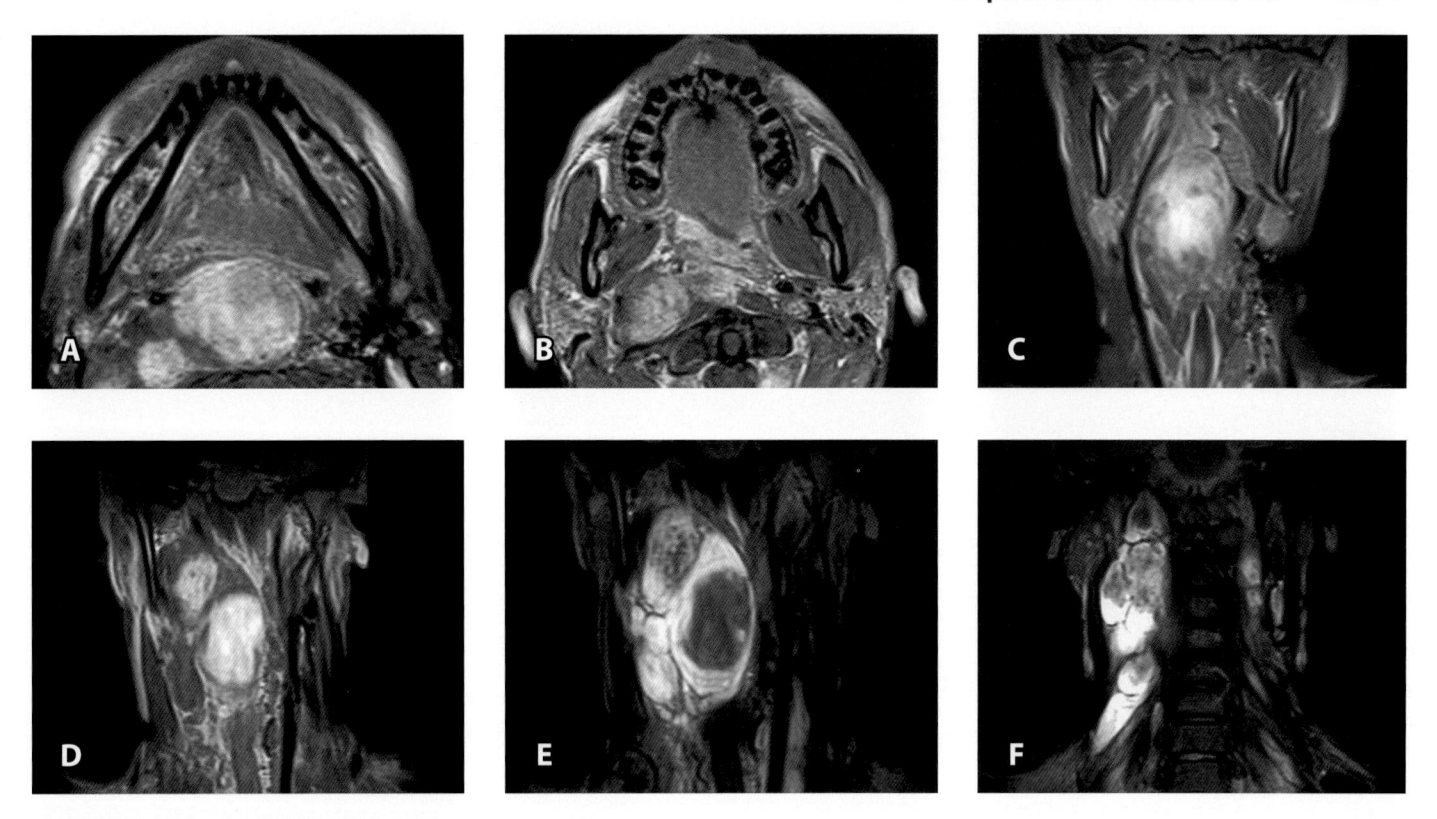

Figure 9-3 CN X Plexiform Neurofibroma
Large plexiform neurofibroma of CN X. Axial (**A–B**) and coronal (**C–F**) T1W postcontrast MR images show a large, cystic, heterogeneously enhancing mass in the regions of the right carotid space, retropharyngeal soft tissues, and superior neck. The strong enhancement with occasional cystic hypointensities is typical of peripheral nerve sheath tumors. Also note the undulating and multifocal nature of the lesions, helping to differentiate it from schwannomas and other regional pathologies.

Schwannoma

Schwannomas are benign, slow-growing tumors of myelinating schwann cells of the peripheral nervous system that account for 7% to 10% of intracranial tumors and arise from cranial nerves in approximately 60% of cases. Sensory schwannomas are more common than are motor schwannomas.[16,17] The vast majority of schwannomas arise from the vestibular branch of CN VIII and occupy the internal auditory canal and cerebellopontine angle. The most common initial presenting symptom is unilateral hearing loss. However, schwannomas have been reported in all cranial nerves. **Table 9-5** outlines the frequency and symptoms of the various cranial nerve schwannomas.[18]

Schwannomas of the cranial nerves may arise spontaneously, but are frequently associated with NF-2 and less commonly with NF-1.[13,16] NF-1 accounts for only 5% of vestibular schwannomas, but is most associated with rare malignant degeneration of the tumors.[19,20] NF-2 is associated with bilateral vestibular schwannomas in 95% of cases.[14] Schwannomas may also be caused by schwannomatosis, a sporadic genetic condition distinct from NF-1 and NF-2. The diagnosis of schwannomatosis is suggested in the event of multiple or recurrent schwannomas in the absence of vestibular nerve involvement[13] (**Fig. 9-5**).

Depending on the location of the schwannoma, CT may show an isodense smooth bone expansion. Low MR T1 signal, high T2 signal and intense enhancement are characteristic of smaller lesions, which is consistent with the histology of the compact, elongated Antoni type A cells that most commonly comprise these lesions. Larger lesions may contain foci of lipid-laden Antoni type B cells and may therefore show cystic heterogeneity up to 25% of the time. All schwannomas enhance strongly with contrast administration[16,21,22] (**Table 9-6**).

Meningioma

Meningioma is the most common extra-axial intracranial neoplasm in adults, accounting for 13% to 26% of all intracranial tumors.[23,24] It may occur at any place within the neuraxis, but is most common at the cranial base and sites of dural reflection. Presenting signs and symptoms of meningiomas include seizures, hydrocephalus, and cranial nerve palsies[24] (**Table 9-7**).

CT imaging of meningiomas most often shows hyperdense lesions with occasional calcifications and hyperostosis.[23] The best diagnostic clue, however, is an enhancing extra-axial mass on MR imaging with broad dural tail, representing peritumor inflamed non-neoplastic dura. It is important to note that though the dural tail sign is highly suggestive of a meningioma, it is neither sensitive nor specific for this diagnosis. The mass is usually isointense to hypointense on T1 and isointense to hyperintense on T2 imaging. Meningiomas will also enhance intensely with

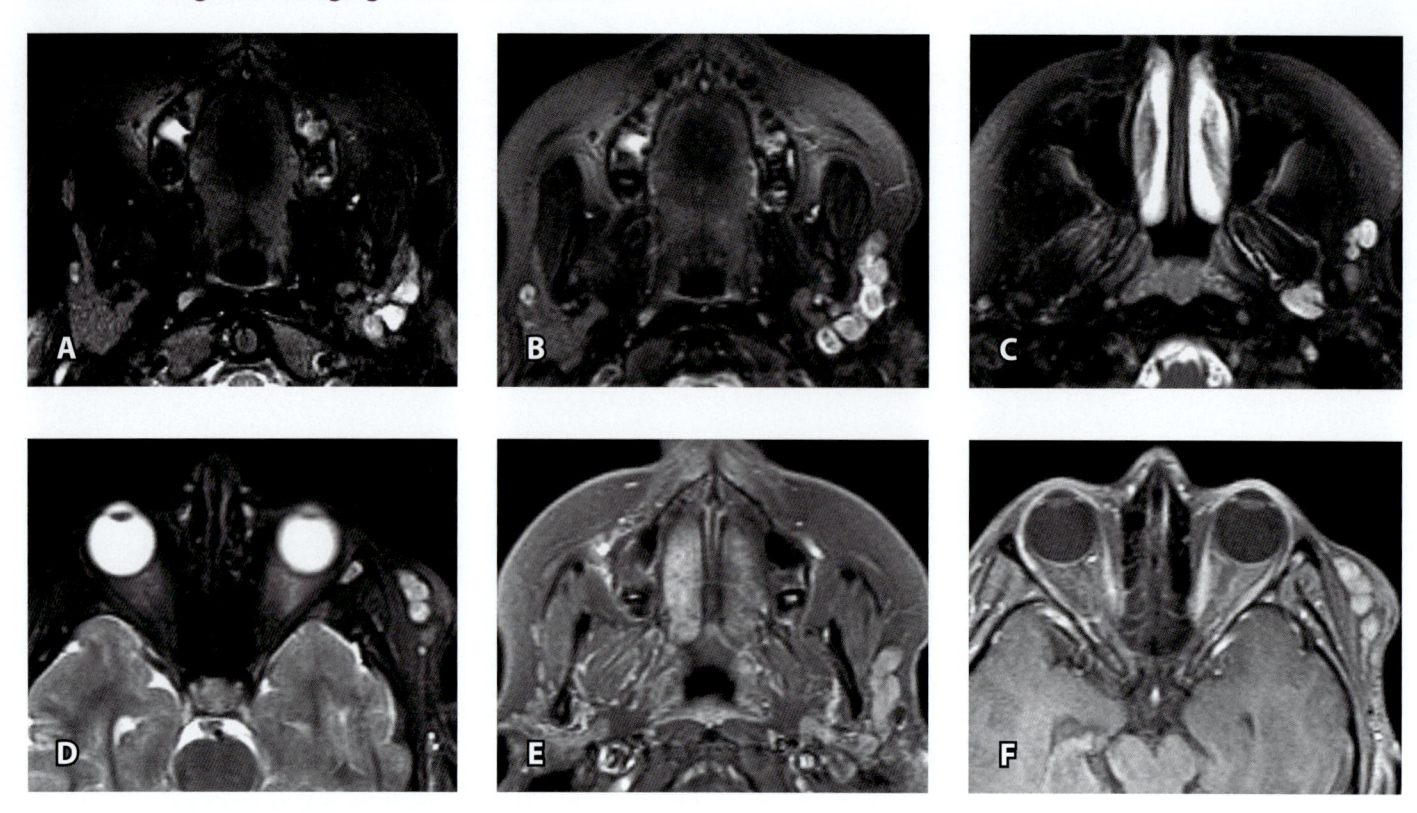

Figure 9-4 CN VII Plexiform Neurofibroma
Plexiform neurofibroma of CN VII. Axial T2W MR images (**A–D**) show hyperintense loculated lesions at the levels of the stylomastoid foramen, parotid gland, and temporal branch of CN VII (**D**) on the left side. Axial T1W postcontrast images (**E–F**) demonstrate heterogeneous enhancement of these lesions, resembling a "bag of worms."

contrast administration (**Table 9-6**). Relative cerebral blood volume (rCBV) ratios on dynamic perfusion enhanced MR imaging are typically elevated with meningiomas, a finding that may help differentiate them from schwannomas, which typically have an rCBV ratio approximating 3.[23] Several treatment options, including observation, microsurgery, external beam radiation, and stereotactic interventions are used to manage meningiomas.[19,24,25]

Metastatic Spread to the Cranial Nerves

Metastasis causing cranial nerve palsies most often result from adjacent osseous lesions and mass effects (**Table 9-6**). However, direct neural invasion may occur through hematogenous spread via the vasa nervorum or by meningeal carcinomatosis. Finally, aggressive perineural spread of certain neurotropic cancers of the head and neck may also produce focal cranial nerve deficits.[26]

Perineural Spread

Perineural spread is a rare complication of various head and neck cancers in which tumor infiltrates and spreads along the perineural sheaths of the cranial nerves. Perineural spread has been documented in neurotropic mucosal variants of squamous cell and adenoid cystic carcinoma, desmoplastic melanoma, lymphoma, and rhabdomyosarcoma. It most commonly affects divisions of CN V, though parotid malignancies may affect smaller branches of CN VII and nasopharyngeal carcinoma may spread along CN IX, X, XI, and XII. Although most perineural spread occurs in a retrograde fashion, anterograde transmission may be seen once progression to regions such as Meckel's cave and the cavernous sinus have been reached. CN VII involvement has also been reported following perineural spread from CN V via the greater petrosal nerve[27] (**Figs. 9-6–9-8**).

Symptoms of perineural spread are most often nonspecific, but may include pain, paresthesia, muscle weakness, and muscle atrophy. Facial pain, burning, and paresthesias are often noted with involvement of CN V. Facial twitching or palsy are rare complications of perineural spread in CN VII, but may be more common in recurrent disease.[26] Denervation atrophy is another known complication of perineural spread and is most often seen in the muscles of mastication, innervated by the mandibular nerve, and the tongue muscles innervated by CN XII[26] (**Fig. 9-9**).

MR imaging is most sensitive in the detection of perineural spread and will often show perineural thickening and replacement of bright perineural fat by intermediate density tumor. Fat suppression sequences and contrast administration may help to highlight more subtle lesions. Intracranial involvement is often visualized as an enhancing mass in Meckel's cave or lateral bulging of the cavernous sinus (**Fig. 9-10**). CT imaging may show widening of the bony foramen that transmit cranial nerves in late stages of the disease (**Fig. 9-11**). Denervation atrophy is often visualized as fatty infiltration of the muscles of mastication and tongue muscles (**Table 9-6**). Apparent

Table 9-5 Cranial Nerve Schwannomas

Type of Schwannoma (descending order of occurrence)	CN Involved	Symptoms	Incidence
Vestibular Schwannoma	CN VIII	• Ipsilateral hearing loss > tinnitus • CN V, VII palsy	common
Trigeminal Schwannoma	CN V	• Sensory trigeminal dysfunction • CNVI > II > III > VII, III, and IV palsy • Cerebellar involvement	rare
Facial Schwannoma	CN VII	• Facial nerve weakness • Hearing impairment • CN IX and X palsy • Cerebellar impairment	rare
Jugular Foramen Schwannomas	CN IX	• Pulsatile tinnitus (CN VIII) • Hearing impairment (CN VIII) • Gait ataxia, nystagmus (cerebellar & brainstem compression) • Palate hypoesthesia (CNIX) • Hoarseness, dysphagia (CNX) • CN VI impairment • Facial hypoesthesia (CN V)	rare
	CN X, XI	• Pulsatile tinnitus, hearing impairment (CN VIII) • Facial hyperesthesia (CN V) • Cerebellar involvement • CN IX, X, XI palsy	
	CN XII	• Tongue wasting, CN IX and X involvement, neck pain	
Other Schwannomas	CNI, III, IV, VI	• Respective nerve palsy; cavernous sinus and orbital apex syndromes	very rare

Adapted with permission from Sarma S, Sekhar LN, Schessel DA: Nonvestibular schwannomas of the brain: a 7-year experience. Neurosurgery 2002;50:437–448; discussion 438–439.

posterior displacement of the tongue may also be a sign of CN XII denervation atrophy.[26–28]

Invasive Nasopharyngeal Carcinoma

Nasopharyngeal carcinoma (NPC) is a pathologically distinct cancer from squamous cell carcinoma of the pharynx. Unlike pharyngeal squamous cell carcinoma, NPC has not been linked to alcohol or tobacco use, but has been associated with prior Epstein-Barr infection. NPC most often presents as a neck mass due to early nodal metastasis and has a propensity for skull base invasion, which may cause palsies of CN II, III, IV, V, VI, VII, IX, X, XI, and XII.[29] Cranial nerve involvement in NPC carries a particularly poor prognosis.[30] MRI is recommended for staging of the lesions.[30] Nodal metastases are the most diagnostic early MRI sign of NPC and include striations of lymphoid crypts on T1, T2, and T1 postcontrast sequences. Larger lesions are apparent as enhancing lesions affecting the retropharynx and skull base[29] (**Fig. 9-12**). Cranial nerve deficits are recovered following radiotherapy in some patients.[30]

Neurosarcoidosis

Sarcoidosis is a multisystem granulomatous disease of unknown etiology with a possible genetic component. Neurologic complications (neurosarcoidosis) are present in approximately 10% of cases and may be among the presenting symptoms of the disease. Cranial nerve involvement is common in neurosarcoidosis. The constellation of cranial neuropathy, uveitis, parotid enlargement, and fever is known as Heerfordt's syndrome, which is highly suggestive of neurosarcoidosis. Cranial nerve palsies are thought to be caused by mass effect from meningeal granulomas, but may also be caused by direct nerve involvement or increased intracranial pressure.[31]

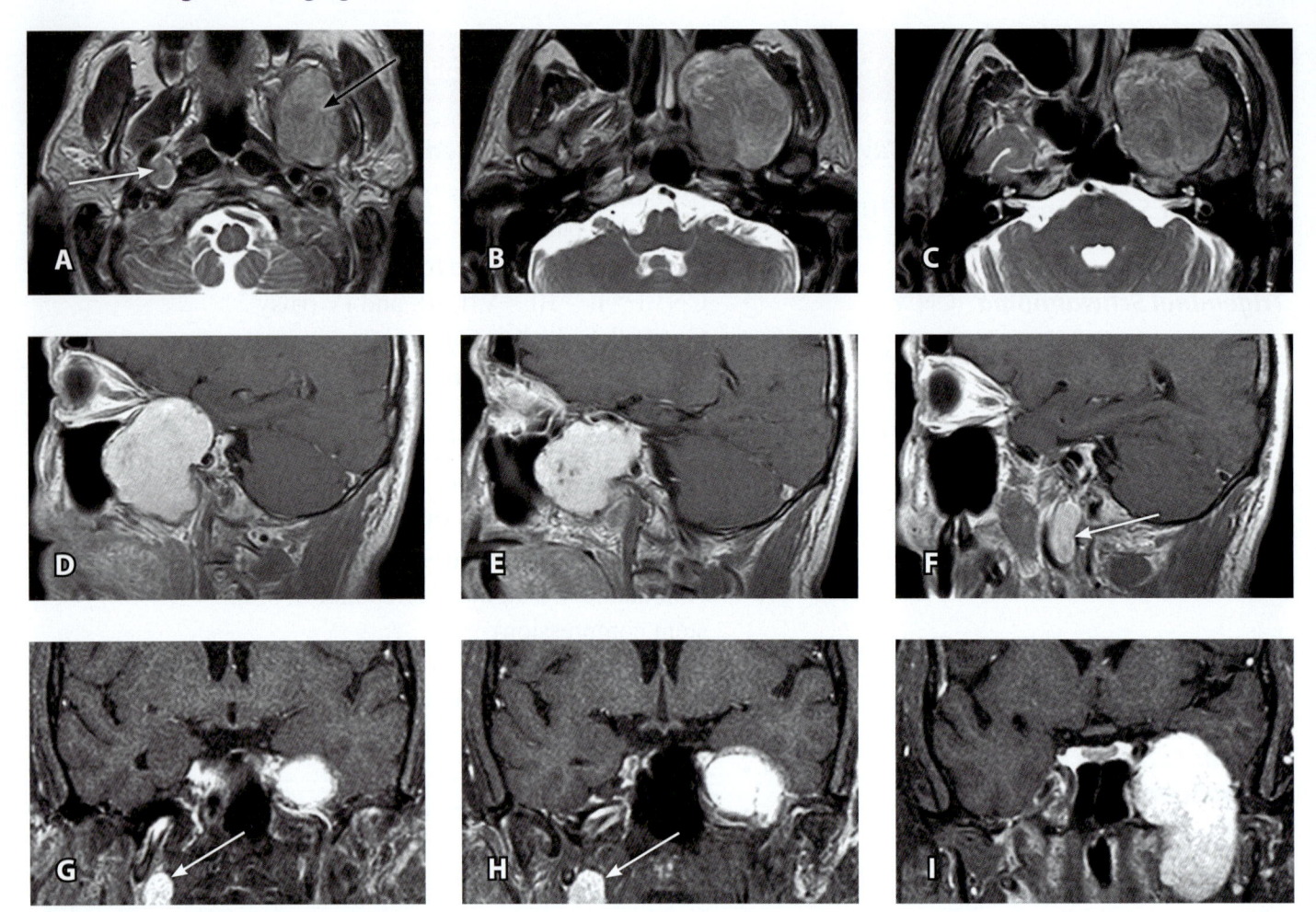

Figure 9-5 Schwannomas of CN V3 and X
Schwannoma in a 57-year-old male with prior history of a resected schwannoma and complaints of headaches, vertigo, and tinnitus. Axial T2W MR images (**A–C**), sagittal T1W postcontrast MR images, and coronal T1W postcontrast images show a large CN V3 schwannoma eroding through the anterior skull base into the left maxillary sinus (*black arrow*, **A**) and a CN X schwannoma extending inferiorly from an enlarged right jugular foramen (*white arrow*, **A**). Sagittal T1W postcontrast images (**D–F**) show the large intensely enhancing CN V3 tumor extending through the left skull base and a smaller right CN X lesion located in the right neck just below the skull base (*arrow*, **F**). Coronal T1W postcontrast images (**G–I**) document the mass in the left cavernous sinus expanding downwards into the foramen ovale and a small right upper neck similarly enhancing tumor (*arrows*, **G–H**.) The hyperintense appearance on T2 imaging, strong enhancement, smooth bony erosion, and cystic heterogeneity is typical of larger schwannomas. This patient had a history of two prior resected schwannomas and a cavernous hemangioma. Such history, coupled with concurrent schwannomas of more than one cranial nerve suggests genetic disorders such as schwannomatosis.

Cranial nerve manifestations of neurosarcoidosis most commonly involve CN VII and facial paralysis may be bilateral in up to 35% of cases.[31] However, palsies of any cranial nerve, but especially CN VIII, II, and V, may be caused by neurosarcoidosis. CN palsies in neurosarcoidosis often present with rapid onset and resolve spontaneously.[31–33] CN II involvement may present with vision loss and mimic optic sheath meningioma on MR imaging.[34] Mainstay treatment includes corticosteroids and immunosuppression.

Imaging findings of neurosarcoidosis are varied and nonspecific, but may include periventricular white matter changes on T2 FLAIR, enhancing leptomeningeal lesions on contrast enhanced T1 imaging, isolated cranial nerve enhancement, infiltrated extraocular muscles, and hydrocephalus (**Table 9-6**).

Systemic involvement, including hilar adenopathy and erythema nodosum and biopsied liver granulomas may support the diagnosis.[31]

Cavernous Malformation
Cavernous malformations (cavernomas, cavernous hemangiomas, or cavernous angiomas) of the nervous system consist of dilated capillary spaces surrounded by gliotic capsules and contain no intervening neural tissue. They occur in approximately 0.5% of the population and may either manifest in sporadic or familial patterns. Though more than 80% of cavernous malformations are supratentorial, a minority may involve the brainstem and affect the nuclei of various cranial nerves. Large suprasellar lesions may impinge on CN II and in extremely rare

Table 9-6 Imaging Findings of Common Cranial Nerve Pathologies

Pathology	CT Findings	MR Findings
Schwannoma	• Isodense • Smooth bone expansion	• Hypointense T1 • Hyperintense T2 • May be heterogenous in larger lesions • Strongly enhance
Meningioma	• Possible calcifications • Possible hyperostosis	• Variable T1 and T2 • Strongly enhance
Sarcoidosis	• Nonspecific	• Periventricular white matter changes on T2 FLAIR • Enhancing leptomeningeal lesions T1 + C • Cranial nerve enhancement
Perineural Spread	• Bony foramen widening in late disease	• Loss of perineural fat on T1 • Enhancement • Denervation atrophy
Cranial Neuritis	• Nonspecific	• Nerve enhancement

circumstances, these lesions may directly affect the cranial nerve fibers. CN VII and CN VIII may be involved secondarily by large cavernomas at the cerebellopontine angle (CPA) or primarily by intrinsic cranial nerve cavernomas. Primary cavernous malformations of CN III and CN IV are very rare. On imaging, cavernous malformations are angiographically occult, but may be visualized on MR. Bright T2 images with a peripheral rim of hypodense hemosiderin are the best diagnostic clue for cavernous malformations. CT may show bony erosion and stippled edges, especially at the internal auditory canal.[35–37]

Cranial Neuritis

Various autoimmune and infectious processes may affect the cranial nerves, producing clinically apparent palsies. Cranial neuritis is best imaged with contrast enhanced T1 MR imaging and generally shows enhancement in areas of neural involvement (**Table 9-6**). Enhancement is thought to arise from increased contrast perfusion through focal deficits in the blood–brain barrier produced by inflammatory demyelinating processes.[38] **Table 9-8** contains a summary of immune and infectious disease processes causing cranial neuritis.[38–59]

Guillain-Barré and Its Variants

Guillain-Barré syndrome is a complex of symptoms that includes a progressive motor neuropathy resulting from acute peripheral motor neuron demyelination in 95% of cases. The syndrome may be a postinfectious immune response, as it has been found to occur in conjunction with recent *Campylobacter jejuni*, hepatitis A, hepatitis C, cytomegalovirus, Mycobacterium pneumoniae, and Epstein-Barr virus infections.[49,60] Maximal symptomatic involvement usually occurs at 4 weeks; complete resolution usually follows within weeks to months. The syndrome typically responds to IV IG therapy. Cranial nerve involvement is common in Guillain-Barré and manifests as ophthalmoplegia (CN III, IV, VI) most frequently, though CN V and CN VII may also be involved (**Fig. 9-13**).[38]

Polyneuritis cranialis and Miller Fisher syndrome are rare forms of acute Guillain-Barré syndrome. As its name suggests, polyneuritis cranialis affects multiple cranial nerves with rare spinal nerve involvement. Concurrent palsies of at least 8 cranial nerves, including CN III, IV, V, VI, VII, IX, X, XI, and XII have been reported.[40] Miller Fisher syndrome is characterized by ophthalmoplegia, ataxia, and areflexia. Facial nerve and lower cranial nerves may also be involved in the syndrome. Miller Fisher syndrome is particularly associated with recent *C. jejuni* infection.[61]

Chronic inflammatory demyelinating polyradiculopathy is often considered a chronic form of Guillain-Barré syndrome that may be associated with genetic defects related to myelin production, including hypertrophic Charcot-Marie-Tooth disease, Dejerine-Sottas disease and Refsum's disease. Onion bulb malformations seen at pathologic examination and MR imaging

Table 9-7 Locations and Cranial Deficits of Meningiomas

Meningioma Location	Possible CN Palsies
Olfactory Groove	CN I
Optic Sheath	CN II
Sphenoidal Wing, Parasellar Region	CN I, III, IV, VI
Petroclival Region	CN V, VII, VIII, IX, X, XI, XII

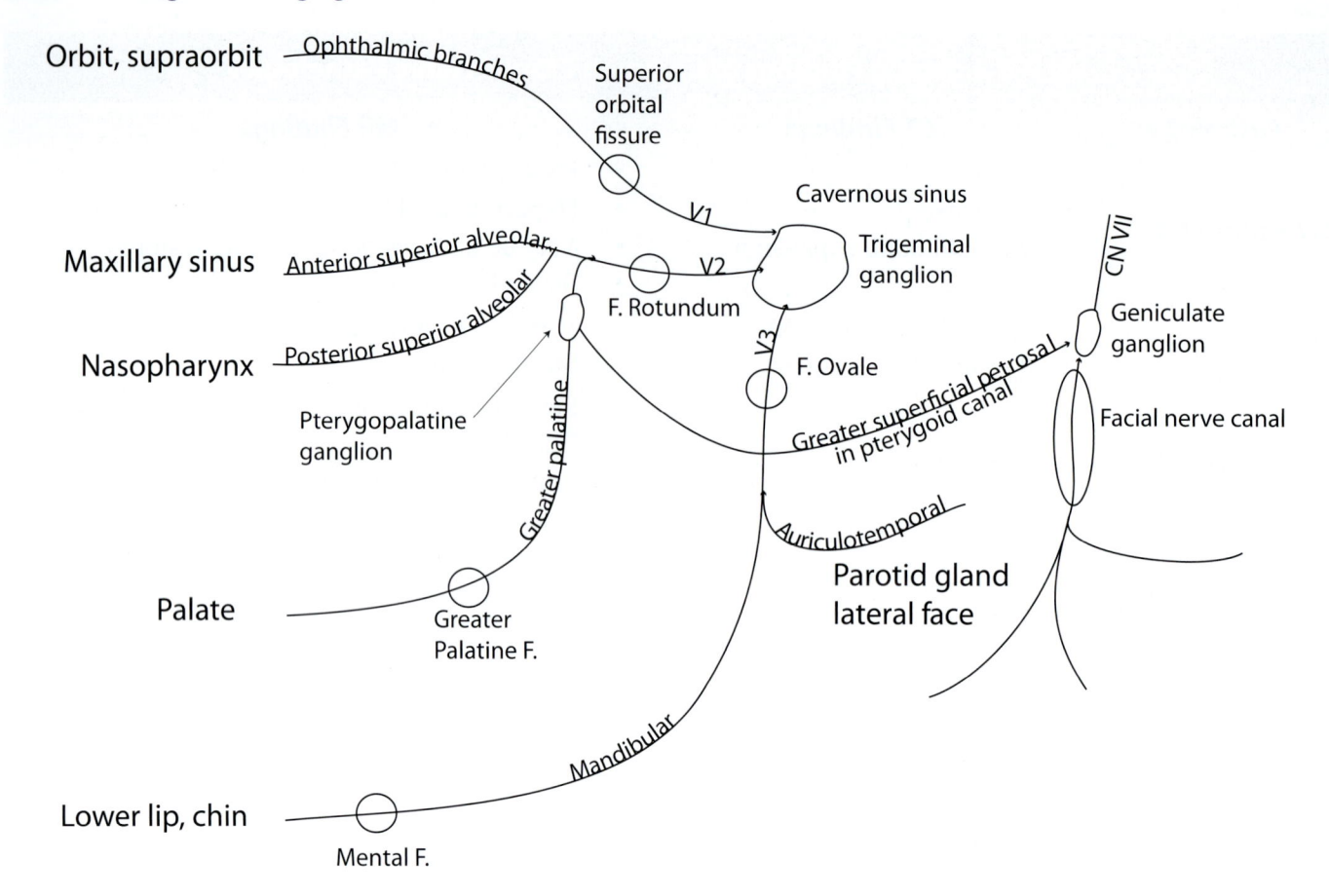

Figure 9-6 Routes of Perineural Spread of Head and Neck Cancers
Schematic representing routes of perineural spread of head and neck malignancies from a lateral view. Neurotropic carcinomas often spread along the regional nerve providing sensory and motor innervation to the respective area. Most head and neck cancers of the orbit, maxillary sinus, nasopharynx, palate, lower lip and chin, and parotid gland will spread along the three branches of the trigeminal nerve in a retrograde fashion toward the trigeminal ganglion. CN VII may become involved through either spread of tumor from the pterygopalatine ganglion to the geniculate ganglion via the greater superficial petrosal nerve or by direct tracking from parotid malignancies. The foramina through which the cranial nerves traverse may show smooth expansion on computed tomography in more advanced lesions.

often shows cranial nerve hypertrophy, which results from the chronic demyelination and remyelination characteristic of this disease process.[62] Concurrent involvement of CN III, IV, V, VI, X, XI, and XII has been reported.[41]

Multiple Sclerosis

Multiple sclerosis (MS) is a chronic demyelinating disease of the CNS that is thought to be autoimmune mediated. The chronic relapsing-remitting symptoms of the disease may manifest as intermittent combined cranial nerve palsies, resulting from demyelination of the oligodendrocyte-encased CN II or of CN nuclei in the brainstem. Visual disturbances may include diplopia, nystagmus, internuclear ophthalmoplegia, gaze palsies, and oculomotor palsies.[43] Brainstem lesions leading to isolated cranial nerve palsies occur in approximately 1.6% of new onset MS, but have been reported in decreasing order of incidence: CN V, CN VII, CN VI.[42] Isolated involvement of CN III, CN VIII, or CN IV are very rare. Finally, in very unusual cases, MS may affect the PNS of the cranial nerves, which has been reported as enhancing lesions of peripheral segments of CN II, V, and VI.[43]

Neuromyelitis Optica

Neuromyelitis optic consists of bilateral severe optic neuritis with concurrent transverse myelitis of three or more spinal cord segments. The disease typically affects young women and has been linked to antibodies against aquaporin 4, located on the astrocyte foot processes. Impaired functionality of these foot processes is thought to be the cause of a breakdown in the blood–brain barrier and resultant demyelination of the optic nerves. Imaging clues include enhancing optic nerves and cord cavitation or swelling. The diagnosis may also be supported by CSF pleocytosis and the absence of oligoclonal bands, distinguishing it from MS.[63]

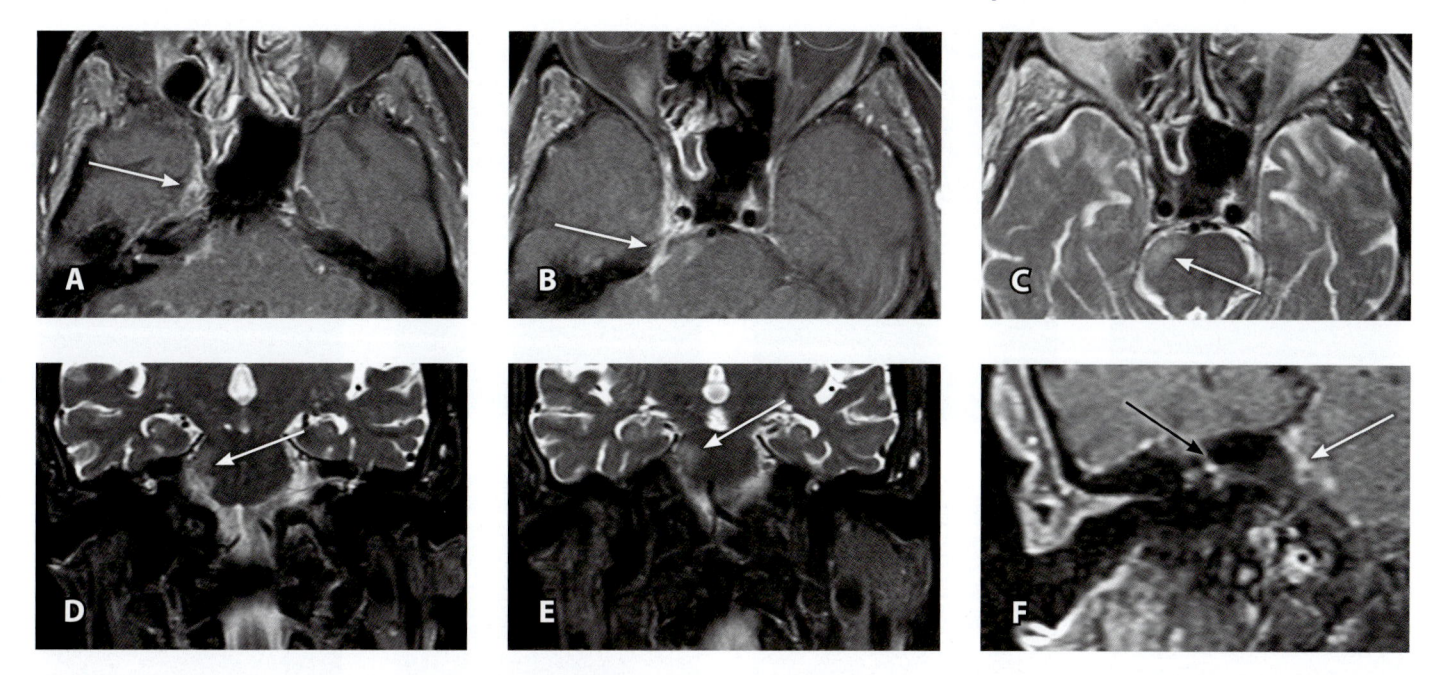

Figure 9-7 Perineural Spread along CN V and CN VII
A 79-year-old male with recurrent squamous cell carcinoma of the face and perineural spread along CN V and VII. Axial T1W postcontrast images (**A–B**) at the level of the cavernous sinus show enhancement of the right trigeminal ganglion (*arrow*, **A**) and root entry zone (*arrow*, **B**). Axial (**C**) and coronal (**D–E**) T2W MR images highlight tumor spread to the lateral pons at the level of the cerebellopontine angle (*arrows*). Coronal T1W postcontrast image (**F**) shows enhancement of the geniculate ganglion (*black arrow*) and patchy enhancement within the left cerebellopontine angle cistern (*white arrow*).

Acute Disseminated Encephalomyelitis

Acute disseminated encephalomyelitis (ADEM)[64] is an inflammatory demyelinating process of the CNS and PNS that most commonly affects children and young adults. The disease typically manifests in days to weeks following febrile reaction to measles, mononucleosis, mumps, varicella, or vaccination. Cranial nerve palsy has been reported in nearly half of cases, in addition to pyramidal tract lesions, hemiparesis, consciousness impairment, and cerebellar ataxia. Optic neuritis with clinically evident vision impairment is a common cranial nerve manifestation of ADEM (**Fig. 9-14**). In addition to enhancement of the nerve, imaging of ADEM lesions may also show multifocal tumefactive lesions of the CNS and PNS, resembling those of multiple sclerosis. Multisystemic involvement and more frequent bilateral cranial nerve involvement help to distinguish ADEM from multiple sclerosis. Furthermore, unlike multiple sclerosis, most cases of ADEM resolve without relapse, though clinical deficits may persist and relapse has been reported in rare instances.[58,59]

Lyme Disease

Lyme disease is a multisystem syndrome caused by the bacterium Borrelia burgdorferi that may manifest with peripheral nervous system complications in up to 25% of untreated cases. Meningitic CNS involvement in Lyme disease is rare, occurring in a reported 10% to 15% of cases.[65] Of those with PNS involvement, approximately 10% to 15% will manifest with cranial nerve palsies, often visible on MR as cranial nerve enhancement. 80% of cranial nerve palsies include CN VII, manifesting as Bell's palsy; bilateral facial nerve paralysis is not uncommon. In addition to CN VII, palsies of CN II, III, V, VI, and XII have also been reported in neuroborreliosis. The acute onset of this disease may mimic Guillain-Barré syndrome, but can be differentiated based on CSF pleocytosis and prominent inflammatory infiltrates common in Lyme disease. Most cranial nerve manifestations of Lyme disease resolve with prompt antibiotic treatment.[44,45,66]

Syphilis

Syphilis is caused by the bacterium Treponema pallidum. In addition to causing tabes dorsalis, both secondary and tertiary syphilis commonly cause cranial nerve palsies. Mechanisms of cranial nerve involvement are thought to occur either by infiltration in secondary syphilis or via obliterative endarteritis-induced ischemia in tertiary syphilis. CN II is most commonly involved, but CN VII and CN VIII involvement have also been reported. MR findings include nerve enhancement, hypertrophy, and occasional enhancement of the associated meninges.[46–48,66]

Varicella Zoster Virus and Herpes Simplex Virus

Varicella zoster virus (VZV) is known to infect and lie dormant in several cranial nerves. It most commonly infects CN V,

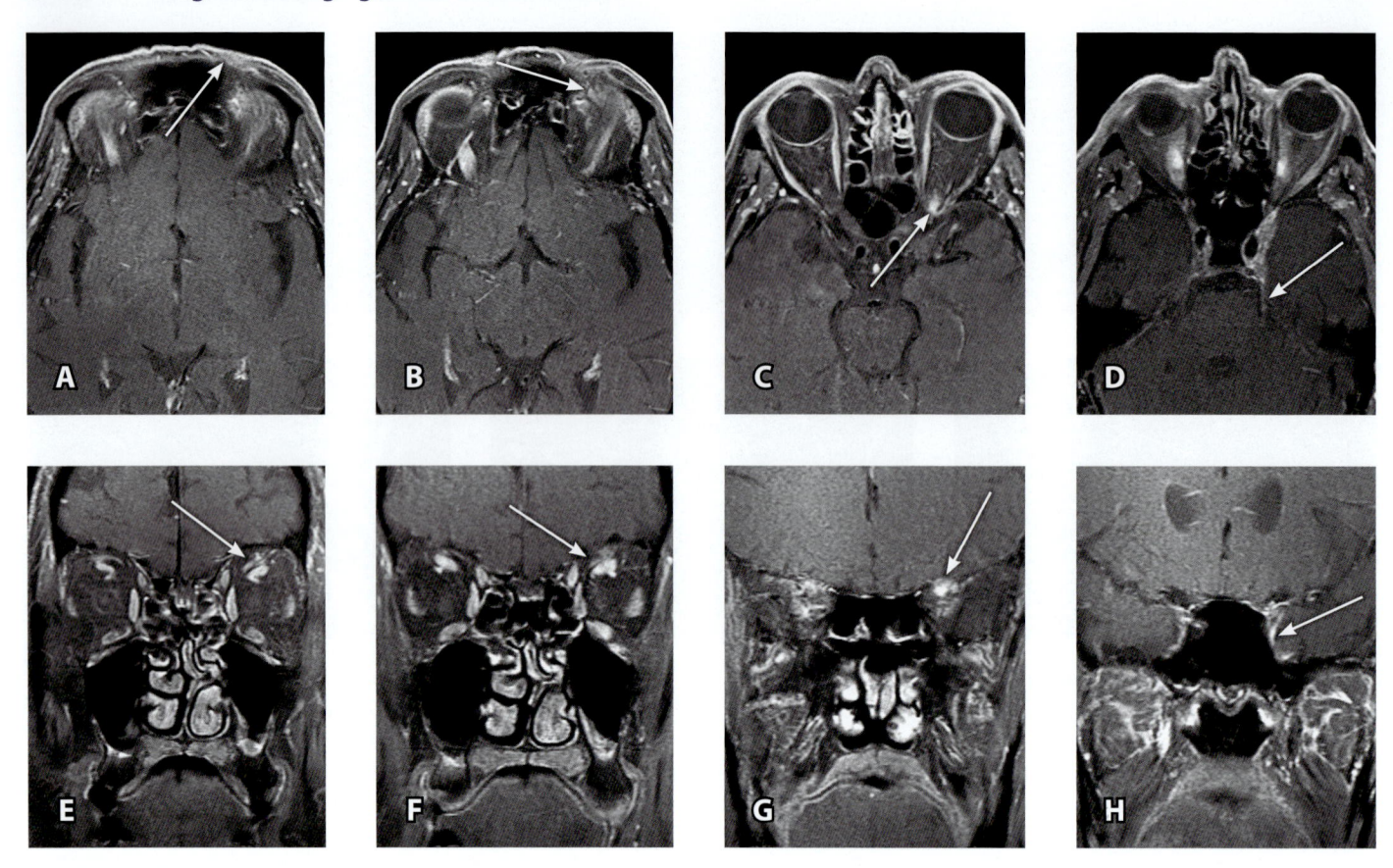

Figure 9-8 Cranial Nerve V1 Perineural Spread
Recurrent melanoma in a 75-year-old male with perineural spread. Axial (**A–D**) and coronal (**E–H**) T1W postcontrast MR images show a lesion in the frontal bone just above the left orbit with tracking along the frontal branch of V1 (*arrows*). The melanoma is visualized as a slight enhancement within the medulla of the left frontal bone (*arrow*, **A**). Enhancement of the frontal branch of V1 is seen as it traverses the orbit (*arrows*, **B, E, F**), the superior orbital fissure (*arrows*, **C, G**), and in the cavernous sinus and root entry zone (*arrow*, **D**). Notice the anterograde involvement of the left V2 branch just distal to Meckel's cave (**H**).

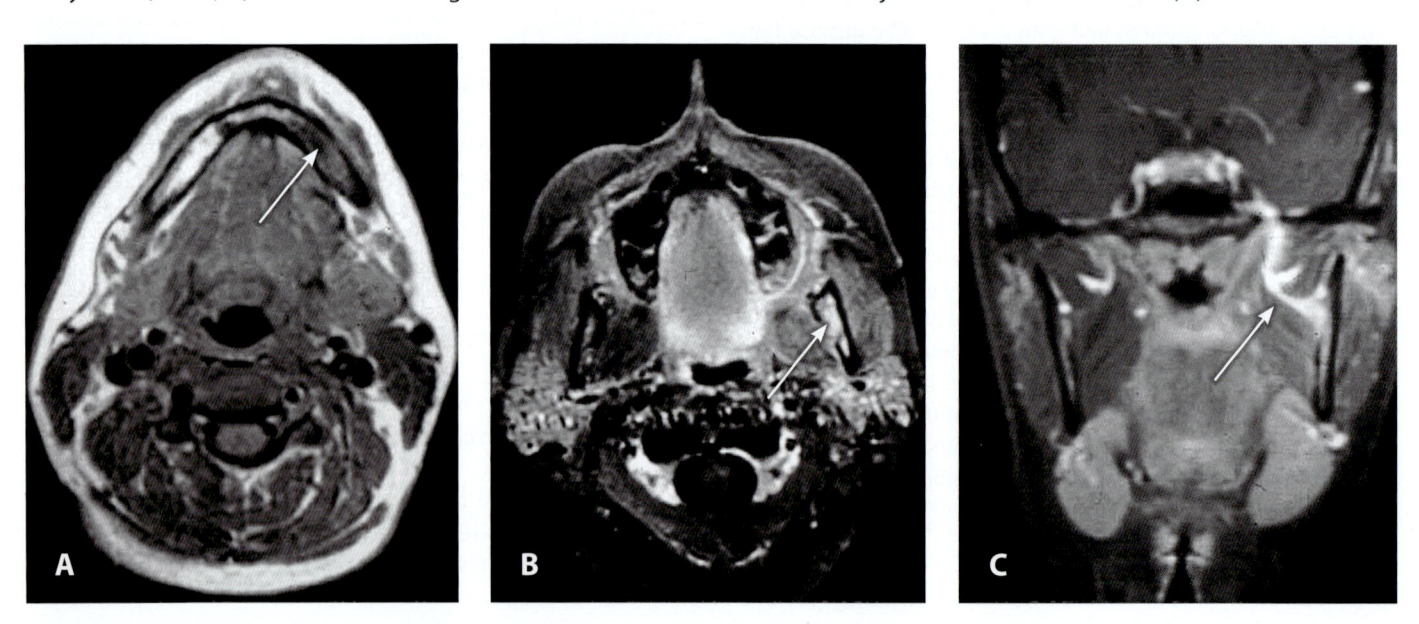

Figure 9-9 Cranial Nerve V3 Perineural Spread
Melanoma of the lip with perineural spread along V3. Axial (**A–B**) and coronal (**C**) T1W postcontrast images show enhancement along the left V3 branch at the mental foramen and mandible (*arrows*, **A–B**), in foramen ovale (*arrow*, **C**), in Meckel's cave (**C**), and in the temporal lobe (**C**). Notice that the left muscles of mastication show acute denervation atrophy with increased fat and enhancement (**B, C**).

Chapter 9: The Cranial Nerves   **369**

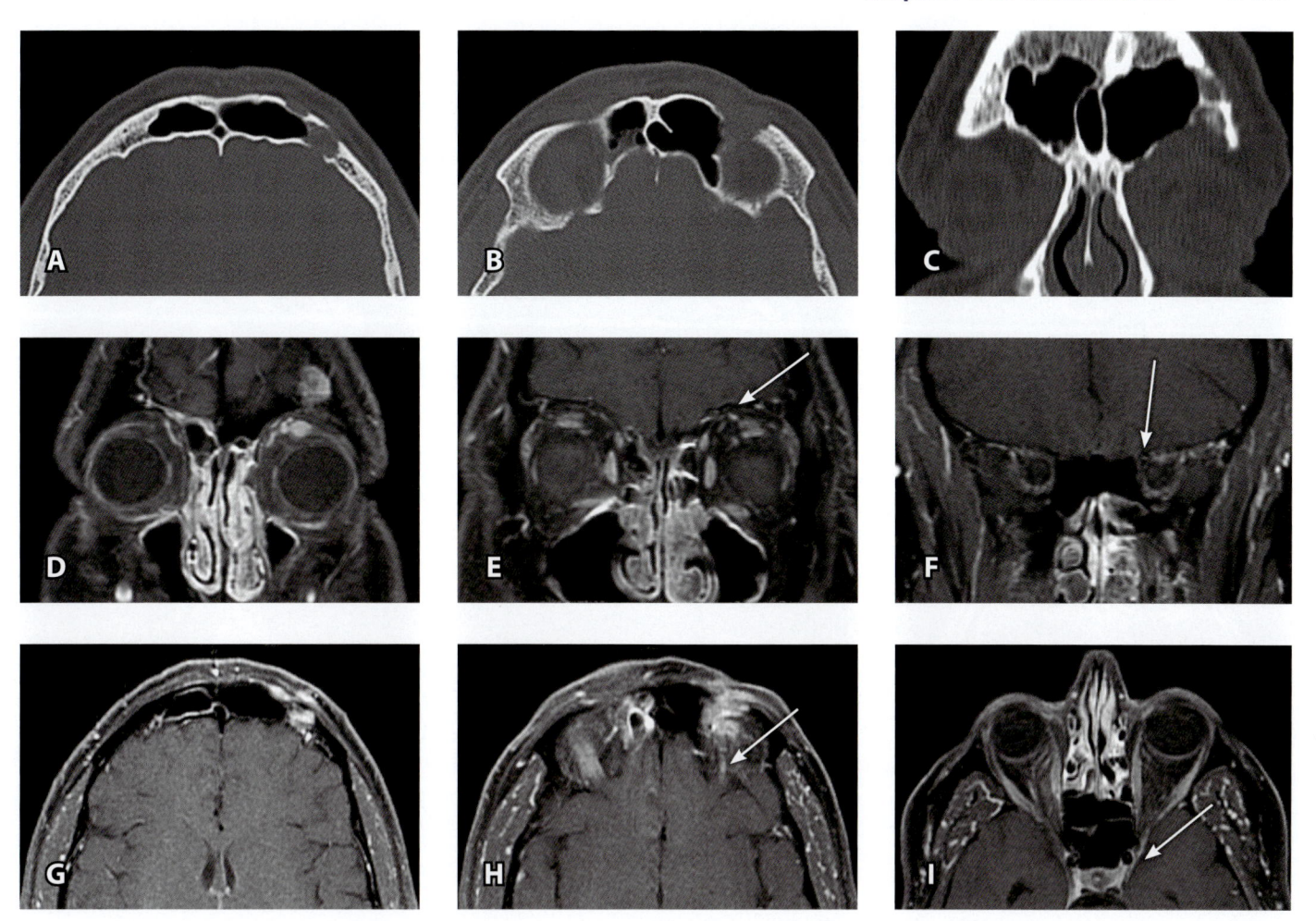

Figure 9-10 Cranial Nerve V1 Perineural Spread
A 47-year-old male with squamous cell carcinoma of the scalp and perineural spread along CN VI. Axial (**A–B**) and reformatted coronal (**C**) NECT images show lytic bone lesions in the superior wall of the left orbit and frontal bone. Coronal (**D–F**) and axial (**G–I**) T1W postcontrast MR images show an enhancing lesion in the frontal bone, superior to the left orbit with inferior spread along the medial portion of the left orbit in the region of the frontal branch of CN V1. Note the tumor mass in the superior portion of the left orbit (**D, H**) and enhancing portions of the intraorbital portion of the frontal nerve as it passes through the superior orbital fissure (*arrows*, **E, F, H**). Also note the enhancement of V1 in the cavernous sinus and Meckel's cave (*arrow*, **I**).

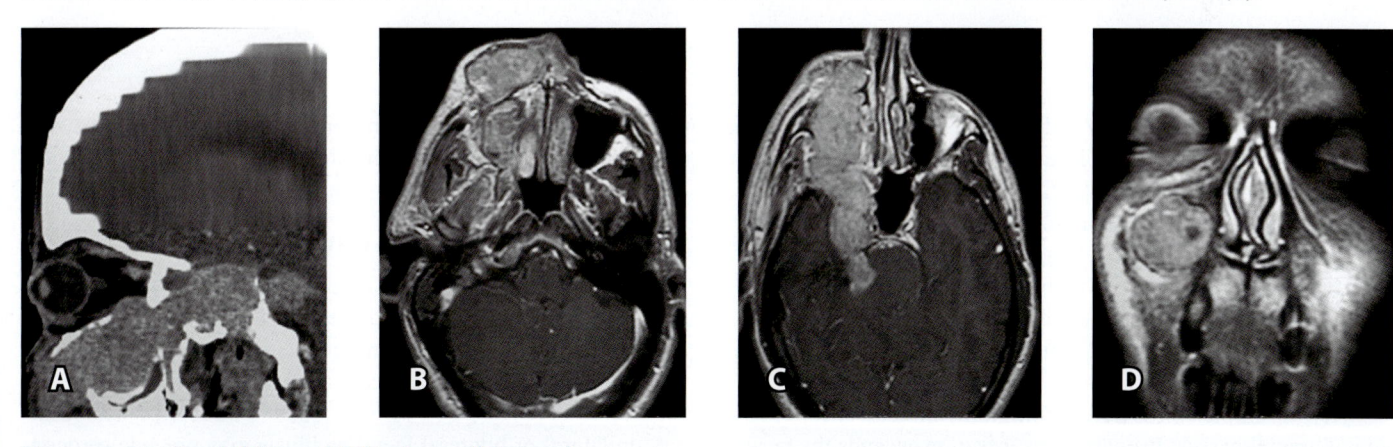

Figure 9-11 Cranial Nerve V2 Perineural Spread
Squamous cell carcinoma perineural spread along the anterior superior alveolar branch of CN V2. Sagittal NECT (**A**) depicts the tumor as a heterogenous mass hyperdense to soft tissue that has invaded through the zygomatic bone, the maxillary sinus, and the inferior orbital wall. Also note the expansion of foramen rotundum and foramen ovale. Axial T1W postcontrast MR images (**B–C**) show the extracranial portion of the tumor in the right maxilla (**B**) and along the course of the nerve through the cavernous sinus, Meckel's cave, root entry zone of CN V, and into the brainstem (**C**). Coronal T1W postcontrast MR image (**D**) shows a central necrotic area within the tumor as it courses through the maxillary sinus.

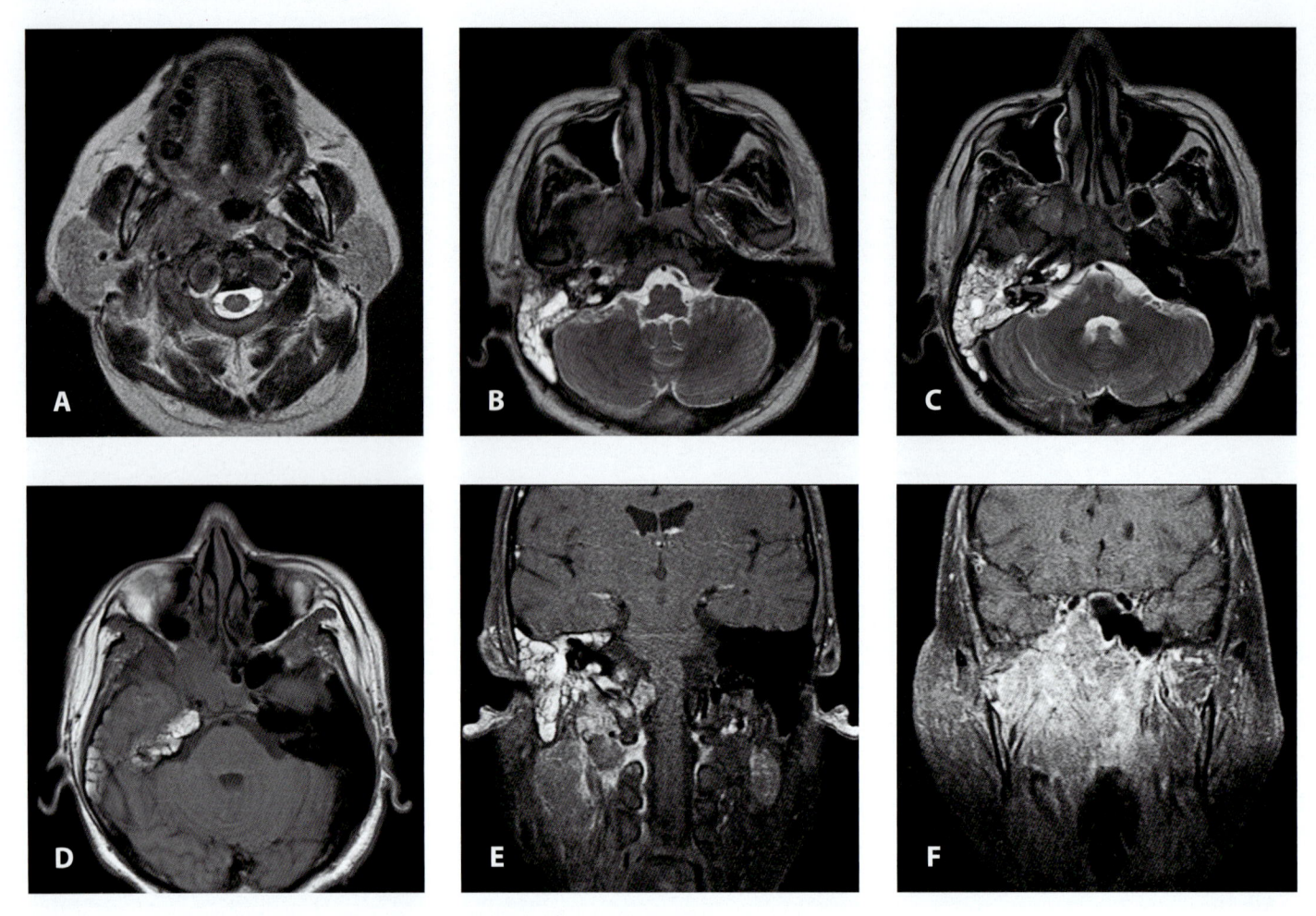

Figure 9-12 Nasopharyngeal Carcinoma Invasion into Skull Base
Invasive nasopharyngeal carcinoma (NPC) in a 32-year-old male with CN XI and CN XII deficits (Tapia syndrome). Axial T2W images (**A–D**) show extensive local invasion of a soft tissue mass into the right pharyngeal space. Note the blocked drainage of the mastoid air cells (**B, C, E**), paranasal sinuses (**B–C**), and tympanic cavity (**E**). The tumor completely encases the cervical (**B**) and petrous (**C**) internal carotid artery. There is extensive bilateral cervical adenopathy. Image F shows the extensive retropharyngeal spread of the tumor upward into the skull base. The propensity of NPC to invade the temporal bone, coupled with cervical adenopathy often cause combined neuropathy of the lower cranial nerves.

particularly the ophthalmic (V1) division. However, active VZV infection of CN VII and CN VIII can result in Ramsay Hunt syndrome, which consists of lower facial nerve palsy and herpetic eruptions of the ear. VZV may also cause ophthalmoplegia by infecting CN III, IV, and to a lesser extent, CN VI. Infection of CN IX and X have also been reported, but are extremely rare.[50] Generally, primary or reactivated VZV infections are visualized as enhancing portions of neural ganglia in affected cranial nerves.[67]

Herpes simplex virus (HSV) commonly infects sensory ganglia of cranial nerves. Primary virus infection ascends the nerve until it reaches the ganglia, where it lies dormant. Reactivation of HSV results in dermatome-specific complications. CN V is most commonly involved, resulting in gingivostomatitis, cold sores, and corneal infections. CN VII and CN VIII are involved less frequently, but are often indistinguishable from Bell's palsy or Ramsay Hunt syndrome on contrast-enhanced MR. Acyclovir treatment is helpful in controlling HSV reactivation in most cases.[39,51,52]

Acute Retroviral Syndrome (HIV)

Acute retroviral syndrome is a recognized complication of recent HIV infection and often manifests with flu-like symptoms, lymphadenopathy, aseptic meningitis, encephalopathy, neuropathy, and myelopathy. The process appears to have a predilection for motor nerves and CN VII is frequently affected.[53] The resultant unilateral or bilateral facial paralysis may precede seroconversion by 4 to 6 weeks.[68] MRI shows contrast enhancement of affected portions of CN VII, including tympanic and labyrinthine portions of the nerve.[53] In addition to CN VII involvement, HIV also can cause optic neuritis, visible as contrast enhancing segments along the nerve.[66]

Table 9-8 Causes of Cranial Neuritis

	Condition	Cranial Nerves Involved
Immune or Idiopathic Demyelinating Cranial Neuropathies	• Guillain-Barré • Polyneuritis cranialis • Miller Fisher syndrome	• Most common: CN VII • Less common: CN III, IV, VI, V, VII, may involve all CN
	Multiple sclerosis	• Most common: Brainstem lesions affecting CN II, III, IV, and VI. • Rare isolated cranial neuropathies • CN V > CN VII > CN VI > CN III, CN VIII, CN IV
	Neuromyelitis optica	• Bilateral CN II palsy • Transverse myelitis
	Acute disseminated encephalomyelopathy	• Most common: CN II
	Ophthalmoplegic migraine	• Most common: CN III • Less common: CN IV and VI • Resolved CN enhancement when asymptomatic
	Erdheim Chester disease and Langerhans cell histiocytosis	• Any
	Vasculitis and ischemia	• Any
Infectious Cranial Neuritis	Lyme disease (neuroborreliosis)	• CN VII in 80% of cases • Less common: CN III, V, VI, VIII, XII
	Syphilis	• Most common: CN II, VII, VIII
	Leprosy	• Most common: CN VII, V
	Varicella zoster	• Most common: CN VII (Ramsay Hunt syndrome) • Less common: CN VIII • Rare: CN III, IV, VI, IX, X
	Herpes simplex	• Most common: CN VII, VIII
	HIV	• Most common CN VII, II
	Cytomegalovirus	• Rare in immunocompetent • Immunocompromised: any CN
Other Causes of Cranial Neuritis	Metachromatic leukodystrophy	• Rare CN enhancement seen on MR
	Radiation-induced neuritis	• Most common: CN VI, XII, II

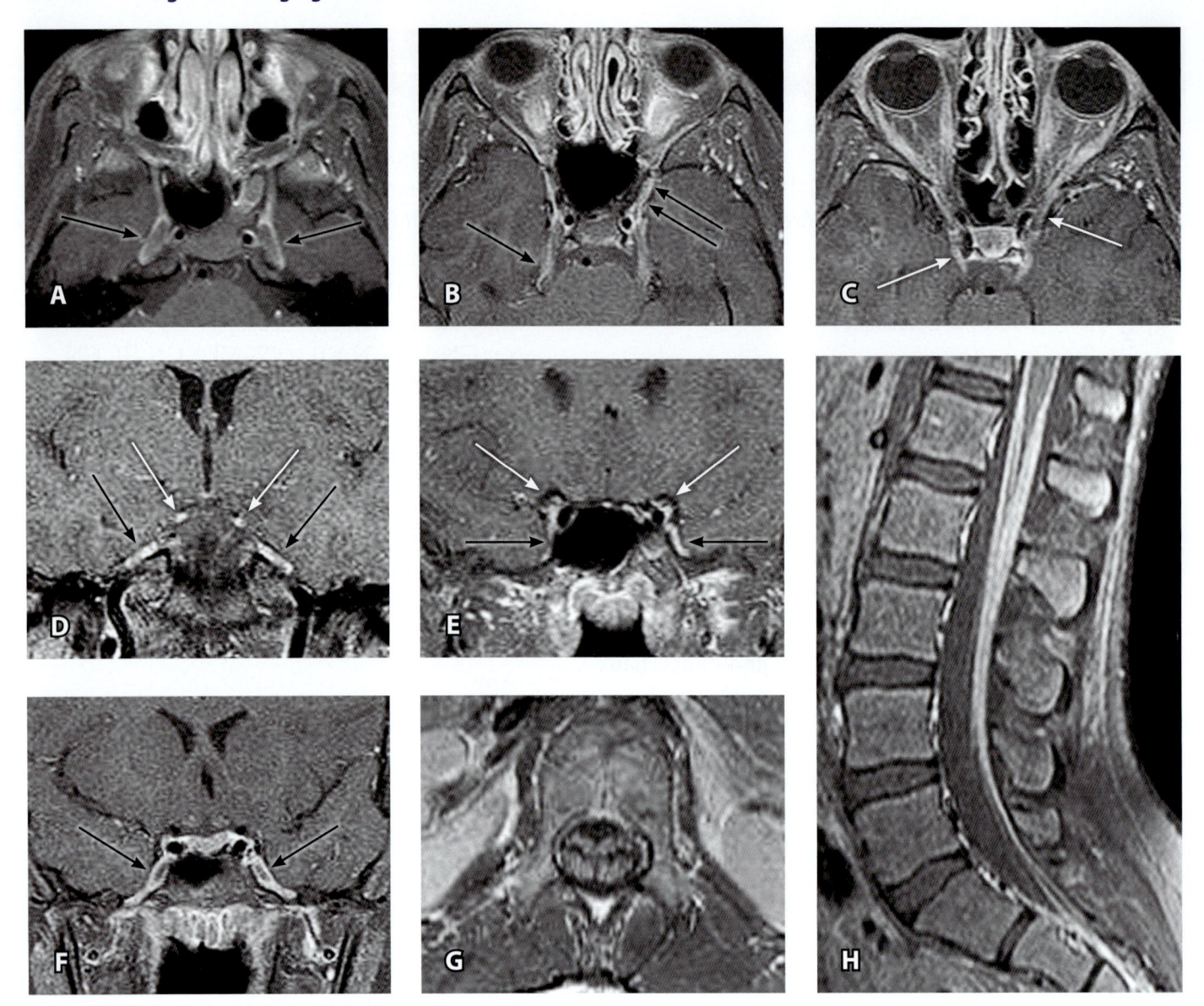

Figure 9-13 Guillain-Barré Syndrome with Polyneuritis Cranialis
Guillain-Barré syndrome with polyneuritis cranialis. Axial (**A–C**) and coronal (**D–F**) T1W postcontrast MR images at the level of the cavernous sinus show enhancement of CN III (*white arrows*) and CN V (*black, arrows*). Enhancement of CN V is seen at the root exit zone (*black arrows*, **B, D**), trigeminal ganglion (*black arrows*, **A**), V2 branch (*black arrows*, **B, E, F**), and V1 branch (*double black arrows* **B**). CN III enhancement is seen in the prepontine cistern (*white arrow*, **D**), in the lateral wall of the cavernous sinus (*white arrow*, **E**) and in the superior orbital fissure (*white arrow*, **C**). Axial (**G**) and sagittal (**H**) T1W postcontrast MR images at the level of the conus medullaris show intense enhancement of the spinal nerves of the cauda equina.

Radiation Neuritis

Radiation neuritis is much less common in cranial nerves than in the CNS, presumably because of large diameter blood vessels, dual arterial supply, and abundant vascular anastomoses feeding these nerves. CN VI is most commonly involved following radiation to the skull base, though radiation neuritis may also affect CN XII. Radiation-induced neuritis of CN II often results in gradual, but irreversible deterioration of vision. Imaging show variable enhancement along portions of the nerve (**Fig. 9-15**).[26]

OLFACTORY NERVE – CN I

CN I is solely responsible for the chemoreceptive transmission of smell. Lesions along the course of the nerve in the anterior skull base and nasal cavities can produces various degrees of anosmia and olfactory dysfunction [69] (**Fig. 9-16, Table 9-9**).

Smell is consciously perceived in the gray matter covering the medial and lateral striae of the olfactory gyri. The lateral

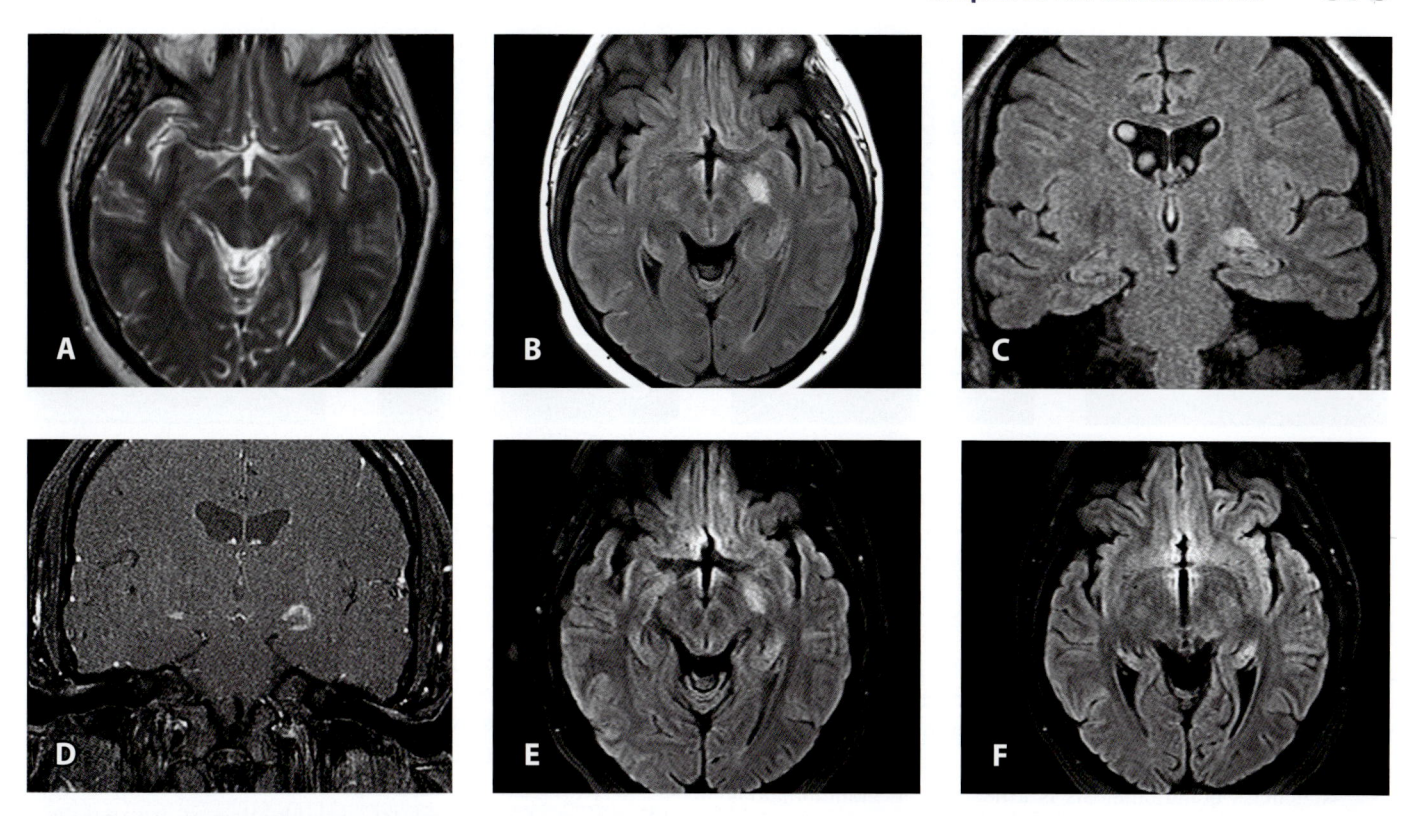

Figure 9-14 ADEM of the Optic Tract
Acute disseminated encephalomyelitis (ADEM) in a 19-year-old female presenting with headache and right visual field deficits following a sinus infection 3 weeks prior. Axial T2W (**A**), T2 FLAIR (**B**), and coronal T2 FLAIR (**C**) MR images show a diffuse area of bright T2 signal in the left optic radiation and posterior to the temporal horn (**B**). Coronal T1W postcontrast MR image shows a tumefactive rim enhancing lesion in the region of the left optic radiation, consistent with an acute demyelinating neuropathy such as ADEM or MS. Followup axial T2 FLAIR MR images at 1 month (**E**) and 6 months (**F**) show decreased signal intensity of the lesions at one month and complete resolution of signal abnormalities and visual disturbances by 6 months. Young age, complete resolution of symptoms, and lack of relapse in this patient is more consistent with ADEM versus MS.

striae travel from the inferior medial aspect of the temporal lobe (pyriform area) and the medial striae from the medial and inferior aspects of the frontal lobe (subcallosal region) to the olfactory trigone located at the anterior perforated substance. The intermediate stria is not significant in humans, but joins the lateral and medial striae at the trigone to extend anteriorly as the olfactory tract. The olfactory tract terminates on the olfactory sulci. The olfactory sulci separate the gyri rectus from the medial orbitofrontal gyri.[70] Sensory nerve bundles exit the olfactory bulbs via the cribriform plate of the skull to separate into multiple neurosensory cells which reside in the nasal epithelium (**Fig. 9-16**).

CN I Pathology

Sinonasal Polyposis

Sinonasal polyposis is the most frequent cause of CN I pathology.[69] The prevalence is 1% to 2% in the overall population with peak incidence in the sixth decade.[71,72] The condition is closely associated with asthma (40% of cases) and aspirin hypersensitivity (25% of cases). The polyps arise from inflammatory processes in the mucous membranes of the middle turbinate and middle meatus at their origin. Inferior turbinate involvement is rare.[73] The condition appears to be mostly clinically silent.[73] However, up to 17% of patients with sinonasal polyposis may present with symptoms including anosmia. Other more common presenting symptoms include nasal stuffiness, rhinorrhea, facial pain, and headache.[74]

Coronal CT is the preferred imaging modality and most commonly shows hypocellular polypoid fluid-densities and pansinus opacification. Other findings include infundibula enlargement, attenuated ethmoid trabeculae, ethmoid sinus opacification, convex lateral walls, and air-fluid levels.[74,75] Medical management is preferred, though endoscopic sinus surgery may be of benefit in severe obstructive cases. However, surgery does not appear to be effective in correcting hyposmia.[76,77]

Sarcoidosis and Wegener's Granulomatosis

Granulomatous disease of the sinonasal cavities is another leading cause of CN I dysfunction. Sarcoidosis of the nasal cavity and neurosarcoidosis of the anterior skull base have both been

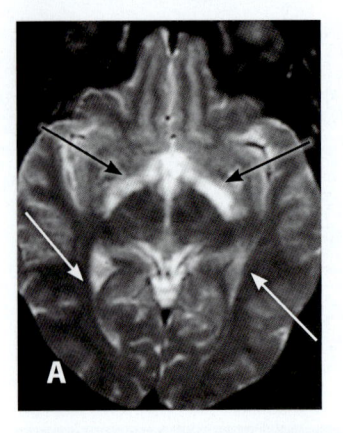

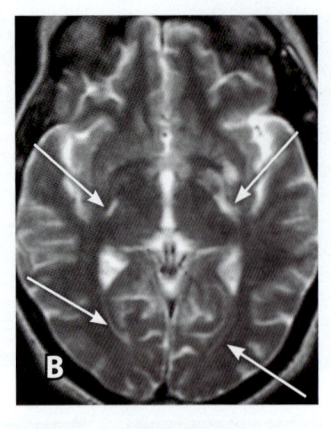

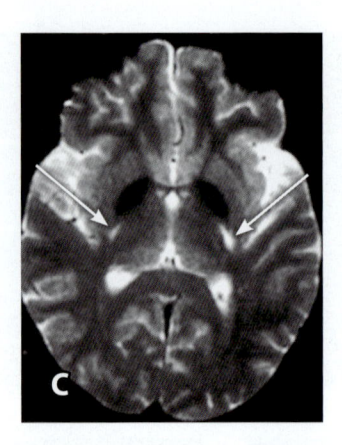

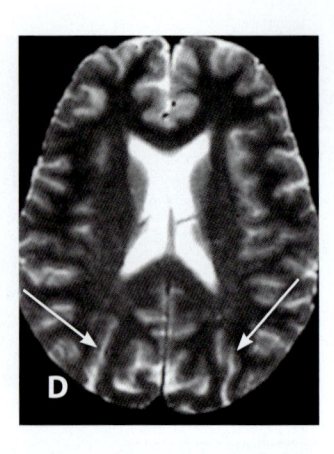

Figure 9-15 Postradiation Optic Tract Degeneration
Radiation-induced degeneration of the optic tract. Axial T2W MR images show abnormal high signal along the optic tracts (*white arrows*, **A–D**), subsequent to axonal degeneration. Notice the moustache appearance of the optic tract demyelination immediately distal to the optic chiasm (*black arrows*, **A**).

shown to cause anosmia (**Fig. 9-17**). In fact, up to 70% of patient cases with sinonasal sarcoidosis complain of anosmia in addition to stuffiness and rhinorrhea.[78,79]

Wegener's granulomatosis is a necrotizing granulomatous condition that affects the sinonasal cavity in up to 80% of cases and may be the sole site of clinical pathology in up to 30% of cases. In addition to the sinonasal cavities, the disease may also affect skin, kidney, and lung. The etiology remains unclear, but autoimmune processes have been implicated in the pathogenesis of Wegener's granulomatosis.[80] Though anosmia has been associated with sinonasal Wegener's granulomatosis, foul-smelling rhinorrhea and epistaxis are more common manifestations.[81] CT is the preferred imaging modality and will show bony destruction especially in the nasal septum. MR findings may include obliteration of periantral fat or infiltration of the maxillary nerve.[82]

Kallmann Syndrome

Kallmann syndrome, comprising combined hypogonadotropic hypogonadism and anosmia, is the result of primary failure of

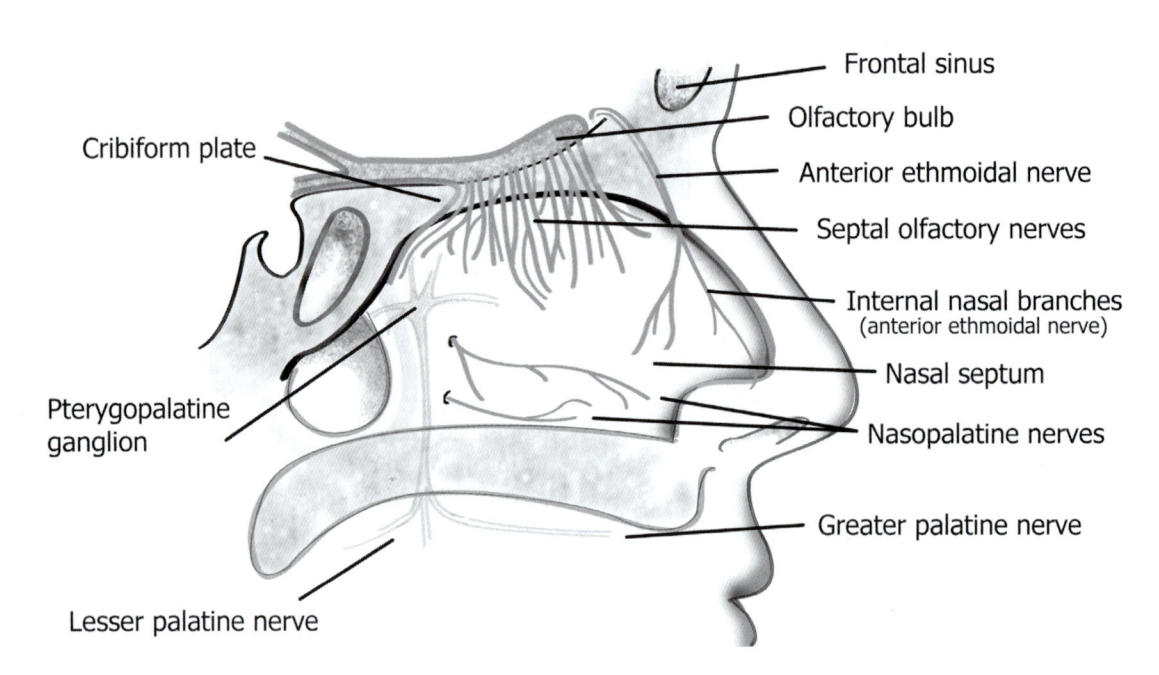

Figure 9-16 Olfactory Nerve and Nasal Septum
Sagittal schematic of the olfactory nerve fibers leaving the olfactory bulb, penetrating the cribriform plate into the superior nasal cavity. Other neural structures, including the branches of V1 and V2, are also depicted as they course through the region.

Table 9-9 CN I Function, Dysfunction, and Pathology

Function	Dysfunction	Pathology
Olfaction	**Anosmia** • Complete lack of olfaction **Hyposmia** • Reduced sense of olfaction **Hyperosmia** • Exaggeration of olfactory perception **Cacosmia** • Extremely unpleasant olfactory perception **Parosmia** • Perversion of sense of smell (perception of a smell other than that with which the stimulus was classically registered) **Phantosmia** • Olfactory hallucination **Other Pathologic Symptoms** • Nasal swelling • Epistaxis	**Sinonasal Cavities** • Sinonasal polyposis • Intranasal sarcoidosis • Wegener's granulomatosis • Non-Hodgkin's lymphoma • Sinonasal adenocarcinoma • Sinonasal melanoma • Olfactory neuroblastoma • Herpes, viral hepatitis infection **Anterior skull base** • Neurosarcoidosis • Aneurysm of anterior communicating artery • Schwannoma • Meningioma **Traumatic lesions** • Skull base fracture • Occipital blow • Surgical trauma during traction of frontal lobes **Congenital** • Kallmann syndrome • CHARGE syndrome **Toxic** • Tobacco, benzene, cement, ammonia, cocaine, nasal sprays, aminoglycosides, tetracyclines

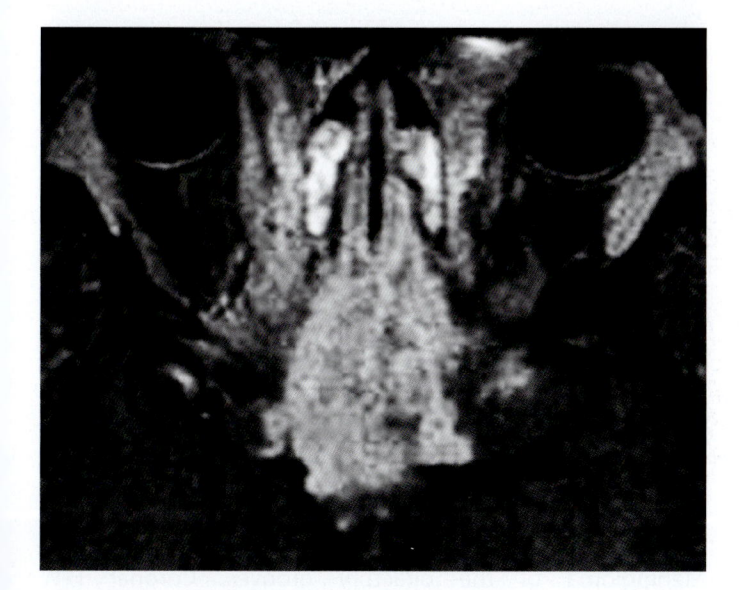

Figure 9-17 Olfactory Neurosarcoidosis
Axial T1W postcontrast MR image show a midline diffusely enhancing mass that occupies the nasal cavities and infiltrates the skull base in the area of the cavernous sinus.

olfactory nerve cell migration during development. Both olfactory neural tissue and luteinizing hormone-releasing hormone (LHRH) producing cells originate from the nasal placode during early embryologic period. Migration of olfactory neural tissue to the forebrain is necessary to induce olfactory bulb formation and also to guide migrating LHRH producing cells to their final destination in the hypothalamus. Failure of this initial migration results in primary anosmia and hypogonadotropic hypogonadism.[20,83] The prevalence of Kallmann Syndrome is 1 in 10,000 men and 1 in 50,000 women and may either be sporadic or inherited.[20] Mutations in fibroblast growth factor receptor-1 (FGFR1) have also been implicated in both inherited and sporadic cases.[84,85] Synkinesia and renal agenesis are also seen in some familial patterns of Kallmann Syndrome.[86]

Diagnosis of Kallmann syndrome involves documented clinical manifestations of anosmia, delayed puberty, micropenis, undescended testicles, and primary amenorrhea. Confirmation involves a gradated smell test to document complete anosmia and/or MRI to document absence of olfactory bulbs. Coronal high resolution fast spin echo T2W and T1W images show hypoplasia of both the olfactory sulci and the olfactory bulbs[87,88] (**Fig. 9-18**).Coronal CT imaging is not considered sensitive

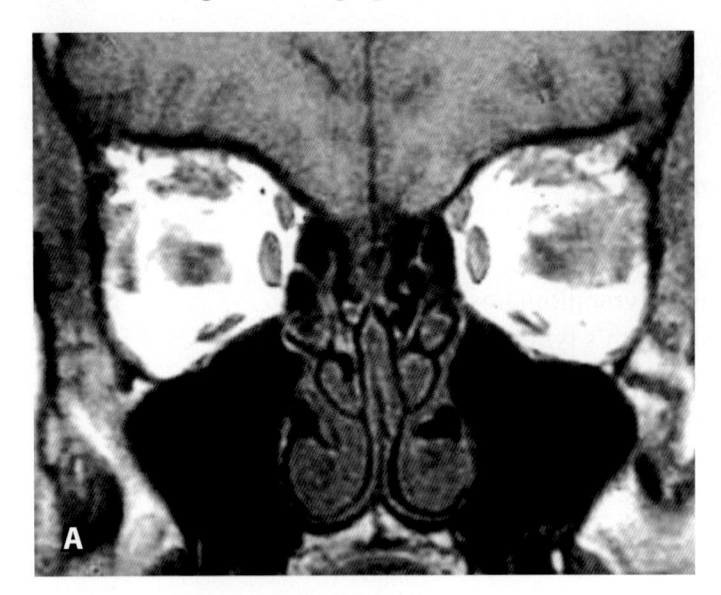

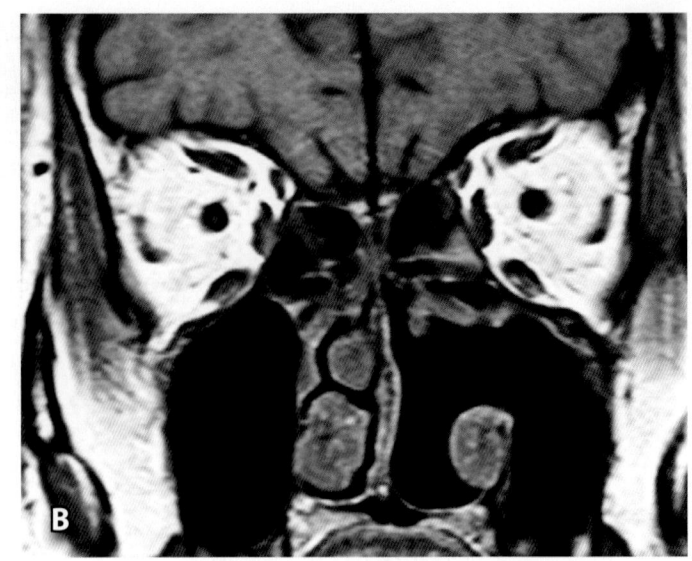

Figure 9-18 Kallmann Syndrome
Olfactory bulb aplasia in Kallmann syndrome. Coronal T1W MR image in an individual with Kallmann syndrome (**A**) shows absence of olfactory bulbs, as well as hypoplastic right olfactory gyrus. There is confirmatory absence of the olfactory sulci. Coronal T1W MR image in a normal individual for comparison (**B**) shows the normal bilateral olfactory sulci and olfactory nerves as they run inferiorly along the cribriform plate in the anterior skull base.

for detecting intracranial olfactory pathology. Fertility can be achieved in patients with Kallmann syndrome with pulsatile GnRH and maintenance hormone therapy.[20]

Neoplasia Affecting CN I

Neoplasia may affect CN I function either from within the sinonasal cavity or from the anterior skull base. Neoplasia affecting the sinonasal cavity includes olfactory neuroblastoma (esthesioneuroblastoma), non-Hodgkin's lymphoma, adenocarcinoma, and melanoma.

Common neoplastic processes that affect the anterior skull base include schwannoma and meningioma. Schwannomas of the olfactory nerve are rare, accounting for less than 4% of cranial nerve schwannomas. In addition to anosmia, olfactory nerve schwannomas may also present with nasal obstruction and epistaxis. Intracranial extension has also been observed.[16,89] See **Table 9-6** for imaging features of schwannomas. Meningiomas of the ethmoid, sphenoid wing, and olfactory grove account for approximately 10% of intracranial meningiomas and may cause anosmia[90] (**Fig. 9-19**).

Esthesioneuroblastoma

Olfactory neuroblastoma (esthesioneuroblastoma) is a rare malignant tumor of the olfactory neuroepithelium and makes up approximately 3% of tumors of the paranasal cavity. The tumor is locally destructive and may invade the ethmoid sinus, orbits, or cribriform plate. Presenting symptoms include nasal obstruction, rhinorrhea, epistaxis, and hyposmia or anosmia in more than half of patients. On CT and MR, esthesioneuroblastomas will often show a mass centered on the cribriform plate. The tumor is often hypointense on T1 images and isointense of hyperintense on T2. Focal areas of hemorrhage may be present and the tumor enhances intensely with contrast (**Fig. 9-20**). Cysts are often seen along the superior margins of the tumor and the anterior cranial fossa.[91] Treatment options include excision, chemotherapy, and radiation.[92]

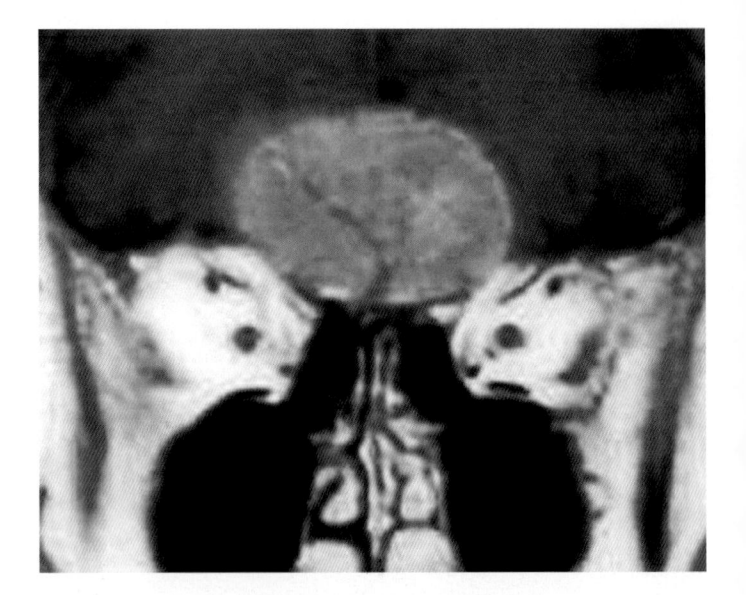

Figure 9-19 Olfactory Groove Meningioma
Meningioma of the olfactory grooves. Coronal T1W postcontrast image shows a symmetric, diffusely enhancing midline mass along the anterior skull base, with cephalad projection. Note that the lesion does not penetrate the nasal cavities and is sharply demarcated from brain parenchyma.

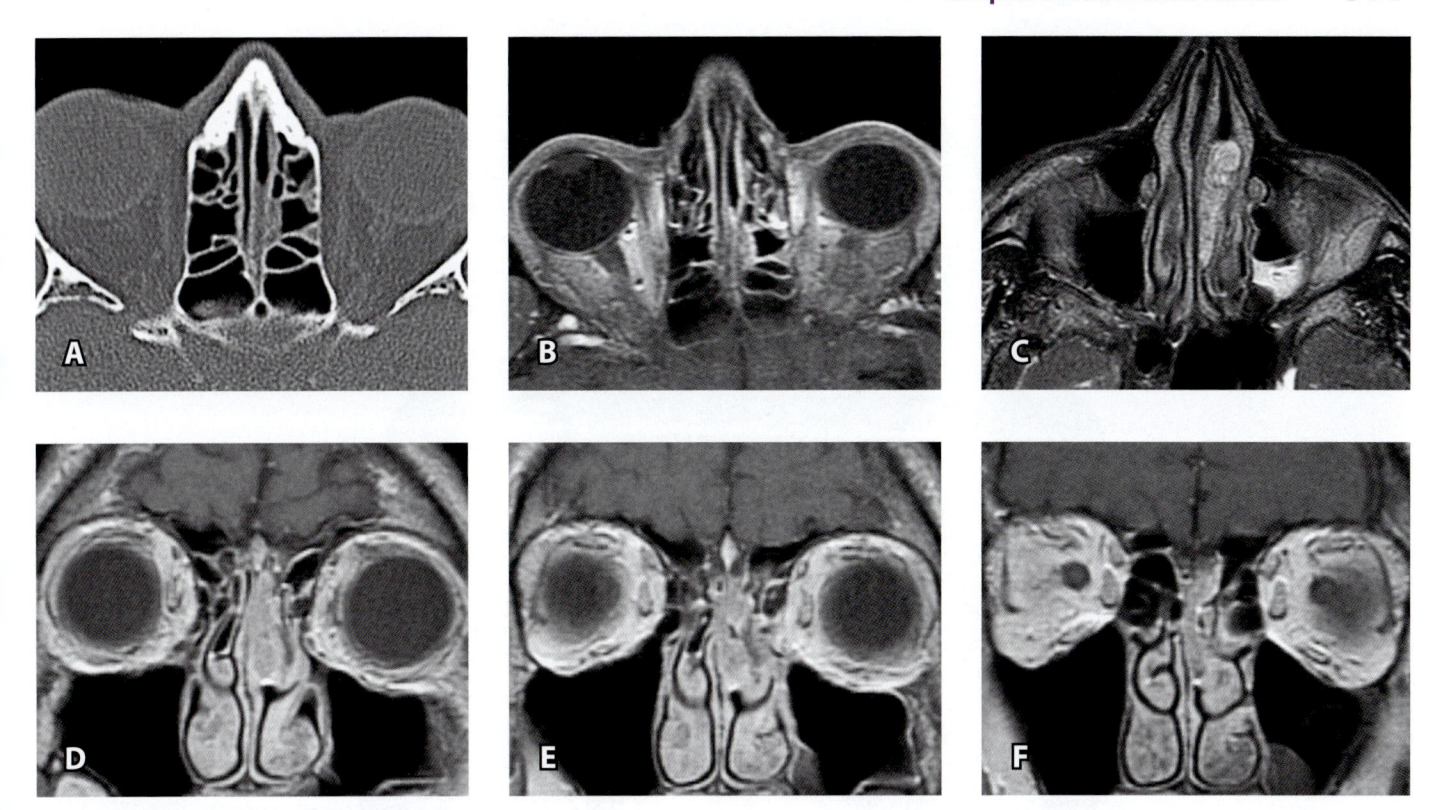

Figure 9-20 Esthesioneuroblastoma
Esthesioneuroblastoma in a 55-year-old male complaining of left-sided headaches and epistaxis. Axial NECT scan (**A**) and T1W postcontrast MR scans (**B–C**) show an enhancing soft tissue density mass in the left superoposterior portion of the olfactory recess at the level of the cribriform plate (**A–B**) with inferior extension into the nasal cavity (**C**) and little associated bony destruction (**A**). Coronal T1W contrast-enhanced MR scans (**D–F**) show the mass at the level of the cribriform plate with inferior extension into the nasal cavity (**D**). In the posterior segments of the nasal cavity, contiguous intracranial extension through the cribriform plate can be appreciated (**E–F**).

Other CN I Pathologies

CN I hypoplasia and aplasia are commonly associated with a syndrome comprising coloboma, heart disease, atresia choanae, retarded growth and mental development, genital anomalies, and ear malformation (CHARGE syndrome). It has been reported in some studies that all children with CHARGE syndrome have deficits in olfaction ranging from hyposmia to complete anosmia.[93] Fetal MRI has documented cranial absence of olfactory sulci and bulbs in up to 25% patients with CHARGE syndrome.[94]

Other lesions affecting CN I include aneurysm of the anterior communicating artery, skull base fractures, surgical trauma, and herpes or viral hepatitis infections. Toxic damage to CN I also accounts for cases of anosmia and may be caused by tobacco, benzene, cement, ammonia, cocaine, nasal sprays, aminoglycosides, or tetracyclines.[69]

OPTIC NERVE – CN II

The optic nerve is solely responsible for carrying visual information to the calcarine cortex and is unique among the cranial nerves in that its oligodendrocyte myelination and meningeal coverings classify it as a forward extension of the CNS, rather than a component of the PNS. Lesions anywhere along the course of the nerve may present with varied degrees of visual field loss (**Fig. 9-21**).

The optic fibers originate in the calcarine portion of the occipital cortex and travel superiorly, inferiorly, and laterally to the occipital horn of the ventricle. The optic fibers then become the optic radiations as they course over the temporal horn of the lateral ventricle and the tail of the caudate nucleus to enter the lateral geniculate body of the thalamus. Bilateral optic tracts then exit the lateral geniculate bodies and meet in the midline to form the optic chiasm. From the optic chiasm ventrally, the optic fibers then divide into bilateral optic nerves coursing initially into the cranial openings of the optic canals. The optic nerves exit the orbital openings of the optic canals and extend forward in a sinusoidal manner to enter the globes at the optic nerve heads.

Pathology of CN II

Pathology of CN II can arise from a variety of processes, both intrinsic and extrinsic to the nerve. Intraorbital optic neuropathy encompasses a wide variety of possible CN II lesions that

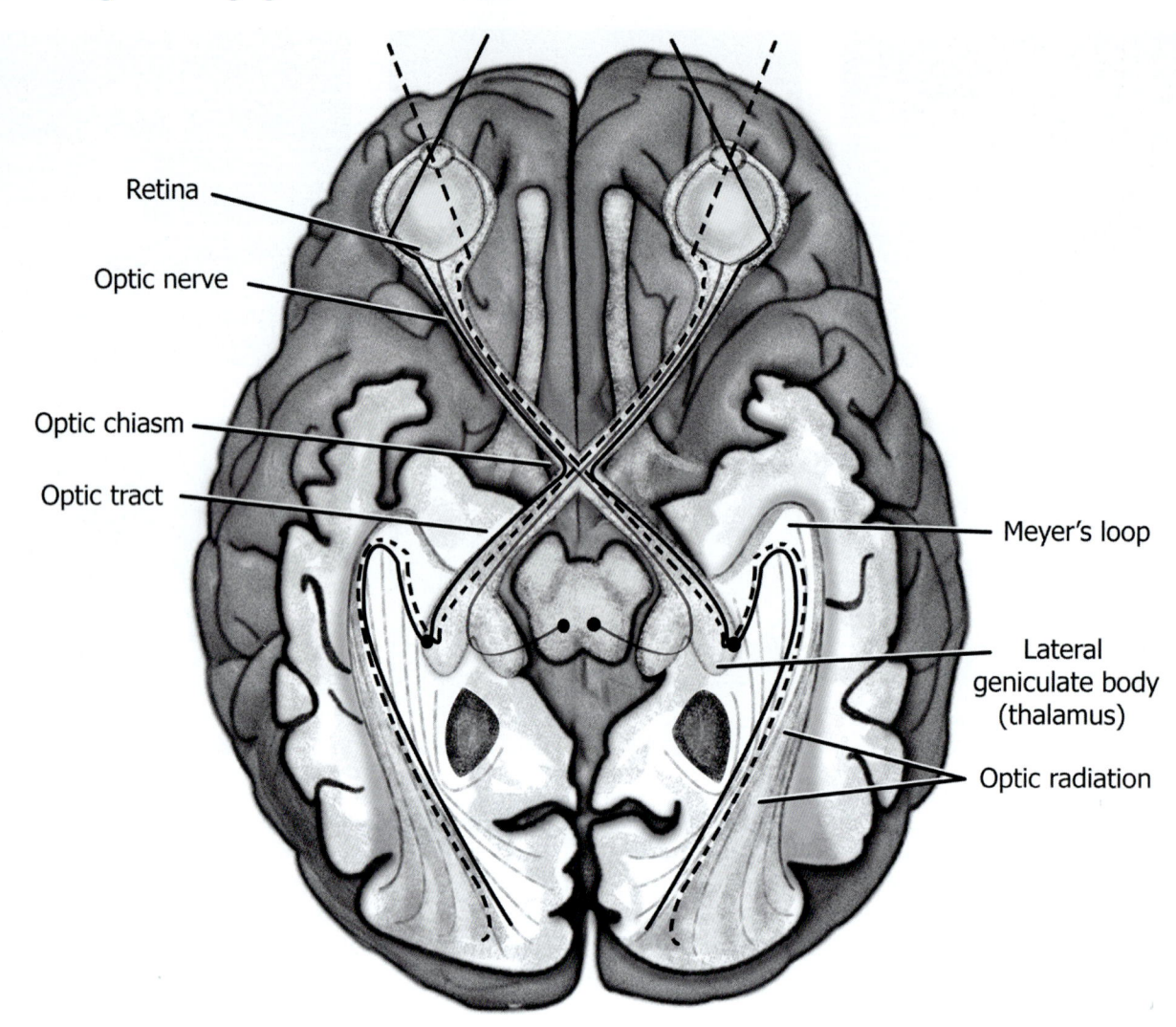

Figure 9-21 Visual Pathway
Axial view schematic depicting the optic nerves and intra-axial visual pathways.

are outlined in detail in Chapter 2. Common causes of CN II pathology include congenital septo-optic dysplasia, optic nerve glioma, optic sheath meningioma, pituitary tumor mass effect, Meyer's loop involvement by intra-axial processes, and radiation-induced optic neuritis (**Fig. 9-15**). Optic neuritis caused by multiple sclerosis, neuromyelitis optica, and other pathologies listed in **Table 9-8** are also commonly visualized on MRI as enhancing optic nerve lesions. **Table 9-10** outlines common pathologies by region of optic nerve and resultant clinical manifestation.[95]

NERVES OF THE EXTRAOCULAR MUSCLES – CN III, IV, VI

CN III, IV, and VI are responsible for coordinating the movements of the six extraocular muscles functioning in the elevation, depression, abduction, adduction, intorsion, and extorsion of the eye. Palsies of any of the oculomotor nerves result in varying combination of ophthalmoplegias as described in **Table 9-11**.[43,96,97]

Function of the Nerves of the Extraocular Muscles

CN III Anatomy and Function

CN III, or the oculomotor nerve, is responsible for the majority of the six eye movements by supplying motor innervation of the medial rectus, superior rectus, inferior rectus, and inferior oblique ocular muscles. Furthermore, parasympathetic innervation to the pupillary and ciliary muscles in the eye, as well as sympathetic innervation to the levator palpebrae superioris, course with the nerve. Dysfunction of any portion of the nerve will present with combinations of oculomotor palsy, pupil dilation, and ptosis (**Table 9-11**). The motor component of cranial nerve III originates in the motor cortex of the cerebrum. The fibers then travel centrally through the internal capsule to the

Table 9-10 Segmental Pathology of CN II

Segment	Pathology Symptoms	Pathology Etiology
Prechiasmal	loss of monocular vision loss of parasympathetics	• Demyelinating neuritis (Table 9-8) • Meningioma • Glioma • Metastases • Retinoblastoma • Sarcoidosis • Pseudotumor • Orbital sarcoidosis • Orbital lymphoproliferative disease • Orbital tuberculosis • Retinoblastoma • Wegener's granulomatosis • Histiocytosis
Chiasmal Lesions	bitemporal hemianopsia	• Pituitary tumor • Craniopharyngioma • Septo-optic dysplasia
Postchiasmal Lesions	homonymous hemianopsia	• Intra-axial space-occupying lesion
Temporal (Meyer's Loop)	contralateral quandrantopia	

ipsilateral superior colliculus. The fibers cross between the red nuclei in the dorsal tegmental decussation and continue distally in the paramedian raphe to synapse in the pontine reticular formation. The fibers then ascend in the medial longitudinal fasciculus to the oculomotor nucleus, which is situated in the paramedian midbrain tegmentum ventral to the aqueduct of Sylvius, at the level of the superior colliculus. At this level, additional fibers from the parasympathetic nucleus, paramedian nucleus, Perlia's nucleus, and Edinger–Westphal nucleus join the motor fibers. These combined fibers bow laterally to extend through the medial aspect of the red nucleus and cerebral peduncle. Fibers then exit from the brainstem anteriorly at the pontomedullary junction near the midline, where the two nerves form parallel structures in a "V" configuration as they extend through the interpeduncular fossa.[70] The oculomotor nerves then travel between the superior cerebellar and posterior cerebral arteries through the prepontine cistern. As CN III enters the cavernous sinus along the superolateral margin, it courses though a dura and arachnoid lined, CSF-filled, avascular cuff known as the oculomotor cistern along the lateral wall of the cavernous sinus [98] (Fig. 9-22). The oculomotor nerve rises superiorly along the lateral wall of the cavernous sinus adjacent to the fourth cranial nerve and above the sixth cranial nerve and ophthalmic division of the fifth cranial nerve. The parasympathetic and motor fibers are in close proximity, and together the fibers penetrate the superior orbital fissure to reach the orbital structures.

CN IV Anatomy and Function

CN IV is also known as the trochlear nerve because it innervates the superior oblique muscle, which courses through the trochlea of the superior orbit. Dysfunction of this nerve causes paralysis of the superior oblique muscle and associated difficulty with intorsion and elevation of the globe (Table 9-11). The motor impulses of cranial nerve IV originate in the motor cortex and then extend centrally via the internal capsule to the ipsilateral superior colliculus. The fibers cross between the red nuclei in the dorsal tegmental decussation and travel caudally in the paramedial raphe to synapse in the pontine reticular formation. The fibers then ascend in the medial longitudinal fasciculus to reach the motor nucleus. The fourth cranial nerve nucleus is located in the tegmentum of the mesencephalon at the level of the inferior colliculus, immediately caudal to the third nerve nucleus. Fibers from the nucleus loop posteriorly to decussate in the tectum of the lower midbrain beneath the inferior colliculi. This pathway forms a sickle-shaped arch around the aqueduct of Sylvius. The trochlear nerve exits from the dorsal aspect of the brainstem, emerging from the superior medullary vellum just beneath the inferior colliculus. The trochlear is the only cranial nerve that exists on the dorsum of the brainstem and crosses to innervate the contralateral side. The nerve extends around the cerebral peduncle between the superior cerebellar and posterior cerebral arteries, just lateral to the third cranial nerve. The nerve then enters the cavernous sinus along the superolateral margin and courses inferior to CN III and superior to CN V1 along the

Table 9-11 Function, Dysfunction, and Isolated Pathologies of the Nerves of the Extraocular Muscle Nerves

CN	Muscle	Function	Dysfunction	Isolated Pathology Causes
CN III — Second most common involvement	superior rectus	globe elevation	unopposed superior oblique and lateral rectus drive: • Downward, laterally displaced, intorted eye "down and out"	microvascular disease > aneurysm > trauma > neoplasia
	medial rectus	globe adduction		
	inferior rectus	globe depression		
	inferior oblique	globe extorsion globe elevation globe abduction		
	levator palpebrae superioris	superior lid retraction	ptosis	
	pupillary sphincter and ciliary muscle (parasympathetics)	pupillary constriction accommodation.	pupillary dilation	aneurysm > microvascular disease > trauma and neoplasia
CN IV	superior oblique	globe intorsion globe depression globe abduction	• Vertical or torsional diplopia, worse with downward contralateral gaze. • Compensating head tilt away from affected lesion.	head trauma > microvascular disease > neoplasia and idiopathic causes

CN VI — Most frequent isolated cranial neuropathy	lateral rectus	globe abduction	lateral rectus palsy, convergent strabismus, esotropia
			• Inability of lateral deviation of eye on lateral gaze
				• Aneurysm > neoplasia > trauma, cavernous aneurysm, carotid-cavernous fistula, petrous apex pathology, and increased intracranial pressure
				• "Pseudolesions"
				  • Myasthenia gravis
				  • Pseudotumor
				  • Orbital thyroid disease

			intranuclear ophthalmoplegia • Defect in adduction of contralateral eye on conjugate lateral eye gaze	• Multiple sclerosis • Brainstem lesions (also commonly coinfect CN VII)

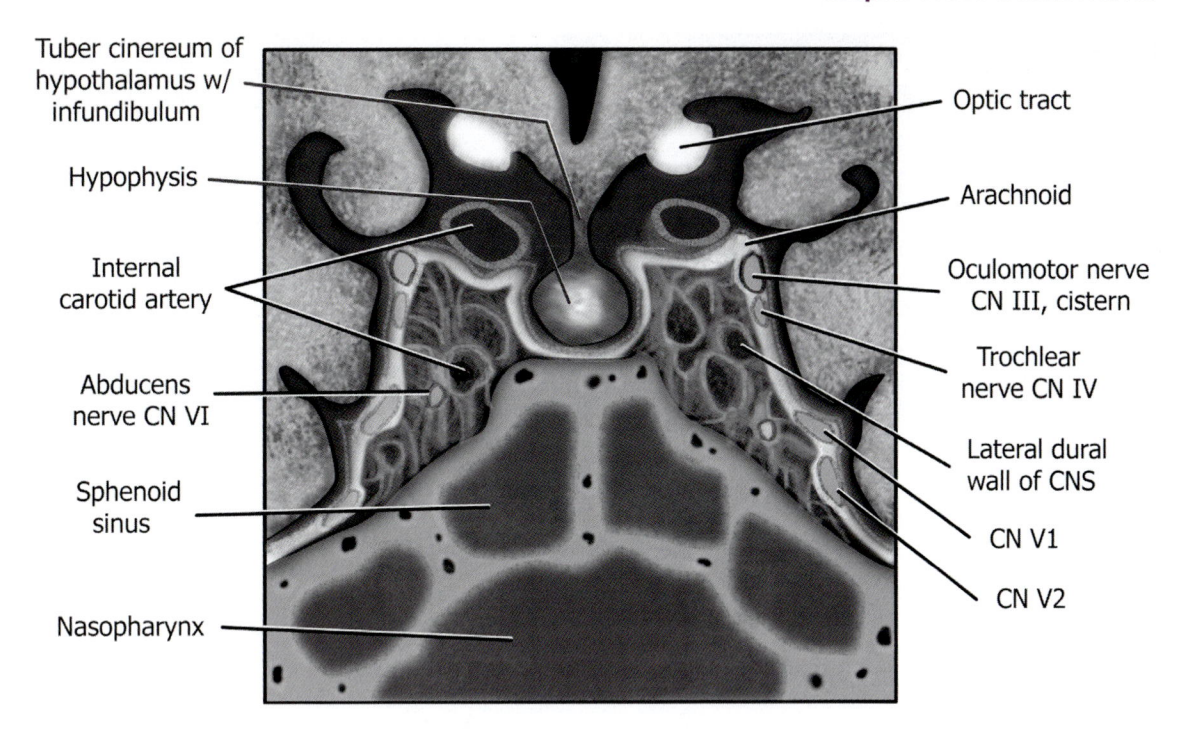

Figure 9-22 Cavernous Sinus
Coronal schematic in a posterior-anterior view showing the course of CN III, IV, V, VI as they traverse the cavernous sinus. Note that the only CN to freely course through the cavernous sinus is CN VI, while the others course in the lateral wall of the sinus.

lateral wall of the cavernous sinus en route to the superior orbital fissure[70,98] (**Fig. 9-22**).

CN VI Anatomy and Function

CN VI, or abducens nerve, is provides the innervation of the lateral rectus muscle. Dysfunction of the nerve leads to lateral rectus palsy and difficulties with lateral gaze (**Table 9-11**). The impulses of cranial nerve VI originate in the motor cortex of the cerebral hemisphere. The fibers extend through the internal capsule and the corticobulbar tract to the ipsilateral superior colliculus. At this point, the fibers cross between the red nuclei in the dorsal tegmental decussation, extending caudally in the paramedian raphe of the brainstem to synapse in the pontine reticular formation. Both ipsilateral and contralateral fibers ascend in the medial longitudinal fasciculus to reach the brainstem nucleus of the abducens nerve, which lies in the pons immediately anterior to the fourth ventricle. These fibers pass through the pontine tegmentum and exit anteriorly from the brainstem at the pontomedullary junction. The abducens nerve then courses superiorly and slightly laterally along the clivus. At the base of the dorsum sella, the sixth cranial nerve courses anteriorly, piercing through the dura at Dorello's canal to enter the cavernous sinus. The nerve then extends obliquely through the cavernous sinus just inferior and medial to CN III and IV, immediately adjacent to the cavernous portion of the internal carotid artery. CN VI and is the only cranial nerve to directly penetrate and travel through the cavernous sinus [98] (**Fig. 9-22**). The nerve then enters the superior oblique fissure en route to the lateral rectus muscle. Coordination between CN III, IV, and VI is mediated through the medial longitudinal fasciculus (MLF), which is located anterior to the floor of the fourth ventricle.[70]

Pathology of the Nerves to the Extraocular Muscles

Syndromes of the Nerves to the Extraocular Muscles

Despite several causes of isolated oculomotor nerve palsies outlined in **Table 9-11**, most clinically evident oculomotor nerve lesions present in combination. Because the oculomotor nerves are intimately associated throughout much of their course, specific constellations of symptoms are helpful in localizing pathology involving these nervous structures; syndromes describing these symptoms are contained in **Table 9-12**. The region of the orbital apex includes the most posterior portion of the orbit, the optic nerve, the annulus of Zinn, and branches of CN III, IV, VI, and the ophthalmic branch of CN V as they penetrate the superior orbital fissure. The superior orbital fissure lies posterior to the orbital apex and thus pathology at this location affects all the structures contained in the orbital apex, but does not involve the optic nerve, which is separated from the fissure by the optic strut. Pathology of the cavernous sinus may affect all of the nervous structures penetrating the superior orbital fissure, as well as CN V2 and the oculosympathetic nerves that traverse the sinus. Because the orbital apex, superior orbital fissure, and cavernous sinus are contiguous, syndromes may progress from one region to another. Common regional pathologies of the ocular cranial nerves are contained in **Table 9-13** [99] (**Fig. 9-23**).

Table 9-12 Extraocular Muscle Nerve Syndromes

Syndrome	Brainstem Lesions	CN II Visual Impairment	CN III Diplopia	CN IV Downward gaze weakness	CN VI Lateral rectus palsy	CN V1 Retrobulbar pain	CN V2 Facial pain and numbness	Ocular Sympathetics Ptosis, miosis
Weber Syndrome (anterior midbrain lesion)	hemiparesis		X					
Benedikt Syndrome (red nucleus lesion)	contralateral tremor		X					
Orbital Apex Syndrome		X	X	X	X	X		
Superior Orbital Fissure Syndrome			X	X	X	X		
Cavernous Sinus Syndrome			X	X	X	X	X	X

Aneurysm

Aneurysm of the posterior communicating artery (PCA) is a common cause of isolated painful CN III pathology. It is estimated that over 90% of patients will present with oculomotor palsy prior to aneurysm rupture. Aneurysms are thought to affect 5% of the population and may grow larger than 25 mm before rupturing. Clinically, anisocoria is observed more frequently in aneurysm than with microvascular disease. Pain may be present in both conditions. Less frequently, palsies of CN III may result from aneurysm or dolichoectasia of the posterior cerebral, superior cerebellar, or basilar arteries.[100]

Table 9-13 Pathology of the Nerves to the Extraocular Muscles by Location

Midbrain	Cavernous Sinus	Intraorbital	Intrinsic Nerve

• Multiple sclerosis
• Midbrain infarct
• Meningeal carcinomatosis
• Brainstem glioma
• Cavernous malformation
• Fourth ventricle pathology
  • Ependymoma
  • Papilloma
• Pinealoma
	• Meningioma
	• Primary CNS lymphoma
	• Metastases
	• Cavernous sinus thrombosis
	• Carotid-cavernous fistula
	• Cavernous carotid aneurysm
	• Pituitary apoplexy
	• Tuberculosis
		• Idiopathic orbital inflammatory disease
		• Orbital pseudotumor
		• Orbital lymphoproliferative lesions
		• Orbital metastasis
		• Orbital cellulitis
		• Mucormycosis
		• HSV
			• Neurofibromatosis 1
			• Schwannoma
			• Demyelinating neuritis (Table 9-8)
			• Leukemia
			• Cavernous malformation

HSV = herpes simplex virus.

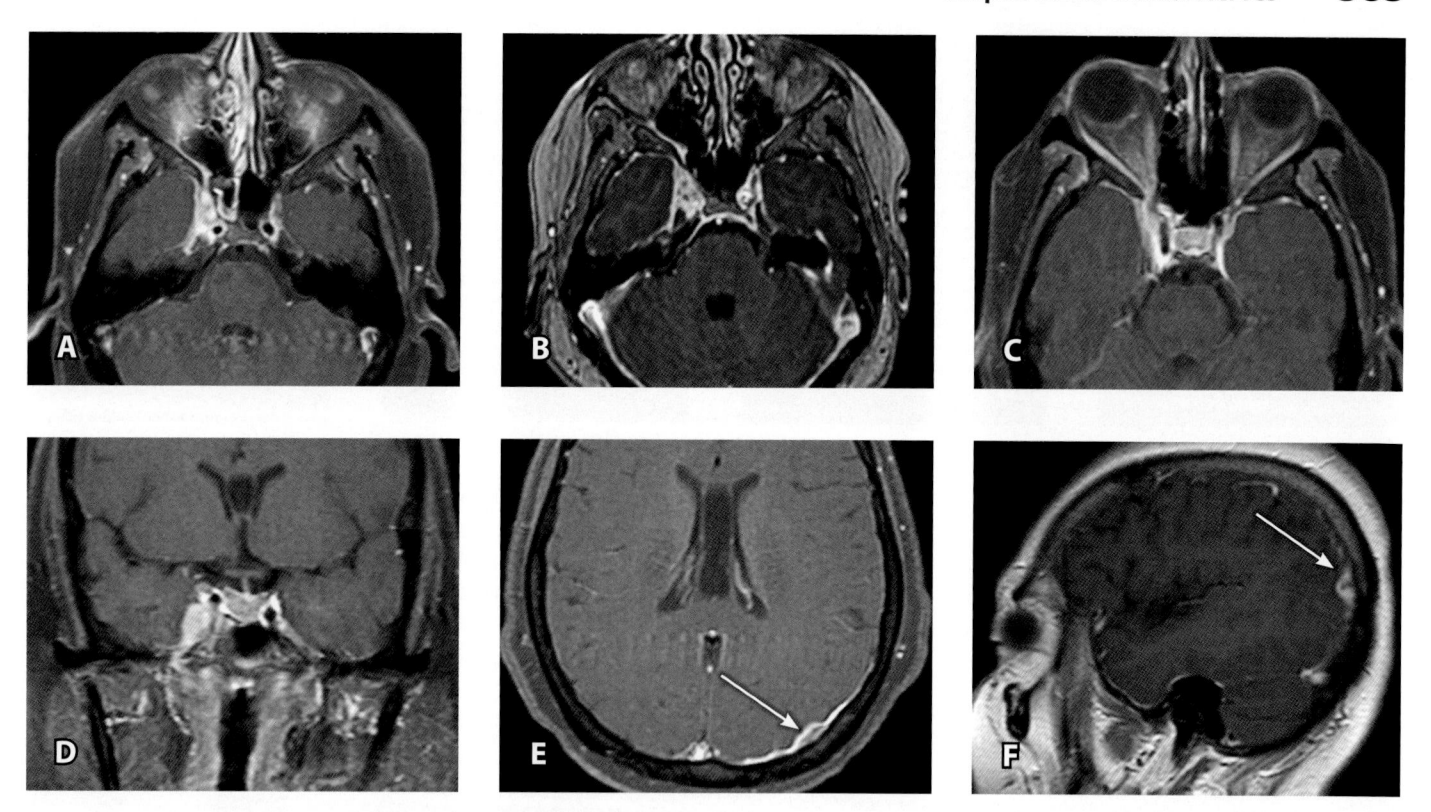

Figure 9-23 Cavernous Sinus and Dural Based Tuberculosis
Intracranial tuberculosis in a patient with right cavernous sinus syndrome. Axial (**A–C**), coronal (**D**), and sagittal (**F**) T1W postcontrast images show multifocal enhancing lesions of the meninges and brain parenchyma. Particularly affected is the cavernous sinus, which has compressed and irritated cranial nerves as they traverse it. Dural biopsy confirmed tuberculous (*white arrows*, **E** and **F**).

In addition to PCA aneurysm, fusiform dilations of the cavernous carotid artery may also cause cranial nerve palsies. Because of the close proximity of CN VI to the carotid artery in the cavernous sinus, lateral rectus palsy is often the presenting symptom of an aneurysm of this vessel (**Fig. 9-24**).

MRI and MRA are often used to screen for aneurysms, but may miss smaller lesions. CTA is considered more sensitive than MRA, but digital subtraction angiography is still the gold standard for diagnosing aneurysms, especially those less than 5 mm in diameter [100] (**Fig. 9-25**).

Microvascular Disease

Microvascular disease secondary to diabetes and hypertension is a common cause of nerve atrophy and demyelination in the population older than 50-years-old. Vascular ischemia affects the core of the nerve before the outer segments, perhaps accounting for the usual pupil-sparing presentation and negative MR imaging on early lesions. Microvascular disease is most common in CN III, but may also be present in CN IV.[101]

Trauma

Traumatic injuries to CN III, IV, and VI are among the leading three causes of isolated cranial nerve palsy.[96] Among all of the cranial nerves, CN IV is most frequently damaged as a result of even slight trauma. It is generally accepted that the narrow 1,500 axon diameter of the nerve, its long course, and its close relationship to other intracerebral structures including the tentorium predispose this nerve to traumatic injury. CN IV takes the longest course of any of the ocular muscle nerves and is the only cranial nerve to exit the dorsal brainstem. As the nerve fibers turn caudally, they pass directly under the tentorium, located superolaterally to the pons. It is thought that this site of intimate relationship with the fibrous tentorium is the location of most injuries to CN IV.[102] Other traumatic ocular nerve injuries may occur in cases of hemorrhagic brainstem injury or fractures of either the petrosal bone or the small wing of the sphenoid. Nerve compression and stretching by petroclival neoplasia may also predispose all ocular nerves to traumatic injury.[101]

Increases in intracranial pressures due to trauma, meningitis, or other causes may manifest as ocular nerve palsies. Though papilledema of CN II and bilateral CN VI nerve palsies are the most frequent manifestations of increased intracranial pressure, palsies of CN III and IV may also be seen. In cases of severe increased intracranial pressure and frank herniation, nerve roots may be compressed by supratentorial cerebrum as they exit the brainstem.[102]

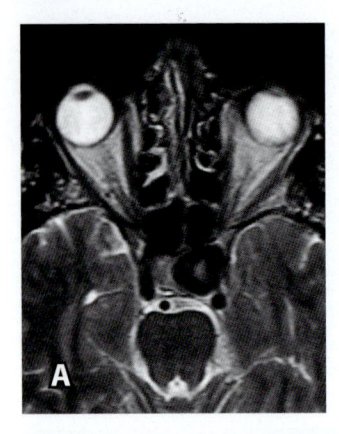

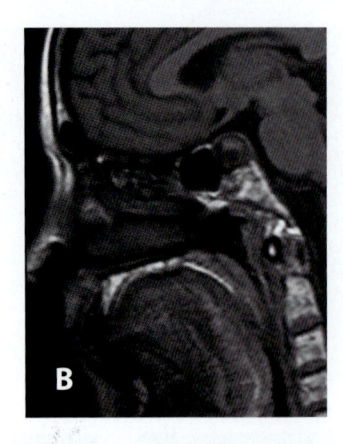

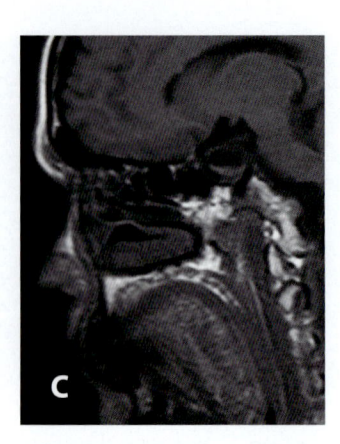

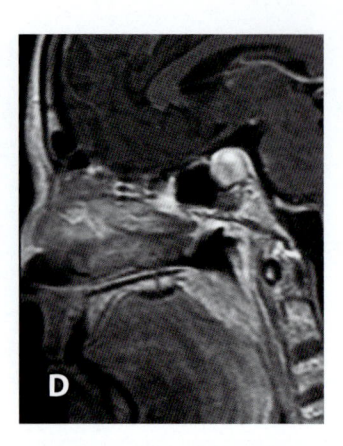

Figure 9-24 Cavernous Carotid Aneurysm with CN VI Palsy
Cavernous–carotid aneurysm in a patient with lateral rectus palsy. Axial T2W (**A**), sagittal T1W (**B–C**), and sagittal T1W with contrast (**D**) MR images show a large saccular aneurysmal dilatation of the left internal carotid artery as it traverses the posterosuperior portion of the cavernous sinus. Heterogenous enhancing signal (**D**) with flow voids (**A**) suggests the presence of intraluminal thrombus. The aneurysm directly abuts the lateral wall of the cavernous sinus (**A**) in the region of CN VI and displaces the posterior genu of the cavernous carotid posterolaterally.

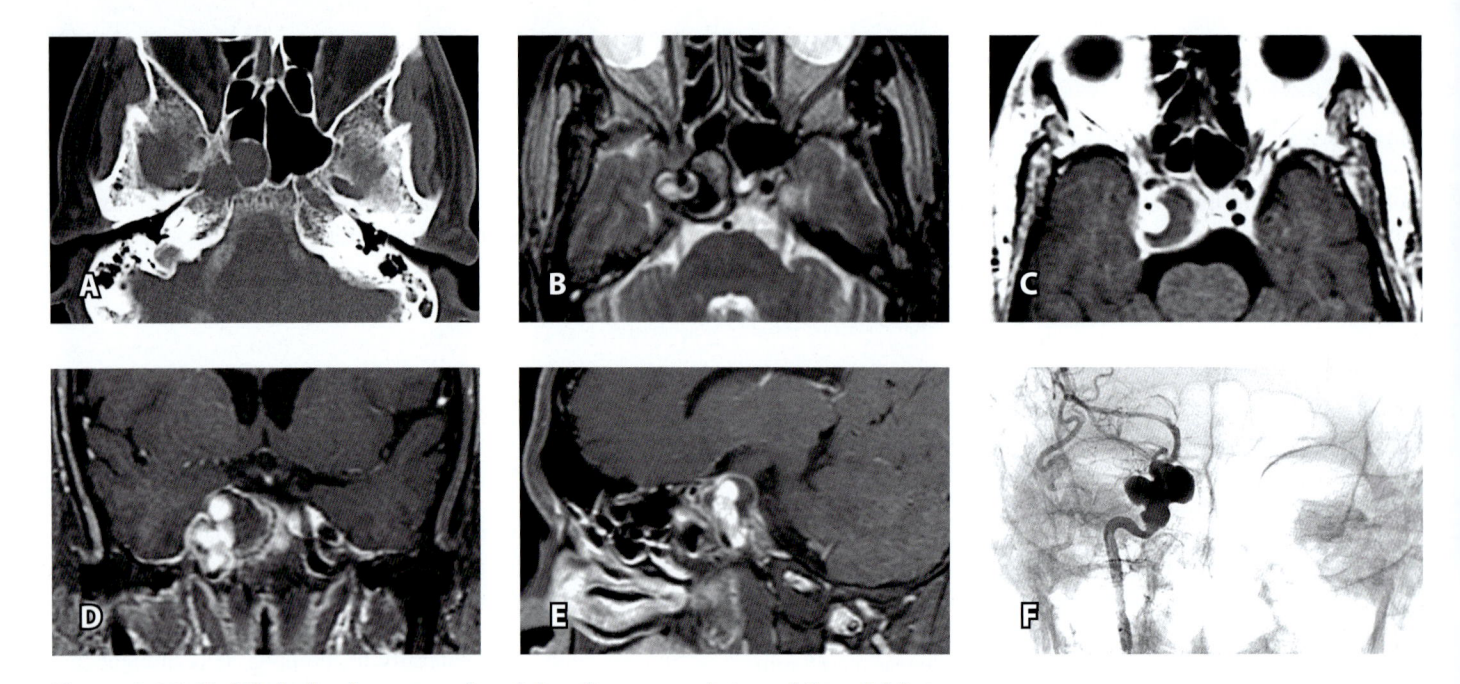

Figure 9-25 Multilobular Aneurysm Involving Cavernous Internal Carotid Artery
Multilobular aneurysm involving cavernous internal carotid artery of mycotic origin in a patient with cavernous sinus syndromes. Axial NECT (**A**) shows a smooth expansion on the anterior wall of the internal carotid canal, expanding into the sphenoid sinus. Axial T2W (**B**) and T1W MR (**C**) images show a complex, heterogenous signal in the lumen of the aneurysm with small patent flow voids. Coronal (**D**) and sagittal (**E**) T1W postcontrast MR images reveal areas of organized thrombus in the medial wall of the aneurysm and multilobar patent walls of the lateral part of the aneurysm. The mass is also seen expanding into the contralateral part of the cavernous sinus (**D**), posteriorly to the brainstem (**E**), and superiorly to the level of the optic chiasm (**E**). DSA of the right internal carotid artery (**F**) confirms a large, multilobulated lesion, consistent of infectious pseudoaneurysm caused by multifocal vessel wall weakening and expansion.

Ophthalmoplegic Migraine

Ophthalmoplegic migraine is a rare migraine variant that also causes paresis of CN III, IV, or VI during symptomatic episodes. The disease most commonly affects children and its exact etiology has not been determined, though it is hypothesized to be a demyelinating neuropathy.[103] Enhancement of CN III at the root exit zone during symptomatic episodes, followed by resolution of enhancement during asymptomatic episodes has been documented.[103] Focal swelling of CN III, IV, and VI have also been reported. Patients typically respond to steroid treatments.[103]

Tolosa-Hunt Syndrome

Tolosa-Hunt syndrome is a rare idiopathic granulomatous cause of pathology at the cavernous sinus or orbital apex and is characterized by unilateral orbital pain with ipsilateral ophthalmoplegia involving CN III, CN IV, or CN VI.[104] In addition to the concurrent onset of orbital pain and ophthalmoplegia for a duration of 2 weeks, the International Headache Society guidelines for Tolosa-Hunt diagnosis require MR or biopsy proven granuloma in the region of the orbital apex, in addition to clinical response to corticosteroids within 72 hours.[105] MRI is more sensitive than CT in the diagnosis of Tolosa-Hunt syndrome and usually reveals a soft tissue lesion that is isointense to gray matter on T1 and T2 imaging and may be viewed as a convexity of the lateral wall of the cavernous sinus. Granulomas will also enhance moderately with contrast administration. Compression of the cavernous internal carotid artery may also be noted. Resolution of the granuloma following corticosteroid treatment can also be visualized with follow-up MRI and may be necessary in the differentiation of the painful ophthalmoplegia from other conditions, including meningioma and pituitary adenoma, or carotid pathology.[106–109]

Petrous Apex Pathology

Pathology at the petrous apex of the temporal bone may affect CN VI as it passes through Dorello's canal and CN V in the region of Meckel's cave. In addition to CN V and CN VI pathology, lesions may cause CN VII and CN VIII palsies in the lateral portions of the petrous apex. The diverse causes of pathology involving the petrous part of the temporal bone have been covered extensively in Chapter 11, and are summarized in **Table 9-14** (**Fig. 9-26**).

CRANIAL NERVES OF THE CEREBELLOPONTINE ANGLE – CN V, VII, VIII

The CPA is a subarachnoid space bounded by petrous temporal bone, the pons, and the anterior part of the cerebellum. The cistern includes CN V superiorly and extends caudally to the level of the jugular foramen nerve complex (CN IX, X, and XI). CN VII, CN VIII, and the AICA loop traverse this CSF-enclosed space (**Fig. 9-27**).

CN V Anatomy and Function

CN V is also known as the trigeminal nerve and is the source of sensory innervation to most of the face, in addition to providing

Table 9-14 Common Causes of Petrous Apex Pathology

- Petrous apicitis
- Cholesterol granuloma
- Cholesteatoma
- CSF/arachnoid cyst
- CSF cephalocele
- Mucocele
- Petrous carotid aneurysm
- Chondroid tumor
- Chordoma
- Meningioma
- Metastasis

motor innervation to the muscles of mastication. Dysfunction of the sensory portion of this nerve often causes facial burning or numbness, while motor symptoms may include weakness of the muscles of mastication (**Fig. 9-28**, **Table 9-15**).

Sensory Trigeminal Division

The sensory impulses from the upper, middle, and lower part of the face extend to the gasserian ganglion via the ophthalmic (V1), maxillary (V2), and mandibular (V3) branches of cranial nerve V. These branches enter the skull via the superior orbital fissure, foramen rotundum, and foramen ovale, respectively. The ophthalmic and maxillary divisions usually extend along the lateral wall of the cavernous sinus, while the mandibular branch bypasses the cavernous sinus and directly enters the trigeminal (gasserian) ganglion.[98] This ganglion lies in the inferior portion of Meckel's cavity and contains the cell bodies of numerous afferent sensory fibers. Sensory impulses from the face then leave the trigeminal ganglion to enter the midlateral pons through the prepontine cistern. As they enter the brainstem, branches go to the three sensory nuclei: The principal sensory nucleus, the mesencephalic nucleus, and the spinal nucleus. Pain and temperature fibers descend to the C2 to C3 cord level where they synapse in the spinal nucleus of cranial nerve V. These fibers then cross the midline ascending in the ventral trigeminal lemniscus to reach the ventral posteromedial nucleus of the thalamus. The thalamocortical tract then carries the fibers via the internal capsule to the sensory cortex. The sensory impulses that mediate proprioception from the face, particularly of the mandible, synapse in the mesencephalic nucleus of cranial nerve V, which extends superiorly into the periaqueductal gray matter of the midbrain. This portion of the sensory nucleus is composed of the sensory neurons that travel with the mandibular nerve. Sensory nerves that mediate touch and pressure from the face synapse in the principal sensory nucleus of cranial nerve V and travel to the ventral posteromedial nucleus of the thalamus via the contralateral dorsal trigeminal lemniscus. The extension to the sensory cortex is via the thalamocortical tract, which passes through the internal capsule.[70]

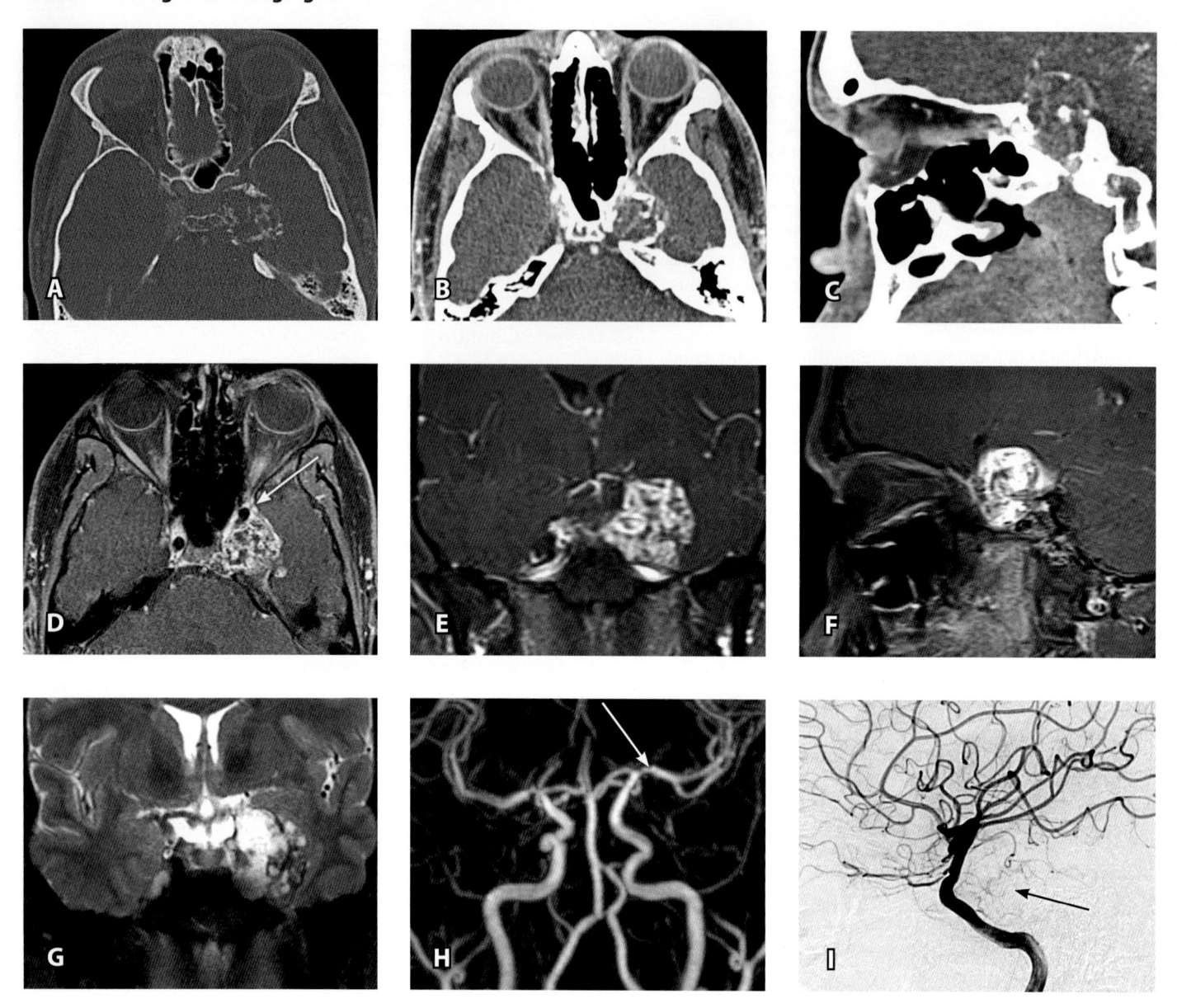

Figure 9-26 Chondrosarcoma of the Petrous Apex
A 15-year-old male with chondrosarcoma of the left petrous apex, presenting with cavernous sinus syndrome and left proptosis. Axial NECT bone algorithm (**A**), axial soft tissue window NECT (**B**), and sagittal NECT soft tissue window (**C**) show paramedian destructive, sclerotic bone lesions at the level of the left cavernous sinus with superior extension into the region of the left frontal lobe (**C**). Axial (**D**), coronal (**E**), and sagittal (**F**) T1W postcontrast MR images show heterogeneous enhancement of the tumor, highlighting its bony matrix. Also note the anterior displacement of the anterior genu of the left internal carotid (*arrow*, **D**). Coronal T2W MR image (**G**) shows a large cystic component of the tumor, as well as mass effect exerted by the tumor, manifesting as compression of the left lateral ventricle. MR angiogram (**H**) and lateral left internal carotid digital subtraction angiogram (DSA) (**I**) show superior elevation of the supraclinoid segment of the left internal carotid (*arrow*, **H**) and a small vascular blush in the region of the tumor core (*arrow*, **I**).

Motor Trigeminal Division

The impulses for the motor components of cranial nerve V originate in the motor cortex of the cerebral hemisphere. The pathway then extends through the genu of the internal capsule and the cerebral peduncle (along the corticobulbar tract) to the motor nucleus, which is situated medial to the principal sensory nucleus. The fused motor and sensory components of the fifth nerve emerge from the ventrolateral pons, coursing through the anterior portion of the CPA cistern near the apex of the medial petrous ridge. The nerve fibers then pierce the dura of Meckel's cavity and enter the trigeminal ganglion. At the distal aspect of Meckel's cavity, the motor fibers of the mandibular nerve exit at the inferolateral surface and extend through the foramen ovale. The motor division of the mandibular nerve supplies the

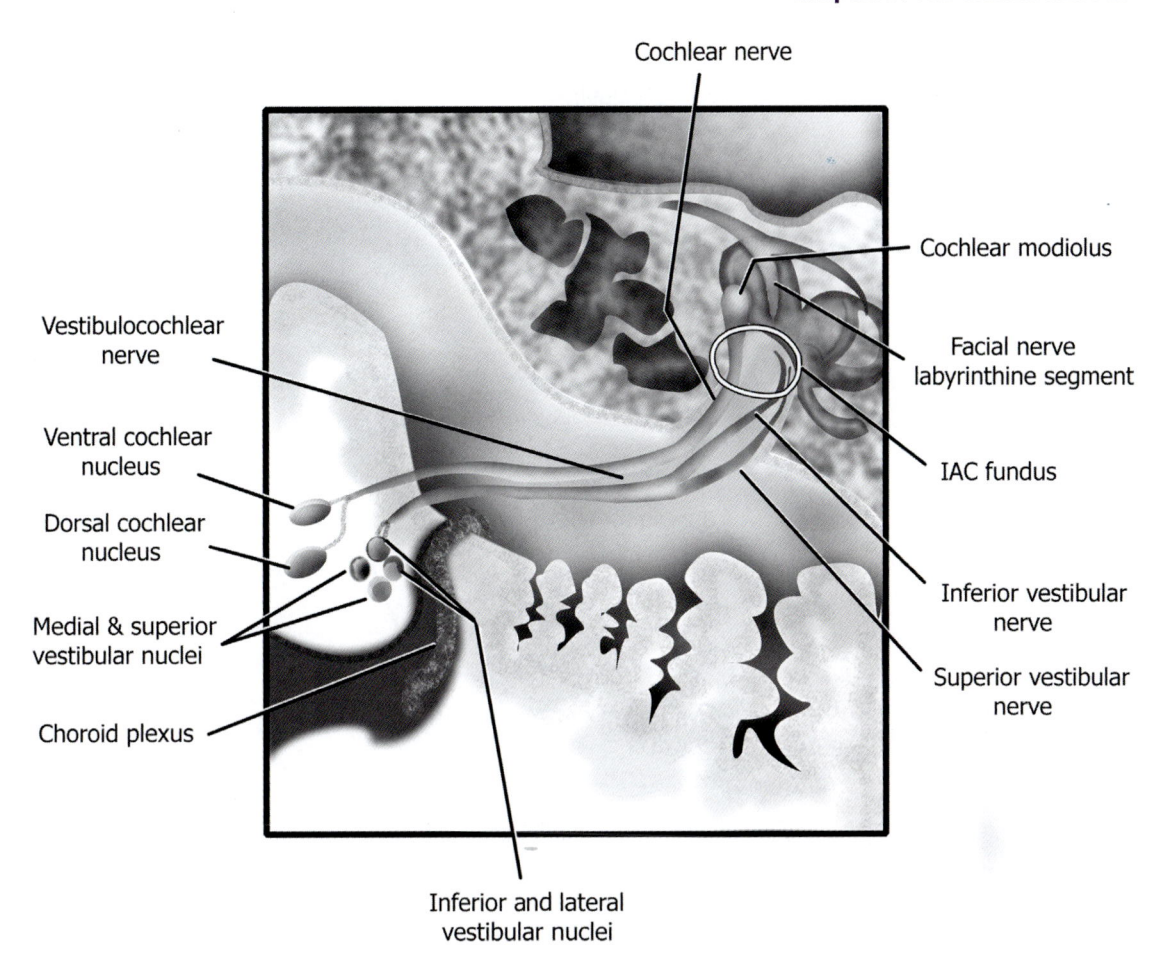

Figure 9-27 Cerebellopontine Angle Cistern and Internal Auditory Canal
Axial schematic of the left cerebellopontine angle (CPA) and internal auditory canal (IAC). CN VII and CN VIII traverse the region of the CPA and are commonly affected by pathology at this region. CN VII and VIII continue into the IAC and may be affected by intracanalicular lesions.

muscles of mastication plus other small muscles (tensor villi palatini, mylohyoid, anterior belly of the digastric, and tensor tympani). The exit point of the motor trigeminal nerve from the brainstem is also the entry point of the sensory trigeminal nerve. This area is termed the "root entry zone" of the sensory trigeminal nerve.

Anatomy and Function of CN VII

Cranial nerve VII has three major functions, including motor innervation to the stapedius muscle and muscles facial expression, taste and sensory innervation to the anterior two-thirds part of the tongue, and parasympathetic efferents to the lacrimal gland. Dysfunction of the various branches of CN VII commonly manifests as hyperacusis and loss of taste to the anterior tongue (**Table 9-16**).

The motor impulses of cranial nerve VII originate in the motor cortex of the cerebral hemisphere and extend via the genu of the internal capsule and cerebral peduncle to the brainstem nucleus. The motor nucleus of cranial nerve VII is situated in the caudal one-third of the ventral pontine tegmentum. Fibers from the ipsilateral and contralateral sides meet in this brainstem nucleus. From the nucleus, the fibers extend posteriorly toward the floor of the fourth ventricle and loop around the nucleus of cranial nerve VI (abducens). Cranial neuropathies of the abducens and facial nerve often occur concurrently due to this close anatomical approximation. This portion of the facial nerve contributes to the facial colliculus, a mound of tissue that protrudes internally toward the floor of the fourth ventricle. Extending from the loop, cranial nerve VII emerges from the brainstem at the anterolateral aspect of the pontomedullary junction. The nerve then extends laterally in the CPA cistern, reaching the anterior-superior quadrant of the internal auditory canal. The facial nerve extends through the temporal bone to the fundus of the internal auditory canal. The facial nerve then exits to join the geniculate ganglion within the roof of the petrous bone. At this point, there is a synapse with the sensory neurons for taste to the anterior two-thirds of the tongue and the cutaneous fibers for light touch in the region of the external ear.[70]

The superior salivatory nucleus in the pons is the site of origin of the parasympathetic fibers that terminate in and stimulate

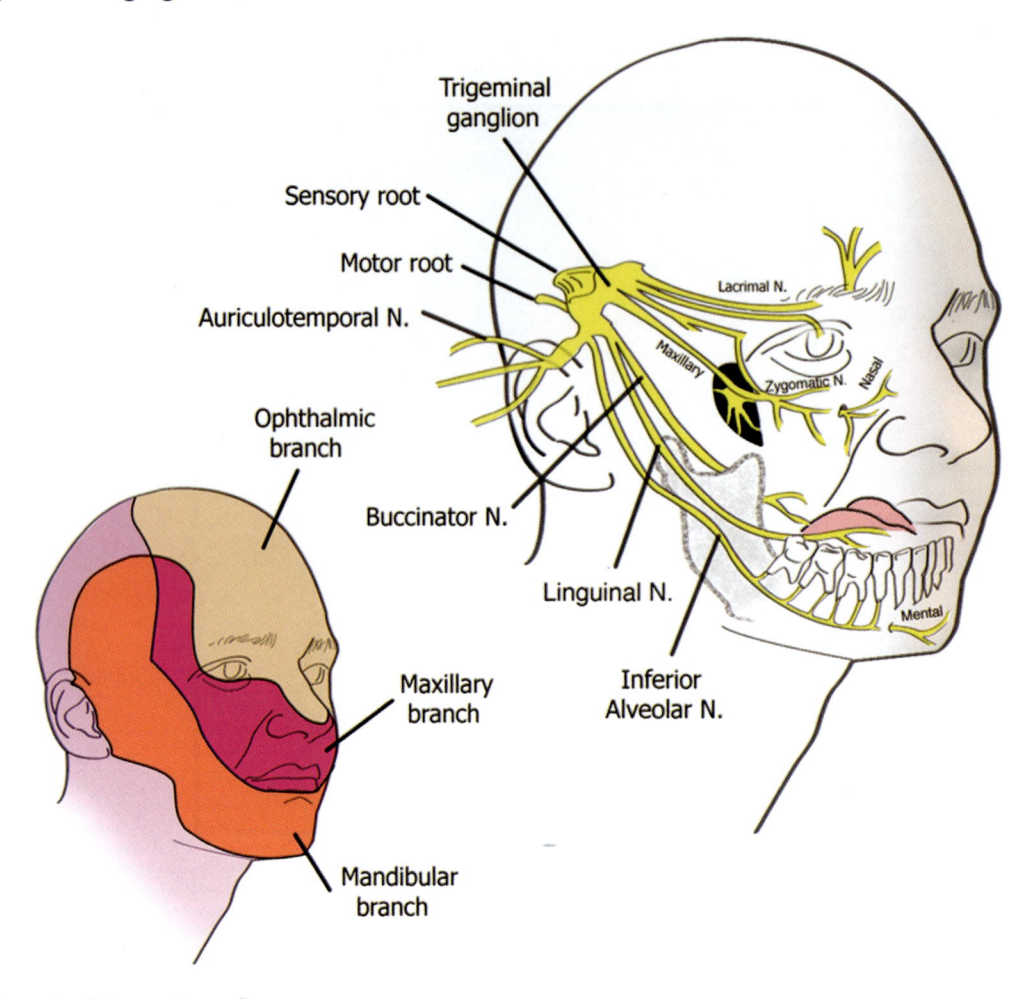

Figure 9-28 Trigeminal Nerve Branches
Schematic demonstrating the neural pathways and dermatome sensory distribution of the ophthalmic (V1), maxillary (V2), and mandibular (V3) branches of the trigeminal nerve.

the lacrimal, sublingual and submandibular glands. The nucleus solitarius represents the end-point of the fibers that convey taste sensation from the anterior two-thirds (via cranial nerve VII) and the posterior third (via cranial nerve IX) of the tongue. The cell bodies of these taste fibers are found in the geniculate ganglion. The impulses from these nuclei form the intermediate nerve fibers, which join the motor root of the facial nerve as it exits the brainstem.

From the region of the geniculate ganglion, the secretomotor fibers project forward as the greater superficial petrosal nerve, which joins some parasympathetic fibers from the carotid artery to enter the pterygoid (vidian) canal. The pterygoid canal will transmit the nerve to the pterygopalatine fossa, from where the parasympathetic components synapse and fibers extend to affect lacrimation and salivation.

From the geniculate ganglion, the facial motor fibers and taste fibers form a 180-degree turn and are directed posteriorly, at the anterior genu of the facial nerve. Extending posteriorly, these fibers lie at the medial aspect of the tympanic cavity medial to the ossicular chain and below the lateral semicircular canal. At the posterior aspect of the middle ear, the motor and taste fibers extend inferiorly at the posterior genu of the facial nerve to enter the stylomastoid foramen. At this point, the stapedial nerve exits to supply the stapedial muscle, which controls the mobility of the ossicles. The chorda tympani fibers for taste also separate from the seventh nerve within the stylomastoid foramen, extending via the petrotympanic fissure and eventually joining the lingual branch of the mandibular nerve to participate in the sensory fibers for taste to the anterior two-thirds of the tongue. The seventh nerve then exits the stylomastoid foramen into the parotid gland and extends anteriorly to innervate the muscles of facial expression as well as the posterior belly of the digastric, the stylohyoid, and the platysma muscles.

Anatomy and Function of CN VIII

CN VIII is also named the vestibulocochlear nerve for its two divisions. The vestibular division provides sensory innervation to the

Table 9-15 Function and Dysfunction of CN V

Branch	Motor Trigeminal		Sensory Trigeminal	
	Function	Dysfunction	Function	Dysfunction
Ophthalmic (V1)	none		**ophthalmic branch** sensory to globe **lacrimal branch** sensory to scalp **frontal branch** sensory to forehead **nasociliary branch** sensory to nose	• Facial pain • Facial numbness • Facial burning • Trigeminal neuralgia
Maxillary (V2)	none		**maxillary branch** sensory to cheek and upper teeth	
Mandibular (V3)	**masticator branch** motor to muscles of mastication **mylohyoid branch** motor to mylohyoid and anterior belly of digastric	• Weakness of muscles of mastication • Denervation atrophy (not always present)	**inferior alveolar** sensory to lower teeth **lingual branch** sensory to tongue **auriculotemporal branch** sensory to lateral head	

Table 9-16 Function and Dysfunction of CN VII and VIII

CN	Branch	Function	Dysfunction
CN VII	greater superficial petrosal nerve	parasympathetics to the lacrimal gland	dry eye
	stapedius nerve	motor innervation to stapedius muscle	hyperacusis
	chorda tympani nerve	taste fibers to anterior two-thirds of tongue	inability to taste
	terminal motor branches	muscles of facial expression	paresis of muscles of facial expression
CN VIII	vestibular branch	sensory from semicircular canals	vertigo
	cochlear branch	sensory from cochlea	sensorineural hearing loss; tinnitus

semicircular canals, while the cochlear division transmits acoustic information from the cochlea. Dysfunction these branches may produce a combination of tinnitus, sensorineural hearing loss, and vertigo (**Table 9-16**).

Vestibular Branch

Movement impulses are modulated by the hair cells within the utricle, saccule, and three semicircular canals and transmitted through the superior and inferior vestibular nerves. The combined vestibular nerve courses along with the cochlear nerve and facial nerve within the internal auditory canal. The superior and inferior vestibular divisions enter the brainstem at the pontomedullary junction after crossing the cerebellopontine angle cistern. These fibers extend into the vestibular nuclear complex with postganglionic fibers carrying information regarding equilibrium to many coordination sites, including the flocculonodular lobe of the cerebellum, the vestibulospinal tract, both medial longitudinal fasciculi, and other pathways, which affect the control of the eyes and the muscles of balance.

Cochlear Branch

Sound waves from the external environment are converted in the inner ear in the form of vibratory impulses at the oval window of the vestibule. The kinetic impulses are propagated as fluid waves in the cochlea. These impulses are then converted to electrical impulses along the spiral organ of Corti. The auditory signals are then transmitted via the spiral ganglion in the cochlear nerve, through the internal auditory canal and cerebellopontine angle to the origin of cranial nerve VIII at the ventrolateral pontomedullary junction. There are two cochlear nuclei (dorsal and ventral) located lateral to the inferior cerebellar peduncles in the upper medulla. The dorsal cochlear nucleus carries high frequencies, while the ventral cochlear nucleus connects low frequencies. Somewhat more than half of the fibers from these nuclei cross to the contralateral superior olivary nucleus to form the trapezoid body. From the trapezoid body, the fibers enter the posteriorly located lateral lemniscus to ascend to the inferior colliculus in the midbrain. From the inferior colliculus, the fibers travel to the medial geniculate body of the thalamus and then via the auditory radiations to the superior temporal gyrus.[70]

Dysfunction and Pathology of the Cerebellopontine Angle Nerves

The anatomic position of cranial nerves V, VII, and VIII makes them susceptible to lesions at the superior orbital fissure, cavernous sinus, the petrous apex of the temporal bone (CN VII and VIII), the cerebellopontine angle, internal auditory canal, intratemporal masses, and large lesions of the jugular foramen with superior extension[18,21,23,110,111] (**Table 9-17, Fig. 9-29**). Pathology at these areas often manifests as trigeminal neuralgia, hemifacial paralysis, facial spasm, sensorineural hearing loss, and tinnitus (**Tables 9-15–9-17**).

Trigeminal Neuralgia (Tic Douloureux)

Trigeminal neuralgia describes a condition involving intense lancinating or burning pain anywhere in the trigeminal nerve distribution that is brief but recurrent in short intervals. The pain is often accompanied by facial twitching, from which its synonym, tic douloureux, French for "painful twitch", is derived.[112] The episodes are usually elicited by stimulation of light touch nerves by physical touch, wind, talking, or eating.[113] The most common cause of trigeminal neuralgia is neurovascular compression of the trigeminal root entry zone, though the disease has been associated with demyelinating disease and other intracranial processes [113] (**Table 9-18**). The syndrome most commonly occurs in middle-aged adults and has a reported incidence of 4.3 per 100,000. However, it has a higher incidence rate among those with multiple sclerosis or hypertension. The condition is usually sporadic, but there have been familial cases reported in connection with Charcot-Marie-Tooth disease.[113] MR imaging is recommended in new cases of unilateral facial pain to examine for vascular compression, tumor, or other intracranial pathology.[112]

It has been postulated the demyelination of the trigeminal nerve causes ephaptic transmission of nerve impulses, in which impulses from light touch nerve fibers ectopically stimulate pain nerve fibers at sites of myelin breakdown.[113] The maxillary branch (V3) is most often involved, followed by the mandibular branch (V2) and the ophthalmic branch (V1). The right side of the face is more frequently involved than the left side, which has been postulated to be caused by the more narrow foramen ovale and rotundum on the right.[112]

Vascular Conflict Syndromes (Vascular Loop Syndromes)

Vascular conflict or vascular loop syndromes typically involve CN V, causing trigeminal neuralgia, and CN VII causing hemifacial spasm, in the region of the CPA, though neurovascular compression may affect any nerve.[113] The syndrome is caused by aberrant or aneurysmal vasculature that compresses CN V and CN VII, most commonly at the root entry (CN V) or exit (CN VII) zone of the nerves. It has been theorized that the nerves may be most susceptible to injury at the root entry and exit zones due to the transition from CNS oligodendroglia myelination to that of Schwann cells in the PNS.[114]

Neurovascular compression is the most frequent cause of trigeminal neuralgia. Furthermore, it has been reported that specific trigeminal branch symptoms are highly correlated with the region of trigeminal compression at it enters the brainstem[115] (**Fig. 9-30**).

Aneurysm, aberrant course, or age-related elongation of the various vascular structures traversing the CPA are the most common causes of neurovascular compression of CN V and CN VII. Superior cerebellar artery, followed by AICA, basilar artery, PICA and veins at the root entry zone are frequently involved vascular structures in trigeminal vascular compression.[115] AICA is the most common cause of hemifacial spasm, though it may also be caused by PICA, vertebral artery, internal auditory artery, and veins of the root entry/exit zone.[116] AICA may particularly affect distal regions of the nerves as they traverse the cistern[116] (**Figs. 9-31–9-33**). In rare cases, a persistent

Chapter 9: The Cranial Nerves

Table 9-17 Pathology of CN V, VII, and VIII by Location

CPA-IAC Pathology Commonly affected CN: V, VII, VIII	Intratemporal Pathology Commonly affected CN: VII and VIII
• Cranial neuritis (Table 9-8) • Schwannoma • Meningioma • Epidermoid cyst • Lipoma • Metastases • Vascular conflict syndromes • Cavernous malformation • AV malformation • Sarcoidosis • Dermoid cyst • Neurenteric cyst • Choristoma • Giant vertebrobasilar aneurysm • Ependymoma • Papilloma • Medulloblastoma	• Cranial neuritis (Table 9-8) • Schwannoma • Temporal bone fracture • Bell's palsy • Ramsay Hunt syndrome • CN VII perineural spread • Endolymphatic sac tumor • Acute mastoiditis • Cochlear osteonecrosis • Labyrinthitis • Paget's disease • Fibrous dysplasia • Rhabdomyosarcoma • Histiocytosis
Superior-extending Jugular Foramen Lesions **Commonly affected CN: IX, X, and XI** **Less Commonly affected CN: VII, VIII, and XII**	**Petrous Apex Lesions Pathology** **Commonly affected CN: V, VI, VII, and VIII**
• Glomus jugulare/tympanicum paraganglioma • Schwannoma of lower cranial nerves	• See (Table 9-14)

CPA = cerebellopontine angle; IAC = internal auditory canal.

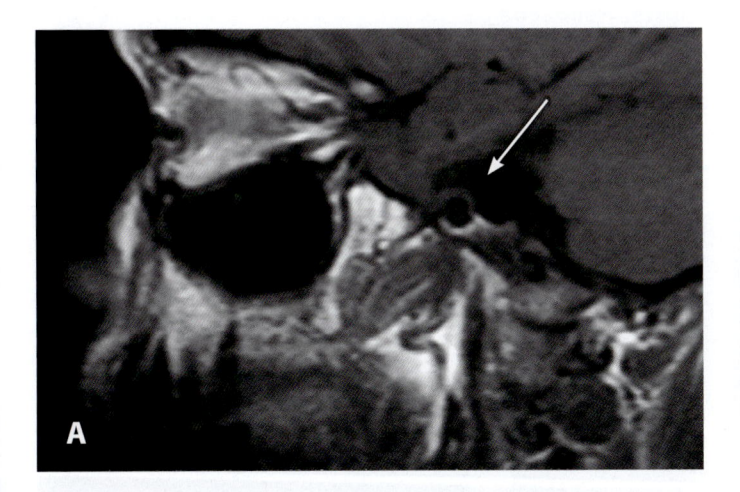

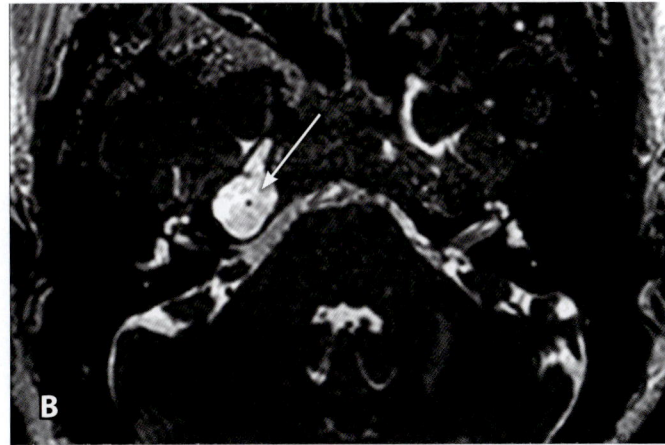

Figure 9-29 Meckel's Cave CSF Cephalocele
CSF cephalocele in Meckel's cave, aka Meckel's diverticulum, in a 56-year-old woman with sudden onset right-sided V2 and V3 trigeminal neuralgia 7-years prior. Sagittal T1W image shows the typical low signal of CSF within Meckel's cave of the petrous apex (*arrow*, **A**). Axial 3D heavily T2-weighted cisternography MR image (**B**) confirms the presence of a fluid-filled cystic cavity on the right side (*arrow*, **B**), consistent with CSF herniation into Meckel's cave with subsequent compression of the trigeminal ganglion.

Table 9-18 Common Causes of Trigeminal Neuralgia

Brainstem Lesions
- Cavernous malformation
- Infarct

Nerve Root Compression
- Vascular conflict – 80%–90% of all causes
- Vestibular and facial schwannomas
- Trigeminal schwannoma
- CPA meningioma
- CPA epidermoid cyst
- Tumor of the CPA
- Postsurgical hardening of prosthetic material from previous trigeminal neuralgia surgeries
- Bony tumors
- Perineural spread

Demyelination Disorders
- Multiple sclerosis
- Charcot-Marie-Tooth

Intrinsic Nerve Lesions
- Carcinomatous deposits within nerve
- Trigeminal amyloidosis
- Perineural metastatic spread

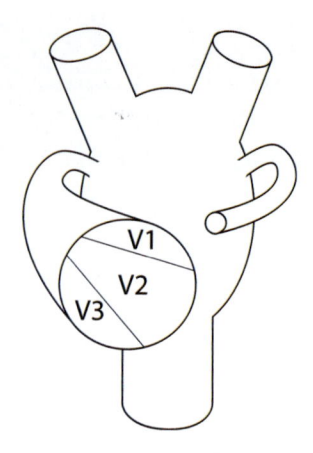

Figure 9-30 Trigeminal Root Anatomy
Anterior-posterior schematic representation of trigeminal nerve as it exits the pons. Segmental nerve fibers travel in a distinctive pattern in CN V, consisting of CN V1 fibers cranially, V2 fibers medially, and V3 fibers caudally. Vascular compression in any of these regions will often cause trigeminal neuralgia symptoms in the respectively innervated facial regions.

primitive trigeminal artery, visualized as a large caliber artery branching from cavernous carotid proximal to the level of the PCA on angiography, may encroach on the trigeminal nerve and cause trigeminal neuralgia.[117] Symptoms caused by vascular conflict syndromes are usually unilateral.[116]

Heavily T2-weighted 3D high resolution MR is the preferred imaging modality as it provides the best spatial resolution of the CPA, allowing differentiation from vascular structures, seen as flow voids from filamentous-appearing neural structures. However, MR angiography may also be of benefit in locating neurovascular compression.[115,116] Some cases of neurovascular compression observed on MR imaging may be asymptomatic and require no treatment. However, surgical microvascular decompression is the treatment of choice for symptomatic individuals and has been reported to reduce or eliminate symptoms in up to 90% of individuals with trigeminal neuralgia due to neurovascular compression.[115,118,119]

Sphenopalatine (Sluder's) Neuralgia and Cluster Headache

Sluder's Neuralgia was described by Sluder in 1908 as a symptom complex of pain, motor, sensory, and gustatory involvement, which he attributed to irritation of the sphenopalatine ganglion.

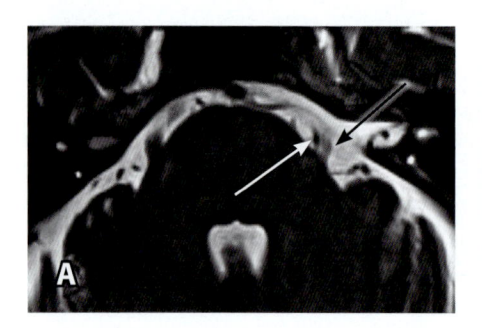

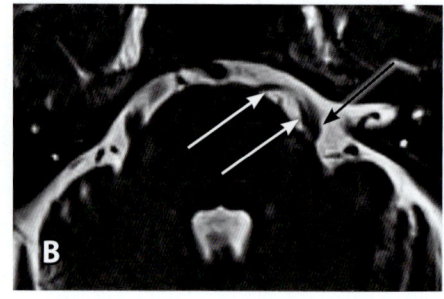

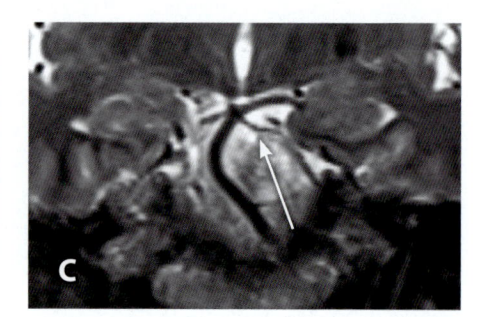

Figure 9-31 Trigeminal Vascular Conflict
Trigeminal conflict in a 58-year-old female with 6-year history of weakness, burning pain, and spasm of the left hemiface. Axial 3D heavily T2W MR cisternograms of the cerebellopontine angle (**A–B**) show a vessel (*white arrows*) originating anterior to the pons and looping posteriorly, impinging the medial aspect of the left trigeminal root entry zone (*black arrow*). Coronal T2W image (**C**) of the vertebrobasilar vasculature confirms the loop as an aberrant loop of the left superior cerebellar artery (*arrow*).

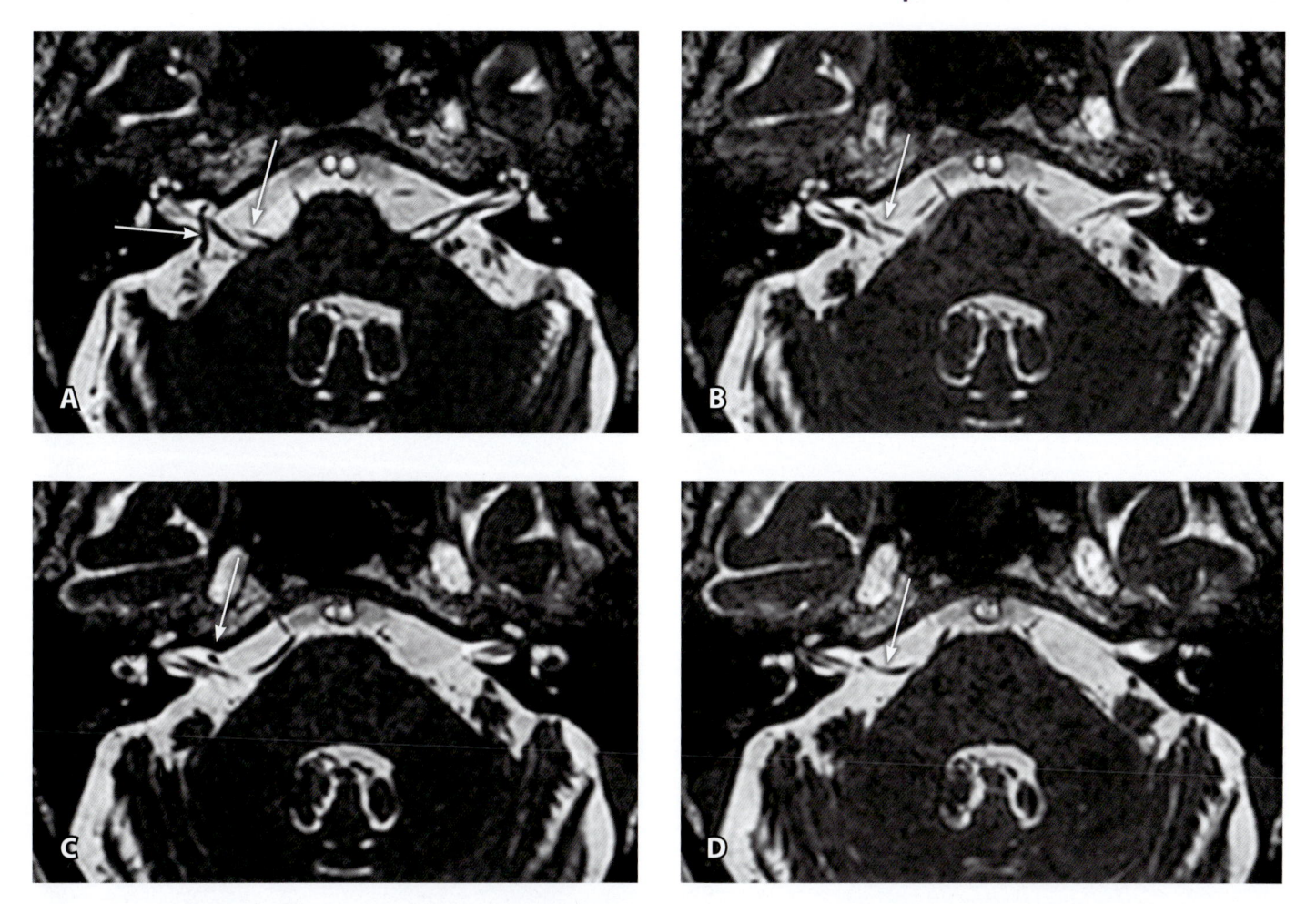

Figure 9-32 Vascular Conflict at the Internal Auditory Canal
Series of four axial 3D heavily T2W cisternogram MR images (**A–D**) at the level of the internal auditory canal in a patient with pulsatile tinnitus. The right anterior inferior carotid artery is visualized as it branches from the basilar in the brainstem (*arrow*, **D**) and then proceeds along an aberrant course, acutely looping around CN VII and VIII at the level of the porus acusticus (*arrows*, **A–C**).

Intense pain was described as unilateral, involving the orbit, maxilla, the mandible, the teeth, and the mastoid area. Occasionally, pain could extend to the neck and axilla in severe cases. Sluder also reported some patients with gustatory hallucinations of a metallic or acidic nature, hyperesthesia in the trigeminal distribution, and hypoesthesia of the soft palate, lower nose, and tonsils. Motor signs reported with the complex included ipsilateral elevation of the soft palate. Parasympathetic symptoms, including increased salivation and ipsilateral nasopharyngeal swelling and discharge were also observed in conjunction with the disorder. Sluder noted that this sphenopalatine ganglion neuralgia often occurred following inflammation of the sphenoid and ethmoid sinuses. He advocated sphenopalatine ganglion blocks or ablations and reported success in controlling or curing symptoms of sphenopalatine ganglion neuralgia with anesthetic or chemical fixatives to the lateral nasal wall at the level of the sphenopalatine foramen.[120] Attempts to reproduce Sluder's success in sphenopalatine ganglion blocks and ablations in modern times, however, have shown mixed and transient results.[121,122] It is now thought that the symptom complex originally described by Sluder is a complex neurovascular process involving not only the sphenopalatine ganglion, but the trigeminal nerve, vasoactive peptides, and the hypothalamus. The symptom complex most closely resembles that of a cluster headache and is classified as such by the International Headache Society.[120] Nevertheless, discrete inflammatory or mass lesions in the region of the pterygopalatine ganglion are known to produce the retro-orbital, maxilla, mandibular, and mastoid pain common in cluster headaches (**Fig. 9-34**).

Bell's Palsy

Bell's palsy is the acute nerve palsy of CN VII, causing paresis of all facial muscles on the affected side. It is important to note that Bell's palsy results from peripheral paralysis of CN VII, as suprabulbar lesions of CN VII present with clinically different signs and often concurrently involve CN VI, due to the intimate association of the nuclei of CN VI and VII in the brainstem (**Fig. 9-35**). Because Bell's palsy is usually unilateral, bilateral CN VII palsies

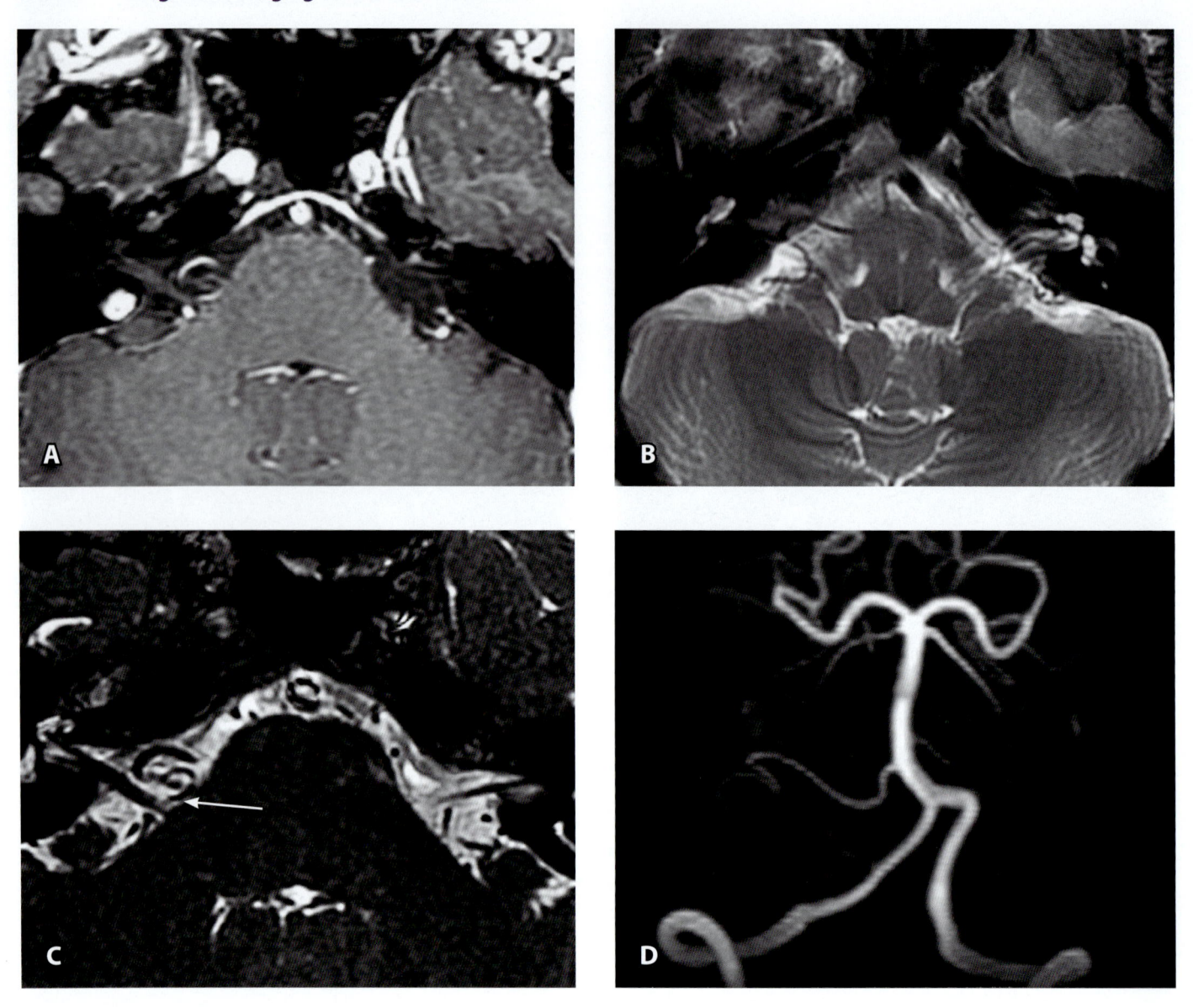

Figure 9-33 CN VII Vascular Conflict
Vascular conflict in a patient presenting with right hemifacial spasm. Axial T1W postcontrast (**A**), T2W (**B**), and heavily T2-weighted 3D cisternogram MR images (**C**) demonstrate an aberrant serpentine loop of vasculature connecting the medial brainstem and the cerebellum in the region of the cerebellopontine angle. As seen on the cisternogram (**C**), the vessel seems to selectively loop around CN VII and indents the nerve at the root exit zone (*arrow*, **C**). Vertebrobasilar MR angiogram (**D**) shows an aberrant left anterior inferior carotid artery branch traveling laterally and making several acute loops in the region of the right internal auditory canal.

may suggest other pathology[44,68] (**Table 9-19**). The incidence of Bell's palsy is estimated at up to 30 per 100,000, is most common in the fifth decade, and has an increased incidence in diabetics and pregnant women.[123] It is generally accepted that inflammation, ischemia, and demyelination of the geniculate ganglion is responsible for the condition. Formally, Bell's palsy is an idiopathic condition, though herpes simplex virus, Epstein-Barr virus, measles, rubella, and cytomegalovirus have been hypothesized as causing the disorder.[124]

Because 90% of Bell's palsy cases resolve spontaneously in fewer than two months, MR imaging is usually not clinically warranted. However, in cases of anticipated decompression surgery, unresolved palsy, recurrent Bell's palsy, other concurrent cranial nerve lesions, disproportionate ear pain, or twitching and hyperfunctionality of the muscles of facial expression, MRI is often performed to rule out other pathology.[125]

Thin section temporal bone T1 contrast-enhanced imaging is the preferred method for evaluating Bell's palsy. CN VII enhancement in the distal intratemporal and labyrinthine portions of CN VII are considered diagnostic for CN VII lesions associated with Bell's palsy (**Figs. 9-36** and **9-37**). Enlargement of CN VII, most frequently visible on higher contrast dosing,

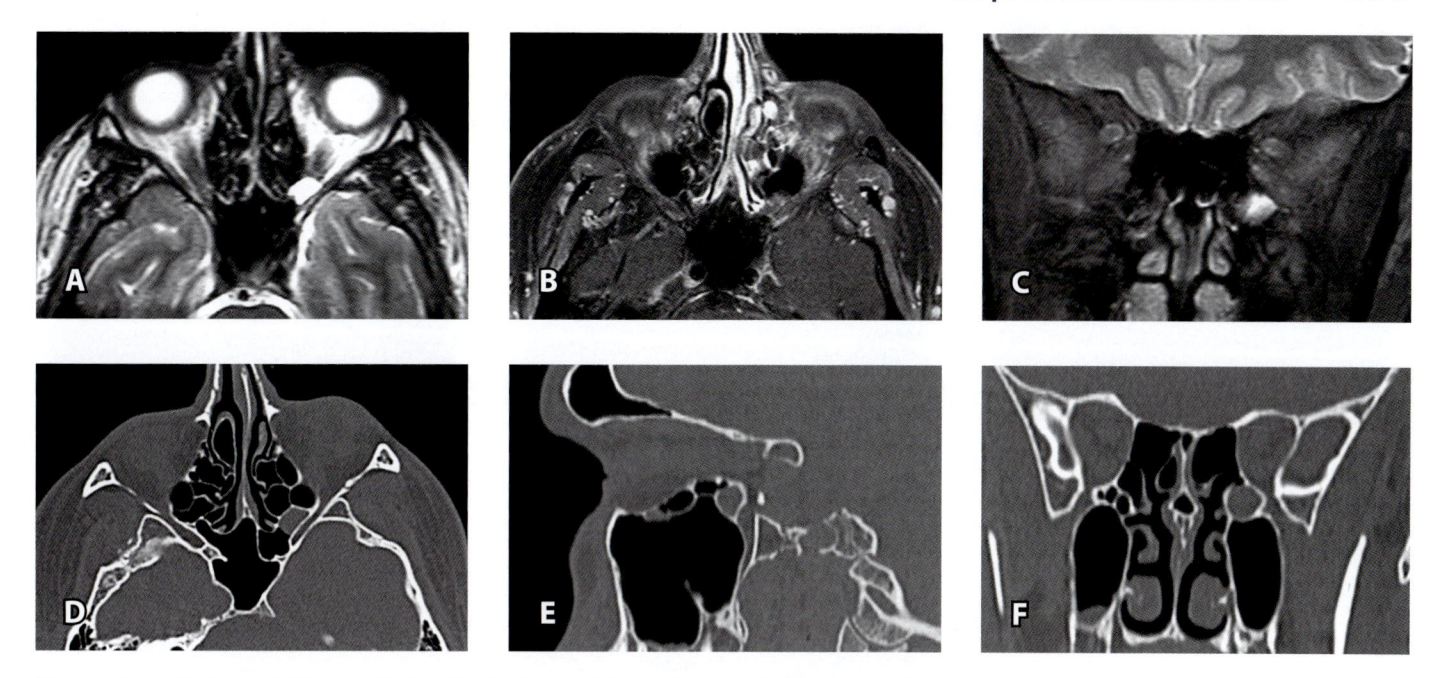

Figure 9-34 Sphenoid Mucocele in the Region of the Sphenopalatine Ganglion
Sphenoid mucocele in a 28-year-old male patient complaining of constant and severe pain in the left mandible, teeth, and maxilla. Axial T2W (**A**), axial T1W postcontrast (**B**), and coronal T2W (**C**) images show a cystic, nonenhancing lesion below the inferior orbital fissure in the region of the sphenopalatine fossa. Axial (**D**), sagittal (**E**), and coronal (**F**) NECT bone window images show a fluid collection and smooth bony expansion in the region of the left pterygopalatine fossa. Compression or irritation of the left sphenopalatine ganglion in this location is the likely cause of the left hemifacial pain in this patient.

is not a typical feature of Bell's palsy and is more suggestive of neoplasia.[123] The geniculate ganglion usually enhances in cases of Bell's palsy, though significant overlap between normal and pathologic enhancement exists at the region. As opposed to Ramsay Hunt syndrome, CN VIII is not involved in Bell's palsy[67] (**Table 9-20**).

Nonpathologic enhancement has been observed in the cavernous segments of CN III and CN VI, the trigeminal ganglion of CN V, and CN VII. The geniculate, tympanic, and mastoid segments of the facial nerve are the most frequent sites of nonpathologic enhancement, while the cisternal, labyrinthine, and mastoid segments of the facial nerve do not normally enhance. Contributing to the normal enhancement seen in certain CN VII segments is the rich vascular arteriovenous plexus surrounds the facial nerve, which is particularly rich at the geniculate ganglion (**Fig. 9-36**). Arterial supply of this plexus is composed of the anterior tympanic branch of the internal maxillary or middle meningeal artery anteriorly, by the ascending pharyngeal artery medially, and by stylomastoid branch of the occipital artery posteriorly. Furthermore, increased vascular permeability, particularly in the area of ganglia and external nerve sheath has been demonstrated.[126–128]

Ramsay Hunt Syndrome

In 1907, Ramsay Hunt hypothesized that facial nerve paralysis with herpes zoster eruptions around the ear was caused by reactivation latent varicella zoster virus in the geniculate ganglion of the facial nerve. Strict definition of Ramsay Hunt syndrome includes peripheral facial nerve palsy accompanied by herpes zoster eruptions in the ear or mouth. Ramsay Hunt syndrome is the second most common cause atraumatic peripheral facial paralysis, accounting for approximately 12% of cases. Presenting symptoms are often more severe and long-lasting than those of Bell's palsy.[129]

Variant symptom complexes of Ramsay Hunt syndrome have been described, including abrupt hearing loss, vertigo, and tinnitus. PCR studies have shown VZV DNA not only in the geniculate ganglion, but also in the facial nerve sheath and the spiral and vestibular ganglion of CN VIII as well, perhaps

Table 9-19 Causes of Bilateral CN VII Palsy

- Lyme disease
- Syphilis
- Guillain-Barré and variants
- Sarcoidosis
- HIV
- Benign intracranial hypertension
- Leukemia
- Meningitis and encephalitis

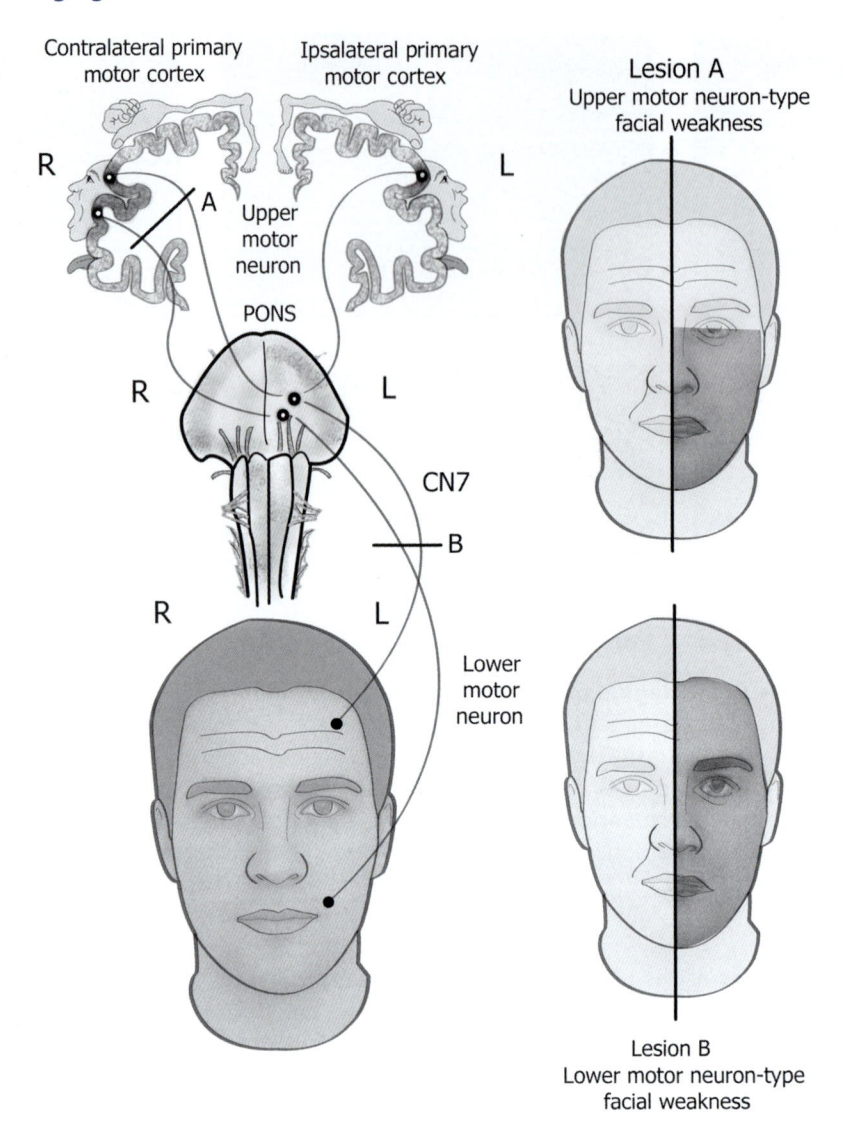

Figure 9-35 Central and Peripheral CN VII Palsy
Schematic representing the clinical differences of central (upper motor neuron, lesion A) and peripheral (lower motor neuron, lesion B) lesions. The muscles of the forehead receive bilateral cortical innervation that is carried through the ipsilateral lower motor neuron, while the rest of the muscles of facial expression are innervated by the contralateral cerebral cortex. Thus, central brain lesions causing facial nerve palsy will cause facial palsy with sparing of the frontal region due to bilateral cortical innervation of the frontal muscles. Conversely, a peripheral or lower motor neuron lesion to CN VII, such as Bell's palsy, will cause complete ipsilateral facial hemiparesis, including the frontal muscles.

explaining the variant vestibulocochlear symptoms.[130] Furthermore, anti VZV antibody spikes have been demonstrated in up to 20% patients with active Bell's palsy but no herpetic eruptions, suggesting that peripheral facial nerve paralysis in this subset of patients may be due to latent VZV reactivation.[131] Most patients with VZV-associated peripheral CN VII palsy with and without herpetic manifestations respond well to prednisone and acyclovir, particularly if administered early in the attack.[129]

Intense enhancement seen on MRI in the area of the geniculate ganglion and labyrinthine segment of CN VII, in addition to occasional enhancement of portions of CN VIII may help to distinguish Ramsay Hunt syndrome from Bell's palsy (**Fig. 9-38**)

(**Table 9-20**). Proteinaceous infiltrate in the vestibule may be seen in some patients with CN VIII symptoms on FLAIR imaging.[67,126,130,132]

Pathology of the Nerves of the Cerebellopontine Angle

The vast majority of pathology involving nerves of the cerebellopontine pathology (70%–80%) is due to vestibular schwannomas, while 10% to 15% is caused by meningiomas and 5% of epidermoid cysts. However, a wide variety of pathology may affect the CPA and cause CPA syndrome, including those listed in **Table 9-17**.[23]

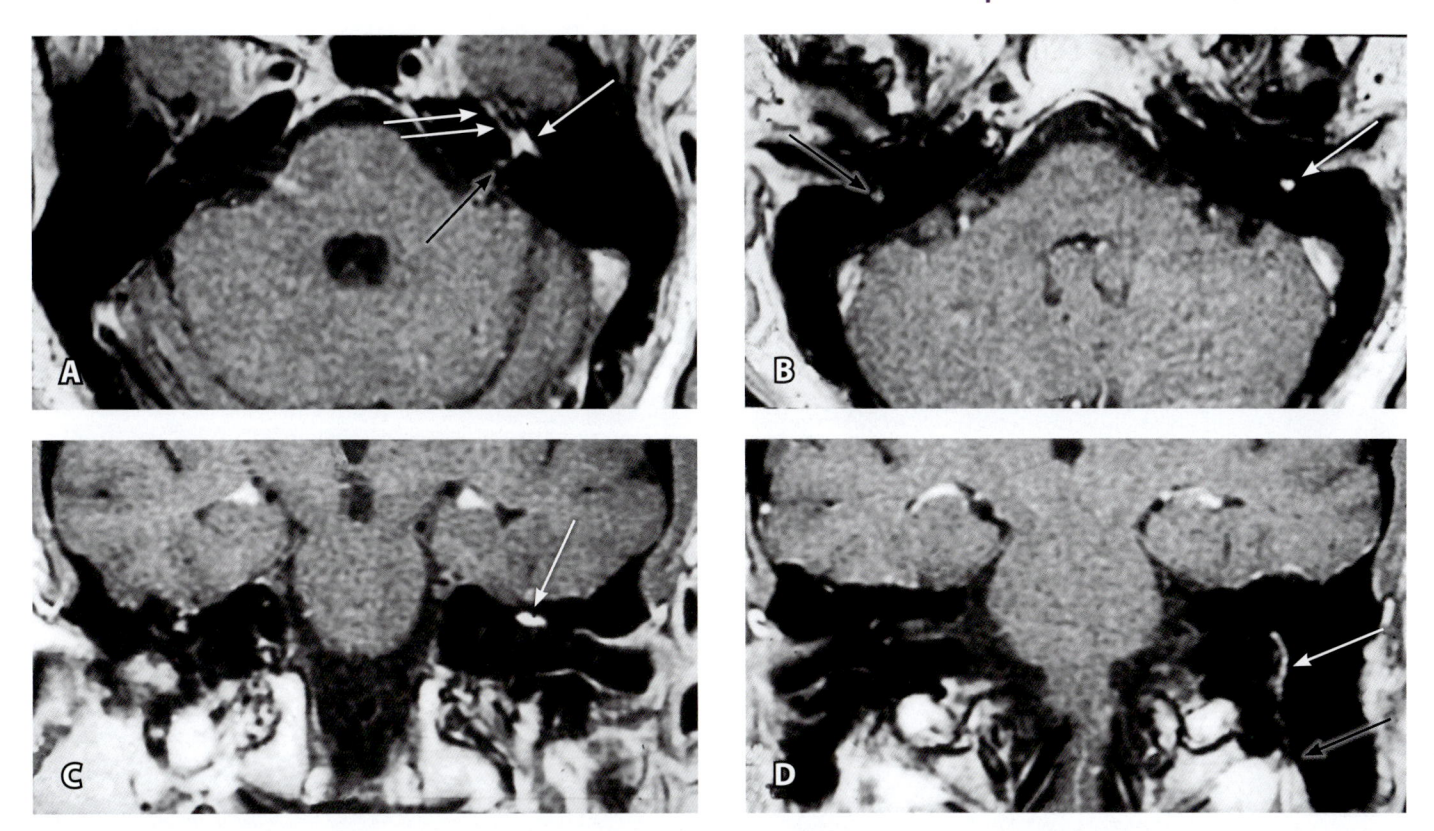

Figure 9-36 Bell's Palsy
Axial (**A–B**) and coronal (**C–D**) T1 postcontrast MR images show intense enhancement of the left facial nerve in the fundus of the internal auditory canal (*black arrow*, **A**) geniculate ganglion (*white arrow*, **A–B**), and greater superficial petrosal nerve (*double white arrows*, **A**). Enhancement of CN VII is also noted in the tympanic (*arrows*, **B,C**), mastoid (*arrow*, **D**), and stylomastoid foramen (*black arrow*, **D**) portions segments of the nerve. Note the mild physiologic enhancement of the geniculate ganglion of the unaffected right side (*arrow*, **B**), compared to the more hyperintense enhancement on the affected left side (*white arrow*, **B**). Though physiologic enhancement of the IAC fundus and labyrinthine segment of CN VII is rare, normal enhancement of CN VII often occurs at the geniculate ganglion and between the anterior and posterior genu of the temporal portions of CN VII.

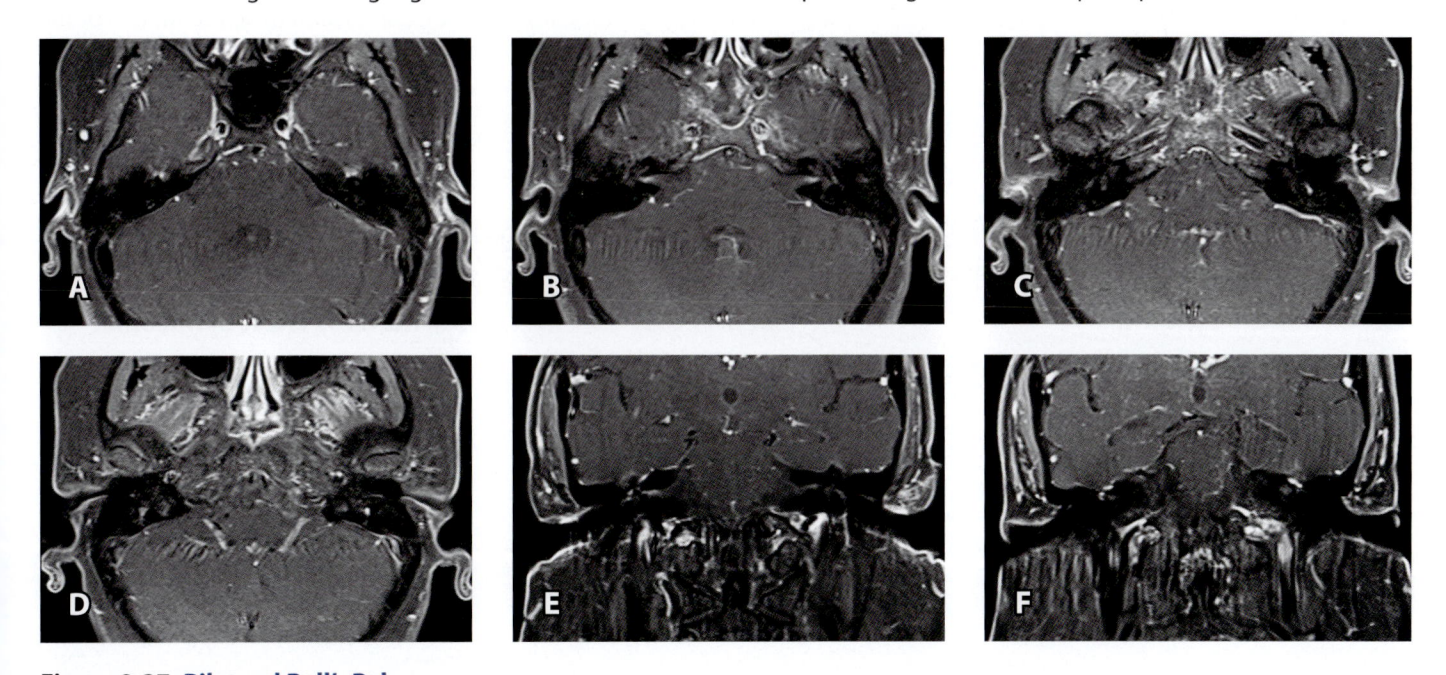

Figure 9-37 Bilateral Bell's Palsy
Axial (**A–D**) and coronal (**E–F**) T1 postcontrast MR images show bilateral enhancement of CN VII at the fundus of the internal auditory canal (**B**), labyrinthine segment (**F**), geniculate ganglion (**A**), tympanic segment (**C–D**), and peripheral nerve segments (**E–F**).

Diagnostic Imaging of the Head and Neck

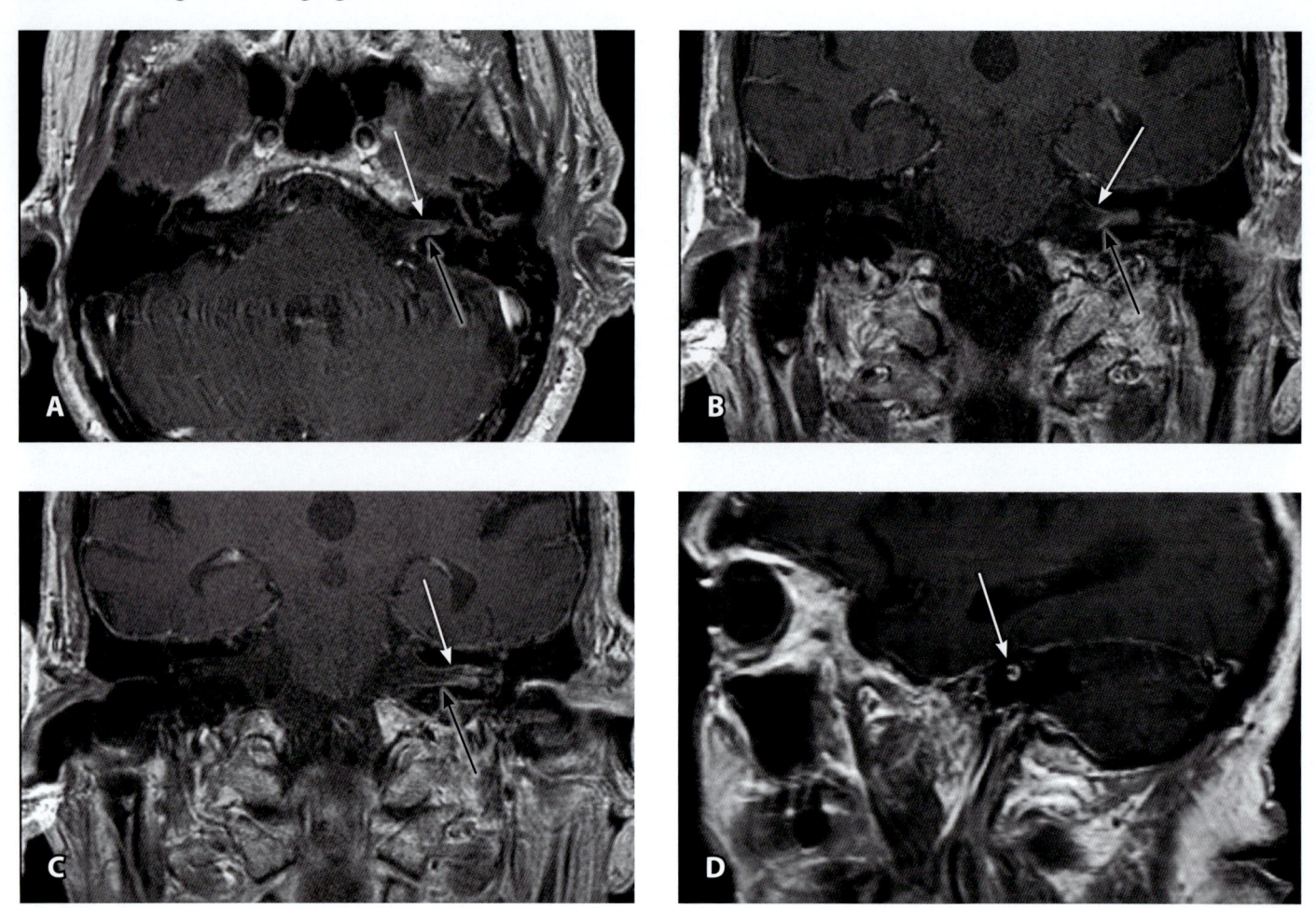

Figure 9-38 Ramsay Hunt Syndrome
Ramsay Hunt syndrome in a patient presenting with hemifacial paralysis. Axial (**A**), coronal (**B–C**), and sagittal (**D**) T1W postcontrast images show enhancement of the neural structures within the left internal auditory canal and left middle ear. Distinct enhancement of both CN VII and CN VIII is visualized (*white and black arrows*, **A–C**). Enhancement of the fundus of the internal auditory canal (*arrow*, **D**) is also a common finding in Bell's palsy, though co-involvement of CN VIII, a common finding in Ramsay Hunt, is very rare in Bell's palsy.

Table 9-20 Differential Diagnosis of Bell's Palsy and Ramsay Hunt Syndrome

Finding	Bell's Palsy	Ramsay Hunt Syndrome
Geniculate ganglion enhancement	moderate	intense
CN VIII enhancement	none	common
Membranous labyrinth enhancement	rare	common
Auricular vesicular eruptions	none	common

Schwannoma

Vestibular Schwannoma

Cranial nerve VIII schwannomas usually involve the vestibular, rather than the cochlear division of the nerve. Though these lesions may arise spontaneously, they are frequently associated with the neurocutaneous syndromes neurofibromatosis 1 (NF-1) and neurofibromatosis 2 (NF-2). Twenty-five percent of CN VIII schwannomas are associated with neurofibromatosis 2 (NF-2) and 95% of individuals with NF-2 develop bilateral vestibular schwannomas. Multiple schwannomas associated with NF-2 may arise concurrently on both sides and may coalesce into larger "collision" tumors.[14] Because vestibular schwannomas typically arise in the third decade in patients with NF-2, MR screening is recommended in this population.

Hearing loss, most often presenting with loss of speech discrimination, is the most common initial clinical presentation of vestibular schwannoma. Horizontal nystagmus and vertigo may also be present early in the course of the pathology. Advanced cases may also involve CN VII and present with decreased sensation over the pinna and external auditory canal (Hitselberger's sign), as well as facial weakness or spasm. CN V palsy causing retrobulbar and facial pain is less commonly associated with the lesion. Intention tremor and vertical nystagmus usually indicate cerebellar and brainstem compression in large schwannomas.[19]

Vestibular schwannomas may have three general morphologic patterns, depending on their location. The most common variant is a combined internal auditory canal and cerebellopontine angle (IAC-CPA) schwannoma. These neoplasms are thought to arise within the IAC and progress medially into the CPA, often eroding the posterior edge of the porous acusticus as they progress. This gives the lesions a typical "ice cream cone" appearance on neuroimaging.[23] Additionally, purely intracanalicular schwannoma may also exist. Though these tumors do not invade the CPA, they do have a tendency to involve the cochlea and/or vestibule taking on a dumbbell appearance on MR imaging. Finally, purely intracisternal schwannomas are the least common type and are less commonly associated with hearing loss. However, because they more commonly compress the cerebellum and fourth ventricle, they are usually larger when they become symptomatic and more often present with vertical nystagmus and intention tremor.[23]

CT may show vestibular schwannomas as isointense, well-delineated, noncalcified, strongly enhancing lesions. MRI, however, is the modality of choice for diagnosis. Lesions typically have an intermediate T1 signal, though they may show low signal foci in instances of intratumor cystic components or hemorrhage in larger tumors (**Fig. 9-39**). High-resolution heavily T2-weighted MR cisternography helps to demonstrate CSF and vasculature between the lesion and the brain parenchyma, confirming the extra-axial nature of peripheral schwannomas. Furthermore, high-resolution T2 cisternography helps to delineate the tumor edge as a hypointense filling defect within the IAC. 100% of acoustic schwannomas will strongly enhance on MR imaging. They are also associated with arachnoid cyst in 0.5% of cases, which are thought to arise from elevation of and adhesions in the leptomeninges as the tumor spreads through toward the brainstem[19] (**Fig. 9-40**).

Because meningiomas at the CPA may mimic vestibular schwannomas, differences in tumor morphology, spread patterns, dynamic MR perfusion, and MR spectroscopy may aid in diagnosis (**Table 9-21**). Furthermore, a schwannoma of CN VII may be impossible to differentiate from a vestibular schwannoma unless it extends through the facial canal.[19] Accurate tumor measurements and evaluation for the involvement of vestibular structures and facial nerve involvement aid in surgical planning and prognosis.[23] Mainstay treatment consists of surgical removal of the tumor with variable preservation of hearing. Postsurgical changes may enhance on MRI and mimic recurrent tumor at followup.[19]

Facial Nerve Schwannoma

Schwannomas of CN VII arise much less frequently than those of CN VIII and most frequently occur in the intratemporal portions of the nerve, though CPA and intracanalicular involvement are also observed. Approximately 10% of facial nerve schwannomas occur in the intraparotid segment, accounting for less than 2% of pathology at that region.[133] Masses originating in the CPA and internal auditory canal often cause sensorineural hearing loss, tinnitus, CN VII paralysis, and hemifacial spasm, while those originating near the parotid gland may present with a slow-growing parotid mass and no CN VIII symptoms.

Generally, schwannomas of CN VII appear as enhancing fusiform dilations along the nerve as it runs through the facial nerve canal (**Table 9-6**). However, distinct patterns are typically visible on imaging, depending on the location of the lesions. Lesions arising in the CPA or internal auditory canal are often indistinguishable from vestibular schwannomas at the same area, except for cases of intralabyrinthine extension of the mass. A dumbbell-shaped enhancing lesion is often seen when imaging canalicular schwannomas that have spread through the narrow labyrinthine portion of CN VII and into the larger geniculate fossa (**Fig. 9-41**). Schwannomas may also track along the greater superficial petrosal nerve into the middle cranial fossa; scalloped bone lesions from the pterygoid canal on CT imaging may suggest this pattern of spread. Schwannomas of the tympanic and mastoid segment of CN VII are characteristically more lobulated and may invade the middle and mastoid cells, respectively, due to the less rigid temporal bone structure in these areas. Finally, enhancement of facial nerve schwannomas running through the parotid segment is similar in appearance to schwannomas involving the proximal facial nerve, though they are often quite large at the time of presentation (**Fig. 9-42**).[23,134]

CN V Schwannoma

Schwannomas of CN V are very rare CPA lesions, but typically arise in younger population. They may arise from any part of the nerve, including the root entry zone, the trigeminal ganglion, and the three peripheral branches (V1, V2, and V3) (**Fig. 9-43**). Imaging findings for trigeminal schwannomas are similar as those in other cranial nerves (**Table 9-6**). Larger lesions can erode the bony foramina, including ovale, rotundum, and the superior orbital fissure. Surgical resection is the preferred treatment option.[135]

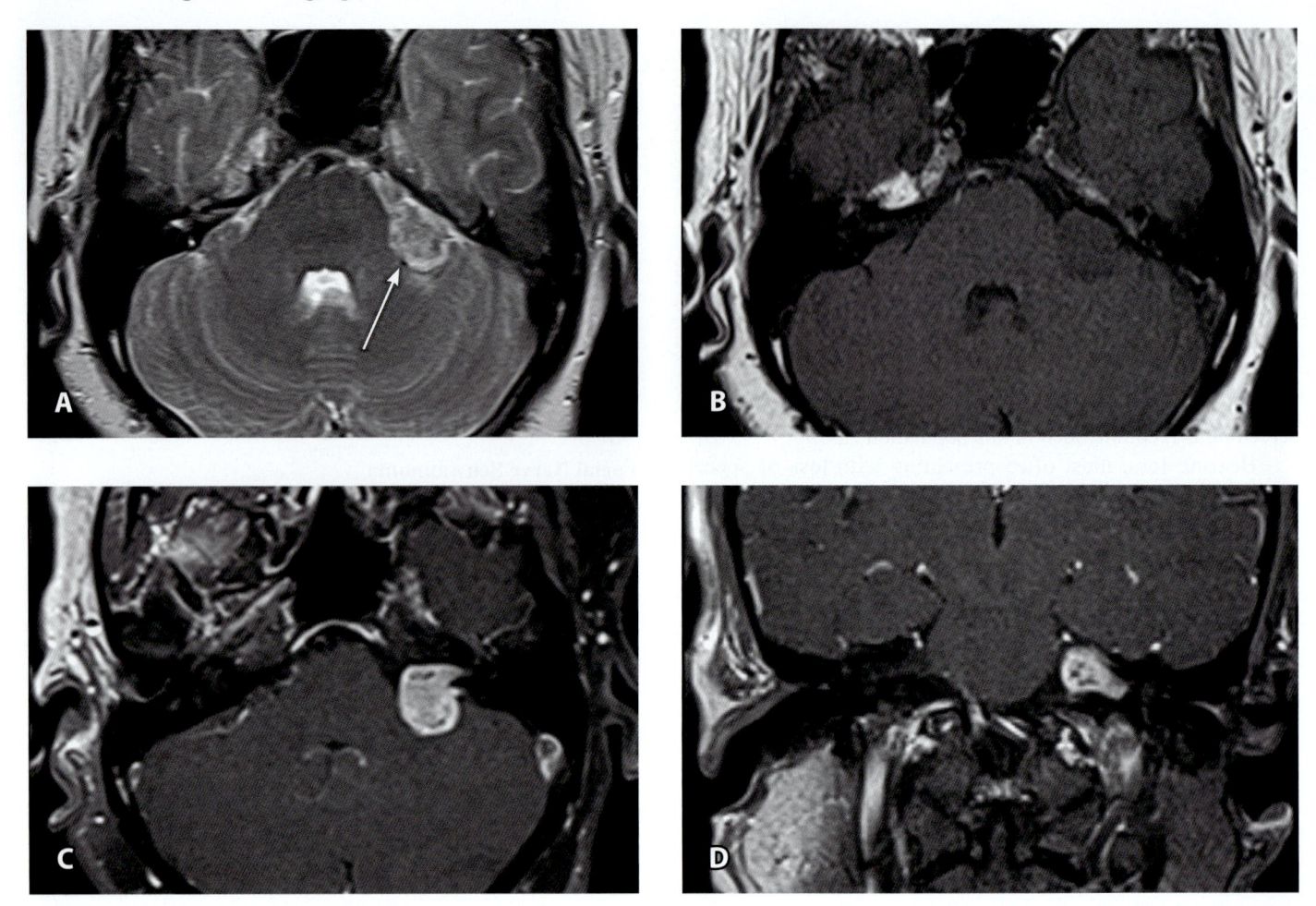

Figure 9-39 Vestibular Schwannoma
Vestibular schwannoma in a 58-year-old female. Axial T2W (**A**), T1W (**B**), T1W postcontrast (**C**), and coronal T1W postcontrast (**D**) MR images show the "ice cream cone" appearance of a mass in the cerebellopontine angle (ice cream) with extension into the left internal auditory canal (cone). The typical intermediate to high T2 signal (**A**), low T1 signal (**B**) and strong enhancement (**C–D**) are typical of schwannomas. Also note the flow void on the T2 image between the mass and the brain stem (*arrow*, **A**). Perforating vasculature and CSF between the lesion and the brainstem helps to distinguish this lesion as extra-axial.

Table 9-21 Differential Diagnosis of Vestibular Schwannomas and Meningiomas at the CPA-IAC

Imaging Finding	Schwannoma 70%–80%	Meningioma 10%–15%
MR Findings	isointense on T1, variable T2 appearance; strongly enhance	
Erosion of posterior porus acusticus of IAC	common	rare
Spread to middle cerebral fossa	rare	common
Calcifications	rare	20%
Direction of displacement of CN VII	anteriorly	posteriorly
rCBV	2–4.4	6 to 9
MR spectroscopy	elevated alanine, elevated glutamate, elevated glutamine	elevated myoinositol

IAC = internal auditory canal.

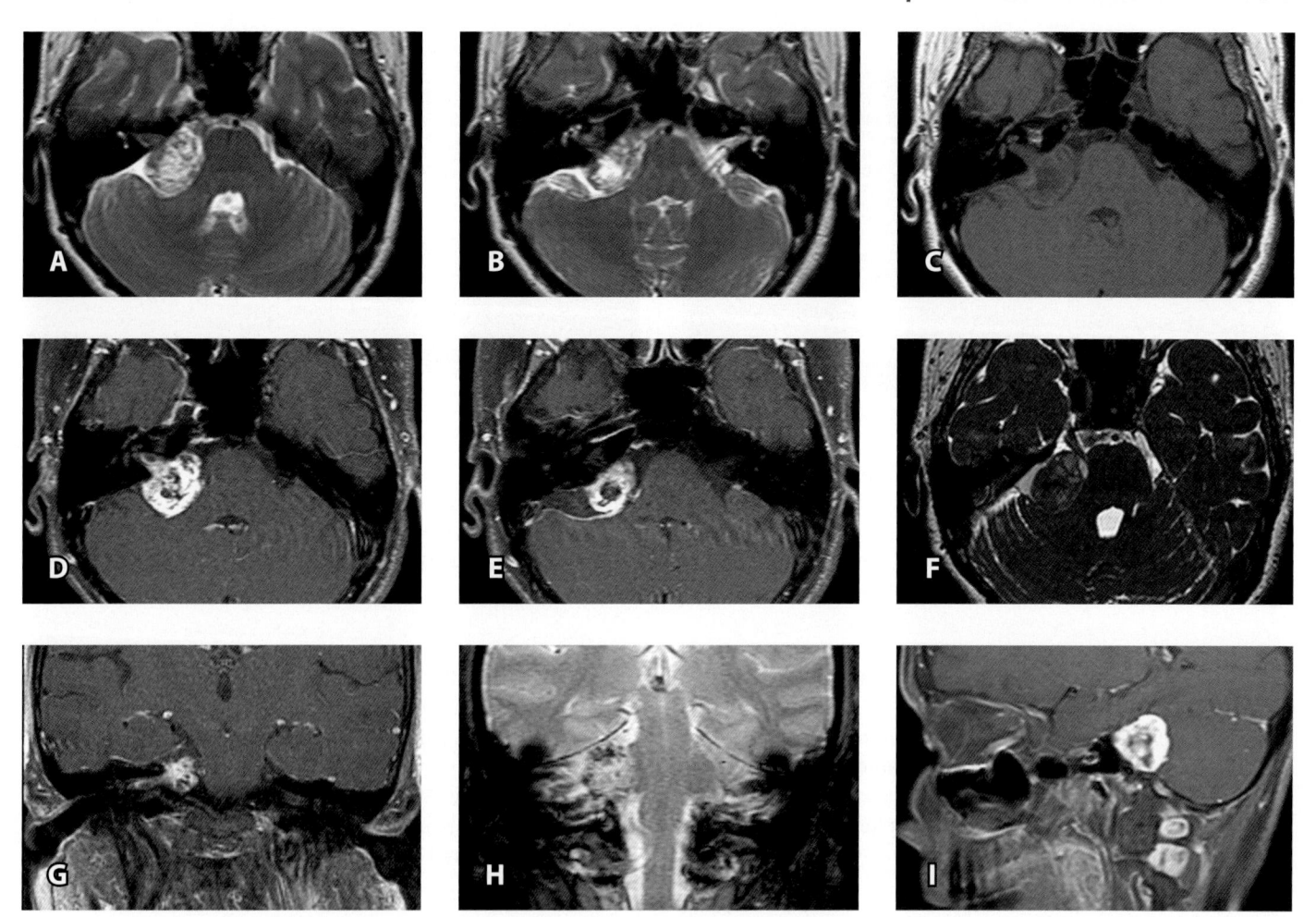

Figure 9-40 Vestibular Schwannoma and Associated Arachnoid Cyst
Large cystic/hemorrhagic vestibular schwannoma in 59-year-old female complaining of unilateral facial pain. Axial T2W (**A–B**), T1W (**C**) and T1W postcontrast (**D, E, G**) MR images depict a large, heterogeneous, extra-axial mass in the right cerebellopontine angle with extension into the right internal auditory canal. The "ice cream cone" shaped mass with low T1 signal, moderate to high T2 signal, and strong enhancement with contrast are typical of schwannomas at the cerebellopontine angle. 3D high-resolution heavily T2-weighted MR cisternography (**F**) shows the close proximity of the tumor to CN V, which is partially displaced by the mass as it exits the pons. Coronal T1W postcontrast image shows the intracanalicular extension of the mass, in addition to CN V enhancement as it courses just medial to the tumor. T2 GRE image (**H**) shows low signal in parts of the tumor, suggesting blood products. Sagittal T1W postcontrast MR image (**I**) displays the mass compressing posterior fossa structures. Also note the large peritumor CSF collection, representing an associated arachnoid cyst (**B, E**). Surgical decompression of associated arachnoid cysts often aids in isolating and resecting schwannomas.

Meningioma at the CPA

Meningioma is led only by vestibular schwannoma as the most common lesion of the CPA.[23,24] A meningioma of the skull base most often causes deficits in of CN VIII, leading to hearing loss and vertigo. However, it can also affect CN V and CN VII, producing symptoms of headache, retrobulbar pain, and facial paresthesias or spasms. CT imaging shows hyperdense lesions with calcifications in 20% of cases, as well as possible hyperostosis.[23] The best diagnostic clue, however, is an enhancing extra-axial mass on MR imaging with broad dural component and a possible dural tail (**Fig. 9-44**). The mass may extend into the external auditory canal, but typically will not enlarge the porus acusticus, a finding commonly associated with vestibular schwannomas. The mass is usually isointense to hypointense on T1 and isointense to hyperintense on T2 imaging. rCBV ratios on dynamic perfusion enhanced MR imaging are typically elevated with meningiomas, a finding that may help differentiate them from acoustic schwannomas, which typically have an rCBV ratio approximating 3[23] (**Table 9-21**).

Epidermoid Cyst of the CPA

Cerebellopontine angle epidermoid cysts are the cause of approximately 5% of regional lesions, following vestibular schwannoma and meningioma as the third most common

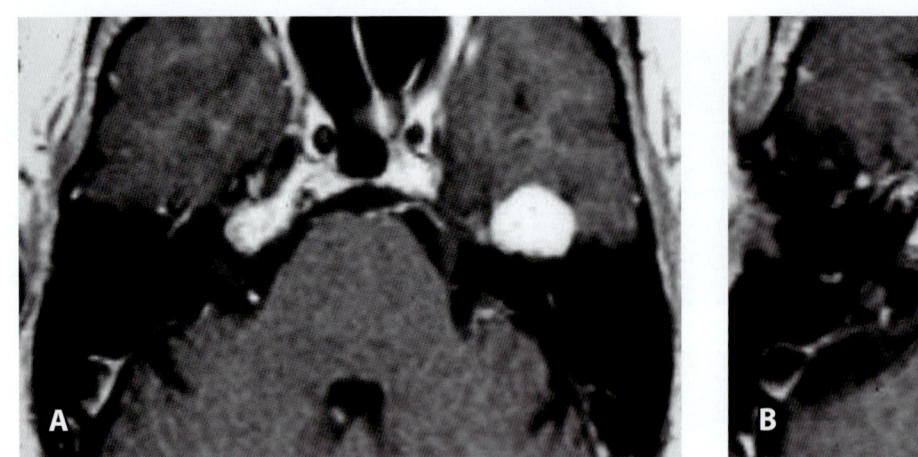

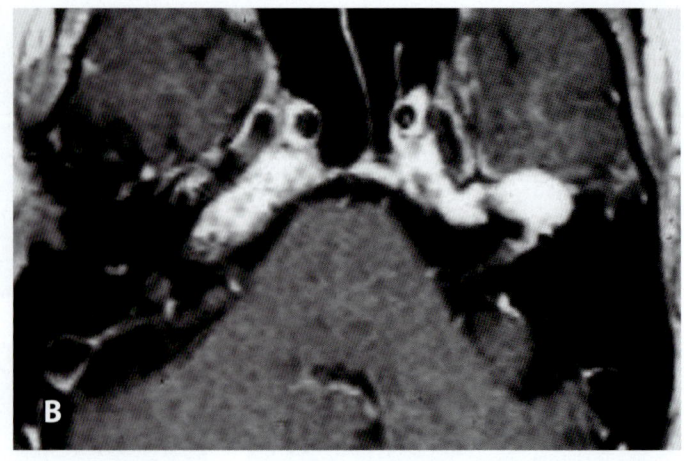

Figure 9-41 Geniculate Ganglion and Facial Nerve Schwannoma
Axial T1W postcontrast images (**A–B**) show an intensely enhancing mass in the left anterior part of the left temporal bone. The localization of the base of the tumor in the region of the geniculate ganglion and the retrograde tumor extension through the labyrinthine segment of CN VII and into the fundus of the internal auditory canal (**B**) help differentiate this left facial nerve schwannoma from the more common acoustic schwannoma.

pathology in the CPA. Approximately 50% of epidermoid cysts are located in the CPA and are the result of desquamation and keratin accumulation arising from heterotopic epithelial tissue. The noninvasive benign lesions enlarge slowly over time over paths of least resistance and may cause cranial neuropathy by encapsulating them, compromising their vascularization. Most epidermoid cysts are the result of congenital trapping of epithelial tissue within the cranium during development, though some may form as the result of intracranial epithelial growth during healing of tympanic membrane rupture. Symptomatic epidermoid cysts are usually large and have low T1 and high T2 signal, consistent with CSF and arachnoid cysts. However, the lesions will typically not attenuate on FLAIR imaging and show fluid restriction on DWI imaging, differentiating them from

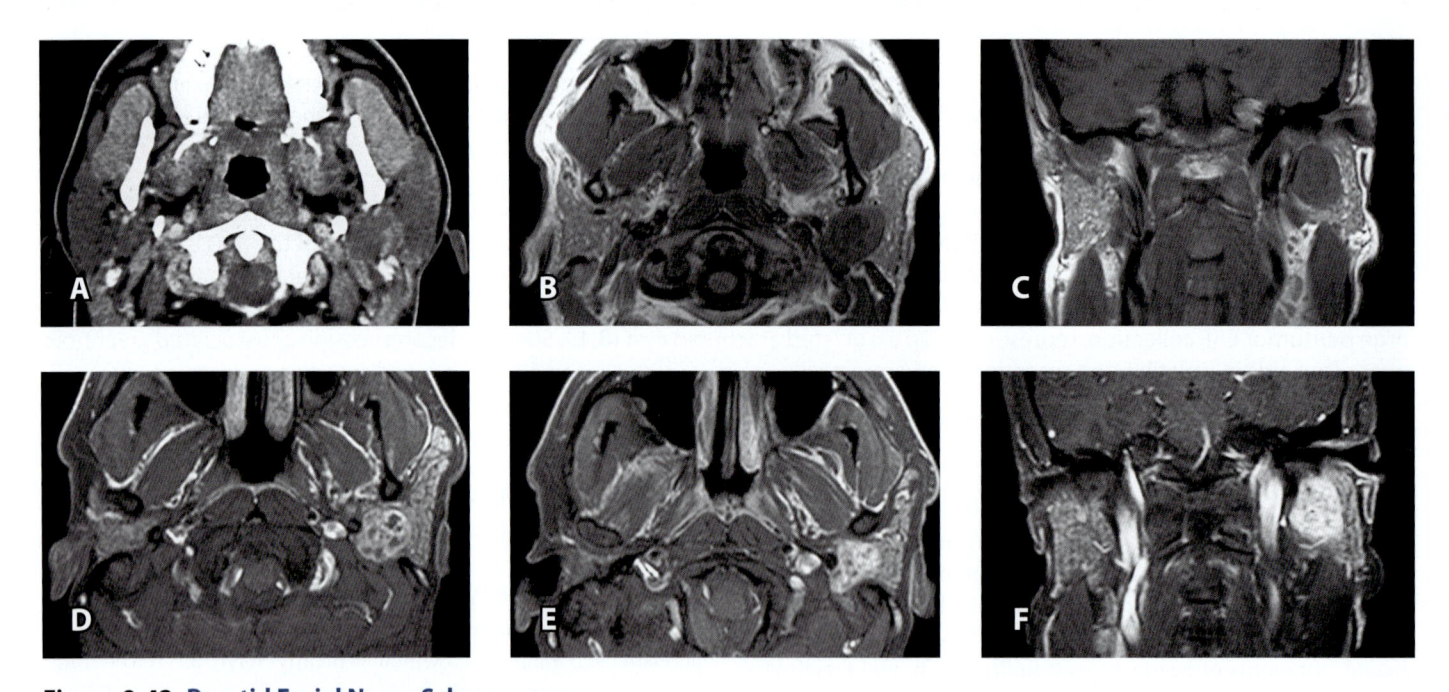

Figure 9-42 Parotid Facial Nerve Schwannoma
Facial nerve schwannoma in the parotid region of the left face. Axial NECT image (**A**) shows a homogenous mass isodense to soft tissue posterior to the angle of the jaw on the left. Axial (**B**) and coronal (**C**) T1W MR scans (**B–C**) show homogenous mass isointense to soft tissue mass with distinct boarders. Axial (**D–E**) and coronal (**F**) T1W postcontrast MR scans show a heterogeneously enhancing mass with some cystic areas, typical of larger schwannomas. Note the posterior local invasion of the tumor into the temporal bone (**E**).

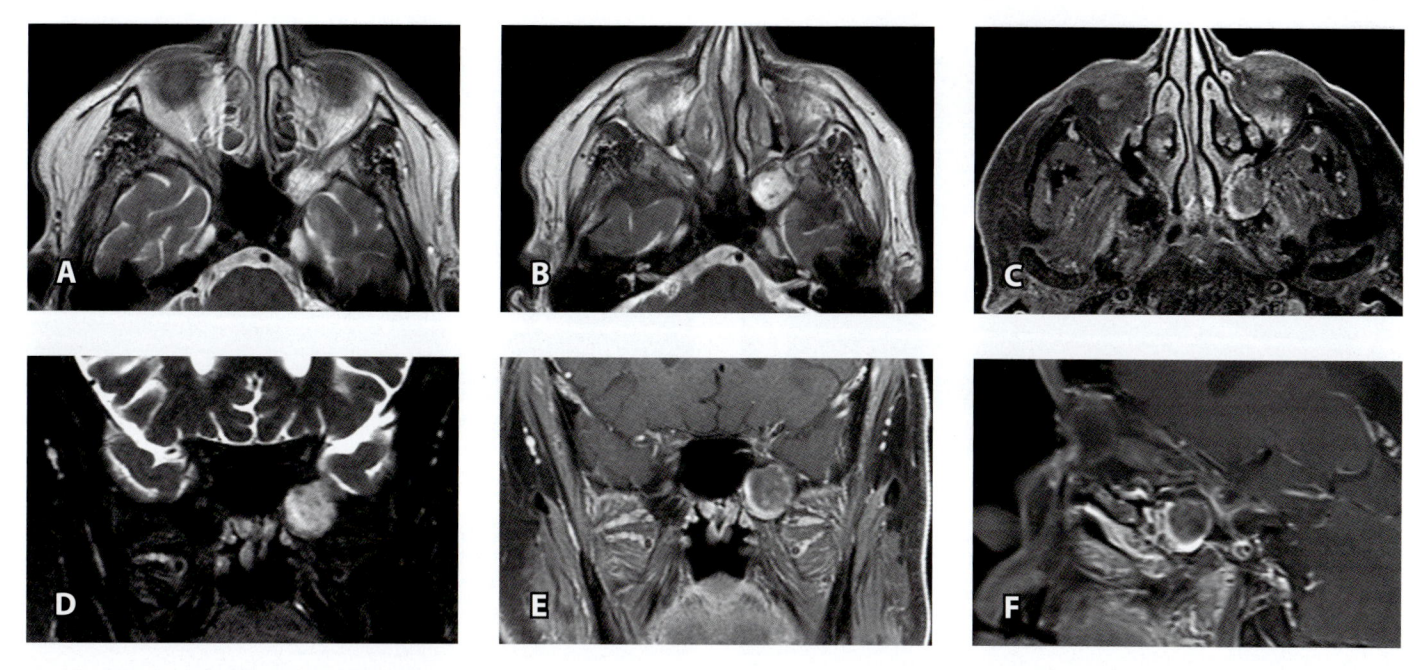

Figure 9-43 Schwannoma of CN V2
CN V2 schwannoma in a 75-year-old patient complaining of headaches, left ear fullness, and occasional vertigo. Axial T2W (**A–B**) and T1W postcontrast (**C**) MR images show a cystic, rim enhancing lesion just below the left inferior orbital fissure in the region of the pterygopalatine fossa. Coronal T2W (**D**), T1W postcontrast (**E**), and sagittal T1W postcontrast (**F**) MR images show the large cystic lesion in an enlarged foramen rotundum.

arachnoid cysts.[19] MR spectroscopy typically shows elevated lactate levels as the only abnormality.[110] Cisternography with 3D heavily T2-weighted high-resolution MR imaging is useful to characterize the exact location of the tumor, in order to plan for surgical excision.

Metastases to the CPA

Metastatic lesions account for less than 1% of pathology at the CPA-IAC. However, imaging patterns may mimic other lesions of the area, including meningioma and schwannoma. The most common metastatic cancers to the CPA-IAC include breast, lung, melanoma, colon, renal cell. Generally, metastasis causing cranial nerve symptoms at the CPA-IAC have four patterns of spread. Metastasis to the flocculus may exert mass effect on the root exit zone of CN VII and root entry zone of CN VII. Pia or arachnoid involvement, on the other hand, may track along the cranial nerves of the IAC, mimicking schwannomas of the nerves. Dural or pachymeningeal metastasis may show dural thickening, enhancement, and possibly the dural tail sign also commonly associated with meningiomas. Involvement of the choroid plexus as it exits the fourth ventricle may mimic either schwannoma or meningioma. Similar to schwannomas and meningiomas of the CPA-IAC, metastatic lesions are typically isointense on T1 and T2 imaging and enhance with contrast. However, eccentric lesions in the IAC, aggressive lytic bony destruction, or nodular parenchymal infiltration may

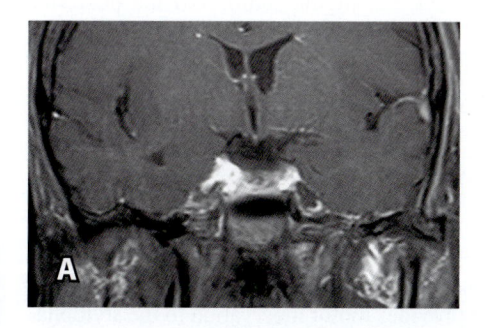

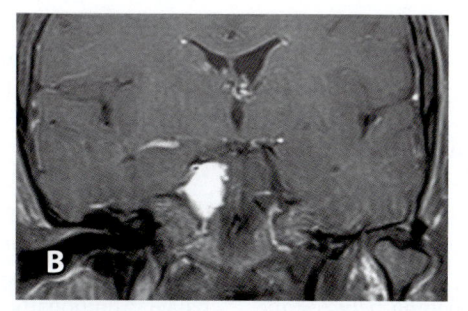

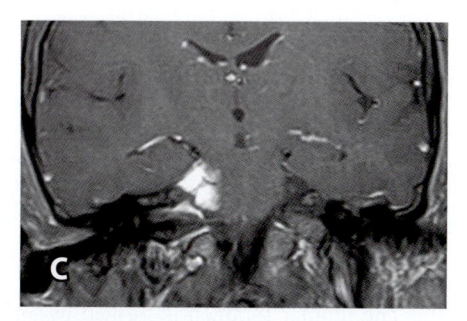

Figure 9-44 Cerebellopontine Angle Meningioma
Meningioma at the cerebellopontine angle. Coronal T1W post contrast images (**A–C**) show an intensely enhancing mass in the right cerebellopontine angle with extension to the contralateral cistern (**A**). Notice that the mass extends superiorly and exhibits a mass effect on the right cerebral hemisphere, seen as a concavity of the right lateral ventricle. Furthermore, a dural "tail" is seen in the right internal auditory canal, suggesting meningioma over other pathologies at the cerebellopontine angle.

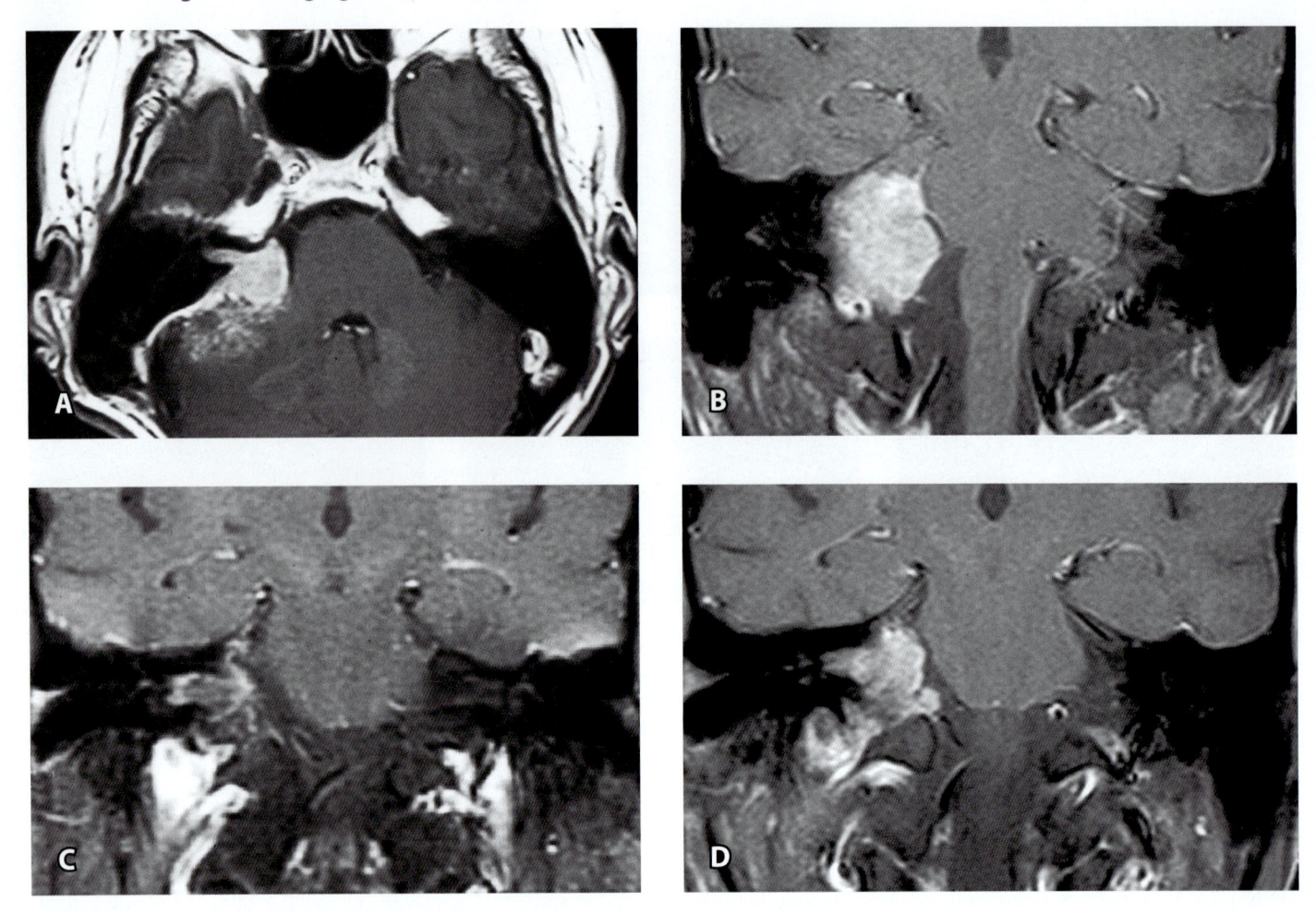

Figure 9-45 Melanoma Metastasis to the Cerebellopontine Angle
Axial (**A**) and coronal (**B–D**) T1W postcontrast MR images show a large, heterogeneously enhancing mass at the right cerebellopontine angle with extension into the right internal auditory canal (**A, C**). Note the enhancing leptomeningeal tail that may mimic that of a meningioma. Nodular infiltration of the ipsilateral brain parenchyma suggests metastases over other common lesions at the cerebellopontine angle.

suggest metastatic lesions (**Fig. 9-45**). Finally, rapidly progressive cranial symptoms may also differentiate these lesions from the slower growing meningiomas and schwannomas.[136]

NERVES TRAVERSING THE JUGULAR FORAMEN

The jugular foramen is located in the posterior skull base, lateral to the foramen magnum, and transmits CN IX, X, and XI in addition to the jugular bulb, inferior petrosal sinus, and posterior meningeal artery (**Fig. 9-46**). Regional pathology in the area often causes concurrent deficits in CN IX, X, and XI.

The jugular foramen is formed by an opening between the occipital and inferior edges of the temporal bone, just medial to the foramen magnum. It is partially divided by a bony protuberance of the temporal bone known as the jugular spine into the pars nervosa anteromedially and the larger pars jugularis posterolaterally. The pars nervosa transmits CN IX, the tympanic branch of CN IX (Jacobson's nerve), and the inferior petrosal sinus. The par jugularis is contiguous with the pars nervosa at its medial edge and transmits CN X, the auricular branch (Arnold's branch) of CN X, CN XI, the jugular bulb, and the posterior meningeal artery. CN XII passes through its own hypoglossal canal, located along the lateral edge of the foramen magnum, inferior to the jugular foramen.

CN IX Anatomy and Function

CN IX is also known as the glossopharyngeal nerve and is the embryologic remnant of the third brachial arch nerve. CN IX supplies sensory fibers to middle ear, posterior oropharynx, and soft palate. Additionally, it provides motor innervation to the stylopharyngeus and taste and sensation to the posterior one-third of the tongue. A summary of the various branches, functions, and clinical signs and symptoms of dysfunction are contained in **Table 9-22**.

Impulses from the motor cortex of the cerebral hemisphere extend to the genu of the internal capsule and subsequently

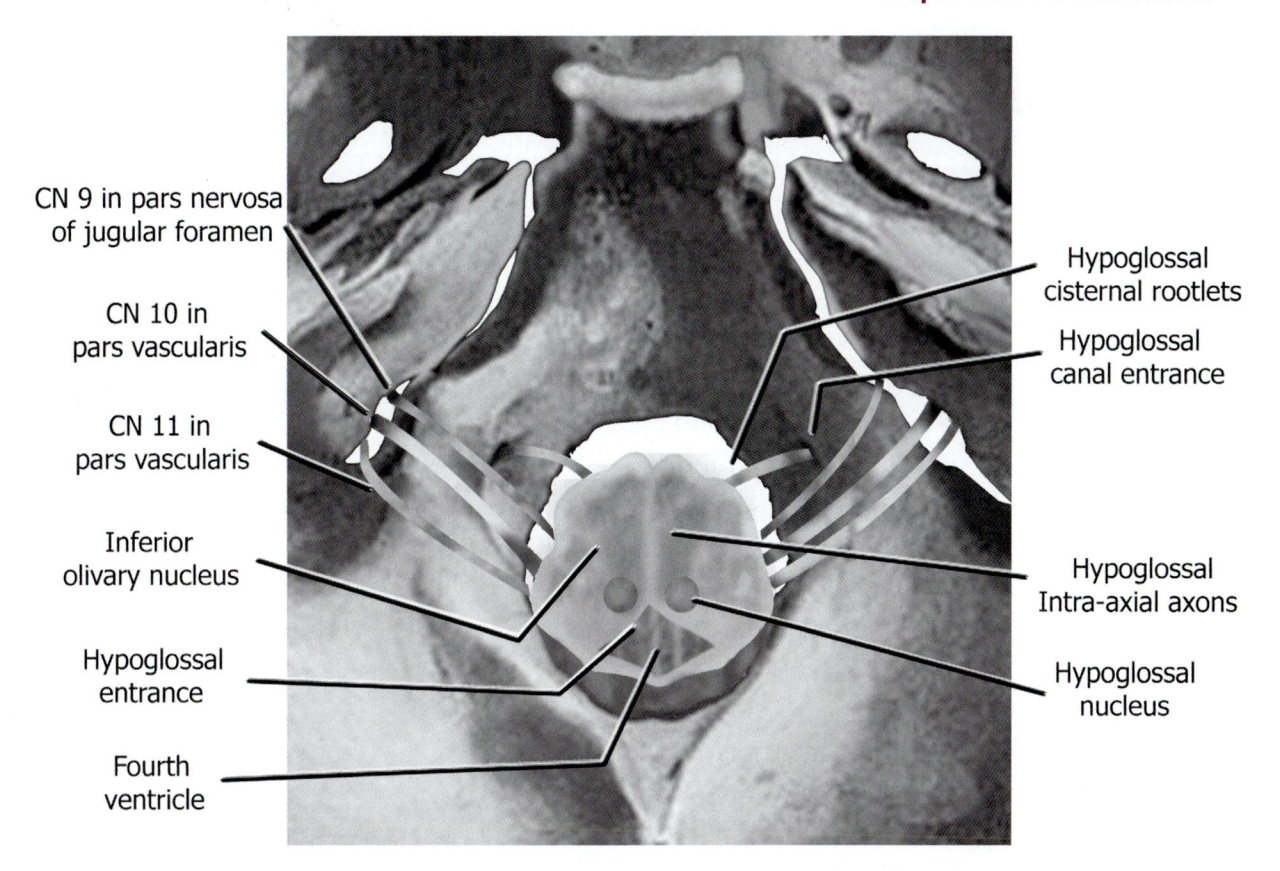

Figure 9-46 Lower Cranial Nerves IX to XII
Schematic of a superior-inferior view of CN IX to XII as they exit the lower brainstem and penetrate the skull base. CN IX to XI penetrate the jugular foramen, a space in the occipitotemporal junction, which also transmits the jugular vein as it exits the skull. The jugular spine, a bony prominence of the mastoid bone, partially separates the jugular foramen anteriorly into the pars nervosa and posteriorly into the pars vascularis. CN IX passes through the pars nervosa while CN X, CN XI, and the jugular vein pass through the pars vascularis. CN XII passes through its own hypoglossal foramen, which is located medially in the occipital bone just superior to the foramen magnum.

follow the corticobulbar tract through the midbrain to the nucleus ambiguous. The fibers extend to the posterior olivary sulcus, leaving the medulla at this point to extend anterolaterally to the superior and inferior glossopharyngeal ganglia situated in the jugular foramen. The fibers then travel inferiorly to supply the stylopharyngeus and constrictor muscles of the pharynx. In addition to this motor component to the muscles, there is a solitary nucleus for sensory fibers and a salivatory nucleus for parasympathetic fibers. These nuclei represent the primary sensory neurons for general visceral and special sensation, including taste for the posterior third of the tongue.

The sensory portion of the glossopharyngeal nerve joins the motor portion, which then extend together into the pars nervosa of the jugular foramen. There is a small tympanic branch (Jacobson's nerve) which supplies sensation to the middle ear and eustachian tube, as well as parasympathetic fibers to the parotid gland. A small visceral branch supplies the carotid body, which controls the pressor and chemoreceptor functions. Pharyngeal sensory branches supply the posterior oropharynx and soft palate. The lingual branch includes fibers for both sensation and taste for the posterior third of the tongue.[70]

CN X Anatomy and Function

CN X or vagus nerve is the nerve of the embryologic lower pharyngeal arches. It persists with motor and sensory functions of the head and neck, in addition to parasympathetic functions in the thorax and abdominal viscera. **Table 9-22** outlines the basic function and dysfunction of the branches of CN X in the head and neck. Impulses from the motor cortex of the cerebral hemisphere travel through the genu of the internal capsule and cerebral peduncle via the corticobulbar tract to the nucleus ambiguous. The fibers extend to the posterior olivary sulcus slightly more lateral than cranial nerve IX exiting the medulla in the groove between the inferior peduncle and olive. Cranial nerve X continues an anterolateral course with its companion nerves (cranial nerve IX and the bulbar portion of cranial nerve XI) through the perimedullary cistern. The vagus nerve and bulbar portion of the eleventh cranial nerve enter the anterior aspect of the pars vascularis of the jugular foramen. As previously

Table 9-22 Function of the Jugular Foramen Cranial Nerves

Cranial Nerve	Branch	Function	Dysfunction
CN IX Glossopharyngeal	tympanic branch (Jacobson's nerve)	• Sensation to middle ear and middle half of the tympanic membrane • Parasympathetics to parotid gland • Parasympathetics to tympanic plexus	• Otalgia • Paresthesia of the eustachian tube
	sinus nerve	• Sensory to carotid sinus • Sensory to carotid body	• Tachycardia or bradycardia with hypotension
	pharyngeal branches	• Sensory to posterior oropharynx • Sensory to soft palate	• Loss of afferent limb of gag reflex
	lingual branch	• Taste and sensation in posterior one-third of tongue	• Loss of taste and sensation in posterior one-third of tongue
	stylopharyngeal branch	• Motor to stylopharyngeus muscle	• Dysphagia
CN X Vagus	auricular branch (Arnold's nerve)	• Sensory to external segment of tympanic membrane, external auditory canal, and external ear	• Paresthesia of external auditory canal and external ear
	pharyngeal branches	• Sensory to epiglottis, trachea, and esophagus • Motor to soft palate, except for tensor veli palatini (CN III) • Motor to pharyngeal constrictor muscles	• Aspiration • Loss of efferent limb of gag reflex; uvula deviation contralateral to side of lesion
	superior laryngeal nerve	• Motor to cricothyroid muscle	• Mild hoarseness
	recurrent laryngeal nerve	• Motor to all laryngeal muscles except cricothyroid • Sensory to inferior glottis	• Unilateral: hoarseness • Bilateral: respiratory distress • Cervical dysphagia
CN XI Accessory	sternomastoid branch	• Motor to sternocleidomastoid	• Downward, lateral rotation of the scapula; • Ipsilateral compensatory hypertrophy of levator scapulae muscle
	trapezius branch	• Motor to trapezius	• Shoulder droop

discussed, the ninth cranial nerve enters the pars nervosa of the jugular foramen. After exiting the jugular foramen, the vagus nerve plunges like a plumb line along the posterolateral aspect of the carotid artery to the aortopulmonic window of the mediastinum on the left side, and to the clavicle on the right side. The right recurrent laryngeal branch turns cephalad around the right subclavian artery, while the left recurrent laryngeal branch turns cephalad by looping through the aortopulmonic window. Both recurrent laryngeal nerves reach the larynx via the tracheoesophageal groove. Sensory fibers of the vagus nerve begin in the thoracoabdominal viscera and chemoreceptors at the aortic arch. These then synapse in the solitary nucleus (pure sensory fibers) and the dorsal motor nucleus (parasympathetic secretomotor fibers).[70]

Table 9-23 Imaging Patterns in Common Jugular Foramen Lesions

Pathology	CT Findings	MR Findings	Angiography Findings
Glomus Tumor	• Aggressive bone erosion/destruction	• Low T1, high T2 signal • Flow voids "salt and pepper" • Intense enhancement	• Vascular blush • AV fistulae • Early venous drainage
Meningioma	• Sclerotic bone erosion	• Low T1, mid-high T2 signal • Heterogenous T2 in larger lesions • Intense enhancement	• Vascular blush • No AV fistulae • No early venous drainage
Schwannoma	• Smooth bone erosion	• Low T1, high T2 signal • Cystic T2 possible in larger lesions • Intense enhancement	• Nondiagnostic
Metastasis	• Lytic, eccentric bone destruction	• Variable	• Nondiagnostic

AV = arteriovenous.

CN XI Anatomy and Function

CN XI is also known as the accessory nerve; its only functionality is motor innervation to the trapezius and sternocleidomastoid muscles. Impulses from the motor cortex of the cerebral hemisphere extend through the genu of the internal capsule and cerebral peduncle via the corticobulbar tract to the nucleus ambiguous. The motor fibers of the bulbar portion of the spinal accessory nerve are joined by additional fibers which arise from the anterior horn cells of the first five cervical cord segments. The fibers from the spinal nucleus have ascended through the foramen magnum. Together, the combined fibers from the bulbar and spinal portions of the spinal accessory nerve pass anteriorly to exit from the medulla at the posterior olivary sulcus. The XIth cranial nerve joins the companion cranial nerves IX and X to pass through the perimesencephalic cistern. The spinal accessory nerve then leaves the skull via the posterior portion of the pars vascularis of the jugular foramen. From the skull base, the XIth cranial nerve enters the carotid space and then quickly diverges posterolaterally to descend along the medial aspect of the sternocleidomastoid muscle. The nerve then continues its course across the posterior triangle of the neck to terminate in the trapezius muscle.[70]

Pathology of Cranial Nerves Traversing the Jugular Foramen

CN IX, X, and XI traverse the jugular foramen and are often concurrently affected by pathology at this region. Glomus jugulare paraganglioma is the most lesion at this location, followed by schwannoma of CN IX, X, or XI, and meningioma[18,21,22,137-139] (Table 9-23). Additionally, metastatic lesions and various other primary and secondary tumors can rarely affect the jugular foramen[18] (Table 9-24). Because of the long intrathoracic course of the vagus nerve and its recurrent laryngeal branches, pathology of the lower neck and thorax may cause palsy of the CN X motor functions, manifesting as hoarseness (Table 9-25). Finally, there may be several congenital asymptomatic lesions mimicking pathology at the jugular foramen, including flow artifacts, high riding and dehisced jugular bulbs, and jugular diverticula.

Lower Cranial Nerve Syndromes

Lower cranial nerve syndromes consist of various combinations of palsies in CN IX, X, XI, and XII. Because CN IX, X, and XI traverse the same foramen, they are often affected by the same disease processes. The clinical presence of palsies of CN IX, X, and XI is known as Vernet or jugular foramen syndrome. Concurrent involvement of the jugular foramen nerves with CN XII is less frequent, considering that CN XII traverses the hypoglossal foramen in the lateral border of the foramen magnum. Furthermore, the sympathetic chain is even less frequently involved

Table 9-24 Uncommon Pathology of the Jugular Foramen

- Peripheral primitive neuroectodermal tumor
- Chondrosarcoma
- Chordoma
- Chondroblastoma
- Giant-cell tumor
- Endolymphatic sac tumor
- Cholesterol granuloma
- Reactive myofibroblastic tumor
- Temporal bone carcinoma

Table 9-25 Infrahyoid Pathology of CN X

- Metastatic neck carcinoma (infrahyoid)
- Thyroid goiter
- Malignant nodes
- Lymphoma
- Angiopathic
- Aortic aneurysm

due to its position below the level of the jugular foramen. However, large lesions or low lesions may also affect CN XII and the sympathetic chain, in addition to the jugular foramen nerves. A list of cranial nerves involved in various lower cranial nerve syndromes, along with the likely location of their pathology is contained in Table 9-26.[140–142]

Glomus Paragangliomas

Glomus bodies or paraganglia of the head and neck are neural crest derived chemoreceptors that respond to differences in blood oxygen and carbon dioxide levels. Tumors of this tissue are referred to as paragangliomas, glomus tumors, or chemodectomas. They are highly vascular, benign in 90% of cases, and embryologically related to the catecholamine-releasing sympathetic-derived chromaffin tumors found mostly in the adrenal medulla (pheochromocytoma), Zuckerland body, the sympathetic plexus of the urinary bladder, the heart, the kidneys, and the sympathetic ganglia of the mediastinum.[137,143] However, most head and neck paragangliomas are derived from parasympathetic nervous tissue and thus do not secrete catecholamines.[139,144]

Paragangliomas in the region of the head and neck usually arise from six locations and are classified by region[138,143] (Table 9-27). Of note, most structures involved in paraganglioma are embryologically derived from the third pharyngeal arch in that most neural structures carry parasympathetics fibers of CN IX and the carotid bifurcation derives from the third arch vasculature.[138]

Unilateral hyperplasia of the carotid bodies has been documented in populations living at high altitudes and is thought to be caused by chronic hypoxic conditions, supported by the finding that the condition is 8 times more common in women who

Table 9-26 Lower Cranial Nerve Syndromes

Syndrome	Pathology Location	CN IX Loss of afferent gag reflex; dysphagia	CN X Hoarseness; loss of efferent gag reflex; uvula deviation	CN XI Shoulder Droop	CN XII Tongue paralysis	Sympathetics Horner Syndrome
Vernet, jugular foramen	Jugular foramen	X	X	X		
Collet-Sicard	Retroparotid space	X	X	X	X	
Villaret's	Retroparotid, retropharyngeal space	X	X	X	X	X
Schmidt's	Pars vascularis of jugular foramen		X	X		
Jackson	Brainstem		X	X	X	
Tapia	High neck			X	X	

Adapted with permission from Brazis PW, Masdeu JC, and Biller J: Localization in Clinical Neurology, 5th ed. Philadelphia: Lippincott Williams & Wilkins, 2007:xiii, 594.

Table 9-27 Classification of Paragangliomas of the Head and Neck

Paraganglioma Location	Paraganglioma Classifications		Symptoms and Signs
Carotid Body afferent branches of CN IX located between carotid branches at their bifurcation	carotid body paraganglioma; glomus body tumor		painless cervical mass, possible CN X palsy
Tympanic branch of CN IX (Jacobson's nerve) contains parasympathetic branches travelling to otic ganglion	glomus tympanicum paraganglioma	glomus jugulotympanicum paraganglioma	pulsatile tinnitus conductive hearing loss
Jugular Bulb Adventitia	glomus jugulare paraganglioma		hoarseness (CN X palsy) dysphagia (CN IX palsy) shoulder weakness (CN XI palsy)
Auricular branch of CN X (Arnold's nerve) contains parasympathetic branches of CN IX traveling to otic ganglion			
Nodose ganglia of CN X contains parasympathetic tributaries of CN IX	glomus vagale		painless mass, possible Horner syndrome
Superior of Inferior Laryngeal Paraganglia rare	laryngeal paraganglioma		dysphonia, stridor, dysphagia, dyspnea

have lower hemoglobin counts.[138] MEN-I, NF-1, and von Hippel-Lindau may predispose to the disease. Multicentric tumor foci are more common in genetically-linked paragangliomas. Early radiographic screening and surgery is recommended in populations with genetic conditions predisposing to paraganlgiomas.[137,139]

MR imaging shows low T1 signal and high T2 signal. Dark areas within the tumor represent high flow voids of feeding arteries, giving it a "salt and pepper" appearance. Due to the highly vascular nature of the tumor, these lesions will intensely enhance with contrast. Angiography is considered the gold standard of diagnosing small paragangliomas and typically shows enlarged feeding arteries with an associated vascular blush and early draining veins. Bone CT may also show destructive bony changes in the area of the jugular foramen in paragangliomas arising at that location, helping to differentiate them from other lesions of the jugular foramen, including schwannoma and meningioma (**Table 9-23**). Glomus vagale tumors cause anterior displacement of the internal and external arteries and may cause splaying of these vessels in some cases (**Figs. 9-47–9-49**). Carotid body tumors, on the other hand, will splay the internal and external branches of the carotid artery laterally at its bifurcation.[137–139]

Jugular Foramen Schwannomas

Schwannomas are the second most common jugular foramen lesion, but account for only 2.9% to 4% of intracranial schwannomas.[21] The tumors may be spontaneous, presenting most commonly in the fourth decade. However, the lesion is commonly associated with neurocutaneous syndromes, most notably NF-2, in which earlier age of onset is seen.[17] Schwannomas of the jugular foramen typically arise most frequently from CN IX, followed by CN X and CN XI. However, it is often not possible differentiate jugular foramen tumor origins to any particular nerve based on exam or imaging.[17]

Of note, most jugular foramen schwannomas do not present with lower CN palsies, but with pulsatile tinnitus and sensorineural hearing loss, similar to vestibular schwannomas. Such symptoms are thought to be caused by mass effect on the posterior fossa.[21,22] Cerebellar involvement, palsies of CN IX, X, VI, VI and V, and papilledema are usually only present with larger lesions.[17] A middle ear mass is rarely seen on otoscopy.[21]

High-resolution CT and MR with contrast are recommended to diagnose jugular foramen schwannomas.[21] Low T1 signal, high T2 signal, and intense enhancement are characteristic of smaller lesions. Larger lesions may demonstrate cystic heterogeneity up to 25% of the time[21,22] (**Table 9-23**). If the

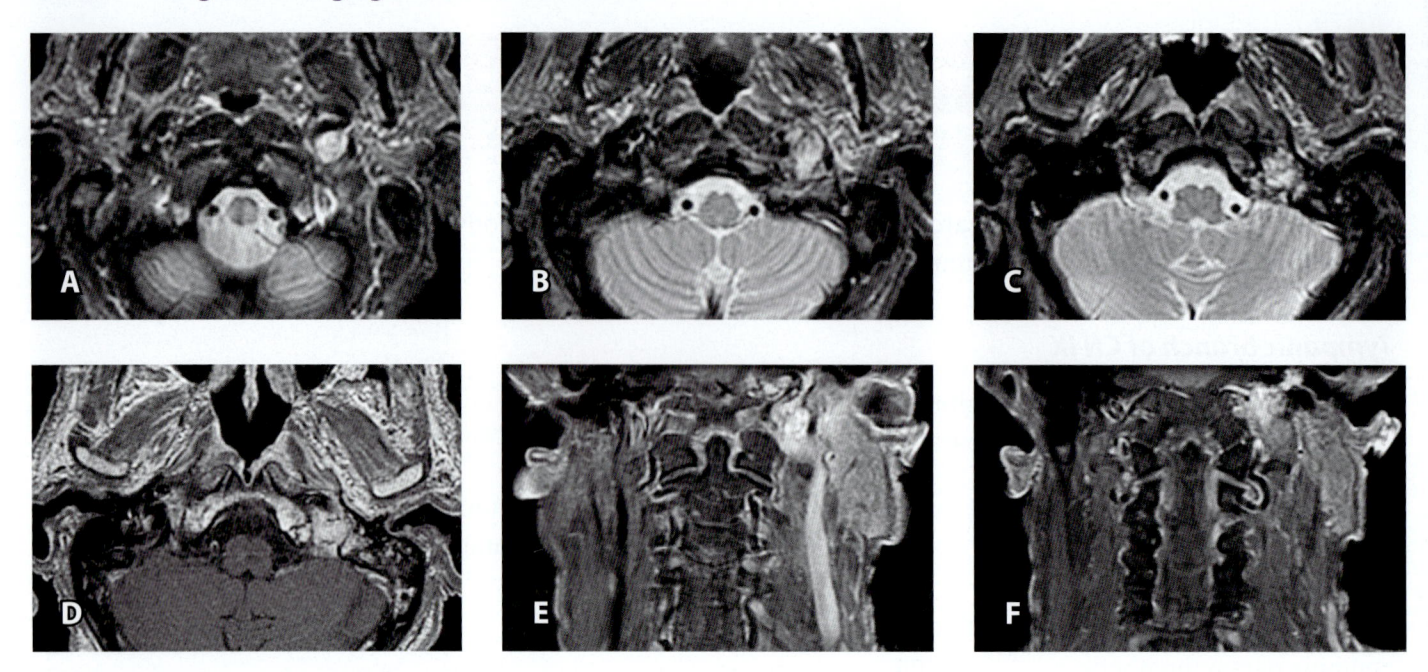

Figure 9-47 Glomus Jugulare Paraganglioma
Axial T2W (**A–C**), axial T1W fat saturated (**D**), and coronal T1W fat-saturated (**E–F**) MR images depict a glomus paraganglioma extending from the inferior portion of the left jugular foramen (**A**) to the jugular bulb (**C–F**). Note the "salt and pepper" appearance of the tumor on T2W images, depicting the highly vascular nature of the lesion with accompanying dilated feeder vessels, producing hypointense flow voids. (Case courtesy of Lubdha Shah, MD.)

lesion extends superiorly into the cerebellopontine angle, it may be difficult to distinguish from vestibular and facial nerve schwannomas unless there are concurrent cranial nerve symptoms (**Fig. 9-50**).[17]

Gross tumor may be visualized within the jugular foramen, as an intracranial mass, as an extracranial mass, or as intracranial and extracranial masses separated by a narrow bridge of tumor as it traverses the jugular foramen, giving the tumor a dumbbell appearance (**Fig. 9-51** and **Fig. 9-52**). The tumor may displace the carotid arteries anteriorly and medially if it descends low enough into the carotid space.[21] Surgery is the mainstay treatment, with varying degrees of CN preservation, depending on the approach.[21]

Jugular Foramen Meningioma

Meningiomas of the jugular foramen may extend secondarily into the jugular foramen from other areas or may arise primarily from the arachnoid of the jugular foramen itself.[145] Primary lesions may originate within the jugular foramen, may extend superiorly into the posterior fossa or may extend inferiorly

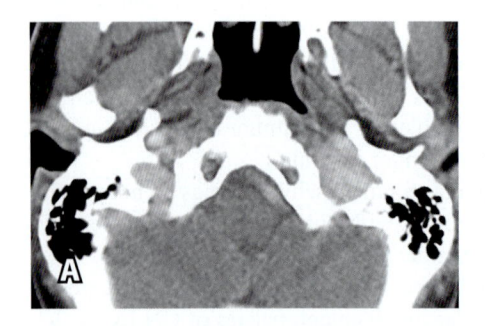

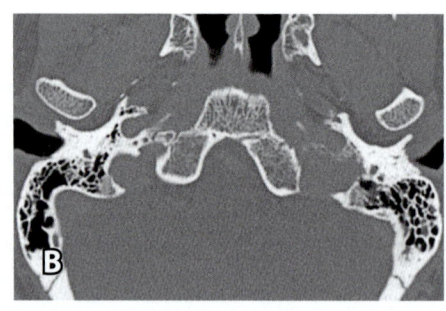

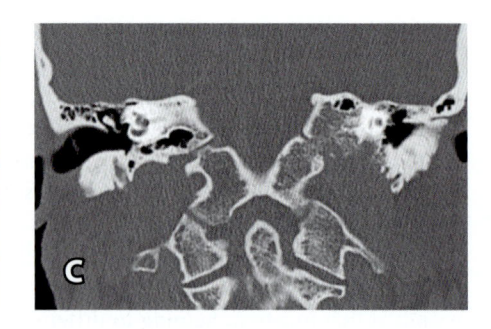

Figure 9-48 Glomus Jugulare Paraganglioma
Biopsy proven glomus paraganglioma of the left jugular foramen. Axial soft tissue (**A**), axial bone (**B**), and coronal bone (**C**) CT scans show an attenuating tumor (**A**) expanding the left jugular foramen. Note the concentric, moth-eaten appearance of the surrounding bone of the left jugular foramen, compared to the normal smooth corticated canalicular bone on the right (**B–C**). The aggressive nature of the bone destruction helps to differentiate this lesion from jugular foramen schwannoma or meningioma. However, metastatic lesions to the region may be difficult to differentiate from glomus jugulare paragangliomas on CT imaging alone. (Case courtesy of Lubdha Shah, MD.)

Chapter 9: The Cranial Nerves 411

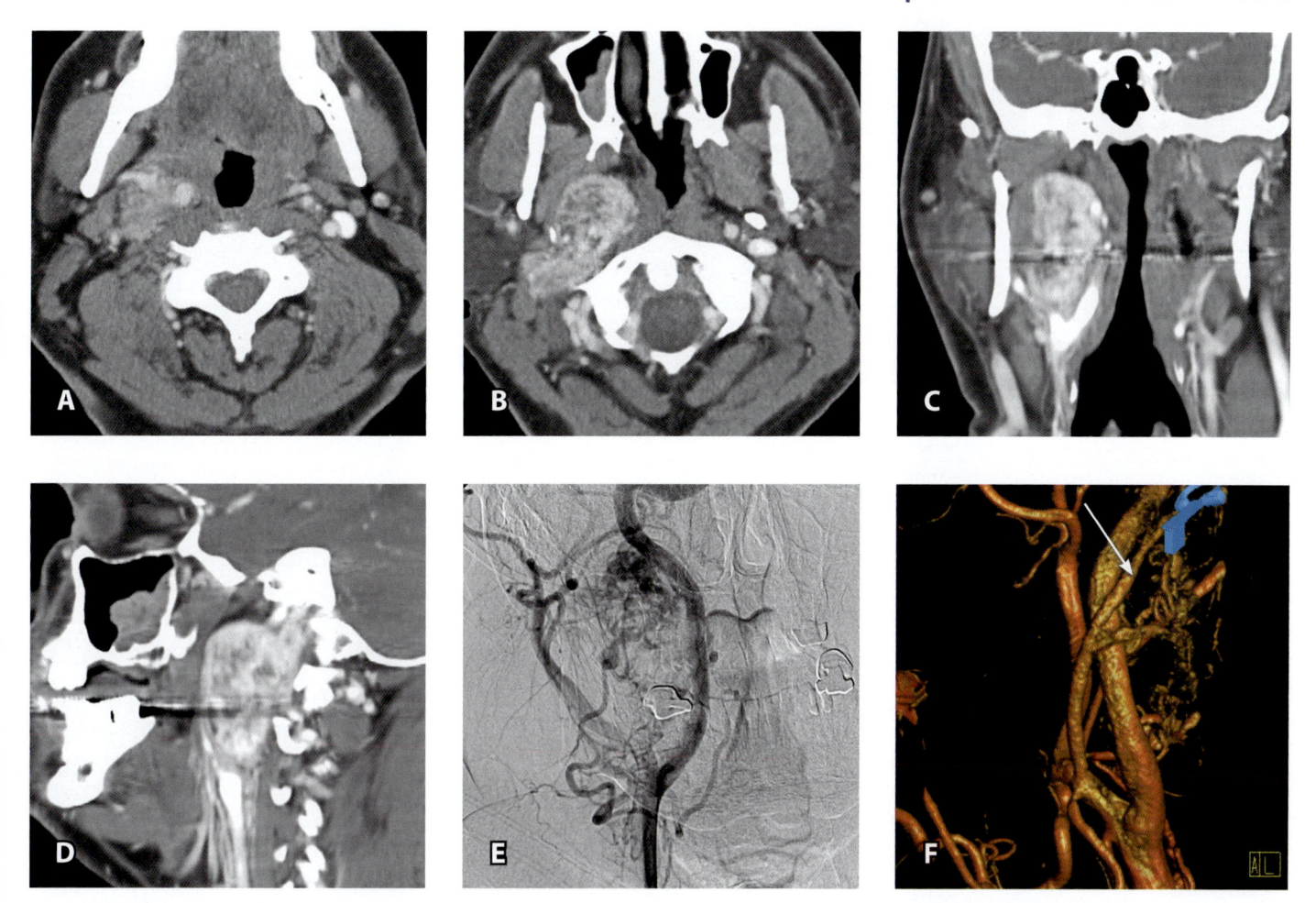

Figure 9-49 Glomus Vagale Tumor
A 44-year-old male with glomus vagale tumor complaining of facial weakness and a neck mass. Axial CECT scans (**A–B**) show a large, heterogeneously enhancing mass at the level of the left carotid bifurcation. Note that the internal and external branches of the left carotid are splayed and anteriorly displaced by the mass. Coronal CECT scan (**C**) shows the mass at the level of the left carotid bifurcation, causing narrowing of the pharyngeal space via mass effect. Sagittal CECT scan (**D**) shows the lesion extending upward into the jugular foramen, though there is no particular widening of the jugular canal. AP DSA (**E**) shows splaying of the internal and external carotid artery branches with a large vascular blush starting at the superior margin of the mass. Oblique 3D angiographic reconstruction (**F**) shows a grossly enlarged left ascending pharyngeal artery (*arrow*) as the main vascular supply of the tumor, typical of glomus tumors at this region.

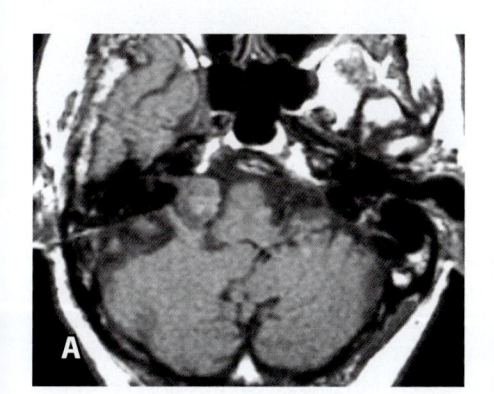

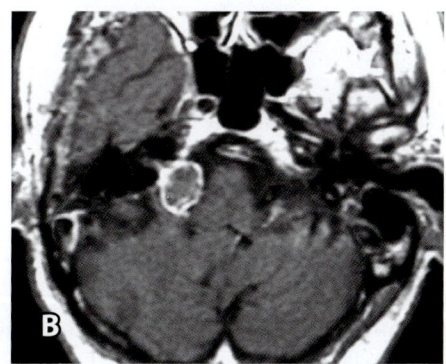

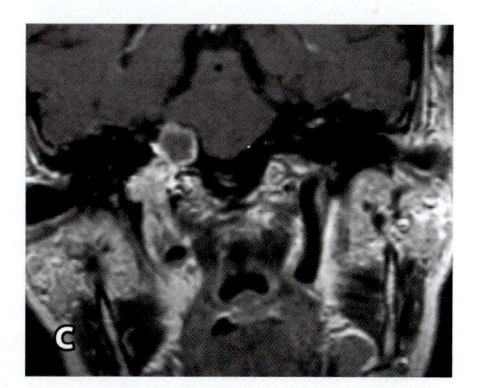

Figure 9-50 CN X Schwannoma in the CPA
Schwannoma of CN X within the cerebellopontine angle. Axial T2 FLAIR (**A**) and axial T1W postcontrast (**B**) show an extra-axial lesion in the right cerebellopontine angle with peripheral enhancement and extension into the internal auditory canal, mimicking a vestibular schwannoma. Coronal T1W postcontrast image (**C**) shows the caudal fusiform expansion of the tumor to the region of the jugular foramen. Strong enhancement of the body of the tumor with cystic heterogeneity is common in large schwannomas.

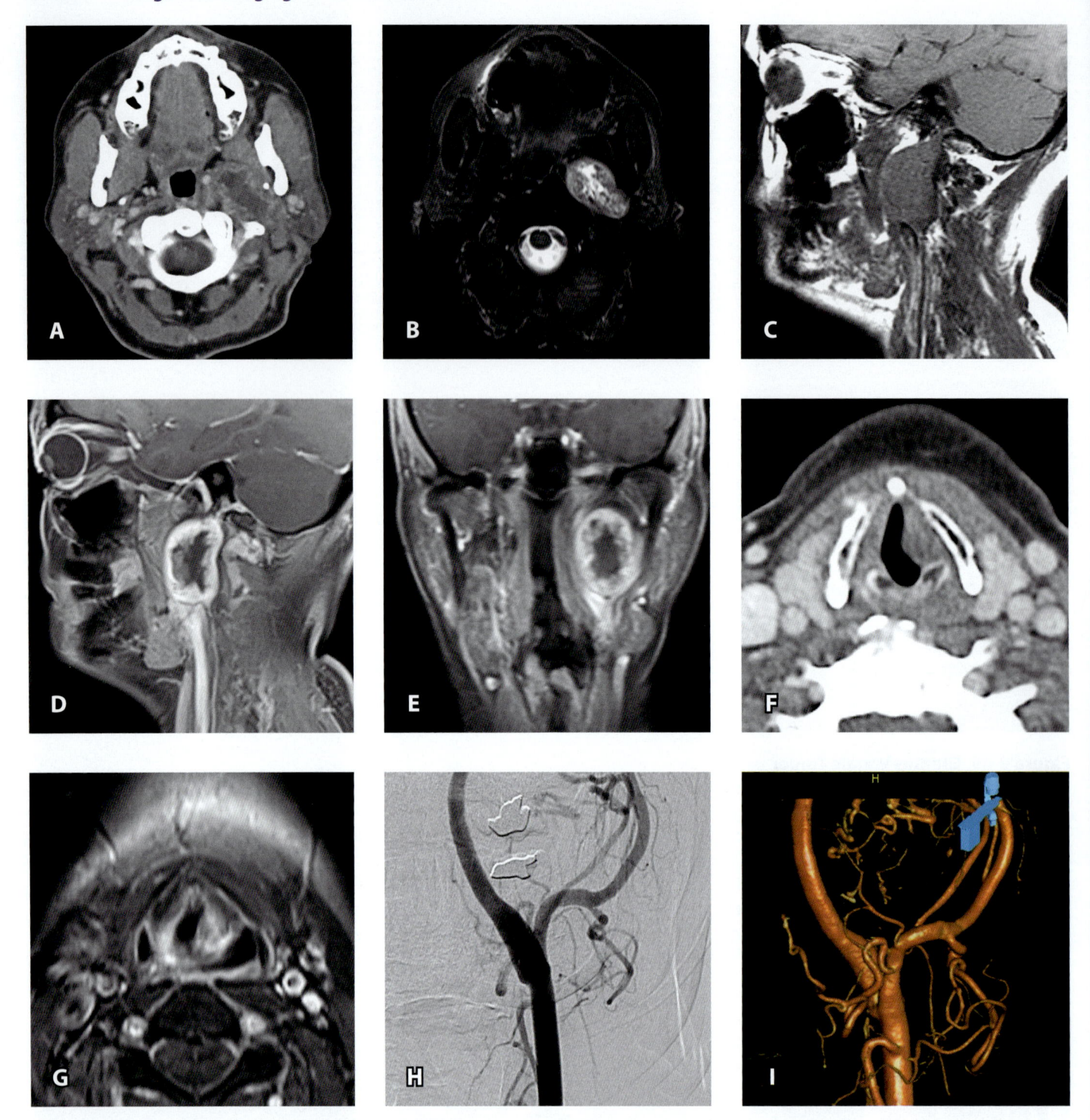

Figure 9-51 Extracranial Schwannoma of CN X
Extracranial schwannoma of CN X in a 54-year-old female complaining of hoarseness. Axial CT scan with contrast (**A**) shows a large mass in the left carotid space just inferior to the skull base with a central cystic cavity. T2W MR image with fat saturation (**B**) shows the large hyperintense mass with a central cystic cavity and the absence of vascular flow voids. Sagittal T1W image (**C**) confirms the location of the mass just inferior to the skull base at the level of the jugular foramen with a possible intraforaminal extension. Sagittal (**D**) and coronal (**E**) T1 postcontrast images show a strongly enhancing mass with a large cystic component at the level of the left common carotid bifurcation. Axial contrast-enhanced CT scan (**F**) and T1W MR image (**G**) at the level of the vocal cords show left vocal cord paralysis with thickening of the ipsilateral aryepiglottic fold and enlargement of the piriform sinus, consistent with ipsilateral CN X palsy. Digital subtraction angiogram (**H**) and 3D angiogram reconstruction with volume rendering (**I**) at the level of the left common carotid bifurcation show a wide splaying of the internal and external branches of the left common carotid artery in the region of the mass. Note the lack of early blushes AV fistulas, early venous drainage (**H**) and vascular flow voids on MR imaging (**B**), helping to differentiate the mass from a glomus tumor.

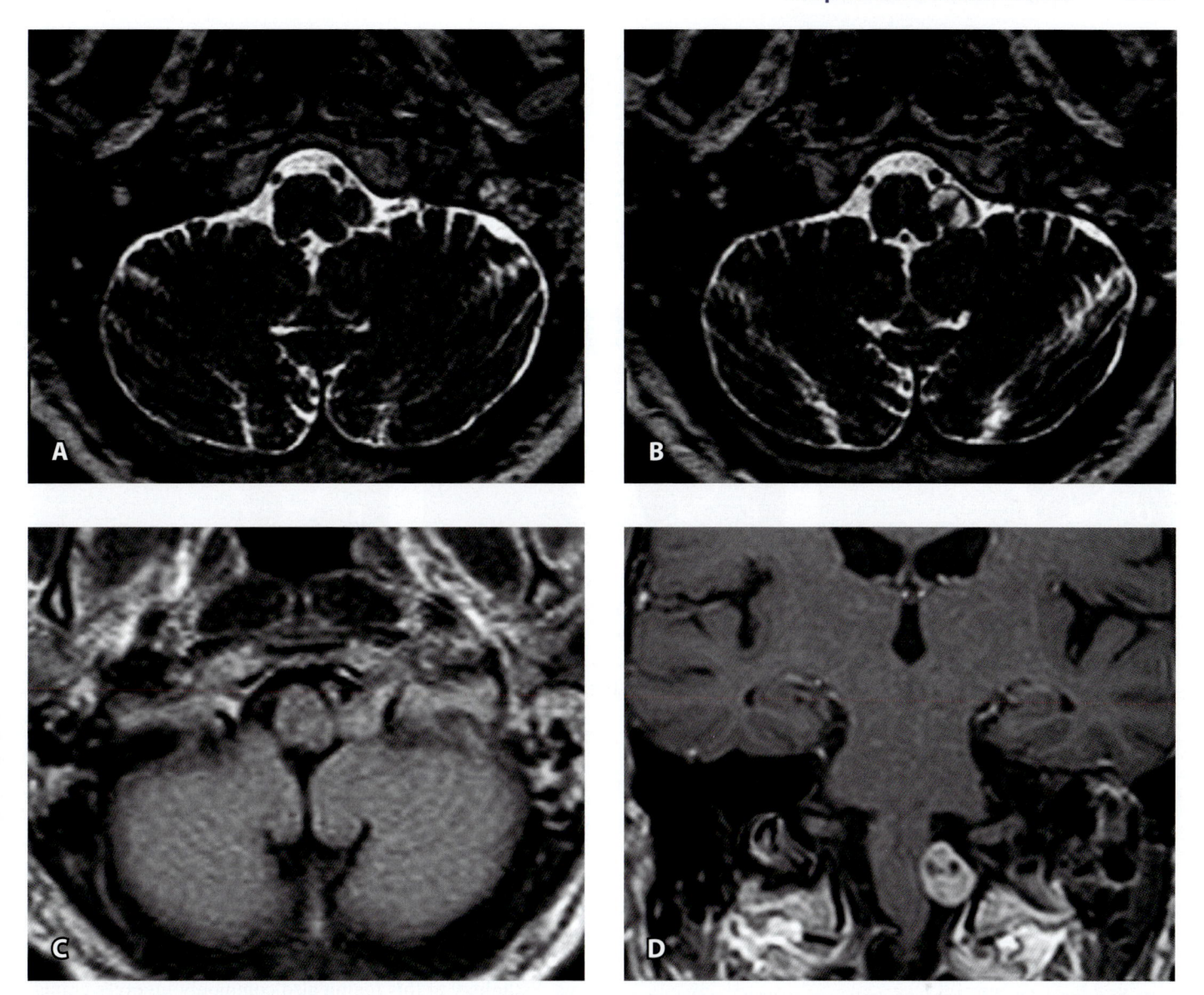

Figure 9-52 CN IX Schwannoma
Glossopharyngeal schwannoma in a 73-year-old male. Axial 3D heavily T2-weighted cisternograms (**A–B**) highlight the extra-axial nature of the lesion and demonstrate its cystic appearance. Axial T2 FLAIR MR image (**C**) shows a homogenous mass in the left prepontine cistern with lateral extension into the jugular foramen. Coronal T1 postcontrast MR image (**D**) shows strong enhancement with cystic hypointensities, typical of larger schwannomas. Note the dumbbell shape of the lesions, characterized by narrow enhancing extension of the tumor inferiorly through the jugular foramen and the connected larger cystic enhancing infratemporal portion of the tumor (**D**).

into the carotid space.[18] Presenting symptoms most commonly include hearing loss, vertigo, and tinnitus. Dysphagia (CN X), shoulder weakness (CN XI), headache, aural fullness, and tongue paresis (CN XII) are less common manifestations.[18,146]

CT imaging typically shows only mild bony infiltration with a relative preservation of architecture, differentiating this lesion from the typically extensive bony destruction common of glomus jugulare paragangliomas. MR findings are typical for meningioma, including hypointense T1 signal, intermediate T2 signal, intense enhancement, and an accompanying dural tail in many cases (**Table 9-23**). Arteriography shows a vascular blush, but not the AV fistulae that are characteristic of glomus jugulare paragangliomas. Surgical management is recommended in most symptomatic cases.[18]

Metastases to the Jugular Foramen

The most common primary site of metastasis involving the jugular foramen is the head and neck, followed by breast, lung, and prostate tumors.[18] Imaging findings are typically nonspecific, but may include lytic bony changes on CT, coupled with circumferential expansion without regard to bony or fibrous boundaries and heterogenous enhancement[21] (**Table 9-23, Fig. 9-53**).

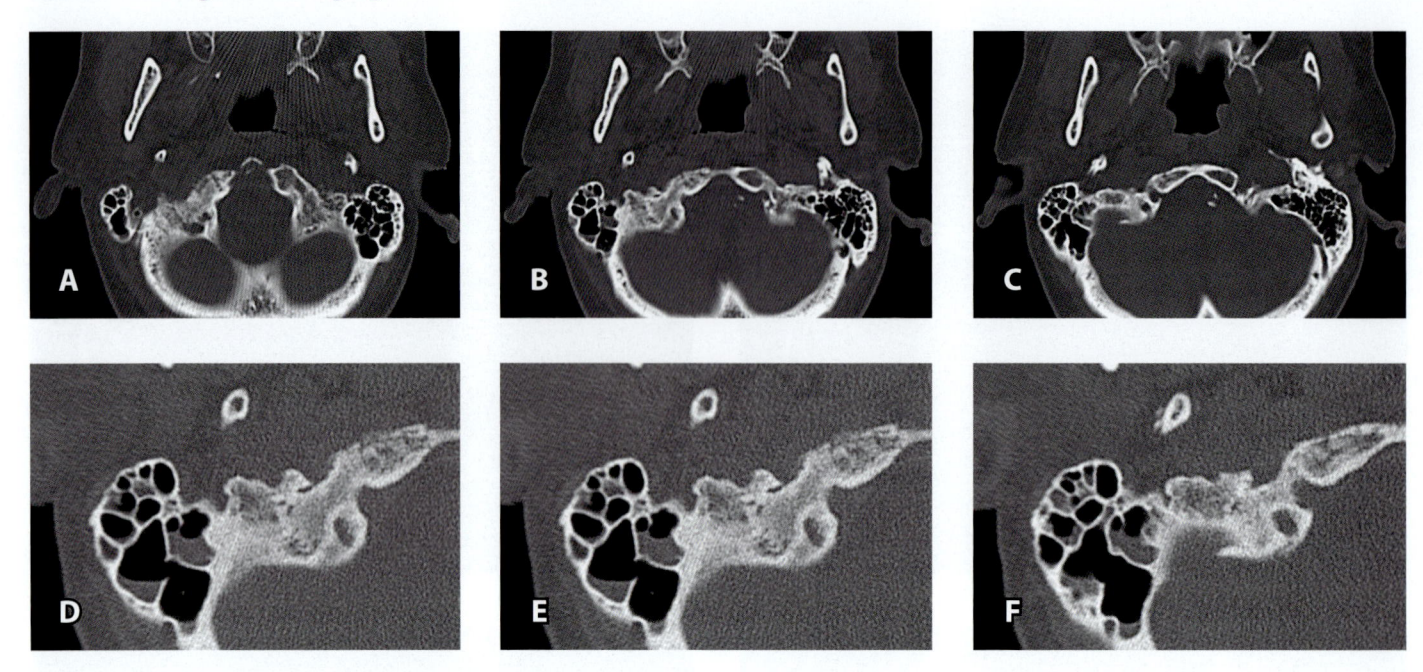

Figure 9-53 Sclerotic Prostate Cancer Metastasis to the Occipital Condyle
Metastatic temporal bone disease in a 68-year-old male with prostate cancer, presenting with tongue paralysis, deviation of tongue to the right, and right sternocleidomastoid atrophy. Axial bone CT scans (**A–C**) and right temporal bone thin slice scans (**D–F**) show eccentric, lytic, bone lesions of the occipital condyle in the region of CN XII. Right temporal bone thin slice scans (**D–F**) depict the sclerotic changes in the jugular foramen. Also note the pathologic fracture in the left occipital condyle, as well as the patchy infiltrates in the left mastoid air cells.

Developmental Abnormalities of the Jugular Foramen

The formation of jugular bulbs happens in the postnatal period and is usually not complete until after the age of 2. They are thought to arise from reverse pressure waves from the right atrium. A more direct venous pathway from the right atrium to the right jugular bulb may explain why the right jugular bulb is often larger than the left. Certain developmental processes have been postulated to produce unilateral variants in the jugular bulbs, including high-riding jugular bulbs, dehisced jugular bulbs. Though they are typically symptomatic, complex blood flow and morphology may mimic pathology on imaging and may rarely present with hearing loss or lower cranial nerve palsies.[147]

HYPOGLOSSAL NERVE – CN XII

CN XII, or the hypoglossal nerve, has the primary function of innervating the intrinsic and extrinsic muscles of the tongue (Table 9-28). Impulses from the motor cortex travel via the corona radiata through the genu of the internal capsule and cerebral peduncle via the corticobulbar tract to reach the hypoglossal nucleus, which is found in a paramedian location in the floor of the fourth ventricle. Hypoglossal nerve root fibers as well as fibers from the nucleus ambiguous exit forward from the medulla, passing lateral to the medial lemniscus. Pathology at this region also commonly involves cranial nerve XI.

The fibers of cranial nerve XII exit from the brainstem in the sulcus, between the pyramid and olive as multiple small rootlets. The rootlets extend anteriorly to form the hypoglossal nerve extending anterolaterally through the hypoglossal canal. Once outside the skull base, the fibers descend inferiorly in the carotid space lying medial to cranial nerves IX, X, and XI and passing lateral to the carotid bifurcation. The hypoglossal nerve then continues forward to enter the posterior portion of the sublingual space of the oral cavity. From here, it curves upward medially

Table 9-28 CN XII Function and Dysfunction		
Branch	**Function**	**Dysfunction**
Motor Branch	extrinsic and intrinsic muscles of the tongue	• Ipsilateral tongue fasciculations • Deviation of the tongue toward side of paralysis on protrusion • Denervation atrophy of tongue muscles

Table 9-29 Common CN XII Pathology

Brainstem Lesions
- Ischemia
- MS
- Aneurysm
- Basilar invagination
- Chiari malformation

Hypoglossal Canal Lesions
- Invasive Nasopharyngeal Carcinoma

Suprahyoid Neck Lesions
- Squamous Cell Carcinoma of the Floor of the Mouth.

Intrinsic Nerve Lesions
- Schwannoma
- Guillain-Barré and Variants (**Table 9-8**)

to the submandibular salivary glands to supply the intrinsic and extrinsic muscles of the tongue and infrahyoid strap.[70,148]

CN XII Pathology

The majority of causes of isolated CN XII neuropathy occur as a result of nodal mass effects or direct invasion from metastatic lesions from the floor of the mouth or the nasopharynx[69] (**Table 9-29**). Nasopharyngeal carcinoma may also directly invade CN XII as it traverses the hypoglossal canal in the skull base.[30] Congenital Chiari malformation may also cause CN XII as the herniated cerebellar tonsil compresses the nerve entering the hypoglossal canal at the lateral boarder of foramen magnum. Often, CN XII involvement occurs in conjunction with the other lower cranial nerves in pathology at the brainstem or skull base (**Table 9-26**). Finally, intrinsic cranial nerve lesions, including schwannoma and neuritis may also affect CN XII.

REFERENCES

1. De Carlos JA, Lopez-Mascaraque L, and Valverde F: The telencephalic vesicles are innervated by olfactory placode-derived cells: a possible mechanism to induce neocortical development. Neuroscience 1995;68(4): 1167–1178.
2. Sadler TW, Langman J: Langman's medical embryology. 9th ed. Philadelphia: Lippincott Williams & Wilkins; 2004:x, 534 p.
3. Cartwright MM and Smith SM: Increased cell death and reduced neural crest cell numbers in ethanol-exposed embryos: partial basis for the fetal alcohol syndrome phenotype. Alcohol Clin Exp Res 1995;19(2):378–386.
4. Jiang X, Rowitch DH, Soriano P, McMahon AP, and Sucov HM: Fate of the mammalian cardiac neural crest. Development 2000;127(8):1607–1616.
5. Krisht A, Barnett DW, Barrow DL, and Bonner G: The blood supply of the intracavernous cranial nerves: an anatomic study. Neurosurgery 1994;34(2):275–279.
6. Lapresle J and Lasjaunias P: Cranial nerve ischaemic arterial syndromes. A review. Brain 1986;109(Pt 1):207–216.
7. Lee H, Ahn BH, and Baloh RW: Sudden deafness with vertigo as a sole manifestation of anterior inferior cerebellar artery infarction. J Neurol Sci 2004;222(1–2):105–107.
8. El-Khouly H, Fernandez-Miranda J, Rhoton AL, Jr.: Blood supply of the facial nerve in the middle fossa: the petrosal artery. Neurosurgery 2008;62:ONS297–ONS303.
9. Ozanne A, Pereira V, Krings T, Toulgoat F, and Lasjaunias P: Arterial vascularization of the cranial nerves. Neuroimaging Clin N Am 2008;18(2):431–439.
10. d'Avella E, Tschabitscher M, Santoro A, and Delfini R: Blood supply to the intracavernous cranial nerves: comparison of the endoscopic and microsurgical perspectives. Neurosurgery 2008;62:ONS305–ONS310.
11. Poussaint TY, Jaramillo D, Chang Y, and Korf B: Interobserver reproducibility of volumetric MR imaging measurements of plexiform neurofibromas. Am J Roentgenol 2003;180:419–423.
12. Ball JR and Biggs MT: Operative steps in management of benign nerve sheath tumors. Neurosurg Focus 2007;22:E7.
13. Mrugala MM, Batchelor TT, and Plotkin SR: Peripheral and cranial nerve sheath tumors. Curr Opin Neurol 2005;18(5):604–610.
14. Ferner RE: Neurofibromatosis 1 and neurofibromatosis 2: a twenty first century perspective. Lancet Neurol 2007;6(4):340–351.
15. Fisher LM, Doherty JK, Lev MH, and Slattery WH, IIIrd: Distribution of nonvestibular cranial nerve schwannomas in neurofibromatosis 2. Otol Neurotol 2007;28(8):1083–1090.
16. Sarma S, Sekhar LN, and Schessel DA: Nonvestibular schwannomas of the brain: a 7-year experience. Neurosurgery 2002;50(3):437–448.
17. Agrawal A, Pandit L, Bhandary S, Makannavar JH, and Srikrishna U: Glossopharyngeal schwannoma: diagnostic and therapeutic aspects. Singapore Med J 2007;48:e181–e185.
18. Lowenheim H, Koerbel A, Ebner FH, Kumagami H, Ernemann U, and Tatagiba M: Differentiating imaging findings in primary and secondary tumors of the jugular foramen. Neurosurg Rev 2006;29:1–11.
19. Swartz JD: Lesions of the cerebellopontine angle and internal auditory canal: diagnosis and differential diagnosis. Semin Ultrasound CT MR 2004;25(4):332–352.
20. Fechner A, Fong S, and McGovern P: A review of Kallmann syndrome: genetics, pathophysiology, and clinical management. Obstet Gynecol Surv 2008;63(3):189–194.
21. Wilson MA, Hillman TA, Wiggins RH, and Shelton C: Jugular foramen schwannomas: diagnosis, management, and outcomes. Laryngoscope 2005; 115(8):1486–1492.
22. Eldevik OP, Gabrielsen TO, and Jacobsen EA: Imaging findings in schwannomas of the jugular foramen. Am J Neuroradiol 2000;21(6):1139–1144.
23. Bonneville F, Savatovsky J, and Chiras J: Imaging of cerebellopontine angle lesions: an update. Part 1: Enhancing extra-axial lesions. Eur Radiol 2007;17(10):2472–2482.
24. Whittle IR, Smith C, Navoo P, and Collie D: Meningiomas. Lancet 2004;363(9420):1535–1543.
25. Isaacson B, Kutz JW, and Roland PS: Lesions of the petrous apex: diagnosis and management. Otolaryngol Clin North Am 2007;40(3):479–519.
26. Chong V: Imaging the cranial nerves in cancer. Cancer Imaging 2004;4 Spec No A:S1–S5.
27. Chang PC, Fischbein NJ, McCalmont TH, et al.: Perineural spread of malignant melanoma of the head and neck: clinical and imaging features. Am J Neuroradiol 2004;25:5–11.
28. Nemec SF, Herneth AM, and Czerny C: Perineural tumor spread in malignant head and neck tumors. Top Magn Reson Imaging 2007;18:467–471.
29. Glastonbury CM: Nasopharyngeal carcinoma: the role of magnetic resonance imaging in diagnosis, staging, treatment, and follow-up. Top Magn Reson Imaging 2007;18:225–235.
30. Chang JT, Lin CY, Chen TM, et al.: Nasopharyngeal carcinoma with cranial nerve palsy: the importance of MRI for radiotherapy. Int J Radiat Oncol Biol Phys. 2005;63:1354–1360.
31. Joseph FG and Scolding NJ: Sarcoidosis of the nervous system. Prac Neurol 2007;7:234–244.
32. Palacios E, Rigby PL, and Smith DL: Cranial neuropathy in neurosarcoidosis. Ear Nose Throat J 2003;82:251–252.
33. Arias M, Iglesias A, Vila O, Brasa J, and Conde C: MR imaging findings of neurosarcoidosis of the gasserian ganglion: an unusual presentation. Eur Radiol 2002;12:2723–2725.

34. Jennings JW, Rojiani AM, Brem SS, and Murtagh FR: Necrotizing neurosarcoidosis masquerading as a left optic nerve meningioma: case report. Am J Neuroradiol 2002;23:660–662.
35. Deshmukh VR, Albuquerque FC, Zabramski JM, and Spetzler RF: Surgical management of cavernous malformations involving the cranial nerves. Neurosurgery 2003;53:352–357.
36. Mathiesen T, Edner G, and Kihlstrom L: Deep and brainstem cavernomas: a consecutive 8-year series. J Neurosurg 2003;99:31–37.
37. Samii M, Nakamura M, Mirzai S, Vorkapic P, and Cervio A: Cavernous angiomas within the internal auditory canal. J Neurosurg 2006;105:581–587.
38. Fulbright RK, Erdum E, Sze G, and Byrne T: Cranial nerve enhancement in the Guillain-Barre syndrome. Am J Neuroradiol 1995;16:923–925.
39. Simmons A: Clinical manifestations and treatment considerations of herpes simplex virus infection. J Infect Dis. 2002;186 Suppl 1:S71–S77.
40. Pavone P, Incorpora G, Romantshika O, and Ruggieri M: Polyneuritis cranialis: full recovery after intravenous immunoglobulins. Pediatr Neurol 2007;37:209–211.
41. McCann EL, Smith TW, Chad DA, and Sargent J: Severe cranial nerve involvement in longstanding demyelinating polyneuropathy: a clinicopathologic correlation. Acta Neuropathol 1996;91:309–312.
42. Zadro I, Barun B, Habek M, and Brinar VV: Isolated cranial nerve palsies in multiple sclerosis. Clin Neurol Neurosurg 2008;110(9):886–888.
43. Bhatti MT, Schmalfuss IM, Williams LS, and Quisling RG: Peripheral third cranial nerve enhancement in multiple sclerosis. Am J Neuroradiol 2003;24:1390–1395.
44. Halperin JJ: Nervous system Lyme disease. Infect Dis Clin North Am 2008;22:261–274.
45. Lell M, Schmid A, Stemper B, Maihofner C, Heckmann JG, and Tomandl BF: Simultaneous involvement of third and sixth cranial nerve in a patient with Lyme disease. J Neuroradiol 2003;45:85–87.
46. Hadrane L, Waterkeyn F, Ghijselings L, Dhaene N, and Gille M: Neurosyphilis revealed by a multiple cranial neuropathy: magnetic resonance imaging findings. Rev Neurol 2008;164:253–257.
47. Offiah CE and Turnbull IW: The imaging appearances of intracranial CNS infections in adult HIV and AIDS patients. Clin Radiol 2006;61:393–401.
48. Smith MM and Anderson JC: Neurosyphilis as a cause of facial and vestibulocochlear nerve dysfunction: MR imaging features. Am J Neuroradiol 2000;21:1673–1675.
49. de Freitas MR: Infectious neuropathy. Curr Opin Neurol 2007;20:548–552.
50. Mueller NH, Gilden DH, Cohrs RJ, Mahalingam R, and Nagel MA: Varicella zoster virus infection: clinical features, molecular pathogenesis of disease, and latency. Neurol Clin 2008;26:675–697.
51. Suzuki F, Furuta Y, Ohtani F, Fukuda S, and Inuyama Y: Herpes virus reactivation and gadolinium-enhanced magnetic resonance imaging in patients with facial palsy. Otol Neurotol 2001;22:549–553.
52. Lavi ES and Sklar EM: Enhancement of the eighth cranial nerve and labyrinth on MR imaging in sudden sensorineural hearing loss associated with human herpesvirus 1 infection: case report. Am J Neuroradiol 2001;22:1380–1382.
53. Abboud O and Saliba I: Isolated bilateral facial paralysis revealing AIDS: a unique presentation. Laryngoscope 2008;118:580–584.
54. Tran C, Du Pasquier RA, Cavassini M, et al.: Neuromyelitis optica following CMV primo-infection. J Intern Med 2007;261:500–503.
55. Maia AC, Jr., da Rocha AJ, da Silva CJ, and Rosemberg S: Multiple cranial nerve enhancement: a new MR imaging finding in metachromatic leukodystrophy. Am J Neuroradiol 2007;28:999.
56. Lachenal F, Cotton F, Desmurs-Clavel H, et al.: Neurological manifestations and neuroradiological presentation of Erdheim-Chester disease: report of 6 cases and systematic review of the literature. J Neurol 2006;253:1267–1277.
57. D'Ambrosio N, Soohoo S, Warshall C, Johnson A, and Karimi S: Craniofacial and intracranial manifestations of langerhans cell histiocytosis: report of findings in 100 patients. Am J Roentgenol 2008;191:589–597.
58. Bangsgaard R, Larsen VA, and Milea D: Isolated bilateral optic neuritis in acute disseminated encephalomyelitis. Acta Ophthalmol Scand 2006;84:815–817.
59. Tenembaum S, Chamoles N, and Fejerman N: Acute disseminated encephalomyelitis: a long-term follow-up study of 84 pediatric patients. Neurology 2002;59:1224–1231.
60. Hughes RA and Cornblath DR: Guillain-Barre syndrome. Lancet 2005;366:1653–1666.
61. Morosini A, Burke C, and Emechete B: Polyneuritis cranialis with contrast enhancement of cranial nerves on magnetic resonance imaging. J Paediatr Child Health 2003;39:69–72.
62. Quan D, Pelak V, Tanabe J, Durairaj V, and Kleinschmidt-Demasters BK: Spinal and cranial hypertrophic neuropathy in multiple sclerosis. Muscle Nerve 2005;31:772–779.
63. Irani S and Lang B: Autoantibody-mediated disorders of the central nervous system. Autoimmunity 2008;41:55–65.
64. Guermazi A, Lafitte F, Miaux Y, Adem C, Bonneville JF, and Chiras J: The dural tail sign—beyond meningioma. Clin Radiol 2005;60:171–188.
65. Halperin JJ: Nervous system Lyme disease. J Neurol Sci 1998;153:182–191.
66. Bhatti MT: Optic neuropathy from viruses and spirochetes. Int Ophthalmol Clin 2007;47:37–66.
67. Sugiura M, Naganawa S, Nakata S, Kojima S, and Nakashima T. 3D-FLAIR MRI findings in a patient with Ramsay Hunt syndrome. Acta Otolaryngol 2007;127:547–549.
68. Serrano P, Hernandez N, Arroyo JA, de Llobet JM, and Domingo P: Bilateral Bell palsy and acute HIV type 1 infection: report of 2 cases and review. Clin Infect Dis 2007;44:e57–e61.
69. Doyon D, Marsot-Dupuch K, and Francke JP: The cranial nerves. 1st English ed. Teterboro, NJ: Icon Learning Systems; 2004:255.
70. Hirbawi I and Hasso A: Cranial nerves: normal anatomy and pathology. In: Stark D, Bradly W, eds. Magnetic resonance imaging. St. Louis: Mosby, 1999:1209–1224.
71. Larsen K and Tos M: The estimated incidence of symptomatic nasal polyps. Acta Otolaryngol 2002;122:179–182.
72. Bachert C, Hormann K, Mosges R, et al.: An update on the diagnosis and treatment of sinusitis and nasal polyposis. Allergy 2003;58:176–191.
73. Larsen PL and Tos M: Origin of nasal polyps: an endoscopic autopsy study. Laryngoscope 2004;114:710–719.
74. Drutman J, Harnsberger HR, Babbel RW, Sonkens JW, and Braby D: Sinonasal polyposis: investigation by direct coronal CT. Neuroradiology 1994;36:469–472.
75. Liang EY, Lam WW, Woo JK, Van Hasselt CA, and Metreweli C: Another CT sign of sinonasal polyposis: truncation of the bony middle turbinate. Eur Radiol 1996;6:553–556.
76. Blomqvist EH, Lundblad L, Anggard A, Haraldsson PO, and Stjarne P: A randomized controlled study evaluating medical treatment versus surgical treatment in addition to medical treatment of nasal polyposis. J Allergy Clin Immunol 2001;107:224–228.
77. Batra PS, Kern RC, Tripathi A, et al.: Outcome analysis of endoscopic sinus surgery in patients with nasal polyps and asthma. Laryngoscope 2003;113:1703–1706.
78. Aubart FC, Ouayoun M, Brauner M, et al.: Sinonasal involvement in sarcoidosis: a case-control study of 20 patients. Medicine 2006;85:365–371.
79. Kieff DA, Boey H, Schaefer PW, Goodman M, and Joseph MP: Isolated neurosarcoidosis presenting as anosmia and visual changes. Otolaryngol Head Neck Surg 1997;117:S183–S186.
80. Gubbels SP, Barkhuizen A, and Hwang PH: Head and neck manifestations of Wegener's granulomatosis. Otolaryngol Clin North Am 2003;36:685–705.
81. Chapelon C, Ziza JM, Piette JC, et al.: Neurosarcoidosis: signs, course and treatment in 35 confirmed cases. Medicine 1990;69:261–276.
82. Benoudiba F, Marsot-Dupuch K, Rabia MH, Cabanne J, Bobin S, and Lasjaunias P: Sinonasal Wegener's granulomatosis: CT characteristics. Neuroradiology 2003;45:95–99.
83. Schwanzel-Fukuda M, Bick D, and Pfaff DW: Luteinizing hormone-releasing hormone (LHRH)-expressing cells do not migrate normally in an inherited hypogonadal (Kallmann) syndrome. Brain Res 1989;6:311–326.
84. Dode C, Levilliers J, Dupont JM, et al.: Loss-of-function mutations in FGFR1 cause autosomal dominant Kallmann syndrome. Nat Genet 2003;33:463–465.

85. Ayari B and Soussi-Yanicostas N: FGFR1 and anosmin-1 underlying genetically distinct forms of Kallmann syndrome are co-expressed and interact in olfactory bulbs. Dev Genes Evol 2007;217:169–175.
86. Tsai PS and Gill JC: Mechanisms of disease: insights into X-linked and autosomal-dominant Kallmann syndrome. Nat Clin Pract Endocrinol Metab 2006;2:160–171.
87. Truwit CL, Barkovich AJ, Grumbach MM, and Martini JJ: MR imaging of Kallmann syndrome, a genetic disorder of neuronal migration affecting the olfactory and genital systems. Am J Neuroradiol 1993;14:827–838.
88. Madan R, Sawlani V, Gupta S, and Phadke RV: MRI findings in Kallmann syndrome. Neurol India 2004;52:501–503.
89. Yu E, Mikulis D, and Nag S: CT and MR imaging findings in sinonasal schwannoma. Am J Neuroradiol 2006;27:929–930.
90. Snyder WE, Shah MV, Weisberger EC, and Campbell RL: Presentation and patterns of late recurrence of olfactory groove meningiomas. Skull Base Surg 2000;10:131–139.
91. Das S and Kirsch CF: Imaging of lumps and bumps in the nose: a review of sinonasal tumours. Cancer Imaging 2005;5:167–177.
92. Constantinidis J, Steinhart H, Koch M, et al.: Olfactory neuroblastoma: the University of Erlangen-Nuremberg experience 1975–2000. Otolaryngol Head Neck Surg 2004;130:567–574.
93. Blake KD, Hartshorne TS, Lawand C, Dailor AN, and Thelin JW: Cranial nerve manifestations in CHARGE syndrome. Am J Med Genet 2008; 146A:585–592.
94. Azoulay R, Fallet-Bianco C, Garel C, Grabar S, Kalifa G, and Adamsbaum C: MRI of the olfactory bulbs and sulci in human fetuses. Pediatr Radiol 2006;36:97–107.
95. Smith MM and Strottmann JM: Imaging of the optic nerve and visual pathways. Semin Ultrasound CT MR 2001;22:473–487.
96. Akagi T, Miyamoto K, Kashii S, and Yoshimura N: Cause and prognosis of neurologically isolated third, fourth, or sixth cranial nerve dysfunction in cases of oculomotor palsy. Jpn J Ophthalmol 2008;52:32–35.
97. Rose JW, Digre KB, Lynch SG, and Harnsberger RH: Acute VIth cranial nerve dysfunction in multiple sclerosis. Evaluation by magnetic resonance imaging. J Clin Neuroophthalmol 1992;12:17–20.
98. Everton KL, Rassner UA, Osborn AG, and Harnsberger HR: The oculomotor cistern: anatomy and high-resolution imaging. Am J Neuroradiol 2008; 29(7):1344–1348.
99. Yeh S and Foroozan R: Orbital apex syndrome. Curr Opin Ophthalmol 2004;15:490–498.
100. Vaphiades MS, Cure J, and Kline L: Management of intracranial aneurysm causing a third cranial nerve palsy: MRA, CTA or DSA? Semin Ophthalmol 2008;23:143–150.
101. Blake PY, Mark AS, Kattah J, and Kolsky M: MR of oculomotor nerve palsy. Am J Neuroradiol 1995;16:1665–1672.
102. Jacobs DA and Galetta SL: Neuro-ophthalmology for neuroradiologists. Am J Neuroradiol 2007;28:3–8.
103. Bharucha DX, Campbell TB, Valencia I, Hardison HH, and Kothare SV: MRI findings in pediatric ophthalmoplegic migraine: a case report and literature review. Pediatr Neurol 2007;37:59–63.
104. La Mantia L, Curone M, Rapoport AM, and Bussone G: Tolosa-Hunt syndrome: critical literature review based on IHS 2004 criteria. Cephalalgia 2006;26:772–781.
105. Colnaghi S, Versino M, Marchioni E, et al.: ICHD-II diagnostic criteria for Tolosa-Hunt syndrome in idiopathic inflammatory syndromes of the orbit and/or the cavernous sinus. Cephalalgia 2008;28:577–584.
106. Cakirer S: MRI findings in Tolosa-Hunt syndrome before and after systemic corticosteroid therapy. Eur J Radiol 2003;45:83–90.
107. Haque TL, Miki Y, Kashii S, et al.: Dynamic MR imaging in Tolosa-Hunt syndrome. Eur J Radiol 2004;51:209–217.
108. Yeung MC, Kwong KL, Wong YC, and Wong SN: Paediatric Tolosa-Hunt syndrome. J Paediatr Child Health 2004;40:410–413.
109. Schuknecht B, Sturm V, Huisman TA, and Landau K: Tolosa-Hunt syndrome: MR imaging features in 15 patients with 20 episodes of painful ophthalmoplegia. Eur J Radiol 2009;69(3):445–453.
110. Bonneville F, Savatovsky J, and Chiras J: Imaging of cerebellopontine angle lesions: an update. Part 2: Intra-axial lesions, skull base lesions that may invade the CPA region, and non-enhancing extra-axial lesions. Eur Radiol 2007;17:2908–2920.
111. Connor SE, Leung R, and Natas S: Imaging of the petrous apex: a pictorial review. Br J Radiol 2008;81:427–435.
112. Krafft RM: Trigeminal neuralgia. Am Fam Physician 2008;77:1291–1296.
113. Love S and Coakham HB: Trigeminal neuralgia: pathology and pathogenesis. Brain 2001;124:2347–2360.
114. Ryu H, Yamamoto S, Sugiyama K, Uemura K, and Miyamoto T: Hemifacial spasm caused by vascular compression of the distal portion of the facial nerve. Report of seven cases. J Neurosurg 1998;88:605–609.
115. Yoshino N, Akimoto H, Yamada I, et al.: Trigeminal neuralgia: evaluation of neuralgic manifestation and site of neurovascular compression with 3D CISS MR imaging and MR angiography. Radiology 2003;228:539–545.
116. Naraghi R, Tanrikulu L, Troescher-Weber R, et al.: Classification of neurovascular compression in typical hemifacial spasm: three-dimensional visualization of the facial and the vestibulocochlear nerves. J Neurosurg 2007;107:1154–1163.
117. Li MH, Li WB, Pan YP, Fang C, and Wang W: Persistent primitive trigeminal artery associated with aneurysm: report of two cases and review of the literature. Acta Radiol 2004;45:664–668.
118. Monstad P: Microvascular decompression as a treatment for cranial nerve hyperactive dysfunction—a critical view. Acta Neurol Scand 2007;187: 30–33.
119. Satoh T, Onoda K, and Date I: Fusion imaging of three-dimensional magnetic resonance cisternograms and angiograms for the assessment of microvascular decompression in patients with hemifacial spasms. J Neurosurg 2007;106:82–89.
120. Ahamed SH and Jones NS: What is Sluder's neuralgia? J Laryngol Otol 2003;117:437–443.
121. McGeeney BE: Cluster headache pharmacotherapy. Am J Ther 2005; 12:351–358.
122. Felisati G, Arnone F, Lozza P, Leone M, Curone M, and Bussone G: Sphenopalatine endoscopic ganglion block: a revision of a traditional technique for cluster headache. Laryngoscope 2006;116:1447–1450.
123. Tiemstra JD and Khatkhate N: Bell's palsy: diagnosis and management. Am Fam Physician 2007;76:997–1002.
124. Becelli R, Perugini M, Carboni A, and Renzi G: Diagnosis of Bell palsy with gadolinium magnetic resonance imaging. J Craniofac Surg 2003; 14:51–54.
125. Gilden DH: Clinical practice. Bell's palsy. N Engl J Med 2004;351:1323–1331.
126. Kinoshita T, Ishii K, Okitsu T, Okudera T, and Ogawa T: Facial nerve palsy: evaluation by contrast-enhanced MR imaging. Clin Radiol 2001; 56:926–932.
127. Tabuchi T, Nakao Y, Sakihama N, and Kobayashi T: Vascular permeability to fluorescent substance in human cranial nerves. Ann Otol Rhinol Laryngol 2002;111:736–737.
128. Martin-Duverneuil N, Sola-Martinez MT, Miaux Y, et al.: Contrast enhancement of the facial nerve on MRI: normal or pathological? Neuroradiology 1997;39:207–212.
129. Sweeney CJ and Gilden DH: Ramsay Hunt syndrome. J Neurol Neurosurg Psychiatry 2001;71:149–154.
130. Kuhweide R, Van de Steene V, Vlaminck S, and Casselman JW: Ramsay Hunt syndrome: pathophysiology of cochleovestibular symptoms. J Laryngol Otol 2002;116:844–848.
131. Murakami S, Honda N, Mizobuchi M, Nakashiro Y, Hato N, and Gyo K: Rapid diagnosis of varicella zoster virus infection in acute facial palsy. Neurology 1998;51:1202–1205.
132. Gupta J, Hutchins T, and Palacios E: Ramsay Hunt syndrome, type I. Ear Nose Throat J 2007;86:138–140.
133. Salemis NS, Karameris A, Gourgiotis S, et al.: Large intraparotid facial nerve schwannoma: Case report and Review of the Literature. Int J Oral Maxillofac Surg 2008;37:679–681.
134. Wiggins RH, 3rd, Harnsberger HR, Salzman KL, Shelton C, Kertesz TR, and Glastonbury CM: The many faces of facial nerve schwannoma. Am J Neuroradiol 2006;27:694–699.
135. Kouyialis AT, Stranjalis G, Papadogiorgakis N, et al.: Giant dumbbell-shaped middle cranial fossa trigeminal schwannoma with extension to the infratemporal and posterior fossae. Acta Neurochir 2007;149: 959–963.

136. Warren FM, Shelton C, Wiggins RH 3rd, Herrod HC, and Harnsberger HR: Imaging characteristics of metastatic lesions to the cerebellopontine Angle. Otol Neurotol 2008;29(6):835–838.
137. Gujrathi CS and Donald PJ: Current trends in the diagnosis and management of head and neck paragangliomas. Curr Opin Otolaryngol Head Neck Surg 2005;13:339–342.
138. van den Berg R: Imaging and management of head and neck paragangliomas. Eur Radiol 2005;15:1310–1318.
139. Isik AC, Erem C, Imamoglu M, Cinel A, Sari A, and Maral G: Familial paraganglioma. Eur Arch Otorhinolaryngol 2006;263:23–31.
140. Dickman CA, Spetzler RF, and Sonntag VKH: Surgery of the craniovertebral junction. New York: Thieme, 1998:xx, 828.
141. Lee KJ: Essential otolaryngology: Head and neck surgery. 8th ed. New York: McGraw-Hill Medical Pub. Division; 2003:xv, 1136.
142. Brazis PW, Masdeu JC, and Biller J: Localization in clinical neurology. 5th ed. Philadelphia: Lippincott Williams & Wilkins; 2007:xiii, 594.
143. Plouin PF and Gimenez-Roqueplo AP: Pheochromocytomas and secreting paragangliomas. Orphanet J Rare Dis 2006;1:49.
144. Lee JA and Duh QY: Sporadic paraganglioma. World J Surg 2008;32:683–687.
145. Macdonald AJ, Salzman KL, Harnsberger HR, Gilbert E, and Shelton C: Primary jugular foramen meningioma: imaging appearance and differentiating features. Am J Neuroradiol 2004;182:373–377.
146. Sanna M, Bacciu A, Falcioni M, Taibah A, and Piazza P: Surgical management of jugular foramen meningiomas: a series of 13 cases and review of the literature. Laryngoscope 2007;117:1710–1719.
147. Kobanawa S, Atsuchi M, Tanaka J, and Shigeno T: Jugular bulb diverticulum associated with lower cranial nerve palsy and multiple aneurysms. Surg Neurol 2000;53:559–562.
148. Voyvodic F, Whyte A, and Slavotinek J: The hypoglossal canal: normal MR enhancement pattern. Am J Neuroradiol 1995;16:1707–1710.

The Craniocervical Junction   10

Anton N. Hasso, MD, FACR
Ramana V. Yedavalli, MD
Danh T. Nguyen, MD
Henry W. Pribram, MD

INTRODUCTION

Certain aspects of the craniocervical junction (CCJ) fall into the realm of neuroradiology, musculoskeletal radiology, head and neck radiology, and/or pediatric radiology. It is therefore essential to ensure that the imaging examination of choice depicts aspects of the CCJ that are of interest to these various subspecialties. Plain film radiography is required to assess bony pathology and craniometric measurements, but has been largely replaced by computed tomography (CT) and magnetic resonance imaging (MRI). In the majority of cases, MRI serves as the definitive imaging study. Conventional or CT myelography may be utilized to assess the spinal cord over several levels, demonstrate cord cavitation or extra dural lesions. Most traumatic lesions and some congenital anomalies still require conventional plain film radiography. Catheter angiography may be indicated in the evaluation of complex vascular malformations or fistulas. However, magnetic resonance angiography (MRA) has replaced conventional angiography as a noninvasive tool to assess vascular lesions in many cases.

ANATOMY

The anatomic boundaries of the CCJ include portions of the lower cranial cavity and upper cervical spine. A line drawn from the spheno-occipital synchondrosis (junction between the basiocciput and the sphenoid bone) across the posterior fossa to the internal occipital protuberance will depict the superior boundary of the CCJ. A second line drawn posteriorly from the C2 to C3 interspace through the cervical spinal canal will outline the inferior boundary of the CCJ (Fig. 10-1).

The CCJ includes several intrinsic neural structures such as the lower brainstem, the upper cervical cord, the fourth ventricle, the inferior cerebellar hemispheres and vermis, the cerebellar tonsils, and the cervicomedullary junction. The extrinsic structures include the lower cranial and upper cervical nerves and their foramina, the vertebrobasilar vessels, the atlanto-occipital and tectorial membranes, and the anterior longitudinal, posterior longitudinal and cruciate ligaments. Several bony structures are recognized as key elements of the CCJ. The nasion, tuberculum sella, basion, opisthion, and posterior pole of the hard palate are structures in the skull base. The anterior and posterior arches of the atlas (C1) and the odontoid process are the key structures in the cervical spine (Fig. 10-2).

The complex articular anatomy of the craniocervical junction is well visualized by MR. There are four joints included within this junction and include the atlanto-occipital joints and lateral atlantoaxial joints which are paired and the singular anterior median atlantoaxial and posterior median atlantoaxial joints. All of these joints are true synovial joints. The transverse

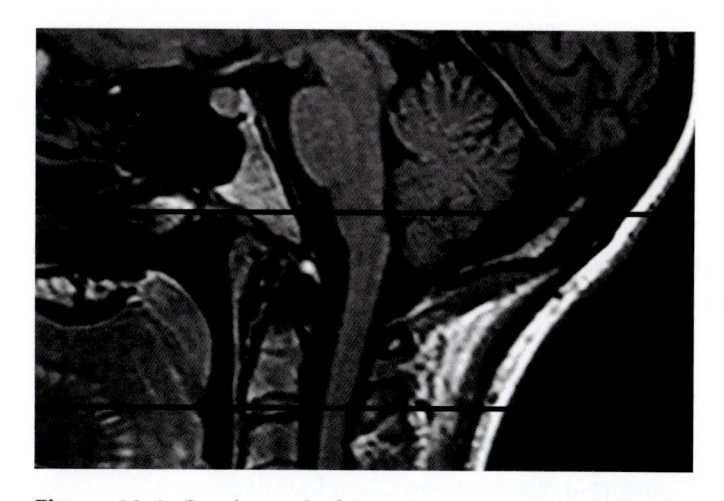

Figure 10-1 Craniocervical Junction Normal Landmarks
Sagittal T1W MR scan. The superior boundary is depicted by a line drawn from the spheno-occipital synchondrosis across the posterior fossa to the internal occipital protuberance. The inferior boundary is depicted by a line drawn from the C2 to C3 interspace through the cervical spinal canal. (Reprinted with permission from Hasso AN: MRI Atlas of the Head and Neck, 1st ed. London: Martin Dunitz, 1993:41.)

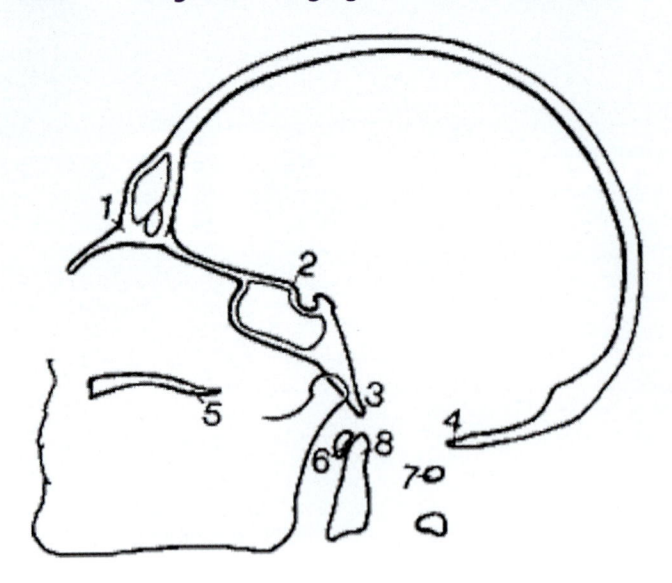

Figure 10-2 CCJ Landmark Schematic
Normal landmarks on lateral view need to assess CCJ relationships and perform basic craniometric measurements. Diagram illustrates nasion (1), tuberculum sella (2), basion (anterior margin of the foramen magnum) (3), opisthion (posterior margin of the foramen magnum) (4), posterior pole of the hard palate (5), anterior arch of the atlas (6), posterior arch of the atlas (7), and odontoid process (8). (Reprinted with permission from Smoker WRK: Craniovertebral Junction: Normal Anatomy, Craniometry, and Congenital Anomalies. Radiographics 1994;14:258.)

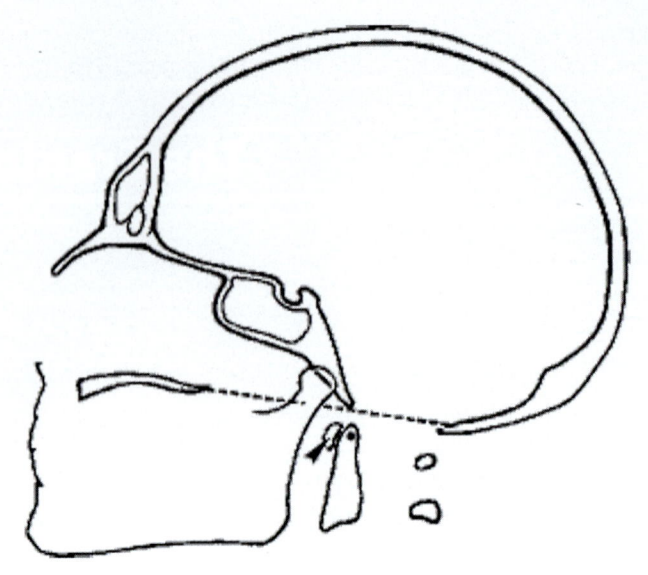

Figure 10-3 Chamberlain Line
The diagram illustrates Chamberlain's line (*dashed* and *solid line*) drawn between the posterior pole of the hard palate and the opisthion. The anterior arch of the atlas (*arrowhead*) and the odontoid process (*dot*) lie below this line. (Reprinted with permission from Smoker WRK: Craniovertebral Junction: Normal Anatomy, Craniometry, and Congenital Anomalies. Radiographics 1994;14:259.)

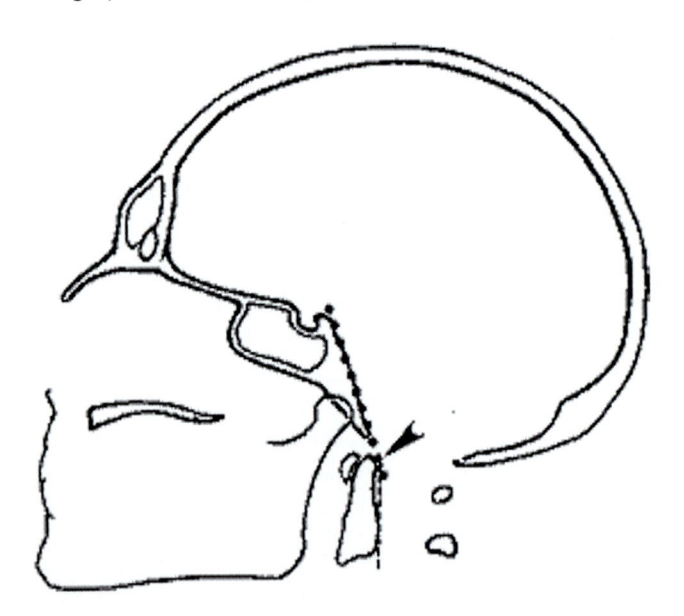

Figure 10-4 Wackenheim Clivus Baseline
The diagram illustrates the Wackenheim line (*dotted line*), which is drawn along the clivus and extrapolated inferiorly (*dashed* and *solid lines*). The line falls tangent to the posterior aspect of the odontoid process. The clivus-canal angle (*arrowhead*) should range between 150 degrees to 180 degrees. (Reprinted with permission from Smoker WRK: Craniovertebral Junction: Normal Anatomy, Craniometry, and Congenital Anomalies. Radiographics 1994;14:260.)

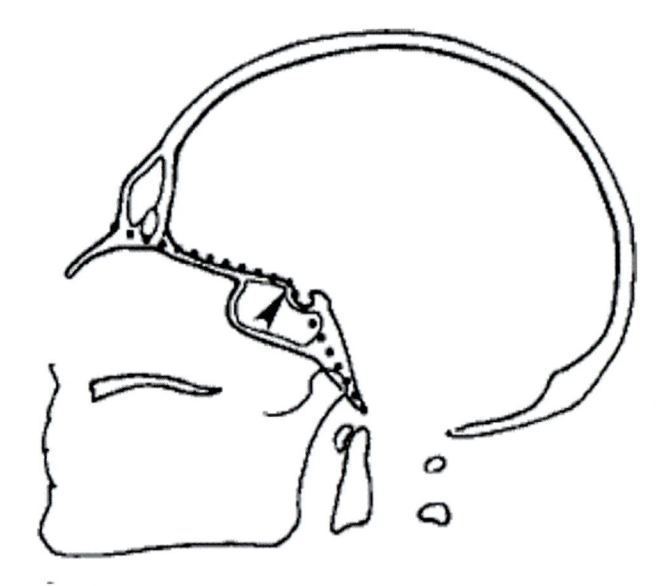

Figure 10-5 Welcher Basal Angle
The diagram illustrates the Welcher basal angle (*arrowhead*) formed between the nasion-tuberculum and tuberculum-basion lines (*dotted lines*). The angle should be 140 degrees or less. (Reprinted with permission from Smoker WRK: Craniovertebral Junction: Normal Anatomy, Craniometry, and Congenital Anomalies. Radiographics 1994;14:260.)

ligament has low to intermediate signal intensity and along with its fasciculi make up the cruciform ligament. The transverse ligament extends between two tubercles on either side of the inner aspect of the atlas. The vertically oriented extensions with lower signal make up the fasciculi.[1] The transverse ligament with a concave anterior border is seen contrasted with the high signal synovium of the dens anteriorly and the high signal cerebrospinal fluid (CSF) posteriorly. Without the integrity of the transverse ligament, the largest and strongest ligament of the craniocervical junction, atlantoaxial stability is lost.[2,3]

The bony structures that are important to the craniocervical junction include the foramen magnum, atlas, and axis and are best visualized on sagittal T1-weighted MR. The foramen magnum has both anterior and posterior margins referred to as the basion and opisthion, respectively. The basion is best identified by the marrow containing clivus and the area of high signal just superior to the odontoid due to fatty soft tissue. The opisthion is best identified by the contrast between the thin layer of low signal cortical bone along the exterior and inferior occiput and the suboccipital fatty soft tissue, which has a high signal. The high signal marrow surrounded by the low signal contrasting cortical bone identifies the anterior arch of the atlas. The axis includes the odontoid process, which has a lower signal than the body of C2.[4,5]

There are two other channels of significance in the area of the craniocervical junction besides the foramen magnum. The hypoglossal canal is discussed in Chapter 9. The condylar canal also known as the condyloid canal, condylar foramen, and posterior condylar canal is a normal channel through the occipital bone.[6–9] Two structures traverse this channel; an emissary vein that passes from the sigmoid sinus to the vertebral veins in the neck and a meningeal branch of the ascending pharyngeal artery.[6–9] This emissary vein, frequently seen on CT or MR imaging, can be mistaken for pathology such as tumor or an abnormal lymph node. It is often asymmetric on CT scans, being present 50% of the time unilaterally and only 31% of the time bilaterally.[8] Of the unilateral cases, 21.6% were right sided and 28.4% were left sided. It is identified on CT scans overall only 81% of the time.

Craniometric Measurements

Craniometric measurements have been developed to assess anatomic relationships which, when abnormal, may be an indication of pathology. There are several important measurements, which are useful to evaluate the CCJ, including Chamberlain's line, Wackenheim's clivus baseline, Welcher basal angle, and atlanto-occipital joint axis angle.[10–12]

Chamberlain's line is illustrated on a sagittal or lateral view of the skull and runs between the posterior pole of the hard palate and opisthion. The odontoid may be several millimeters above or below this line and the anterior arch of the atlas is usually below the line (**Fig. 10-3**). The Wackenheim clivus baseline is a line that is visualized on the sagittal or lateral view and runs along the edge of the clivus extrapolated to the upper cervical spinal canal behind the odontoid (**Fig. 10-4**). When a line is drawn along the posterior surface of the axis body and odontoid process to meet the Wackenheim clivus baseline, the craniocervical or clivus-canal angle is formed. This angle ranges from 150 degrees in flexion to 180 degrees in extension. If this angle

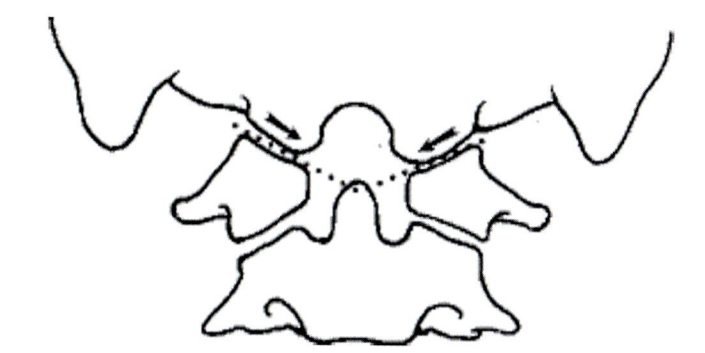

Figure 10-6 Atlanto-occipital Joint Axis Angle
The diagram illustrates the atlanto-occipital joint axis angle formed at the intersection of lines drawn through the atlanto-occipital joints (*dotted lines*). The angle should range between 124 degrees and 127 degrees. If the mastoid tips were connected (*bimastoid line*), the entirety of the odontoid process would lie below this line. The skull base should descend as it approaches midline (*arrows*). (Reprinted with permission from Smoker WRK: Craniovertebral Junction: Normal Anatomy, Craniometry, and Congenital Anomalies. Radiographics 1994;14:261.)

is less than 150 degrees, the spinal cord may be compressed on the ventral aspect.[10–12]

The Welcher basal angle viewed in the sagittal plane or lateral view is formed when the nasion-tuberculum line and tuberculum-basion line intersect. This angle averages 132 degrees and if greater than 140 degrees indicates skull base flattening (**Fig. 10-5**). The atlanto-occipital joint axis angle is formed when lines drawn parallel to the atlanto-occipital joints meet at the center of the odontoid process. If these lines do not meet in the center of the odontoid or the angle is larger than the range 124 degrees to 127 degrees it may be an indication of occipital condyle hypoplasia[9,10,11] (**Fig. 10-6**).

EMBRYOLOGY

The embryological development of the CCJ depends on the development of the adjacent skull base and cervical spine. The enchondral structures that later ossify to form the CCJ are the exoccipital, basioccipital, and supraoccipital bones along with Kerckning's process and the upper three cervical sclerotomes. Fusion and ossification of the occipital bone components form the boundaries of the foramen magnum and adjacent skull base. (**Fig. 10-7**). The atlas (C1) develops from one anterior and two lateral ossification centers. The axis (C2) has seven ossification centers, two of which form the odontoid process. The five other ossification centers form the remainder of C2.[10]

CLINICAL FINDINGS

Patients with CCJ lesions typically have symptoms that begin insidiously and progress slowly. There may be signs of dysfunction of the cerebellum, brainstem, cervical cord, and nerve

Table 10-1 Symptomatology of the CCJ

- Decreased hearing
- Soft palate paralysis
- Dysphagia
- Tongue atrophy
- Dysphasia
- Vertigo
- Tinnitus

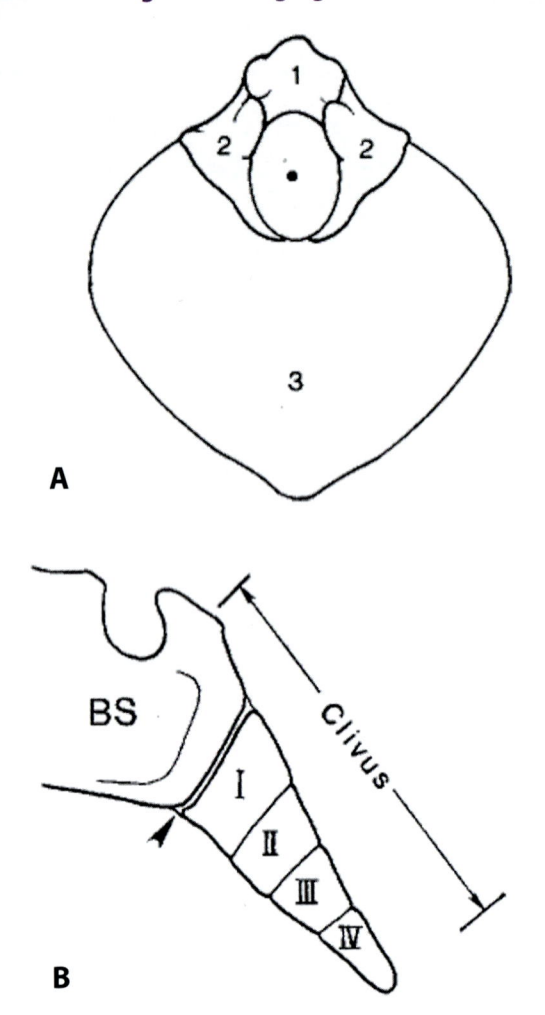

Figure 10-7 Occipital Bone
The diagram (**A**) illustrates the components of the occipital bone: basioccipital portion (1), exoccipital portion (2), and supraoccipital portion (3). The foramen magnum lies in the center (*dot*). The diagram (**B**) illustrates the contribution of the basiocciput, formed by four occipital sclerotomes, to the lower portion of the clivus. The upper portion is formed by the basisphenoid (BS). The sphenooccipital synchondrosis (*arrowhead*) lies in between. (Reprinted with permission from Smoker WRK: Craniovertebral Junction: Normal Anatomy, Craniometry, and Congenital Anomalies. Radiographics 1994; 14:263.)

roots, or of the vascular supply to these structures. Weakness may be manifested as lack of endurance, mild paresis, or major motor myelopathy. Motor myelopathy may be quite subtle and nonspecific. Sensory abnormalities typically represent posterior column dysfunction, although there may be spinothalamic tract dysfunction with hypalgesias. Occasionally, there may be bladder dysfunction with downbeat or horizontal nystagmus, ataxia, dysmetria, or even apnea may be evident. Cranial nerve dysfunction may be present with decreased hearing, dysphasia, soft palate paralysis, trapezius muscle weakness, or tongue atrophy. There may be vascular symptoms with syncope, vertigo, or intermittent paresis[9–11] (Table 10-1).

CONGENITAL AND DEVELOPMENTAL LESIONS

Stenoses of the foramen magnum or segmentation anomalies of the osseous components of the CCJ are critical, congenital, or developmental anomalies of the CCJ to recognize. These lesions are well depicted on MR scans of the region. The role of conventional X-rays is diminished. The amount of bony encroachments along with what is happening to the brainstem and/or cervical cord may be directly visualized with MRI.

Platybasia

Platybasia is defined as abnormal flattening of the skull base. Platybasia can occur in a variety of congenital disorders (e.g., craniocleidodysostosis, Arnold-Chiari malformation, osteogenesis imperfecta, craniofacial anomalies, Klippel-Feil syndrome) or may develop in conjunction with acquired diseases (e.g., Paget disease, osteomalacia, rickets, senile atrophy, hyperparathyroidism, trauma). Platybasia occurs when there is abnormal flattening, or increase, of the Welcher basal angle, greater than 140 degrees. The assessment for platybasia was originally performed with the use of plain radiography and was first described by Schuller in 1911. There are limitations with the use of plain film radiography because of ambiguity in discerning midline structures and because slight rotation in position can produce significant changes in the measurement of the Welcher basal angle. MRI is now considered the study of choice in the assessment and quantification of the degree of platybasia. Platybasia often occurs in conjunction with basilar invagination, or the inward and upward migration of the cervical spine through the foramen magnum. When platybasia occurs in conjunction with basilar invagination, signs and symptoms of compression of the brainstem and upper cervical spine can result.[5,13]

Basilar Invgination

There are three key alterations that affect the craniocervical junction. These are basilar invagination, basilar impression, and platybasia. The terms basilar invagination and basilar impression are often confused. Basilar invagination occurs when the vertebral column is shifted superiorly and incorporated into the skull base. It is a developmental anomaly and should not be used synonymously with the term basilar impression, which

Table 10-2 Basilar Impression

- An acquired form of basilar invagination
- Invagination of the cervical spine in the base of the skull due to softening of bone

Causes of Basilar Impression

- Rheumatoid arthritis
- Paget disease
- Pseudogout (CPPD)
- Osteomalacia
- Hyperparathyroidism
- Rickets
- Hurler syndrome
- Osteogenesis imprefecta

is the acquired form of basilar invagination. Basilar impression is the term used in reference to secondary, or acquired, basilar invagination and is typically caused by processes that soften the skull base such as, rheumatoid arthritis, Paget disease, pseudogout (CPPD), severe osteomalacia, hyperparathyroidism, rickets, Hurler syndrome, and osteogenesis imperfecta (Table 10-2). The term platybasia may also be confused with basilar invagination and refers to a flattening of the skull base demonstrated by an increase in the Welcher basal angle (greater than 140 degrees) as described in the previous section.

Basilar invagination is a radiographic finding and is caused by basiocciput hypoplasia, occipital condyle hypoplasia (Fig. 10-8), and atlanto-occipital assimilation (Table 10-3, Fig. 10-9). Basiocciput hypoplasia is due to the failure of formation of one or more primary cranial vertebrae resulting in a shortened clivus. The condyles will appear flattened and the atlanto-occipital joint axis angle will be widened when occipital condyle hypoplasia is present. There may be vertebral artery compression or a limited range of motion of the neck as a consequence (Fig. 10-10).

The finding of atlanto-occipital assimilation results from failure of segmentation between the skull and C1. There can be a

Table 10-3 Basilar Invagination

- Developmental anomaly
- Abnormally high vertebral column indenting the base of the skull
- A radiographic finding not a diagnosis
- Associated with low hairline, short neck, mental disturbances
- Occipital condyle hypoplasia
- Basiocciput hypoplasia
- Fusion abnormalities

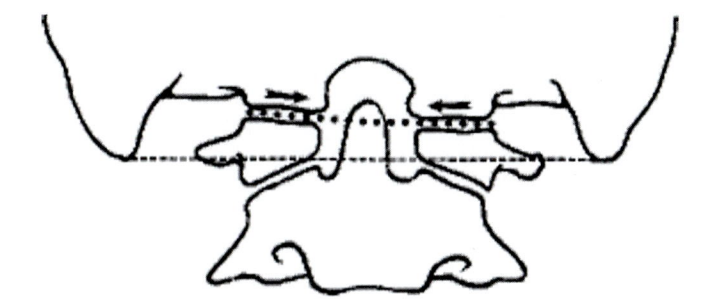

Figure 10-8 Condylar Hypoplasia
The diagram illustrates marked widening of the angle formed by lines traversing the atlanto-occipital joints (*dotted line*). Flattening of the skull base is evident (*arrows*). Note how far cephalad the tip of the odontoid process lies above a line drawn between the tips of the mastoid processes (*dashed line*). (Reprinted with permission from Smoker WRK: Craniovertebral Junction: Normal Anatomy, Craniometry, and Congenital Anomalies. Radiographics 1994;14:264.)

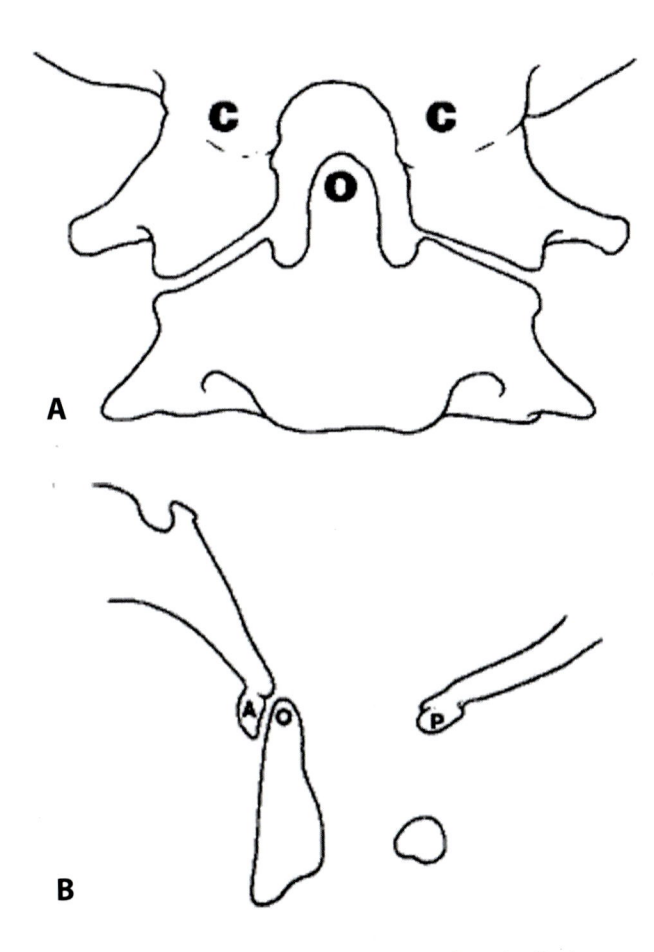

Figure 10-9 Complete Atlanto-occipital Assimilation
Coronal (**A**) and midsagittal (**B**) diagrams illustrate the occipital condyles (C), odontoid process (O), anterior atlas arch (A), and posterior atlas arch (P). (Reprinted with permission from Smoker WRK: Craniovertebral Junction: Normal Anatomy, Craniometry, and Congenital Anomalies. Radiographics 1994; 14:266.)

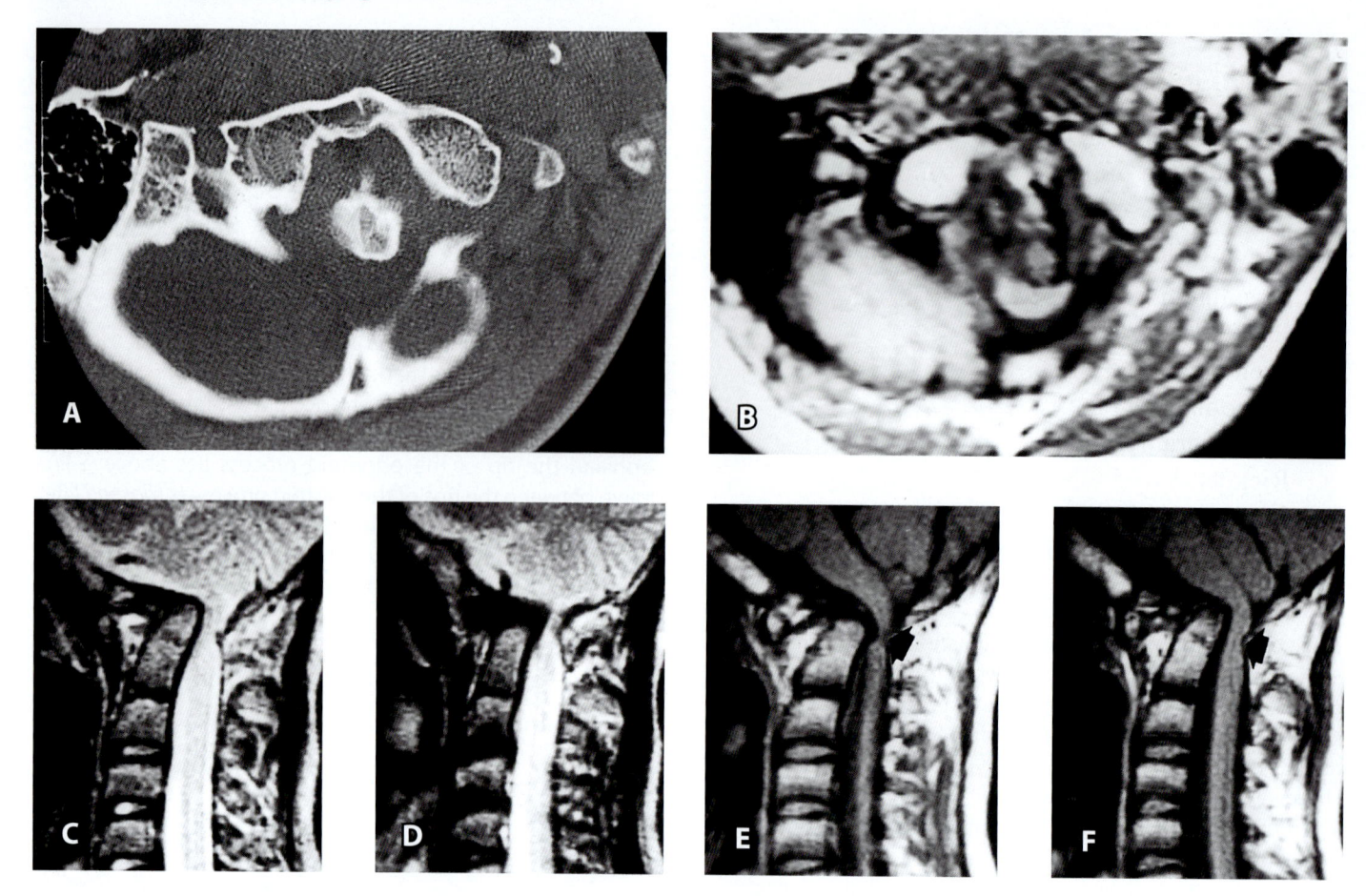

Figure 10-10 Basilar invagination Secondary to Occipital Assimilation
Basilar invagination secondary to occipital assimilation in a 12-year-old boy. There is a history of progressive myelopathy and occasional loss of bladder control. Axial CT scan (**A**) shows atlas assimilation into the basiocciput, the anterior portion of C1 is fused to the occipital condyles. Posterior and superior displacement of the dens to the level of the occipital condyles and severe narrowing of the foramen magnum is also demonstrated. Sagittal T2W MR scans (**B**) show assimilation of the atlas with only a small anterior ring of C1 visible and no rear spinous process visible. Sagittal T2W MR scan (**C–D**) shows the atlanto-occipital condyles and the cord compressed into a half moon shape. Sagittal T1W MR scan (**E–F**) shows compression of the cord at the craniocervical junction (*arrows*). (Reprinted with permission from Hasso AN: MRI Atlas of the Head and Neck, 1st ed. London: Martin Dunitz, 1993:41.)

total or partial failure and clinically the patient may have limited range of motion of the neck. There can be associated findings of C2 to C3 fusion, low hairline, and short neck. If there is an associated C2 to C3 fusion, progressive atlantoaxial subluxation may occur with a risk of sudden death.[5,10]

Os Odontoideum

Chronic atlantoaxial subluxation may be due to anomalies of the odontoid process or incompetence of the C1 to C2 ligaments. Os odontoideum is the most common developmental odontoid anomaly. Os odontoideum is defined as an ossicle with smooth circumferential cortical margins representing the odontoid process that has no osseous continuity with the body of C2. It may represent either a failure in fusion of the ossification centers of the odontoid process (dens) or the sequelae of trauma in early childhood.[8,9] Odontoid process dysplasia can be found in many syndromes including pseudoachondroplasia, metaphyseal chondrodysplasia, dystrophic dwarfism, spondyloepiphyseal dysplasia congenita, mucopolysaccharidosis, spondylometaphyseal dysplasia, Scott's syndrome, cartilage hair hypoplasia, and Down's syndrome[10-15] (**Fig. 10-11**).

Os odontoideum can present with a wide range of clinical symptoms and signs; it can also often be an incidental on imaging. Generally speaking, symptomatic patients have been categorized into three groups in the literature: 1) those with occiptocervical pain, 2) those experiencing myelopathy, and 3) those with intracranial symptoms or focal neurologic signs resultant from vertebrobasilar insufficiency. Patients with os odontoideum and myelopathy have been further subclassified: 1) those with transient myelopathy, 2) static myelopathy, and 3) progressive myelopathy.[14-16]

Two types of os odontoideum have been described: orthotopic and dystopic. An orthotopic os is one in which the ossicle moves in conjunction with the anterior arch of C1.

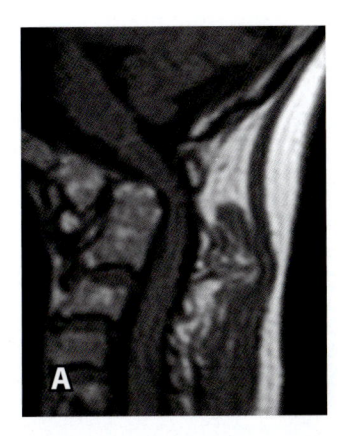

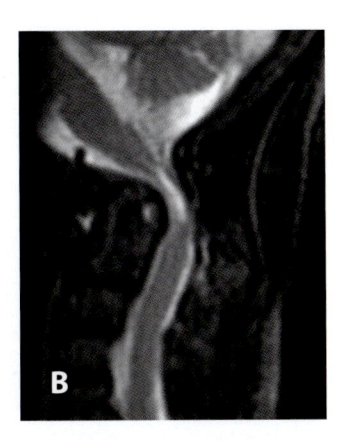

Figure 10-11 Os Odontoideum
Os odontoideum in a 6-year-old boy with Down syndrome. **(A)** Sagittal T1W MR scan shows the anteriorly displaced odontoid beneath the clivus. The remainder of C2 is displaced posteriorly due to the known laxity in patients with Down syndrome. The spinal cord is compressed. **(B)** Sagittal T2W MR scan shows high signal intensity within the markedly compressed spinal cord at the CCJ.

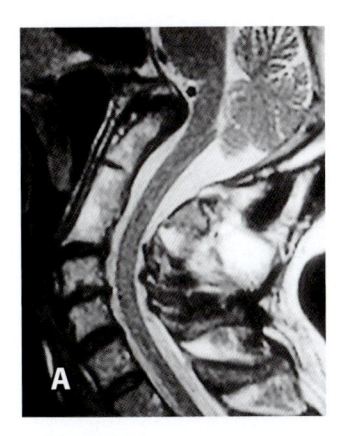

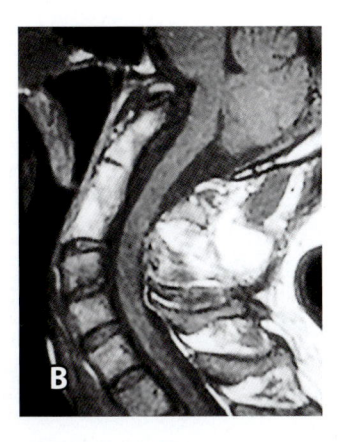

Figure 10-12 Condylus Tertius With Pseudogout
Condylus tertius in a patient complaining of limited range of motion in the neck. Sagittal T2W MR scans **(A)** demonstrate an ossified remnant superior to the dens at the base of the clivus. Sagittal T1W MR scans **(B)** show the ossified remnant in close proximity to the dens, pseudojoint formation can sometimes occur between these two structures limiting range of motion. There is also fusion of C2 to C3.

A dystopic ossicle is one that is functionally fused to the basion. Most often, there is anterior instability with anterior subluxation of the os odontoideum with respect to the body of C2. However, cases have been described where there is either no visible instability or there is movement of the os odontoideum posteriorly with respect to the body of C2 into the spinal canal during neck extension. Reports in the literature show that the degree of neurological dysfunction associated with os odontoideum is not well correlated with the degree of C1 to C2 instability.[14–16]

Dysplasia of the dens becomes significant when it causes chronic subluxation. Acquired causes of subluxation include degenerative joint disease, inflammatory arthritides, infectious subluxation,[14–16] and trauma (**Fig. 10-11**).

Condylus Tertius

Os odontoideum can be associated with condylus tertius or "third occipital condyle." When the hypochordal bow of the fourth occipital sclerotome, the proatlas, persists or when it has failed to integrate, an ossified remnant may be present at the distal end of the clivus. In other cases, multiple, small, or large supernumerary ossicles may be present around the foramen magnum. A condylus tertius is found in the median or slightly paramedian plane attached at the anterior rim of the foramen magnum. A condylus tertius may end freely or – if fully developed – form an articulated connection with the anterior arch of the atlas or the dens of axis. In single cases, a condylus tertius remains isolated between basiocciput and the anterior arch of the atlas. There may be more than one ossified remnant and at times there will be a joint formed between a remnant and the dens or anterior arch of the atlas. This may cause limited range of motion of the neck[5,10,17] (**Fig. 10-12**).

Chiari I and II Malformations

The Chiari I malformation has classically been described as a defect of the cerebellum with downward displacement of the cerebellar tonsils into the upper cervical canal. Tonsillar herniation of greater than 5 mm below the plane of the foramen magnum is diagnostic of the Chiari I malformation. The posterior fossa is also quite shallow and is most often less than 30 mm in height. Syringomyelia is often seen in patients with Chiari I malformation. Various series in the literature have reported syringomyelia occurring in up to 50% of patients with Chiari I malformations. Chiari I malformation associated osseous abnormalities involving the craniocervical junction include basioccipital hypoplasia with associated basilar invagination in up to 50% of patients, atlanto-occipital assimilation in up to 10% of patients, nonsegmentation of the C2 to C3 vertebrae in 18% of patients, and extensive Klippel-Feil associated anomalies in 5% of patients. The level of descent of the tonsils, evidence of occipital assimilation of C1 or basilar invagination, the size of the precervical cord space, and the size and shape of an associated syringohydromyelic cavity are all well seen by standard T1-weighted MR scans (**Figs. 10-13** and **10-14**).

The Chiari II malformation is a complex anomaly that can involve many portions of the central nervous system (CNS). The abnormality at the CCJ consists of a hindbrain hernia containing the tonsils, vermis, and fourth ventricle. The Chiari II malformation is a dysgenesis of the hindbrain that is characterized by herniation of the inferior portions of the cerebellar vermis, fourth ventricle, and medulla into the superior portion of the cervical spinal canal. This hindbrain hernia may be impacted within the foramen magnum. A discrepancy between the diameter of the foramen magnum and the ring of C1 causes additional impaction of the hindbrain. This leads to the entrapment of a "peg" of cerebellum between the lower surface of the skull base and the

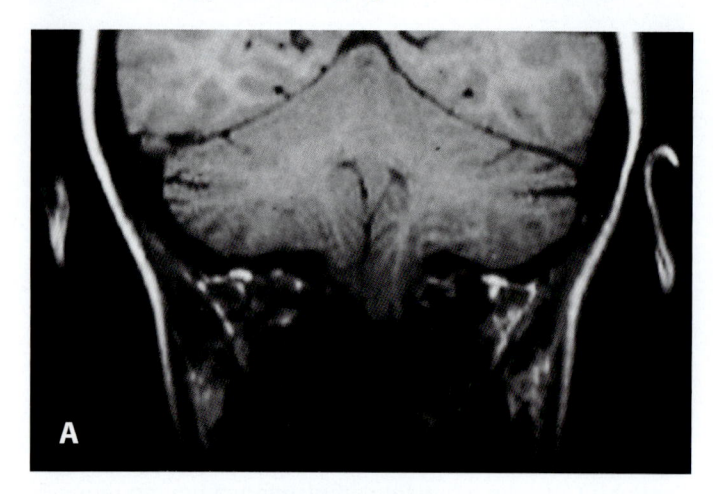

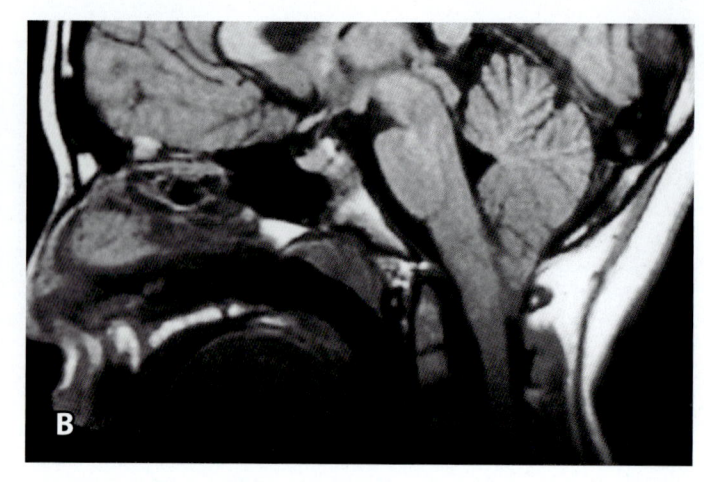

Figure 10-13 Chiari I Malformation
Chiari I malformation in a 10-year-old girl presenting with apneic spells. Coronal T1W MR scan (**A**) shows downward herniation of the cerebellum into the spinal canal. Sagittal T1W MR scan (**B**) clearly depicts the downward cerebellar herniation and mild cord compression anteriory which was the probable cause of apnea in this child.

posterior arch of C1. There may be dural bands or adhesions, which trap the herniated fourth ventricle leading to hydrocephalus with further downward compression of the hindbrain. The impaction of the structures in the foramen magnum causes obliteration of the precervical cord space and obstruction of the craniocervical veins. This venous engorgement leads to gliosis of the neural tissues in the hindbrain hernia. There may be syringohydromyelia and/or syringobulbia, which further compress the contents of the foramen magnum. Patients with a Chiari II malformation often have associated spina bifida aperta and myelomeningoceles of the lower lumbar spine and

syringohydromyelia of the cervical spinal cord is present in up to 70% of cases. Chiari II associated CCJ abnormalities also include thinning of the basiocciput with resultant concavity of the clivus and scalloping of the posterior aspect of the odontoid process. The scalloping of the posterior aspect of the odontoid process may be due to pressure effects or osseous dysplasia. Also seen is widening of the foramen magnum with notching of the opisthion. Rachischisis of the posterior arch of C1 occurs in up to 70% of patients with the Chiari II malformation; spina bifida aperta of the lower cervical spine occurs in up to 20% of patients.[4,5,10]

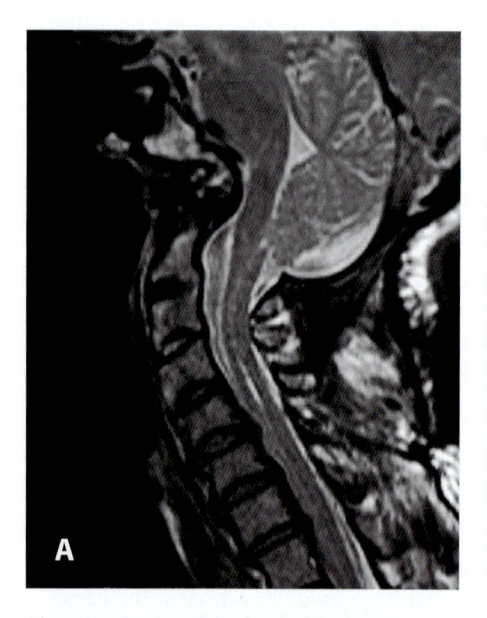

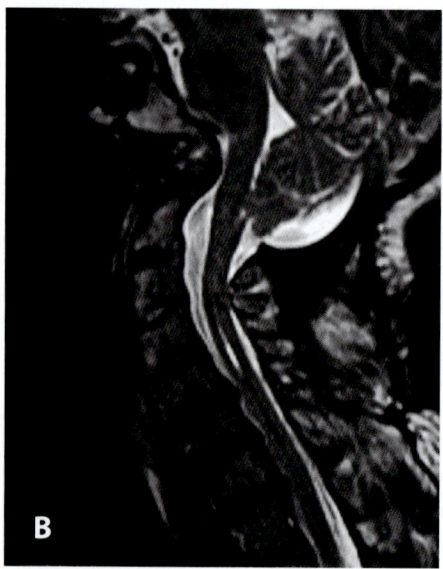

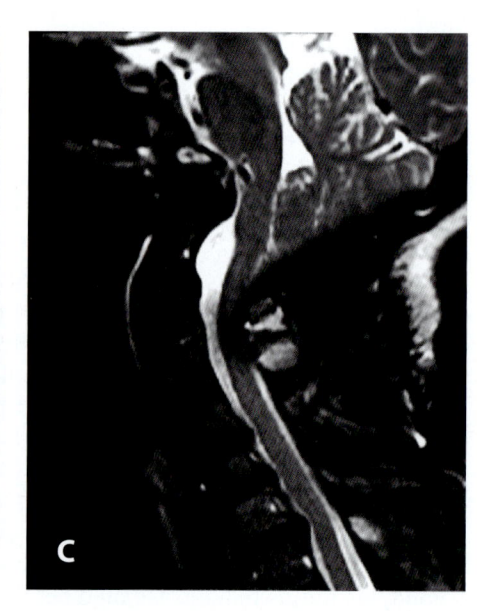

Figure 10-14 Chiari I Malformation, Cervical Syrinx, Condylus Tertius
Complex anomaly at the CCJ with a Chiari I malformation, small cavitation in the cord at C4 to C5 and a condylus tertius at the anterior rim of the foramen magnum. Sagittal PDW image (**A**) shows the short clivus with a protuberance along its caudal end and tonsillar ectopia posterior to the medulla. (**B**) T2W image shows the accessory bone beneath the focus of increased signal within the atlanto-occipital junction. FSE T2WI (**C**) shows the protuberant bone that represents the condylus tertius at the CCJ.

Both the T1- and T2-weighted images will show all these changes. MRI is most useful in the evaluation of patients following surgical decompression of the foramen magnum and upper spinal canal.[17] Unlike the Chiari I malformation, basiooccipital hypoplasia with basilar invagination and atlanto-occipital assimilation are not characteristic of the Chiari II malformation.[5,10]

Achondroplasia

Achondroplasia is the most common of the heritable skeletal dysplasias and is the most frequently occurring form of short-limbed dwarfism. It is inherited in an autosomal dominant fashion and is characterized by short stature, macocephaly with frontal bossing, midface hypoplasia, and rhizomelic shortening of the limbs. Inhibition of endochondral bone formation leads to achondroplasia or a small skull base. Radiologic findings in achondroplasia include platybasia with a small foramen magnum and caudad narrowing of the lumbar interpediculate distance. This is best evaluated with MR imaging. On axial images there will be a stenosis of the foramen magnum with a triangular shape to the opening. There can be evidence of cord compression seen as foci of abnormal signal intensity in the cervicomedullary region, narrowing of the subarachnoid space at the level of the foramen magnum, and a concave and short clivus. These findings are best represented in the sagittal view. Cervico-medullary compression is a frequently encountered complication. It can be progressive and is potentially fatal. Sudden death can occur by encroachment upon the respiratory center in the medulla oblongata by the narrowing of the foramen magnum, resulting in central respiratory failure. Clinically, the patients often lead a normal life, but may have hydrocephalus, cervicomedullary junction compromise, unexplained apnea, and death[22–25] (**Figs. 10-15** and **10-16**).

Down's Syndrome

Down's syndrome, or trisomy 21, is the most common chromosomal abnormality and is seen in approximately 1 in 700 live births. Patients with Down's syndrome commonly have abnormalities of the craniocervical junction. These abnormalities include C1 hypoplasia or assimilation, hypoplasia of the dens, basiooccipital hypoplasia with invagination, hypoplasia of the posterior aspect of the arch of C1, and ligamentous laxity of the atlanto-occipital and atlantoaxial articulations. As a result of these malformations, there can be anterior or posterior subluxation, narrowing of the dural space, and spinal cord compression.[19,20] These patients may be asymptomatic or have severe spinal compression that could be potentially worsened if more than one of these malformations is present at the same time. However, symptomatic instability is thought to occur in less than 1% of patients with Down's syndrome.

The plain radiographic measurement which best correlates with clinical risk of cord compression is the actual neural canal width, instead of the atlas-dens interval or Wackenheim's clivus baseline. This is correlated best with the width of the subarachnoid space on MR imaging[26–30] (**Fig. 10-11**).

Klippel-Feil Syndrome

Klippel-Feil syndrome was first described in 1912 by Klippel and Feil. Although there has been disagreement in the past regarding the minimum number of nonsegmented vertebrae needed for the diagnosis of Klippel-Feil syndrome, it is now generally agreed that the diagnosis can be made when there is failure of segmentation of at least two cervical vertebrae. The etiology is unknown and cases are usually rare and sporadic, but the syndrome has been known to occur in siblings. Along with nonsegmented cervical vertebrae, other anomalies of the CCJ associated with Klippel-Feil syndrome include basilar invagination, odontoid process hypoplasia, platybasia, Chiari I malformations, and atlanto-occipital assimilations. The classical findings are those of short neck, low hairline, restriction of neck motion, and fusion of at least two cervical segments. There have been many reported associated anomalies, including scoliosis greater than 20 degrees in more than 50% of patients, Sprengel's

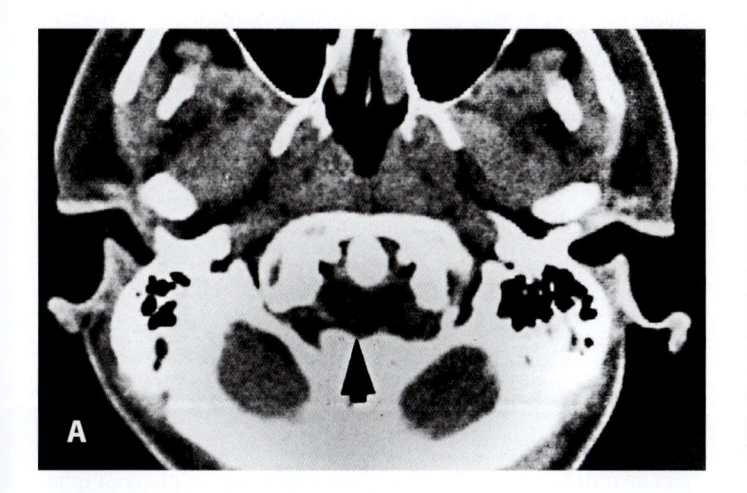

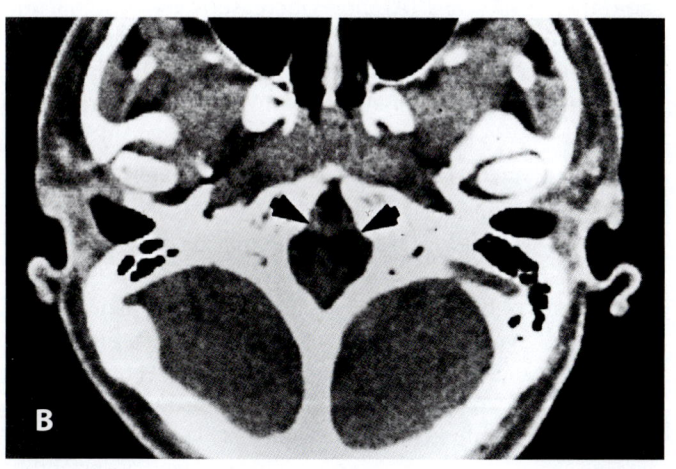

Figure 10-15 Achondroplasia
Achondroplasia in a young child. Axial CT scans. (**A**) shows narrowing of the foramen magnum with cord compression. Posteriorly C1 is seen superiorly displaced into the canal causing further narrowing (*arrow*). In (**B**) the characteristic triangular shape of the foramen magnum with a narrow sagittal diameter is clearly demonstrated (*arrows*).

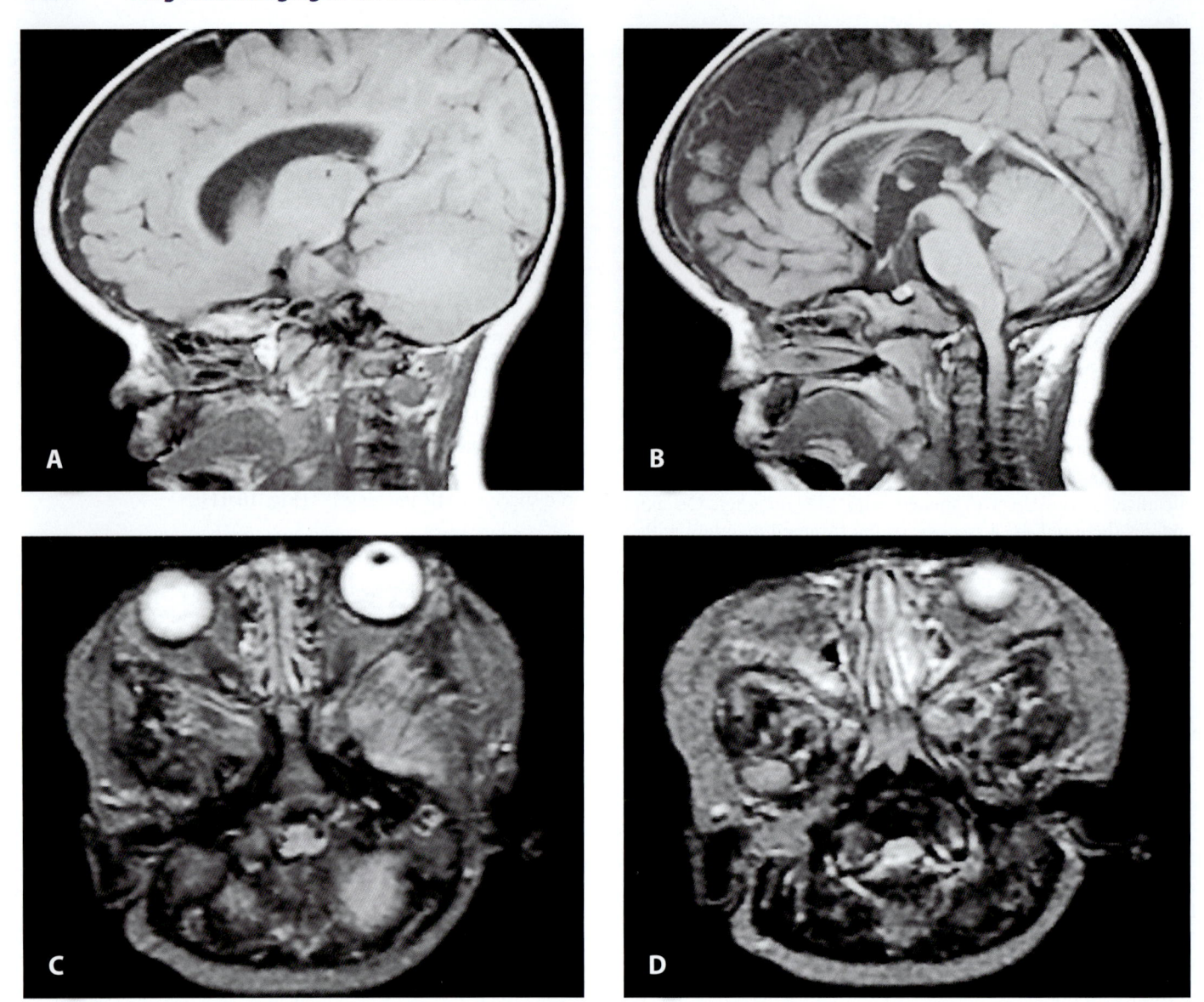

Figure 10-16 Achondroplasia
Sagittal T1W MR scans. (**A**) shows increased cerebrospinal fluid and hydrocephalus. (**B**) shows apparent upward displacement of the brainstem secondary to chondrocranium shortening. Axial T1W MR scans (**C** and **D**) show narrowing of the foramen magnum and a triangular shape with cord compression. This deformity is the usual cause for the hydrocephalus observed on the sagittal images as the cerebrospinal fluid pathways are compressed by the narrowed foramen magnum.

deformity in 33% of patients, ventriculoseptal defects in up to 14% of patients, deafness, and sykinesis. Cases of cervical diastematomyelia have also been reported in patients with Klippel-Feil syndrome. Several visceral anomalies are seen including genitourinary abnormalities in greater than 66% of patients with Klippel-Feil syndrome; these include vaginal agenesis, unilateral renal agenesis, renal malrotation, and renal ectopia. There is a tendency to compensate for the cervical fusion by increased mobility at the unfused cervical segments. This hypermobility can cause accelerated cervical spondylosis as well as instability or osteoarthritis over time. This hypermobility can also cause severe cervical cord injury with relatively minor trauma. There can also be associated odontoid abnormalities, basilar invagination, and/or cervical stenosis.

Conventional c-spine series and flexion/extension lateral views show flattening and widening of the vertebrae, hemivertebrae, or block vertebrae with instability. The presence of subluxation and cord compression can best be assessed with MR imaging[31,32] (**Fig. 10-17**).

Mucopolysaccharidosis Type II (Hunter's Syndrome)

Hunter's syndrome is a x-linked recessive disorder in which there is a deficiency of the enzyme iduronate sulphate sulphatase. As a result of this enzyme deficiency, there is deposition of glycosarninoglycans (GAG) in the tissues including the skeleton and central nervous system. There is both a mild and severe form of this condition. Patients with the mild form are typically

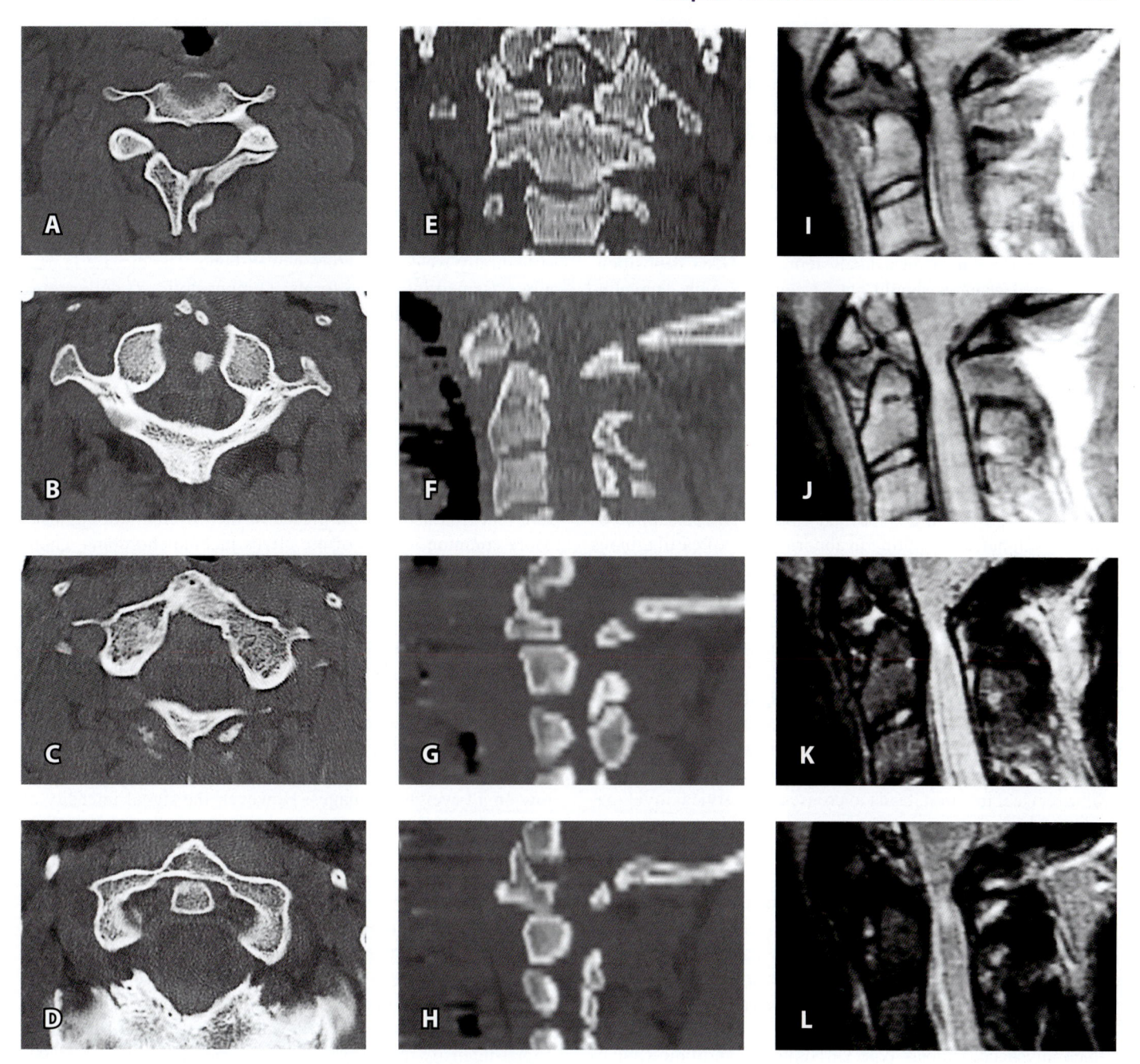

Figure 10-17 Klippel-Feil Syndrome with Os Odontoideum
Cervical vertebrae fushion with susceptibility to fracture are characteristic of this congenital syndrome. Patient presented with mild upper neck pain after a motor vehicle accident without focal neurological deficits. Axial CT scans. (**A**) shows a bifid C3 and (**B**) shows C1 without abnormality at this level. The C1 anterior arch is larger on the left than right in (**C**) and nonarticulating. In (**D**) the C1 dens relationship is demonstrated. Reformatted coronal CT scan (**E**) shows the lateral mass on the left larger than the right, there is partial assimilation and a C1 to C2 fracture dislocation. Reformatted sagittal CT scans. Midsagittal scan (**F**) also shows separation of the dens. Right parasagittal scan (**G**) shows the separation of the dens from C2 with probable fibrous union and bony overgrowth. Left parasagittal scan (**H**) shows the larger left anterior arch of C1. Sagittal T2W MR (**I** and **J**) and T1W MR (**K** and **L**) images show fushion of C1 to the occiput and assimilation.

of normal intelligence and live a normal life span, but craniocervical junction involvement can manifest as a chronic cervical myelopathy. In the severe form, there is mental retardation.

At the craniocervical junction there is thickening of the soft tissues posterior to the odontoid with resultant canal stenosis and cord compression. The thickened soft tissues have an intermediate signal on T1W MR and a low signal on T2W MR. The compressed spinal cord shows changes of compression, but there has also been a report of more diffuse signal changes with cord expansion which most likely represent GAG deposition. These signal changes should not be confused with demyelination or intramedullary tumor. Platyspondyly and disc dehydration have also been observed.[33,34]

Mucopolysaccharidosis Type IV (Morquio's Syndrome)

Morquio's disease (mucopolysaccharidosis type IV) is an autosomal recessive disorder of glycosaminoglycan metabolism due to deficiency of the lysosomal enzyme galactosamine-6-sulphate sulphatase, resulting in abnormalities of cartilaginous bone and ligamentous tissue. Definitive descriptions of this condition were given simultaneously and independently in 1929 by Morquio in Uruguay and Brailsford in Birmingham. It is usually diagnosed during the second year of life when the short trunk and thoracic kyphosis become evident. The radiological hallmarks are platyspondyly and central vertebral beaking, which predate the clinical deformities. Odontoid process hypoplasia is virtually always present in the severely affected individual and this, with other abnormalities of the craniocervical junction, leads to progressive cervical myelopathy, a major cause of morbidity and mortality. Ligamentous laxity and abnormal ossification of the dens are associated with a soft-tissue mass around the hypoplastic dens. This, and posterior indentation from the arch of the atlas, lead to varying degrees of compromise of the spinal canal and cord. In contrast to the majority of mucopolysaccharidosis disorders, Morquio's disease does not impair intelligence. Severe changes on MR scanning correlate well with the mental retardation that occurs in other mucopolysaccharidoses such as Hurler syndrome (mucopolysacccharidosis type I), Hunter's syndrome (mucopolysacccharidosis type II), and Sanfilippo syndrome (mucopolysacccharidosis type III).

High spinal cord compression is the major cause of complications and death in Morquio's disease. Chronic low-grade compression can give rise to spastic quadriparesis, posterior column signs of mild degree and, less frequently, spinothalamic signs. The earliest symptom is usually reduced exercise tolerance, frequently occurring before development of neurological signs. Apnea and sudden death can occur, usually following relatively minor trauma. The clinical course is usually slowly progressive. All patients with classical Morquio's disease type A have odontoid peg hypoplasia or aplasia. This, and the presence of ligamentous laxity, lead to atlanto-axial subluxation. However, severe subluxation is uncommon and demonstrating this can be difficult and unreliable using plain radiographs. Assessment of the presence and extent spinal cord compression is best assessed using MRI. The periodontoid soft-tissue mass seen in Morquio's syndrome has been reported in the literature to have intermediate signal on T1-weighted imaging and low signal on T2-weighted imaging.[35–37]

Fibrous Dysplasia

Fibrous dysplasia is a developmental disorder that can affect any bone in the body and is caused by abnormal proliferation and maturation of fibroblasts resulting in replacement bone by structurally weak, immature woven bone. The disease is usually classified into three forms: 1) monostotic, 2) polyostotic, and 3) McCune-Albright syndrome. The skull and facial bones are affected in 10% to 25% of patients with monostotic fibrous dysplasia and in 50% of patients with polyostotic fibrous dysplasia. The common craniofacial sites affected in the monostotic form include the frontal bone, ethmoid bone, sphenoid bone, orbit, zygoma, maxilla, mandible, and temporal bones. There have been three reports in the literature of monostotic fibrous dysplasia of the clivus. Involvement of the clivus is so rare that it is usually not placed in the differential diagnosis. More common lesions of the clivus include chordoma, chondrosarcoma, giant cell tumor, cavernous hemangioma, lymphoma, and metastases. Craniopharyngiomas may also involve the clivus.

The CT findings of fibrous dysplasia generally consist of three varieties: 1) ground-glass pattern, 2) homogeneously dense pattern, and 3) the cystic variety. Localized fibrous dysplasia can often be confused with tumor on MR imaging due to the brilliant enhancement after intravenous injection. The signal intensity of fibrous dysplasia has been reported to be low on T1-weighted images. However, the signal intensity of fibrous dysplasia on T1-weighted images may be intermediate, thus resembling that of a soft-tissue tumor. The signal intensity of fibrous dysplasia on T2-weighted images is often variable, ranging from low to high signals in some patients. These high signal intensities on T2-weighted images correspond to nonmineralized areas and regions of cystic changes seen on CT. In some areas within the bone affected by fibrous dysplasia, there may be collections of bone marrow to produce high signal intensities on T1-weighted images. These high-signal-intensity regions show corresponding low signals in fat-suppressed contrast-enhanced images, thus verifying the presence of fatty marrow. When T2-weighted images show high signal intensities, the differential diagnosis should include an inflammatory lesion or a neoplastic process. A destructive pattern is not usually a feature of uncomplicated fibrous dysplasia. Because fibrous dysplasia is typically a painless anomaly, the presence of pain should also alert the radiologist to a more sinister process. The confidence in making a correct MR imaging diagnosis of fibrous dysplasia is high when the signal intensities on both T1- and T2-weighted images are low in spite of enhancement after the injection of contrast material. Confusion arises when fibrous dysplasia shows intermediate signal intensities on T1-weighted images and high signal intensities on T2-weighted images and enhances vividly after the injection of contrast material. Under such circumstances, CT should be performed to resolve the problem.[38–42]

INFLAMMATORY/INFECTIOUS LESIONS

Both infections and noninfectious processes of the CCJ may develop and cause neurovascular compression or spinal deformities. MRI without and with gadolinium enhancement may be used in the evaluation of the level and extent of such infectious and inflammatory diseases. Serial scans are essential for determining the response of diseases to surgical or medical treatment. Evidence of spinal column instability due to destruction of the bones or ligaments by an infectious process or compression of the neural tissues following the deposition of collagenous material by a noninfectious disease may be readily seen.

Rheumatoid Arthritis

Rheumatoid arthritis (RA) is a systemic inflammatory disease that is characterized by chronic inflammation and proliferation of the synovial lining of bursae and articular capsules. This is often associated with destruction of articular cartilage and subchondral bone. Women are affected more commonly than men (at a ratio of 3:1). The prevalence has been estimated to be 1% to 2% of the world's adult population. Although men represent only about 25% of the patient population, they have a greater risk of advanced cervical involvement. RA is a symmetric arthritis of the appendicular skeleton, particularly the small joints of the hand, foot, and wrist. The synovial joints of the axial skeleton also may be affected, especially the apophyseal and atlantoaxial joints of the cervical spine.

The incidence of rheumatoid involvement of the cervical spine is second only to that of the hands. It is the most common inflammatory disorder of the cervical spine. Cervical spine involvement is common in rheumatoid arthritis and affects 60% to 80% of the cases. Typically, it involves the atlantoaxial complex, causing a variety of subluxations: horizontal atlantoaxial subluxation, nonreducible head tilt, and vertical translocation. Subaxial involvement may coexist with these abnormalities (**Fig. 10-1**). The sequelae of cervical spine involvement ranges from pain and paralysis to death. In patients with rheumatoid arthritis, the incidence of neck pain has been reported to be 40% to 88%. Cervical subluxations have been observed in 43% to 86% on radiographic evaluation. However, a neurologic deficit is reported in only 7% to 34% of patients. Some patients with significant radiographic evidence of disease may be entirely asymptomatic.[25]

Three deformities occur most commonly in the rheumatoid cervical spine: 1) Atlantoaxial instability or subluxation is the most common and represents 65% of all cervical subluxations, 2) superior migration of the odontoid process is the second most common deformity in the rheumatoid spine, and 3) subaxial subluxation occurs in approximately 15% of rheumatoid patients and frequently occurs at multiple levels. The majority of atlantoaxial deformities result in anterior subluxation, although in as many as 20% of cases, it may be lateral and in 7% of cases, posterior. Rotatory subluxations have been reported but are rare. Atlantoaxial subluxation can be reducible, partially reducible, or fixed; this determination is important in planning treatment.

Superior migration of the odontoid process is caused by erosion of the occiput – C1 and C1 to C2 joints which causes diminution in the vertical distance between the brainstem and the odontoid process. This is seen in up to 20% of rheumatoid patients and is also described as cranial settling, atlantoaxial impaction, and pseudobasilar invagination. Superior migration of the odontoid process can lead to direct compression of the brainstem or cause neurologic injury or death by placing the cervicomedullary junction into excessive kyphosis. Subaxial subluxation may produce a "stepladder" type of deformity with associated kyphosis. Subaxial subluxation has also been reported to occur after previous upper cervical fusions.

A soft-tissue pannus consisting of inflamed and hypertrophic synovial tissue commonly surrounds the odontoid process. The eroding pannus and hyperemic effects cause ligamentous laxity leading to instability and atlantoaxial subluxation of all types in 40% to 80% of cases.[25] If the pannus occurs in the predental space it may prevent full reduction of the subluxation. Flexion and extension views are useful in demonstrating the degree of subluxation and instability.

On MR imaging, the mass has intermediate signal intensity on T1-weighted images and slight increased signal intensity on T2-weighted images. The pannus usually enhances with intravenous contrast, and can simulate active infections or neoplasms.[26,27] Widening of the predental space can often be seen on lateral plain film views of the cervical spine.

There is erosion and eventual obliteration of the odontoid process as the disease progresses. The erosions predominately occur in the synovial lined spaces between the posterior aspect of the anterior arch of C1 and the anterior aspect of the odontoid process, in addition to the posterior surface of the odontoid process and the transverse process. Cord compression is common and is caused not only by atlantoaxial subluxation but also by the periodontoid pannus[26,27] (**Fig. 10-18**). Compression of the medulla and spinal cord may cause increased signal intensity of the spinal cord at the level of the compression. The pannus may be partly due to an abnormal response to chronic subluxation because it has been shown to decrease in size when stabilization by cervical fusion is performed.[43–49]

Other Arthritides

Psoriatic arthritis is a chronic inflammatory disease. Most patients have a long history of psoriatic skin disease and arthritis is more common in patients with moderate or severe skin involvement. Cervical spine involvement with psoriatic arthritis may be ankylosing in nature up to 35% of patients.[28] This pattern consists of syndesmophytes, apophyseal joint ankylosis, and ligamentous calcifications. Psoriatic arthritis can also involve the cervical spine in a pattern similar to RA with apophyseal and odontoid erosions, and atlantoaxial subluxation.

On CT scans, there may be multiple small globular and linear calcifications within these masses.[32] The masses are isointense on T1-weighted images and there is mixed signal intensity with hypo and hyperintense areas on T2-weighted MR images.[32] There is marked enhancement in the periphery of the masses on gadolinium-enhanced T1-weighted images[50–54] (**Fig. 10-19**).

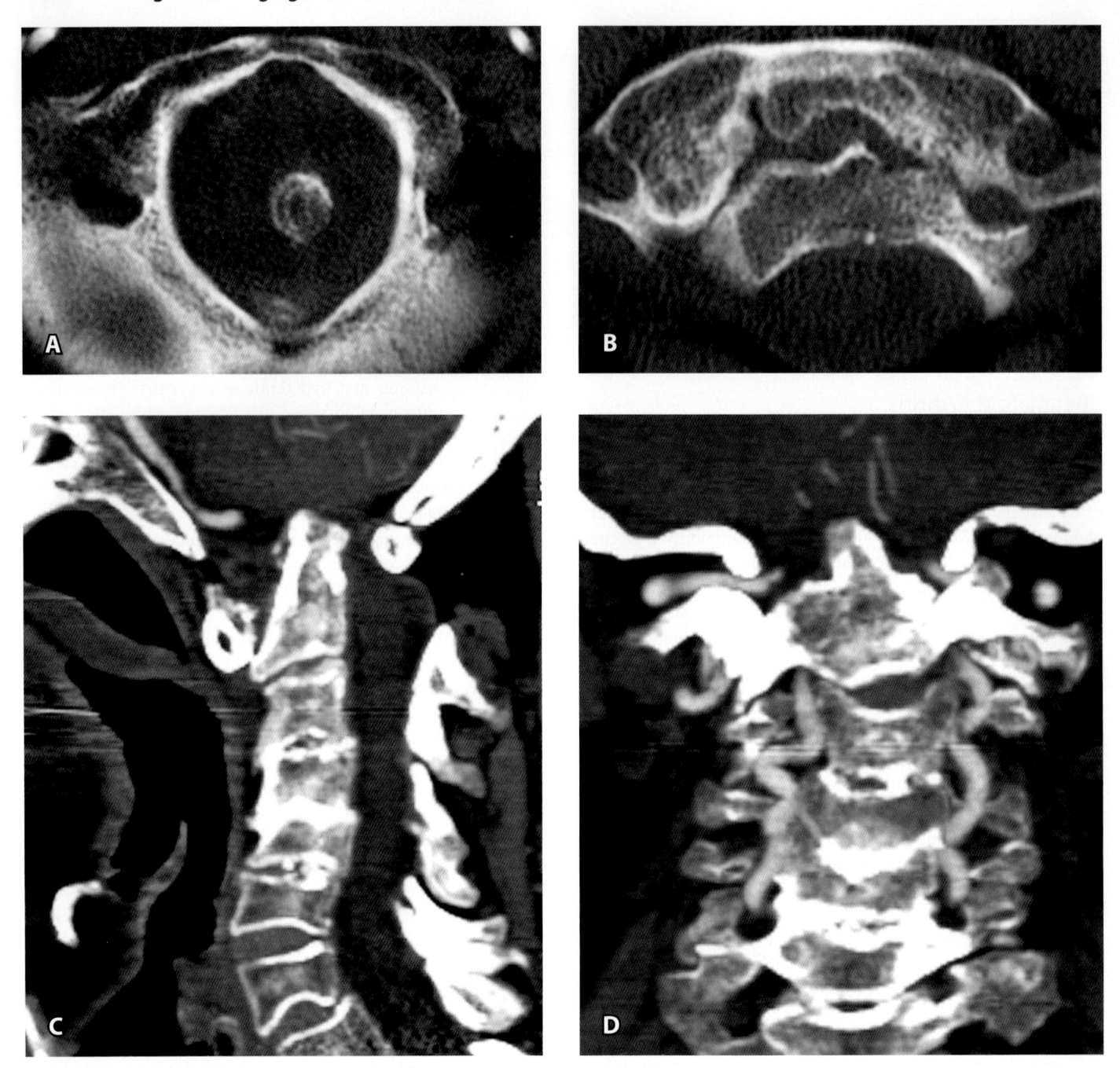

Figure 10-18 Rheumatoid Arthritis with Cranial Settling at the CCJ
Middle-aged male with severe rheumatoid arthritis and progressive quadriparesis. Axial CT scans through the foramen magnum (**A, B**) show severe settling of the odontoid posteriorly to the center and slightly to left of the foramen magnum (**A**), the body of C2 is displaced cephalad and lies adjacent to the occipital condyl on the right side and to the hypoglassal canal to the left side (**B**). Reformatted CT scans from a CT angiogram (**C, D**) optimally show the degree of cephalad migration of the odontoid and C1 vertebra. On the sagittal image (**C**), the cervical cord lies posterior to the odontoid and anterior to C1, which is narrowed to approximately 6 mm. In addition to the cranial settling, the coronal image (**D**) shows the tilting of the odontoid toward the right, indicating rotational instability. The tip of the odontoid is amputated, secondary to erosion from the rheumatoid arthritis.

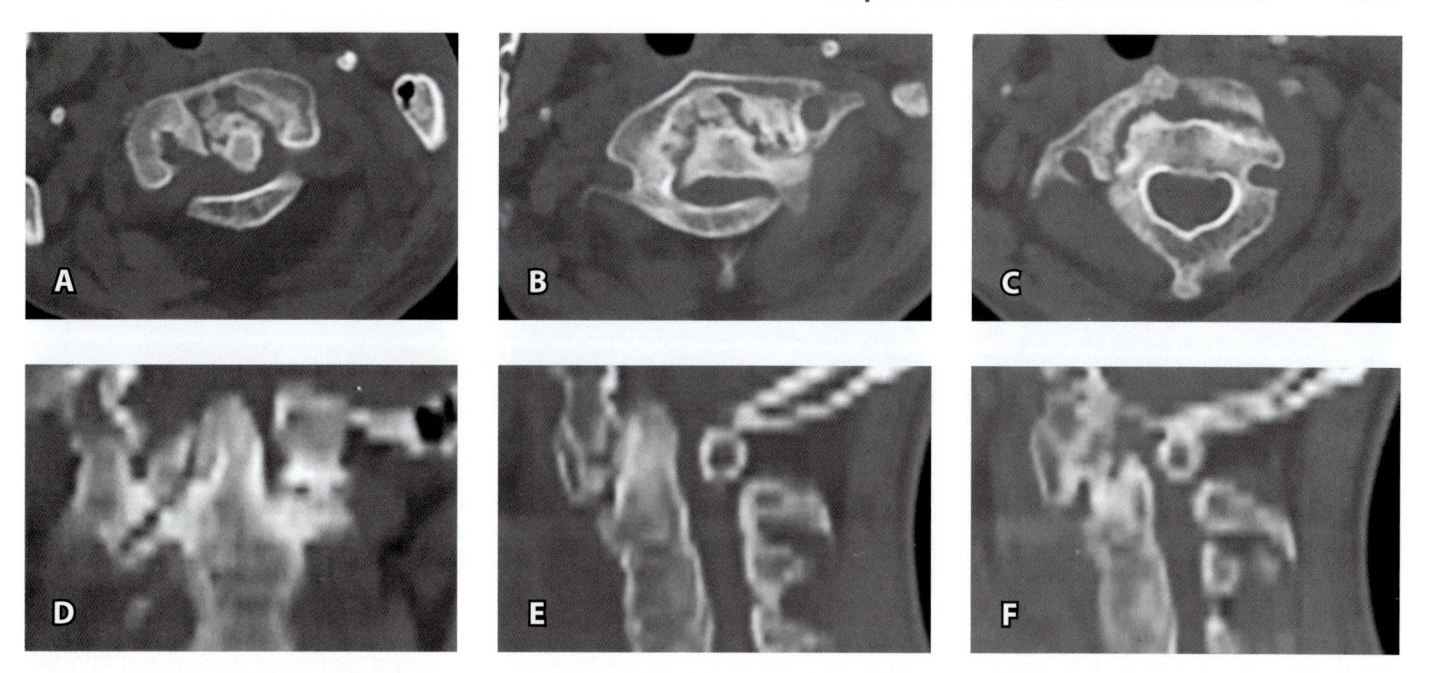

Figure 10-19 Psoriasis of the CCJ
Axial CT scans. (**A**) shows displacement of the dens posterolaterally to the left. In (**B** and **C**) there is axial subluxation and erosive changes at the atlantoaxial joint. Reformatted coronal CT scan (**D**) shows the dens displaced superiorly with sclerotic bony overgrowth and cranial settling. Reformatted sagittal CT scans (**E** and **F**) show the spinal stenosis as a result of the displaced dens.

Pseudogout

Calcium pyrophosphate dihydrate deposition (CPPD) disease is considered to be one of the most common forms of crystal induced arthritis. The prevalence of CPPD increases with age to reach a rate of 45% of patients 85 years or older. CPPD crystal deposition disease is an inflammatory arthropathy characterized by the deposition of weakly positively birefringent crystals in articular and periarticular structures. It is also referred to as pseudogout and articular chondrocalcinosis. CPPD crystal deposition can be seen in various spinal structures, such as intervertebral disks, ligaments, bursae, articular cartilage synovium, and joint capsules. Although CPPD deposition disease frequently manifests as a primary arthropathy unassociated with any disorder, it can be associated with several endocrine or metabolic disorders, including hemochromatosis, diabetes mellitus, hyperparathyroidism, hypothyroidism, Wilson's disease, gout, and rheumatoid arthritis.

CPPD involvement of the cervical spine and the craniocervical junction is usually asymptomatic. To date, there have been only 12 reported cases of symptomatic CPPD deposition involving the C1 to C2 articulation and the majority have been reported in older women. Signs and symptoms of CPPD deposition disease involving the cervical spine include neck pain, stiffness, and myelopathy. One of the ligaments that may be involved by CPPD crystal deposition is the transverse ligament of the atlas, which is a thick, strong band of collagen fibers that arches behind the odontoid process and maintains contact between the odontoid process and the anterior arch of C1 (**Fig. 10-12**). When disrupted, atlantoaxial subluxation may result. CT will typically show speckled calcification within the transverse atlantal ligament and, if present, a retro-odontoid mass. These lesions are most often isointense to healthy neural tissue on T1-weighted MR images and are of mixed intensity on T2-weighted MR images. On gadolinium-enhanced MR imaging, these lesions will typically show peripheral enhancement (**Fig. 10-20**). CT may also show subchondral cysts erosions of the odontoid process. MR imaging is less sensitive for the detection of calcification than CT. However, MR is much better at determining the degree of of involvement of the spinal cord and at determining the degree of ligamentous and cartilaginous involvement. Subchondral cyst formation is usually especially prominent. It has been postulated that CPPD crystal deposition within the transverse atlantal ligament may be associated with odontoid process erosion. It has also been postulated that there is increased risk of odontoid process fracture with the presence of atlantoaxial involvement in CPPD crystal deposition disease.

Symptomatic patients with retro-odontoid CPPD deposition will often require surgical decompression. Decompression is usually performed via a transoral approach. Posterior stabilization of the cervical spine is also usually required. Often, the occiput will be incorporated into the posterior fusion construct. In addition to CPPD deposition disease, the differential diagnosis of a retro-odontoid calcified mass includes rheumatoid pannus, Paget disease, and acromegaly.[55–60]

Gout

Gout is a disorder of urate metabolism characterized by the deposition of monosodium urate crystals in the joints and soft tissues. Gout is the most common cause of inflammatory arthritis in men over 40 years of age and affects 0.5% to 1% of men in

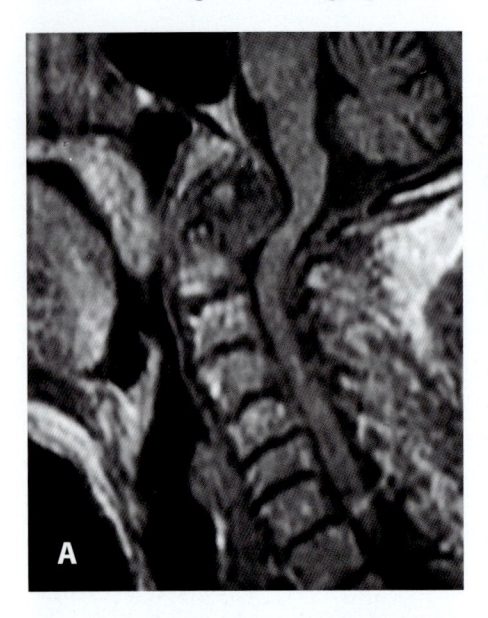

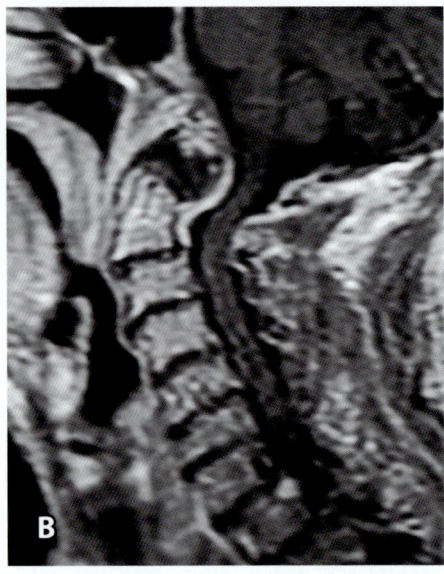

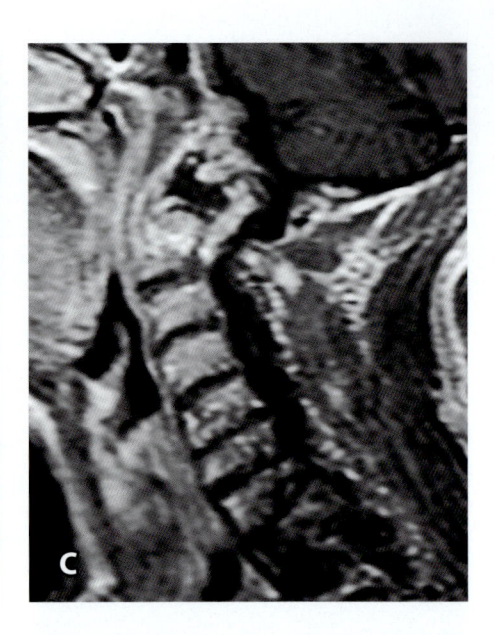

Figure 10-20 Pseudogout of the CCJ
Pseudogout at the craniocervical junction in an 84-year-old man with left hand numbness and weakness. Parasagittal T1W MR scan (**A**) view shows a mass isointense to neural tissue at the base of the clivus. Sagittal T1W MR scan with contrast (**B**) shows the mass posterior to the odontoid compressing the medulla. The dura is thickened and enhances, as opposed to true gout in which the dura would not enhance. Parasagittal T1W MR scan with contrast (**C**) demonstrates the peripheral enhancement of the mass and areas of hypointensity within the mass which may represent calcification.

Western countries. The disease affects men predominantly and has a male:female ratio of 7 to 9:1.

Tophaceous gout typically affects the appendicular skeleton and gouty involvement of the axial skeleton is uncommon and urate deposition in the spine is rare. To date, only 15 cases of gout affecting the cervical spine have been described in the world literature. Characteristically, gouty tophi on MRI are isointense to muscle on T1 and low-intermediate signal intensity on T2 with homogeneous enhancement. Metastatic lytic bony lesions and infective processes are generally hypointense on T1 and hyperintense on T2. The low T2 signal on gouty tophi is thought to be due to the fibrous tissue and crystalline structures, and the enhancement reflects the presence of vascularized reactive tissue within the lesion but does not help differentiate from neoplastic or infective lesions. Many tophaceous deposits in the spine are asymptomatic. Only three case of spinal compression due to tophaceous gout has been reported. Patients with long-standing polyarticular gout have a higher risk of spinal involvement. Deposition of tophaceous material may cause sclerosis or destruction of the odontoid process.[61-63]

Multicentric Reticulohistiocytosis (Lipoid Dermato-Arthritis)

Multicentric reticulohistiocytosis is a systemic disease of unknown etiology. It predominately affects middle-aged patients, particularly three times more often in women than in men. Clinical manifestations are symmetric polyarthritis involving mainly the interphalangeal joints and nodules in skin, mucosa and subcutaneous tissue.[64,65] In 60% to 70% of cases, polyarthritis precedes the skin lesions.

Early subluxation at the atlantoaxial joint can occur with eventual osseous destruction of the atlas, the axis including the odontoid process, and the base of the skull[64,65] (**Figs. 10-21** and **10-22**). MRI findings at the CCJ have not been previously described. However, the MRI findings in the knee joint include severe joint destruction with well-defined marginal erosions and bulky masses within the joint space with intermediate intensity on T1 weighted images and relatively high intensity on T2 weighted images[65] (**Fig. 10-23**). These masses represent marked proliferation of synovial tissue in the joint space. Scattered tiny spots of decreased signal intensity on both T1- and T2-weighted images may be seen and are due to hemosiderin deposits.[65]

Pyogenic Infections

Infectious masses caused by a variety of organisms can involve the CCJ, pyogenic organisms may reach the spine by direct extension from a contiguous site or by hematogenous dissemination from a distant focus of infection.[66] Pyogenic osteomyelitis of the cervical spine is less common than in the lumbar or thoracic spine and osteomyelitis confined to the CCJ is rare.[67] The most common pathogen is *Staphylococcus aureus*, but osteomyelitis may be caused by any organism including *Streptococcus* and gram negative organisms.[66-68] Most patients have some underlying chronic disorder, such as diabetes or intravenous drug abuse.

Radiologic findings include a destructive process involving the axis and odontoid process. Typically, T1-weighted images show low signal intensity within the vertebral body and a periodontoid soft-tissue mass of decreased signal intensity, both of which usually have high signal intensity on T2-weighted images. Contrast enhancement often obliterates the low signal

Chapter 10: The Craniocervical Junction 435

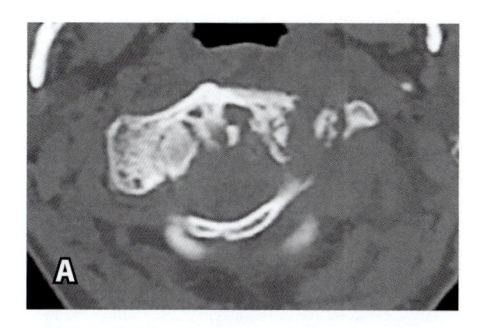

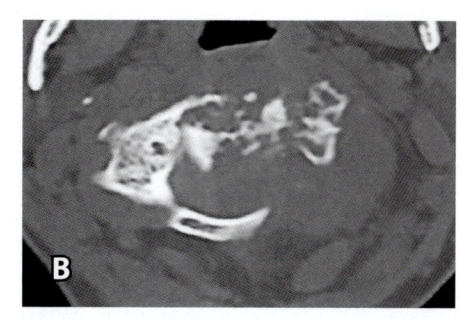

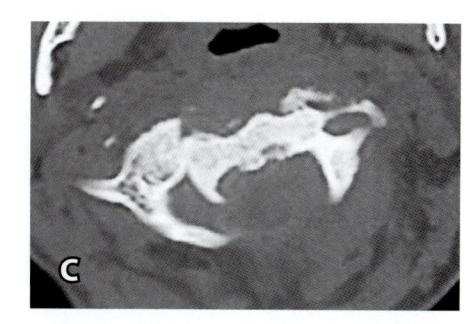

Figure 10-21 Multicentric Reticulohistiocytosis of the CCJ
Multicentric reticulohistiocytosis of the craniocervical junction in a 56-year-old female with symptoms of nerve compression. Axial CT scans. (**A** and **B**) show bony destruction of dens, and left anterior arch and lateral mass of the atlas. (**C**) shows lateral subluxation of C1 to the right relative to C2.

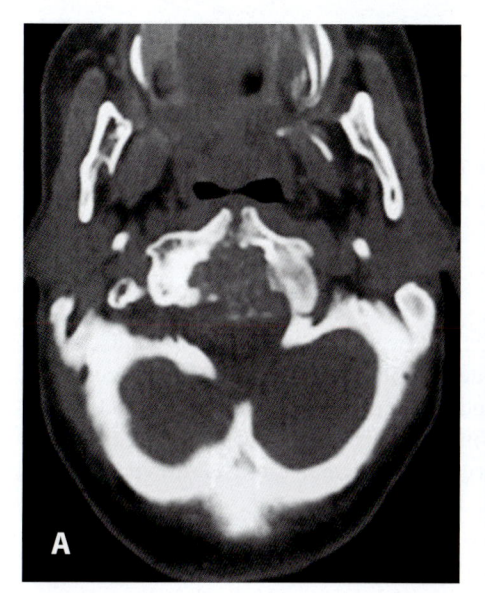

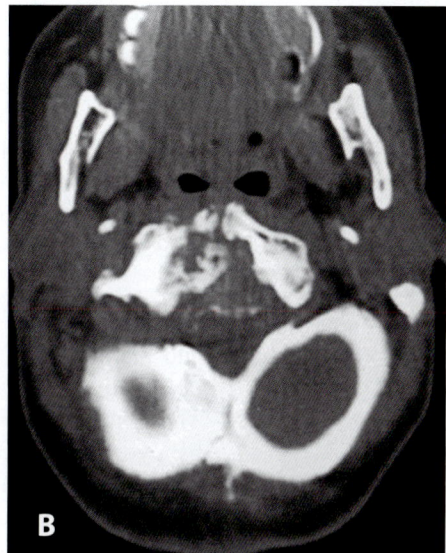

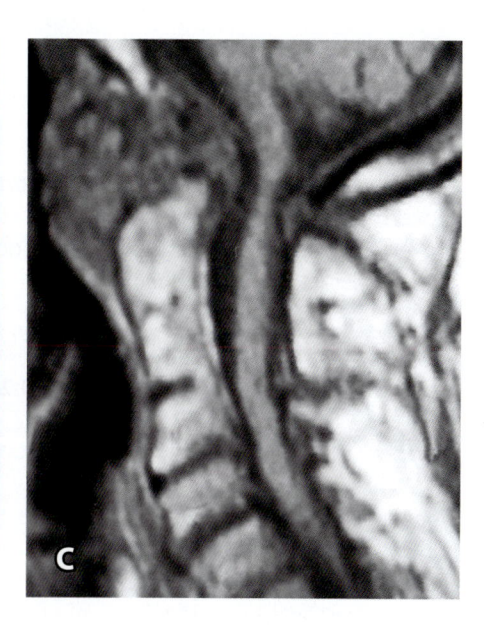

Figure 10-22 Multicentric Reticulohistiocytosis of the CCJ
Axial CT scans (**A** and **B**) show dense sclerotic bone and bony destruction of the C1 to C2 junction. Sagittal T1W MR scan (**C**) shows a fibrous pseudotumor of intermediate to low signal intensity at the base of the clivus most likely representative of synovial cell proliferation. The mass is impinging upon the spinal canal anteriorly and posteriorly.

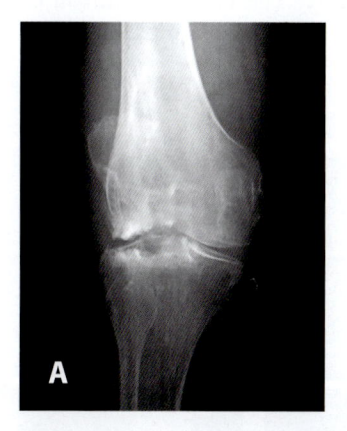

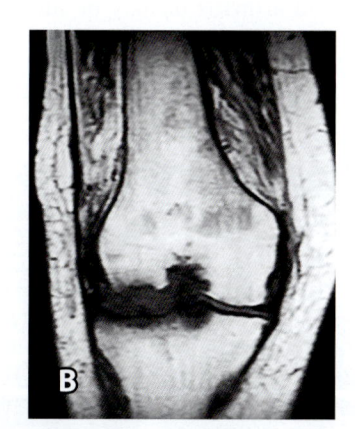

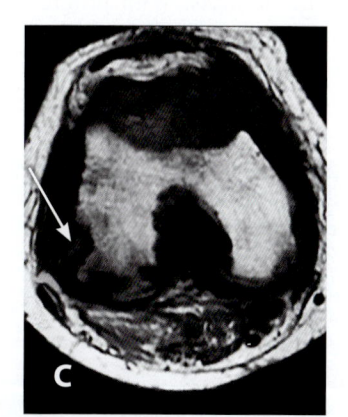

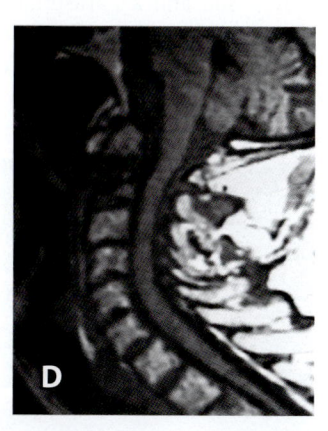

Figure 10-23 Multicentric Reticulohistiocytosis of the CCJ and Right Knee
Plain film of the right knee (**A**) shows marginal erosions. Coronal T1W MR scan of the right knee (**B**) shows a low intensity irregular mass in the joint and marginal erosions of both the femur and tibia. Axial T1W MR scan of the right knee (**C**) shows distinctive marginal erosions (*arrow*). Sagittal T1W MR scan (**D**) shows synovial cell proliferation exemplified by the low density mass inferior to the dens and anterior arch of C1.

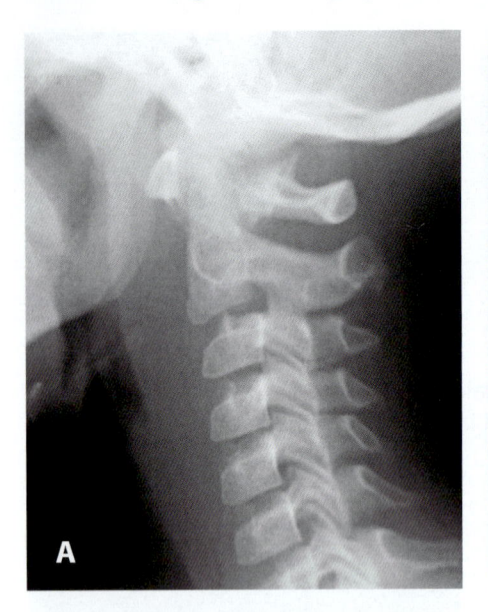

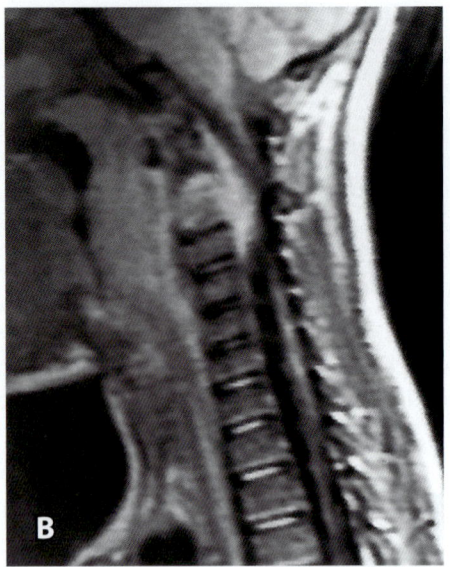

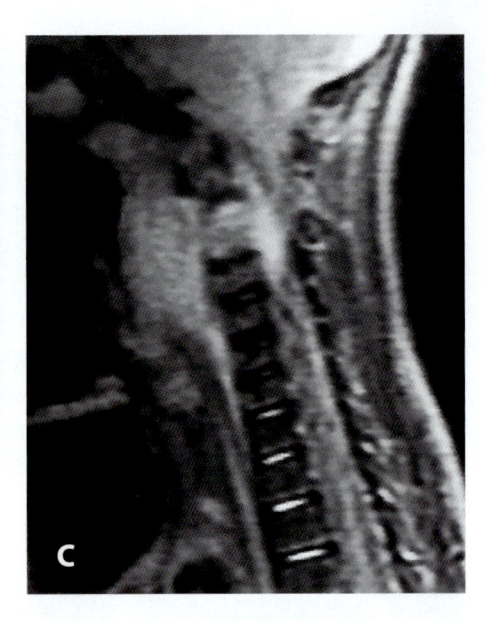

Figure 10-24 Osteomyelitis of the CCJ
Osteomyelitis of the craniocervical junction in a 6-year-old girl with fever and torticollis. Plain film lateral c-spine (**A**) demonstrates prevertebral soft-tissue swelling. At this stage, there is no evidence of disk space narrowing. Sagittal T1W MR scan (**B**) shows prevertebral and prespinal suppurative adenitis extending through the disk space.

intensity in the vertebral body and enhances the soft-tissue mass on T1-weighted images[69] (**Figs. 10-24 –10-26**).

Nonpyogenic Infections

Nonpyogenic causes are most likely due to tuberculosis, but may also caused by *Coccidioides*, *Aspergillus*, and *Brucellosis*. Spinal tuberculosis affects, in descending order, the lumbar, thoracic, and cervical spine. Involvement of the odontoid is uncommon, the incidence ranging from 0% to 2%.[70] It may take 2 to 5 months after the onset of illness for radiologic abnormalities to develop.

The earliest finding is widening of the retrophmyngeal soft tissue and a paraspinal soft-tissue mass. With progression, there is increasing ligamentous involvement resulting in anterior subluxation of C1 on C2 and minimal bony involvement. This is followed by narrowing of the disc space and marked bony destruction which may result in complete obliteration of the odontoid process and anterior arch of C1.[71] These findings are indistinguishable from the changes caused by pyogenic infection, except that there is slower progression[70] (**Fig. 10-27**).

With nonpyogenic infections, there may be associated meningitis, which typically involves the dura (pachymeningitis). When the dura becomes involved it may appear inflamed and fibrotic. This finding is seen as areas of hypointensity with hyperintense edges on T2-W MR imaging and typically enhances intensely and homogeneously. Such evidence of pachymeningitis may also be caused by rheumatoid arthritis or may be idiopathic. The involvement can be severe enough to cause cervicomedullary compression and hydrocephalus.[72]

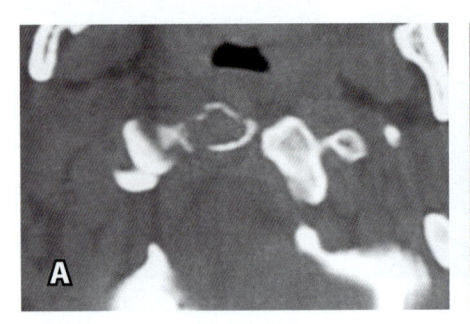

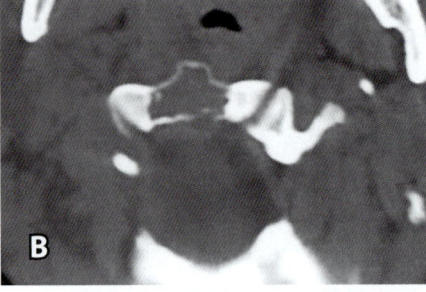

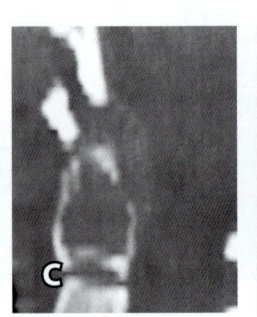

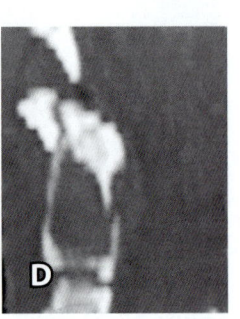

Figure 10-25 Osteomyelitis of the CCJ
Osteomyelitis of the craniocervical junction in a 26-year-old female with fever and complaints of neck pain for several weeks. Axial CT scans. (**A**) shows a bubbly bone lesion with an unusually preserved cortex at the level of the dens and extending into the body of C2 (**B**). Reformatted sagittal CT scans (**C–D**) shows the bubbly lesion in the right lateral mass of C2.

Chapter 10: The Craniocervical Junction **437**

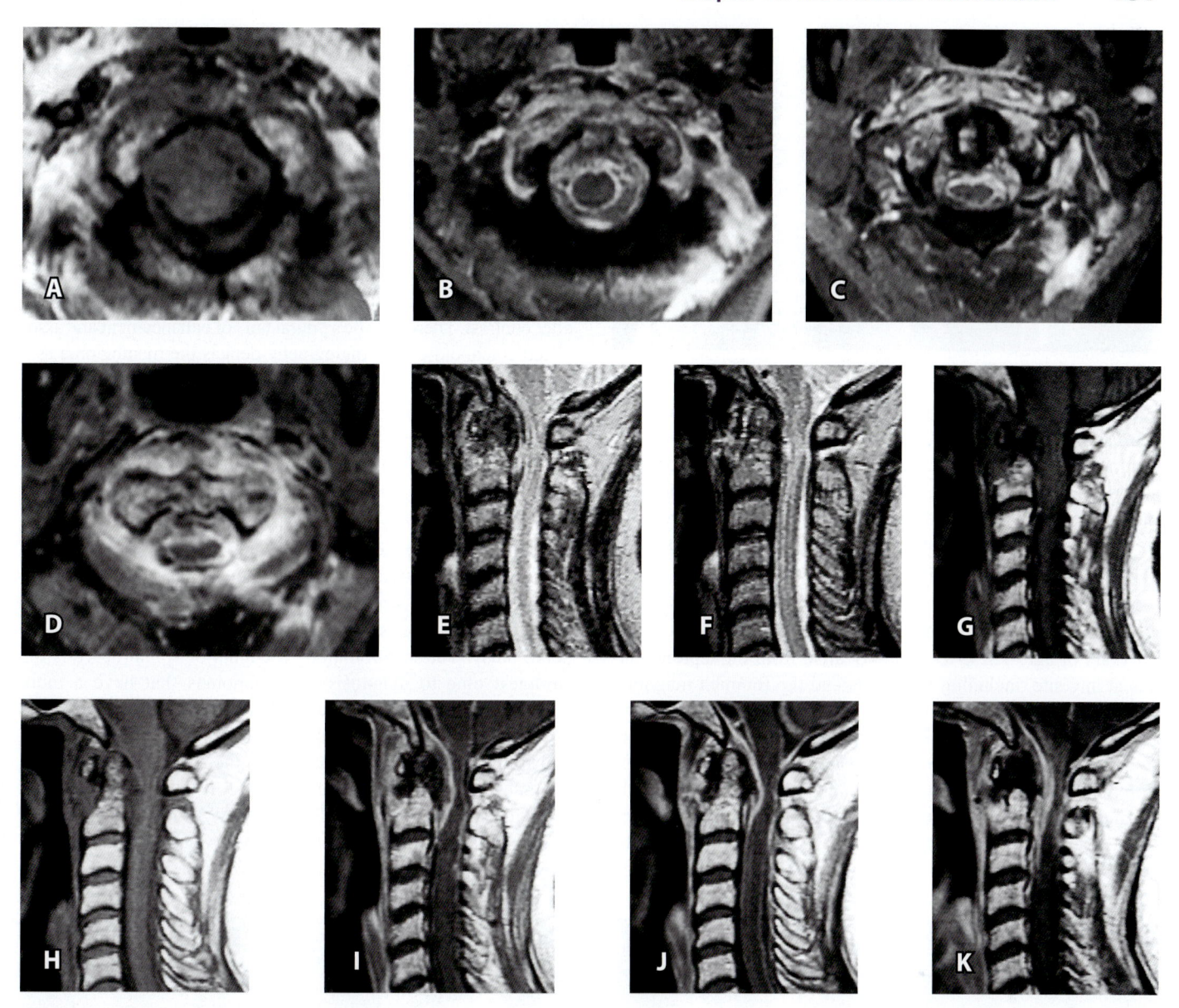

Figure 10-26 Pyogenic Empyema at the CCJ
Pyogenic empyema at the craniocervical junction in a diabetic patient on steroids. Axial T1W MR scan (**A**) shows spinal cord centrally, compare with postcontrast scans (**B, C,** and **D**) where the cord and vertebral arteries show peripheral enhancement and increasing compression with progression down the cord. There is enhancement surrounding the dens representing pus. Sagittal T2W MR scans (**E** and **F**) show a soft-tissue mass at the C1 to C2 level consistent with fibrous pseudotumor. Sagittal T1W MR scans (**G** and **H**) show diffuse bright signal of the bone marrow secondary to a history of radiation therapy. Sagittal T1W MR scans (**I–K**) with gadolinium show enhancement of the epidural margin from the posterior fossa to the upper cervical spine. Note the presence of the lesion in all three images shows the lesion in the paramedian on both sides extending across the midline.

NEOPLASTIC LESIONS

A variety of intramedullary, intradural-extramedullary and extradural tumors may be seen at the CCJ. MRI without and with gadolinium enhancement is the procedure of choice for the examination of these neoplasms. Tumors that straddle the foramen magnum may be both intra- and extracranial. This distinction is readily depicted by multiplanar MR images. Cystic changes or cord cavities that may be associated with some neoplasms are easily shown on the T1- and T2-weighted spin-echo images. MR angiography or conventional angiography may be required in order to differentiate between a vascular tumor and an arteriovenous malformation (AVM).

Benign Neoplasms

Meningiomas

Meningiomas arise from meningoendothelial cells and tend to occur in the adult age group. There is a 2:1 female predominance. They represent 15% to 20% of intracranial neoplasms. Approximately 35% of meningiomas occur along the skull base,

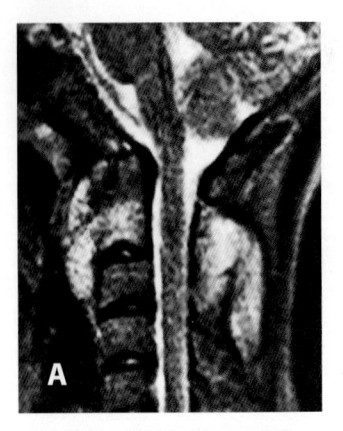

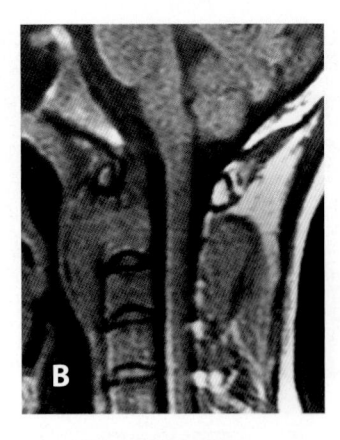

Figure 10-27 Tuberculous Abscess of the CCJ
Sagittal T2W MR scan (**A**) shows a high intensity lesion in the retropharyngeal space extending into the area of the C1 to C2 junction and following posteriorly into the posterior cervical space. Sagittal T1W MR scan (**B**) shows the same lesion with homogeneous intermediate signal intensity. (Reprinted with permission from Hasso AN: MRI Atlas of the Head and Neck, 1st ed. London: Martin Dunitz, 1993:54.)

primarily affect women, and have a peak incidence at about 40 years of age. These lesions may arise from the leptomeninges at any site, including the clivus and the foramen magnum. Clinically, they present with symptoms of neurological compression. Neurofibromatosis II and a history of previous radiation therapy predispose to the development of a meningioma. Foramen magnum meningiomas usually are located anteriorly or anterolaterally and become symptomatic by compression of the cervico-medullary junction or by compression of the lower cranial nerves. In this location they are well visualized by traditional techniques such as myelography; however, most lesions are currently diagnosed by CT or MR imaging.

On CT scans, there is a hyperdense (compared to gray matter) mass with or without calcifications (**Fig. 10-28**). If present, the calcifications typically follow two patterns; fine and evenly distributed representing psammoma bodies and larger and scattered calcifications. There is uniform enhancement of the mass after contrast injection and there may be hyperostosis adjacent to the tumor at the site of bony attachment or sclerosis. Using MR imaging the mass most often appears isointense to gray matter on T1- and T2-weighted imaging. Meningiomas tend to enhance markedly and uniformly after contrast. There may be a "dural tail" of enhancement and associated arachnoid cysts. Angiography depicts the meningioma as a hypervascular honeycomb or solid lesion with a characteristic "sunburst" appearance at the capillary phase. Dilated feeding arteries may also be demonstrated. Treatment for meningiomas is surgical resection with or without prior embolization.[73–75]

Schwannomas

Schwannomas may be seen in the craniocervical region originating typically from the lower cranial and upper cervical nerves. Patients may show symptoms of progressive myelopathy, headache, and long tract signs. The tumor may also present with a nerve palsy. The location along a cranial or spinal nerve is the strongest clue to diagnosis. Schwannomas that have a more anterior location are more likely to have the lower cranial nerves as their origin, in contrast to those lesions that are more posterior and are likely to have originated from the upper cervical nerves.

Schwannomas will enhance on both CT and MR imaging, and will give a low signal on T1-weighted MR images. There may be bony erosion along the course of the nerve tumor and the lesion may straddle the foramen magnum[76] (**Figs. 10-29** and **10-30**).

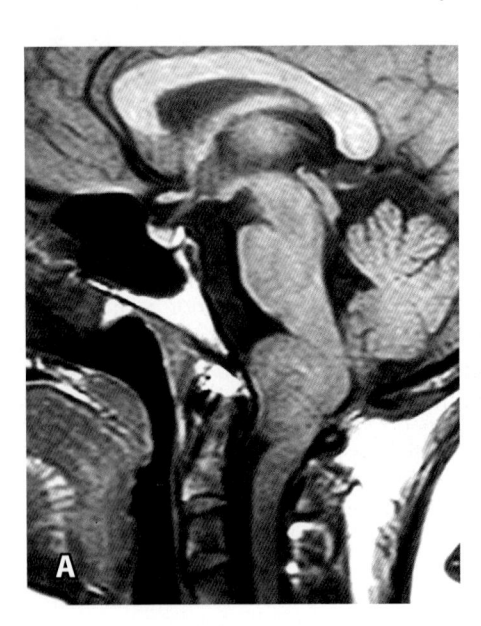

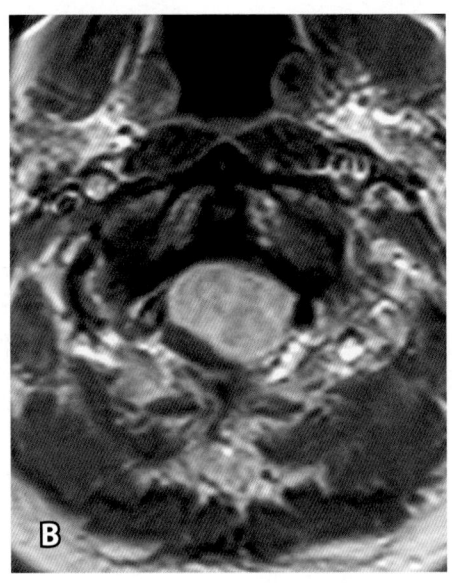

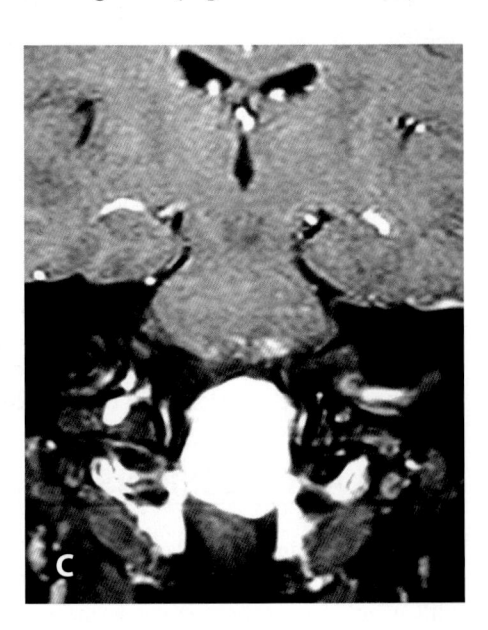

Figure 10-28 Clivus Meningioma
30-year-old woman complaining of neck pain and extremity weakness. (**A**) Sagittal T1W MR scan shows a rounded mass anterior to the brainstem and spinal cord at the CCJ. The mass has a broad dural base anteriorly. (**B**) Axial PDW image without contrast shows a large mass behind the C2 that nearly fills the spinal canal. (**C**) Coronal postcontrast T1W MR scan shows intense enhancement throughout this tumor.

Chapter 10: The Craniocervical Junction **439**

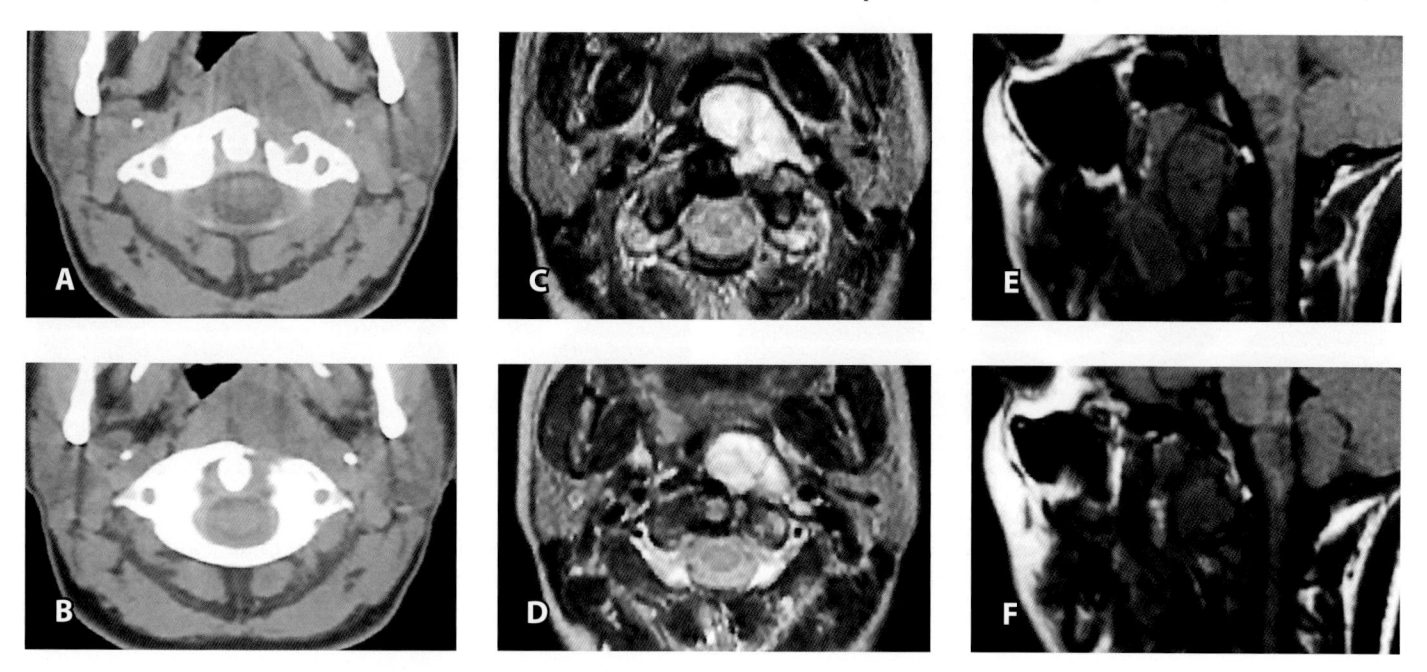

Figure 10-29 Schwannoma of the Vagus Nerve at the CCJ
Axial CT scans. (**A** and **B**) show destruction of the left anterior arch of C1 and asymmetric shape of the nasopharynx as the mass extends into the anterior nasopharynx. Axial proton density MR scans show the mass eroding bone and the mass appearing to originate from the root of the vagus nerve (**C**). The oropharynx is markedly compressed in (**D**) and the mass is more clearly surrounding the area of the carotid. Sagittal T1W MR scans show a mass of intermediate signal intensity anterior to the dens (**E–F**). (**F**) shows the mass anterior and superior to the anterior ring of C2.

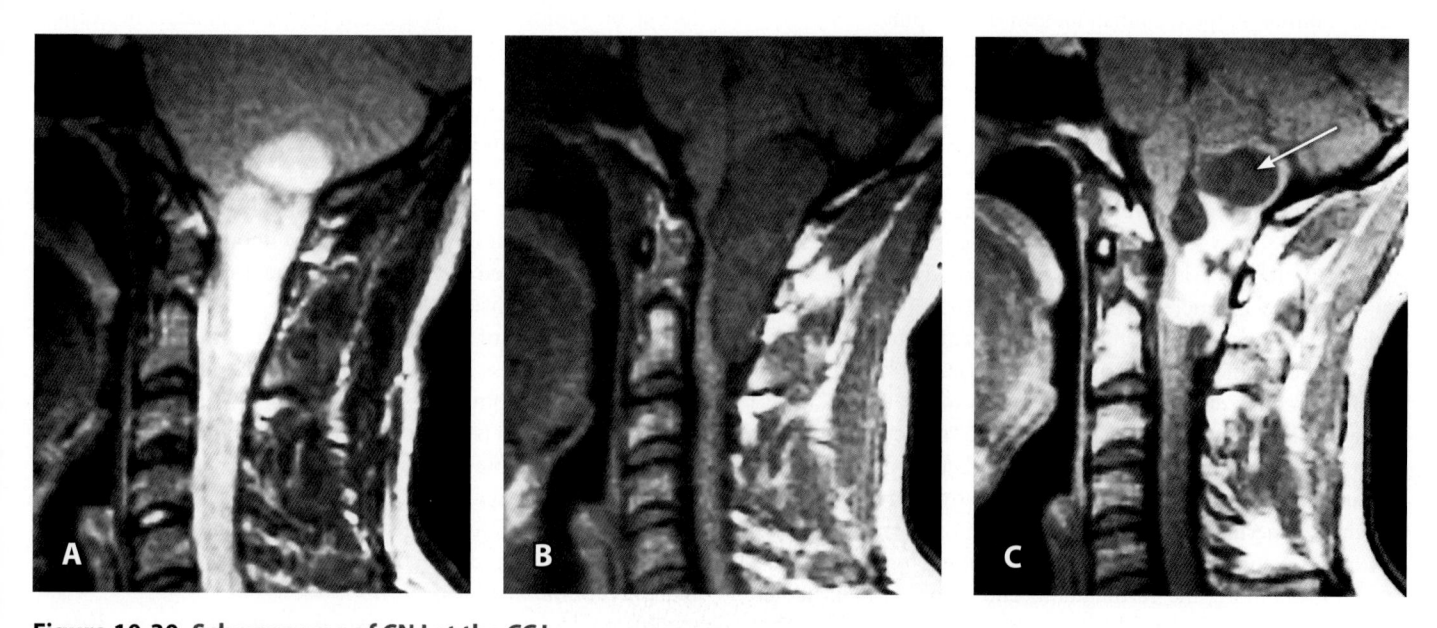

Figure 10-30 Schwannoma of CN I at the CCJ
Sagittal T2W MR scan (**A**) shows the lesion with high signal, although not as high as CSF and the distinction between solid and cystic components is not demonstrated. Sagittal T1W MR scan (**B**) shows a mass lesion extending through the foramen magnum straddling the craniocervical junction compressing the cord anteriorly. Sagittal T1W MR scan with gadolinium (**C**) shows the lesion to have heterogeneous enhancement. There are low signal areas representing cystic regions with peripheral enhancement (*white arrow*). Other areas of the mass with enhancement and a homogeneous pattern represent solid components. (Modified from Hasso AN: MRI Atlas of the Head and Neck, 1st ed. London: Martin Dunitz, 1993:51.)

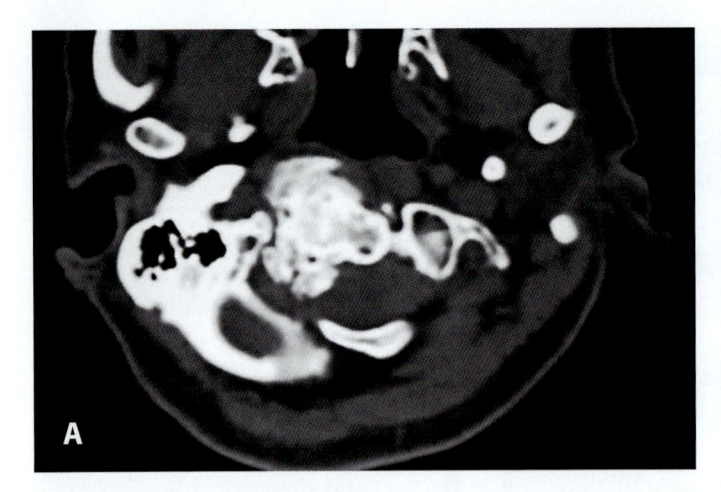

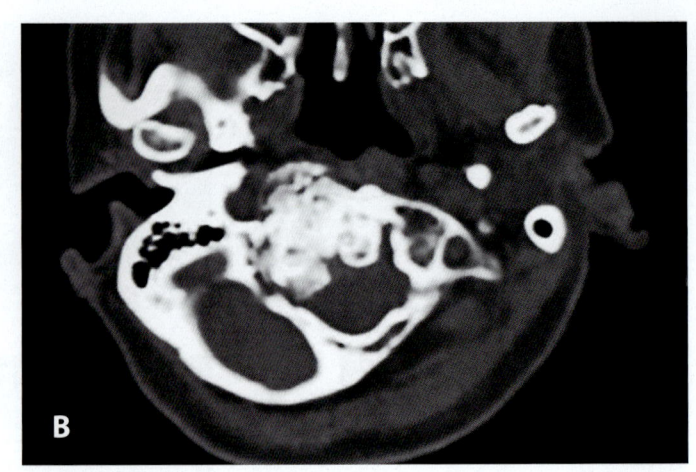

Figure 10-31 Osteochondroma at the CCJ
Axial CT scans. (**A** and **B**) show a mostly high density heterogeneous mass in the area of the right occipital condyle and dens consistent with a myxofibrous makeup. There is much bony overgrowth, but little bony destruction consistent with a benign lesion.

A wide variety of benign primary bone and soft-tissue neoplasms can involve the CCJ. They are typically similar as those affecting other areas of the spine. These include osteochondroma, osteoid osteoma, osteoblastoma, aneurismal bone cysts, giant cell tumors, and eosinophilic granuloma. Unusual tumors include ganglion or synovial cysts, hemangiopericytoma, and infantile myofibromatosis. However, some of these lesions are more common in the CCJ than the rest of the spine.

Osteochondromas are common benign lesions usually occurring in the metaphysis of long bones with spinal involvement being uncommon. In hereditary multiple exostoses, only 7% to 9% have a spinal lesion.[78,79] Despite the multiplicity of lesions, there is usually only one spinal osteochondroma. Spinal osteochondromas are more common in the cervical spine particularly C2. Most lesions arise from the posterior element but may uncommonly arise from the vertebral body.[80]

They are characterized radiographically by a sessile or pedunculated osseous protuberance. Spinal osteochondromas can only be diagnosed in the minority of cases (21%) from radiographic findings due to the complex anatomy at the CCJ.[79] CT is the most important imaging modality for detecting the lesion as well as demonstrating its exact size and location (**Fig. 10-31**). MR imaging is able to demonstrate the yellow marrow centrally, which is hyperintense on T1-weighted and intermediate intensity on T2-weighted images with a surrounding hypointense cortex.[79] Furthermore, the cartilaginous cap is low to intermediate signal intensity on T1-weighted images and high signal intensity on T2-weighted images.[79]

Osteoid osteoma is a benign osteoblastic tumor consisting of a central core of vascular osteoid tissue and peripheral zone of sclerotic bone. The presenting complaint is usually pain that is worse at night and is relieved with salicylates. Patients are usually affected between the ages of 10 to 35 years and there is a male predominance.[83] Although frequently located in the femur and tibia, 10% of the cases involve the axial skeleton.[81] The majority of these lesions occur in the lumbar spine (59%), followed by the cervical (27%), thoracic (12%), and sacral (2%) spine.[83] The majority of axial osteoid osteomas are located in the posterior elements (75%) and only 7% are in the vertebral body.[51] Involvement of the C2 vertebra is unusual, but has been described.[84]

An osteoid osteoma is characterized by an oval or round nidus, which is generally 1.5 cm or less in diameter, which is lucent on radiography. When the lesion is located in cortical bone the nidus is often associated with a prominent surrounding zone of sclerosis.[83] In cancellous bone, this zone of sclerosis is much less prominent or may be absent.[83] Central calcification may be present within the nidus. Bone scintigraphy is very sensitive and demonstrates marked increased uptake by the nidus.[83] CT is the definitive study, demonstrating a well-defined oval or round low attenuation nidus, with or without central calcification, and surrounded by a variable amount of bony sclerosis.[83] MR imaging is considerably less useful in detecting the nidus. The MRI findings of bone marrow edema, synovitis, or a reactive soft-tissue mass may be misleading and simulate a malignant tumor or osteomyelitis.[83]

Osteoblastoma is a rare benign primary bone tumor that histiologically resembles osteoid osteoma. They are less frequent than osteoid osteoma. Patients present with dull localized pain, which rarely interferes with sleep and is not relieved by salicylates. They occur in the second and third decades of life, with a male predominance.[85]

Osteoblastoma affects the spine in approximately 30% to 40% of the cases[81,83,85,86] and appear to occur more or less equally in the cervical, thoracic, and lumbar segments.[81,83,86] They are rarely found in the odontoid process.[87] The lesions are often greater than 1.5 to 2 cm in diameter. Unlike osteoid osteoma, which tends to be stable or regress over time, osteoblastoma tend to increase in size. Lesions involve the posterior elements and rarely arise from the vertebral bodies.[81,85]

There are three radiographic patterns of osteoblastoma.[83] The lesions may be almost identical radiographically to osteoid osteoma, but are larger than 1.5 cm. The second pattern has an aggressive appearance that may simulate a malignant lesion, consisting of osseous expansion, bone destruction, infiltration of surrounding soft tissue, and intermixed matrix calcification. The third pattern is the most common appearance of spinal osteoblastoma appearing as an expansile lesion with multiple small calcifications and a peripheral sclerotic rim. Bone scintigraphy demonstrates marked radionuclide uptake.[83]

CT is the most useful imaging modality in the diagnosis of osteoblastoma. The lesions are expansile with a thin sclerotic rim, with cortical disruption, matrix ossification, and extension into the surrounding soft tissue.[85,86] The MR imaging appearance is nonspecific with low to intermediate signal intensity on T1-weighted images and intermediate to high signal intensity on T2-weighted images.[83] The lesion may have peripheral enhancement on the postgadolinium T1-weighted images.

Aneurysmal bone cysts (ABC) are expansile, lytic bone lesions that pathologically consist of multiloculated blood filled spaces. The etiology is unclear but may be related to other primary bone lesions such as giant cell tumors, chondroblastoma, osteoblastoma, chondromyxoid fibroma, osteosarcoma, and fibrous dysplasia.[81,88,89] These lesions typically affect patients in their second decade and there is a slight female predominance.[81,90] Patients typically present with local back pain and neurologic symptoms resulting from encroachment of the spinal canal. About 3% to 20% of ABCs involve the spine and are equally distributed between cervical, thoracic and lumbar spine.[90] When the incidence per vertebral body is considered, they are more frequent in the lumbar spine.[90] ABC may rarely involve the odontoid process.[89] They affect the vertebral bodies in 40% of cases and the posterior elements in 60% of cases.[90]

Radiograph of a spinal ABC shows an osteolytic expansile lesion containing fine septations and surrounded by a thin cortical shell.[90,91] CT and MRI may demonstrate the fluid-fluid levels characteristic of ABCs.[81,91,92] MRI findings include a hypointense rim on both T1- and T2-weighted images, multiple internal septations, and cysts with fluid-fluid levels of varying signal intensities on T1- and T2-weighted images.[91,92]

Primary giant cell tumors mainly originate in the metaphyseal region of long bones in the appendicular skeleton. They are rarely seen before the closure of the epiphyseal plate and mostly occur in the epiphyseal-metaphyseal regions of long bones, especially around knee joint. A tendency toward local recurrence and late malignant change with metastases has been reported. The recurrence rates are as high as 50% if curettage or any other treatment short of complete removal is employed and the tumor usually recurs within 4 years of treatment. Malignant transformation is usually seen only after radiation therapy. Giant cell tumors are quite rare. They comprise 4% of all primary bone tumors in one series at the Mayo Clinic (195 of 3,987). Seventy-five percent were found primarily in the long bones and a 25% were in the sacrum, carpus, patella, vertebrae, and skull. Only three cases of giant cell tumor were found in the skull. Although it is infrequent, cranial giant cell tumors can involve the skull and if situated over the skull base, most commonly involve the sphenoid bone, followed by the petrous temporal bone. Giant cell tumors have a female preponderance and young adult prevalence with a peak incidence between 20 and 30 years of age. Giant cell tumors of the head and neck are uncommon, accounting for approximately 2% of all giant cell tumors. Giant cell tumors of the craniocervical juction present with lytic localized bone lesions, where cranial lesions preferably arise from the skull base rather than the vault. Giant cell tumors involving the cervical spine are rare. Involvement of the body of C2 and the odontoid process has been reported.[93–96]

In patients with skull base lesions, pain, swelling, and neurological symptomatologies are the most common initial complaints. Frontal headaches, diplopia, proptosis, and visual disturbances are frequent symptoms with sphenoid involvement. A so-called "typical presentation" of patients with giant cell tumor involving the skull base has previously been defined by Watkins et al.: a woman in her 20s or 30s having headache, ocular palsy, and visual loss with erosion of the body of sphenoid, but with normal endocrine function.[93–96]

The giant cell tumor is gray to yellow-brown, soft or firm, and friable mass at gross pathology and may contain dark red hemorrhagic areas. Small cystic areas and gray-white necrotic foci are also seen, with a variable amount of vascularity. In some cases, angiography of the external carotid artery has demonstrated supply from branches of the internal maxillary artery.[94]

On imaging, giant cell tumor usually has the nonspecific appearance of expansile, destructive soft-tissue mass. The major radiological differential diagnosis includes giant cell reparative granuloma and brown tumors of hyperparathyroidism. However, giant cell granulomas are often preceded by a history of tooth extraction or trauma, while brown tumors are usually multiple and demonstrate other radiographic and laboratory evidence of hyperparathyroidism. The plain film characteristics of giant cell tumors are indistinguishable from other radiolucent lesions of the skull.[93–96]

At CT, giant cell tumors tend to expand and attenuate the bony cortex rather than actually erode through it. CT demonstrates an expansile, lytic mass of soft-tissue attenuation with an expanded, thinned cortex often associated with a large paraspinal mass. Intravenous contrast administration demonstrates relatively homogeneous enhancement of the tumor reflecting the vascularity of the lesion. Giant cell granulomas and brown tumors also enhance. Therefore, CT alone is not sufficient for differentiation of giant cell tumors from these lesions.[88,94,95]

Giant cell tumors on MRI demonstrate heterogeneity with low-to-intermediate signal on both T1- and T2-weighted sequences. Infusion of intravenous gadolinium elicits brisk enhancement. Giant cell tumors often can have regions of hemorrhage and necrosis. These hemorrhagic areas will have very low signal on T2-weighted sequences and intermediate-to-high signal on T1-weighted images. This is related to the presence of hemosiderin in these areas from prior hemorrhage.[94,95] There may be evidence of fluid-fluid levels, focal cystic areas, and a low signal intensity pseudocapsule.[81] With a well-defined, expansile bony lesion of significant hypointensity on T2-weighting and no abundant matrix calcifications on CT, and given the location of the lesion one should consider giant cell tumor in the differential diagnosis.

Langerhans cell histiocytosis (LCH) is a disorder characterized by abnormal focal or systemic proliferation of Langerhans cells. The most common sites of involvement include the skeleton, skin, lymph nodes, lungs, liver, and central nervous system. There are three forms: 1) Letterer-Sieve, an acute form; 2) Hand-Schuller-Christian, a severe chronic form; and 3) Eosinophilic Granuloma (EG), the mildest form. EG is characterized by single or multiple skeletal lesions, and represent 70% of the total cases of Histiocytosis X.[100,102] Overall, LCH has an incidence of approximately 1 in 200,000 children per year and a male-to-female ratio of 1.8:1 with a high prevalence of the cases (80%) in Caucasians.[97]

A monostotic lesion is the most common presentation of this disease with a predilection for the vertebral bodies, ribs, long bones, and calvaria, and 75% of these cases occur before the age of 20.[97] The spine is often involved as part of the broad spectrum of bony involvement and is usually discovered during a skeletal survey in patients with known LCH.[102–104] Spine lesions may produce pain, muscle stiffness, or neurologic symptoms.[102–104] The mean age of presentation in patients with symptomatic LCH is 12 years.[97,98] LCH most often affects the lumbar, thoracic, and cervical spine in descending order of frequency.[102] However, the incidence of symptomatic LCH is highest for the cervical spine followed by the lumbar and then the thoracic spine.[102] Presentation with a unifocal cervical lesion is uncommon and solitary involvement of C2 is rare.[102,103] Most lesions involve the vertebral body.[102]

LCH is rarely seen at the skull base. This may be related to the fact that in contrast to the calvarium that originates from the mesenchymal membranous neurocranium by intramembranous ossification, the clivus, petrous bone, and the rest of the skull base develop from cartilaginous neurocranium by endochondral ossification. The rarity of the skull base lesions may also be because of underdiagnosis, since a painful calvarial swelling is likely to be detected much earlier than a skull base swelling. Brisman et al. distinguished two forms of the skull base LCH: a) the extracranial base lesions that are confined to the petrous temporal bone, do not extend into the middle cranial fossa, and that mainly present with otorrhea and postauricular swelling; and b) the intracranial base lesions that extend from the petrous temporal bone or the clivus into the middle cranial fossa and most often present with cranial nerve palsies, as seen in the present case. Only 10 previous cases of the latter variety have been reported. Of these, three occurred at the clivus, three at the petrous apex, two at the mastoids and the lateral sinus (one also involved the facial canal and the jugular foramen, while the other also involved the middle cranial fossa), one at the foramen rotundum; and finally, one with the involvement of the parasellar region, sphenoid sinus, and sella.[97–100]

Radiographically, the initial vertebral lesion is an osteolytic lesion that progresses to vertebral collapse and to the classical vertebrae plana.[102–104] However, in the cervical spine most lesions are osteolytic without evidence of collapse, probably because of early presentation.[64] Infiltration of the soft tissue adjacent to the involved vertebra may occur.[64] On MRI, the lesions are hypointense on T1-weighted images and hyperintense on T2-weighted images, which is nonspecific and is similar to other bone lesions.[66] The extent of soft-tissue infiltration by LCH is best documented by MRI and, in particular, with gadolinium-enhanced T1-weighted imaging. CT is useful in evaluating the extent of bone erosion. Once the diagnosis is suspected, a limited skeletal survey is recommended, including a chest radiograph, frontal views of the long bones and pelvis, and lateral views of the cervical and thoracolumbar spine.[97,101,105]

In the reported literature, MRI has been performed in three of the 10 cases with an intracranial skull base LCH and showed a lytic lesion in two and a marrow replacing lesion of the clivus in one. Krishna et al. report a case of a patient with LCH of the clivus with parasellar and petrous extension. The MR images revealed a heterogeneous mixed intensity lesion with relatively higher signal intensity on T2-weighted images. The enhancement of the lesion on gadolinium administration contrasted with the absent signal of the cortical bone, the low signal of the surrounding cerebrospinal fluid cisterns and the moderate intensity of the underlying brain on contrast-enhanced T1-weighted MR images. Clivus invasion was revealed by the enhancing mass within and outside its cortical margins. The presence of the enhancing mass within the clival cortical margins may perhaps represent marrow replacement by LCH. In this region, the other radiological differential diagnoses that must be considered include chordoma, chondrosarcoma, meningioma, fibrous dysplasia, tubercular or fungal osteomyelitis, metastatic disease from neuroblastoma or from leukemic deposits, primary Ewing's sarcoma, plasmacytoma, hemangioblastoma, giant cell tumor of the sphenoid, local extension from nasopharyngeal carcinoma and pituitary tumors or less likely a cavernous haemangioma, epidermoid cyst or chondroma. An extensive clinoid and/or alar meningiomas would be less likely in a young child, but should be considered in an adult.[97–101]

Synovial cysts or ganglion cysts are benign cystic lesions that are found in close proximity to a tendon sheath or joint space. Synovial cyst and ganglion cyst are often used interchangeably when referring to a cystic lesion adjacent to the facet joints. However, they differ in that the former is lined with synovial cells containing clear fluid while the latter is lined with fibrous connective tissue and contains gelatinous and highly viscous fluid.[106–108] Both are uncommon and are usually found in the lumbar spine but may occur at the CCJ.[106–108] Ganglion cysts may arise intraosseously in the odontoid process.

Plain radiographs and CT reveals a well-defined low-density lesion.[108] Synovial cysts usually present as a well-circumscribed homogenous mass posterior to the odontoid process. The mass has intermediate signal intensity on T1-weighted images and low signal intensity on T2-weighted images[107,108] (**Fig. 10-32**). This appearance may mimic a meningioma. However, a synovial cyst only shows a thin rim of enhancement while a meningioma homogeneously enhances on gadolinium-enhanced T1 images.[106,107,109]

Hemangiopericytoma is an uncommon tumor that arises from Zimmerman's pericytes and may occur where there are capillaries. It may affect, in decreasing order, the lower extremity, pelvis, retroperitoneum, head and neck region, trunk, and upper extremity.[110] Primary hemangiopericytoma of the vertebra is rare. It mostly affects the lumbosacral spine. Involvement of

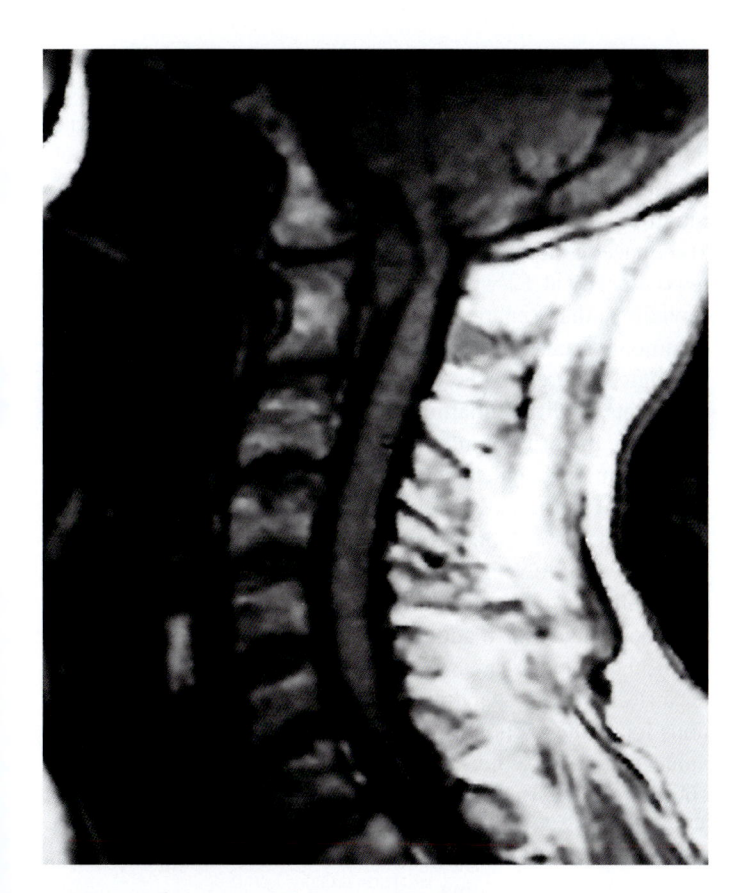

Figure 10-32 Synovial Cyst at the CCJ
Synovial cyst at the craniocervical junction in a 61-year-old female complaining of neck pain. Sagittal T1W MR scan shows a homogeneous lesion of intermediate signal intensity anterior to the cord and posterior to the vertebrae. The adjacent joint is destroyed and there is overgrowth of the bony margins.

the odontoid is extremely rare.[110] On radiograph, the lesion is osteolytic. MR imaging reveals a hypointense lesion with moderate enhancement on T1-weighted images.[111]

A rare lesion that may affect the odontoid process is infantile myofibromatosis.[112] It is a benign proliferation of fibrous tissue. There are solitary and multicentric forms. The solitary form is more common in males (69%) and affects the soft tissues of the head and neck region, and the trunk. The multicentric form is more common in females (63%) and involves the soft tissue, bone, and viscera.[113] Lesions in the odontoid are osteolytic. The lesions are inhomogeneous and hypointense on both T1- and T2-weighted MR images.

Malignant Neoplasms

Extradural neoplasms may account for more than 50% of spinal tumors depending on the series and patient population studied.[115] The great majority of these will be metastatic disease to bone. Primary malignant tumors of the spine such as chordoma, chondrosarcoma, osteosarcoma, and Ewing's sarcoma are much less common. Lesions that originate intracranially can also straddle the craniocervical junction as they extend extracranially.

Intracranial chordoma is a locally aggressive and relatively rare tumor of the skull base that is thought to originate from embryonic remnants of the primitive notochord. Both CT and MRI are usually required for evaluation of intracranial chordomas due to bone involvement and the proximity of these tumors to many critical soft-tissue structures.[116] Chordomas are considered locally invasive, but are thought to infrequently metastasize. However, certain case series have shown that 10% to 43% of patients have distant metastasis.[116,121,122] They arise from embryonic remnants of the primitive notochord, a primitive cell line around which the skull base and the vertebral column develop. Remnants of the notochord usually remain in or close to the midline, entrapped within bone. Chordomas account for 1% of intracranial tumors and 4% of all primary bone tumors. They may occur at any age but are usually seen in adults, with peak prevalence in the fourth to fifth decades of life. Chordomas have a 2:1 male predilection and affect whites more than blacks.[116] About 50% of chordomas arise from the sacrum, 35% from the clivus, and 15% from the spine.[116,121,122] The cervical spine, particularly C2, and the lumbar spine are the most common sites of spinal involvement.[49,75-77] Intracranial chordomas most often originate from the spheno-occipital synchondrosis of the clivus. The site of origin may be along the upper clivus (basisphenoid) or along the caudal margin of the clivus (basiocciput). Occasionally, intracranial chordomas may arise unilaterally from the petrous apex, a finding that was seen in up to 15% of cases in one series.[116]

Generally, chordomas grow slowly and produce symptoms insidiously. Symptoms of intracranial chordomas vary with lesion location and proximity to critical structures, reflecting the specific sites of extension from the clivus (i.e., the sellar, parasellar, and retroclival areas and, occasionally, the sphenoid sinus). The most common initial complaint is diplopia related to cranial nerve palsy and headache. Among cranial nerves, the abducent nerve is the most commonly affected. Headache is usually reported in an occipital or retro-orbital location. Although intracranial chordomas are generally slow growing, their intimate relation to critical structures and extremely high local recurrence rate have often resulted in high mortality rates in the past. However, recent advances in skull base surgery and radiation therapy now provide greater opportunity for cure. The excellent imaging capabilities of MRI and CT allow precise delineation of the tumors with respect to volume and relation to adjacent neural structures, thereby helping to increase cure rates.[116-119]

Before addressing the radiological characteristics of chordomas, a brief note should be made regarding the gross and histopathological features of chordomas. At gross examination, chordomas appear as gelatinous, multilobulated, semitranslucent grayish tumors with the majority of lesions 2 to 5 cm in size. Chordomas have been divided into two histopathologic subtypes: typical chordomas and chondroid chordomas. In typical chordomas, the cells tend to be arranged in cords set in a pale matrix of mucopolysaccharide with a characteristic physaliphorous appearance. In addition, typical chordomas contain areas of necrosis, recent and old hemorrhage, and entrapped bone trabeculae. In chondroid chordomas, the stroma resembles hyaline cartilage with neoplastic cells in lacunae. This variant is more commonly seen in the skull base, constituting up to one-third of cases in that region, and usually has a better prognosis. Chondroid chordomas may resemble low-grade chondrosarcomas.[116]

Both CT and MRI are used in the diagnosis, and the delineation of the extent, of chordomas. High-resolution CT with a bone and soft-tissue algorithm has proved to be sensitive for detecting lesions of the skull base. Thin-section axial and coronal unenhanced and contrast material-enhanced images are usually obtained for assessment. CT is very accurate in the depiction of bone abnormalities; however, due to beam-hardening artifacts, it is somewhat limited in its capacity to show soft-tissue structures in the posterior fossa. The classic appearance of intracranial chordoma at CT is that of a centrally located, well-circumscribed, expansile soft-tissue mass that arises from the clivus with associated extensive lytic bone destruction. The bulk of the tumor is usually hyperdense relative to the adjacent neural structures. Intratumoral calcifications usually appear irregular at CT and are thought to represent sequestra from bone destruction rather than dystrophic calcifications within the tumor itself. The chondroid variant is more likely to demonstrate true intratumoral dystrophic calcifications. There is moderate to marked enhancement following administration of iodinated intravenous contrast material. Solitary or multiple low-attenuation areas are sometimes seen within the soft-tissue mass and probably represent the myxoid and gelatinous material seen at gross examination.[116,117,119,120]

While CT is excellent at examining the extent of bony involvement and destruction, MR is far superior at determining extent of the tumor and the extent of soft tissue spread. MR imaging is deficient relative to CT only in the evaluation of calcification and cortical bone.[116,120] Because cortical bone has few mobile protons, it manifests as an area of low signal intensity with all sequences. Osseous destruction is implied by replacement of the signal void of cortical bone with the soft-tissue signal intensity of tumor. However, even so the definition of fine cortical structures such as the carotid canal wall is limited. In addition, soft tissues adjacent to a thin bone can demonstrate enough signal intensity that a signal void is not present, resulting in a false positive picture of cortical involvement. Use of contrast-enhanced imaging can solve this problem if the tissue on the opposite side of the bone (e.g., dura mater) shows abnormal enhancement, which confirms bone involvement even though the cortex is not actually visualized.[116,120,122,123]

Sagittal MR images are generally the most valuable in defining the posterior margin of the tumor, showing the relation between the tumor and brainstem, and depicting nasopharyngeal extension of the tumor. Sagittal imaging is also useful in disclosing transdural transgression by a tumor, an important factor in surgical planning. Coronal MR images, on the other hand, are helpful in detecting tumor extension into the cavernous sinus and depicting the position of the optic chiasm and tract.[116,117,120,122,123]

On conventional spin-echo T1-weighted MR images, intracranial chordoma has intermediate to low signal intensity and is easily recognized within the high signal intensity of the fat of the clivus. Small foci of T1 hyperintensity can sometimes be visualized in the tumor, a finding that represents intratumoral hemorrhage or a mucus pool. The presence of hemorrhagic foci can be confirmed with gradient-echo imaging at which the foci appear as dark areas. Classic intracranial chordoma has high signal intensity on T2-weighted images, a finding that likely reflects the high fluid content of vacuolated cellular components. The intratumoral areas of calcification, hemorrhage, and a highly proteinaceous mucus pool usually demonstrate heterogeneous hypointensity at T2-weighted imaging. Low T2-signal-intensity septations that separate high T2-signal-intensity lobules are commonly seen, corresponding to the multilobulated gross morphologic features of the tumor. Also, T2-weighted imaging is excellent for differentiating tumor from adjacent neural structures. The majority of intracranial chordomas demonstrate moderate to marked enhancement following intravenous contrast injection. Occasionally, the enhancement pattern of the tumor sometimes has a "honeycomb" appearance created by intratumoral areas of low signal intensity. Fat suppression is useful for differentiating enhanced tumor margins from adjacent bright fatty bone marrow. In addition, small intraclival chordomas are often better demarcated with this technique. Sze reported that because a watery, gelatinous matrix is replaced by cartilaginous foci/matrix, chondroid chordomas have shorter T1 and T2 values than do typical chordomas. Consequently, chondroid chordomas may not be as bright as typical chordomas on T2-weighted MR images. This finding is an important prognostic factor due to the significantly better survival rate of patients with chondroid chordoma.[116,117,120,122,123]

Chondrosarcoma is the third most common primary malignant tumor of bone, exceeded in frequency only by multiple myeloma and osteosarcoma. Chondrosarcoma accounts for 3.5% of all primary bone tumors that lead to biopsy and 20% to 27% of primary malignant osseous neoplasms.[124] Craniofacial chondrosarcomas account for 2% of all chondrosarcomas and have a predilection for the skull base (probably related to the fact that this portion of the calvarium is preformed in cartilage). As described previously, the bones of the skull base mature predominantly by endochondral ossification, whereas the bones of the skull vault develop primarily by intramembranous ossification. The areas of the petro-occipital, spheno-occipital, and spheno-petrosal synchondrosis, as well as a large part of the petrous portion of the temporal bone, are sites in the mature skull that embryologically underwent endochondral development. It is hypothesized that islands of residual endochondral cartilage may be present in these areas and that chondrosarcoma develops from these chondrocytes. As an alternative, some authors have suggested that chondrosarcoma may arise from pluripotent mesenchymal cells involved in the embryogenesis of the skull base and temporal bone.[124,125]

Although only 6% of skull base tumors are chondrosarcomas, benign chondroid tumors of the skull base are rare. Therefore, solitary intramedullary cartilaginous tumors at this site, similar to lesions in the pelvis, ribs, sternum, and spine, should always be regarded as malignant.[124–126] Facial lesions most commonly involve the maxilla and may affect younger patients. The differential diagnosis for CSA of the temporal bone and skull base includes chordoma, chondroid chordoma, chondroma osteogenic sarcoma, meningioma, enchondroma, and glomus jugulare.[124,125] Skull base chondrosarcomas involving the clivus may be confused with chordomas. Chordoma is a more common tumor in the skull base than chondrosarcoma. Differentiation between these two skull base neoplasms is very important because chondrosarcoma has a much better prognosis. The major clinical distinctions between chordomas and chondrosarcomas of the skull base are patient age and rate of growth. Chordomas tend to occur, on average, in patients a decade older than chondrosarcomas and grow much more rapidly. Unfortunately, these distinctions are not true for mesenchymal chondrosarcomas involving the craniofacial region that also grow rapidly. Skull base chondrosarcomas have also been confused with meningiomas and metastases, the latter usually having a much worse prognosis than chondrosarcomas. Skull base chondrosarcomas are often very large at presentation, compressing the brainstem and invading adjacent areas such as the cavernous sinus, and are usually low-grade lesions histologically. In a series of 17 cases, the age range of patients with skull base chondrosarcomas was 14 to 65 years, with a mean age of 36 years. The majority of patients (59%) were between 30 and 44 years of age, and the male-to-female ratio was 2.4:1. The majority of these tumors (71%) were located in the petrous apex. The second most frequent site was the clivus (12% of cases). The maxilla, orbit, and foramen magnum were each the site of the tumor in one patient (6%).[124,126]

Plain radiographs reveal bone destruction with extension into the soft tissue. Chondroid matrix calcification may be seen within the soft tissue component. CT is most useful in demonstrating bone destruction and tumor calcification. The typical appearance of chondrosarcoma on CT scan is a destructive lesion with patchy infiltration. A rim of calcification can be seen in many cases, although calcification within the tumor matrix is often absent. Nonmineralized areas show high water content on CT and MR images. As is true for chondrosarcomas in other regions, MR imaging is optimal for depicting areas of tumor involvement but not subtle matrix mineralization. MR imaging is nonspecific revealing low to intermediate signal intensity on T1-weighted images and very high signal intensity on T2-weighted images.[124,128] The tumor is usually heterogeneous due to areas of calcification. Both CT and MR imaging performed after administration of contrast material show mild peripheral and septal enhancement typical of chondroid lesions, which have been described as variegated or having a "salt-and-pepper" appearance. This appearance corresponds to a lack of perfusion at MR angiography, a feature that helps distinguish these lesions from other more vascular skull base tumors, such as metastases and meningiomas. Similarly, skull base chondrosarcomas appear relatively avascular at digital subtraction angiography.[124,125]

Osteosarcoma is the second most common malignant primary tumor arising from bone, after myeloma. Its greatest predilection is for the metaphyses of long bones, most often the distal femur or proximal tibia. Osteosarcoma of the extragnathic (outside the jaws) craniofacial bones is exceedingly rare. Most arise de novo. Secondary osteosarcoma occurs in the setting of prior radiation therapy or of benign bone disorders, such as Paget disease, fibrous dysplasia, multiple osteochondromatosis, osteomyelitis, myositis ossificans, and trauma. Craniofacial osteosarcoma constitutes a minority of all osteosarcomas, accounting for 8.6% of the Mayo Clinic's series of 1,274 osteosarcomas. The majority of osteosarcomas about the head and neck, between 88% and 75%, arise in the mandible and maxilla.[129]

Osteosarcoma of the spine is rare, accounting for only 0.85% to 3% of all primary osteosarcoma.[130,131] Primary osteosarcoma of the spine tends to occur in older patients than those with osteosarcoma of the extremity.[130] Spinal osteosarcoma may be induced by exposure to radiation or Paget disease.[130,131] Most cases involve the vertebral body. There is equal distribution between the thoracic and lumbar spine, with rare involvement of the cervical spine.[131,132] Involvement of the CCJ has been reported.[130] Most lesions are predominantly blastic with lytic areas, but purely lytic lesions may occur. Loss of vertebral body height and soft tissue involvement is frequently seen.[130-132]

CT is useful in demonstrating the calcifications within the lesion and cortical destruction.[133] T1-weighted MR images are superior to demonstrate replacement of the normally hyperintense bone marrow by the more hypointense tumor involvement. T2-weighted MR images are useful in evaluating the extension into adjacent soft tissues, because tumor is hyperintense to muscle.[133] MR imaging is also sensitive in detecting epidural extension and cord compression.

Ewing's sarcoma is a poorly differentiated, highly aggressive neoplasm found primarily in the long bones, occurring in the first three decades of life. The spine is frequently involved in metastatic Ewing's sarcoma; primary involvement of the spine is much less frequent, occurring in 3.5% to 8.5% of cases.[84] Patients usually present with local pain, neurological deficit, or a palpable mass. Most lesions are in the sacrum followed in frequency by the lumbar, thoracic and then cervical spine.[84-86] In the cervical spine, the axis is the most commonly involved vertebra.[87-89]

Radiographically, spinal Ewing's tumors are mostly lytic lesions, with sclerotic or mixed lesions being much less common.[84,85,87] The vertebral body is typically involved, but there is a tendency to extend into the odontoid process, posterior elements, paravertebral soft tissues, and extradurally around the spinal cord. Calcification within the tumor is rare. The MRI findings are similar to other malignant tumors, but are valuable to visualize tumor spread to the bone marrow, paraspinal soft tissues, epidural space, and cord compression.[83,90]

In addition to primary malignant tumors of the osseous structure, blood-borne metastasis is the most common neoplasm of the spine. Metastasis is seen in all age groups, depending on the origin of the neoplasm. The location of metastatic disease to the vertebra is dependent on the distribution of red marrow. The vertebral bodies, particularly the pedicles, are therefore more often involved than the posterior elements. Metastatic disease most commonly involves the thoracic spine (66%), followed by the lumbar spine (20%), and then the cervical spine.[115] The most common metastatic disease to the odontoid process is from breast and lung cancer.[142] Other metastatic diseases that can involve the odontoid process include lymphoma,[143] multiple myeloma, nasopharyngeal carcinoma, colon carcinoma, rhabdomyosarcoma, renal cell carcinoma, and esophageal adenocarcinoma.[144] Metastases to the skull base also occur. Those patients affected by breast cancer, prostate cancer, lymphoma, and lung cancer (in descending order of frequency) are particularly prone to metastasis in this region.[141] Clinical manifestations depend upon the metastatic site. In a retrospective study of 43 patients treated for base-of-skull metastasis, Greenberg et al. identified five clinical syndromes of different frequencies: the orbital (7%), parasellar (16%), middle-fossa (35%), jugular foramen (16%), and occipital condyle syndromes (21%).[142] Others have found a predominance of the parasellar and sellar syndromes (29%), whereas middle-fossa and jugular foramen syndrome were less common (6% and 3.5%, respectively).[141]

Plain radiographs will show an osteolytic lesion or destruction of the vertebral body and possible loss of height. Radionuclide bone scans are the most sensitive imaging procedure to detect metastatic disease, but lack specificity and are limited in detecting myeloma. CT is more specific in demonstrating osteolytic lesions as well as cortical destruction and extraspinous extension. MR imaging, however, is the modality of choice in evaluating metastatic disease to the spine, as both the soft tissue extent is evident along with neurovascular compression.[144,146]

MRI is extremely sensitive in detecting replacement of the marrow within the vertebrae by tumor.[146] Because of the high fat content, normal bone marrow is usually high signal intensity on T1-weighted images and intermediate signal intensity on T2-weighted images. Any process, including metastatic disease that replaces the fat results in a decrease in signal on the T1-weighted images and an increase in signal on the T2-weighted images. The lesions tend to become isointense to surrounding bone marrow on T1-weighted images after gadolinium-enhancement.[147] Because of this, contrast-enhanced images need to be combined with precontrast images to improve the detection and characterization of the lesions. Gadolinium-enhanced T1-weighted images are useful in evaluating epidural extension of tumor where the lesion becomes hyperintense to CSF signal and to distinguish the lesion from disc herniation.[115]

VASCULAR LESIONS

The vascular supply to the lower brainstem and upper cervical cord has a common origin from the vertebrobasilar system. Therefore, an arteriovenous malformation (AVM) at the CCJ may straddle the foramen magnum, despite supply from only one vascular pedicle. MRI without and with gadolinium infusion can identify these lesions, provided there is flow through the AVM and/or breakdown of the blood-brain barrier.

AVMs can be either intra or extra medullary. Intramedullary AVMs typically take their origin from the anterior blood supply and often occur in young patients which present with acute hemorrhage. Extramedullary AVMs which are typically dural fistulas usually take their origin from the posterior blood supply, occur in elderly men, and present with progressive neurological deficits. These deficits are thought to be caused by congestive hypoxia of the cord secondary to raised perimedullary venous pressure.

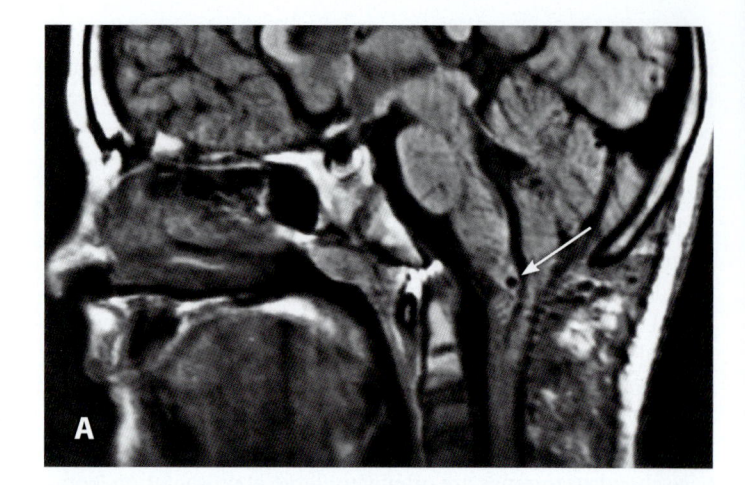

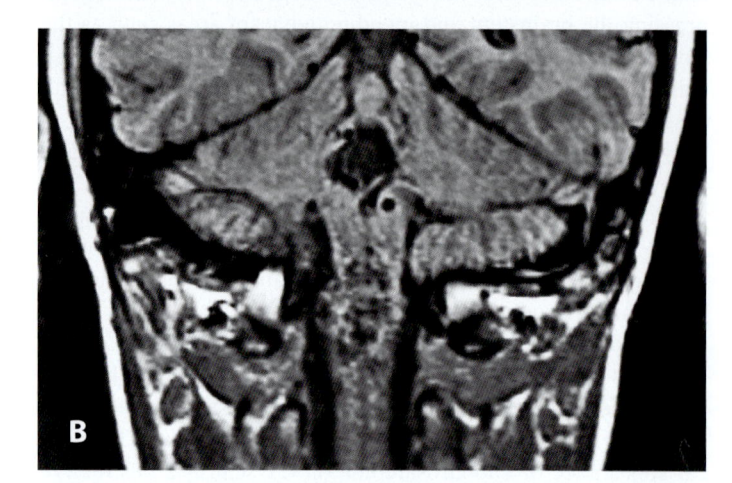

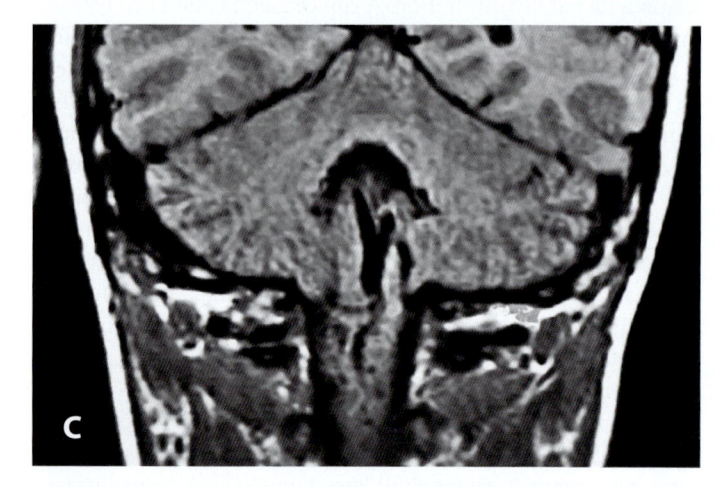

Figure 10-33 Cervicomedullary Arteriovenous Malformation
Cervicomedullary arteriovenous malformation in a 5-year-old boy discovered after an intracranial bleed. Sagittal T1W MR scan (**A**) shows an irregular heterogeneous area within the medulla at the craniocervical junction with a prominent vessel demonstrated by a flow void (*arrow*). Coronal T1W MR scans. (**B**) shows the lesion with cord expansion at the level of foramen magnum and (**C**) shows several prominent serpentine vessels demonstrated by the significant flow voids in a central location suggesting an intramedullary process.

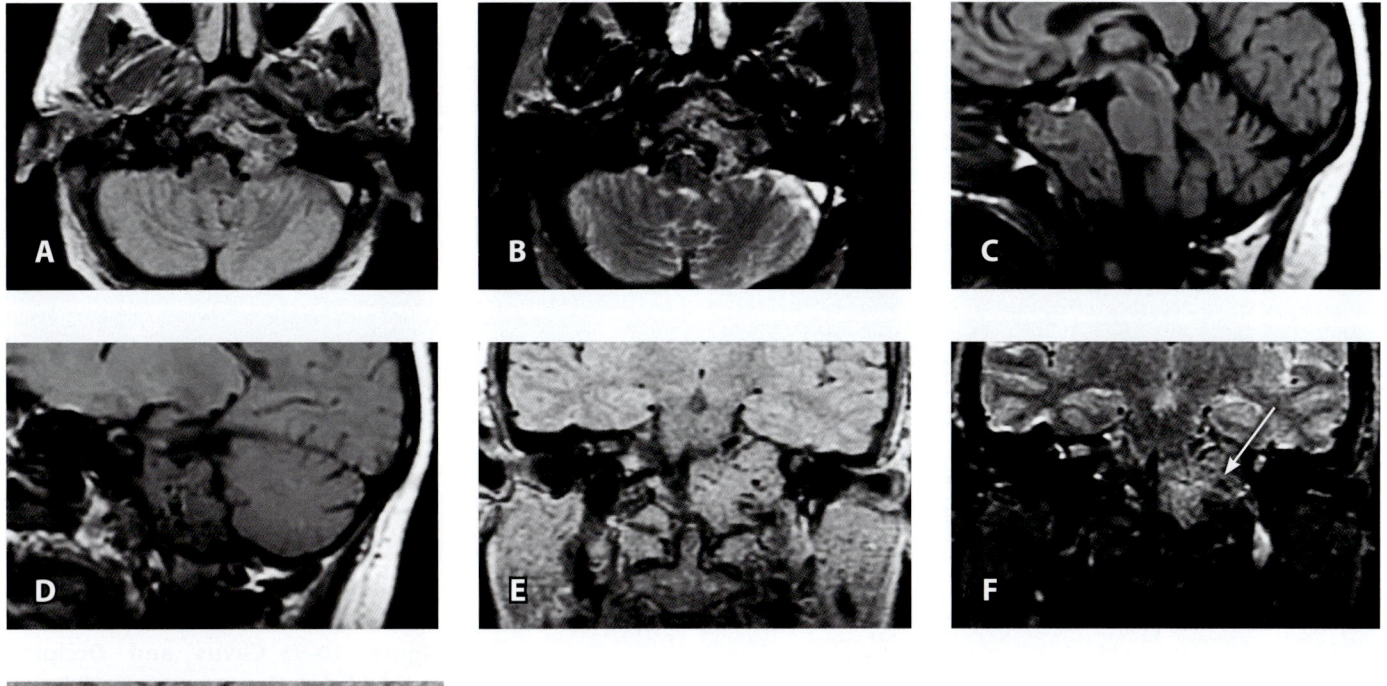

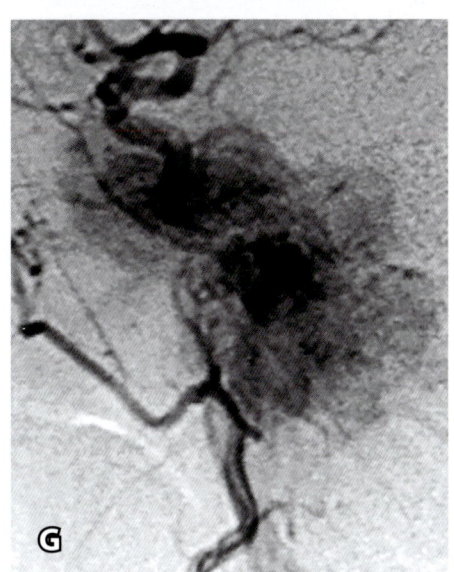

Figure 10-34 Paraganglioma at the CCJ
Paraganglioma extending across the craniocervical junction in a 70-year-old female. Axial proton density (**A**) and T2W (**B**) MR scans show the mass left anterolateral to the cavernous sinus with an irregular margins. Sagittal T1W MR scans show (**C**) the mass extending posteroinferiorly from the sphenoid sinus around the borders of the clivus into the craniocervical junction. There are areas of low signal representing flow voids (**D**) in the otherwise isointense mass. Coronal proton density (**E**) and T2W (**F**) MR scans demonstrate the mass transcranially extending through the posterior fossa to the level of C1. There are mini flow voids (*arrow*) present throughout the mass demonstrating the vascular nature of this mass. Left lateral common carotid angiogram (**G**) shows an extensive multilobular vascular blush emanating from the internal carotid artery and extending from middle skull base to the CCJ. The intense blush is characteristic of a paraganglioma that has spread upward from the region of the temporal bone and downward through the foramen magnum.

An excavated medulla or spinal cord with large perimedullary vessels is characteristic of an intramedullary AVM on MR imaging. MR imaging of extramedullary AVMs will demonstrate serpentine low intensity vessels around the cord on T1-W images and cord scalloping suggestive of dilated perimedullary vessels. Pusatile artifact will be seen on T2-W images. The spinal cord may show changes consistent with both reversible and irreversible damage such as myelomalacia and edema[96–98] (**Fig. 10-33**).

Although typically a lesion of the lumbar region, a dural arteriovenous fistula (DAVF) can also occur in the craniocervical junction region and may present with subarachnoid hemorrhage. Differentiation of a DAVF from an intramedullary AVM is by the arteriovenous connection, which lies outside the cord substance within the dura.[96–98] Thrombosed AVMs may be recognized, although they may be difficult to differentiate from a vascular neoplasm. As is the case with neoplasms, AVMs may be extra- or intraaxial. Multiplanar imaging may be required to make this differentiation. Gradient echo images greatly facilitate the recognition of blood or blood products.

Several other types of vascular lesions may also occur at the craniocervical junction including aneuysms, vertebrobasilar dolichoectasia, and vascular tumors (**Fig. 10-34**). Vertebrobasilar dolichoectasia is a dilatation and elongation of the vertebrobasilar artery. Patients present with symptoms of cervicomedullary compression. Magnetic resonance angiography (MRA) is the method of choice to evaluate this lesion, but digital subtraction angiography should be performed to reduce the risk of occluding small pontine vessel branches with stagnant contrast.

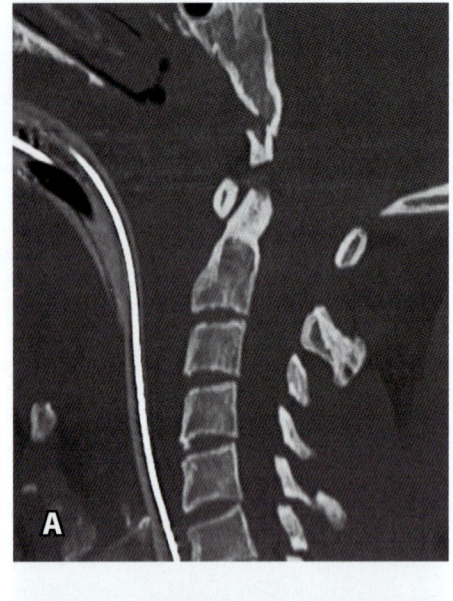

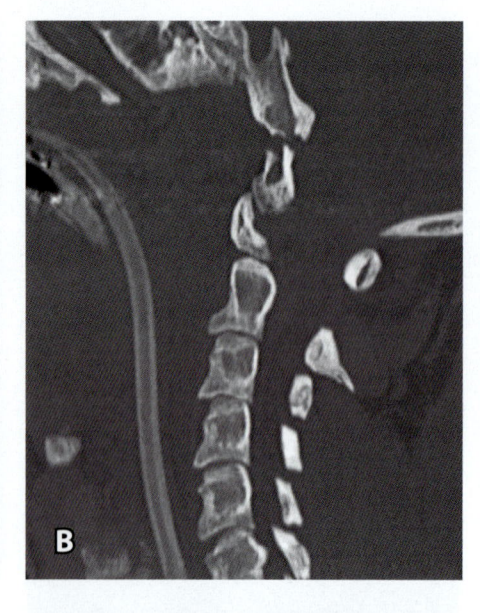

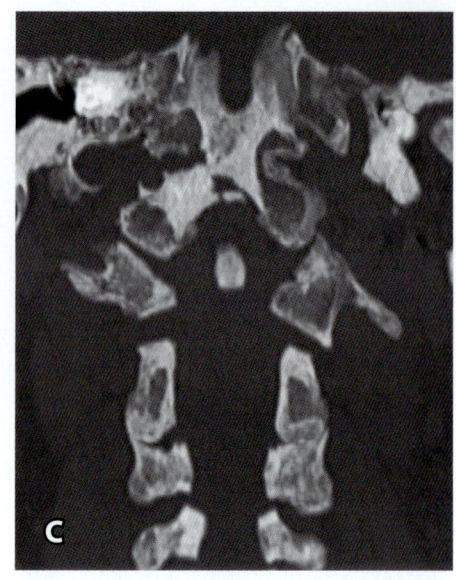

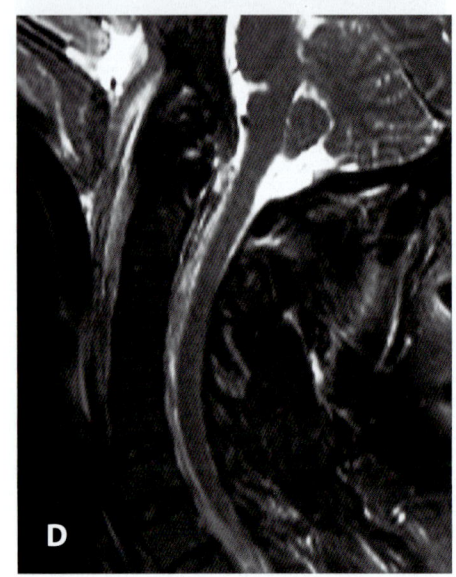

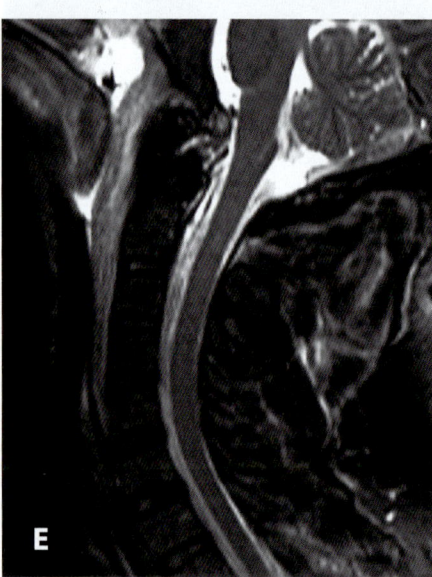

Figure 10-35 Clivus and Occipital Condyl Fractures
Young adult male victim of severe trauma. Sagittal reformatted CT scans (**A, B**) show wide separation between the fracture of the distal portion of the clivus and the C1. There is also a fracture of the right occiptal condyl that has separated from the skull base. (**C**) Coronal reformatted CT scan clearly shows the fracture fragment involving the distal clivus and right occipital condyl. Sagittal T2W MR scans (**D, E**) show hemorrhagic products positioned vertically behind the sites of injury in the spinal canal. There is also disruption of the ligaments at the CCJ.

TRAUMATIC LESIONS

A variety of spinal cord injuries can be seen about the CCJ. With the use of MRI, all serious traumatic injuries including swelling, hemorrhage, compression, or transection of the cord can be detected. In addition, the diagnosis of traumatic intervertebral disc herniation, fracture-dislocation, ligamentous rupture, or extra-axial hemorrhage is significantly improved with MRI. The ability to directly visualize ligamentous disruptions is vital and greatly improves the evaluation of cervical spine instability. This information aids in determining the preferred surgical approach (anterior to posterior) needed to stabilize an injury. A combination of spin-echo and gradient-echo images are essential sequences in the examination of patients with acute or subacute injuries to the CCJ.

The true incidence of occipital condyle fractures is unknown, but was noted to be as high as 19% in a small series of patients with high-energy trauma to the CCJ.[99] Clinically, the patients may complain of neck pain and limited range of motion, torticollis, or lower cranial nerve palsies. There may be compromise of the vertebrobasilar circulation. With associated ligamentous injury, atlanto-occipital dissociation may occur and can result in death.[100,101] Occipital condyle fractures can be placed into three types: 1) comminuted and nondisplaced, 2) linear and extending from a basilar skull fracture, and 3) avulsion with displacement and fractures at the insertion of the alar ligaments. Type 1 fractures result from axial compression injury and are associated with ipsilateral alar ligament injury. Type 2 fractures result from a direct blow injury and are not associated with ligamentous injury. Rotation injuries cause type 3 fractures, which are associated with both tectorial membrane and bilateral alar ligament injury, and are potentially unstable.

CT imaging is the method of choice to identify fractures of the occipital condyle and treatment is dependent upon

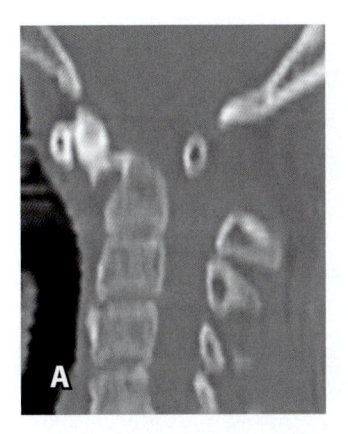

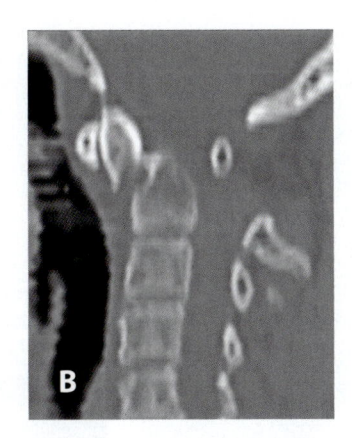

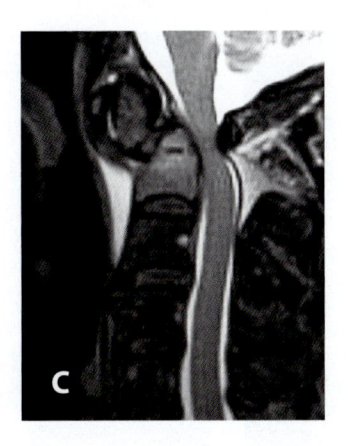

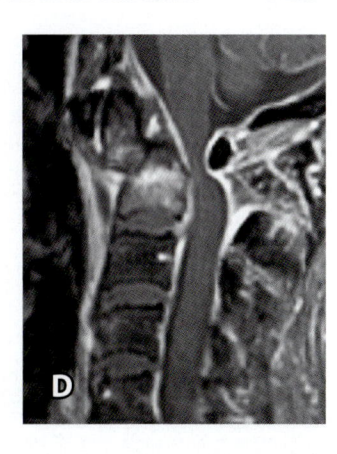

Figure 10-36 Odontoid Pathologic Fracture and Dislocation
Elderly female with known breast cancer who sustained a MVA. (**A–B**) Sagittal reformatted CT scans show that the odontoid is completely fractured and displaced anteriorly in front of the body of C2. C1 is also displaced anteriorly with marked narrowing of the spinal canal. (**C**) Sagittal T2W MR scan clearly shows the fracture dislocation and cord compression. There is no abnormal signal within the spinal cord. (**D**) Sagittal T1W postcontrast fat-saturated image shows enhancement of the margins of the fractured odontoid consistent with preexisting metastatic breast cancer, which was later confirmed during surgery.

neurological involvement ranging from placement of a hard cervical collar to surgical stabilization.[100–103] MR imaging is necessary to identify any associated ligamentous injury. A ligament tear will appear of high intensity on T2W images in general, but using MRI appearances to detect the integrity of the tectorial membrane and alar ligaments have not been thoroughly tested and can only be assessed indirectly at this time[102,104] (**Figs. 10-35** and **10-36**).

In cases of chronic injuries, the status of spine instability is no longer an issue. Instead, it is essential to be able to differentiate an area of myelomalacia from a cystic cavity. Myelomalacia will be seen as localized regions of CSF-like signal intensity with cord atrophy due to the presence of devitalized tissues. Cavitation will be seen as an area of CSF-like signal intensity extending along several segments associated with an expanded cervical cord. Surgical drainage of these syrinx cavities may be necessary in order to prevent progressive neurological deficits.[105]

DEGENERATIVE LESIONS

Fibrous Pseudotumor

Chronic atlantoaxial subluxation may be associated with masses posterior to the odontoid process composed of fibrous granulation tissue. These masses are referred to as fibrous pseudotumors, as the process may cause cord compression.[148] These "masses" are hypointense on both T1- and T2-weighted magnetic resonance (MR) images.[148] Chronic subluxation, ligamentous degeneration, chronic hemodialysis, or disc herniation can cause fibrous pseudotumors. Elderly patients with degenerative disease of the cervical spine may develop fibrous pseudotumors posterior to the odontoid process.[149] Histologically, these masses consist of degenerate ligament and fibrocartilage.[149] It is speculated that these masses may be due to degeneration and partial tear of the transverse ligament with subsequent mass formation.

Plain radiographs show degenerative changes with osteophytes at C1/C2, with no evidence of subluxation.[149] Computed tomographic (CT) findings consist of a smooth occasionally lobulated mass behind the odontoid process, which may contain small calcifications. There may be well-corticated erosions of the atlas at the sites of attachment of the transverse ligament and erosion of the posterior surface of the odontoid.[149] These masses are low to intermediate signal intensity on T1-weighted MR images and heterogeneous, with areas of low and areas of high signal intensity on T2-weighted MR images.[149] They may cause cord compression and mimic a meningioma (**Figs. 10-37** and **10-38**).

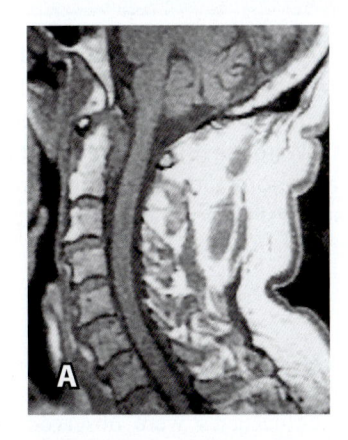

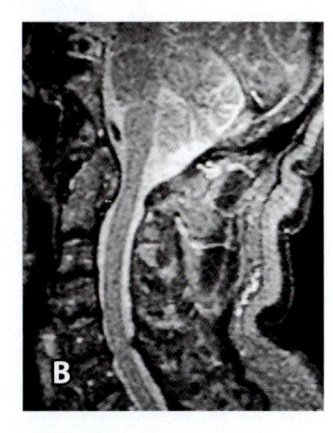

Figure 10-37 Fibrous Pseudotumor of the CCJ
Elderly patient with no specific symptoms relating to the CCJ. Sagittal T1W (**A**) and T2W (**B**) MR scans show a low signal lesion compressing the ventral cord representing fibrocartilage formation which was confirmed at surgery. This pathology arises from chronic C1 to C2 subluxation secondary to ligamentous laxity.

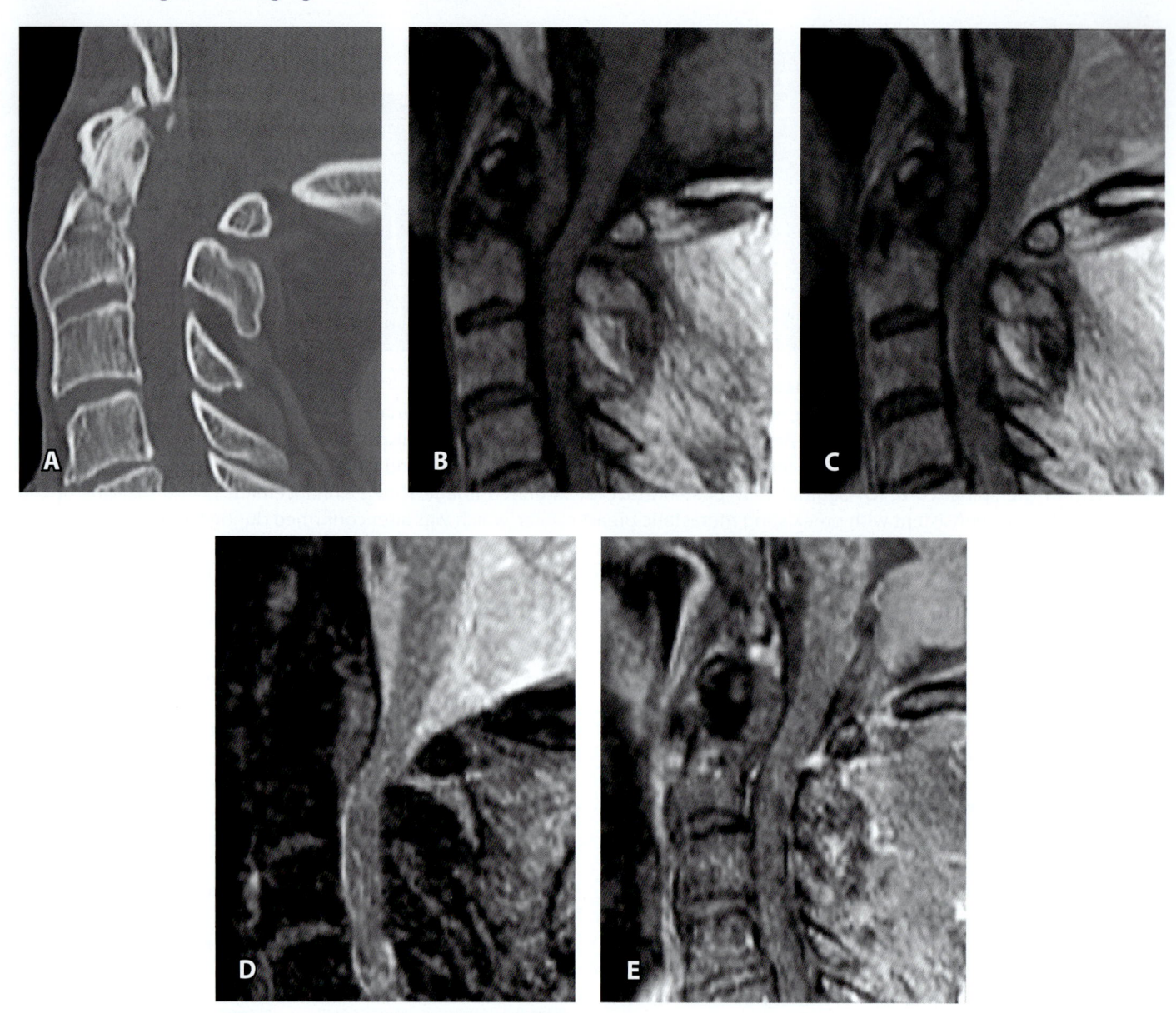

Figure 10-38 Chronic Fibrous Pseudotumor of the CCJ with Acute C1 to C2 Fracture
Elderly patient with history of recent trauma sustained in a fall. (**A**) Sagittal reformatted CT scan shows a fracture at the base of the odontoid extending into the body of C2 without significant displacement. Sagittal MR scans (**B–E**) show a soft-tissue mass dorsal to the fracture at C1 to C2. T1W image (**B**) shows the soft tissue indenting the CCJ with slight narrowing of the spinal canal. PDW image (**C**) shows focal signal abnormality in the cord representing injury, secondary to the cord compression. GRE image (**D**) shows no blood products to suggest hemorrhage. Postcontrast T1W image (**E**) shows isointense mass without enhancement, consistent with fibrous pseudotumor.

Abnormal periodontoid soft-tissue masses have been found in 28% of patients receiving long-term hemodialysis.[51,150] In 20% of these patients, cystic radiolucencies were observed in the atlas and axis.[150] These lesions are hypointense on both T1- and T2-weighted images.[150] These findings are found only in patients who have evidence of amyloid arthropathy and it is postulated that these masses are due to hemodialysis related amyloidosis.[149] In one patient switching from hemodialysis to peritoneal dialysis and administration of steroids dramatically reduced the fibrous pseudotumor in size.[151] Massive amyloid deposition in the odontoid due to plasma cell dyscrasia has also been described.[152]

Herniated intervertebral disc material may lodge posterior to the odontoid and present as a fibrous pseudotumor.[153] MR imaging demonstrates the lesion as intermediate signal intensity on T1-weighted images with peripheral enhancement.

Parenchymal atrophy due to a variety of congenital or acquired degenerative processes may be evident at the CCJ. The tissue loss may be diffused or selectively involve only one structure. T1-weighted images can show morphological alterations. T2-weighted images are used to show alterations in signal intensities. Instability during movements of the cervical spine may be demonstrated by dynamic maneuvers such as flexion and extension views.

Basilar impression is the acquired form of basilar invagination. There are many causes which all lead to bony softening of the skull base. The result is an abnormally high positioned vertebral column in relation to the skull base. This abnormal positioning can cause both cord or brainstem compression and obstructive hydrocephalus. Craniometric measurements are useful to assess basilar impression as they are in basilar invagination.[154]

REFERENCES

1. Schweitzer ME, Hodler J, Cervilla V, et al.: Craniovertebral Junction: normal anatomy with MR correlation. Am J Roentgenol 1992;158:1087.
2. Mamourian AC, Dickman CA, Wallace R, et al.: Magnetic resonance appearance of the transverse ligament: an in vitro and in vivo anatomical and imaging study. BNI Quarterly 1994;10(1):27.
3. Pfirrmann CWA, Binkert CA, Zanetti M, Boos N, and Hodler J: MR morphology of alar ligaments and occipito-atlantoaxial joints: study in 50 asymptomatic subjects. Radiology 2001;218:133–137.
4. Hasso AN: MRI atlas of the head and neck. 1st ed. London: Martin Dunitz; 1993:34.
5. Smoker WRK: MR imaging of the craniovertebral junction. Magn Reson Imaging Clin N Am 2000;8(3):635–650.
6. Takahashi S, Sakuma I, Omachi K, Otani T, Tmura N, Watarai J, and Mizoi K: Craniocervical junction venous anatomy around the suboccipital cavernous sinus: evaluation by MR imaging. Eur Radiol 2005;15:1694–1700.
7. Weissman JL: Condylar canal vein: unfamiliar normal structure as seen at CT and MR Imaging. Radiology 1994;190(1):81.
8. Ginsberg LE: The posterior condylar canal. Am J Neuroradiol 1994;15:969.
9. Caruso RD, Rosenbaum AE, Chang JK, and Joy SE: Craniocervical junction venous anatomy on enhanced MR images: the suboccipital cavernous sinus. Am J Neuroradiol 1999;20:1127–1131.
10. Smoker WRK: Craniovertebral junction: normal anatomy, craniometry, and congenital anomalies. Radiographics 1994;14:255.
11. El Gammal T, and Brooks BS: Anatomy of the craniovertebral junction. Chapter 78, Neuroradiology of the head and neck, from radiology, diagnosis, imaging, intervention. Taveras JM eds. Philadelphia, PA: JB Lippincott;1988:1–8.
12. Prescher A: The craniocervical junction in man, the osseous variations, their significance and differential diagnosis. Ann Anat 1997;179:1–19.
13. Koenigsberg RA, Vakil N, Hong TA, Htaik T, Faerber E, Maiorano T, Dua M, and Gonzales C: Evaluation of platybasia with MR imaging. Am J Neuroradiol 2005;26:89–92.
14. Fielding JW, Mensinger RN, and Hawkins RJ: Os odontoideus. J Bone Joint Surg Am 1980;62(3):376.
15. Shirasaki N, Okada K, Oka S, Hosono N, Yonenobu K, and Ono K: Os odontoideum with posterior atlantoaxial instability. Spine 1991;16:706.
16. Hadley MN: Os odontoideum. Neurosurgery 2002;50(3):409.
17. Van Ludinghausen M, Schindler G, Kageyama I, and Pomaroli A: The third occipital condyle, a constituent part of a median occipito-atlanto-odontoid joint: a case report. Surg Radiol Anat 2002;24:71–76.
18. Clements WD, Mezue W, and Mathew B: Os odontoideum: congenital or acquired? That's not the question. Injury 1995;26:640–642.
19. Caldarelli M and Di Rocco C: Diagnosis of chiari I malformation and related syringomyelia: radiological and neurophysiological studies. Childs Nerv Syst 2004;20:332–335.
20. Adamsbaum C, Moutard ML, Andre C, Merzoug V, Ferey S, Quere MP, Lewin F, and Fallet-Bianco C: MRI of the fetal posterior fossa. Pediatr Radiol 2005;35:124–140.
21. Richards PS, Bargiota A, and Corrall RJM: Paget's disease causing an Arnold-Chiari Type I malformation: radiographic findings. Am J Roentgenol 2001;176:816–817.
22. Ho NC, Guarnieri M, Brant LJ, Park S, Sun B, North M, Francomano CA, and Carson BS: Living with achondroplasia: quality of life evaluation following cervico-medullary decompression. Am J Med Genet 2004;131A:163–167.
23. Kao SCS, Waziri MH, Smith WL, et al.: MR Imaging of the craniovertebral junction, cranium, and brain in children with achondroplasia. Am J Roentgenol 1989;153:565.
24. Kopits SE: Orthopedic complications of dwarfism. Clin Orthop 1976;114:153.
25. Kopits SE, Perovic MN, McKusick V, et al.: Congenital atlantoaxial dislocations in various forms of dwarfism. J Bone Joint Surg 1972;54A:1349.
26. Quintanilla JS, Biedma BM, Rodriguez MQ, Mora MTJ, Cunqueiro MMS, and Pazos MA: Cephalometrics in children with down's syndrome. Pediatr Radiol 2002;32:635–643.
27. El-Khoury GY, Clark CR, Dietz FR, et al.: Posterior atlantoccipital subluxation in down syndrome. Radiology 1986;159:507.
28. Martich V, Ben-Ami T, Yousefzadeh DK, et al.: Hypoplastic posterior arch of C-1 in children with down syndrome: a double jeopardy. Radiology 1992;183:125.
29. White KS, Ball WS, Prenger EC, et al.: Evaluation of the craniocervical junction in down syndrome: correlation of measurements obtained with radiography and MR imaging. Radiology 1993;186:377.
30. Hreidarsson S, Magram G, and Singer R: Symptomatic atlantoaxial dislocation in Down syndrome. Pediatrics 1982;69:568.
31. Tracy MR, Dormans JP, and Kusumi K: Klippel-Feil syndrome: clinical features and current understanding of etiology. Clin Orthop 2004;(424):183–190.
32. Curcione PJ and Mackenzie W: Klippel-Feil Syndrome. Case presentation. Wilmington, DE: The Alfred I. Dupont Institute; Available from: http://gait.aidi.edel.edu/res695/homepage/pd_ortho/educate/clincase/klipfeil.htm:1995.
33. Parsons VJ, Hughes DG, and Wraith JE: Magnetic resonance imaging of the brain, neck and cervical spin in mild Hunter's syndrome (mucopolysaccharidosis type II). Clin Radiol 1996;51:719.
34. Parsons VJ, Hughes DG, Wraith JE, et al.: Magnetic resonance imaging of the brain, neck, and cervical spine in mild hunter's syndrome (mucopolysaccharidoses Type II). Clin Radiol 1996;51:719.
35. Hughes DG, Chadderton RD, Cowie RA, Wraith JE, and Jenkins JPR: MRI of the brain and craniocervical junction in morquio's disease. Neuroradiology 1997;39:381–385.
36. Stevens JM, Kendall BE, Crockard HA, and Ransford A: The odontoid process in Morquio-Brailford's. J Bone Joint Surg 1991;73B:851.
37. Taccone A, Tortori Donati P, Marzoli A, Dell'Acqua A, Gatti R, and Leone D: Mucopolysaccharidosis: thickening of dura mater at the craniocervical junction and other CT/MRI findings. Pediatr Radiol 1993;23:349.
38. Itshayek E, Spector S, Gomori M, and Segal R: Fibrous dysplasia in combination with aneurysmal bone cyst of the occipital bone and the clivus: case report and review of the literature. Neurosurgery 2002;51:815–818.
39. Sirvanci M, Karaman K, Onat L, Duran C, and Ulusoy OL: Monostotic fibrous dysplasia of the clivus: MRI and CT findings. Neuroradiology 2002;44:847–850.
40. Adada B and Al-Mefty O: Fibrous dysplasia of the clivus. Neurosurgery 2003;52:318–323.
41. Chong VFH, Khoo JBK, and Fan YF: Pictorial essay: fibrous dysplasia involving the base of the skull. Am J Roentgenol 2002;178:717–720.
42. Stompro BE, Alksne JF, and Press GA: Diagnosis and treatment of an odontoid fracture in a patient with polyostotic fibrous dysplasia: case report. Neurosurgery 1989;24:905.
43. O'Brien MF, Casey ATH, Crockard A, Pringle J, and Stevens JM: Histology of the craniocervical junction in chronic rheumatoid arthritis: a clinicopathologic analysis of 33 operative cases. Spine 2002;27(20):2245–2254.
44. Kroft LJM, Reijnierse M, Kloppenburg M, Verbist BM, Bloem JL, van and Buchem MA: Rheumatoid arthritis: epidural enhancement as an underestimated cause of subaxial cervical spinal stenosis. Radiology 2004;231:57–63.
45. Bouchaud-Chabot A and Liote F: Cervical spine involvement in rheumatoid arthritis. a review. Joint Bone Spine 2002;69:141–154.
46. Nguyen HV, Ludwig SC, Silber J, Gelb DE, Anderson PA, Frank L, and Vaccaro AR: Contemporary concepts review: rheumatoid arthritis of the cervical spine. Spine J 2004;4(3):329–334.
47. Resnick D and Niwagama G: Rheumatoid arthritis. In Resnick D, Niwayama G, Eds. Diagnosis of bone and joint disorders. Philadelphia: Saunders;1994.
48. Anda S, Nilsen G, and Roysland P: Periodontoid changes in rheumatoid arthritis; MRI observations. Scand J Rheumatol 1988;17:59.

49. Pettersson H, Larsson EM, Holtas S, et al.: MR imaging of the cervical spine in rheumatoid arthritis. AJNR Am J Neuroradiol 1988;9:573.
50. Laiho K and Kauppi M: The cervical spine in patients with psoriatic arthritis. Ann Rheum Dis 2002;61:650–652.
51. Theodorou DJ, Theodorou SJ, and Resnick D: Imaging in dialysis spondyloarthropathy. Semin Dial 2002;15(4):290–296.
52. Yeadon C, Dumas JM, and Karsh J: Lateral subluxation of the cervical spine in psoriatic arthritis: a proposed mechanism. Arthritis Rheum 1983;26:109.
53. Blau RH and Kaufman RL: Erosive and subluxing cervical spine disease in patients with psoriatic arthritis. J Rheumatol 1987;14:111.
54. Lee ST and Lui TN: Psoriatic arthritis with C1-C2 subluxation as a neurosurgical complication. Surg Neurol 1986;26:428.
55. Kakitsubata Y, Boutin RD, Theodorou RD, et al.: Calcium pyrophosphate dihydrate crystal deposition in and around the atlantoaxial joint: association with type 2 odontoid fractures in nine patients. Radiology 2000;216:213–219.
56. Griesdale DEG, Boyd M, and Sahjpaul RL: Pseudogout of the transverse atlantal ligament: an unusual cause of cervical myelopathy. Can J Neurol Sci 2004;31:273–275.
57. Feydy A, Liote F, Carlier R, Chevrot A, and Drape JL: Cervical spine and crystal-associated disease: imaging findings. Eur Radiol 2005;16(2):459–468.
58. Zunkeler BZ, Schelper R, and Menezes AH: Periodontoid calcium pyrophosphate dihydrate deposition disease: pseudogout mass lesions of the craniocervical junction. J Neurosurg 1996;85:803.
59. Dirheimer Y, Wackenheim C, and Dietemann JL: Calcification of the transverse ligament in calcium dihydrate deposition disease (CPPD). Neuroradiol 1985;27:87.
60. Dirheimer Y, Bensimon C, Christmann D, et al.: Syndesmo-odontoid joint and calcium pyrophosphate dihydrate deposition disease (CPPD). Neuroradiol 1983;25:319.
61. Cabot J, Mosel L, Kong A, and Hayward M: Tophaceous gout in the cervical spine. Skeletal Radiol 2005;34(12):803–806.
62. Jacobs SR Edeiken J, Rubin B, et al.: Medically reversible quadriparesis in tophaceous gout. Arch Phys Med Rehabil 1985;66:188.
63. Sequeira W, Boutfard A, Salgia K, et al.: Quadriparesis in tophaceous gout. Arthritis Rheum 1981;24:1428.
64. Gold RH, Metzger AL, Mirra JM, et al.: Multicentric reticulohistiocytosis (lipoid dermatoarthritis). Am J Roentgenol 1975;124:610.
65. Yamada T, Kurohori YN, Kashiwazaki S, et al.: MRI of multicentric reticulohistiocytosis. J Comput Assist Tomogr 1996;20:838.
66. Ruskin J, Shapiro S, McCombs M, et al.: Odontoid osteomyelitis. Western J Med 1992;156:306.
67. Limbird TJ, Brick GW, Boulas HJ, and Bucholz RW: Osteomyelitis of the odontoid process. J Spinal Disord 1988;1:66.
68. Keogh S and Crockard A: Staphylococcal infection of the odontoid peg. Postgrad Med J 1992;68:51.
69. Post MJD, Sze G, Quencer RM, et al.: Gadolinium-enhanced MR in spinal infection. J Comput Assist Tomogr 1990;14:721.
70. Levin MF, Vellet AD, Munk PL, et al.: Tuberculosis of the odontoid bone: a rare but treatable cause of quadriplegia. Canad Assoc Radiol J 1992;43:199.
71. Lifeso R: Atlanto-axial tuberculosis in adults. J Bone Joint Surg 1987;69B:183.
72. Botella C, Orozco M, Navarro J, et al.: Idiopathic chronic hypertrophic craniocervical pachymeningitis:case report. Neurosurgery 1994;35(6):1144.
73. Akalan N, Seckin H, Kiliç C, et al.: Benign extramedullary tumors in the foramen magnum region. Clin Neurol Neurosurg 1994;96(4):284.
74. Taverns JM: Neuroradiology. 3rd ed. Baltimore: MD: Williams & Wilkins; 1996:780–781,1161.
75. Tsuchiya K, Hachiya J, Mizutani Y, et al.: Three-dimensional helical CT angiography of skull base meningiomas. Am J Neuroradiol 1996;17(5):933.
76. Filho MBL, Borges G, Ferreira A, Franca D, and Mello P: Schwannoma of the craniocervical junction: surgical approach of two cases. Arq Neuropsiquiatr 2003;61(3-A):639–641.
77. Levine DN: The pathogenesis of syringomyelia associated with lesions at the foramen magnum: a critical review of existing theories and proposal of a new hypothesis. J Neurol Sci 2004;220:3–21.
78. Sato K, Kodera T, Kitai R, and Kubota T: Osteochondroma of the skull base: MRI and histological correlation. Neuroradiology 1996;38(1):41–43.
79. Murphey MD, Andrews CL, Flemming DJ, et al.: From the archives of AFIP. Primary tumors of the spine: radiologic-pathologic correlation. Radiographics 1996;16:1131.
80. Tully RJ, Pickens J, Oro J, et al.: Hereditary multiple exostoses and cervical cord compression: CT and MR studies. J Comput Assist Tomogr 1989;13:330.
81. Murphey MD, Andrews CL, Flemming DJ, et al.: From the archives of AFIP. Primary tumors of the spine: radiologic-pathologic correlation. Radiographics 1996;16:1131.
82. Tully RJ, Pickens J, Oro J, et al.: Hereditary multiple exostoses and cervical cord compression: CT and MR studies. J Comput Assist Tomogr 1989;13:330.
83. Greenspan A: Benign bone forming lesions: osteoma, osteoid osteoma, and osteoblastoma. Skeletal Radiol 1993;22:485.
84. Bucci MN, Feldenzer JA, Phillips WA, et al.: Atlantoaxial rotational limitation secondary to osteoid osteoma of the axis. J Neurosurg 1989;70:129.
85. Nemoto O, Moser RP, Van Dam BE, et al.: Osteoblastoma of the spine. Spine 1990;15:1272.
86. Kroon HM and Schurmans J: Osteoblastoma: clinical and radiologic findings in 98 new cases. Radiology 1990;175:783.
87. Hladky JJP, Lejeune JP, Singer B, et al.: Osteoblastoma of the odontoid process. Pediatr Neurosurg 1994;21:260.
88. Ito H, Kizu O, Yamada K, and Nishimura T: Secondary anuerysmal bone cyst derived from a giant-cell tumor of the skull base. Neuroradiology 2003;45:616–617.
89. Andersen BJ, Goldhagen P, and Cahill DW: Aneurysmal bone cyst of the odontoid process; case report. Neurosurgery 1991;28:592.
90. Hay MC, Paterson D, and Taylor TK: Aneurysmal bone cysts of the spine. J Bone Joint Surg 1978;60B:406.
91. Beltran J, Simon DC, Levy M, et al.: Aneurysmal bone cysts: MR imaging at 1.5 T. Radiology 1986;158:689.
92. Munk PL, Helms CA, Holt RG, et al.: MR imaging of aneurysmal bone cysts. Am J Roentgenol 1989;153:99.
93. Zorlu F, Selek U, Soylemezoglu F, and Oge K: Malignant giant cell tumor of the skull base originating from clivus and sphenoid bone. J Neurooncol 2006;76(2):149–152.
94. Tang JY, Wang CK, Su YC, Yang SF, Huang MY, and Huang CJ: MRI appearance of giant cell tumor of the lateral skull base, a case report. Clin Imaging 2003;27:27–30.
95. Lee HJ and Lum C: Giant-cell tumor of the skull base. Neuroradiology 1999;41:305–307.
96. Schwimer SR, Bassett LW, and Mancuso AA: Giant cell tumor of the cervicothoracic spine. Am J Roentgenol 1981;136:63.
97. Hurley ME, O'Meara A, Fogarty E, and Hayes R: Langerhans' cell histiocytosis of the clivus: case report and literature review. Pediatr Radiol 2004;34:267–270.
98. Krishna H, Behari S, Pal L, Chhabra AK, Banerji D, Chhabra DK, and Jain VK: Solitary langerhans-cell histiocytosis of the clivus and sphenoid sinus with parasellar and petrous extensions: case report and a review of literature. Surg Neurol 2004;62:447–454.
99. Boston M and Derkay CS: Langerhans' cell histiocytosis of the temporal bone and skull base. Am J Otolaryngol 2002;23(4):246–248.
100. Brisman JL, Feldstein NA, Tarbell NJ, Cohen D, Cargan AL, Haddad J Jr., and Bruce JN: Eosinophilic granuloma of the clivus: case report, follow-up of two previously reported cases, and review of literature on cranial base eosinophilic granuloma. Neurosurgery 1997;41(1):273–279.
101. Prayer D, Grois N, Prosch H, Gadner H, and Barkovich AJ: MR imaging presentation of intracranial disease associated with langerhans cell histiocytosis. AJNR Am J Neuroradiol 2004;25:880–891.
102. Ferguson L and Shapiro CM: Eosinophilic granuloma of the second cervical vertebra. Surg Neurol l979;11:435.
103. Sanchez RL, Llovet J, Moreno A, et al.: Symptomatic eosinophilic granuloma of the spine. Orthopedics 1984;1721.
104. Osenbach RK, Youngblood LA, and Menezes AH: Atlantoaxial instability secondary to solitary eoginophilic granuloma of C2 in a 12 year old girl. J Spinal Disord 1990;3:408.
105. Graif M and Pennock JM: MR imaging of histiocytosis X in the central nervous system. Am J Neuroradiol 1986;7:21.
106. Choe W, Walot I, Schlesinger C, et al.: Synovial cyst of dens causing spinal cord compression. Case report. Paraplegia 1993;31:803.

107. Miller JD, Al-Mefty O, and Meddleton TH: Synovial cyst at the craniovertebral junction. Surg Neurol 1989;31:239.
108. Tabaddor K, Sachs D, and Llena JF: Ganglion cyst of the odontoid process. Spine 1996;21:2019.
109. Eustacchio S, Trummer M, Unger F, and Flaschka G: Intraspinal synovial cyst at the craniocervical junction. Zentralbl Neurochir 2003;64:86–89.
110. Lorigan JG, David CL, Evans HL, et al.: The clinical and radiologic manifestations of hemangiopericytoma. Am J Roentgenol 1989;153:345.
111. Lin YJ, Tu YK, Lin SM, et al.: Primary hemangiopericytoma in the axis bone: case report and review of literature. Neurosurgery 1996;39:397.
112. Asirvatham R, Moreau PG, and Antonius JL: Solitary infantile myofibromatosis of axis. Spine 1994;19:80.
113. Chung EB and Enzinger FM: Infantile myofibromatosis. Cancer 1981;48:1807–1818.
114. Lustrin ES, Karakas SP, Ortiz AO, et al.: Pediatric cervical spine: normal anatomy, variants, and trauma. Radiographics 2003;23(3):539–560.
115. Zimmerman RA and Bjlanjuk LT: Imaging of tumors of the spinal canal and cord. Radiol Clin North Am 1988;26:965.
116. Erdem E, Angtuaco EC, Van Hemert R, Park JS, and Al-Mefty O: Comprehensive review of intracranial chordoma. Radiographics 2003;23(4):995–1009.
117. Kitai R, Yoshida K, Kubota T, et al.: Clival chordoma manifesting as nasal bleeding. A case report. Neuroradiology 2005;47:368–371.
118. Mehnert F, Beschorner R, Kuker W, Hahn U, and Nagele T: Retroclival ecchordosis physaliphora: MR imaging and review of the literature. AJNR Am J Neuroradiol 2004;25:1851–1855.
119. St. Martin M and Levine SC: Chordomas of the skull base: manifestations and management. Curr Opin Otolaryngol Head Neck Surg 2003;11:324–327.
120. Soo MYS: Chordoma: review of clinicoradiological features and factors affecting survival. Australas Radiol 2001;45:427–434.
121. Sundaresan N, Galicich JH, Chu FCH, et al.: Spinal chordomas. J Neurosurg 1979;50:312.
122. Meyer JE, Lepke RA, Lindfors KK, et al.: Chordomas: their CT appearance in the cervical, thoracic and lumbar spine. Radiology 1984;153:693.
123. Sze G, Uichanco LS, Brant-Zawadzki MN, et al.: Chordomas: MR imaging. Radiology 1988;166:187.
124. Murphey MD, Walker EA, Wilson AJ, Kransdorf MJ, Temple T, and Gannon FH: From the archives of the AFIP. Imaging of primary chondrosarcoma: radiologic-pathologic correlation. Radiographics 2003;23(5):1245–1278.
125. Schmidinger A, Rosahl SK, Vorkapic P, and Samii M: Natural history of chondroid skull base lesions – case report and review. Neuroradiology 2002;44:269–271.
126. Neff B, Sataloff RT, Storey L, Hwakshaw M, and Spiegel JR: Chondrosarcoma of the skull base. Laryngoscope 2002;112:134–139.
127. Camins MB, Duncan AW, Smith J, et al.: Chondrosarcoma of the spine. Spine 1978;3:202.
128. Kretzschmar HA and Eggert HR: Mesenchymal chondrosarcoma of the craniocervical junction. Clin Jeurol Neurosurg 1990;92:343.
129. Whitehead RE, Melhem ER, Kasznica J, and Eustace S: Telangiectatic osteosarcoma of the skull base. Am J Neuroradiol 1998;19:754–757.
130. Shives TC, Dahjjn DC, Sim FH, et al.: Osteosarcoma of the spine. J Bone Joint Surg 1986;68A:660.
131. Patel DV, Hammer RA, Levin B, et al.: Primary osteogenic sarcoma of the spine. Skeletal Radiol 1984;12:276.
132. Mnaymneh W, Brown M, Tejada F, et al.: Primary osteogenic sarcoma of the second cervical vertebra. J Bone Joint Surg 1979;61A:460.
133. Boyko OB, Cory DA, Cohen MD, et al.: MR imaging of osteogenic and Ewing's sarcoma. Am J Roentgenol 1987;148:317.
134. Sharafuddin MJ, Haddad FS, Hitchon PW, et al.: Treatment options in primary Ewing' sarcoma of the spine: report of seven cases and review of the literature. Neurosurgery 1992;30:610
135. Grubb MR, Currier BL, Pritchard DJ, et al.: Primary Ewing's sarcoma of the spine. Spine 1994;19:309.
136. Pilepich MV, Vietti TJ, Nesbit ME, et al.: Ewing's sarcoma of the vertebral column. Int J Radiat Oncl Biol Phys 1981;7:27.
137. Siegal GP, Oliver WR, Reinus WR, et al.: Primary Ewing's sarcoma involving the bones of the head and neck. Cancer 1987;60:2829.
138. O'Connell JE, Calder C, Raafat F, et al.: Ewing's sarcoma of the retropharynx. J Laryng Oto 1994;108:363.
139. Martin Garcia G, Cruz Hernandez JJ, Sanchez P, et al.: Ewing's sarcoma in the second cervical vertebra. Ann Oncol 1991;2:521.
140. Frouge C, Vanel D, Coffre C, et al.: The role of magnetic resonance imaging in the evaluation of Ewing sarcoma. Skeletal Radiol 1988;17:387.
141. Laigle-Donaday F. Taillibert S, Martin-Duverneuil N, Hildebrand J, and Delattre J-Y: Skull-base metastases. J Neuro-Oncol 2005;75:63–69.
142. Greenberg HS, Deck MD, Vikram B, Chu FC, and Posner JB: Metastasis to the base of the skull: clinical findings in 43 patients. Neurology 1981;31:530–537.
143. Sundaresan N, Galicich JR, Lane JM, et al.: Treatment of odontoid fractures in cancer patients. J Neurosurg 1981;54:187.
144. Fertakos RJ, Swayne LC, Yablonsky TM, et al.: Gallium SPECT detection of lymphomatous involvement of the cervical dens. Clin Nucl Med 1995;1:70.
145. Walsh IK, Wilson RH, and Moorehead RJ: Odontoid peg metastasis from an oesophageal adenocarcinoma. Ulster Med J 1993;63:177.
146. Daffner RH,Lupetin AR, Dash N, et al.: MRI in the detection of malignant infiltration of bone marrow. Am J Roentgenol. 1986;146(2):353.
147. Sze G, Krol G, Zimmerman RD, et al.: Malignant extradural spinal tumors: MR imaging with Gd-DTPA. Radiology 1988;167:217.
148. Sze G, Brant-Zawadzki MN, Wilson, Norman D, and Newton TH: Pseudo tumor of the craniovertebral junction associated with chronic subluxation: MR imaging studies. Radiology 1986:161:391.
149. Crockard HA, Sett P, Gedes JF, Stevens JM, Kendall BE, and Pringle JAS: Damaged ligaments at the craniocervical junction presenting as an extradural tumor: a differential diagnosis in elderly. J Neurol Neurosurg Psych 1991;54:817.
150. Rousselin B, Helenon O, Zingraff L, Delons S, Drueke T, Bardin T, and Moreau JF: Pseudotumor of the craniocervical junction during long-term hemodialysis. Arthritis Rheum 1990;33:1567.
151. Hatakeyama A, Fujinaga H, Togo T, et al.: Remarkable improvement of activity by CAPD in a hemodialysis patient with a pseudotumor of the craniocervical junction. Adv Perit Dial 1992;8:116.
152. Manz HJ and Bauer H: Pathologic fracture of odontoid process secondary to amyloid deposition. J Neurol 1981;225:277.
153. Rosenberg WS, Rosenberg AE, and Poletti CE: Cervical disc herniation presenting as a mass lesion posterior to the odontoid process. J Neurosurg 1991;75:954.
154. El Gammal T and Brooks BS: Radiologic evaluation of the craniovertebral junction. Chapter 79. In Taveras JM, eds. Neuroradiology of the head and neck from radiology, diagnosis, imaging, intervention. Vol. III. Philadelphia, PA: JB Lippincott;1987:1–16.

The Temporal Bone 11

Anton N. Hasso, MD, FACR
Wende N. Gibbs, MS, MD
Max Cho, MD
Sahar Farzin, MD
Christopher R. Trimble, MD, MBA

NORMAL ANATOMY

Major Divisions of the Temporal Bone

Squamous Part

The squama is a smooth, vertical plate that forms part of the lateral wall and floor of the middle cranial fossa. It forms the posteroinferior segment of the temporal fossa, and as such provides muscular attachment for the temporalis muscle, an important muscle of mastication. Its superior and posterior borders articulate with the parietal bone and its anteroinferior border with the greater wing of the sphenoid bone. The temporal surface of the slightly convex shell of squama is grooved by the middle temporal artery, and similarly by the middle meningeal artery on its cerebral surface. Laterally, the lower part of the squama gives rise to an arch that extends anteriorly and forms the zygomatic process. The zygomatic process articulates with the temporal process of the zygomatic bone forming the zygomaticotemporal suture located at the midpoint of the zygomatic arch. The medial surface of this zygomatic arch provides a muscular origin to another muscle of mastication, the masseter muscle. The zygomatic process widens as it approaches the squama posteriorly and bifurcates into two roots: an anterior and posterior root. The anterior root gives rise to the articular tubercle of the temporal bone, and the posterior root extends backward and upward as the supramastoid crest, the posteroinferior boundary of the temporal fossa. The articular tubercle marks the anterior limit of the mandibular fossa, and lends attachment for the lateral temporomandibular ligament that reinforces the lateral aspect of the temporomandibular joint (TMJ).[1,2]

Mastoid Part

The mastoid is the posterior-most segment of the temporal bone located behind the external auditory canal (EAC). Externally it has a rough texture owing to the attachments of the auricularis posterior and occipitalis muscles. The extension of the mastoid anteriorly and inferiorly forms a lateral protrusion known as the mastoid process. The mastoid process lends attachment to the sternocleidomastoid, splenius capitis, and longissimus capitis muscles on its lateral surface. Medial to the mastoid process the posterior belly of the digastric muscle inserts into the deep groove formed by the mastoid notch. Slightly more medial to this groove, is the occipital groove. The occipital artery traverses this groove as it passes posteriorly and upward to supply the occipital region of the skull.

An inconstant mastoid foramen may pierce the intracranial or cerebral surface of the mastoid near or within the occipitomastoid suture. This foramen (if present) serves as an anastomotic channel between the intracranial sigmoid sinus and mastoid emissary veins, as well as intracranial cerebral arteries and the mastoid branch of the occipital artery. The adjacent sigmoid sinus indents the cerebral surface of the mastoid forming the deep groove for the sigmoid venous sinus on its way route to exit the jugular foramen.

The internal cavity of the mastoid process is pneumatized in the adult. However, pneumatization begins to occur in postnatal development and is completed by about the second year. The mastoid air cells that form within the mastoid process vary in size and shape, but generally are smallest in the apex of the process, and become larger toward the upper, anterior part. These air cells are continuous with the mastoid antrum, the single large chamber located in the posterior tympanic cavity. The antrum communicates with the epitympanic recess and the greater tympanic cavity through a small aperture, the aditus ad antrum.[1,2]

Petrous Part

The petrous portion of the temporal bone mimics a three-sided pyramid that is lying on one side, with its apex pointing anteromedial and its base facing posterolateral adjacent to the internal surfaces of the squamous and mastoid parts. Within the inner cavity of the petrous bone lie the acoustic apparatus, which includes the ossicular chain within the tympanic cavity laterally, and the highly convoluted acoustic labyrinth medially. The anterior face of the pyramid contributes to flooring the middle cranial fossa and delineating its posterior limit. Continuous with the anterior face, the posterior face is a vertical plane that forms the anterior wall of the posterior cranial fossa and contains the openings of the internal acoustic meatus and the vestibular aqueduct.

The anterior surface of the pyramidal petrous bone contains a fairly large opening for the carotid canal at its apex. Just lateral to this opening, the apex of the petrous bone forms the posterior limit of the foramen lacerum, together with the posteromedial border of the greater wing of the sphenoid that forms the anterior limit. Behind the carotid canal is the impression of the trigeminal (semilunar) ganglion, from which the three divisions of the fifth cranial nerve (CN) emerge. At about midpoint along the anterior surface, the superior semicircular canal bulges out into the middle cranial fossa as the arcuate eminence. Adjacently, the petrous bone becomes the substantially thinner tegmen tympani roofing the mastoid antrum and tympanic cavity. At its lateral margin, the paper-thin tegmen tympani fuses with the squama at the petrosquamous suture. Anterior to the tegmen an oblique groove extends posterolateral from the foramen lacerum to the hiatus for the greater petrosal nerve. Just lateral to this, a less pronounced groove traverses the petrous bone, leading to the hiatus for the lesser petrosal nerve.

The posterior surface of the petrous bone forms the anterior wall of the posterior cranial fossa, and meets the intracranial mastoid surface laterally at the petromastoid suture. At and near the apex, the posterior surface is fused to the occipital component of the clivus, lateral to the basilar part of the occiput. Near the midpoint of the posterior surface, the opening to the internal acoustic canal (the porus acusticus) transmits the facial and vestibulocochlear nerves, along with the artery for the internal auditory canal. A minute opening for the vestibular aqueduct occurs just posteroinferior to the internal auditory canal (IAC), and transmits the endolymphatic duct along with its corresponding blood supply.

The inferior surface of the pyramidal petrous bone is sandwiched between the sphenoid and occipital bones, in an oblique orientation. Medially, it has a blunt margin due to the adjacent opening of the foramen lacerum. Its external surface has a rugged texture, as it contributes to the external cranial base along with the occipital bone. It contains the external opening for the carotid canal, situated in approximately the same coronal plane as the external acoustic meatus. Behind this external opening, a tiny tympanic canaliculus perforates the petrous bone on the ridge separating the carotid canal from the jugular fossa posteriorly. The tympanic canaliculus transmits the tympanic branch of the glossopharyngeal nerve as it exits the jugular foramen anterior to the internal jugular vein. The tympanic nerve runs through the canaliculus emerging onto the floor of the tympanic cavity. Just posterolateral to this minute opening, the auricular branch of the vagus nerve pierces the (lateral) roof of the jugular fossa exiting through the mastoid canaliculus. The jugular fossa is a smooth depression roofing the jugular foramen, and it marks the posterior margin of the inferior face of the petrous bone. CN IX, X, and XI, in addition to the internal jugular vein and the posterior meningeal artery exit the cranium through the jugular foramen.[1,2]

Styloid Process

Lateral to the jugular fossa, on the inferior surface of the petrous bone, the styloid process projects anteroinferiorly with varying degrees of curvature. With a length of approximately 2.5 cm, the process lend attachment for muscles and ligaments of the hyoid, pharyngeal, and glottic regions. In between the styloid process and the mastoid process, the stylomastoid foramen transmits the facial nerve just before it enters the substance of the parotid gland.[1,2]

Tympanic Part

The tympanic bone forms the anterior, inferior, and part of the posterior wall of the osseous external auditory canal. It is situated below the squamous part and anterior to the mastoid process. Its anterior wall from the lateral edge of the EAC up to the tympanosquamous fissure medially, forms the posterior part of the condylar fossa. Posteriorly, the tympanic bone fuses with the squamosa part and the mastoid process, at their squamomastoid suture. At its medial end the concave tympanic plate is grooved by the narrow tympanic sulcus, which is absent superiorly and houses the tympanic annulus (thickened periphery of tympanic membrane).[1,2]

External Ear

External Auditory Canal and Pinna

The external ear, which is responsible for funneling sound waves through the ear canal and onto the eardrum, is composed of the pinna (auricle) and the EAC (meatus). The pinna and outer one-third of the EAC have a cartilaginous skeleton with overlying perichondrium that is tightly attached to the subcutaneous tissue and skin. The inner or medial two-thirds of the EAC has an osseous skeleton lined with a stratified squamous epithelium that is continuous with the outer layer of the tympanic membrane. In the adult, the EAC is approximately 2.5 cm from the concha to the tympanic membrane. As compared with the relatively thick epithelial lining, or skin, covering the cartilaginous part, the bony canal has much thinner skin measuring on average at 0.2 mm in thickness. The skin of the cartilaginous part of the canal (although variable) averages between 0.5 and 1.0 mm in thickness, resembling much of the skin throughout the rest of the body. Only within this outer, cartilaginous canal can integument specializations, such as hair follicles, sebaceous and ceruminous glands, be found. Sebaceous and ceruminous glands together secrete the substance of earwax, an evolutionarily protective sticky seal that repels and entraps insects, dust, bacteria, and other potential harms.[3,4]

Course of the External Auditory Canal

The EAC of the adult ear does not take a simple transverse course from the concha of the pinna to reach the eardrum. Instead, the route through the canal is directed in three continuous segments (from lateral to medial): the pars externa courses medially, anteriorly, and superiorly, the pars media courses medially, posteriorly, and superiorly, and the medial-most pars interna courses medially, anteriorly, and inferiorly. In contrast to the EAC in adults, children and newborns have much shorter and more horizontally directed EACs.[3,4]

Innervation

The sensory innervation of the adult ear includes branches of three different CNs and sensory afferents from the cervical plexus. In the region of the external ear, the pinna and EAC both receive sensory information from the auriculotemporal branch of CN V3 and the auricular branch of CN X. In addition, the pinna also receives cervical sensory fibers from the great auricular (C2, C3) and lesser occipital nerves (C2), and the EAC receives a minor contribution from a somatic sensory component of CN VII traveling with the auricular branch of CNX (Arnold's nerve).[3,4]

Vessels

The blood supply to the external ear arrives via one of the major arteries of the head and neck, namely, the external carotid artery. The pinna receives its principal supply from several branches of the external carotid artery including, the posterior auricular branch, the anterior auricular branch (from the superficial temporal branch), and the mastoid branch (from the occipital branch). The EAC receives the posterior auricular branch and anterior auricular branch (of the superficial temporal branch) of the external carotid artery, and in addition, the deep auricular branch of the maxillary artery. All venous systems accompany their respective arteries.[3,4]

Middle Ear

Tympanic Membrane

The tympanic membrane, or eardrum, is composed of three layers. An outer stratified squamous epithelial layer that is contiguous with the inner two-thirds of the EAC; a middle layer of dense fibrous tissue; and an inner layer of mucous membrane, contiguous with the mucosa of the middle ear cavity. Circumscribing the eardrum is a peripheral fibrous thickening called the annulus, which anchors the membrane into the tympanic sulcus (of the tympanic bone). This fibrous annulus is slightly perforated at its superior pole where it meets the notch of Rivinus (or tympanic incisura) of the tympanic bone. Also within this superior region is the triangular pars flaccida, the portion of the tympanic membrane above the lateral process of the malleus. Nearly the entire eardrum is tense and semitransparent except for this small patch. The pars tensa is the extended, more prominent part of the tympanic membrane below the lateral process. The pars flaccida and pars tensa are similar in their outer epithelial and inner mucosal layers; however, they differ in the composition of their intermediate layers. The pars flaccida, as its name suggests, is lax and flaccid due to irregularly organized elastic fibers in its middle layer; contrarily, the pars tensa is the very tense and taut portion of the tympanic membrane. This difference is due to tensa's inner-circular and outer-radial distributions of fibrous tissue, without substantial elastic fibers.

Medial to and behind the tympanic membrane is the tympanic cavity, which houses the auditory ossicles. Upon otoscopic examination of the eardrum, a silhouette of the handle of the malleus and its lateral process can be viewed fairly clearly. Where the tip of the handle of the malleus contacts the tympanic membrane, there is a puckering of the membrane that gives it a conical shape, with its apex known as the umbo. At the superior end of the handle of the malleus is its lateral process, which is another point of attachment of the malleus to the eardrum. This attachment forms a prominence in the membrane, from which anterior and posterior malleal folds extend to the tympanic bone. The significance of these malleal folds is their delineation of the two parts of the tympanic membrane: the pars flaccida above and the pars tensa below.

At the distal end of the EAC, the outer-most layer of the tympanic membrane is lined with the same thin epithelium as the bony segment of the ear canal. Correspondingly, the sensory fibers that supply the eardrum include the auriculotemporal nerve (CN V3) and the auricular branch of CN X, both of which also innervate the EAC. The tympanic membrane also receives somatic sensory fibers from the tympanic branch of CN IX, which innervates the middle ear cavity and thus the innermost layer of the eardrum.

The first two branches of the maxillary artery, namely, the deep auricular and the anterior tympanic arteries, and the stylomastoid branch of the posterior auricular artery, together supply the delicate membrane of the eardrum.[3–6]

Tympanic Cavity

The tympanic cavity is a mucosal-lined chamber within the petrous part of the temporal bone that houses a chain of auditory ossicles responsible for transmitting sound energy from the tympanic membrane to the acoustic labyrinth (**Fig. 11-1**). The cavity is situated in between the tympanic membrane laterally, and the petrous encasement of the inner ear structures, medially. Its average dimensions measure to be about 15 mm both vertically and anteroposteriorly. In the horizontal plane, it measures to be approximately 6 mm superiorly and 4 mm inferiorly.

Four distinct spaces contribute to the overall unique contour and orientation of the tympanic cavity: the mesotympanum, epitympanum (epitympanic recess), hypotympanum, and protympanum. These air-filled spaces communicate with the mastoid antrum and mastoid air cells posteriorly, and with the nasopharynx (and thus external environment) via the pharyngotympanic (auditory) tube, anteriorly.

The mesotympanum is the principal cavity of the middle ear, adjacent to, and at about the same level as, the tympanic membrane. It contains the handle and lateral process of the malleus, and the long process of the incus, both of which extend upwards into the attic, or epitympanic recess. The epitympanic recess is a hollowed cavity within the roof of the middle ear, or tegmen (tympani), which contains the head of the malleus and the body and short crus of the incus, and is continuous with the mastoid antrum posteriorly. A horizontal plane transecting the tympanic cavity at the superior margin of the tympanic membrane laterally and the prominence of the facial canal medially designates the boundary between the mesotympanum and the epitympanic recess.

The epitympanum measures at approximately one-third of the vertical length of the tympanic cavity. It is bound medially

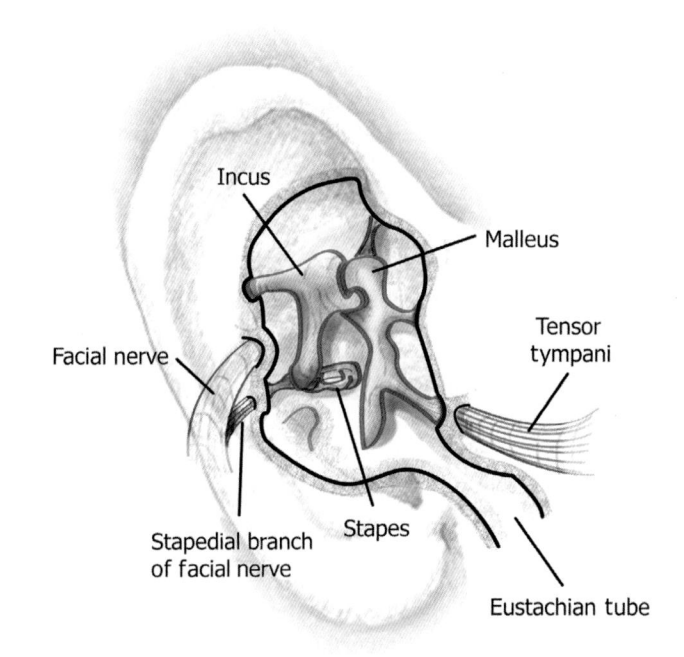

Figure 11-1 Middle Ear Schematic
Diagram of structures of the middle ear. The auditory ossicles span the width of the tympanic cavity. The facial nerve descends along the posterior wall of the tympanic cavity in its vertical segment. It gives rise to a branch to the stapedius just behind the pyramidal eminence. The tensor tympani is contained in the bony canal above the osseous portion of the Eustachian tube and ends in a tendon which inserts on the manubrium of the malleus.

by the prominences of the lateral semicircular and facial canals and laterally by the squamous part of the temporal bone. The inferior-most part of the lateral wall has a spiny process, the scutum, which is also the bony indentation at the superior margin of the tympanic annulus.

A smaller, highly variable space, the hypotympanum is located below a horizontal plane transecting the cavity at the inferior margin of the tympanic membrane. A significant degree of anatomic variation exists in the area of the hypotympanum, particularly with differences found in its depth. This natural variation may be due to the embryological development of the hypotympanum, which results from the fusion of the tympanic bone, otic capsule, and petrous. In individuals with a larger than average jugular bulb, the hypotympanic space may be significantly reduced with the impression of a bulge in its floor. Thus, for the purposes of radiological imaging and in prescribing differential diagnosis, these variations in the hypotympanum are very critical.

The fourth space within the tympanic cavity is attributed to the protympanum, the area which lies in front of a coronal plane drawn through the anterior margin of the tympanic membrane. The protympanum is continuous with the hypotympanum inferiorly, and the pharyngotympanic (Eustachian or auditory) tube anteromedially.[3]

Roof of Tympanic Cavity

Viewed from within the middle cranial fossa, the rocky, irregular texture of the petrous bone diminishes along its posterolateral extension, becoming especially smooth and thin above the tympanic cavity, where it gives rise to the tegmen tympani or tegmental wall. Here, the tegmen tympani forms the roof for the tympanic cavity centrally, the canal for the tensor tympani muscle anteriorly, and the mastoid antrum posteriorly. This thin plate of bone separates these cavities from the middle cranial fossa above. As it is part of the petrous bone, the tegmen tympani, as aforementioned in the description of the petrous part of the temporal bone, is fused with the squamous part at its lateral margin forming the petrosquamous suture.[1,4,7]

Floor of Tympanic Cavity

The tympanic cavity is separated from the underlying jugular bulb and internal jugular vein by the jugular fossa, which thereby forms its floor. The jugular fossa has two surfaces: a tympanic surface, which forms the jugular wall or floor of the tympanic cavity, and an external cranial surface, which forms the roof of the jugular foramen. The tympanic floor, or jugular wall, is composed of a thin plate of petrous bone containing numerous tiny air cells that are continuous with air cells within the bony external auditory canal. The jugular wall is limited at its angle with the posterior wall of the carotid canal, which corresponds to the anterior wall of the tympanic cavity. A tiny opening for the tympanic canaliculus perforates the bony ridge located in between the jugular fossa and the opening of the carotid canal. As the glossopharyngeal nerve exits the skull through the jugular foramen, its tympanic branch, carrying somatic sensory fibers for the tympanic cavity, loops around and re-enters the skull through the tympanic canaliculus. It traverses the tympanic canaliculus, ultimately arriving on the floor of the tympanic cavity to supply its mucosal surfaces. The tympanic nerve (nerve of Jacobson) joins the caroticotympanic nerves from the internal carotid plexus, to form the tympanic plexus within the middle ear.[1,4,7]

Anterior Wall of Tympanic Cavity

The anterior wall of the tympanic cavity consists of a thin plate of bone corresponding to the posterior part of the carotid canal, inferiorly, and the openings of the musculotubal canal, superiorly. Sympathetic fibers of the caroticotympanic nerves from the internal carotid plexus (postganglionic sympathetic fibers originating from the superior cervical ganglion), together with the tympanic branch of the internal carotid artery, pierce the anterior wall to supply the tympanic cavity. The musculotubal canal is divided into two semicanals, with one above the other, which open into the superior part of the mesotympanum (tympanic cavity proper). A thin bony septum provides the partition between the two compartments of the musculotubal canal. The distal end of this septum forms a cochleariform process, a blunt edge over which the tendon of the tensor tympani muscle bends. As such, the superior, narrower canal contains the tensor tympani muscle and its tendon just before it exits above the oval window, to insert onto handle of the malleus; and the inferior, larger canal contains the auditory tube (Eustachian tube) that communicates with the nasopharynx. The superior semicanal for tensor tympani makes its entrance into the tympanic cavity just anterior and adjacent to the medial wall covering the bony labyrinth.[1,4,7]

Posterior Wall of Tympanic Cavity

The complexity of the temporal bone in the region of the middle ear is exemplified through a careful study of the posterior wall of the tympanic cavity. The details and intricacies of the posterior mastoid wall are quite numerous, and as such play an important functional and clinical role in the middle ear. Situated behind the EAC and middle ear, the mastoid provides the posterior wall of the tympanic cavity. The epitympanic recess communicates with the mastoid antrum posteriorly through an irregular aperture, the aditus ad antrum. Mastoid air cells are continuous with the mastoid antrum; as such, this aperture provides a link between the mastoid air cells, the greater tympanic cavity, and nasopharynx (by way of the Eustachian tube).

The pyramidal eminence, a hollow mucosal-lined protrusion in the posterior wall, lies on the approximate boundary between the epitympanum and the mesotympanum, anterior to the vertical portion of the facial canal. Situated directly in front of the pyramidal eminence within the medial wall of the tympanic cavity is the oval window, with the stapes sealing its orifice. A tiny stapedius muscle originates in the posterior wall within the pyramidal eminence. An opening at the tip of the eminence transmits the slender tendon of the stapedius muscle, which then projects straight ahead and inserts on the neck of the stapes. The nerve to the stapedius muscle, a branch of the facial nerve, pierces the thin bony plate separating the facial canal from the posterior wall and enters the pyramidal eminence to innervate the muscle belly within. Lateral to this eminence is another bony protrusion, the chordal eminence, which transmits the chorda tympani nerve through a tiny foramen at its tip. The chordal eminence occurs anterior to the facial canal as well, and medial to the posterior edge of the fibrous annulus surrounding the eardrum. The chorda tympani nerve branches off of the facial nerve within the vertical portion of the canal and courses anteriorly through the chordal eminence to traverse the tympanic cavity. It courses forward on the medial side of the tympanic membrane, in between the incus and malleus to ultimately exit the tympanic cavity through a canal in the petrotympanic (Glaserian) fissure.

Within the posterior wall, there are two depressions that form clinically significant recesses: the sinus tympani and the facial recess. The sinus tympani is bound by the pyramidal eminence laterally, and the bony labyrinthine wall medially and extends posteriorly, medial to the facial nerve.

The facial recess lies within the valley formed in between the pyramidal and cochlear eminences, and just as the sinus tympani its posterior extent is highly variable. Both the sinus tympani and facial recess pose as potential sites for extension and prolongation of diseases, such as cholesteatoma of the middle ear. The facial recess is of particular importance from a surgical perspective, for it is the route utilized to reach the tympanic cavity from the mastoid in a posterior tympanotomy (canal wall up tympanoplasty).

Situated above both recesses, and just below the aditus ad antrum within the posterior wall of the epitympanic recess, is the incudal fossa. It contains the short process of the incus, held in place by the posterior incudal ligament and its inferior margin forms the upper limit for the facial recess.[4,7]

Lateral Wall of Tympanic Cavity

The inner mucosal layer of the tympanic membrane together with the thin circumscribing margin of the tympanic ring, form the lateral (membranous) wall of the tympanic cavity proper. Superiorly, the tympanic bone is deficient at the notch of Rivinus, where the pars flaccida contributes a small slice to complete the eardrum. The tympanic membrane is tethered to the tympanic sulcus at an angle of approximately 140 degrees with respect to the roof of the external auditory canal. Internally, this oblique orientation translates into a slanted lateral wall for the mesotympanum. The manubrium of the malleus attaches firmly to the tympanic membrane near its center at a site called the umbo, thereby pulling it inward. Externally, this puckers the membrane creating a tent-like effect with the umbo at the tent's peak.[1,4,7]

Medial Wall of Tympanic Cavity

The lateral face of the bony acoustic labyrinth that casts the inner ear structures forms the medial wall of the tympanic cavity. The medial labyrinth wall is characterized by the several prominent bulges and depressions, which outline its tympanic surface. These structures extend up past the mesotympanum into the epitympanic recess.

The largest of these bulges, the promontory, occurs within the mesotympanum in the center of the medial wall, and is produced by the bony labyrinth overlying the basal turn of the cochlea. Branches of the tympanic plexus run over the promontory within its mucosal lining, providing sensory innervation to the tympanic cavity and carrying autonomic fibers to their extra-acoustic destinations.

Located just posteroinferior to the promontory and anteroinferior to the sinus tympani, is the round window niche, which leads to the round window, medially. A bony ridge, the subiculum, separates the round window niche from the superoposterior sinus tympani, thereby forming the common superior and inferior boundary for each, respectively. At the medial end of the round window niche, lies the round window or fenestra cochlea, closed off in life by a membrane. The sole function of the round window membrane is to permit compensatory movements of the inner ear fluids associated with movements of the stapes footplate at the oval window.

Superior to the promontory in the medial wall, the base of the stapes lies within the fossa for the oval (vestibular) window, leading to the vestibule of the inner ear. The oval window niche is bound by the canal for the facial nerve superiorly, the promontory inferiorly, the pyramidal eminence and sinus tympani posteriorly, and the cochleariform process anteriorly. It is hidden in the posterior part of the medial labyrinthine wall within the mesotympanum. Above the oval window niche, the prominence of the facial canal marks the superior margin of the mesotympanum, above which lies the prominence of the lateral semicircular canal in the epitympanic recess. The tympanic portion of the facial nerve produces the prominence of the facial canal as it courses backward from the geniculate ganglion after it has given off the greater petrosal branch. Located anterior to this prominence, the cochleariform process of the musculotubal canal marks the approximate site of the geniculate ganglion, just above. Superior to the prominence of the facial canal, within the epitympanic recess and bordering the aditus ad antrum, is the prominence of the lateral semicircular canal.[1,4,7]

Contents of Tympanic Cavity

The key players in the functional anatomy of the middle ear are the auditory ossicles, their ligaments and muscles, located within the tympanic cavity. With lesions to any of these components of the middle ear, the conductive pathway for sound to reach the inner ear is obstructed, and may lead to hearing deficits.

Auditory Ossicles and Ligaments

The auditory ossicles consist of three small bones, which linked together extend across the tympanic cavity from the eardrum to the labyrinthine oval window. Beginning at the tympanic membrane, the malleus consists of a head, neck, anterior process, lateral process, and manubrium. Its head resides within the epitympanic recess, where it articulates with the body of the incus at the incudomalleal articulation/joint. Superior and anterior suspensory ligaments fix the head of the malleus into the roof and anterior wall of the epitympanum, respectively. The neck extends just below the plane separating the mesotympanum from the epitympanum, at the superior margin of the tympanic membrane. A lateral suspensory ligament tethers the neck into the bony margin of the notch of Rivinus, in the tympanic sulcus. Jutting straight ahead from the neck is the anterior process of the malleus, which courses together with the medial chorda tympani nerve as they make their way into the petrotympanic (Glaserian) fissure in the anterior wall. The anterior process is secured into the petrotympanic fissure by the anterior malleal ligament, a dense fibrous tissue that is continuous with the periosteum of the malleus. The lateral process is a short bony stub that attaches to the tympanic membrane in its anterosuperior quadrant, with the pars flaccida immediately superior to it. Anterior and posterior malleal folds extend superiorly from the point of contact between the lateral process and the mucosal layer of the tympanic membrane. The manubrium, or handle, of the malleus is its long inferior extension, which firmly attaches to the tympanic membrane at the umbo. The tendon of the tensor tympani muscle also contributes to stabilizing the manubrium within the tympanic cavity, by attaching onto its anterior surface.

The second ossicle in the conductive chain is the incus. It is situated behind the malleus, bound to it via the saddle-shaped incudomalleal articulation, a diarthrodial joint. The incus contains a body, a short and long process, and a lenticular process. The body and short process are located within the epitympanic recess, while the long process projects inferiorly, parallel to the manubrium, into the mesotympanum. The articular surface for the head of the malleus is a deep concavity within the anterior body. A superior incudal ligament parallels the superior suspensory ligament of the malleus, and anchors the body of the incus into the tegmen tympani. Posteriorly, the short process extends back into the incudal recess, firmly held in place by the posterior incudal ligament. Two anteriorly directed ligaments, the medial and lateral incudomalleal ligaments contribute to the diarthrodial joint capsule between the body of the incus and head of the malleus. The malleoincudal joint is typically described as an "ice cream cone" on axial computerized tomography images. With temporal bone trauma, there can be malleoincudal dislocation, seen as derangement of the "ice cream cone" appearance. The long process of the incus descends into the mesotympanum and ends in the lenticular process, a rounded, cartilaginous convexity that articulates with the corresponding concave surface of the head of the stapes.

The stapes completes the ossicular chain medially, by connecting to the incus and extending inward to seal the oval window at the labyrinth. The stirrup-shaped stapes is slightly deviated downward from its axial orientation, assuming the stirrup is lying on its side. The incudostapedial articulation consists of a diarthrodial synovial joint between the cartilaginous surfaces of the head of the stapes and the lenticular process of the incus. Adjacent to the head, a subtle constriction marks the neck of the stapes. Its posterior surface provides insertion for the tendon of the stapedius muscle as it emerges from the pyramidal eminence. Joining the head and neck to the base of the stapes are the anterior and posterior crura. The anterior crus is slightly shorter and less curved than the posterior. They form an asymmetrical arch, with each crus ending at opposite poles of the base, which is a flattened oval plate, called the footplate of the stapes. Its cartilaginous rim is fixed into the margins of the oval window by the annular ligament, forming the tympanostapedial or stapediovestibular syndesmosis.[1]

Muscles

The tendons of the tensor tympani and stapedius muscles proceed from opposite poles of the tympanic cavity to insert on their respective ossicles. Under loud conditions, they contract reflexively to produce a protective dampening effect. The tensor tympani muscle originates from the superior division of the musculotubal canal, with the septum forming its floor. Near the lateral end of the semicanal, the muscle fibers converge into a tendon, which emerges into the tympanic cavity. The tendon hooks over the cochleariform process at a right angle and traverses the cavity posterolateral to insert on the superior part of the manubrium of the malleus. This enables the tensor tympani muscle to draw the manubrium medially, thereby tensing the tympanic membrane and reducing the amplitude of oscillation of the malleus. It receives its innervation from a branch of the mandibular nerve that passes through the otic ganglion.

On the opposite pole of the tympanic cavity, the tendon of the stapedius muscle juts out of the pyramidal eminence and courses anteriorly to insert on the neck of the stapes. The muscle belly takes its origin within the hollowed cavity of the pyramidal eminence anterior to the vertical facial canal, in the posterior wall of the tympanic cavity. As the stapedius muscle contracts it tugs on the posterior aspect of the neck of the stapes. This creates a partial rotating-door effect with respect to the stapes and the oval window. The footplate is situated in an almost-vertical plane, within the oval window niche. The stapedius tendon pulls on the posterior neck of the stapes, which causes the footplate to rotate around its vertical axis. The posterior crus swing inward toward the vestibule as the anterior crus pulls outward, tilting the stapes and stretching the annular ligament. The facial nerve gives a branch to the stapedius muscle as it descends in the vertical portion of the facial canal just behind the pyramidal eminence.

Sound produces gaseous movements that result in alternating air pressures around the ears. The changes in pressure cause the tympanic membrane to vibrate, which in turn initiates the oscillatory chain of events within the tympanic cavity. The vibration is transmitted from the eardrum first to the malleus, then to the incus and ultimately through the stapes, to the fluid within the vestibular apparatus. The tensor tympani and stapedius muscles play an important protective role against loud, damaging sounds. The tensor tympani will pull the eardrum medially, tensing the membrane and thereby retarding the vibration at the malleus. The contraction of the stapedius rotates the footplate of the stapes out of the plane of the oval window niche, reducing the effective area of the footplate that is in contact with the inner ear fluid. This mechanism reduces the extent of vibration that is ultimately transmitted to the vestibule.[1]

Nerves

The tympanic cavity receives its innervation from branches of the tympanic plexus. The glossopharyngeal nerve gives a tympanic branch (nerve of Jacobson) as it exits the skull through the jugular foramen. The tympanic branch immediately re-enters the cranium via the tympanic canaliculus, a small opening situated between the carotid canal and the jugular fossa. The course of the canaliculus eventually leads the tympanic nerve onto the floor of the tympanic cavity through an internal opening. It provides general sensory innervation to the tympanic membrane and tympanic cavity. In addition, the tympanic nerve gives rise to preganglionic parasympathetic fibers. Together with the caroticotympanic nerves, these fibers give rise to the tympanic plexus that lies on the cochlear promontory.

The caroticotympanic nerves are postganglionic sympathetic fibers from the internal carotid plexus that enter the tympanic cavity by piercing through its anterior wall. The pre- and postganglionic autonomic fibers from the tympanic plexus coalesce, as the lesser petrosal nerve, and exit the tympanic cavity through a small canal in the anterior wall. The lesser petrosal nerve surfaces within the middle cranial fossa from the hiatus for the lesser petrosal nerve. It continues forward and medially within its own sulcus and ultimately exits the skull through the foramen ovale. The preganglionic parasympathetic fibers eventually synapse in the otic ganglion and give rise to postganglionic parasympathetic secretomotor fibers.

Within the posterior wall, the facial nerve gives rise to the chorda tympani, as it descends in the vertical canal. The chorda tympani emerges into the tympanic cavity through a tiny foramen at the tip of the chordal eminence, at the posterior edge of the fibrous annulus of the eardrum. It courses anteriorly adjacent to the medial side of the tympanic membrane, running in between the long process of the incus and manubrium of the malleus. Along with the anterior process of the malleus, the chorda tympanic enters the petrotympanic (Glaserian) fissure; however, unlike the anterior process, it exits the tympanic cavity through a canal within the petrotympanic fissure. The chorda tympani nerve only traverses the tympanic cavity, and is not a source of its innervation.[4]

Vessels

The blood supply of the middle ear is predominantly derived from the external carotid artery, with a few caroticotympanic branches from the internal carotid artery. The vessels originating from the external carotid artery include: 1) the deep auricular artery, 2) the anterior tympanic artery, 3) the inferior tympanic artery, 4) the stylomastoid artery, 5) the superior tympanic artery, and 6) the petrosal artery.

The deep auricular artery and the anterior tympanic artery are the first and second major branches arising from the internal maxillary artery, respectively; the inferior tympanic artery arises from the ascending pharyngeal artery; the stylomastoid artery arises from the occipital artery; and finally, the superior tympanic artery and petrosal artery both stem from the middle meningeal artery.

Generally, veins accompany their corresponding arteries and drain into the superior petrosal sinus and pterygoid plexus. The former ultimately drains into the internal jugular vein via the sigmoid sinus, and the latter via the maxillary and retromandibular veins.[1,3]

The Inner Ear

Bony Labyrinth

The bony labyrinth of the inner ear derives from the embryological otic capsule, and resides within the petrous part of the temporal bone. Its conspicuous shape and contour correspond to the underlying membranous labyrinth responsible for the functions of balance and hearing. Three major components contribute to the bony labyrinth: the vestibule, cochlea, and semicircular canals. The bony labyrinth is stretched across the long axis of the petrous pyramid, with the cochlea situated anteriorly near the apex and the semicircular canals posteriorly near the base. Along this axis, the bony labyrinth measures at approximately 20 mm in length.

Vestibule

The vestibule is an ovoid cavity located centrally within the bony labyrinth, measuring approximately 4 mm in diameter. Within its lateral wall, it contains the oval window, sealed shut by the footplate of the stapes. Inside the chamber of the vestibule a perilymphatic space filled with fluid, bathes the membranous labyrinth within. This space is continuous with the cochlea anteriorly, and the semicircular canals posteriorly. Three cusplike recesses form concavities within the inferior and medial walls of the vestibule. Anterosuperiorly in the medial wall, the spherical recess contains part of the membranous saccule. Posterosuperiorly, the membranous utricle partially occupies the elliptical recess. The cochlear recess forms the depression within the floor of the vestibule for the basal end of the cochlear duct. Tiny foramina within the medial wall and floor of the vestibule transmit nerve branches from the vestibular nerve to the internal acoustic canal. Within the posteroinferior part of the vestibule, an internal opening for the vestibular aqueduct contains the membranous endolymphatic duct.[1]

Cochlea

The cochlea consists of a snail-shaped bony labyrinth, which spirals around a central axis and makes between two and three turns. It is situated in the anterior part of the inner ear, in front of the vestibule and semicircular canals. The cochlea has a wide base adjoining the anterolateral aspect of the internal auditory canal. Tiny foramina within the base transmit the cochlear nerve from the IAC into the bony labyrinth. The axis of rotation for the 30-mm spiral canal is a central bony core, the modiolus, which is directed anterolateral from the base. The orientation of the cochlea is such that from the base the spiraling canal extends out through the axis and terminates at its apex, or cupula. The cupula is a blunt terminus, resembling the swirling tip of an ice cream cone. It is directed anteriorly, laterally, and inferiorly. The height of the cochlea measures at about 5 mm.

The basal turn of the cochlea produces a large bulge, the promontory, in the medial labyrinthine wall of the tympanic cavity. From there the diameter of the spiraling canal gradually tapers down and ends in the narrow cupula. The internal chamber of the cochlea is continuous with the perilymphatic cavity of the vestibule, posteriorly.

Internally, the cochlear canal is compartmentalized by bony and membranous partitions. A sagittal cross section through its central axis (modiolus) depicts a thin osseous spiral lamina. This bony plate is derived from the modiolus and extends approximately halfway into the canal to partially divide it. It rotates with the cochlear canal, around the modiolus, ultimately ending at the hamulus. A fibrous continuation, the basilar membrane, attaches to the free lip of the osseous spiral lamina, and extends across the canal, to the spiral ligament hugging the bony cochlear wall. The canal is thus divided into an anterior scala vestibuli and posterior scala tympani. These two chambers communicate with each other at the helicotrema, an apical opening between the two compartments, at the hamulus of the spiral lamina. Within the scala vestibuli, a vestibular (Reissner's) membrane arises from the anterior surface of the osseous spiral lamina, and extends laterally toward the bony cochlear wall. These results in the formation of a third compartment, the scala media, of the cochlear duct.

The scala vestibuli is proximally continuous with the vestibule. At the helicotrema, the perilymphatic space of the scala vestibuli communicates with that of the scala tympani. Distally the blind terminus of the scala tympani abuts the membrane of the round window.[1]

Semicircular Canals

Situated behind the vestibule and directly communicating with it are three osseous semicircular canals in the base of the petrous pyramid. The posterior canal lies along the long axis of the petrous pyramid. Perpendicular to this axis and the posterior canal, is the superior semicircular canal. It is the vertex of this superior semicanal that produces the arcuate eminence within the floor of the middle cranial fossa. The lateral semicircular canal lies 30 degrees above the horizontal, that is, with the head tilted downward by 30 degrees, the lateral semicircular canal lies in the horizontal plane.

Each canal has two crura, which together form the half-circular arches. Two crura, one from each end of the posterior limbs of the superior and posterior semicircular canals join to form a common crus, which opens into the posterior aspect of the vestibule. The posterior crus of the lateral semicircular canals opens into the vestibule just inferior to the common opening. The three remaining limbs of the canals terminate anteriorly as dilated ampullae, which drain into the vestibule along its anterolateral surface. The ampullated crus of the superior semicircular canal opens into the supero-lateral aspect of the vestibule. Just below it are the openings for the ampullae of the lateral semicircular canal, and posterior semicircular canal, more inferiorly. Altogether, there are five crural openings within the osseous vestibule.[1,8]

Cochlear Aqueduct

Near the round window membrane and within the basal turn of the cochlea, this narrow canal extends from the scala tympani to an external opening in the inferior surface of the petrous pyramid (**Fig. 11-2**). The cochlear aqueduct connects the perilymphatic space of the scala tympani to the subarachnoid space. Although this provides a raw form of communication between these two spaces, in life, the cochlear aqueduct is filled with arachnoid, fibrous, and connective tissues.[1,8]

Vestibular Aqueduct

Within the depths of the elliptical recess of the vestibule a tiny aperture leads to the vestibular aqueduct. This narrow canal extends from the vestibule to the posterior surface of the petrous pyramid, opening into the subarachnoid space of the posterior cranial fossa. The vestibular aqueduct contains the endolymphatic duct.[1,8]

Membranous Labyrinth

The epithelial lined membranous labyrinth is contained within the bony labyrinth discussed above. The same perilymphatic fluid that flows throughout the otic capsule baths the membranous labyrinth. Inside, endolymph flows within the interconnected vestibular and acoustic structures. These membranous

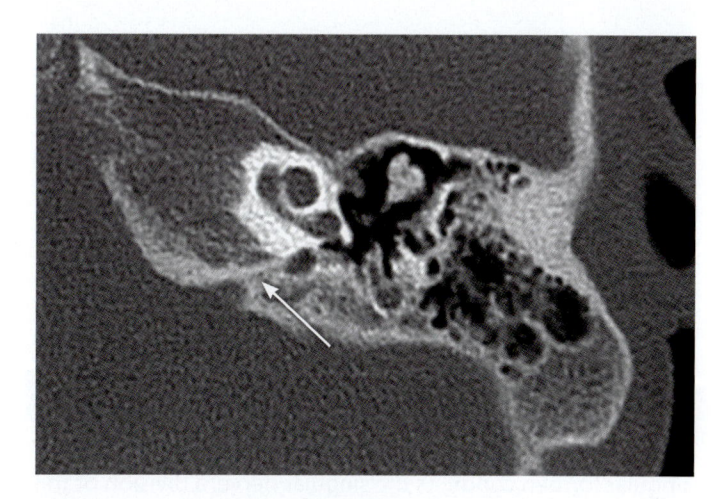

Figure 11-2 Cochlear Aqueduct
Axial bone CT demonstrating the cochlear aqueduct.

structures include: the utricle and saccule, the three semicircular ducts and ampullae, the cochlear duct and the endolymphatic duct and sac.

Vestibular (Otolithic) Sense Organs

The sensory structures reserved for vestibular function reside within the maculae of the membranous utricle and saccule, and the cristae of the ampullary semicircular canals. The maculae and cristae contain the sensory hair cells responsible for vestibular sensory function. Within the maculae, hair cells are lined with ciliary projections, which become embedded in a gelatinous membrane covering their corresponding vestibular organs. Similarly, the cristae also contain ciliated hair cells; however, these cilia project into a gelatinous cupula. Hair cells in the utriculo-saccular complex play a role in linear acceleration. They detect changes in head position with respect to the trunk and limbs, and initiate counteracting muscle reflexes. The ampullary cristae detect angular acceleration of the head.

Nerve fibers from the saccule are contained in the inferior branch of the vestibular nerve. Signals from the utricle, as well as the ampullae of the superior and lateral semicircular canals are conducted via the superior branch of the vestibular nerve. Nerve fibers from the ampulla of the posterior semicircular canal course separately through the singular foramen, which is visible on CT scanning (Fig. 11-3), and unite with the inferior vestibular nerve in the fundus of the IAC.

The utricle and saccule reside within the chamber of the vestibule. The utricle is the larger, more oblong structure, and the saccule is in the shape of a rounded bean. The utricle extends farther superiorly than the saccule, and the two are joined and communicate with each other via the utriculosaccular duct. The superior half of the utricle conforms to the elliptical recess in the medial vestibular wall, and the saccule lies within the more anterior spherical recess. The utriculosaccular duct continues posteriorly as the endolymphatic duct, which exits the vestibule through the vestibular aqueduct. The saccule also communicates with the cochlear duct, where it is situated within the cochlear recess. The narrow isthmus connecting the two-endolymphatic labyrinths is called the ductus reuniens.

The three semicircular ducts encased within the corresponding bony labyrinth, drain into the utricle via five openings. Each duct has a terminal dilation, or ampulla, which opens into the anterior face of the vestibule. The cristae, or ampullary sense organs, reside within the base of each ampulla. The posterior crus of the lateral semicircular canal and the common crus are not dilated by ampullae, and simply open into the posterior surface of the vestibule.[1,4]

Cochlear Duct

The membranous cochlear duct mimics the spiraling course of the osseous labyrinth within which it resides. The endolymphatic tube spans the full length of the cochlear turns distally and communicates with the saccule by way of the ductus reuniens, proximally. Its proximal tail ends blindly in the vestibule and abuts the labyrinth wall immediately below the oval window and above the round window. Its position within the spiraling labyrinth is such that it is wedged in between the scala vestibuli and scala tympani, and contributes to their division together with the osseous spiral lamina. The basilar membrane, extending from the outer edge of the spiral lamina to the outer cochlear wall, forms the floor of the cochlear duct. The roof is supported by Reissner's membrane, and its outer wall by a thickened periosteum called the spiral ligament. Along the floor of the cochlear duct, the specialized hearing apparatus called the Spiral organ of Corti, is supported by the basilar membrane.[1,4]

Endolymphatic Duct and Sac

The endolymphatic apparatus contains a membranous sinus, duct, and sac. The endolymphatic sinus is its vestibular portion arising from the union of the utricular and saccular ducts. The sinus immediately tapers into a narrower endolymphatic duct. The duct is transmitted through the vestibular aqueduct through its internal opening within the elliptical recess. Its initial segment traverses a narrowed isthmus within the proximal aqueduct. It continues posteromedially within the canaliculus toward its external opening in the posterior surface of the petrous pyramid. The membranous duct expands into a flattened sac near its dural opening. It emerges into the posterior cranial fossa, as the endolymphatic sac, which is wedged in between the dura and the periosteum.[1,4]

EMBRYOLOGY AND CONGENITAL ANOMALIES

The temporal bone develops from the pars branchialis and the pars otica. The pars branchialis radiates from the first and second branchial arches, the first branchial groove, and the adjacent mesenchyme, and the pars otica develops from the auditory vesicle and the adjacent mesenchyme. The development of the external ear and the middle ear is independent of the development of the inner ear, and anatomic variations and congenital anomalies reflect the fact that one portion of the ear may be normal although another portion may be grossly

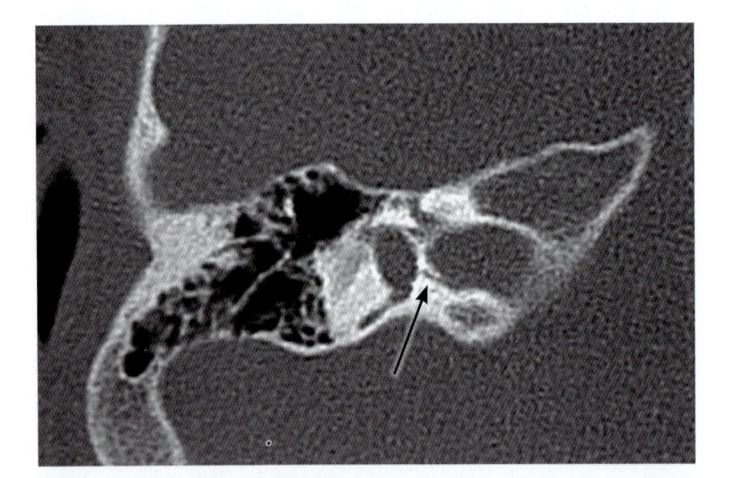

Figure 11-3 Singular Foramen
Axial CT bone CT scan at the level of the internal auditory canal fundus shows a normal singular foramen (*arrow*). The singular formen conducts the singular nerve, a division of the inferior vestibular nerve, which carries fibers from the ampulla of the posterior semicircular canal.

malformed. Because the development of the external and middle ear is closely linked, significant malformations of the external auditory canal are usually accompanied by middle ear deformities and vice versa. By comparison, inner ear anomalies usually occur independently. However, as compared with the normal population, some inner ear anomalies occur more frequently in patients who have concomitant anomalies of the other two ear compartments. Because mesenchyme is involved in the development of all portions of the ear, there are certain situations in which combined malformations can occur. The toxic embryopathy subsequent to maternal ingestion of thalidomide is an example of such a situation, and some of the otocranio-facial dysplasias show similar combined malformations (see **"Appendix 11-1 Congenital Syndromes involving the Ear"**).

The IAC, which is not part of the ear, may be normal in the presence of a grossly deformed inner ear. Conversely, cases of dysplasia or aplasia of the internal auditory canal may occur in the presence of a normal labyrinth, but extreme hypoplasia or aplasia of the IAC more commonly is associated with significant bony malformations of the inner ear. The development of the IAC is distinct from that of the labyrinth, and the underlying mechanism explaining the coexistence of these congenital deformities is not apparent.

Anatomic variations compose the range of dimensions, contours, and spatial orientations of the bony structures within the temporal bone region encountered in a normal population that demonstrates neither functional impairment nor anatomic substrate carrying the potential for imperiling the wellbeing of the individual. These two tests provide the crucial distinction between a "variation" and an anomaly.[9]

Normal Variations

The bony EAC shows considerable variation in both size and configuration. It composes the medial one half to two-thirds of the complete external auditory canal, the lateral portion being cartilaginous. The bony portion is usually narrower than the cartilaginous portion and is directed medially, anteriorly, and slightly inferiorly, forming in its course a slight curve, the convexity of which is posterosuperior in position. There is a wide spectrum of shapes of the external auditory canal, varying from circular to oval to heart shaped to triangular. The long axis of an oval canal may change its orientation, spiraling from medially to laterally. The bone that forms the anterior wall of the EAC and separates it from the temporomandibular joint (TMJ) averages about 1.5 mm in thickness, with a range varying from about 0.2 mm to almost 4 mm in thickness.[9]

The middle ear, including its epitympanic recess, measures 15 mm in its anteroposterior and vertical diameters. The transverse diameter measures about 6 mm above and 4 mm below the tympanic membrane, and opposite the center of the tympanic cavity, its transverse diameter is only about 2 mm. The hypotympanum is the pneumatized inferior extension of the middle ear cavity below the level of the tympanic ring. This is variable both in depth and in medial extension. The bone of the floor of the tympanic cavity, which separates it from the jugular bulb below, is thick when the hypotympanum is underdeveloped and thin when the hypotympanum is deep. Air cells of the mastoid group variably pneumatized this bony separation, particularly if the floor of the cleft is some distance removed from the jugular bulb.[9]

An important variation exists in the depth and angle of the sinus tympani, which forms a bony cavity lying between the bony labyrinth medially and the pyramidal eminence laterally. The sinus tympani is of surgical significance because it may contain diseased tissue, most commonly an acquired cholesteatoma that is not easily visualized by the usual surgical approach to the middle ear. The important surgical variations of the sinus tympani depend on how deeply and in what direction the sinus extends. The retroauricular surgical approach to the sinus tympani requires an entry between the facial nerve and the posterior or lateral semicircular canals or both. The distance between the sinus tympani and the facial nerve is therefore important, as is the distance between the facial nerve and the posterior semicircular canal. The normal measurements for the sinus tympani are a depth of 3 mm (range 0.6 to 6.0 mm) and a width of 2 mm (range 1 to 3 mm). The deepest and widest portion of the sinus tympani usually is located at the level of the round window membrane. The distance between the sinus tympani and the facial nerve is about 1 mm (range 0.1 to 1.6 mm). The distance between the facial nerve and the posterior semicircular canal is about 3 mm (range 2.0 to 3.5 mm) at a distance between 2 and 3 mm below the inferior border of the footplate of the stapes. Although such minute differences may seem to be of interest only to the surgeon, they emphasize the need for precise diagnostics in this field of imaging.[9]

There is essentially no variation in size or shape of the osseous labyrinth, and people of all ages have virtually the same size and shape labyrinthine structures.[9,10] The cochlea is conical, measuring about 5 mm from base to apex, and its breadth across the base is about 9 mm. It normally has 2½ to 2¾ coils or turns. Although minor alterations in the size of the cochlea and minor variation in the number of coils is not significant, a marked reduction of the lumen of the various coils is clinically important. The vestibule is roughly ovoid, flattened transversely, and measures about 5 mm from the front to back, the same from above downward, and about 3 mm across. No normal variants exist for the vestibule.

Each of the semicircular canals is about 0.8 mm in diameter, and each has a dilatation of the anterior most limb called the ampulla. The superior semicircular canal is oriented transversely to the long axis of the petrous temporal bone and measures about 15 to 20 mm in length. The posterior semicircular canal also is vertically placed and is directed backward, nearly parallel with the posterior surface of the petrous portion of the temporal bone. It is the longest canal and measures from 18 to 22 mm. The lateral semicircular canal is the shortest of the three canals, its arch is directed backward and laterally, and it is inclined 30° with the horizontal plane. As with the vestibule, there are no normal variants, although an anatomically abnormal vestibule or semicircular canal may be present without clinical symptoms.[9]

Anomalies of the Outer Ear

Malformations of the outer ear may involve the auricle or the EAC. The auricle develops around the first branchial groove and contains tissues contributed by both the first (mandibular) and second (hyoid) branchial arches.[11] An anomaly of the auricle (microtia) may be an isolated event, but it usually is associated with other anomalies. Severe microtia is typically associated with atresia or stenosis of the external auditory canal.[12]

The EAC is a derivative of the first ectodermal branchial groove between the mandibular and hyoid arches, and this ectodermal tissue comes in contact with adjacent mesoderm and endoderm (from the tympanic cavity lining) to form the tympanic membrane and the tympanic ring.[11] In the adult, ossification of the tympanic ring forms the tympanic portion of the temporal bone.

Stenosis of the External Auditory Canal

Dysplasia of the tympanic ring may lead to the development of stenosis of the EAC. The canal may be diffusely narrowed, or there may be variable focal stenosis. Severe stenosis may trap epithelial debris in the medial end of the canal, and the normal canal squamous epithelium subsequently may form an acquired cholesteatoma of the external canal. As the cholesteatoma enlarges, the medial end of the canal expands, and there can be concomitant pressure on the tympanic membrane and ossicles. In some cases, perforation of the tympanic membrane leads to gross bone destruction, with the predictable consequences of an untreated cholesteatoma.[13]

Atresia of the External Auditory Canal

Atresia of the EAC typically is caused by tympanic ring aplasia and may be complete or partial and unilateral or bilateral. Complete osseous atresia of the EAC consists of a bony plate of variable thickness, across the external auditory canal, where the tympanic membrane is usually located. This deformity is associated with fusion of the neck of the malleus to the atresia plate.[14,15] The short, or anterior, process of the malleus originates from the tympanic ring and may be the only absent portion of the ossicles when there is no concomitant involvement of the first or second branchial arches.[11] With isolated tympanic ring anomalies, the tympanic cavities are normal in size, and the mastoids are well developed (unless there is a history of infection). Fusion of the malleus and incus is also a common middle ear deformity associated with EAC atresia. The ossicles in general are frequently hypoplastic[16] (**Fig. 11-4**). Compared to middle ear malformations, the incidence of inner ear anomalies

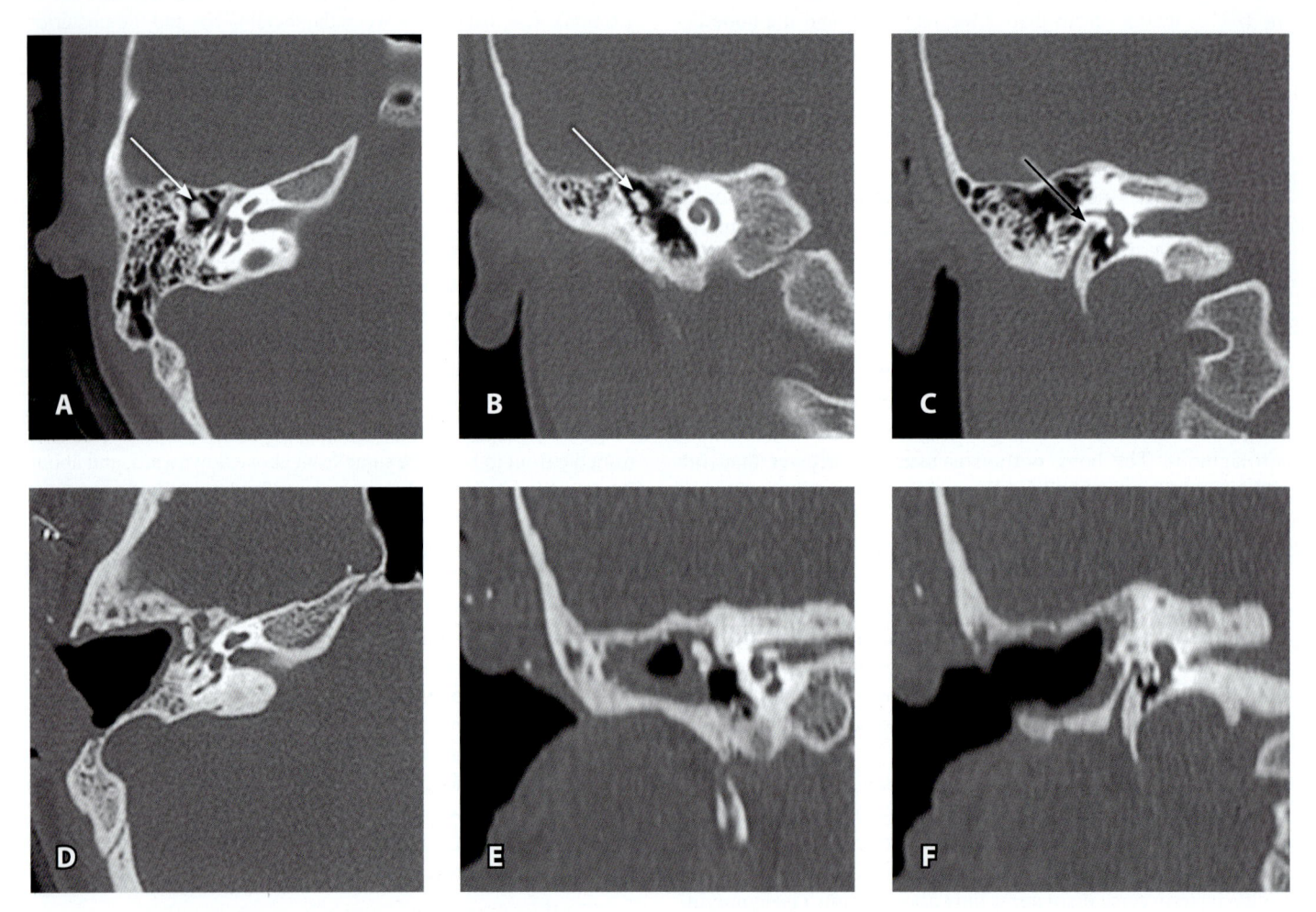

Figure 11-4 Aural Atresia Pre and Postoperative Repair
Preoperative axial (**A**) and coronal (**B–C**) bone CT images of the right temporal bone show a dysplastic pinna, complete atresia of the external auditory canal, dysmorphic ossicles within a small middle ear cavity (*white arrows*, **A, B**), and a medially displaced posterior genu of the facial nerve (*black arrow*, **C**). Postoperative axial (**D**) and reconstructed coronal (**E–F**) images show a surgically reconstructed external auditory canal approximating a preserved middle ear cavity.

Table 11-1 Jahrsdoerfer Grading System for Congenital Aural Atresia

Parameter	Points
Stapes present	2
Oval window open	1
Middle ear space	1
Facial nerve	1
Malleus/incus complex	1
Mastoid pneumatized	1
Incus–stapes connection	1
Round window	1
Appearance of external ear	1
Prognosis	**Total Points**
Good	8
Fair	7
Marginal	6
Poor	5

Adapted from Jahrsdoerfer RA, Yeakley JW, Aguilar EA, Cole RR, Gray LC: Grading system for the selection of patients with congenital aural atresia. Am J Otol 1992;13(1):6–12.

in patients with EAC atresia is relatively low, reflecting the earlier and independent embryonic development of the inner ear.[17] Other middle ear abnormalities frequently seen in patients with EAC atresia include hypoplasia of the middle ear space and a low degree of mastoid aeration.[18] These radiological features are important, since the risk of surgical complications is minimized and chances for successful hearing are increased if the middle ear and mastoid size are at least two-thirds of normal size and if all three ossicles, although deformed, can be identified.[19] Additionally, Jahrsdoerfer has created a scoring system used to quantify the developmental status of the ear and has been shown to predictive postoperative success[20,21] (**Table 11-1**).

In some cases, there may be a fibrous, or "membranous," atresia of the external auditory canal. Instead of the tympanic membrane, a "plug" of soft tissue is located at the site of the tympanic membrane. This relatively mild anomaly is caused by failure of recanalization, with or without fusion of a portion of the malleus to the lateral wall of the tympanic cavity.[9,15]

The facial nerve canal must be carefully examined in patients being considered for surgery with congenital aural atresia. The horizontal segment is often dehiscent, and can be displaced caudally, extending as inferiorly as the round window.[18] The vertical segment is often displaced anteriorly, with the facial nerve exiting the temporal bone early at the level of the round window.[22] These abnormalities are important from a surgical standpoint, as anterior displacement of the vertical segment of the facial nerve restricts access to the middle ear space, reducing the chance for successful hearing result and increasing the chance of facial nerve injury[23] (**Table 11-1**).

Patients with atresia of the EAC cannot be examined otoscopically. It is essential to examine these patients with high resolution computed tomography (HRCT) to rule out the presence of a concomitant dysplasia of the middle ear cleft or the presence of a congenital or acquired cholesteatoma.[15] In such patients, CT shows either a dysplastic nonaerated middle ear or an opaque tympanic cavity with possible erosion of its walls. MRI has been found to be useful in the characterization of a mass in an atretic EAC.[24] A cholesteatoma will appear hyperintense on diffusion-weighted images and inflammatory granulation tissue (GT) will enhance with contrast after gadolinium administration. Patients with cholesteatoma may require early surgery to remove the cholesteatoma and preserve facial nerve function with or without reconstruction of the external auditory canal.

Anomalies of the Temporomandibular Joint

Because the tympanic ring is significantly involved in all anomalies of the outer ear, there also may be alterations in the usual architecture of the TMJ. Deformity of the mandibular condyle frequently is associated with tympanic ring anomalies, along with a shallow joint space.[25] The temporal squama may be pushed downward, and the glenoid fossa may be markedly flattened or even absent.[13] The position of the TMJ is frequently abnormal, being relatively higher and more posterior in relationship to the middle ear.[25] Normally, the distance from the posterior aspect of the ramus of the mandible to the anterior surface of the tympanic bone is approximately 8 mm. In some congenital cases, depending on the degree of hypoplasia or agenesis of the tympanic bone, the distance may reach 40 mm, and the abnormal position of the TMJ may affect the ability of the surgeon to reconstruct the EAC.[13,25] Furthermore, the facial nerve canal may exit in the narrow space between the glenoid fossa and the mastoid process, directly in the surgical field.

Anomalies of the Middle Ear

Anomalies of the middle ear form a continuum with varying degrees of involvement. Minimal middle ear involvement occurs with tympanic ring dysplasia or aplasia. Mild to moderate involvement occurs when there is anomalous development of the first branchial arch. Severe involvement occurs when there is additional involvement of the second branchial arch.

Tympanic Ring Dysplasia

Tympanic ring dysplasia first appears with varying degrees of EAC stenosis, and the size of the middle ear cavity may be completely normal. The ossicles may be normal or may be partially fused to each other or to the lateral wall of the attic or both. Obliteration or erosion of the middle ear and mastoid air cells or both may result from the presence of embryonic debris in these spaces (congenital cholesteatoma) or from an acquired cholesteatoma arising from a stenosis of the external auditory canal.[7,13]

Tympanic Ring Aplasia

Under certain conditions, especially common in the thalidomide malformations, complete aplasia of the tympanic ring may occur.[7] A bony plate forms in place of the tympanic ring and obliterates the external ear canal and tympanic membrane.

This atresia plate redirects the terminal portion of the facial nerve, causing it to course more anteriorly within the plate and to exit at the bottom of the plate near the TMJ.[14,26] The lack of posterior support allows dorsal positioning of the TMJ with abutment of the glenoid fossa against the anterior aspect of the mastoid process.[7,12,15]

A constant finding is fusion of a portion of the malleus to the atretic plate.[14] Most of the malleus develops from Meckel's (first branchial arch) cartilage. The short or anterior process originally forms from the tympanic ring through intramembranous ossification. In later embryologic development, the malleus annexes this small portion of the ring, creating the anterior process.[11] When no tympanic ring forms, the neck of the malleus is fused to the atretic plate. The tympanic cavity may be of normal size or may be slightly smaller than normal, depending on the size of the bony atresia plate.[7,9,12,25] The mastoids are usually well pneumatized.[12] Complete tympanic ring aplasia consists of absence of the EAC and the tympanic membrane, presence of a bony atretic plate including fusion of the neck of the malleus, anterior displacement of the facial nerve, and posterior positioning of the TMJ.

First (Mandibular) Branchial Arch Dysplasia

Maldevelopment of the first branchial arch result in variety of congenital malformations of the eyes, ears, mandible, and palate, which together constitute the first arch syndrome. The complete syndrome is believed to be caused by insufficient migration of cranial neural crest cells into the first branchial arch.[27] Dysplasias of the first branchial arch have characteristic otologic anomalies, the more obvious manifestations resulting from defects of Meckel's (first branchial arch) cartilage. This cartilage forms part of the incus and most of the malleus.[11] These ossicles are usually anomalous with varying maldevelopment of the external auditory canal, middle ear cavity, and mastoid air cells. First arch dysplasias also show mandibular anomalies guided by the first arch cartilage template that plays a role in formation of the mandible.

Second (Hyoid) Branchial Arch Dysplasia

Second branchial arch dysplasias include anomalies of the stapes superstructure, lateral lamina of the stapes footplate, and the facial nerve canal. Normally, the facial nerve migrates anteroinferiorly after exiting the stylomastoid foramen to extend directly to the facial musculature innervated by this nerve. Within the temporal bone, anterior migration of the nerve normally is prevented by the formation of second branchial arch structures such as the bony wall of the facial nerve canal, the stapes superstructure, and the styloid process. The nerve maintains a position posterior and superior to these bony structures, all of which form from Reichert's cartilage of the second branchial arch. As a result of defective formation of the facial nerve canal wall and the stapes superstructure, the facial nerve is unimpeded and the tympanic segment can migrate inferiorly to lie on the stapes or pass across the oval window with the stapes crura attaching partially to the nerve. With further migration the nerve can cross the promontory below the stapes or lie exposed, traveling directly across the floor of the middle ear. The facial nerve may appear as a soft tissue mass within the floor of the tympanic cavity, and the presence of a soft tissue mass seen on the promontory of the cochlea inferior to the oval window, and absence of the normal bony facial canal superior to the oval window (tympanic portion of the nerve) should suggest the diagnosis of an anomalous course of the facial nerve.

An aberrant course of the facial nerve canal should be suspected whenever the structures originating from Reichert's cartilage (i.e., the superstructure and lateral lamina of the stapes footplate, styloid process, stylohyoid ligament, and superior cornu of the hyoid bone) are maldeveloped. However, an isolated migration can occur with minor anomalies involving only the facial nerve canal or the facial canal and stapes.

In general, most congenitally aberrant facial nerves are short and relatively thick.[13] Occasionally, the facial nerve is in normal position but is exposed because of failed development of a complete bony wall of the facial nerve canal. In other cases, the nerve lies exposed in submucosal tissue and may cross an anomalous middle ear cavity in the region of the oval or round windows.[25]

The anomalous facial nerve may be either partially bipartite or tripartite. The most common bifid nerve extends just beneath the lateral semicircular canal as one trunk, splits into two trunks through its vertical course downward in the temporal bone, and unites either at or just outside the stylomastoid foramen into a single trunk. The more lateral of these trunks is usually the larger one, and it is the one that usually receives the chorda tympani.

During development, if the facial nerve is displaced anteriorly, the stapes is prevented from coming in contact with the otic capsule, resulting in a malformed stapes.[28] One example of this is stapes footplate fixation, the most common isolated middle ear anomaly. It must be considered in a child who has a stable conductive hearing loss without other associated middle ear pathology,[29] especially because the associated hearing loss can be corrected by appropriate intervention.[30] CT can define congenital fixation of the stapes only if the footplate is abnormally thickened on CT. Another common stapes anomaly is a single thick, monopolar stapes crus. A combined absence of the stapes superstructure and long process of the incus has been reported, reflecting the two structures' derivation from the second branchial arch.[31]

Another result of aberrant facial nerve development is congenital absence of the oval window. It is thought that the facial nerve acts as a barrier to the stapes, preventing it from inducing development of the oval window where it normally makes contact with the developing oval window.[32] This theory is supported by the association of oval window atresia aberrant course of the facial nerve, malformed incus, and displaced stapes.[33] The stapes superstructure may or may not be present, but there is no footplate or annular ligament.[34]

Anomalies of the Inner Ear

Approximately 20% of patients with congenital sensorineural hearing loss have radiographic anomalies of the inner ear.[35] Various causes that can result in sensorineural hearing loss (SNHL) are listed in (**Table 11-2**). These anomalies represent a broad range of histopathologies. In the past, attempts at classifying

Chapter 11: The Temporal Bone

Table 11-2 Sensorineural Hearing Loss

Condition	Temporal Bone and Ear Anomalies	Critical Features	Imaging
Schwannoma, Vestibular	Benign neoplasm originating from Schwann cells wrapping the vestibulocochlear nerve, particularly its vestibular division; compression of the CN VIII	Grows slowly, arising near or within IAC; majority are medium-sized; fill the funnel-shaped IAC, extending out of the porus acousticus and into the cistern as a spherical mass	MR: "mushroom" configuration with stem conforming to the IAC and the cap protruding into the CPA; T1: intense enhancement post-gadolinium; T2: hyperintense to adjacent brain tissue; CT: occasional flaring of the porus acousticus; CT + C: delineates cystic and/or solid tumor
Arachnoid Cyst, CPA	Arachnoid (meningeal) split forms CSF-containing cyst; compresses cisternal structures, i.e., vestibulocochlear nerve	75% of AC occur in children; commonly congenital	Incidental finding on MRI; MR and CT: well-defined, rounded cyst resembling CSF in signal intensity and density, respectively; T1: low intensity, T2: high intensity; complete fluid attenuation on FLAIR; no enhancement
Arteriovenous Malformation, CPA	Focal compression of vestibulocochlear nerve within CPA-IAC cistern; symptoms may also be caused by hemorrhage	Cranial neuropathy, subjective/objective pulsatile tinnitus	MRI: tangled collection of abnormal vessels; hemorrhage: T1 and T2 scans offer insight on the composition and age of blood
Cochlear Aplasia	Complete lack of cochlea	Arrested development of inner ear, in fifth week of embryogenesis resulting in profound congenital SNHL; vestibule and semicircular canals persist normally or malformed	CT: poorly developed vestibule and semicircular canals (varies), labyrinthine dysgenesis and hypoplastic cochlear cavity
Cochlear Dysplasia or Incomplete Partition (Mondini Malformation)	Cochlea lacks full 2½ turns due to arrested development during seventh week of gestation; interscalar septum and osseous spiral lamina also absent	Congenital, often bilateral, SNHL; timing of developmental cochlear arrest determines severity of disease; possible association with large ELS anomaly	CT or FSE-T2 MR: cystic cochlea, incomplete partition, or apical turn dysmorphism; present severe, moderate, and mild forms; with exception of severe dysplasia, the basal turn of cochlea is developed and visible in both CT and MR
Cochlear Hypoplasia	Small cochlea with one or less turns; extent of membranous labyrinth development dictates severity of SNHL	Arrested development of cochlea during sixth embryogenic week; normal or malformed vestibule and semicircular canals persist	CT: small, underdeveloped cochlea; malformed vestibule and semicircular canals
Otic Capsule Common Cavity	A single, common cystic cavity results from the attenuated differentiation of the cochlea, vestibule and semicircular canals	Severe congenital SNHL results from the arrested development of the otocyst in the fifth embryogenic week; although variable, the ovoid cystic space averages 7 × 10 mm in size, and lacks normal internal architecture	CT: single, large, continuous cavity within bony labyrinth; possible observation: normal middle ear and mastoid development

(Continued)

Table 11-2 Sensorineural Hearing Loss (Continued)

Condition	Temporal Bone and Ear Anomalies	Critical Features	Imaging
Complete Labyrinthine Aplasia (Michel Deformity)	Complete absence of inner ear structures	<1% of all congenital inner ear deformities; profound SNHL results from arrested development of the otic placode in the third gestational week	CT: lack of inner ear labyrinth; dense, bony appearance similar to labyrinthine ossification; differentiation factor: lateral wall remnant of inner ear is flat in MD and convex in LO (due to the lateral semicircular canal)
CPA Aneurysm	Aneurysms involving posterior inferior cerebellar, vertebral, or anterior inferior cerebellar arteries within CPA compress the facial and vestibulocochlear nerves	Partial or complete thrombosis may result in stroke and/or CN palsy; rarely cause subarachnoid hemorrhage	CT: high-density ovoid mass with calcified rim in CPA cistern; with thrombosis, T1: increased signal intensity secondary to methemoglobin; no thrombosis, MR: oval-round flow void; lumen of patent aneurysm enhances homogeneously; only rim enhances in completely thrombosed aneurysms; MRA confirmation necessary
Endolymphatic Sac Tumor	Erosive adenomatous tumor of the ELS spreads through the inner ear	Tumor enlargement invades entire posterior wall, CPA cistern and jugular foramen	T1: high signal intensity foci; T1 + C: heterogenous enhancement; CT: bony spicules within tumor matrix
Epidermoid Cyst, CPA	Congenital, nonneoplastic solid lesion that remains silent until adulthood when vestibulocochlear nerve compression occurs	Results from inclusion of ectodermal epithelia during embryogenesis; "pearly white" lobulated tumor; fills cisternal space, around cranial nerves and vessels	T1: low intensity signal and T2: high intensity signal of cisternal mass with irregular margins; MR and CT: signal close to CSF; T1 + C: no enhancement
Jugular Diverticulum	Impingement on the IAC or vestibular aqueduct	Limited to the postero-medial portion of petrous pyramid, not affecting middle ear cavity	CT: diverticulum protrudes superiorly into petrous pyramid; erosion into the IAC and/or vestibular aqueduct may be observed
Labyrinthine Ossificans	Bilateral ossification of membranous labyrinth following inflammation, infection, trauma, or surgery of the inner ear	Meningitis-induced LO is the primary cause of acquired childhood deafness	CT: bone density within fluid spaces of membranous labyrinth; FSE-T2: early signs of labyrinthine fibrosis, prior to ossification
Otic Capsule Common Cavity	A single, common cystic cavity results from the attenuated differentiation of the cochlea, vestibule, and semicircular canals	Severe congenital SNHL results from the arrested development of the otocyst in the fifth embryogenic week; although variable, the ovoid cystic space averages 7 × 10 mm in size, and lacks normal internal architecture	CT: single, large, continuous cavity within bony labyrinth; possible observation: normal middle ear and mastoid development

AC = arachnoid cyst, CPA = cerebellopontine angle, CN = cranial nerve, CSF = cerebrospinal fluid, ELS = endolym-phatic sac, FSE = fast spin echo, IAC = internal auditory canal, LO = labyrinthine ossification, MD = Michel deformity, SNHL = sensorineural hearing loss.

these anomalies relied heavily on certain restricted categorical types. Because many of the observed anomalies did not fit these defined types, there were many difficulties in classification. A description based on anatomic terms appears to be more accurate and practical. Some of the histologic types are described here because they represent classic descriptions that are widely used in the literature.

Membranous Labyrinth

The membranous labyrinth is the fundamental part of the ear. It is the first to form, preceding the development of other portions of the inner ear. As the acoustic nerve develops, its peripheral process reaches the membranous wall. The epithelium then becomes modified into the neural epithelium for the end organs of hearing and equilibrium.[11]

Many genetically determined anomalies, such as the Bing-Siebenmann and Scheibe types, involve portions of the membranous labyrinth, including the basilar membrane, organ of Corti, or spiral ganglia. Bing-Siebenmann deformity is complete membranous labyrinthine dysplasia and is extremely rare. In Scheibe's dysplasia, abnormalities are limited to the saccule and cochlea due to maldevelopment of the pars inferior. It is believed to be the most frequent cause of congenital deafness.[10,36,37] Radiographic diagnosis is precluded in these anomalies because the osseous labyrinth is normal.[35]

Bony Labyrinth

Semicircular Canals

Malformation of the lateral semicircular canal is one of the most common inner ear anomalies.[35,36,38,39] This occurs because the lateral semicircular canal is the last to develop, after the superior and posterior semicircular canals. Malformation of the superior and posterior semicircular canals without involvement of the lateral canal is unusual. The malformed canals are either narrow or more commonly are short and wide. In extensive malformation the vestibule is dilated and forms a common lumen with the lateral canal. In some cases it may not be possible to identify the canals because the lumen is obliterated or the canals are absent. When the canals are absent, there is typical flattening of the corresponding portion of the otic capsule. The correct diagnosis is readily made on thin gradient echo images, showing a fluid-filled common utriculo–saccular-lateral semicircular duct cavity. Subtle changes like short or wide semicircular ducts and even localized protrusions of the semicircular ducts can be recognized on gradient echo images.

Narrowing or absence of the semicircular ducts may be detected on MR, but the differentiation from a partially or totally calcified or fibrous obliteration is possible only when an additional CT image of the inner ear is performed. In cases of semicircular duct aplasia, no fluid is seen within the ducts on MR, and the semicircular canal is absent on CT. However, partial or total loss of the fluid within a semicircular duct on MR also can be caused by fibrous or calcified obliteration of this duct, and this will correspond to a normal or partially calcified semicircular canal on CT.

The first cases of bilateral semicircular duct aplasia in combination with normal or near normal cochleas were reported by Parnes and Chernoff.[40] If such an anomaly were caused by arrested development, the cochlea should be malformed as well. Thus, occasionally, a specific aberration may take place, halting further development at a confined level.[39] These patients present with vertigo or abnormal findings during vestibular testing, and absence of fluid in the semicircular ducts is seen on the gradient echo images. Confirmation of the absence of the semicircular canals on CT is necessary to differentiate this entity from fibrous or calcified obliteration of the semicircular ducts and canals.

Superior semicircular canal dehiscence is another malformation that affects the semicircular canals. It is an entity which should be sought in patients presenting with vertigo triggered by straining, heavy lifting, or loud noise, known as Tullio's phenomenon[38] (**Fig. 11-5**). Normally, the oval and round windows are the only two openings to the inner ear pressure system. Sound waves are transmitted to the oval window via the ossicular chain, travel through the cochlea, and dissipate through the round window. When there is dehiscence of the roof of the superior semicircular canal, the dehiscence acts as a "third mobile window" through which sound pressure can be transmitted to the vestibular apparatus.[41] This results in unphysiological motion of endolymph in the affected semicircular canal, and thus, sound induced vertigo. Typically, superior semicircular canal dehiscence is identified with high-resolution CT, in which there is an absence of bone forming the roof of the semicircular canal.[42,43] However, reliable identification of the malformation using heavily T2-weighted fast spin-echo MRI has been described.[44]

Vestibule/Utriculosaccular Structures

Anomalies of the vestibule or utriculosaccular structures rarely occur as an isolated event; more frequently, they are present in association with other inner ear anomalies.[45] The vestibular anomalies consist of complete or partial assimilation of the semicircular canals (usually the lateral semicircular canal) into the vestibule.[26] Rarely, an enlarged, globular vestibule may be found. This anomaly of the inner ear has been associated with thalidomide-induced deafness.[45] Occasionally, subtle enlargement or malformation of the utriculosaccular structures and semicircular canals can be reliably detected only on MRI when thin images with high contrast between the intralabyrinthine fluid and the surrounding bone are obtained.

Cochlea

Jackler has advanced a classification of cochlear anomalies based on the hypothesis that the various morphologic patterns result from an arrest of maturation during stages of inner ear embryogenesis.[35] The following represents the spectrum of cochlear abnormalities corresponding to the arrested stage of development (**Fig. 11-6**).

Complete labyrinthine aplasia (Michel's Deformity). In complete labyrinthine aplasia there is no inner ear development. In place of the normal inner ear structures, a small, single cystic cavity or several small cavities are present. This description corresponds to the histopathology classically described by Michel and represents an early failure in development correlating to the third gestational week. It is essentially an aplasia of the inner ear. It is extremely rare.[41] Complete labyrinthine aplasia must be differentiated from labyrinthitis ossificans, which is usually acquired through childhood meningitis. In labyrinthine ossificans,

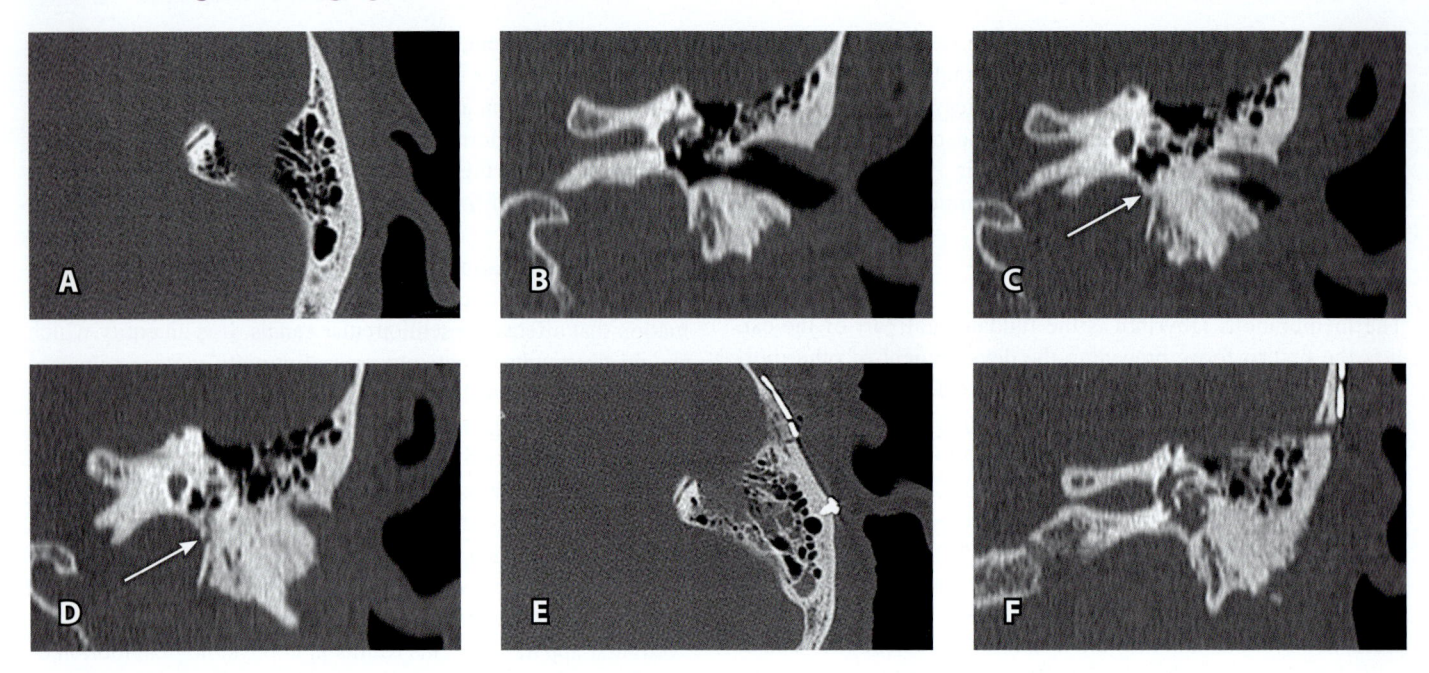

Figure 11-5 Tullio Phenomenon Pre and Postoperative
Axial (**A**) and coronal (**B–D**) preoperative CT images in a patient with superior semicircular canal (SSC) dehiscence (*arrows*, **C, D**). The dehiscence is evident as a lack of cortical bone between the SSC and the superior margin of the temporal bone. Axial (**E**) and coronal (**F**) CT scans following placement of a dural graft over the SSC dehiscence following a squamous temporal craniotomy to gain access to the floor of the middle cranial fossa.

the dense otic capsule is present and is evidenced by the presence of a promontory bulge in the middle ear on CT.[46] In labyrinthine aplasia, the otic capsule is absent, as is the promontory bulge. Also, in labyrinthine aplasia, the petrous bone is hypoplastic.[47] It is important to differentiate complete labyrinthine aplasia from labyrinthitis ossificans because the former is an absolute contraindication for cochlear implantation, while implantation has been successful in some patients with the latter.[28,48,49]

Common cavity
Arrested growth during the fourth fetal week results in a common cavity for the cochlea and vestibule. This is a relatively common malformation, constituting 26% of cochlear malformations.[41] There is a large cystic cavity with no internal architecture. The semicircular canals may be normal or malformed. The labyrinthine segment of the facial nerve can be displaced anteromedially. On axial CT, a common cavity can be differentiated from lateral semicircular canal dysplasia by its anterior position with respect to the IAC[50] (**Fig. 11-7**).

Cochlear aplasia
Arrested development during the fifth week of embryogenesis produces aplasia of the cochlea. The cochlea fails to form and appears as a single cavity. The other elements of the inner ear (i.e., the vestibule and semicircular canal) may be normal or malformed. These patients typically have profound sensorineural hearing loss, and implantation may be contraindicated by the lack of an auditory nerve.[51]

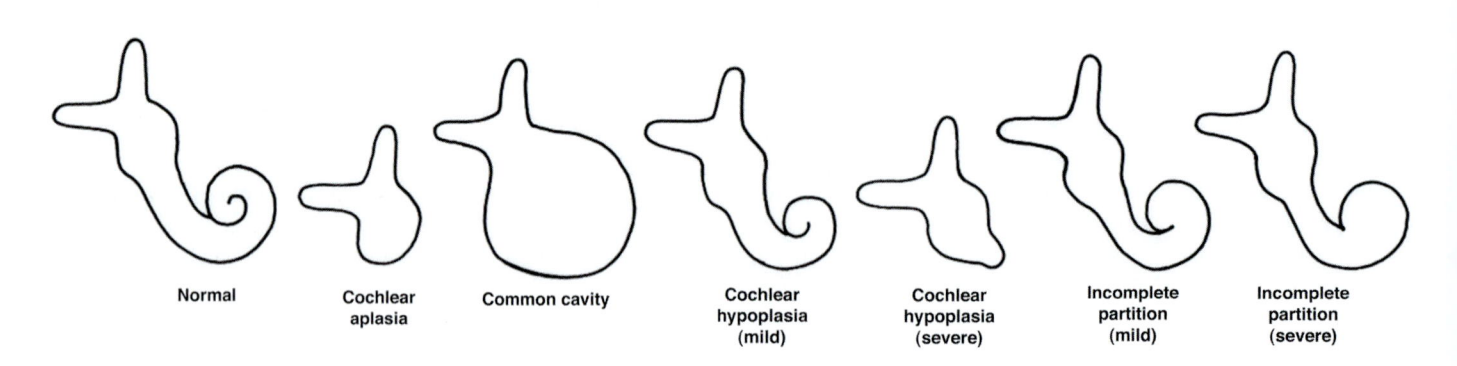

Figure 11-6 Congenital Cochlear Abnormalities
Schematic representation of the radiographic appearance of labyrinth malformations. (From Jackler RK, Luxford WM, House WF: Congenital malformations of the inner ear. Laryngoscope 1987;97:2–14.)

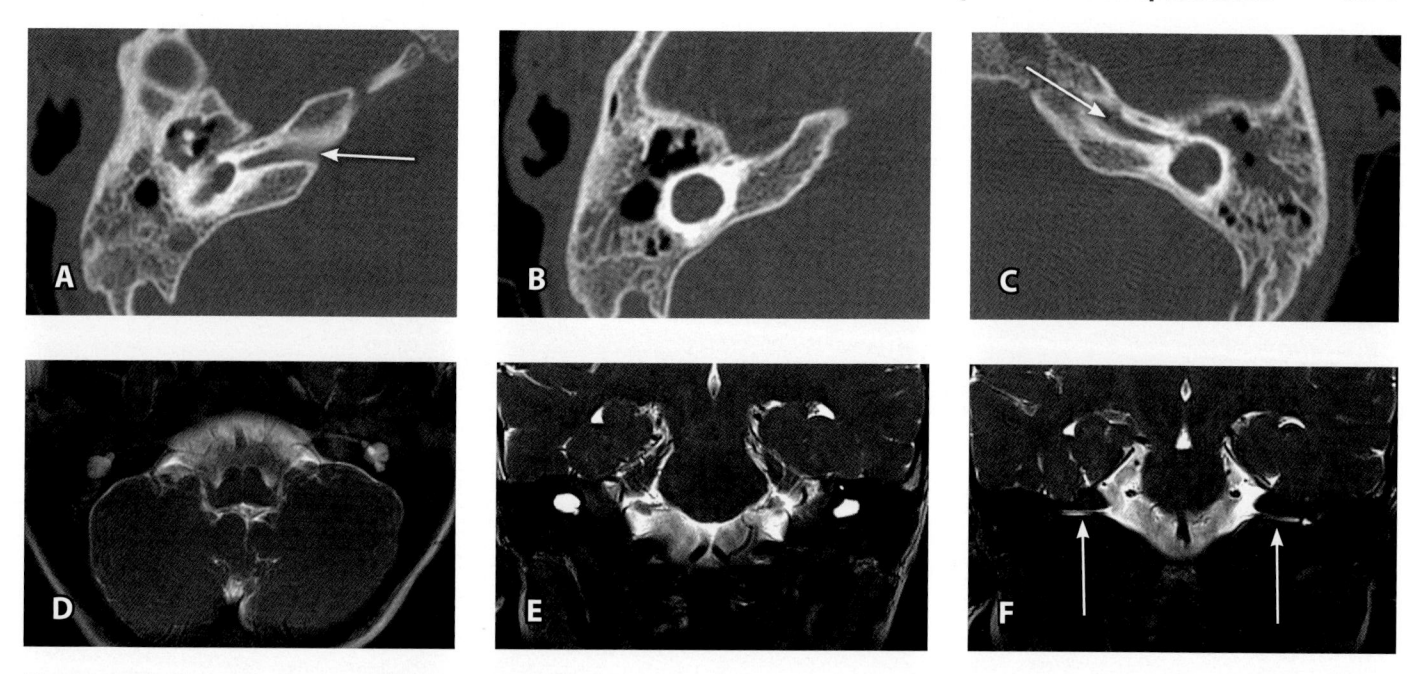

Figure 11-7 Common Cavity with Nerve Aplasia
Common cavities of the inner ears with bilateral vestibulocochlear nerve aplasias, aka cystic cochleovestibular anomaly. Axial CT (**A–C**), axial T2W MRI (**D**), and coronal T2W MRI (**E, F**) of the temporal bone. The cochlea, vestibule, and semicircular canals appear as a single common cavity bilaterally (**A–E**). The middle ear structures are normal (**A, B**). The internal auditory canal is markedly reduced in caliber bilaterally (arrows, **A, C, F**) to accommodate the facial nerves that are uninvolved. On axial (**E**) and coronal (**E**) MR images, the common cavity appears as a high signal intensity fluid within the cystic fused cochleas and vestibules.

Cochlear hypoplasia

Cochlear hypoplasia displays a small rudimentary cochlear bud associated with a normal or malformed vestibule and semicircular canals. A cessation of cochlear development during the sixth week of intrauterine life is the probable cause of this defect. Patients have differing degrees of hearing loss depending on the degree of membranous labyrinthine development within the truncated cochlear lumen.[36]

Incomplete partition (classic Mondini's malformation)

This entity represents a small cochlea with incomplete or no interscalar septa. There is a basilar cochlear turn and a common cloaca or cavity where the middle and apical turns would be. Anomalies of the remaining inner ear, such as dilatation of the vestibular aqueduct, may be present. Arrest of maturation at the seventh week of intrauterine life may result in these findings. Incomplete partition of the cochlea characterizes a classic histologic malformation first described by Mondini in 1791 (**Fig. 11-8**). Mondini documented a flat cochlea, having 1½ turns instead of the normal 2½ to 2¾ turns. He also described a large vestibule with wide, small, or missing semicircular canals and immature sensorineural structures.[52] The vestibular aqueduct is almost always enlarged. The interscalar septal defect and absence of the osseous spiral lamina of the middle and apical turns can best be demonstrated on heavily T2-weighted gradient echo images.[53] The interscalar septal defects of the middle and apical turns results in a scala communis cochleae. Aside from Scheibe's deafness, Mondini's malformation is probably the most common form of genetic deafness.[54]

Internal Auditory Canal and Cochlear Nerve Aplasia

The IAC may be either stenosed or even atretic. A narrow IAC, especially in the presence of IAC stenosis and thickening of the modiolus, is classically associated with aplasia of the vestibulocochlear nerve.[36,41,55,56] However, it should be noted that cochlear nerve aplasia and hypoplasia can be found in normal size IACs,[57] as has been described in up to 39%[58] to 58%[59] of cases. Thus, MRI should be performed in all cases of profound pediatric hearing loss.

Cochlear nerve aplasia is not an uncommon cause of congenital hearing loss. It is best identified with high resolution thin section T2-weighted MR images, using oblique plane sagittal view imaging.[60] There are three types of vestibulocochlear nerve aplasia and hypoplasia. In type 1, there is aplasia of the vestibulocochlear nerve with stenosis of the IAC. In type 2a, there is a aplasia of the cochlear branch in the presence of a labyrinthine malformation (**Fig. 11-9**). Finally, in type 2b, there is aplasia of the cochlear branch in the presence of a normal labyrinth. Cochlear nerve aplasia is one of the few absolute contraindications for cochlear implantation.[61]

Mri of Inner Ear Anomalies

There are several situations in which MRI has gained importance in the study of inner ear anomalies. Patients with isolated inner ear malformations present with SNHL or vertigo. Following childhood and in cases of asymmetric SNHL, congenital inner ear malformations may not be clinically suspected. Such patients are usually referred for MRI, principally to rule out a

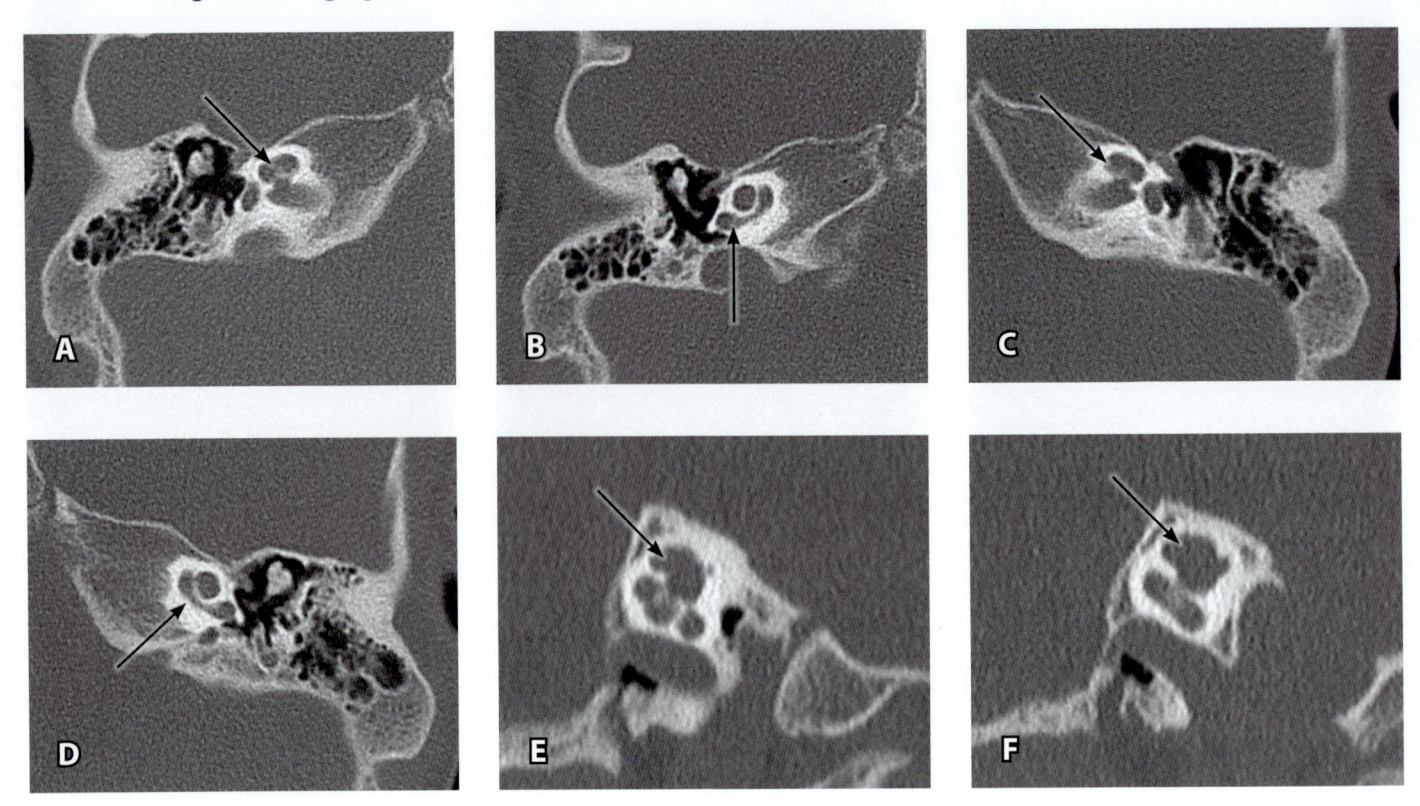

Figure 11-8 Mondini Malformation and CSF Gusher AU
Mondini malformation (incomplete partition): Axial CT of the right (**A, B**) and left (**C, D**) ears and sagittal reconstruction of the right (**E**) and left (**F**) ear demonstrate bilateral classic Mondini malformation. There are normal basilar turns (*arrows*, **B, D**), but cystic cochlear apices (*arrows*, **A, C**) where the middle and apical turns would normally be. There is bilateral deficiency of the modiolus and enlargement of the cochlear aperture seen on the axial images (*arrows*, **A, C**) and on the reformatted sagittal images (*arrows*, **E, F**).

vestibular schwannoma (VS) or other posterior fossa lesions.[62] MRI protocols need to be adapted to include thin gradient echo images to detect clinically unsuspected congenital malformations, which are known to occur in up to 2.3% of inner ear studies.[63]

Gradient echo MRI allows for detailed evaluation of the membranous labyrinth with visualization of the intralabyrinthine fluid spaces. This technique enables excellent visualization of membranous labyrinthine pathology in an otherwise normal bony labyrinth. High spatial-resolution MRI makes it possible to differentiate between the scala tympani and the scala vestibuli. Reissner's membrane and the organ of Corti, structures that are involved in Bing-Siebenmann and Scheibe dysplasias, may be too small to detect with MRI. This technique has shown great value in demonstrating fibrous obliteration of the scala tympani and the scala vestibuli in patients with congenital inner ear malformations requiring cochlear implantation.

The diagnosis of vestibulocochlear nerve aplasia or hypoplasia can be made with thin gradient echo images. These images are able to show the facial nerve, the cochlear nerve, and the superior and inferior vestibular branches of the vestibulocochlear nerve separately inside the IAC. The thickness of individual nerves can be optimally evaluated in the oblique sagittal plane.

A suggested MR protocol for temporal bone imaging is shown below (Table 11-3).

Imaging Techniques

Routine selective 3 mm thick contiguous T1W spin echo images before and after intravenous gadolinium contrast administration and routine serial 7 mm or selective 4 mm thick T2W spin echo images can detect some congenital inner ear malformations. Only thin gradient echo images are sensitive enough to detect all congenital inner ear malformations. The whole membranous labyrinth is approximately 12 mm high and 1 mm thick, and sections less than 1 mm thick must be used to study this small structure. Good in plane spatial resolution (0.7 or 0.8 mm) and optimal contrast between the intralabyrinthine fluid and the surrounding bone and nerves is required. Heavily T2W gradient echo images can provide such images with bright intralabyrinthine fluid and dark surrounding bone and nerves. Several gradient echo techniques like three-dimensional (3D) Fourier transform fast imaging with steady precession (3DFT-FISP) and constructive interference in steady state (3DFT-CISS) have proven to be valuable in the study of the membranous labyrinth and IAC.[64] Pre- and postcontrast 2 mm thick fast spin echo techniques also can be helpful.[65]

In one study, the T1W images only showed portions of the congenital malformations, or the malformations were not visible

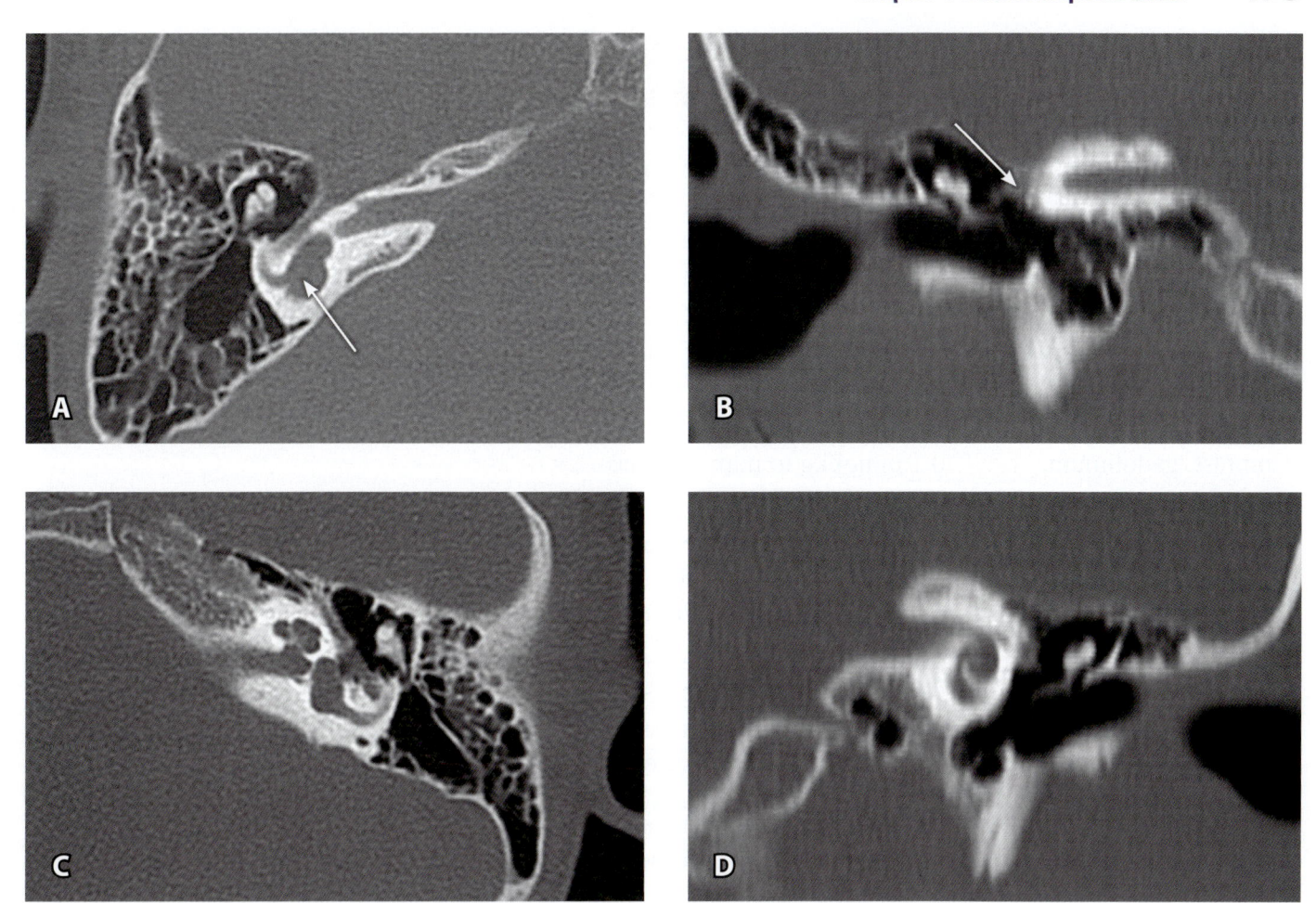

Figure 11-9 Cochlear Aplasia and Semicircular Canal Dysplasia
Axial (**A**) and coronal (**B**) CT images show complete absence of the cochlea and the cochlear nerve with a narrowed internal auditory canal (IAC). The narrowing is less than that seen in **Fig. 11-7**, as the vestibular nerve fibers are encompassed within the lumen of the IAC. The vestibule and semicircular canals are dilated and malformed (*arrow*, **A**). There is absence of the cochlea evident on coronal CT (*arrow*, **B**). Normal left side for comparison Axial (**C**) and coronal (**D**) CT in the left ear show a normal cochlea (*arrow*), vestibule (*arrow*), and semicircular canals.

in 40% of the patients. Nearly all anomalies were recognized on the thin gradient echo images.[63]

The ability to acquire MR images in multiple planes and the use of multiplanar reconstructions further facilitates the detection and detailed evaluation of inner ear malformations. Visualization of the inner ear structures in three dimensions allows better visualization of the complexity of the inner structures and their interrelationships avoiding the need for mental reconstruction using two-dimensional images. Maximum intensity projection (MIP) is one such technique in which high-resolution 512 × 512 matrix gradient echo images provide images with good spatial resolution (0.31 × 0.39 mm). These images can demonstrate the scala tympani and vestibuli separately and have the potential to detect subtle intracochlear pathology, particularly with its ability to visualize the 2.5 windings of the cochlea. In general, MIP has proven to be useful for assessing details in structures with gradual transitions between different surfaces.[66] MIP, however, has partial volume artifacts and poor spatial resolution. Volume reconstruction, a 3D rendering technique by which a simulated source is applied to acquire a 3D perspective by adding light and shadow, allows excellent spatial delineation of the inner ear structures. It was found to allow superior visualization of the three ampullae and give better spatial information regarding the vestibule and semicircular canals when compared with MIP. It is becoming more popular due to improvements in computer power and memory size.[67–69]

Malformations of the Petrous Bone Associated with Meningitis

Cerebrospinal fluid (CSF) leakage from the petrous bone structures is a rare and potentially life-threatening condition.[70] This cryptic condition typically develops as a result of trauma or following the destructive effects of infection. An associated congenital abnormality of the temporal bone should always be suspected in cases of recurrent meningitis, especially when there is hearing impairment. Most of these patients have a history of

Table 11-3 Temporal Bone Imaging MR Protocol

Precontrast brain	Sagittal T1WI, axial T2WI, axial FLAIR, and axial DWI through whole brain
Precontrast temporal bone	Axial T1WI through temporal bone from arcuate eminence through mastoid tip with TR of 300 ms, TE of 12 ms, flip angle of 90 degrees, slice thickness of 3 mm, distance factor of 0.10, matrix of 192–256, and FOV of 180 mm with 2 acquisitions. Imaging time of 3 min and 15 s
Precontrast IAC	Axial CISS or 3D FIESTA through IAC's and pons with TR of 12.25 ms, TE of 5.9 ms, flip angle of 70 degrees, slab thickness of 32 mm, effective thickness of 0.7 mm, 46 partitions, matrix of 230 × 512, FOV of 200 mm. Imaging time of 4 min and 20 s.
Contrast: gadolinium	0.1 mmol/kg to max of 20 cc
Postcontrast brain	Axial T1WI through whole brain
Postcontrast temporal bone (Two interleaved sets)	Axial T1WI through temporal bone with TR of 450 ms, TE of 15 ms, flip angle of 90 degrees, slice thickness of 2 mm, distance factor of 0.1, matrix of 192 × 256, FOV of 170 mm, with 2 acquisitions. Imaging time of 4 min 20 s for each set, total time of 8 min 40 s
Postcontrast IAC	Coronal T1WI through IAC with TR of 450 ms, TE of 15 ms, flip angle of 90 degrees, slice thickness of 3 mm, no gap, matrix of 192 × 256, FOV of 170 mm, with 3 acquisitions. Imaging time of 4 min and 22 s

TR = time to repetition, TE = echo time, FLAIR = fluid attenuated inversion recovery, DWI = diffusion weighted imaging, CISS = constructive interference in steady state, FIESTA = fast imaging employing steady-state acquisition, IAC = internal auditory canal, FOV = field of view.
Caruso P, et al.: Temporal Bone Imaging Technique, in Imaging of the Temporal Bone, Swartz JD and Harnsberger HR, eds. New York: Thieme, 2009.

recurrent meningitis and persistent otorrhea, rhinorrhea, or both; but some may have no otologic symptoms. When suspected, it is essential to document subtle sites of bone dura discontinuities.

CSF fistulas conveniently have been described according to their various entrances and exits that occur across the complex anatomy of the temporal bone.[71] The following discussion classifies these lesions according to their entrances, with identification of their corresponding exits.

Translabyrinthine Fistulas

A CSF fistula commonly associated with recurrent meningitis takes a translabyrinthine route in individuals with inner ear malformations. There are two aberrant communications that must be present for a translabyrinthine fistula to occur: 1) a communication from the subarachnoid space to the inner ear, 2) a communication from the inner ear to the middle ear.[41]

The IAC is one of the most frequently observed entrances of CSF from the subarachnoid space into the inner ear.[7] The canal is normally filled with CSF to its most lateral extent, where it is separated from the vestibule by the thin lamina cribrosa. The vestibular and cochlear nerves penetrate this thin bony layer to enter the inner ear. Defects in the development of the lamina cribrosa[7,45,72] or the existence of patent perineural pathways[70,73] accompanying the nerves piercing this plate can allow communication between the subarachnoid space and the perilymphatic fluid.[7,45,70,72,73]

Symptoms of translabyrinthine fistulas are variable. If the tympanic membrane is intact, the patient will have CSF rhinorrhea. If the tympanic membrane is perforated, the patient will have CSF otorrhea.[74] Other symptoms may include hearing loss, serous otitis media, loss of caloric responses, and pseudo Ménière's disease.[71,75] At times, no clinical evidence of a fistula is present.

This abnormal communication between CSF and perilymph causes the hydrostatic pressure within the inner ear to increase. This state of "perilymphatic hydrops" has been postulated to cause displacement, perforation, or both of the stapes footplate.[10,71] (The round window is involved less frequently.) This defect allows communication to the middle ear, or communication may be established when the surgeon manipulates or removes the stapedial footplate "stapes gusher."[7] This leak is difficult to manage and often results in hearing loss or is complicated by meningitis.

On CT, there will often be an absence of a bony separation between the cochlea/vestibule and IAC. The IAC can have a bulbous shape.[53] Associated with the fistula may be a variety of inner ear malformations, the most common being an enlarged and confluent vestibule and lateral semicircular canal. The cochlea is often cystic and is devoid of internal architecture[7,35] (**Fig. 11-10**). Direct evidence of the CSF fistula route may be difficult to elucidate owing to the complex anatomy and at times the lack of obvious leakage. Various imaging materials have

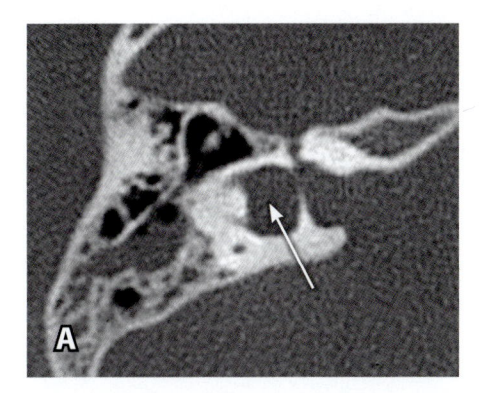

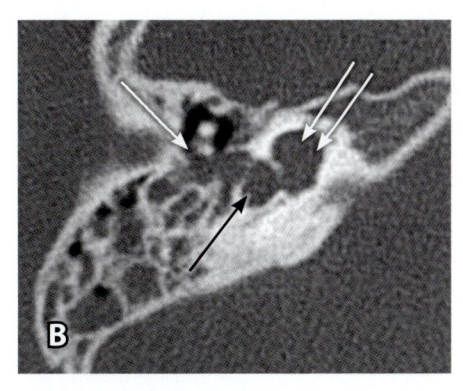

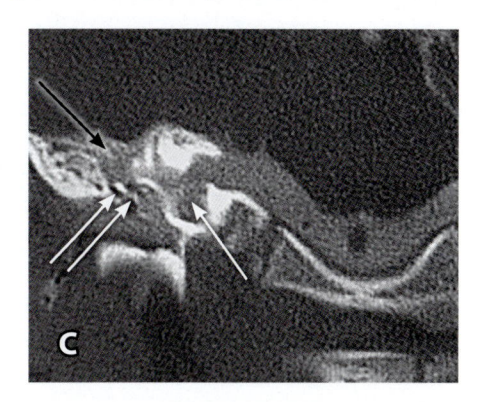

Figure 11-10 Deafness with Recurrent Episodes of Meningitis
Axial CT images through the right temporal bone show opacification and air–fluid levels in the antrum and tympanic cavity (*white arrow*, **B**). The inner ear is dysplastic, the internal auditory canal (IAC) is bulbous (*arrow*, **A**), and there is cystic vestibulocochlear anomaly formed by the cochlea (*double white arrows*, **B**) and the vestibule (*single black arrow*). Coronal CT myelogram after injecting intrathecal contrast shows a normal contrast collection in the CPA and IAC. However, there is abnormal spread to the vestibule (*white arrow*, **C**), as evidence of subarachnoid space-inner ear communication. There is also contrast in the middle ear (*double white arrows*, **C**), mastoid air cells (*black arrow*, **C**), and external auditory canal on the right, evidence of inner ear–middle ear communication.

been injected into the subarachnoid space, usually by lumbar puncture, to document these fistulas. Nuclear-tagged substances (i.e., technetium DTPA, radioactive iodinated serum albumin, or indium) may accumulate in and localize the affected ear.[52,70,75] Dyes such as indigo carmine may be injected and visualized either as leaking into the middle ear or as discoloration of the tympanic membrane, nose, and nasopharynx. An intrathecal injection of a nonionic radiographic contrast agent may be used to outline the defect, and CT of the petrous pyramid has become an integral part of the workup. Defects may be directly visualized (i.e., intrathecally injected contrast material may be seen in the labyrinth), and any associated inner ear abnormalities can be demonstrated simultaneously.

In these situations, MRI may be helpful as a noninvasive way of localizing the route of CSF leak. 3D fast spin echo T2-weighted imaging and 3D FIESTA techniques have proven useful in identifying fistulous routes.[74] Flow-sensitive MRI has been shown to detect flow rates as low as 0.5 cc per second.[76]

Surgical closure of the fistula should be undertaken some time after complete recovery from meningitis.[73] The method of correction is dictated by the functional status of the ear, the size of the fistula, and the quantity of fluid issuing from the fistula. If hearing and vestibular function are to be preserved, a tissue graft of fat, venous wall, or fibrous tissue is placed to inhibit the leakage. If the leakage continues, the stapes can be removed and a graft can be placed to cover the oval window. A stapes prosthesis is then placed to preserve hearing and to hold the graft in place. If preservation of vestibular or auditory function, or both, is not an issue, the fistula may be closed by a tissue implant into the vestibule.[52]

Direct Subarachnoid Space – Middle Ear Fistulas

Direct subarachnoid space–middle ear fistulas include dehiscence of the tegmen tympani, aberrant arachnoid granulation, giant apical air cell, defect in the facial nerve canal, or Hyrtl's fissure.

Dehiscence of the tegmen tympani results from congenital absence of a portion of the tegmen tympani.[71] If there is an associated defect in the adjacent meninges, CSF can reach the middle ear.[12] In contradistinction to IAC defects, these patients tend to be adults. As a result of the lack of inner ear involvement, the patients usually have no inner ear signs.[12,71] Coronal CT of the petrous pyramid typically demonstrates incomplete development of the tegmen tympani. There may be an associated meningocele protruding into the middle ear. Treatment consists of neurosurgical repair of the bone and meningeal defects.

Hyrtl's fissure is a congenital cleft between the posterior fossa and the hypotympanum lying in proximity to the cochlear aqueduct and jugular fossa.[41,77] Like other direct subarachnoid space-middle ear fistulas, the degree of hearing loss is much less than in translabyrinthine fistulas.

Wide Cochlear Aqueduct

Many investigators have confirmed a communication of CSF and perilymph through the cochlear aqueduct.[78] Normally, the flow is directed from the labyrinth through the aqueduct to the cisternal spaces. Some authors believe that the narrow adult aqueduct is not patent at all and that the fluids intermingle by diffusion through the membranous structure of the aqueduct.[36] In contrast to the adult state, the cochlear aqueduct in children is patulous and short and may communicate directly with the subarachnoid space. The persistence of this fetal type wide aqueduct has been postulated as causing a retrograde flow of CSF into the vestibule.[71,73] The pulsating pressure of the CSF transmitted to the perilymphatic spaces sets the stage for "perilymphatic hydrops" with its accompanying lesions in or near the stapes footplate ("stapes gusher"). The pressure can cause an intermittent leak of fluid from inner to middle ear. A patient with such a perilymphatic fistula has progressive, fluctuating mixed hearing loss that was not present earlier in life.[71] Because there is a conductive component, the patient may be considered a candidate

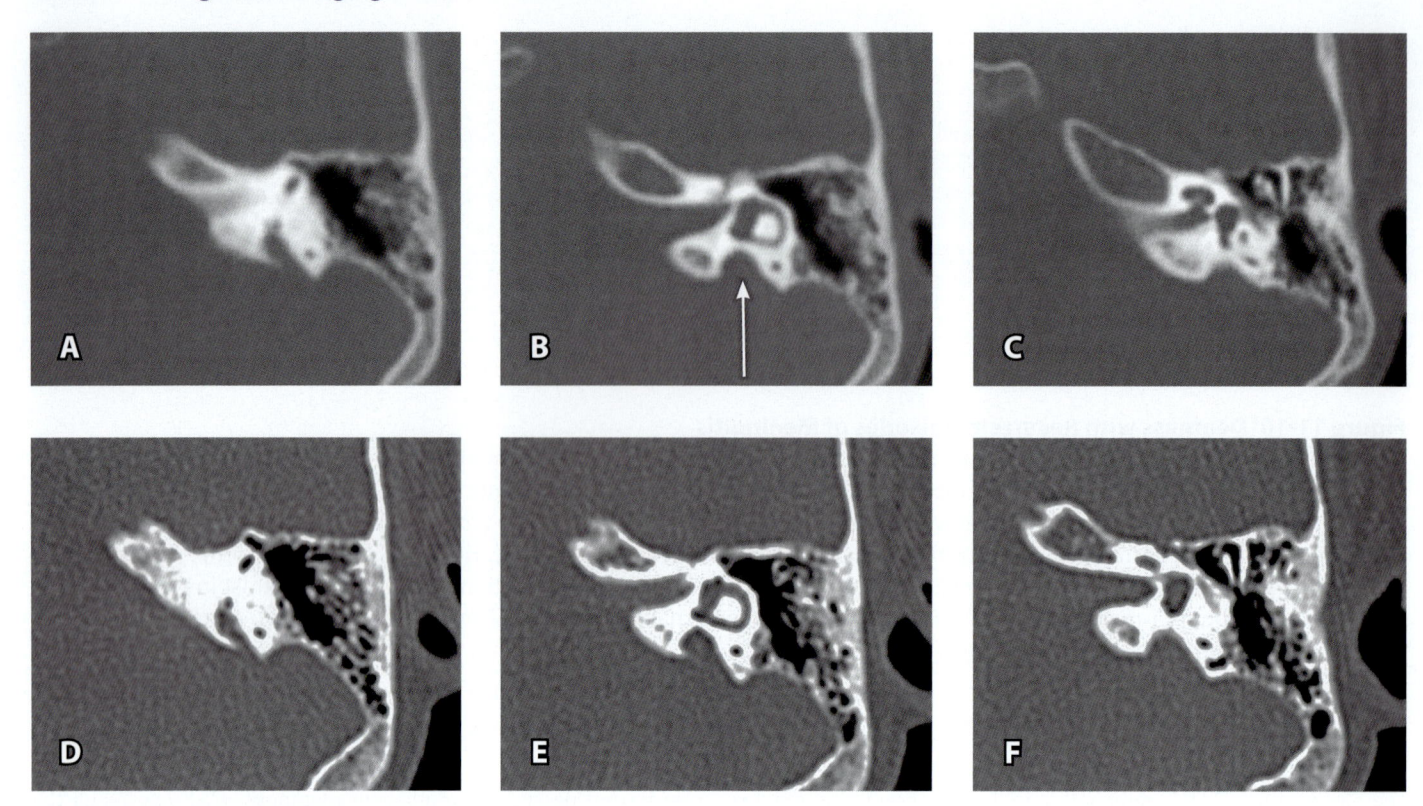

Figure 11-11 Large Endolymphatic Duct and Sac
Comparative images of a patient with recurrent episodes of hearing loss and dizziness following minor head trauma. Axial CT (**A–C**) obtained following the first episode show a markedly enlarged endolymphatic duct sac with expansion of the vestibular aqueduct (*arrow*). Low dose axial CT scans (**D–F**) obtained after the second episode of dizziness and hearing loss five years later.

for stapes footplate surgery such as is done in otosclerosis. If the otologist drills through the stapes, a connection is made between the inner and middle ears, and the perilymph "gushes" into the middle ear. This can cause significant acute hearing loss.

CT demonstrates a short, widely patent cochlear aqueduct (**Fig. 11-11**). This anomaly may be associated with a variety of inner ear malformations as described with IAC fistulas. The concept of CT detection of a dilated cochlear aqueduct is somewhat controversial. The cochlear aqueduct normally tapers laterally toward the labyrinth, and the significance of an isolated dilatation of the medial segment is unclear.

Treatment of a perilymphatic fistula may include ablation of the cochlear aqueduct, tight packing of the vestibule with tissue grafts, or a combination of these approaches.[7]

Perilymphatic Fistula

Perilymphatic fistulas are abnormal paths of communication from the inner ear to the middle ear. They may be congenital, spontaneous, posttraumatic, or secondary to barotrauma or sudden physical exertion.[41] Congenital perilymphatic fistulas occur most frequently at the stapes and at the round window.[79] Pneumolabyrinth, or air bubbles in the inner ear that are demonstrated by CT, are highly suggestive of perilymphatic fistula.[80,81] However, it is a rare finding. Thus, image diagnosis of fluid flow through the fistula into the middle ear is required. Just as in CSF fistula diagnosis, iodinated contrast[82] or radionuclides[83] can be administered into the intrathecal space, usually by lumbar puncture. However, recently, high-resolution T2-weighted MRI has been used to visualize fluid leakage into the tympanic cavity.[84]

Congenital Syndromes Involving the Ear

Syndromes associated with congenital anomalies of the ear are usually the result of an inherited disorder, although substrate damage in utero as a result of an external teratogen may occur in some cases. Hearing loss associated with these syndromes tends to be severe and is less responsive to correction because the onset is early and there are significant architectural anomalies present.

It is convenient to organize these syndromes into major classification groups according to their dominant morphologic features. The clinical and radiographic findings in these syndromes have been collected and categorized into various clinical groups. The groups consist of the otocraniofacial syndromes, otocervical syndromes, otoskeletal syndromes, and miscellaneous syndromes. These groups are described and classified in **"Appendix 11-1 Congenital Syndromes Involving the Ear"**.

Otocraniofacial Syndromes

The otocraniofacial syndromes consist of anomalies of the ear, skull, and face. This group contains dominantly inherited syndromes involving the structures derived from the first and second branchial arches. These arch anomalies invariably involve the EAC with varying degrees of stenosis or atresia. The middle ear is typically involved with ossicular and facial canal abnormalities. Various facial asymmetries, as well as calvarial anomalies, are present in all cases. Occasionally, there may be inner ear anomalies.

Otocervical Syndromes

Otocervical syndromes include anomalies of the ear, neck, and shoulder. The ear anomalies occur less frequently with the otocervical syndromes than with the otocraniofacial syndromes. The dominant features of this group are malformations of the cervical vertebrae, which consist primarily of fusion of one or more of the vertebral bodies. Typically, there tends to be inner ear involvement, with occasional anomalies of the branchial arch systems.

Otoskeletal Syndromes

The otoskeletal syndromes consist of anomalies of the ear, face, and limbs. The common feature is abnormalities involving portions of the osseous skeleton. The otic manifestations of the otoskeletal syndromes portray a bony hyperactivity with osseous infiltration and narrowing of the various bony fissures and foramina. The associated skeletal anomalies tend to repeat this common theme of bony overgrowth.

Other Syndromes

Several other syndromes have associated otic anomalies representing a broad range of morphologic types. The prominent features range from metabolic disorders to purely structural anomalies. The range of otic anomalies crosses over anatomic boundaries to engulf every aspect of the ear, representing a basic mesenchymal defect caused by a particular teratogen, for example, thalidomide.

Recently, the CT findings in the syndrome of "X-linked congenital mixed deafness, fixation of the stapedial foot plate, and perilymphatic gusher" (XDFG) were described. The IAC is large and communicates with the cochlea through a malformed modiolus and defect in the cochlear base. The CSF pressure is transmitted to the perilymph via the defect. When the stapes is perforated surgically, the abrupt pressure change gives an acute drop in hearing.[85]

VASCULAR ANOMALIES

Internal Carotid Artery Anomalies

Aberrant (Lateral) Course

An aberrant course of the internal carotid artery through the middle ear is rare.[86] More than 90% of the cases described in the literature occur in females, with the majority occurring on the right side.[87] No convincing explanation for this predominance in females or of the right side has been presented.[88]

There is no universally accepted etiology for this anomaly.[86] Among the proposed mechanisms is a congenital failure of ossification of the bony limiting wall of the petrous carotid canal. Some authors have reported that the bony plate is frequently less than 0.5 mm thick, and with age, as the vessel elongates and becomes tortuous, it may protrude through the defect into the tympanic cavity.[87,88] Persistence of embryonic vessels also may produce sufficient traction to pull the artery into the middle ear[87] (Fig. 11-12).

In these cases, otalgia has been reported as one of the initial symptoms.[89] Other signs and symptoms include tinnitus, hearing loss (mostly conductive), a red blue pulsatile mass behind the tympanic membrane, vertigo, and the sensation of fullness in the ear.[87,88] The tinnitus may be caused either by the direct mechanical transmission of the vessel's pulsations to the tympanic membrane and ossicles or by the audible sound produced by arterial blood flow emanating from the abnormal vessel within the middle ear. The hearing loss may be the result of the mass effect of the vessel (e.g., the dampening of the tympanic membrane vibrations or encroachment or erosion of the ossicles).[87] Many patients are asymptomatic.

Not infrequently, the red blue mass behind the tympanic membrane has been inadvertently ruptured during therapeutic myringotomy, biopsy for suspected glomus tumors, or both. This has resulted in catastrophic hemorrhage from the middle ear, emergently treated by ear packing.

CT shows an enhancing soft tissue mass in the hypotympanum extending toward the oval window area, indenting the promontory and displacing the tympanic membrane laterally.[87] Grooving of the apical, middle, and basilar turns of the cochlea by the artery also may be seen.[86] A stapedial artery, which is seen as a soft tissue mass in the middle ear with an enlargement of the tympanic portion of the facial canal, is often present. The persistent stapedial artery passes through the crura of the stapes and then passes into the tympanic facial nerve canal. The vessel then passes from the region of the geniculate ganglion to the floor of the middle cranial fossa before continuing as the middle meningeal artery. On coronal views, the limiting lateral wall of the carotid canal is absent, and the enlarged facial canal is visible above the cochlea.[9] On axial views, the bony posterolateral portion of the canal is absent[86] (Fig. 11-13).

Internal carotid angiography documents a large carotid artery that is deviated laterally and buckled beyond the "vestibular line." The vestibular line is a vertical line drawn tangential to the lateral margin of the vestibule on an anteroposterior view.[86,87,89] In an examination of 100 normal patients, none of the normal arteries were found lateral to this line.[90] At the site of the bony defect, the caliber of the artery is normal or dilated.

Asymptomatic aberrant arteries require no treatment. Therapy usually is reserved for patients with pulsatile tinnitus, hemorrhage, or CN palsies. Intervention ranges from the interposition of synthetic material between the artery and ossicles, disarticulation of the ossicular chain, or ligation of the internal carotid artery in cases of hemorrhage.[87]

Partial Absence

A small segment of the intrapetrous portion of the internal carotid artery may be absent, resulting in an aberrant arterial course through the middle ear. Embryologically a variation in flow leads to regression of blood flow through the cervical internal carotid artery with preferential flow through the inferior tympanic artery and hyoid artery, which then joins the horizontal petrous portion of the normal internal carotid artery. Thus, lack of flow results in atrophy of the internal carotid artery up to the

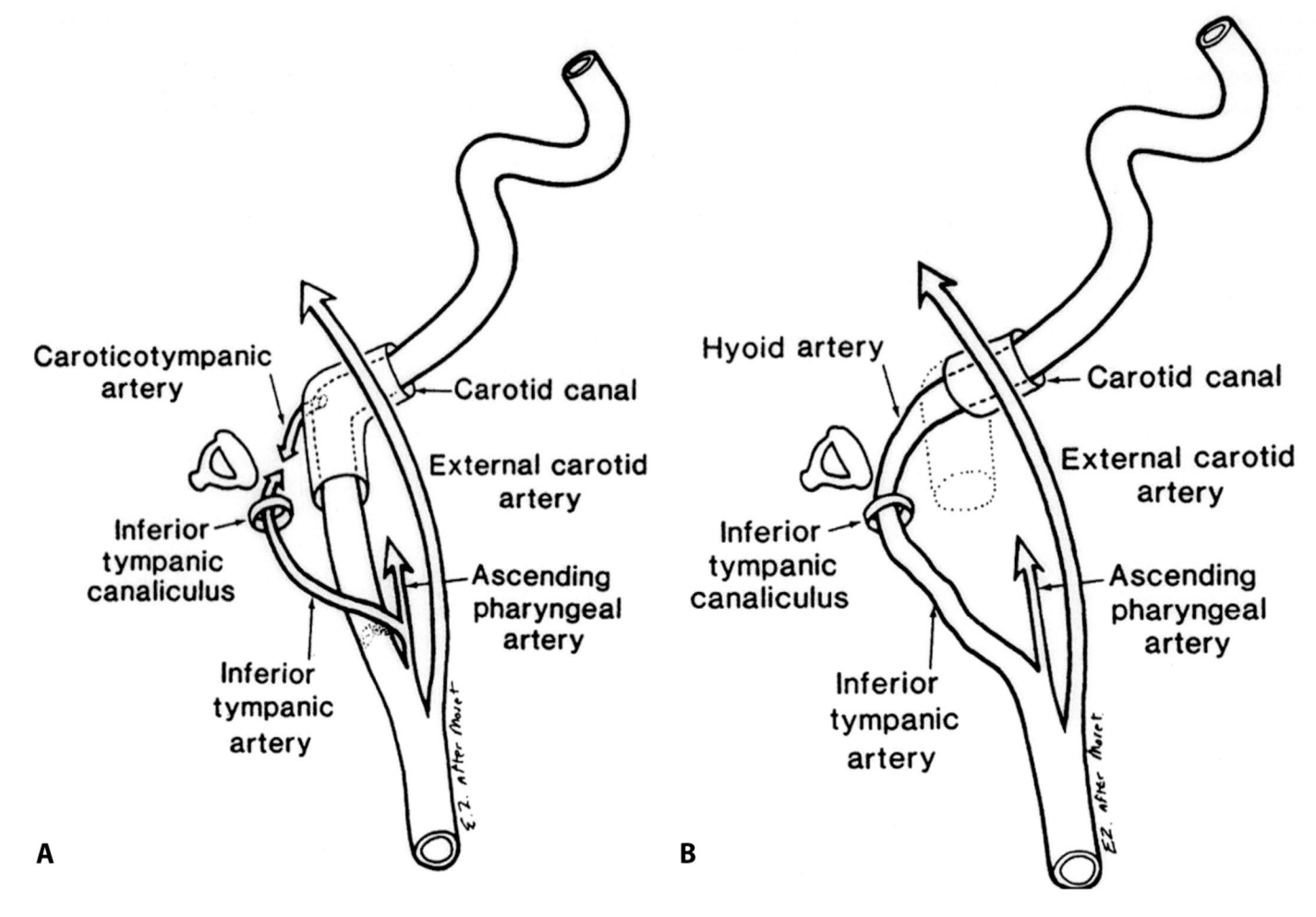

Figure 11-12 Aberrant Internal Carotid Artery Schematic
(**A**) Schematic representation of normal anatomy of the cervical and petrous internal carotid artery. (**B**) Schematic representation of aberrant internal carotid artery (ICA). Absence of the normal vertical petrous segment of the ICA leads to preferential flow through the inferior tympanic artery, which joins with an enlarged the caroticotympanic artery through an enlarged tympanic canaliculus. The aberrant ICA is posterior and lateral to the expected site of the carotid foramen. (From Lo W, Solti-Bohman L, McElveen J: Aberrant carotid artery: radiologic diagnosis with emphasis on high-resolution computed tomography. Radiographics 1985;5(6):985–993.)

horizontal petrous portion. Under such conditions, the tympanic canaliculus transmits an unusually prominent inferior tympanic artery. This vessel appears as an aberrant internal carotid artery in the middle ear, with the associated signs and symptoms described above.

CT shows an enhancing soft tissue mass in the hypotympanum and shows absence of the vertical portion of the bony carotid canal. Internal carotid angiography demonstrates the artery entering the middle ear with a reduced caliber as a result of the bony confines of the tympanic canaliculus. From that point it courses below and against the promontory inferior and anterior to the stapes and proceeds forward to join the horizontal petrous portion of the carotid canal.[12]

Internal Carotid Artery Agenesis

The etiology of congenital absence of the internal carotid artery is unknown. Keen has suggested that unilateral absence of the internal carotid artery may be caused by mechanical causes in early development such as pressure effects, excessive bending of the cephalic end of the embryo from side to side, or the effects of amniotic adhesions.[91] No explanation has been offered for bilateral absence, which is extremely rare.

Symptoms may or may not lead to the discovery of an absent internal carotid artery. The agenesis may be discovered as an incidental finding during the workup of an unrelated problem or, more commonly, it may be discovered during the workup of neurologic symptoms. In 42 reported cases of congenital absence of the internal carotid artery, 12 patients initially had subarachnoid hemorrhage caused by a ruptured intracranial aneurysm. Other clinical presentations include multiple cranial nerve palsies caused by compression of a dilated loop of the basilar artery, hemiparesis after minor head trauma, and various other neurologic signs and symptoms resulting from major head injuries.

CT shows no carotid canal in the petrous bone or a small vertical cleft, possibly representing an abortive carotid canal. Internal carotid angiography demonstrates absence of the internal

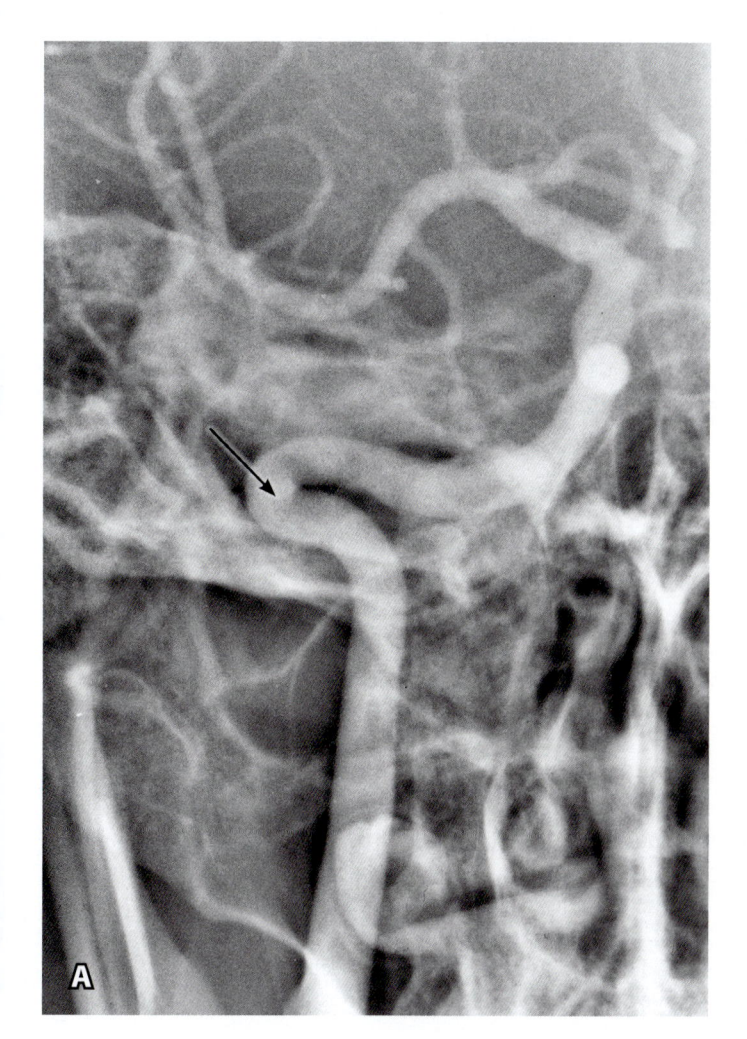

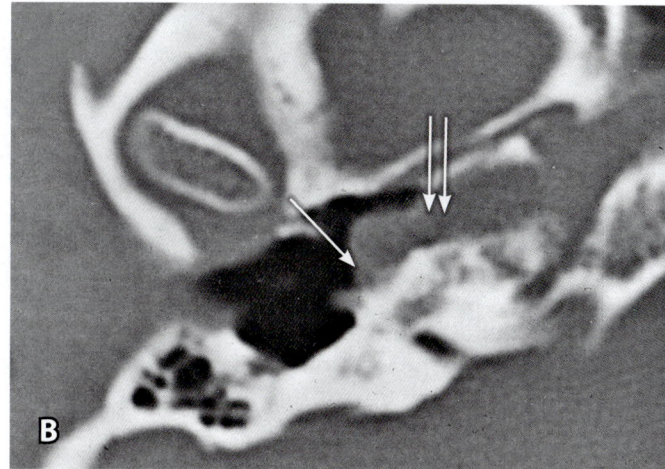

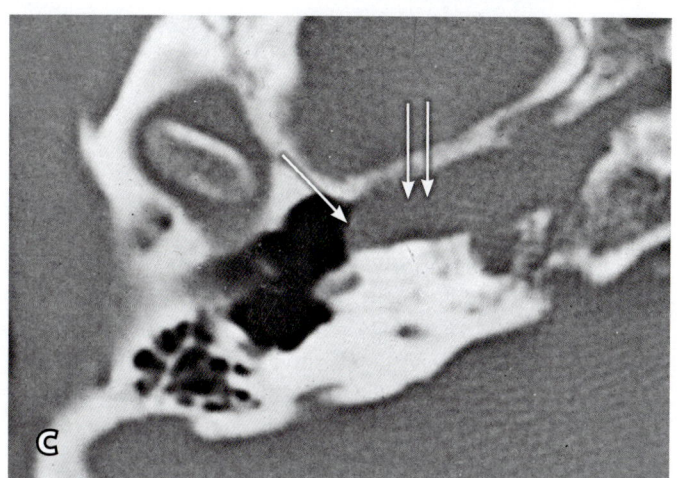

Figure 11-13 Aberrant Internal Carotid Artery
Internal carotid arteriogram (ICA) (**A**) shows a laterally displaced aberrant right internal carotid (*arrow*, **A**). Contiguous axial CT images (**B, C**) show the aberrant right ICA running along the medial aspect of the middle ear (*arrows*, **B, C**) to join the horizontal segment of the petrous portion of the ICA (*double arrows*, **B, C**).

carotid artery. This examination also shows the frequent occurrence of associated anomalies of the remaining vasculature (i.e., dilated basilar artery collaterals, ipsilateral dilation of the posterior communicating artery filling the corresponding anterior or middle cerebral arteries or both, and ipsilateral ophthalmic or anterior cerebral arteries arising from the middle cerebral artery).

Jugular Vein Anomalies

High Jugular Bulb

A high jugular bulb is a jugular bulb located above the level of the bony annulus of the temporal bone.[92,93] Because of this high position, the bony covering of the jugular bulb may be thin, rendering the bulb vulnerable to trauma. In three separate studies, this anatomic variant was found in 7%, 6%, and 3.5% of temporal bones examined histologically, making it the most common vascular anomaly of the petrous portion of the temporal bone.[93]

This entity bears some relation to the degree of pneumatization of the mastoid air cells. In a poorly pneumatized mastoid, the sigmoid sinus is more anterior, the jugular fossa tends to be deep, and the jugular bulb has a correspondingly high dome.[93] The height of the bulb is significant because of the risk of inadvertently entering the vein during myringotomy or middle ear procedures. CT and jugular venography show the high position of the bulb and the thin hypotympanic limiting wall.

Protruding Jugular Bulb

The second most common vascular anomaly of the temporal bone is a dehiscence of the floor of the middle ear and a protrusion of a portion of the jugular bulb through the dehiscence into the hypotympanum (**Fig. 11-14**). Clinically, the jugular bulb often is mistaken as a vascular mass in the middle ear. In one cadaveric study, a bony dehiscence overlying the jugular bulb was found in 7% of the cases.[88]

Patients may have pulsatile tinnitus, headaches, hearing loss (usually conductive, with the jugular bulb impinging on the ossicles, tympanic membrane, oval window, or a combination), a bluish mass behind the tympanic membrane, or hemorrhage

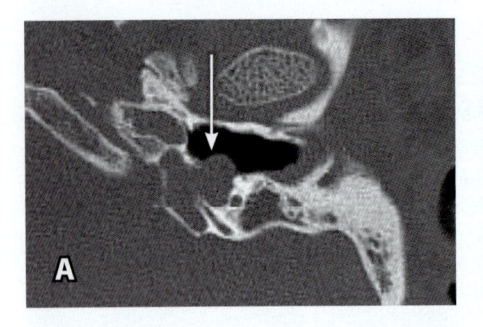

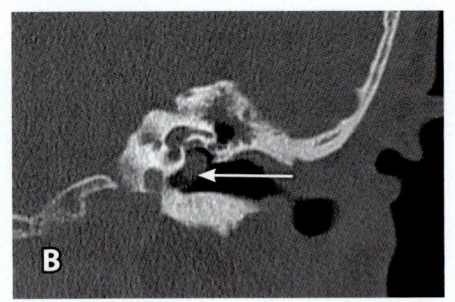

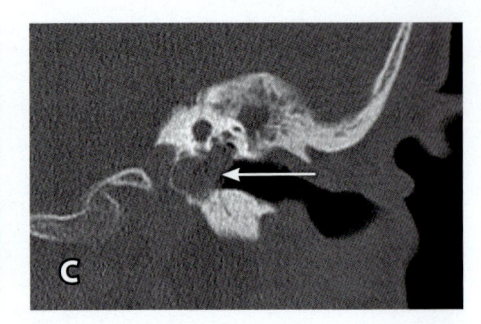

Figure 11-14 Jugular Bulb Dehiscence
Prior middle ear surgery and removal of ossicles: Axial CT (**A**) and contiguous coronal CT images (**B, C**) show a dehiscent left jugular bulb that extends upward into the posterior middle ear (*arrows*).

after myringotomy.[88,92,94,95] CT shows an enhancing soft tissue mass in the middle ear, as well as a bony defect above the jugular bulb in the floor of the hypotympanum. Jugular venography shows the jugular bulb projecting through the defect into the middle ear.

Jugular Diverticulum

A jugular diverticulum is an irregular outpouching of the jugular bulb that rises superiorly and medially in the petrous pyramid. The cause of this venous anomaly is unknown.[93] There are characteristic differences between a jugular diverticulum and a protruding jugular bulb. A jugular diverticulum is situated more medially and posteriorly in the petrous bone than is a protruding jugular bulb. A jugular diverticulum does not invade the middle ear, is not visible on inspection, and is not exposed to surgical trauma from a myringotomy or tympanotomy. The diagnosis of a jugular diverticulum is made only radiographically. A protruding jugular bulb is diagnosed by both radiologic and otoscopic examinations.[93]

The hearing loss from a jugular diverticulum is sensorineural from encroachment on the endolymphatic duct or on the internal auditory canal, and tinnitus, if present, is continuous or intermittent. Patients with a jugular diverticulum may be dizzy or vertiginous, symptoms that are commonly associated with a protruding jugular bulb. Sometimes, a jugular diverticulum may cause signs and symptoms that mimic classic Ménière's disease.[93]

CT demonstrates the irregular diverticulum extending superiorly into the petrous pyramid. The diverticulum may show encroachment on the IAC (**Fig. 11-15**), the vestibular aqueduct, or both. Jugular venography shows the irregular outpouching of the diverticulum extending superiorly into the petrous bone. The most superior extension of the diverticulum lies in a plane higher than the level of a protruding jugular bulb, often reaching the cranial margin of the petrous pyramid. The diverticulum may show encroachment on the IAC, the vestibular aqueduct, or the posterior semicircular canal[9] (**Fig. 11-16**).

Jugular Agenesis

Agenesis of the jugular bulb and sigmoid sinus is extremely rare. In these cases, the absent sigmoid sinus redirects the flow from the transverse sinus into a canal posterior and superior to

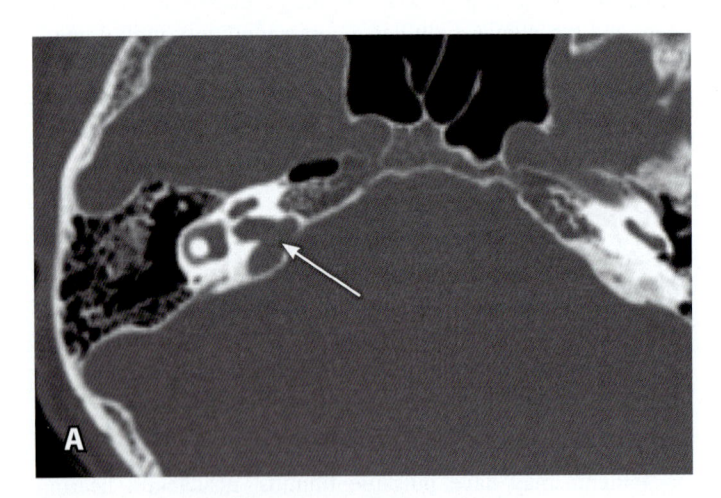

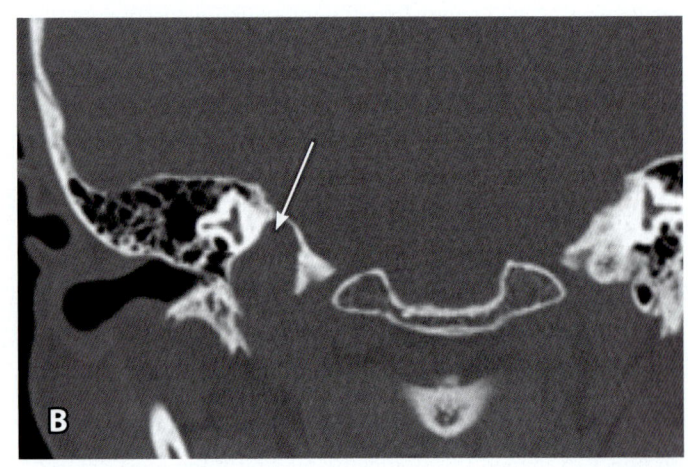

Figure 11-15 Jugular Bulb IAC Diverticulum
Axial (**A**) and coronal (**B**) CT images demonstrate a right jugular bulb diverticulum (*arrow*) invading the internal auditory canal. The coronal image shows the diverticulum (*arrow*) as a finger-like projection off the top of the jugular bulb.

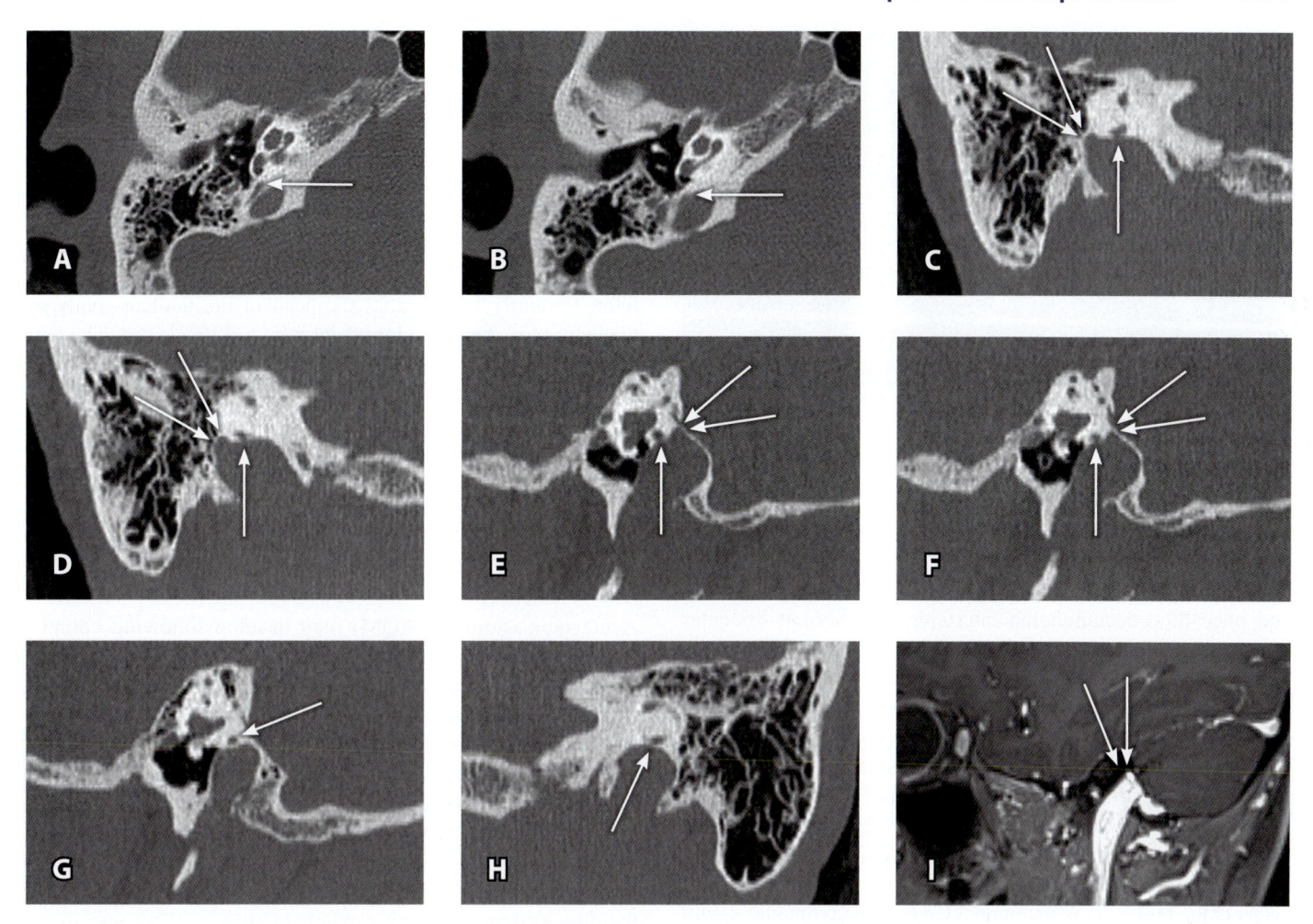

Figure 11-16 Jugular Diverticulum Dehiscence into Posterior Semicircular Canal
Axial (**A–B**), coronal (**C–D**), and sagittal (**E–G**) bone CT scans of the right temporal bone reveal dihescence of the right posterior semicircular canal (*arrows*, **A–F**) into a high riding jugular bulb with a jubular diverticulum (*double arrows*, **C–F**). Coronal bone CT through the left temporal bone CT (**H**) for comparison shows a high riding left jugular bulb that approximates, but does not dehisce the posterior semicircular canal. Sagittal contrast enhanced MR highlights the right jugular diverticulum as a small contrast filled projection at the jugular bulb (*double arrows*, **I**).

the petrous pyramid. This canal then drains directly through the transmastoidian venous channels into adjacent scalp veins. CT of the temporal bone and skull base will document the absent sigmoid sinus and jugular bulb along with the aberrant venous drainage system.

Magnetic Resonance Imaging of Vascular Anomalies

Carotid artery (aberrant course, partial absence, and agenesis) and jugular vein (high jugular bulb, protruding jugular bulb, jugular diverticulum, and agenesis) anomalies all can be recognized on vascular MR images. Unlike CT, MRI does not show the bony changes associated with these vascular anomalies, but it shows the anomalous vessels. Vascular MR is able to demonstrate the occurrence of associated anomalies of the remaining vasculature like the presence of dilated collaterals, and the use of high resolution time of flight MR angiography makes the technique highly sensitive. Even small vascular anomalies can be detected on these images.

INFECTIONS OF THE TEMPORAL BONE AND EAR

Acute Otitis Media

An acute inflammation of the middle ear mucosal lining secondary to an infection. The most common predecessor of acute otitis media (AOM) is an upper respiratory infection, which spreads to the middle ear cavity via the Eustachian tube. A less frequent cause of AOM may be the extension of an EAC infection by way of a ruptured eardrum. The middle ear consists of a continuum between the mesotympanum, hypotympanum, epitympanic recess, and the mastoid antrum and air cells via the aditus ad antrum; as such, AOM may affect any or all of the continuous parts of the middle ear. AOM is especially common in children, for reasons explained by their immature and developing immune system. In the initial stages of the disease, otalgia is the predominant clinical symptom. The steady accumulation of fluid within the middle ear cavity marks the onset of hearing impairment,

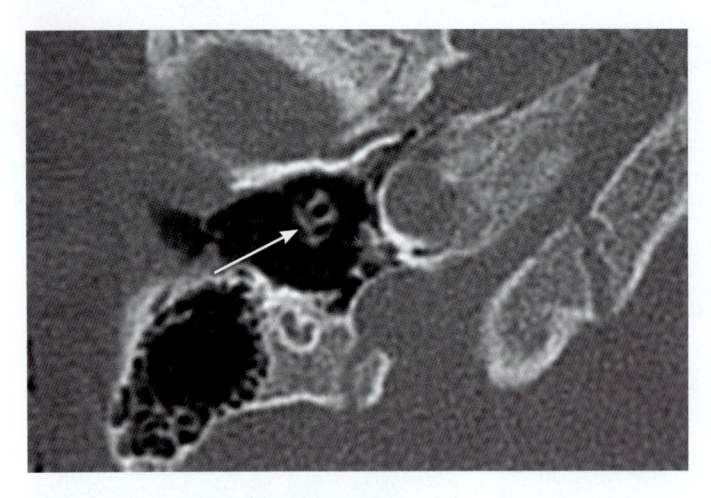

Figure 11-17 Tympanostomy Tube
Axial CT scan of the right temporal bone shows an appropriately placed tympanostomy tube (*arrow*).

and once fluid accumulation interferes with normal ossicular dynamics the patient suffers from conductive hearing loss.

With the spread of infection, the tympanic membrane appears inflamed (erythematous) and begins bulging. The diagnosis for AOM is therefore easily made by otoscopy. However, in the event that high-resolution imaging becomes necessary, CT findings demonstrate patchy opacification of the air-filled cavities of the middle ear, with or without air-fluid levels. Mucosal thickening is evident on CT scans. Tympanostomy tubes placed for recurrent episodes of otitis media are also visualized on CT scans (**Fig. 11-17**). It is recommended that the tympanic cavity be imaged in both the coronal and axial planes for air–fluid level comparison.[96,97]

Chronic Otitis Media

Failure to treat and/or resolve an acute otitis media infection can result in the chronic stage of the disease. Chronic otitis media is divided into two general types: a nonpurulent otitis media with effusion (OME) and a purulent infection involving bony erosion.

In the case of OME, there is retention of mucoid and/or serous fluids within the air spaces of the middle ear cavity. OME is often referred to as "glue ear" and poses as a common cause of childhood conductive hearing loss. Other than its occurrence with chronic otomastoiditis (COM), OME also occur with reductions in intratympanic pressure due to Eustachian tube blockage. OME occur most frequently in children, but it can be monitored otoscopically without imaging intervention; however, in adults radiologic intervention is recommended in order to rule out the possibility of an obstructed Eustachian tube by tumor (neoplasm).

With the spread of a purulent infection in the mastoid and middle ear spaces, bony/ossicular erosion is likely to ensue. Lysosomal enzymes being released by immune cells result in proteolytic destruction of the bony structures, including the ossicles of the middle ear and the bony trabeculae of the mastoid cells. Obliterative labyrinthitis may eventually be the outcome of an advanced infection due to resorption of the labyrinthine walls and structures. CT images demonstrate further opacification of the air-filled cavities, in addition to mucosal thickening. With the onset of conductive hearing loss, bony resorption of the ossicles and/or articular fixation most likely has occurred. A thorough study of both axial and coronal images is necessary to determine the exact site and extent of the bony damage.

Axial CT scans are preferred for identifying the stapes, lenticular process of the incus and their incudostapedial articular joint. Similarly in the attic, the head of the malleus, body of the incus, and their incudomalleal joint can be viewed. The tendon for the tensor tympani muscle can also be visualized just anterior to the incudostapedial joint, coursing laterally to insert on the neck of the malleus. Axial scans are also necessary for viewing the state of the sinus tympani, which can offer valuable information regarding the recommended surgical route in a preoperative case. Coronal scans offer an optimal view of the long process of the incus.[98]

Acute Otomastoiditis

Acute otomastoiditis (AOM) may develop following complications in otitis media, and is therefore caused by a bacterial infection. The extent of the infection and mucosal swelling, in addition to the pneumatization of the mastoid determine the transition from a case of otitis media to AOM. Progression of the disease may lead to several types of complications including coalescent mastoiditis, subperiosteal abscess, petrous apicitis, dural sinus occlusive disease, meningitis, brain abscess and labyrinthitis.

Streptococcus pneumoniae and Haemophilus influenzae are the most common causative agents of such purulent infections. The mucosal swelling within the middle ear cavity may obstruct the aperture of the aditus ad antrum. This will lead to an accumulation of pus within the mastoid antrum and air cells, which lack a drainage outlet. The infection persists within the mastoid and bony resorption begins to occur within the septae or trabeculae. With a drop in pH due to the local hyperemia, decalcification reactions result in erosion of the bone, ultimately yielding one large coalescent mastoid cavity; hence coalescent mastoiditis.

Since detection of subtle bony changes is required for diagnosis, high-resolution CT is the best imaging modality during this interval.[99,100] CT scans demonstrate nonspecific debris throughout the mastoid and generalized opacification of the cavity. The bony trabeculae appear thinned and poorly defined. It is recommended to evaluate both sides for comparison of the diseased coalescent mastoid to the normal; however, diagnosis is generally obvious with imaging techniques (**Fig. 11-18**).

Mastoiditis can spread extracranially to various locations.[101] A subperiosteal abscess may form due to extension of the purulent infection through the thin trabecular bone in the lateral mastoid cortex. The abscess is generally palpable posterior to the EAC; however, with a zygomatic root infection, the palpable abscess can be felt anterior to the EAC/auricle. Extension inferiorly through the mastoid tip into the neck results in the formation of Bezold abscess medial to the sternocleidomastoid muscle. Subperiosteal abscesses present a focal defect in the external mastoid cortex in axial CT scans. Following contrast

Chapter 11: The Temporal Bone **483**

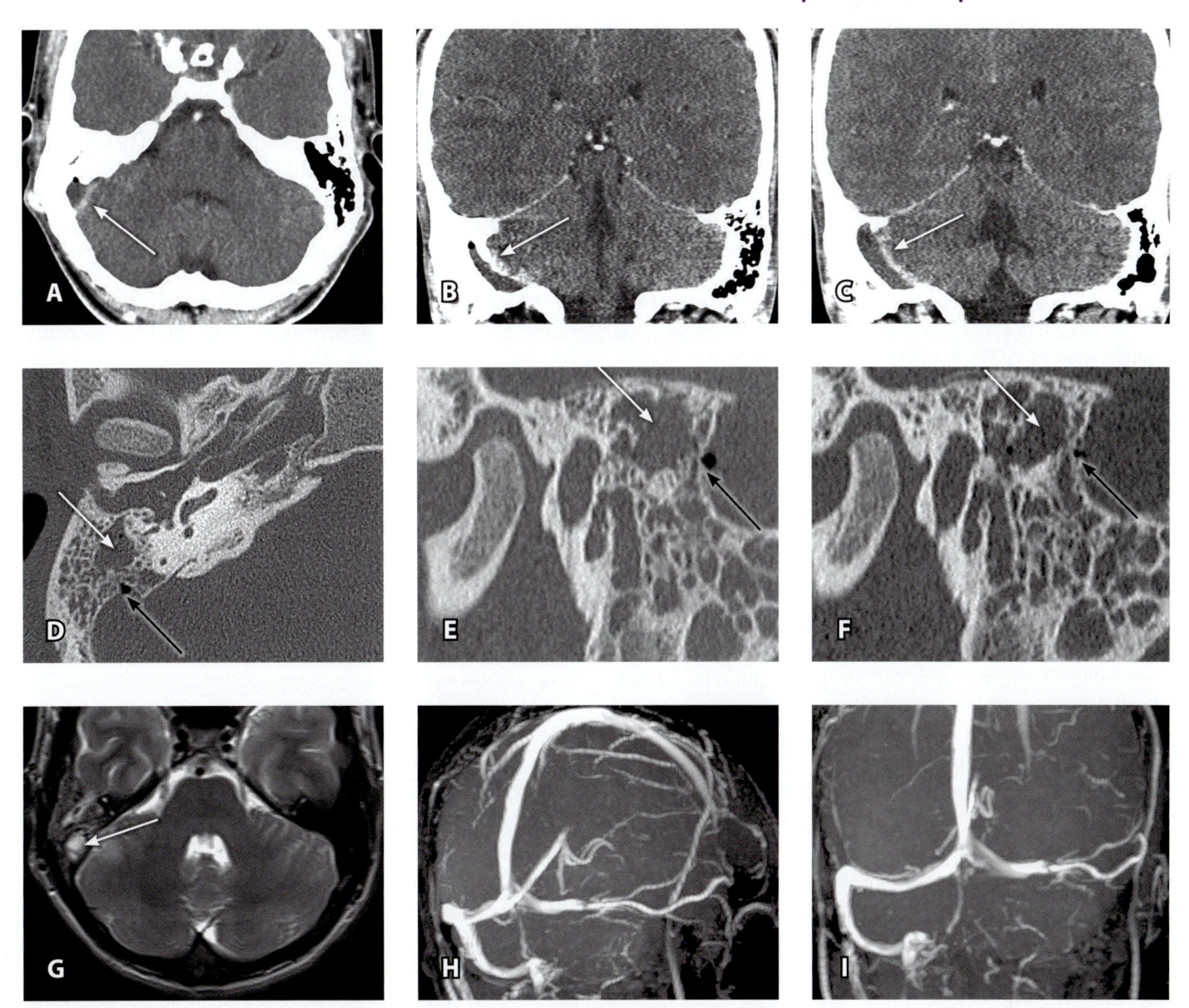

Figure 11-18 Coalescent Mastoiditis with Sigmoid Sinus Thrombosis
Axial (**A**) and reformatted coronal (**B, C**) contrast-enhanced CT images shows a luminal filling defect in the right sigmoid sinus. Enhancement of the inner margin of the dura is consistent with an epidural abscess (*arrows*, **A–C**). On nonenhanced axial (**D**) and reformatted coronal (**E, F**) CT, diffuse mastoid debris is apparent with coalescent changes with loss of mastoid septations (*white arrows*, **D–F**) consistent with coalescent mastoiditis. There is thinning of the sigmoid sinus plate with an adjacent air bubble (*black arrows*, **D–F**). Axial T2W MR scan (**G**) shows hyperintense mastoid debris with abnormal signal in the mastoid air cells and lack of flow void in the sigmoid sinus (*arrow*, **G**). 3D MR venography with contrast (**H, I**) demonstrates narrowing and decreased flow in the right sigmoid sinus and internal jugular vein.

administration, the abscess will appear as a low-density mass in the region of the mastoid. Intracranial complications such as dural venous sinus thrombosis, abscesses, and meningitis are best evaluated by MRI.[61]

Petrous Apicitis

Petrous apicitis can result from a well-pneumatized petrous apex, which communicates with the infected mastoid and middle ear cavity. Because of the close relationship of the ophthalmic branch of the trigeminal nerve and the abducens nerve to the petrous apex, the classic symptoms of petrositis are otitis media, retroorbital pain, and ipsilateral abducens nerve paralysis. This triad, called Gradenigo's syndrome, is present only in a minority of patients.[102] CT of a petrous apicitis case demonstrates septal erosion of the petrous apex as well as diffuse debris within the cavities. There is trabecular breakdown, which leads to a confluent petrous apex. Following a finding such as petrous apicitis with CT, a thorough MRI study is recommended to evaluate the potential intracranial extension of the inflammatory disease. MRI usually shows peripheral meningeal enhancement at the petrous apex as the adjacent dura becomes thickened and covered with granulation tissue. MRI also helps ion differentiating marrow from mucus or CSF.[103] Postcontrast MR findings may demonstrate further complicating factors such as sigmoid sinus thrombosis, meningitis, or brain abscess.

Dural Sinus Thrombosis

Defects in the inner mastoid cortex and spread through the emissary veins may place inflammatory debris in contact with the sigmoid sinus and adjacent dura. With the spread of inflammatory infection to the venous system, there exists the grave risk of thrombus formation leading to thrombophlebitis. This complication of AOM is called dural sinus occlusive disease, or specifically sigmoid sinus thrombosis. This condition may be asymptomatic or associated with intermittently spiking ("picket fence") fever, signs of toxemia, torticollis, and septic embolization. The thrombus may then propagate in antegrade fashion in the internal jugular vein or retrograde into the transverse or superior sagittal and straight sinuses.

MR is ideal for diagnosis and follow-up of dural venous sinus thrombosis.[104] MR imaging findings include the absence of normal flow void on spin echo images and absence of flow related enhancement of gradient echo images. The thrombus may also be directly identified within the sinus. This is best done using T2 and proton density weighted spin echo images to appreciate the deoxyhemoglobin state.[96] MR venography can be used to assess venous flow and permits the distinction between slow venous flow and occlusive thrombus, which may be difficult to determine from spin echo MRI sequences[105] (**Fig. 11-18**). Three-dimensional MR gradient-echo cerebral venography has been shown to be superior to 2D MR.[106] Nonetheless, the diagnosis of dural venous thrombosis remains difficult as aberrant arachnoid granulations appear as filling defects within the sinus and may lead to false positive MR imaging diagnoses.[107]

Thrombosis of the sigmoid and transverse sinuses can result in intracranial hypertension (**Fig. 11-19**). Normally, cerebrospinal fluid from the ventricles is absorbed in the arachnoid villi within the superior sagittal sinus. The majority of individuals have a right dominant venous circulation in which the superior sagittal sinus drains into the right lateral sinus. Occlusion of the sigmoid and transverse sinuses impairs with venous drainage of the superior sagittal sinus.[108] The resulting intracranial hypertension with accompanying papilledema is known as "otitic hydrocephalus," which is actually a misnomer since the ventricles are typically not enlarged in these cases. Since the obstruction to drainage is located at the end of its transport pathway, there is no pressure gradient between the subarachnoid spaces at the surface of the brain and the ventricles.[109]

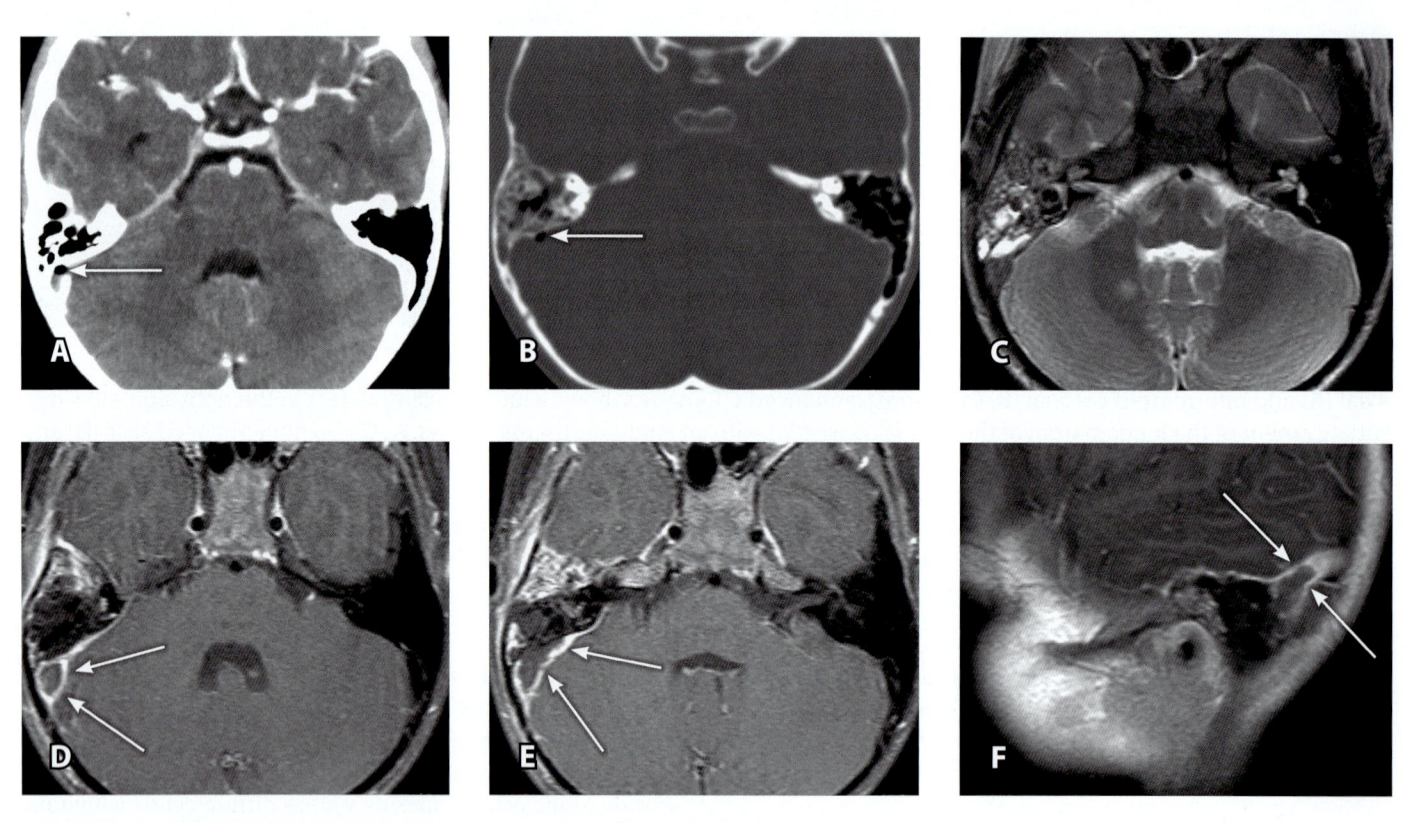

Figure 11-19 Mastoiditis with Septic Sigmoid Sinus Thrombosis
(**A**) Soft tissue and (**B**) bone windows of axial CT show opacification of the right mastoid air cells with a small amount of air within a thrombosed right sigmoid sinus (*arrows*, **A, B**). (**C**) Axial T2-W, and (**E**) axial and (**F**) sagittal T1-W MR images with contrast. The filling defect and enhancement of the inner margin of the dura is consistent with sigmoid sinus thrombosis and an epidural empyema (*arrows*, **D–F**).

Brain Abscess

Medial extension of the extension through defects of the internal mastoid cortex can also result in epidural, subdural, and intracerebral abscess formation. Abscesses can also result from retrograde thrombophlebitis, where the bone is intact.[98] The abscess is a pus collection walled off by a fibrous capsule. When otogenic in origin, it will typically occur in the temporal lobe and cerebellum. Epidural abscesses lie between the dura and the skull bones.[97] Postcontrast CT demonstrates a hypointense center with a hyperintense capsule about a formed abscess.[110] On T2W MRI, there is a hyperintense central area of pus surrounded by a well-defined hypointense capsule and hyperintense surrounding area of edema. MRI is more sensitive than CT for detection of intracranial complications because paramagnetic contrast agents such as gadolinium DTPA cross the blood brain barrier in areas of cerebritis or abscess. Meningeal enhancement is more easily seen with MRI than with CT scanning in which the adjacent bony skull often obscures the image.[102] To distinguish between a brain abscess and other focal-central nervous system lesions such as a tumor, diffusion weighted imaging (DWI) may be of use. Abscesses are usually hyperintense on DWI (indicating restricted diffusion, characteristic of viscous pus)[111] with low ADC while neoplastic lesions are hypointense.[112]

Chronic Otomastoiditis

COM usually results from decreases in intratympanic pressure, secondary to Eustachian tube defects, although there are less frequent occurrences in association with otitis media. The manifestations of COM include granulation tissue, tympanic membrane retraction, acquired cholesteatoma.

Granulation Tissue

GT is a common development in the middle ear as a result of COM. In CT imaging, it presents as diffuse debris in the middle ear. MRI assists in differentiation between GT, cholesteatoma, and a subtype of GT called cholesterol granuloma (CG). Normal GTs and the CG subtype differ in that CGs tend to consist of brownish fluid as a result of spontaneous hemorrhage. Cholesterol crystals form in clefts within the CG as a result of the bleeding vascular mass. Both T1- and T2-weighted MR images of CGs demonstrate bright signal intensities indicating the presence of methemoglobin in the middle ear/mastoid. Normal GTs show bright enhancement post-gadolinium on T1-weighted MR scans, while cholesteatoma does not, providing the radiologist with a marker for differential diagnosis. In addition, CGs show a bright signal in the unenhanced T1-weighted MR images. The use of CT imaging is less yielding for viewing and differentiating GTs and CGs, as both offer more or less the same diffusely opaque fields with signs of patchy debris.

Generally, GTs and CGs do not pose an erosive threat to the surrounding bony structures of the middle ear and mastoid; however, CGs of the petrous apex, also known as giant cholesterol cysts, do have a tendency to erode adjacent bony structures such as the carotid canal, anteriorly. CGs are also known as "chocolate" cysts due to their hemorrhagic brownish fluid consistency and "blue-domed" cysts for their otoscopic appearance through the lining of the tympanic membrane. The hemorrhagic state of a CG could lead to the diagnosis of a paraganglioma (glomus tympanicum); however, CGs unlike paragangliomas do not cause bulging of the tympanic membrane. In addition, history of COM will steer the differential diagnosis toward CG.[98]

Tympanic Membrane Retraction

The formation of medially-directed pockets within the eardrum, also known as tympanic membrane retraction, can be diagnosed without radiologic intervention, using otoscopic surveillance. With an obstructed Eustachian tube, or decreased ventilation through the anterior and posterior tympanic isthmi, the level of oxygenation and aeration of the middle ear and mastoid cavities is reduced. With increased absorption of the oxygen and continued obstruction retraction pockets begin to form in the tympanic membrane. They may form within the greater pars tensa or the smaller, superiorly positioned pars flaccida.

Retraction of the pars flaccida, although less common, may be associated with acquired cholesteatoma of the epitympanum and mastoid antrum; in addition, it may be missed in an otoscopic examination, as it occurs quite superiorly within the eardrum. Pars tensa retractions are more easily viewed both otoscopically and on CT imaging. The degree of tympanic membrane retraction may increase gradually beginning with a minor retraction, followed by ossicular contact, atelectasis of the tympanic cavity, and ultimately adhesion to the labyrinthine wall. Progressive retraction may present as ossicular erosion, especially of the long process of the incus, visible on CT. In severe cases of TM retraction, the ossicular chain can become dismantled with the retracted eardrum in contact with the capitulum of the stapes. This condition is known as "nature's myringostapediopexy," and often even afford normal conductive hearing.[96,113]

Acquired Cholesteatoma

Another manifestation of COM is the formation of an acquired cholesteatoma. A cholesteatoma is essentially a sac filled with keratinized squamous epithelium shed from the mucosal lining of the tympanic membrane, and found in the tympanic cavity. Although a topic of much scientific debate and research, the etiology of acquired cholesteatoma has been narrowed down to involve several epithelial theories.

In patients with pre-existing Eustachian tube defects, it is likely that decreased intratympanic pressures cause formation of tympanic membrane retraction pockets, which in turn are the predecessors of cholesteatoma development. A slightly different explanation suggests that patients with a history of repeated COM can develop scars and perforations in the tympanic membrane. Later, the shedding of keratinized squamous epithelium from the outer layer of the tympanic membrane can get shunted inward through the perforation and into the middle ear.

Regardless of the precise etiology, acquired cholesteatoma can be associated with bony erosion that results in destruction of middle ear structures. As a result, the initial presenting symptom of an acquired cholesteatoma is the onset of conductive hearing loss. With tympanic membrane perforations, there may also be signs of otorrhea. In severe cases in which labyrinthine erosion has occurred in the region of the lateral semicircular canal, the formation of a labyrinthine fistula poses grave complications. If the cholesteatoma erodes the medial labyrinthine wall and arrives in the membranous labyrinth, the disease status is escalated to the potential for SNHL and persistent vertigo.

Pars flaccida cholesteatomas develop from Prussak's space, lateral to the head of the malleus and medial to the epitympanic wall, just beneath the lateral mallear ligament. The cholesteatoma may cause bony erosion of the scutum in the posterosuperior aspect of the tympanic membrane and the head of the malleus and body of the incus, in the attic. It may also displace the malleus medially and extend posteriorly to involve the posterolateral attic and antrum. Pars tensa cholesteatoma commonly results from tympanic membrane retractions and, in some instances, perforation. The sinus tympani and facial recess located in the posterior tympanic cavity are frequent sites of invasion by the ingrowth of the cholesteatoma from the retraction pocket. Cholesteatoma extension into the attic can displace the ossicular chain laterally.

The most characteristic imaging features of cholesteatoma on CT include the identification of a well-marginated soft tissue mass in the middle ear/epitympanum in association with bony erosion of the ossicles, scutum, and/or the cavity walls. Ossicular erosions most commonly involve the long process of the incus, presumably due to its watershed region vascular supply.[114] The differential diagnosis between an acquired cholesteatoma and GT is based on the evidential finding of bone destruction with cholesteatoma. The preferred plane for CT imaging for a pars flaccida cholesteatoma is the coronal, whereas for pars tensa cholesteatoma it is the axial CT plane. When complications such as extension of cholesteatoma intracranially or epidurally, or facial nerve involvement become apparent on CT, MRI imaging is the next recommendation. T1-weighted post-contrast MR images demonstrate a low-intensity mass with bright rim-enhancement of GT clearly delineating the extension of the cholesteatoma.[115] MRI is also useful in differentiating cholesteatoma and associated infection, as cholesteatomas do not enhance with gadolinium unless infiltrated with GT.[116,117] On diffusion-weighted MRI sequences, a cholesteatoma is seen as a hyperintense spot on B 1000 images, probably due to a T2 shine-through effect, whereas inflammation does not display a hyperintense signal[118,119] (**Fig. 11-20**).

Bone Erosion

Most serious complications of cholesteatomas are secondary to bone erosion that may be seen with or without the presence of osteitis. Without osteitis, rarefying bone destruction occurs secondary to proteolytic enzymatic activity as discussed above. The presence of pus causes sequestration and osteitis which leads to additional bone decay. The bone erosion may also be caused by pressure necrosis due to the presence of an expanding soft-tissue mass. The adjacent bone is thinned by the pressure and finally destroyed. Structures within the temporal bone and in the surrounding regions are all subject to involvement by the cholesteatomatous mass. Extensions into the antrum, inner ear, facial nerve canal or mastoid air cells are well known.

High-resolution CT is the procedure of choice in the evaluation of bone erosion particularly of the tegmen tympani, scutum, otic capsule, and ossicles. Horizontal CT scans are particularly suited for defining erosions of the lateral semicircular canal and ossicles. Coronal CT scans are ideal for showing erosions of the tympanic portion of the facial canal (**Figs. 11-21** and **11-22**), tegmen tympani (**Fig. 11-23**), and ossicles. Some of these changes can be picked up on reformatted images; however, it is often desirable to obtain a series of direct coronal images in patients being evaluated for suspected cholesteatomas. If defects are suspected at the tegmen tympani and sigmoid sinus plate, MRI is recommended because there could be associated epidural invasion by the cholesteatoma. MRI can demonstrate middle fossa invasion by showing meningeal enhancement and signal changes in the adjacent temporal lobe.[120] MRI can also define an encephalocele extended through an eroded tegmen.[121]

Labyrinthine Fistula

The lateral semicircular canal, because of its strategic location between the antrum and tympanic cavity, is the portion of the bony labyrinth most readily eroded by a cholesteatoma. Erosion by the mass causes leakage of endolymph out of the membranous labyrinth and alteration of labyrinthine function that is clinically manifested as disequilibrium or vertigo. The fistula may be tamponaded by the eroding mass so that when manual pressure is placed externally on the petrous temporal bone, the patient develops transient vertiginous episodes. Labyrinthine fistulas are seen well with CT, and both axial and coronal sections should be studied carefully.[98] Surgical removal of all the cholesteatoma may actually aggravate the symptoms unless the fistulous orifice is patched up.

Erosions of other portions of the bony labyrinth such as the posterior semicircular canal, vestibule, or cochlea can also lead to the formation of fistulas. Extensive erosion into the cochlea may precede involvement of the IAC. More typically the cholesteatoma erodes above the cochlea and enters the IAC via a supralabyrinthine route.

Infections of the Petrous Apex

Petrous apex infections are defined relative to the presence or absence of pneumatization. Petrous apicitis is defined as spread of suppurative infections to a well-pneumatized petrous apex. When an infectious process extends to a nonpneumatized petrous apex, the term petrous apex osteomyelitis is preferred. The purulent organism travels from the suppurative middle ear infection though the mastoid air cells to the petrous apex. Petrous apicitis, however, may be the result of chronic inflammatory changes following granulomatous or other forms of meningitis. Fungal disease or tuberculosis may cause such granulomas. Fungal infections should be considered in immunosuppressed or chronically ill patients. These fungal infections demonstrate a propensity for invading blood vessels resulting in a purulent arteritis and rapid intracranial dissemination.

Tuberculosis of the petrous apex has an insidious and chronic course and may simulate other noninfectious processes such as carcinomatosis, sarcoidosis, and/or inflammatory pseudotumor. The differential diagnosis is primarily based on

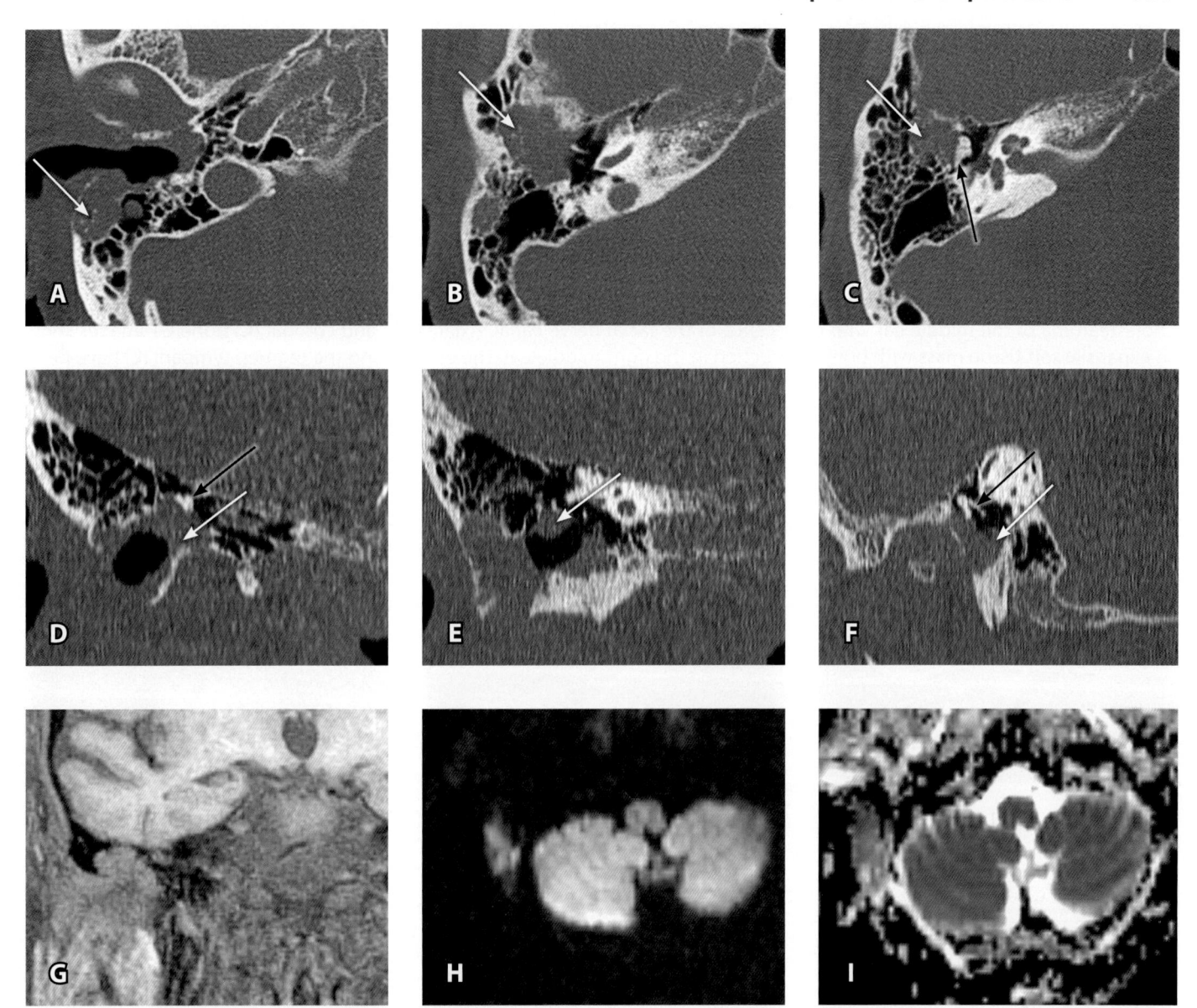

Figure 11-20 Cholesteatomas of the EAC and Middle Ear
Axial (**A–C**), coronal reconstructed (**D–E**), and sagittal reconstructed (**F**) bone CT images show bony destruction of the mastoid air cells located posterior to the external auditory canal (**A, E**). Coronal images (**D–F**) depict the mass encircling the external auditory canal, with extension into the middle ear. There is also a soft tissue density mass located in Prussak's space in the right epitympanum with destruction adjacent to the right mesotympanum (*white arrows*, **B–D**). The tegmen tympani is intact (**F**). Though the soft tissue mass abutts the ossicular chain, the ossicles appear intact (*black arrows* **C, D, F**). Notice the bony flecks (*arrows*, **A, B**), a common finding in cholesteatomas. Coronal T1 fat-saturated MR (**G**), axial DWI (**H**), and axial ADC maps (**I**) show a contiguous soft tissue density mass right external ear and middle ear with restricted diffusion, also consistent with cholesteatoma.

clinical manifestations of meningitis and, in the case of an infection that invades the superior petrosal sinus, signs of an epidural empyema within the petrous apex.

Imaging studies will usually define the extent of involvement. There may be erosive changes in the petrous apex with abnormal thickening and enhancement of the adjacent meninges. CT scans will often demonstrate opacification and destruction of the petrous apex air cell system. MRI may show a hypointense lesion with rim enhancement on T1-weighted images and a hyperintense signal on T2-weighted images[122] (**Fig. 11-24**).

Diffuse meningeal enhancement may be seen with fungal or granulomatous processes. An epidural empyema will show an extraaxial mass that is sharply defined and separate from the brain with linear or convex postcontrast enhancement. An associated osteomyelitis is characterized by the presence of bony sequestrum intermixed with the infectious nidus.

Mucoceles of the petrous apex have been reported as a complication of prior infections. Such mucoceles have a lining of thin cuboidal epithelium and contain mucous. There may be a capsule of fibrous connective tissue around the hydrated or

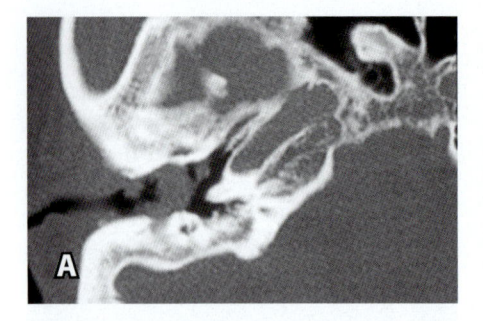

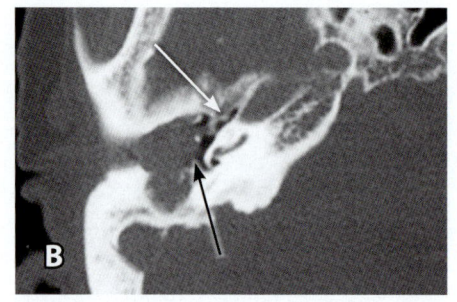

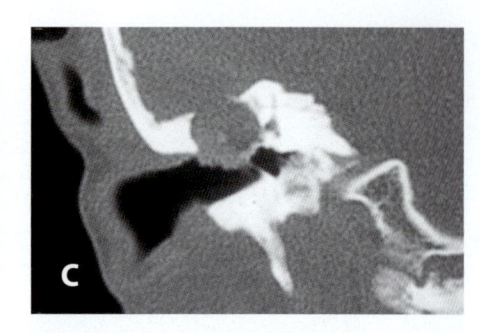

Figure 11-21 Middle Ear Cholesteatoma
Cholesteatoma of the middle ear with dehiscence of the facial nerve canal. Axial (**A–B**) and coronal (**C**) bone CT images show an expansile soft tissue mass with bony destruction in the right middle ear. The ossicles and the tegmen tympani (**C**) have been destroyed. The mass abuts the lateral wall of the inner ear and has caused the dehiscence of the tympanic portion of the facial nerve canal (*white arrow*, **B**) and lateral semicircular canal (*black arrow*, **B**).

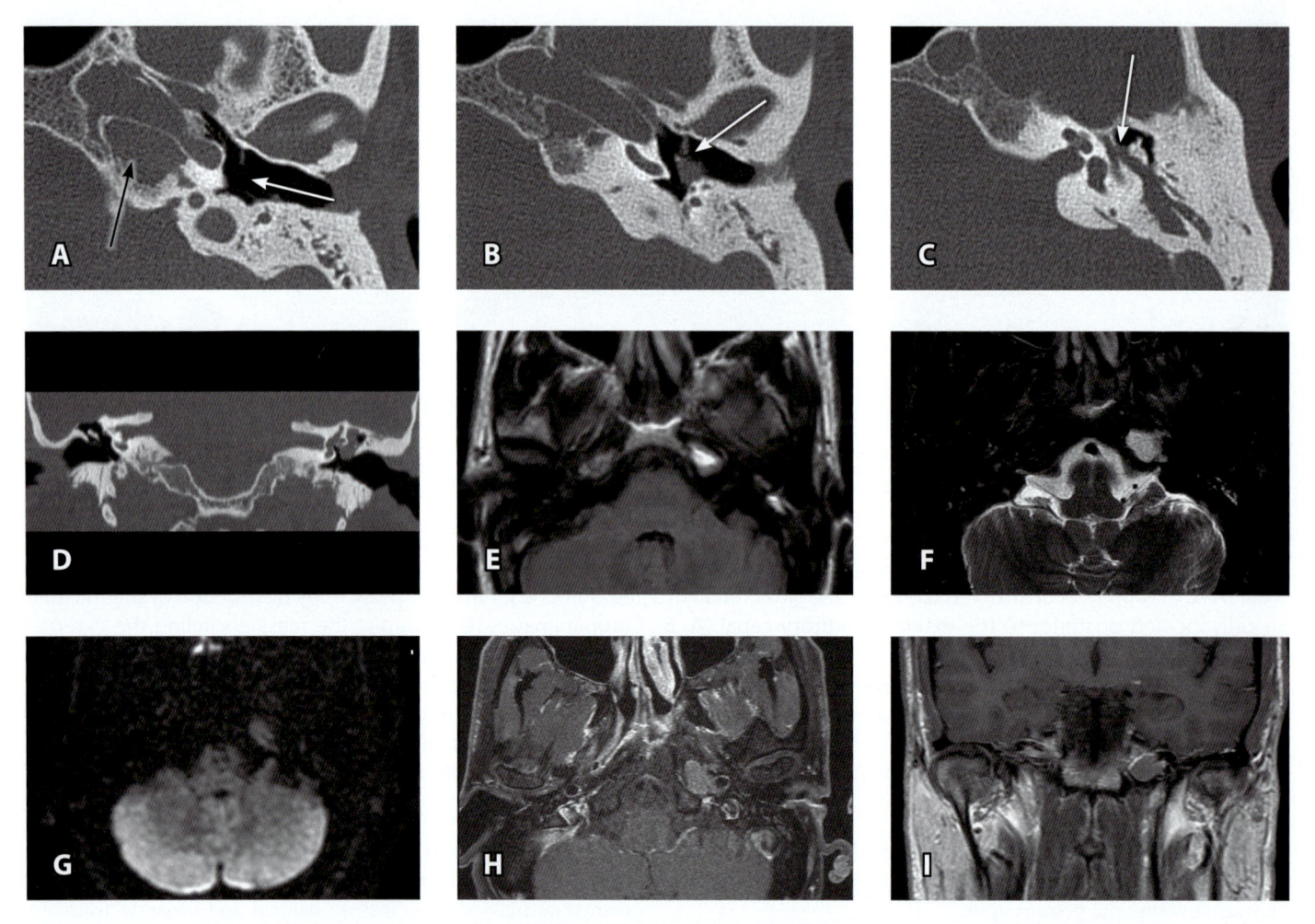

Figure 11-22 Acquired Cholesteatoma of the Middle Ear with a Congenital Cholesteatoma of the Petrous Apex
Axial CT scans (**A–C**). There is a smoothly marginated expansile mass in the left petrous apex (*black arrow*, **A**) and a perforation of the TM (*white arrow*, **A**). There is a soft tissue mass in the left attic and antrum with expansion of the Prussak space (*arrow*, **B**) with likely invasion of the tympanic portion of the facial nerve canal (*arrow*, **C**) consistent with erosion by an atticoantral cholesteatoma. These findings are also seen on the reformatted coronal view (**D**). (**E–I**) MRI scans, (**E**) T1-W, (**F**) T2-W, (**G**) DWI, (**H**) axial, and (**I**) coronal T1-W with contrast enhancement. The lesion in the left petrous apex shows low T-1 and high T-2 signal intensities with mild restricted diffusion and no contrast enhancement consistent with a congenital cholesteatoma.

Chapter 11: The Temporal Bone **489**

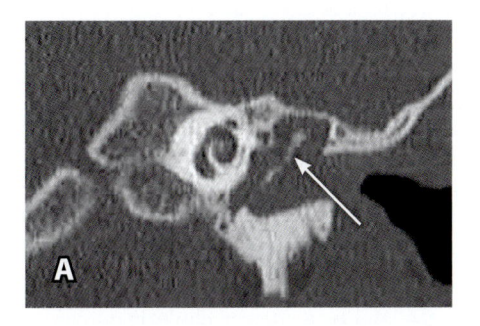

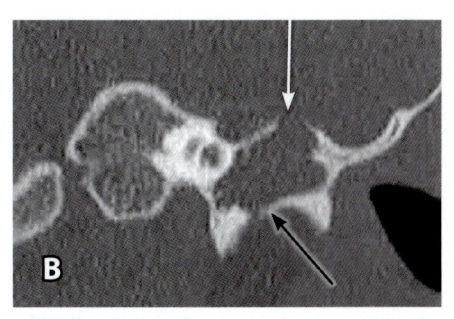

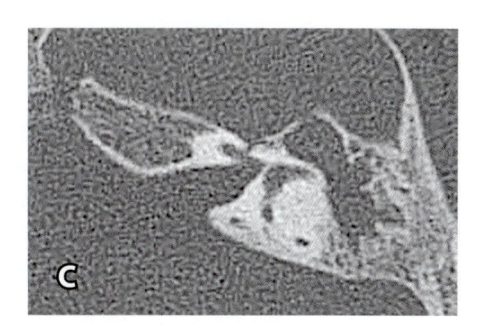

Figure 11-23 Cholesteatoma with Tegmen Tympani Erosion
Coronal (**A–B**) and axial (**C**) bone CT images depict a large soft tissue mass occupying the epitympanum, mesotympanum, and hypotympanum of the left middle ear. The mass has surrounded and partially eroded the ossicles (*arrow*, **A**). There is thinning of the tegmen tympani with a focal area of dehiscence (*arrow*, **B**). Expansion of the cholesteatoma through the aditus and into the mastoid antrum is depicted in the axial plane (**C**).

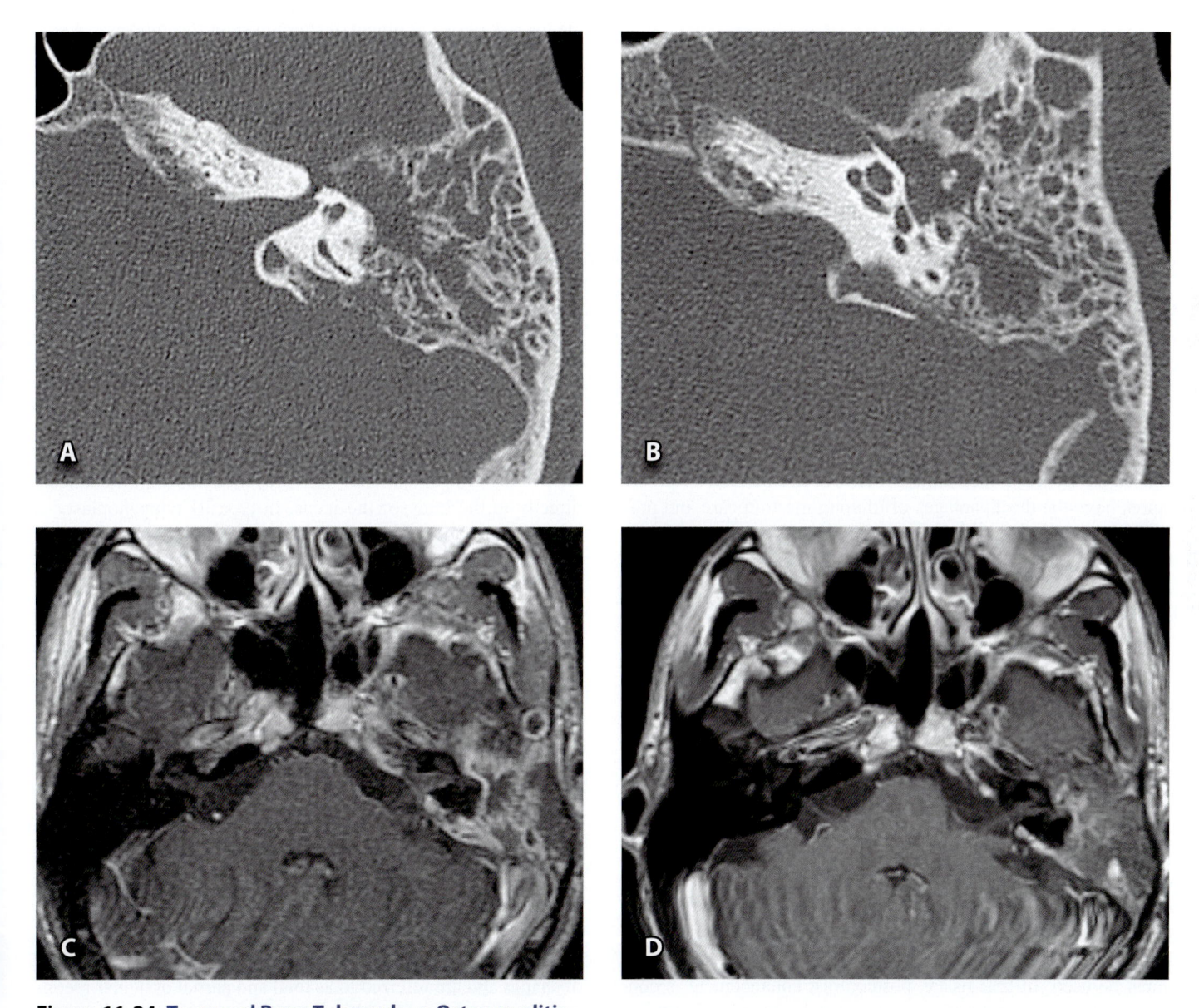

Figure 11-24 Temporal Bone Tuberculous Osteomyelitis
Axial CT (**A, B**) shows trabecular breakdown of multiple opacified left mastoid air cells with soft tissue debris in the middle ear, attic, and antrum. There are coalescent changes in the mastoid air cells extending into the petrous apex secondary to bony destruction of the trabeculae. On axial T1-W MR scans with contrast (**C** and **D**), there are multiple foci of patchy enhancement within the mastoid air cells and petrous apex intermixed with nonenhancing foci that represent collections of dormant granulomas.

inspissated central contents. A petrous apex mucocele may be difficult to differentiate from a cholesteatoma, but is quite different form a CT. Both mucoceles and cholesteatomas have a lytic appearance with sclerotic margins. On CT, there is enhancement of the capsule, which may be secondary to inflammatory and/or granulation tissues in the case of a mucocele, and due to compression of the adjacent vessels in the case of a cholesteatoma. Both lesions show intermediate to low signal intensity on T1-W sequences that does not enhance with gadolinium and high signal intensity on T2-W images.[122] Distinction between the two diagnoses may be facilitated with the use of diffusion-weighted imaging, in which cholesteatomas will appear hyperintense due to restricted diffusion.[118,123] Differentiation from a cholesterol granuloma is readily accomplished as cholesterol granulomas have high signal intensities on both the T1-W and T2-W sequences.

Postoperative Middle Ear and Mastoid

Mastoidectomy

There are a variety of different surgical techniques for treating COM and cholesteatoma, which can be categorized as open cavity (canal wall down) and closed cavity (intact canal wall) mastoidectomy. In cases of medium to large cholesteatoma, open-cavity procedures are used. In such cases, the external auditory canal is removed and the scutum is resected, allowing access to the attic. Most often, the modified radical mastoidectomy is performed, in which the ossicular chain is preserved and reconstructed. Radical mastoidectomies, in which most of the ossicular chain with the exception of the stapes is removed, are now rarely performed. Open cavity procedures offer wide access to the middle ear, epitympanum, and mastoid. Moreover, the rate of recurrence of cholesteatoma are lower (5% to 15%) than with closed cavity mastoidectomies.[124] However, open cavity procedures have the disadvantages of lifelong mastoid care and possible recurrence of discharge. In intact canal wall mastoidectomies, the EAC wall and ossicular chain are spared. Thus, there is a normal EAC and no mastoid cavity. However, the incidence of recurrence of cholesteatoma is high (20% to 50%), so second look operations after 12 to 18 months are necessary in almost all cases.[125-127]

A major role of postoperative imaging is the detection of residual cholesteatoma within the tympanic cavity. CT is essential in this regard due to its ability to demonstrate the complete absence of a soft tissue mass within the cavity or bony destruction. Since CT has a high negative predictive value for residual cholesteatoma,[128] no further imaging may be required. However, CT does not allow a distinction between residual cholesteatoma and postoperative granulation, inflammatory, or scar tissue.[129,130] Contrast-enhanced MRI is useful in this case, as granulation and inflammatory tissue enhance while cholesteatoma does not. To differentiate cholesteatoma from scar tissue, delayed contrast must be used. In scar tissue, postcontrast enhancement is constant but appears only after approximately 30 minutes due to poor vascularization.[131] On the other hand, cholesteatomas never enhance following gadolinium injection. As an additional tool in characterizing residual cholesteatoma, diffusion-weighted imaging has been proposed as an adjunct to T1 and T2 MRI. Venail et al. found DWI to be more specific but less sensitive than delayed postcontrast T1W MRI, supporting its concurrent use in residual cholesteatoma detection.[132] The low sensitivities reported on echoplanar DWI are likely due to its low resolution, slice thickness, and susceptibility artifacts of the sequence which prevent it from reliably detecting cholesteatomas <5 mm in size.[133] New, non-echoplanar based DWI sequences, turbo based DWI sequences, have been described, and found have higher resolution, and the ability to detect cholesteatomas at least >2 mm in size.[134,135]

Perhaps the more important characterization of postoperative debris in the middle ear is the status of the bony margin of the mastoid cavity, which is best demonstrated by CT examination. The regions of the tegmen and sigmoid sinus plate have special importance. Defects next to the sigmoid sinus plate create the risk of development of sigmoid sinus thrombosis.[98] A soft tissue mass protruding through a defect in the tegmen suggests the possibility of a meningocele. The differentiation between a meningocele and a cholesteatoma can best be made by MR, in which a meningocele will have the same characteristics as cerebrospinal fluid.[136] Defects in the integrity of the facial canal and the presence of fistulas must also be sought after, for they may complicate the postoperative course.

Tympanoplasty

Tympanoplasty is a surgical procedure performed to eradicate middle ear infection and restore the function of the middle ear. This is done by reestablishing an intact tympanic membrane and securing a durable connection between the tympanic membrane and the inner ear (**Fig. 11-25**). There are five main types. In type I, also known as myringoplasty, a graft is used to cover defects of the tympanic membrane without altering the ossicular chain. In type II, the tympanic membrane is repaired and a graft connects directly to the body of the incus. In type III tympanoplasty, a graft attaches to the capitulum of the stapes. In type IV tympanoplasty, the graft attaches to the footplate of the stapes. Finally, in type V tympanoplasty, the graft attaches to the oval window.

Ossiculoplasty

Disruption of the integrity of the ossicular chain can result from chronic otitis media in almost any form. However, cholesteatoma is the most common cause. The pathology can be restricted to the incudostapedial joint with loss of the lenticular process. However, there is usually a complete loss of some portion of the distal incus.[137] Such ossicular destruction necessitates ossiculoplasty. Although homograft ossicular implants from cadavers and autograft ossicles sculpted from the patient's own middle ear are used, allograft prosthesis using synthetic materials are currently extremely popular.[96] A variety of biomaterials are used, but currently hydroxyapatite and titanium are currently the most widely used.[129] These substances can be fashioned into a variety of shapes and are referred to as total and partial ossicular reconstructive prosthesis (TORP and PORP, respectively). The TORP and PORP devices transmit sound directly from the tympanic membrane to the oval window. PORP is used when the stapes is intact, with a mobile footplate (**Fig. 11-26**). TORP is used when

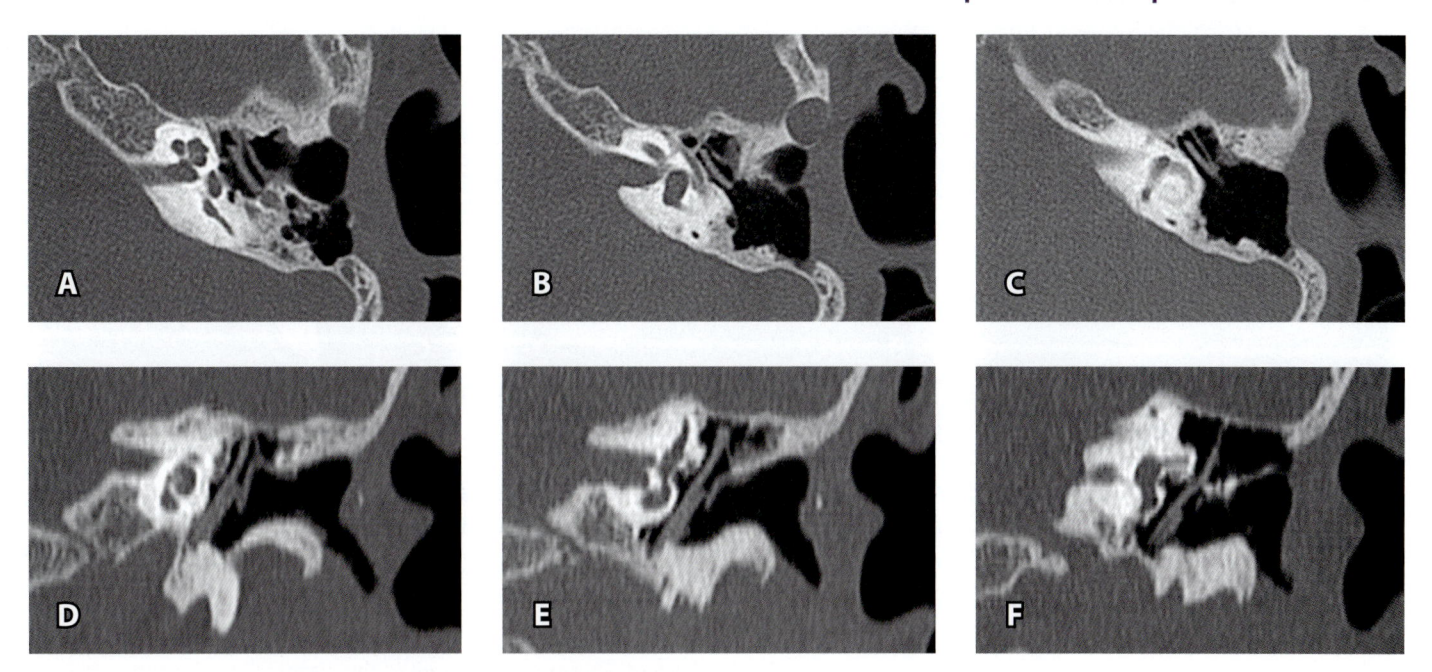

Figure 11-25 Canal Wall Up Tympanoplasty with no Ossicles
Axial (**A–C**) and reformatted coronal (**D–F**) CT scans following canal wall up tympanoplasty. The roof of the external auditory canal has been replaced, that is, canal wall up. Prosthetic material(s) is used to recreate the contiguity of the tympanic membrane, with one layer connecting to the scutum superiorly and the other connecting to the inferior portion of the external canal.

the arch of the stapes is missing with a mobile footplate, with the TORP is interposed between the tympanic membrane and the oval window (**Fig. 11-27**).

CT is useful in evaluating patients with postoperative conductive hearing loss. The most common cause of symptoms is subluxation or dislocation of the prosthesis, seen in 50% to 60% of patients with postoperative hearing loss.[138] Dislocations are well-visualized with high-resolution CT techniques. Native ossicles are characteristically delicate and small, while prosthetic devices are broad and bulbous. In other cases, fibrous adhesions may be seen as postoperative debris near the oval window, or sometimes more laterally at the incal attachment. Fibrous tissue is more likely to occur in patients with preexistent chronic otitis, and typically appears more than 4 to 6 weeks after surgery.[98] Finally, CT may also demonstrate complete opacity of the middle ear, usually representing fluid effusion preventing proper functioning of the prosthesis in a ventilated middle ear.[129]

There have been reports of nonferromagnetic (MRI safe) devices exhibiting movement in vitro in the presence of a strong magnetic field.[139,140] However, these minor displacements have been deemed to be clinically nonsignificant, even at 4.7 T.[141–143] One reason is that movement ex vivo does not necessarily mean there will be movement in vivo, as prostheses are fixed surgically in the ear. Nevertheless, it has been recommended that MRI be "performed with caution" in ossicular implant patients, especially in cases where prosthetic types are not known or have not been determined on CT examination.[129]

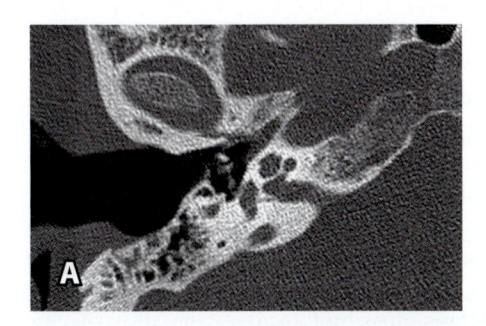

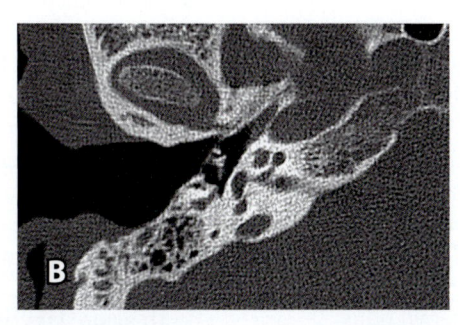

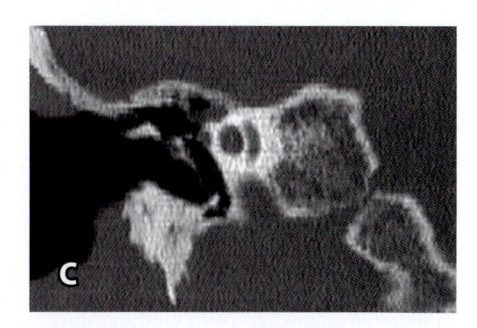

Figure 11-26 Canal Wall Up Tympanoplasty with PORP
Axial (**A, B**) and reformatted coronal (**C**) CT scans following canal wall up tympanoplasty and partial ossicular reconstructive prosthesis (PORP) placement. In addition to an artificial tympanic membrane, there is a residual portion of the native ossicles (malleus and body of incus) and interpostion of the PORP forming the long and lentiform processes of the incus to its articulation with the stapes.

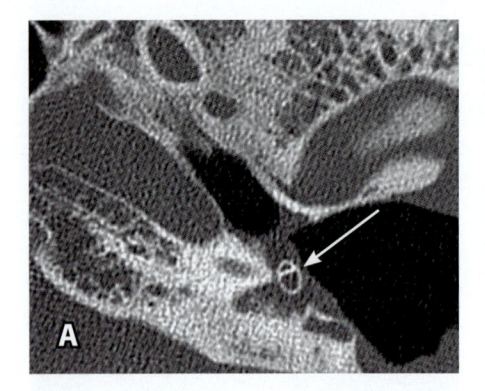

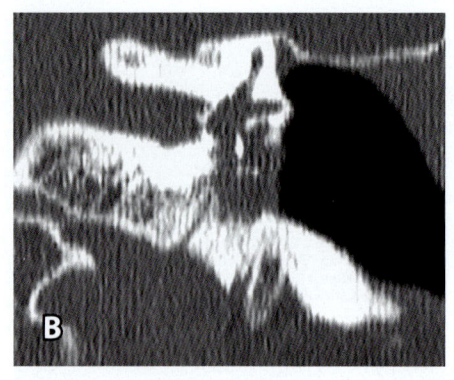

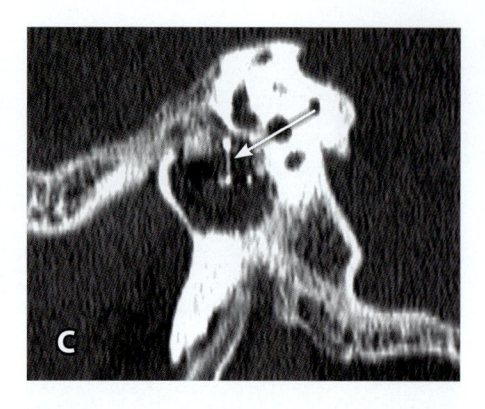

Figure 11-27 Canal Wall Down Tympanoplasty with Titanium TORP (**A**) axial, (**B**) coronal reformatted and (**C**) sagittal reformatted CT scans. There is evidence of tympanoplasty with removal of the roof of the external canal (canal wall down) for treatment of a prior large cholesteatoma. A circular titanium total ossicular reconstructive prosthesis (TORP) device (*arrows*) is interposed between the TM and the oval window. There is extensive soft tissue in the tympanic cavity.

Malignant External Otitis

Malignant external otitis (MEO) is a potentially lethal inflammatory disease of the external auditory canal. It is also known as necrotizing external otitis, and is commonly caused by pseudomonas infection. Classically, MEO infects elderly diabetic and/or immunosuppressed patients. Clinical symptoms include severe otalgia and purulent otorrhea from the EAC. The grave dangers of a persistent MEO infection include its invasion into various soft tissues, and less commonly bony structures. Soft tissue infection can spread into the nasopharynx and the oropharynx by way of the subcranial fissures of Santorini just beneath the EAC. Invasion of the posterior cranial fossa may occur by way of the CNs exiting the temporal bone. The infection may also spread anteriorly to the temporomandibular joint or medially into the middle ear toward the petrous apex.[144] Uncontrolled intracranial infections can lead to meningitis, abscess formation, osteomyelitis of the skull base, and sigmoid sinus thrombosis.

Currently, both CT and MRI are being used complementarily for differential diagnosis of MEO. For delineation of the size and extent of the soft tissue mass, either CT or MRI can be used; however, CT is superior for detection of erosive bony changes, and for this reason may be considered the better front-line technique for initial diagnosis.

CT shows demonstrates subtle bony erosion and involvement of the mastoid and middle ear cavity with less precise information about soft tissue. CT may define subtle bony changes such as erosion of the anterior canal wall with involvement of the TMJ and erosion of the tympanic ring and base of the skull. It may also demonstrate soft tissue thickening and mastoid clouding.[145] Cortical bone erosion or soft-tissue extension beneath the temporal bone or along the skull base have been proposed as diagnostic criteria on either CT scans or MR images in patients suspected of having malignant external otitis.[144]

In advanced stages of the disease when severe bone defects are suspected, MRI detects the edematous appearance skull base osteomyelitis. MRI is slightly superior to CT in this regard due to its ability to delineate changes in the fat content of the marrow.[144] In addition, MRI is the modality of choice in cases of intracranial complications where dural enhancement is necessary to determine the extent of the disease.[98] Underlying cerebral involvement can be easily visualized with gadolinium enhanced MRI. The patency of dural sinuses and great vessels of the neck may be assessed with MR angiography or venography. However, both CT and MRI are not useful in evaluating response to therapy since the erosive and marrow changes caused by inflammation may take up to 6 months to return to normal.[146]

Technetium-99m bone scanning and gallium-67 scanning have been advocated in the evaluation of MEO due to their high sensitivity as early diagnostic tests.[147] However, radionuclide studies are limited by their low specificity and imprecise anatomic localization of disease. Nonetheless, several studies suggest that the combination of gallium citrate with single photon emission computerized tomography (SPECT) scanning is useful in the follow-up of MEO patients.[148,149]

Labyrinthitis

Labyrinthitis, or inflammation of the membranous labyrinth, is usually viral in origin. However, autoimmune disease, neoplasm, trauma, and bacterial infection can also be causative. When bacterial in origin, the damage may result in significant deficits such as extensive inner ear and spiral ganglia cell loss.[110] The condition usually presents as SNHL or vertigo. Tympanogenic and meningogenic labyrinthitis are the two most frequent variants of suppurative labyrinthitis, the former occurring because of passage of microorganisms or toxins from the middle ear to the inner ear through the round, or occasionally the oval, window. Meningogenic labyrinthitis results from spread of infection through the cochlear aqueduct or IAC. Tympanogenic labyrinthitis is usually unilateral while meningogenic labyrinthitis is typically bilateral.

If acute labyrinthitis does not resolve, the disease can progress to a chronic stage, the final stage of which is ossification, or labyrinthitis ossificans. The progression is divided into three stages. In the acute phase, there is purulence and serofibrinous exudate in the perilymphatic spaces.[98] At this stage, CT scanning is normal and the sole imaging finding is

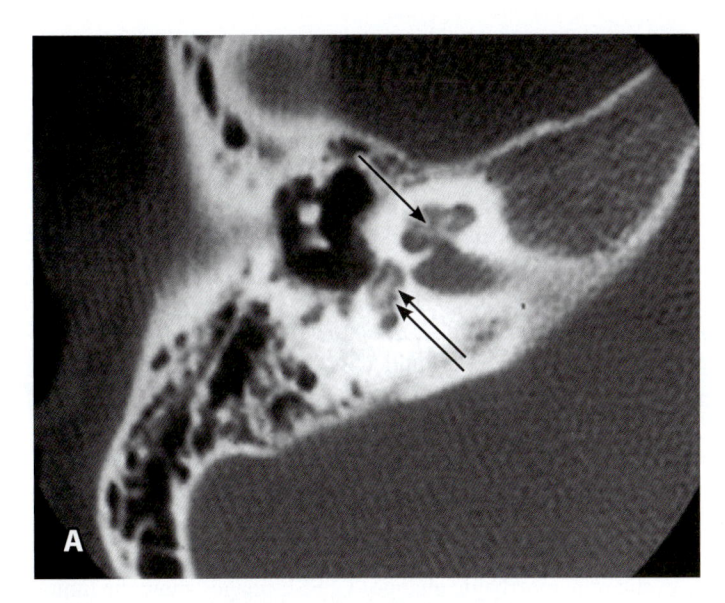

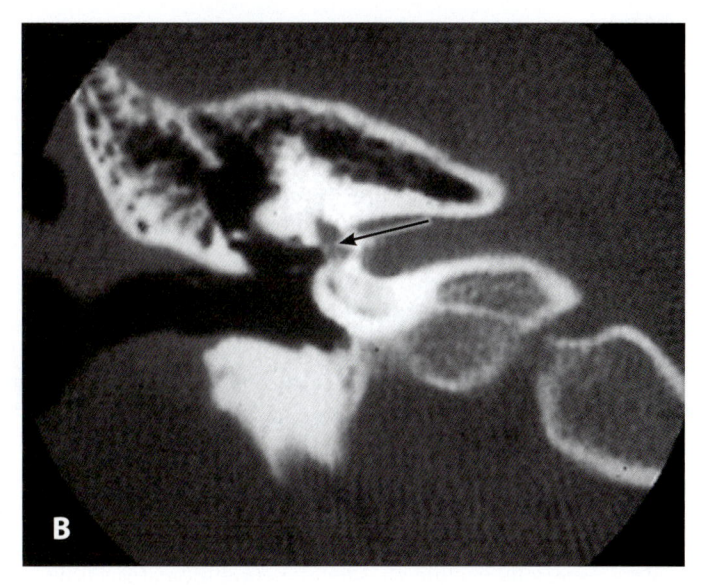

Figure 11-28 Ossifying Labyrinthitis–Early
Axial CT scans of the right temporal bone (**A, B**) demonstrate hazy increase in densities within the fluid space of the cochlear modiolus (*arrows*, **A, B**) consistent with ossific changes, also noted in the vestibule (*double arrows*, **A**).

faint enhancement of the normally nonenhancing fluid-filled spaces of the labyrinth seen on contrast-enhanced T1-weighted images.[150] This finding has to be differentiated from labyrinthine schwannoma in which the enhancement pattern is much more intense.[151] In the second stage, the fibrous stage, fibrous strands replace the endolymph and perilymph in the inner ear, resulting in a decrease of the signal on T2-weighted images. The enhancement of the inner ear after gadolinium injection is not as intense as in the acute stage of the disease.[152] The third stage, labyrinthitis ossificans, includes osteoid deposition and osteoneogenesis within the endolymphatic and perilymphatic spaces.[153] This stage is easily demonstrated by CT, with severe cases resulting in a total "white-out" of the membranous labyrinth (**Figs. 11-28** and **11-29**). On MRI, labyrinthitis ossificans appears as a signal void in the normally high signal strength labyrinth on T2W images.[98]

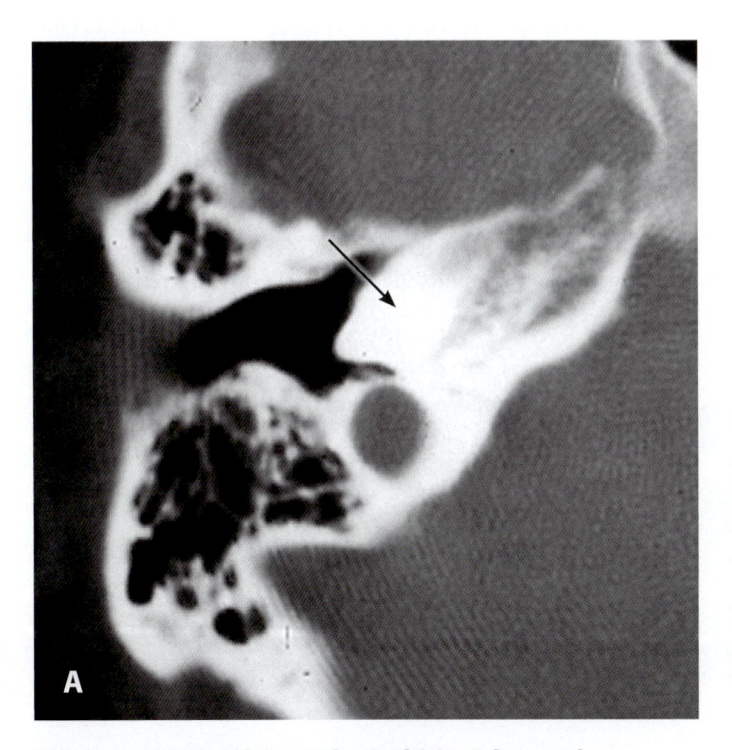

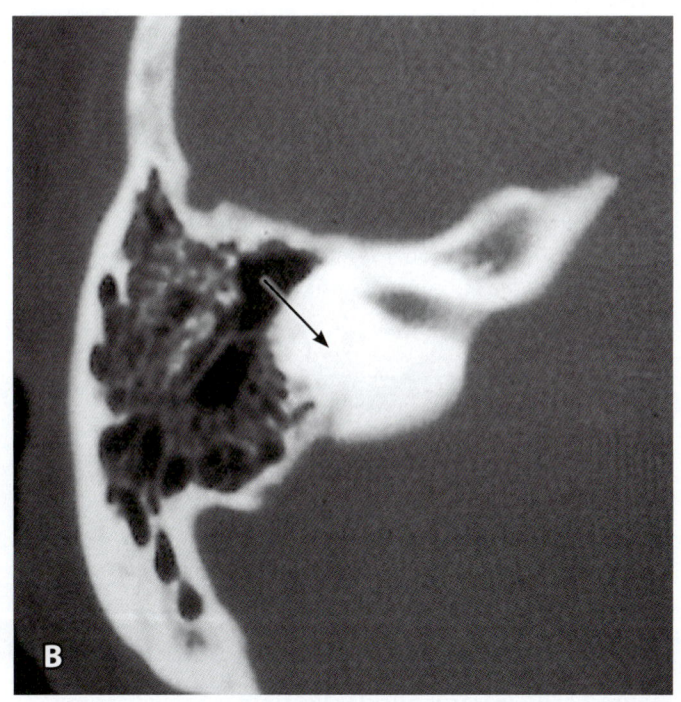

Figure 11-29 Ossifying Labyrinthitis–Advanced
Axial CT images (**A, B**) show complete obliteration of the expected locations of the cochlea (*arrow*, **A**) and vestibule (*arrow*, **B**) representing total bony replacement of the fluid spaces.

TEMPORAL BONE TUMORS AND MIMICS

Cerebellopontine Angle Masses

Vestibular Schwannoma

Schwannomas are benign, slow-growing nerve sheath tumors, which arise from Schwann cells. Vestibular schwannomas comprise 85% to 90% of tumors of the cerebellopontine angle, and 10% of all intracranial tumors. They are also the most common tumor in patients with unilateral SNHL. Eighty-five percent of eighth CN schwannomas involve the vestibular rather than the cochlear portion of the nerve. The tumor typically arises at the transitional zone where myelin produced by oligodendrocytes intersects with myelin from Schwann cells. This area, called the Obersteiner-Redlich zone, is normally located at the level of the porus acousticus.

The tumors are usually unilateral and sporadic. Bilateral tumors, especially in children, suggest neurofibromatosis type 2. In this case, there should be additional investigation for associated lesions, such as meningiomas and spinal tumors.[154] Many centers now perform genetic testing on all patients under the age of twenty presenting with a VS.

VS present with slowly progressive unilateral sensorineural hearing loss, with early impairment of high frequencies and speech discrimination. Acute or episodic hearing loss may occur secondary to cochlear nerve vascular occlusion.[155] Tinnitus is another common symptom. Vertigo is less common, despite involvement of the vestibular nerve. Very large tumors may present with cerebellar dysfunction (ataxia, disequilibrium) or lower cranial neuropathy (hoarseness, dysphagia, sternocleidomastoid weakness), but in general, these CNs are less sensitive to tumor compression.[155]

Grossly, these tumors are encapsulated, nodular, and rubbery, with a variegated cut surface. Yellow and gray areas may be interspersed with hemorrhagic foci or cysts. The nerve may be splayed over the surface of the tumor.[156] Stretching of the nerve over the tumor surface adds to vascular occlusion, accelerating hearing loss.

Histologically, schwannomas comprise variable amounts of compact fibrous stroma (Antoni A), and areas with myxoid stroma (Antoni B). Verocay bodies, parallel rows of nuclei separated by a band of anucleate fibrous tissue, are a hallmark finding. The vessels of these tumors leak plasma proteins, and develop thick hyalinized walls. Typical VS do not invade the nerve, and there are well-defined planes between nerve and tumor. Schwannomas are very vascular, and may contain hemorrhage or thrombosis (see **Fig. 9-40**). They are also prone to fatty degeneration.

On imaging, smaller lesions, 15 mm or less, are primarily intracanalicular, and thus tubular in shape. Larger lesions, greater than 30 mm, are rounded masses in the CPA. The classic "ice cream cone" shape of these lesions results from medium-sized tumors with components in both locations: the CPA portion is the "ice cream" on the canalicular "cone." T1-weighted images without contrast show a lesion isointense to brain that displaces normal CSF signal. Small lesions show uniform contrast enhancement. Larger lesions may be heterogeneous if there is cystic or hemorrhagic change. T2 FSE images show the tumor as a nodule or filling defect in bright CSF. The detail of these images allows for the determination of nerve segment of origin (**Fig. 11-30**). CT images can demonstrate widening of the IAC or erosion of the temporal bone (**Fig. 11-31**).

Epidermoids may also occur in this region, and can be differentiated by low T1-weighted signal, high T2 signal, and no enhancement with contrast. Meningiomas can be differentiated from schwannomas by intratumoral calcification, location eccentric to IAC, and hyperostosis.

Treatment options are based upon tumor size, presence or absence of useful hearing, and medical risk factors. Most small, asymptomatic tumors are observed with serial MR imaging of the brain and cervical spine. Over half of unilateral VS do not enlarge.[157] The optimal treatment of symptomatic tumors is controversial, with the primary options being resection or radiosurgery.[158,159]

Gamma knife radiosurgery (GKR) may be used for the successful treatment of vestibular schwannoma. GKR consists of the focusing of multiple beams on the center of the neoplasm using cobalt sources.[249] It is typically reserved for treatment of small to moderate-sized tumors, especially when hearing is preserved or minimally decreased. Following radiosurgery,

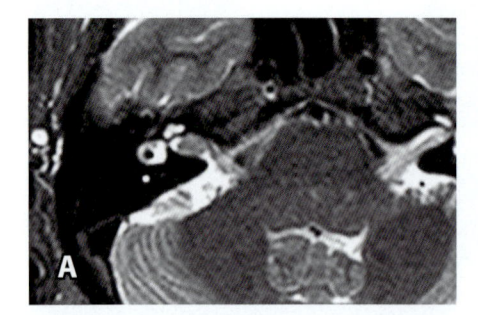

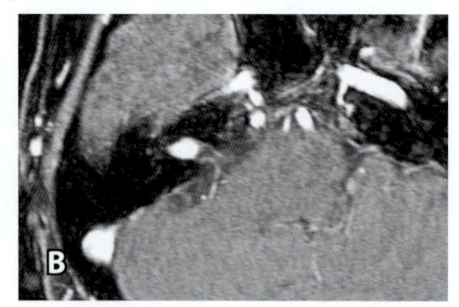

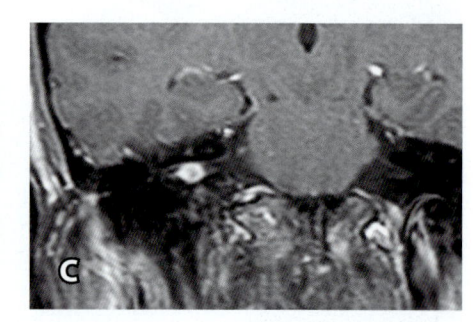

Figure 11-30 Intracanalicular Vestibular Schwannoma
Axial T2 (**A**) and postcontrast axial (**B**) and coronal (**C**) T1W MR images show an enhancing filling defect (**B, C**) in the high signal CSF (**A**) within the right internal auditory canal. Note that the fundus of the internal auditory canal is spared (**A**), suggesting its location is confined solely to the internal auditory canal.

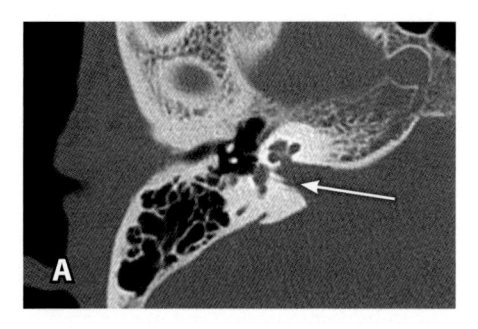

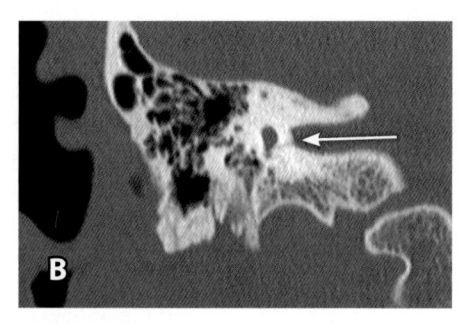

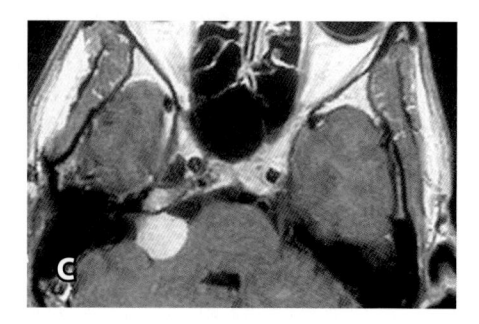

Figure 11-31 Schwannoma of the Inferior Vestibular Nerve
Axial (**A**) and coronal reformatted (**B**) CT show enlargements of both the singular foramen (*arrows*) and of the porus acusticus of the internal auditory canal (IAC). On axial postcontrast T1W MR, there is a focal, enhancing mass of the cerebellopontine angle (CPA) IAC cistern centered on the porus acusticus.

the tumor gradually becomes more heterogeneous and cystic as the center of the lesion undergoes cell death and fibrosis with decrease in the amount of enhancement over the course of 2 years after treatment (**Fig. 11-32**). Temporary enlargement of the tumor and adjacent edema in the brain stem may also be seen following radiation.

Patients with NF-2 usually require surgery because the natural history of these tumors includes continued growth, the involvement of multiple CNs, and greater difficulty with resection secondary to adherence to the nerves.[155]

Postoperative surveillance imaging is scheduled based upon extent of resection and likelihood of recurrence. For those with

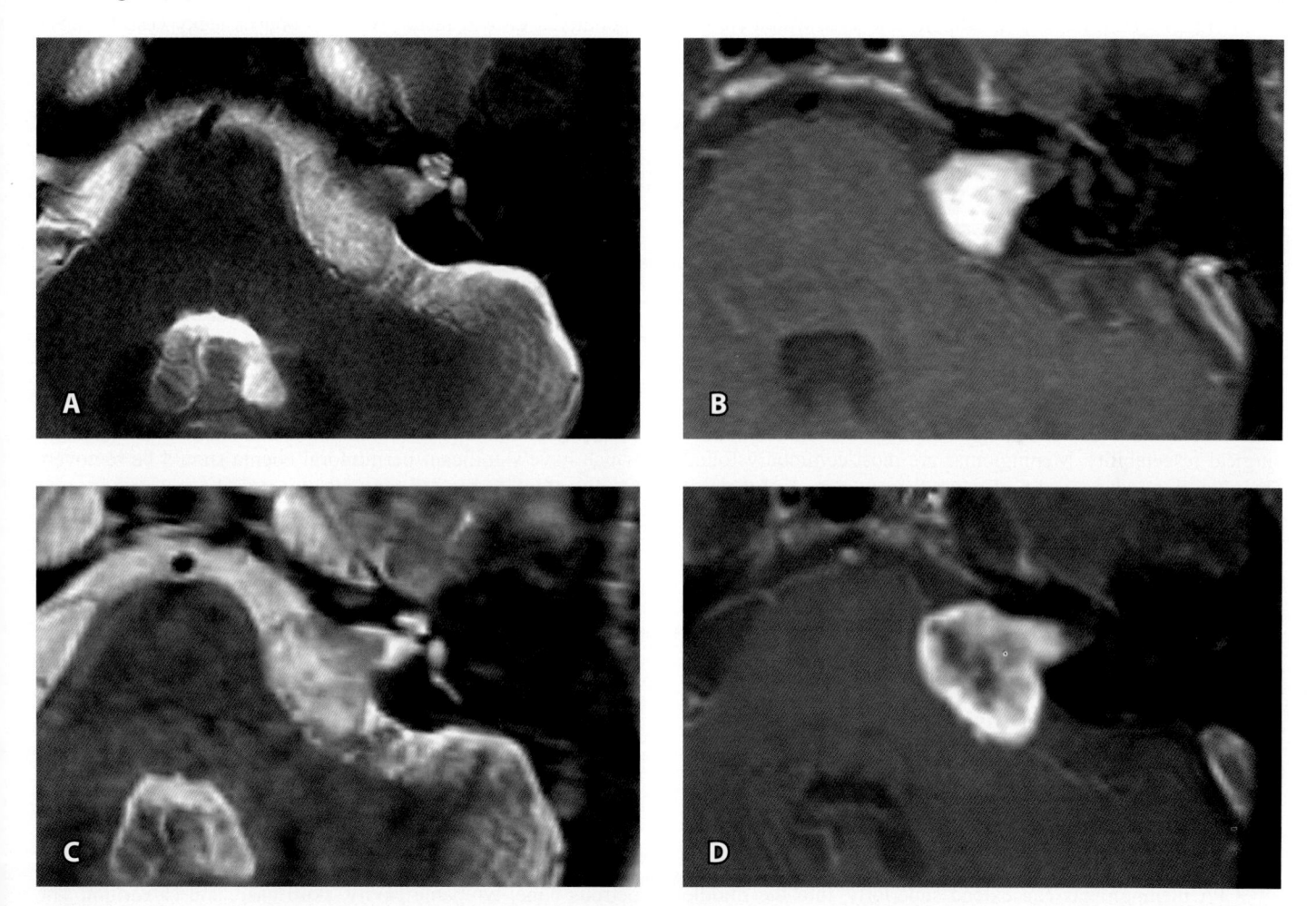

Figure 11-32 Vestibular Schwannoma Pre and Postradiosurgery
Preradiosurgery axial T2 (**A**), axial contrast-enhanced T1 (**B**) and 12-months postradiosurgery axial T2 (**C**) and axial contrast enhanced (**D**) MR scans show a vestibular schwannoma as an "ice cream cone" shaped filling defect in the CPA-IAC. Following treatment, there is greater heterogeneity of the tumor, suggesting hemorrhagic change or cellular debris within the tumor capsule. There is also less enhancement.

complete resection, repeat imaging at three years is reasonable, while subtotal resection may require earlier imaging, perhaps at one year.[160] The surgical approach determines whether a fat or muscle graft was left in the defect. Muscle will enhance and should not be mistaken for recurrence.

Meningioma

Meningiomas are the most common extra-axial tumors, and make up 5% to 10% of CPA masses. Most meningiomas are benign, well-circumscribed tumors that arise from arachnoid membrane. The primary differential diagnosis in the CPA is vestibular schwannoma.

Meningiomas arise at middle age, and more commonly in females by a 3:2 ratio.[161] The incidence increases with age, and many incidental meningiomas are found at autopsy. There is an association with previous radiation therapy and estrogen-dependent neoplasms. Hereditary forms are associated with NF2. Ten percent of sporadic meningiomas are multiple. Five percent are malignant.[161] In children, meningiomas are rare, aggressive, and usually associated with NF2. In this case, they are often multiple and associated with multiple schwannomas.

Meningiomas arise from arachnoid cap cells, which collect in clusters around the tips of arachnoid villi. These meningothelial cells have both epithelial and mesenchymal characteristics, with differentiation toward one or the other leading to a variety of subtypes. The WHO classification system recognizes three grades of meningioma based upon mitotic count, with a number of variants in each category. The WHO grade 1, classic meningioma subtypes include fibrous, angiomatous, and transitional. Approximately 90% of meningiomas are grade 1. WHO grade 2 meningiomas are the more aggressive, atypical variants with a greater propensity for recurrence. WHO grade 3 lesions, which comprise 3%, are anaplastic, with greater propensity for malignant behavior, local invasion, and metastases.[162]

The location of meningiomas and involvement of local structures are the primary prognostic factors, as they affect surgical resectability. Meningiomas are most commonly found along the dural sinuses, their large tributary veins, and the exit foramina of vessels and CNs.[163] In the temporal bone, they occur most frequently at the IAC, the jugular foramen, the geniculate ganglion, and the sulcus of the greater and lesser superficial petrosal nerves.[164] They can be rounded masses, as they displace adjacent brain, but in some regions, such as the sphenoid ridge, they grow en-plaque within the dura. En-plaque meningiomas are more likely to be aggressive and cause hyperostosis, an osteoblastic process in overlying bone. The tumors displace, but do not invade neural tissue. They can invade bone without destruction by spreading through haversian canals. Fifty percent of skull base meningiomas cause hyperostosis in adjacent bone, which appears on imaging as spicules of bone protruding into the tumor.[165]

CPA meningiomas can extend superiorly, into the middle cranial fossa, inferiorly, descending into the foramen magnum, through the jugular foramen into the upper cervical region, or medially to involve the clivus. Tumors of the IAC can spread along nerves into the cochlea, vestibule, and semicircular canals.[163]

Over half of meningiomas present with seizure as their only symptom.[166] Depending upon the location of the tumor, meningiomas may also present with hearing loss, tinnitus, vertigo, cerebellar dysfunction, or obstructive hydrocephalus. The facial nerve is not commonly affected, but symptoms of its involvement would include facial paresis and hemifacial spasm.

Grossly, the tumors are smooth or lobulated, and rubbery. There are a range of microscopic patterns, and a characteristic feature is the psammoma body, a calcified arachnoid villi tip.

Meningiomas are iso- to hypointense to gray matter on T1- and T2-weighted images. Highly fibrous areas and calcification in the tumor will have low signal intensity. Meningiomas enhance intensely with contrast unless there is central necrosis or calcification. Approximately 15% have necrosis, cysts, or hemorrhage, which may make diagnosis more difficult.[166] Meningiomas are well known to possess a dural tail, which likely represents vascular tissue adjacent to tumor. Dural tails suggest meningioma, but are not specific, and can present in other CPA tumors.[167] The CSF cleft sign represents flow voids from pial vessels between tumor and brain. There is often significant peritumoral white matter edema. This may correlate with tumor production of vascular endothelial growth factor, which produces leaky vessels and is variable amongst meningiomas.[168] CT may show hyperostosis, and up to 25% of meningiomas calcify.[169] The tumor is hyperintense on noncontrast CT images. Meningiomas have a broad dural margin, in contrast to vestibular schwannomas which may appear as a spheroid or nodular mass with an acute angle to the adjacent bone. Meningiomas will not widen the IAC, unlike VS, but will invade other neural foramina. It is rare that a meningioma is limited to the IAC, but in this instance, differentiating this lesion from a VS can be very difficult.[170–172]

Treatment of asymptomatic meningiomas is controversial, as these are slow growing tumors which most often occur in older patients. Many tumors are observed with serial imaging for up to a year before decision is made as to treatment. It is generally agreed that tumors which are symptomatic, enlarging, or which have significant peritumoral edema should be removed. Choice of treatment and surgical approach depends upon tumor location at the convexity, parasagittal region, or skull base. Complete resection is preferable, but not always possible, and in these cases, subtotal resection with conventional radiotherapy or radiosurgery can retard tumor progression and prevent recurrence. Fractional conformal radiotherapy has also been shown to be effective as a primary treatment option.[159,173,174]

Epidermoid

Epidermoids, also called congenital cholesteatomas or epidermoid inclusion cysts, develop from congenital rests of ectoderm, most commonly in the CPA cistern. They are the next most common CPA neoplasm after meningioma, comprising up to 10% of masses in the region.[175] They can also occur in the ventricles, petrous bone, tympanic cavity, skull base, and calvarium. The tumor is a solid collection of desquamated keratin debris and cholesterol crystals. These unilocular masses expand slowly, and may produce only mild symptoms.

These tumors are congenital, but commonly do not present until young or middle adulthood. Neuropathies arise secondary to compression effect. Hearing loss, the most common presenting symptom of all CPA tumors, is frequently the presenting symptom for epidermoids, as well. Involvement of the fifth CN is common, resulting in trigeminal neuralgia, facial hypesthesia, or motor deficits. Facial nerve compression produces hemifacial spasm and weakness. Temporal lobe involvement may produce seizures. Typically, symptom onset is gradual, but acute onset of aseptic meningitis can result from cyst rupture. Rarely, acute symptom onset and aggressive tumor behavior represent malignant degeneration to squamous cell carcinoma.

Epidermoids do not displace adjacent structures like most benign CPA tumors, but rather conform to available space, and insinuate into the brainstem and other areas through paths of least resistance. Eventually, they envelop nerves and vessels. Epidermoids adhere to adjacent structures secondary to inflammatory reaction from cyst leakage.

Grossly, the tumor may be nodular or smooth, and has a glistening, pearly appearance. Sectioned surfaces demonstrate soft, coarsely granular debris composed of keratin layers. The cyst wall is a flattened layer of squamous epithelium on a thin band of fibrous tissue. The tumor has a broad, noninvasive interface with adjacent brain.

T1-weighted signal depends upon the relative amounts of keratin and cholesterol in the mass. Most commonly, the epidermoid is hypointense, but brighter than CSF. "Dirty CSF" is the term used to describe the mild heterogeneity. Rarely, an epidermoid will be hyperintense on T1-weighted images and hypointense on T2-weighted images because of significant triglyceride and fatty acid content (**Fig. 11-33**). On T2-weighted images, the tumor is hyperintense. CISS images or 3D FSE images, which are heavily T2-weighted, allow for clear delineation of tumor extent.[176] There is no contrast enhancement, which differentiates this tumor from other CPA tumors. Diffusion weighted imaging can be used in difficult cases, and will show greater restricted diffusion, or a lower apparent diffusion coefficient (therefore, high signal on DWI images) than arachnoid

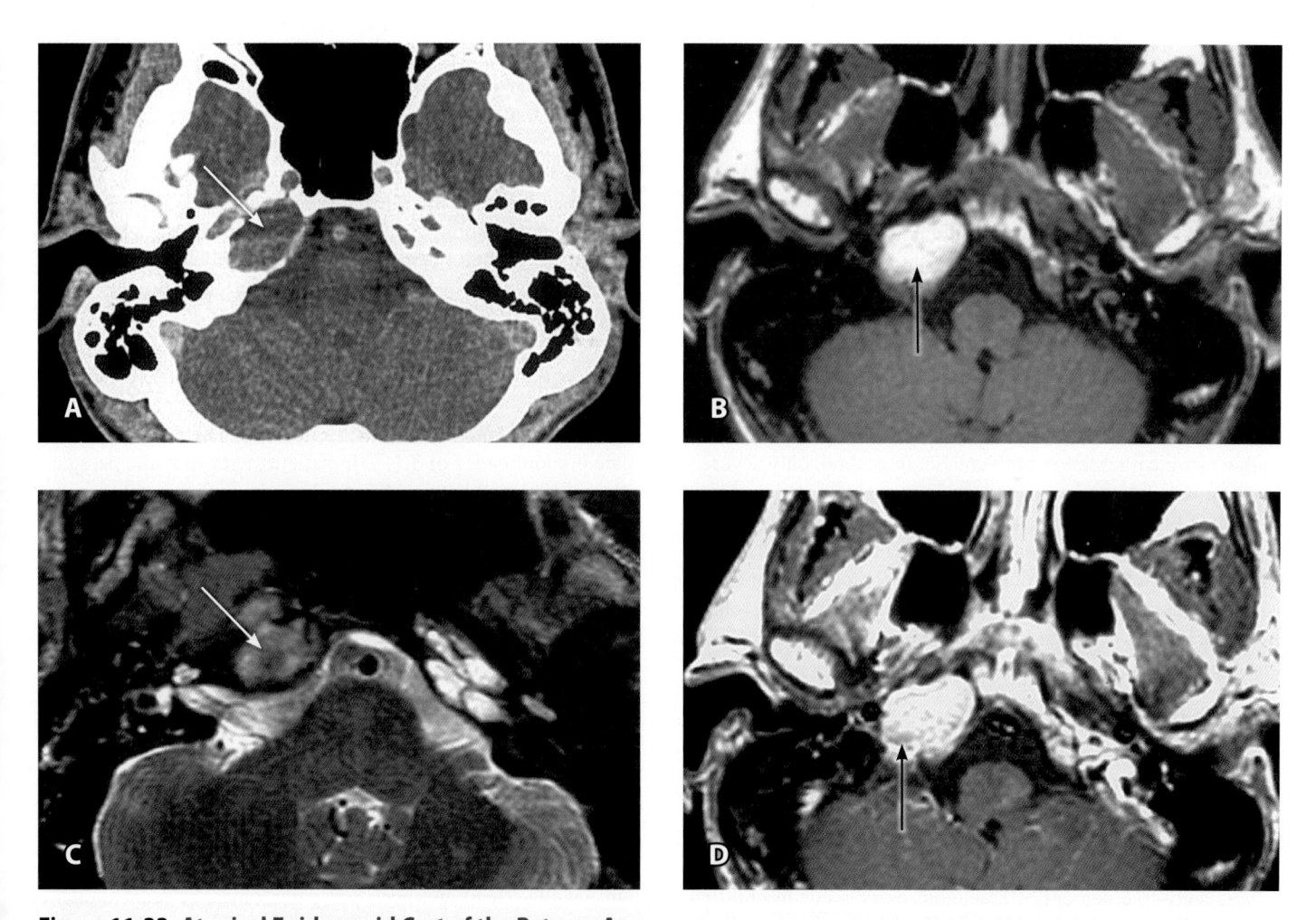

Figure 11-33 Atypical Epidermoid Cyst of the Petrous Apex
Axial contrast-enhanced CT (**A**) shows a nonenhancing cystic mass with smooth bony expansion in the right petrous apex (*arrow*). Axial T1 (**B**), axial T2 (**C**), and contrast-enhanced axial T1 (**D**) MR scans. Please note this atypical or "white" epidermoid cyst shows high T1 signal and low T2 signal, but no post contrast enhancement. A cholesterol granuloma would demonstrate both T1 and T2 increased signal intensities. Also note fluid in the apical air cells on the left side, consistent with mastoid disease without cholesteatoma.

cysts. CT demonstrates a well-defined, homogeneous, lobulated mass that is iso- or mildly hypodense to CSF, secondary to cholesterol and keratin content. Twenty percent of epidermoids will show calcification.[115] The bulk of these cysts are avascular debris, so they will not enhance, except for a thin peripheral rim.

The most common differential diagnosis is arachnoid cyst. On MR images, signal in arachnoid cysts will exactly match CSF, whereas epidermoids may not be completely uniform. In addition, epidermoids will engulf blood vessels, while arachnoid cysts do not. On CT, the presence of rim enhancement or calcification makes epidermoid more likely. Epidermoids may mimic acoustic schwannoma when it extends into the IAC, but can be differentiated by lack of contrast enhancement.

The preferred treatment of epidermoid cysts is surgical resection. Complete resection can be difficult because of the dense adherence to neurovascular structures. Controversy exists as to whether complete removal, with the increased risk of surgical complication while dissecting out the CNs is more efficacious than subtotal resection with its high rate of eventual tumor recurrence.[177] Postsurgical surveillance requires diffusion-weighted imaging.

Lipoma

Lipomas are heterotopias which result from the fatty maldevelopment of the meninx primitiva. Meninx primitiva is a mesenchymal derivative of the neural crest that surrounds the primitive notochord which resorbs in the developing embryo, and persistent reticuloendothelial components are the precursors of lipomas.[178] These masses of ectopic fat are commonly found in the midline in association with callosal abnormalities, but are more rarely found in the CPA,[179] the IAC,[180] and the vestibule.[181]

These lesions are often not symptomatic, and can be observed with serial imaging. If the tumor is symptomatic, it usually presents as mild unilateral SNHL in a young adult. Symptoms result from neurovascular compression by encasing tumor. The fatty tumor often adheres to nerves by fibrous bands, making surgical resection problematic. In general, only severely symptomatic lesions are treated.[182]

On T1-weighted images, images show hyperintense fat signal, which yields contrast-enhancement less useful, but fat saturation is very helpful, demonstrating complete suppression. Signal is intermediate on T2-weighted images, but will remain high on FLAIR. Unenhanced CT images demonstrate signal, and there is no enhancement with contrast.

Arachnoid Cyst

An arachnoid cyst is a congenital split or duplication of the arachnoid membrane which collects CSF. They are less commonly found in the CPA or IAC, with most found in the sylvian, parasagittal, and convexity regions. This lesion will cause SNHL when sufficiently large to compress the vestibulocochlear nerve.

Seventy-five percent of arachnoid cysts occur in children, with a male to female ratio of 2:1.[183] The majority are found incidentally. Symptoms arise secondary to compression or increased intracranial pressure, and are most commonly SNHL, ataxia, and headache.[184]

The walls of the arachnoid cyst are thin; often only a few layers of mesothelial-like cells with an inner lining layer of pseudostratified ciliated epithelial cells. Most small arachnoid cysts do not enlarge, but they can fill secondary to a "ball-valve" mechanism after increases in intracranial pressure.[185]

Arachnoid cysts have MR signal characteristics similar to CSF; low signal intensity on T1 and high signal on T2-weighted images. There is no enhancement with contrast. They are rounded and smooth, with an imperceptible cyst wall. FLAIR and CISS sequences and diffusion weighted imaging can help differentiate arachnoid cyst and epidermoid. In addition, arachnoid cysts can be differentiated by relation to surrounding structures. Arachnoid cysts will displace adjacent structures, while epidermoids will encase them. Arachnoid cysts often erode adjacent bone.

In most cases, small or asymptomatic cysts are not treated. If symptomatic, these lesions can be treated with resection and fenestration or shunted.[184]

Glomus Tympanicum Paraganglioma and Jugular Foramen Tumors

Glomus Tympanicum Paraganglioma

Glomus tympanicum paraganglioma (GTP) is a rare, benign, hypervascular tumor arising from glomus bodies on cochlear promontory. Large paragangliomas located in the jugular foramen – glomus jugulare tumors (see **Fig. 9-47**) can extend through the jugular plate into the middle ear, and are called glomus jugulotympanicum paragangliomas. GTPs arise from the paraganglia along the tympanic branch of the glossopharyngeal nerve (the nerve of Jacobson), while glomus jugular tumors arise from paraganglia on the auricular branch of the vagus nerve (the nerve of Arnold.)

GTPs are the most common tumor of the middle ear, and the second most common temporal bone tumor, after vestibular schwannoma. Paragangliomas can present at any age, but usually between the fourth and sixth decades. There is a female to male predominance of 3:1.[186] In patients with sporadic paraganglioma, 10% will have additional lesions. In those with familial paragangliomas, 30% to 40% will have multicentric tumors.[187] Symptoms relate to tumor location, extension, and vascularity. Tumor in the middle ear can cause conductive hearing loss, and aural discharge. Extension can cause SNHL, vertigo, and cranial neuropathies. Pulsatile tinnitus, the most frequently reported symptom, is caused by the vascular nature of the tumor and early involvement of the umbo with resulting transmission of vascular pulsations.[163] On exam, GTP appears as a vascular, pulsatile, retrotympanic mass in the anterior inferior quadrant of the tympanic membrane.

Paragangliomas arise from widely dispersed chief cells; cells of the diffuse neuroendocrine system, which are of neural crest origin and migrate in association with sympathetic nervous system ganglia. Head and neck paragangliomas, or branchiomeric paragangliomas, most commonly arise at the carotid body, followed by the jugulotympanic region. One percent of head and neck paragangliomas are functional, secreting vasoactive catecholamines. Two percent to 4% of jugulotympanic paragangliomas are malignant.[188] Histologically, one finds clusters of Type I or catecholamine containing chief cells, described as "zellballen," along with unmyelinated nerve fibers and blood vessels in a fibrovascular stroma.[189]

Paragangliomas grow slowly and insidiously. They spread through the temporal bone along pathways of least resistance, including vascular channels, fissures, and through air cells, and can enter the intracranial cavity by following the petrous carotid artery into the middle cranial fossa and cavernous sinus, or enter the nasopharynx via the eustachian tube. Tumor can also spread via the jugular bulb, inferior petrosal sinus, sigmoid sinus, and jugular vein to enter the skull base and the carotid artery. In the middle ear, the tumors can envelop the ossicular chain or erode through the tympanic membrane. The Glasscock-Jackson classification of GTPs allows for description of the tumor extension (Table 11-4).

On CT images, GTPs will appear as well-defined intratympanic soft tissue masses that can fill the tympanic cavity without destroying the ossicular chain. While advanced tumors can destroy bone, which appears "moth eaten", most GTPs present with otologic symptoms early, before extensive remodeling. Jugulotympanic paragangliomas will demonstrate erosion of the jugular plate and carotid spine. T1-weighted MR images demonstrate the highly vascular nature of the tumor. On T2-weighted images, large tumors have a characteristic "salt and pepper" appearance (Fig. 11-34).

Table 11-4 Glasscock-Jackson Classification

Type I	Small mass limited to cochlear promontory
Type II	Tumor completely filling middle ear space
Type III	Filling middle ear and extending into mastoid air cells
Type IV	Filling middle ear, extending into mastoid or through tympanic membrane to fill external auditory canal; may extend anterior to carotid artery

The differential diagnosis for GTP and jugulotympanic paragangliomas includes other vascular anomalies of the middle ear, including an aberrant internal carotid artery, congenital intratympanic ICA aneurysm, or a dehiscent or high-riding jugular bulb. An accurate imaging diagnosis is vital to prevent a potentially disastrous biopsy of the ICA.

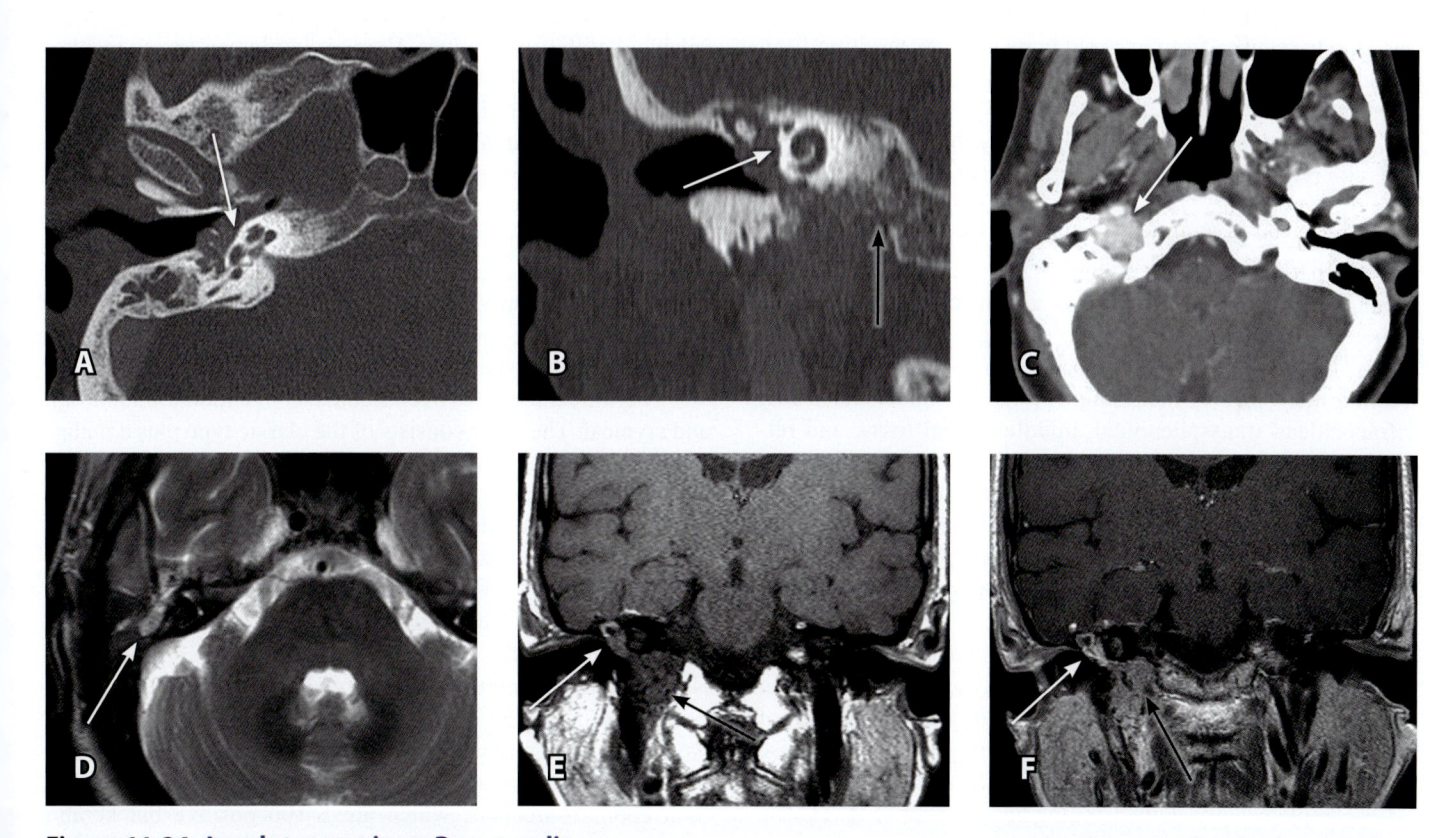

Figure 11-34 Jugulotympanicum Paraganglioma
Axial (**A**), reformatted coronal (**B**) and axial contrast-enhanced CT scans. A soft tissue mass fills the tympanic cavity (*arrow*, **A**) and expands beneath the hypotympanum toward the jugular foramen (*arrows*, **B**) which contains an intensely enhancing tumor (*arrow*, **C**). Axial T2 (**D**), coronal T1 (**E**) and coronal contrast enhanced T1 (**F**) MR scans show the tumor in the middle ear cavity (*arrow*, **A**) and its extension inferiorly into the jugular fossa (*arrows*, **E**) and its characteristic "salt and pepper" pattern of postcontrast enhancement (*arrow*, **F**).

Small GTPs are treated with tympanotomy, while large tumors require mastoidectomy. Prognosis is good with complete resection. Significant bleeding can complicated surgical removal of these highly vascular tumors. Preoperative embolization is favored in large tumors of the jugular foramen and skull base.[163]

Petrous Apex Masses

Cholesterol Granuloma of the Petrous Apex

CGs are smoothly expanding cystic masses with a thin fibrous capsule filled with "crankcase oil" fluid consisting of old blood and cholesterol crystals.

These lesions most often present with sensorineural hearing loss in young or middle age adults. Other symptoms include can tinnitus, dizziness and fifth, sixth, and seventh CN deficits, depending on size and position. Very large lesions can cause intradural erosion, and patients may present with cerebrospinal fluid leak, cerebellopontine angle mass lesion, or chemical meningitis from cyst rupture within the subarachnoid space.

Chronic inflammation and isolation of air cells is believed to cause hemorrhage secondary to mucosal engorgement. Continued obstruction, with recurrent hemorrhage and inflammation incites a granulomatous response, and blood degradation products produce cholesterol crystals.[190] An alternative theory of development has recently been described involving continuous bloody seepage from exposed bone marrow, resulting from breakdown in the bone partition between pneumatic tracts and marrow spaces.[191]

These lesions have a variable growth rate. Aggressive behavior resulting in bony destruction may relate to the robustness of the vascular source of hemorrhage.[192] Asymptomatic patients can be observed followed with imaging.[193] In symptomatic patients, treatment has traditionally involved cyst drainage and stent placement via a transtemporal approach. Reported recurrence rates were as high as 60% in some series.[194] Multiple surgical approaches have been described for treating these lesions including: infralabyrinthine, transcanal infracochlear, transsphenoidal, middle cranial fossa, and retrosigmoid. The approach taken depends on the patients hearing and the site and extent of the lesion. Controversy exists as to which surgical approach is most efficacious, but many prefer the extended middle fossa approach, which allows for complete drainage and obliteration of the cyst cavity to prevent recurrence.[194]

The presence of chronic blood products (methemoglobin) and cholesterol crystals produce a hyperintense signal on T1-weighted images. Contrast-enhanced images show a rim of GT in the periphery, with a nonenhancing center. Hyperintense T2 signal rounds out the characteristic picture of these lesions. CT is complementary, demonstrating bony erosion (**Fig. 11-35**). On MRA, these lesions resemble ICA aneurysms.

Mimics include mucoceles and normal marrow, but these lesions can be differentiated by low signal on T1 for the former, and low signal on T2-weighted images in the later. An ICA aneurysm in the petrous apex will show heterogeneous enhancement with contrast. A nonaggressive lesion which is hyperintense on T1 and T2 and does not enhance, is highly suggestive of cholesterol granuloma.

Chordoma

Chordomas are rare, aggressive tumors that develop from primitive notochord. Most are located in the sacrococcygeal region and clivus.[195] Most chordomas arise in the midline, distinguishing them from skull base chondrosarcomas which arise laterally along the sphenoid wing.

Chordomas that arise in the clivus infiltrate bone along paths of least resistance, and may spread laterally to the petrous apex or cavernous sinus, posteriorly to the posterior cranial fossa and CPA, ventrally to the middle fossa, paranasal sinuses, orbit, nasopharynx, and nasal cavity, or inferiorly to the infratemporal fossa. This low-grade malignant tumor spreads slowly along the surfaces of the skull base, enveloping nerves and blood vessels. Consequently, complete resection is nearly impossible, and recurrence rate is high.

The tumor can present at any age, but most commonly in middle age. Though tumors appear to be more aggressive in young patients, their prognosis is better. Older patients have a 10-year mortality rate of 11%, while in younger patients it is 63%.[196] Patients most commonly present with the insidious onset of headache, diplopia, and sixth CN palsy.

Chordomas tend to arise in the basiocciput along the clivus or inferior to the spheno-occipital synchondrosis or the basisphenoid of the upper clivus. Cranial chordomas arising in other sites are rare but include the nasopharynx, paranasal sinuses, parotid region, petrous bone, nasal cavity, soft palate, hard palate, and alveolar ridge. In embryological development, the notochord begins in the sphenoid bone, posterior to the sella. It exits bone along the clivus in the soft tissue adjacent to the nasopharyngeal mucosa, and then re-enters bone in the basiocciput. The cranial aspect of the cord has stalks which extend into the subendothelium of the nasopharynx and ventral brainstem. Therefore, chordomas may be found in the clivus, or as nasopharyngeal or intracranial soft tissue tumors.[197]

There are three types of chordoma: conventional, chondroid, and atypical. The latter consists of the classic type plus a malignant mesenchymal component such as malignant fibrous histiocytoma, fibrosarcoma, or osteosarcoma.[156] Grossly, chordomas are gelatinous, lobulated, and semitranslucent gray tumors. They are encapsulated, with a variegated appearance and solid and cystic areas.[198] Histologically, they are pseudoencapsulated, and separated into lobules by fibrous connective tissue.[198] They are characterized by irregular, often-branching cords of cells. Nests of cuboidal epithelioid cells and physaliphorous (bubble-bearing) cells appear to float in a myxoid stroma. Chordomas have a unique immunohistochemistry reaction pattern: they are both S-100 and keratin positive. This distinguishes them from both chondrosarcomas, which are S-100 positive but keratin negative, and mucinous adenocarcinomas which are keratin positive and S-100 negative.

Metastases are rare, but can occur late in the disease process, and mainly go to lungs, bone, liver, and lymph nodes.[198] Malignant transformation of chondroma to chondrosarcoma has been reported in association with Maffucci syndrome, a congenital

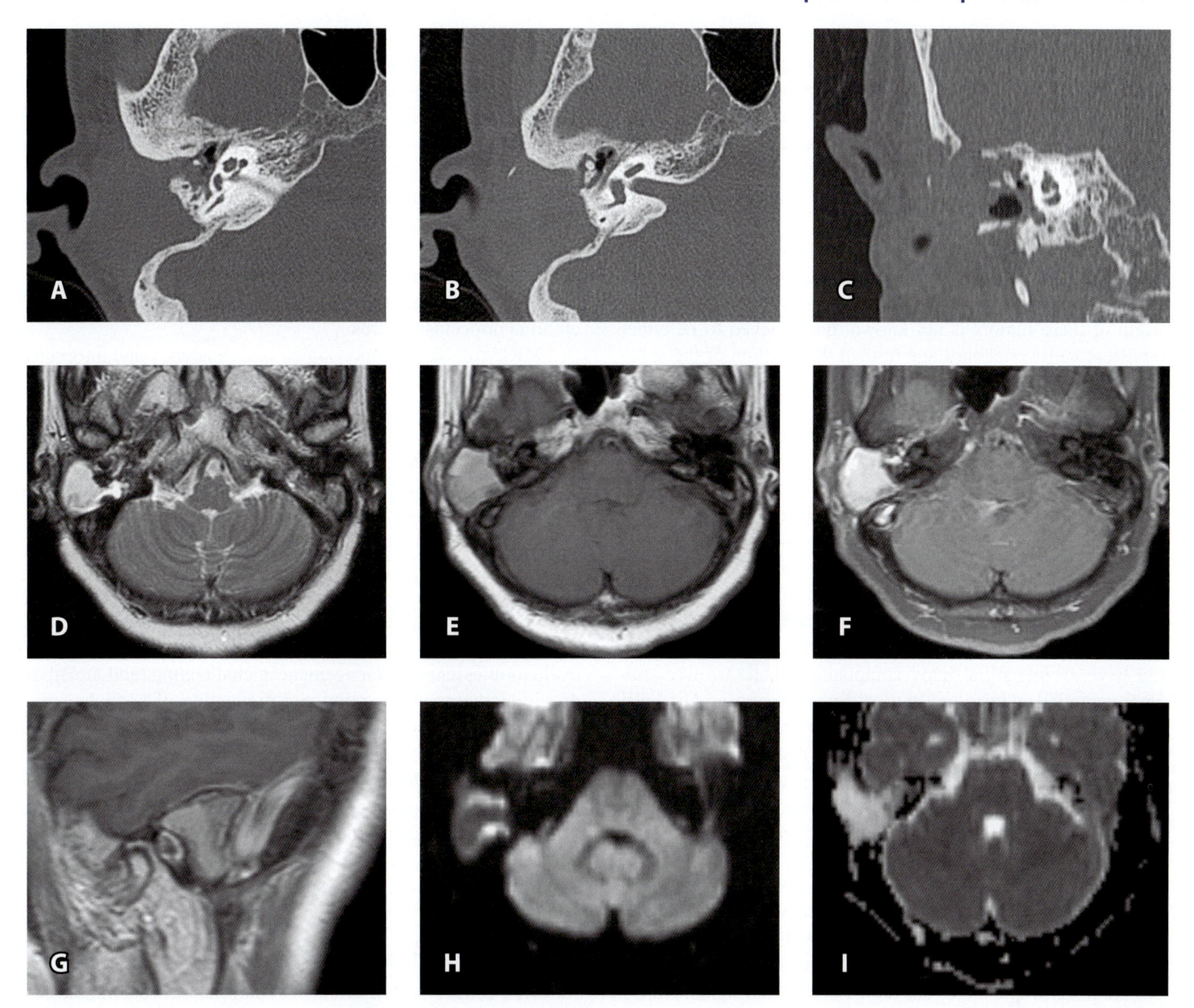

Figure 11-35 Cholesterol Granuloma Post Mastoidectomy
Cholesterol granuloma in a 62-year-old female with prior right mastoidectomy and several months of gradual onset conductive hearing loss. Axial (**A–B**) and coronal reformatted (**C**) bone CT scans show a soft tissue density mass within the postsurgical temporal bone cavity. The mass also extends into the middle ear via the aditus, where there is patchy granulation tissue in Prussak's space and the mesotympanum (**A–B**). There is erosion of the lenticular process of the incus and partial erosion of the stapes (**A**). Also note the focal complete erosion in the tegmen tympani (**C**). Axial T2 FLAIR (**D**), axial T1 without contrast (**E**), axial T1 with contrast (**F**), and sagittal T1 postcontrast (**G**) MR images show a heterogeneous high T1, high T2 signal without enhancement, compatible with old blood product composition of cholesterol granulomas. Axial DWI (**H**) with corresponding ADC map (**I**) show no restricted diffusion, differentiating the lesion from cholesteatoma.

syndrome which includes intracranial vascular lesions and chondroid tumors.[199]

Chordomas are typically seen as midline, expansile, destructive lesions involving the clivus. The tumor contains multiple calcifications or bony fragments of the adjacent destroyed bone. T1-weighted images show a hypo- to isointense mass within the high signal clivus. It may have foci of high signal due to old bleeding or proteinaceous fluid. There is intense contrast enhancement, which can be heterogeneous. Calcifications within the tumor mass will have low signal on T1-, T2-, and gradient echo images. MRA shows vessel displacement and encasement. On CT images, the tumor is homogeneous, isointense to brain, and enhances with contrast. There is bone erosion and destruction without active sclerosis.

The deep location of these tumors makes surgical access difficult, and patterns of spread necessitate the use of various surgical approaches. Resection is the agreed upon treatment. Postoperative conventional radiotherapy does not increase survival, but has been shown to increase disease free survival in patients younger than 40 years.[196] Some have found that stereotactic fractionated photon or proton-beam radiotherapy was associated with significantly less recurrence than conventional radiotherapy.[195]

Chondrosarcoma

Chondrosarcomas are rare, malignant chondroid tumors that are found in the petro-occipital fissure or anterior basisphenoid. The origin of these tumors is not known, but believed to be either persistent embryonal cartilage rests at the junction of the sphenopetrosal, petrooccipital, and sphenooccipital synchondroses, or metaplasia of fibroblasts or pluripotent mesenchymal cells.[200] The paramedian location of these tumors differentiates them from chordomas. Chondrosarcomas grow slowly, and 15% metastasize, commonly to lymphatics, lung, and brain.

The tumor affects men and women equally and most commonly arises at middle age. Headache, hearing loss, hoarseness, and diplopia are frequent presenting symptoms, which are noticed months to years before final diagnosis.

On gross exam, the tumors are variegated, with a gritty texture on cut section. They are lobulated with intratumoral cysts, and have an interstitial bony component. There are five subtypes identified on histology, with different prognoses. Grade III lesions, with increased mitotic activity, are rare in the temporal bone.[200] Subtypes can be identified with fine needle aspiration cytology.

Bone erosion of the petrous apex, with extension into the CPA is a common early finding. The tumor can grow superiorly to involve Dorello's canal and compress the abducens nerve, the most commonly affected CN.

T1-weighted images show a low to intermediate signal mass which may have low signal foci of mineralization or fibrocartilage.[201] Contrast enhancement is heterogeneous, with a ring and-arc pattern. The tumor has high T2-weighted signal. On CT there is bone destruction at the petro-occipital fissure and popcorn calcification.

Surgical excision is the mainstay of therapy. Postoperative radiotherapy may be used in cases of recurrence, or growth of residual tumor in subtotal resections.[202,203]

Petrous Apex ICA Aneurysm

Aneurysms of the petrous ICA are rare lesions, which can be acquired or congenital. They are often discovered incidentally, but may present with unilateral SNHL, most commonly, or pulsatile tinnitus, headaches, cranial neuropathies, or sudden onset of severe otorrhagia or epistaxis from blood down the Eustachian tube.

The congenital fusiform type is most common, presenting in children or adolescents. These lesions occur at the weakened sites of regressed embryonic vessels.[204] Microscopically, these lesions demonstrate a connective tissue pseudo wall around an area of full thickness arterial injury.

Acquired aneurysms can arise in patients with prior head trauma and skull base or temporal bone fracture. Pseudoaneurysms resulting from ICA dissection can result from closed head injury with or without fracture of the carotid canal. A history of infection in these areas in immunocompromised patients, or in patients with COM or cholesteatomas can also predispose to these lesions. The petrous ICA is well-protected and without branches, so acquired lesions are especially uncommon.

Otologic symptoms result from erosion through the posterior carotid canal wall to the middle ear or eustachian tube.[205] Lateral expansion into the inner ear may result in symptoms of pulsatile tinnitus, vertigo, or hyperacusis. With enlargement there is increasing risk of life-threatening hemorrhage or embolic or occlusive stroke.

MRI with MRA demonstrates vessel patency and thrombus extension and aneurysm morphology. T2-weighted images show a mass with complex signal, secondary to turbulent flow within the aneurysm, and peripheral hemosiderin. T2*GRE will show blooming of thrombus. T1-weighted images show a hyperintense ovoid mass that enhances with contrast. Nonenhanced CT can demonstrate a destructive lesion with local extension. The lesion enhances with contrast. Thrombosed aneurysm may look like a solid tumor with an enhancing rim and an isodense, nonenhancing center.

Inadvertent manipulation or biopsy of any aneurysm can result in massive hemorrhage, making careful preoperative evaluation essential. Management is challenging, and aimed at providing symptomatic relief and prevention of hemodynamic compromise, embolism, or hemorrhage. Treatment depends upon symptoms and risks of treatment, therefore the patient's age and medical history must be considered. Treatment options range from conservative management with serial imaging, endovascular balloon occlusion, endovascular coil placement, or surgical trapping and revascularization with extra-intracranial bypass.[205,206] Ruptured aneurysm requires immediate endovascular balloon occlusion with or without bypass.[204]

Aberrant Internal Carotid Artery

Rarely, a congenitally aberrant ICA can present as a middle ear mass, and must not be misdiagnosed as a surgical lesion, in order to prevent the significant complications associated with biopsy. Failure of normal ICA development results in the enlargement of a collateral, the inferior tympanic artery, which will enter the skull through the inferior tympanic canaliculus and course through the middle ear, before joining the petrous ICA.[207,208]

These lesions are often asymptomatic, but may present with subjective or objective pulsatile tinnitus or even conductive hearing loss.[207,209]

The appearance of aberrant ICA on otoscopic exam is of a vascular retrotympanic mass, mimicking glomus tympanicum paraganglioma. Therefore, careful examination with thin section temporal bone CT is crucial. The key features identifying an aberrant ICA are the appearance of an enlarged inferior temporal canaliculus, with a tubular mass which courses anteriorly at the cochlear promontory to the horizontal petrous canal through a dehiscence in the IAC canal. The vertical petrous ICA and carotid foramen are absent.

A more common vascular mass is high-riding jugular bulb, which is characterized by the visualization of a normal carotid canal, but a large jugular fossa, with a very thin or deficient hypotympanic bone plate between the middle ear cleft and jugular fossa.[86]

A persistent stapedial artery is a rare anomaly which may be associated with an aberrant ICA. The stapedial artery is a branch of the hyoid artery, which itself is a branch of the ICA. The persistent artery travels in Jacobson's canal, through the obturator foramen of the stapes, and then into the facial canal and extradural space of the middle cranial fossa.[209] Postembryonic persistence of this vessel give rises to the middle meningeal artery, with the associated absence of the ipsilateral foramen spinosum. While this finding is not specific, it is suggestive in the setting of pulsatile tinnitus and retrotympanic vascular mass.

Inner Ear Masses

Endolymphatic Sac Tumor

Endolymphatic sac tumor (ELST) is a rare, destructive adenomatous tumor arising from the proximal portion of the endolymphatic sac on the posterior face of the petrous temporal bone. The tumors are locally invasive, destroying adjacent bone, with bony spicules demonstrated on imaging. They are hypervascular and tend to fistulize the inner ear.

This tumor can present at any age, but is most common in the fourth and fifth decades. In Mukherji's series of 20 patients, 100% presented with unilateral sensorineural hearing loss, 60% had facial nerve paralysis, 50% had pulsatile tinnitus, and 20% had vertigo.[210]

Eleven percent of patients with Von Hippel-Lindau disease (VHLD) have unilateral or bilateral ELSTs.[211] VHLD is an autosomal dominant disorder with incomplete penetrance, resulting from mutation on the short arm of chromosome 3. It presents with multiple retinal and central nervous system hemangioblastomas, renal cysts and carcinoma, pheochromocytoma, pancreatic cysts, papillary cystadenomas of the epididymis, and ELST. The prevalence is 1 in 40,000. Patients most commonly present in their twenties with retinal lesions. All VHLD patients with hearing loss should be screened for ELST with MR imaging.

Histologically, the tumors contain both papillary and cystic components. The papillary component resembles the normal endolymphatic sac epithelium. The cystic portion contains a proteinaceous material resembling thyroid colloid, and thyroglobulin staining is necessary to distinguish ELST from papillary thyroid carcinoma.[163] Nuclear pleomorphism and mitoses are rare.[197] The tumor stroma contains areas of hemorrhage, fibrosis, and cholesterol clefts. There is an abundant capillary vascular supply. Immunohistochemical staining can differentiate ELST from similar appearing tumors, as it is uniquely positive for cytokeratins and S-100.

The tumor infiltrates adjacent bone, replacing it in some areas with fibrotic tumor.[197] New bone is not produced. Intratumoral bony fragments demonstrated on CT images results from tumor infiltrating and interdigitating with the bone spicules. Extension of the tumor from its origin at the retrolabyrinthine, presigmoid petrous ridge along the endolymphatic duct to the labyrinth, with its resultant destruction, accounts for the SNHL that characterizes the vast majority of these tumors. Larger tumors frequently involve the middle ear, and are seen as a soft tissue mass. From the middle ear, further growth can occur superiorly, in the middle cranial fossa, laterally through the tympanic membrane, or medially to the otic capsule. The tumor can also grow laterally to involve the mastoid, and posteriorly to the posterior cranial fossa, accounting for the high incidence of headaches and ataxia in patients with large tumors.[212] Anterior extension into Meckel's cave and the IAC can involve the trigeminal, facial, and vestibulocochlear nerves.

The location of ELST in the posterior temporal bone makes sampling for histological analysis difficult, therefore imaging analysis is especially important. T1-weighted MR images demonstrate intermediate signal speckled with foci of hyper- and hypointensity. This heterogeneity, which is due to subacute hemorrhage breakdown products, slow flow, and cholesterol clefts, is unusual in more common petrous apex lesions, including meningioma, glomus tumors, metastases, eosinophilic granuloma, chondrosarcoma, and chordoma. The majority of ELSTs have a peripheral rim of increased signal.[210] The tumor is expansile rather than diffusely destructive, which differentiates it from metastatic lesions and chondrosarcoma (**Fig. 11-36**). Contrast enhancement can be homogeneous or heterogeneous. There is homogeneously high T2-weighted signal, with flow voids apparent in larger lesions.

CT images show permeative destruction of the temporal bone and intratumoral bony spicules. Nearly all lesions show a peripheral rim of calcification from expansion of posterior cortex of petrous bone.[210] ELSTs are highly vascular, and angiographic information is useful for requisite presurgical embolization.

The primary differential diagnosis for destructive retrolabyrinthine lesions include metastases, lymphoma, sarcoidosis, rhabdomyosarcoma, histiocytosis X, plasmacytoma, and radiation effect. Clinical history and the distinctive imaging characteristics of this tumor facilitate diagnosis in most cases.

Complete surgical resection with wide margins can result in cure. Radiation therapy and chemotherapy are used for palliative treatment.[212,213]

Intralabyrinthine Schwannoma

Intralabyrinthine schwannoma (ILS) is a rare variant of schwannoma that arises from Schwann cells wrapping the distal branches of the cochlea (**Figs. 11-37** and **11-38**), posterior vestibular, or inferior vestibular nerves within the membranous labyrinth. Patients can present with unilateral hearing loss that is sensorineural, mixed, or both. They may also have vertigo, with nausea and vomiting, tinnitus, and aural fullness, making these patients indistinguishable from those with Mèniére's disease on exam.[214,215] For this reason, ILS should be considered in the differential diagnosis of Mèniére's disease before surgical treatment, and patients should undergo high-resolution contrast-enhanced MR imaging.[215,216]

Endolymphatic hydrops is believed to be the cause of symptoms in Mèniére's disease. Some authors believe that ILS can also cause hydrops, resulting in the identical symptoms.[215] Tumor in the vestibule may interfere with the flow of endolymph, with dilation of the endolymphatic spaces of the saccule and cochlear duct, which results in episodic vertigo and hearing loss.[217]

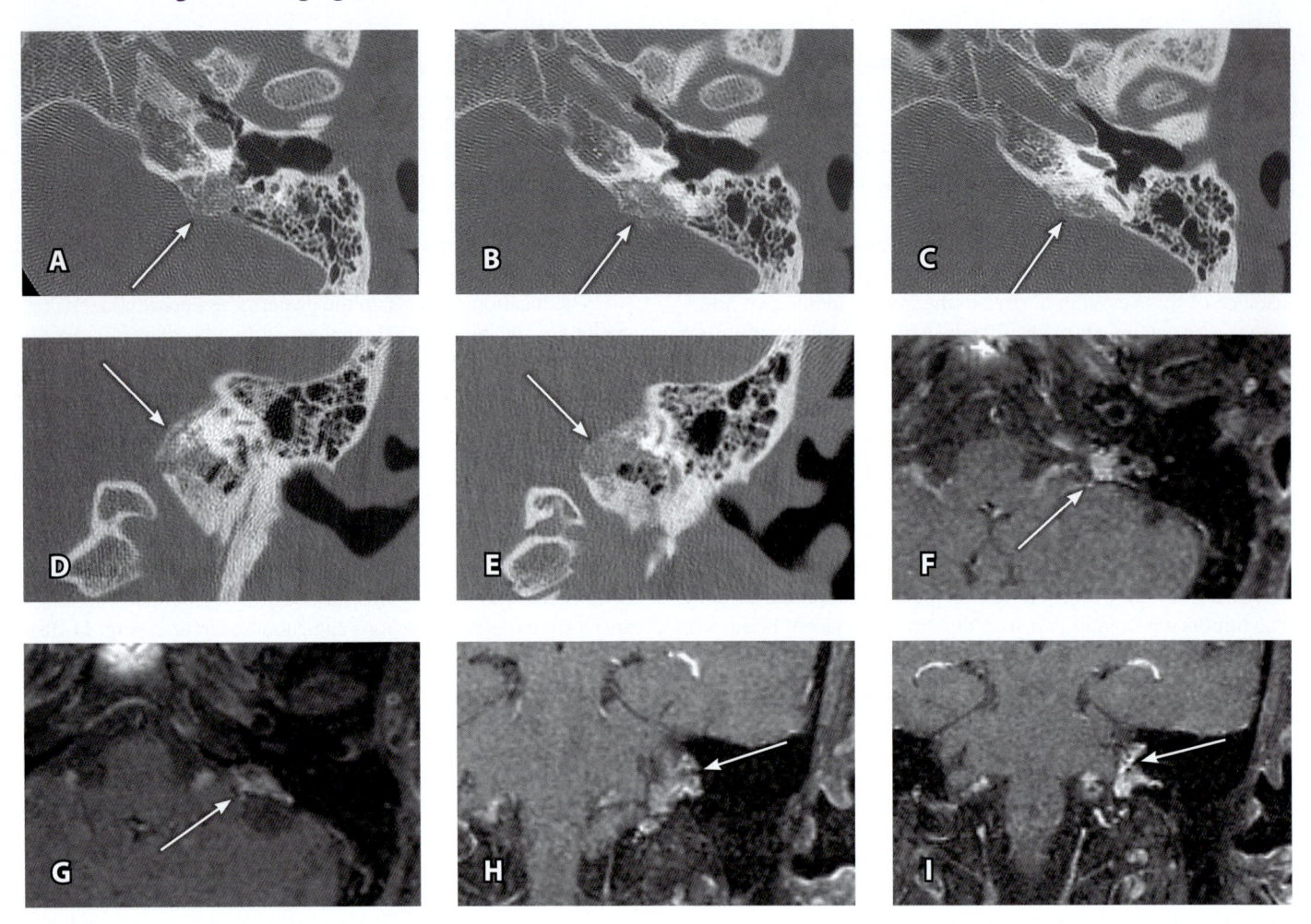

Figure 11-36 Endolymphatic Sac Tumor
Axial (**A–C**) and reformatted coronal (**D, E**) CT scans demonstrate cortical erosions with "smudgy" destruction of the posterior wall of the petrous bone in the region of the endolymphatic sac (*arrows*, **A–E**). Contrast-enhanced axial (**F, G**) and coronal (**H, I**) MR scans document a heterogeneous, ill-defined enhancing mass attached to the posterior wall of the left petrous bone (*arrows*, **F–I**).

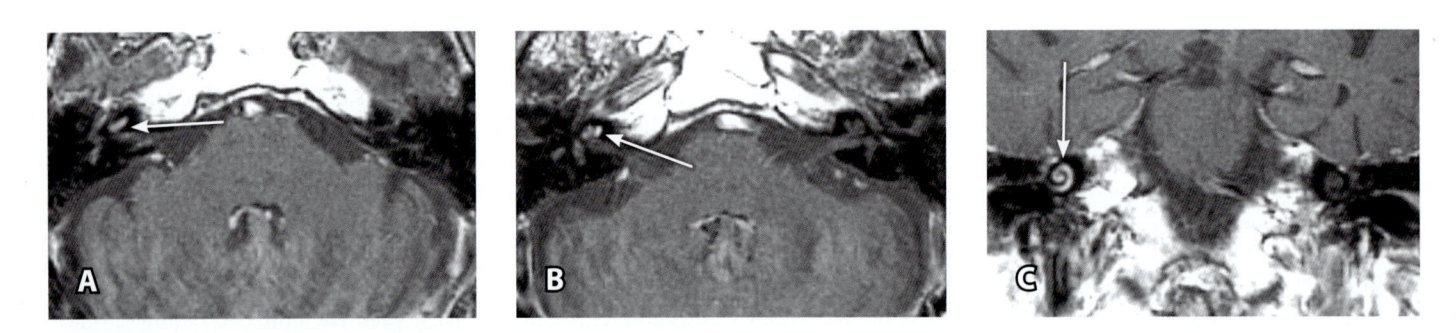

Figure 11-37 Cochlear Neuroma
Axial (**A–B**) and coronal (**C**) postcontrast MR images show enhancement within the first and second turns of the right cochlea (*arrows*). Though there is appreciable enhancement within the first turn of cochlea (*arrows*, **A, B**), the vestibule and the fundus of the internal auditory canal are spared, confirming that the neuroma is isolated to the cochlea.

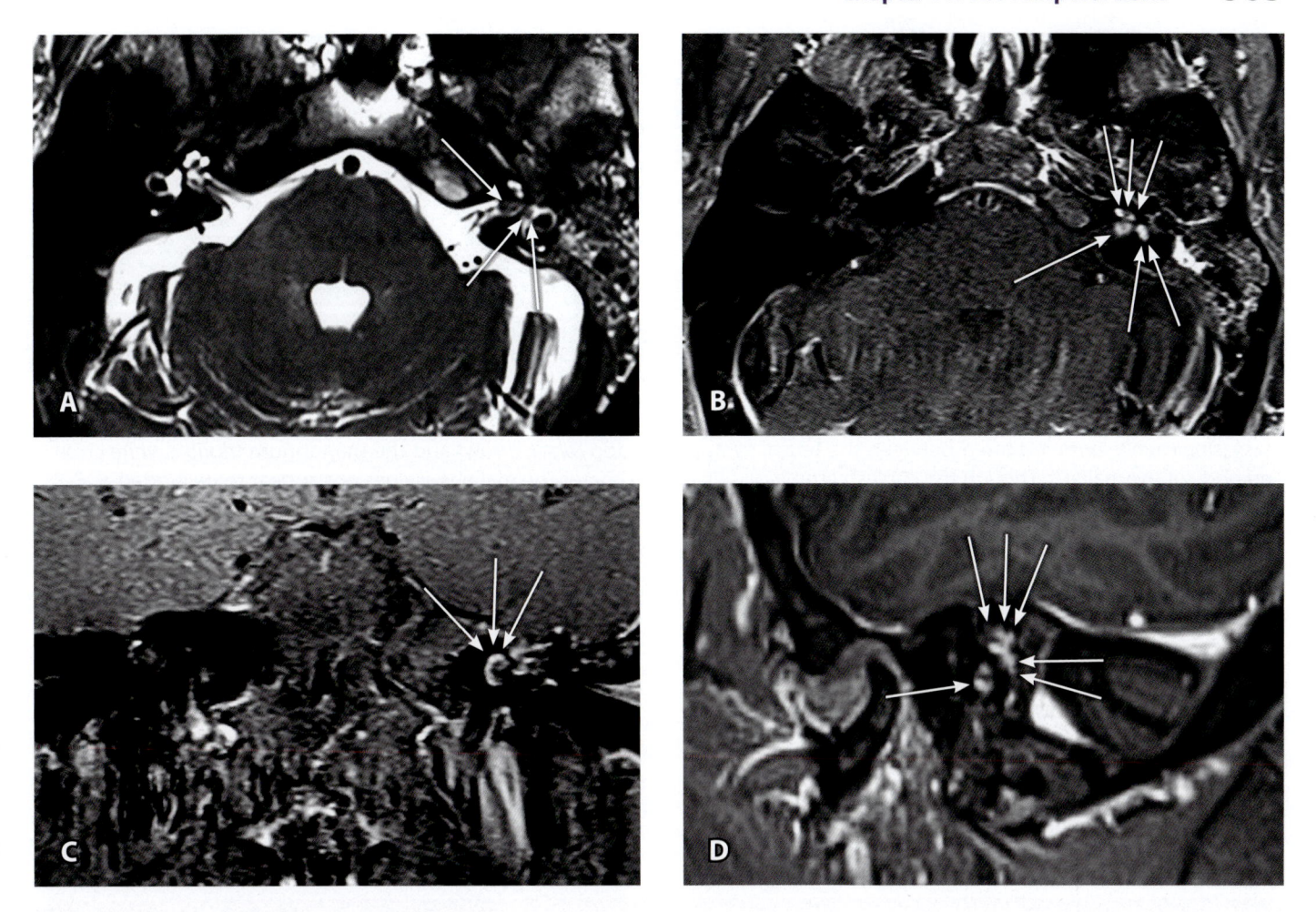

Figure 11-38 Acoustic Neuroma Recurrence
Axial 3D heavily T2-weighted cisternogram (**A**), axial postcontrast (**B**), coronal postcontrast (**C**), and sagittal postcontrast (**D**) MR images at the level of the temporal bone show a mass occupying the fundus of the internal auditory canal (*single white arrows*), membranous vestibule (*double white arrows*), and cochlea (*triple white arrows*) on the left. Note the opacification of the mastoid air cells (**A**) and evidence of mastoid surgery. The enhancing lesion represented recurrence of an excised neuroma.

High-resolution MR imaging has allowed for the increased visualization and diagnosis of these tumors, which were once thought to be rare.[218] On T2-weighted images, the lesion will be seen as a tissue-intensity mass in high-signal perilymphatic fluid. The tumor will show intense enhancement with contrast on T1-weighted images. Intralabyrinthine schwannomas are not easily seen on CT unless large, in which case there may be some bone erosion. Kennedy et al. have further categorized ILS based upon areas of the ear involved in order to facilitate diagnosis and proper treatment. These categories include intravestibular, intracochlear, intravestibulocochlear, transmodiolar, transmacular, transotic, and tympanolabyrinthine.[218]

These tumors are mostly commonly observed with serial imaging, but if symptoms, such as vertigo, become disabling, they can be surgically resected, but at the cost of serviceable hearing. A transotic approach is required for tumors involving the cochlea, while a transmastoid/translabyrinthine approach or transmastoid labyrinthectomy provides access to tumors of the vestibule.[214,217]

Middle Ear Masses

Congenital Cholesteatoma

Congenital cholesteatoma, or epidermoid, is a rare tumor of the middle ear and are due to epithelial rests of embryonic origin. They are far less common than acquired cholesteatomas. They appear otoscopically as whitish globular masses lying medial to an intact tympanic membrane. There is usually no history of antecedent otitis media or otorrhea. On CT, they appear as a well-defined soft tissue mass within the middle ear (**Fig. 11-39**). Congenital cholesteatomas are typically located in the anterosuperior quadrant of the middle ear, near the eustachian tube opening.

Facial Nerve Masses

Facial Nerve Schwannoma

Schwannomas of the facial nerve may occur anywhere along the course of the nerve, from the CPA to the parotid gland, but are most common in the cisternal segment and in the

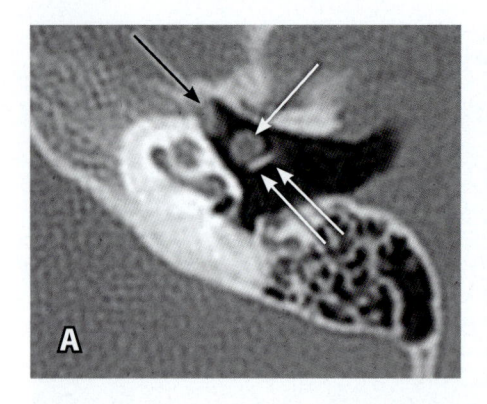

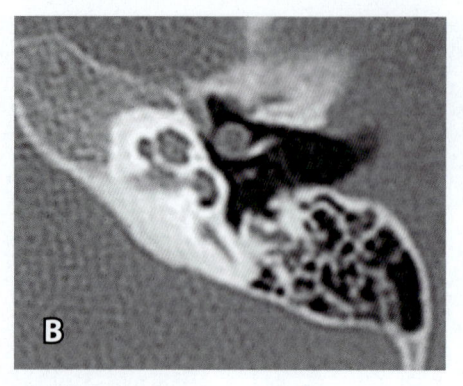

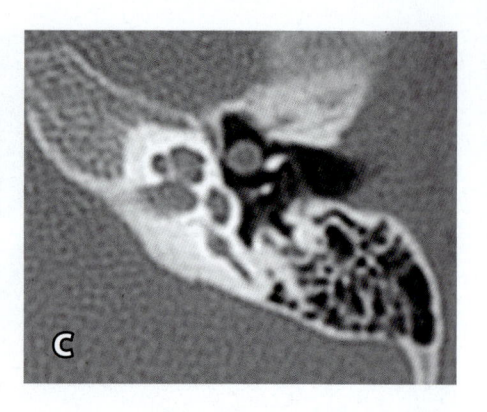

Figure 11-39 Congenital Cholesteatoma
Sequential axial bone CT images (**A–C**) through the left middle ear shown from inferior to superior. There is a well circumscribed mass (*single white arrow*) located between the tensor tympani tendon (*black arrow*) and the manubrium (*double white arrows*) and body of the malleus. Though the cholesteatoma closely approximates the malleus, it does not appear to be eroded.

intratemporal segment of the facial nerve in the region of the geniculate ganglion.[219] These tumors often affect multiple segments of the nerve, likely reflecting the large size they reach before coming to clinical attention.[220] In a series of 20 patients with 24 FNS, Wiggins et al. found that 88% had two contiguous lesions, and 71% involved three contiguous segments.[221] A facial nerve schwannoma restricted to the CPA will appear nearly identical to the more common vestibulocochlear nerve schwannoma.[222] In this case, the clinical presentation can assist in the differentiation of the two lesions.

These tumors are a rare cause of facial nerve palsy, but this is the most common presenting symptom, occurring in approximately half of patients[221] (**Table 11-5**). The onset may be gradual, or less commonly, acute, mimicking viral facial neuritis. When the FNS is located in the IAC, it can cause SNHL. Tumors in the horizontal segment of the nerve may present with conductive hearing loss as they impinge upon the ossicular chain.

On MR imaging, the tumor has signal characteristic identical to those of vestibulocochlear schwannomas. The tumors have low to intermediate signal on T1-weighted images and

Table 11-5 Facial Nerve Palsy

Condition	Temporal Bone and Ear Anomalies	Critical Features	Imaging
Schwannoma, Facial Nerve	Benign Schwann cell tumor wrapped around the facial nerve; temporal bone and ear symptoms vary depending on location of facial nerve symptoms along the course of the nerve.	Most common site: geniculate ganglion; tumors within the CPA-IAC segment of facial canal compress CN VIII producing SNHL; those within tympanic or mastoid segments interfere with ossicles, causing CHL.	CT: smooth focal enlargement at a segment along nerve course; T1 + C: enhance homogeneously.
Hemangioma, Facial Nerve	Benign, anastomotic network of vessels in association with the facial nerve and situated within the facial nerve canal.	Typically, a small lesion (<1 cm) at presentation; ossifying facial nerve hemangiomas contain bony spicules within lesion.	T1 + C: enhancing mass most frequently in region of geniculate ganglion; T2: hyperintense to brain tissue; CT: intrahemangiomal bone spicules.
Bell Palsy	Idiopathic acute onset lower motor neuron facial paralysis; strong evidence supporting association with herpes simplex virus.	Often preceded by a viral prodrome. 70% of patients complain of alterations in taste prior to onset of facial paralysis. 50% have pain in or around ipsilateral ear. 90% of patients spontaneously recover.	MRI T1 + C: uniformly enhancing facial nerve, either normal in size or slightly enlarged. Enhancement pattern is linear; there is no nodularity or focal enlargement present (differentiates from neoplasm).

CHL = congenital hearing loss, CPA = cerebellopontine agle, IAC = internal auditory canal, SNHL = sensorineural hearing loss.

high signal on T2-weighted images. Smaller lesions enhance homogeneously, while larger lesions may be heterogeneous secondary to hemorrhage and cystic change.

CT images show focal expansion of the facial canal as a result of slowly growing tumor. Bony changes in the geniculate fossa and labyrinthine facial canal are useful in differentiating facial schwannomas from other petrous bone lesions.

Asymptomatic lesions are followed with serial MRI and EEMG, to detect subclinical loss of nerve function.[220] If surgery is indicated, the approach depends upon tumor location and hearing status.

Facial Nerve Hemangioma

Hemangioma of the facial nerve is a benign vascular tumor arising from the capillaries surrounding the nerve's epineurium. These lesions can occur anywhere along the course of the nerve, but most commonly occur at the geniculate fossa in the anterior petrous bone because of the rich capillary network surrounding the geniculate ganglion.[223] The labyrinthine facial nerve and distal IAC are less common locations.

There are three types of facial nerve hemangioma: capillary, cavernous, and ossifying, characterized by vascular channel size and production of bony spicules, respectively. Capillary hemangiomas are characterized by small vessels lined by plump to flat endothelial cells, while cavernous lesions have larger, ecstatic, thin-walled vessels, lined by flattened epithelial cells. Ossifying lesions produce new bone in response to the hemangioma, which can be visualized on CT images as stippled calcifications.[207] Batsakis categorized these lesions by stage of development: vascular, in cystic transformation, and sclerosing or osseous.[224] Subclassification is often difficult secondary to fragmentation of the biopsy sample, and does not appear prognostically important.[225] On gross exam, the tumor is red or blue, spongy, and unencapsulated.

The majority of patients present with a slowly progressive facial nerve palsy, which resolves and recurs, or hemifacial spasm. In some cases, the tumor causes an acute facial paralysis, mimicking a Bell palsy.[226] Tumors in the IAC more often cause otologic symptoms, presenting with hearing loss, vertigo, or tinnitus.[227,228] Symptoms may be caused by compression, nerve invasion, or vascular steal, in which the tumor is believed to shunt blood from the nerve, causing local ischemia.[229] Seventh nerve hemangiomas can become symptomatic when the tumor is very small, in contrast to nerve sheath tumors which can reach a large size without clinical signs or symptoms.[230] Over half of non-schwannoma lesions in the IAC present with facial nerve symptoms, as opposed to only 6% of schwannomas.[230] Any age can be affected, but most patients are adults. In children, other entities, such as dermoids of the geniculate fossa should be considered (**Fig. 11-40**).

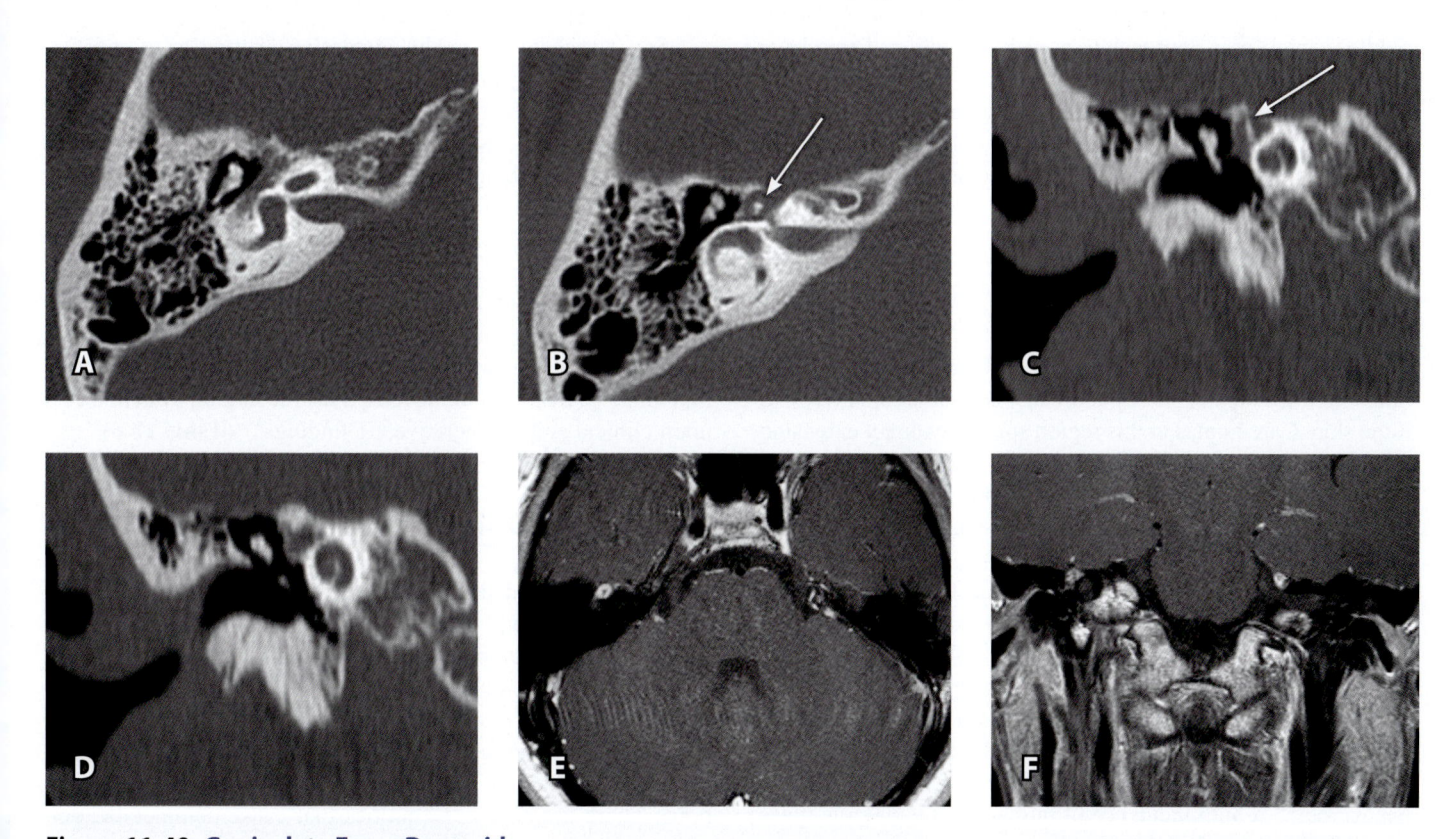

Figure 11-40 Geniculate Fossa Dermoid
Axial (**A, B**) and reformatted coronal (**C, D**) CT scans demonstrate smooth expansion of the right geniculate fossa surrounding a minute focus of calcification (*arrows*, **B, C**). Contrast-enhanced axial (**E**) and coronal (**F**) MR scans demonstrate some enhancement around the focus of calcification. A supra-labyrinthine epidermoid tumor would demonstrate the same findings, except for the enhancement. A supra-labyrinthine hemangioma would demonstrate the same findings, except for homogeneous enhancement throughout the tumor.

Imaging diagnosis requires both high resolution CT and contrast-enhanced MRI.[169] On HRCT imaging, one may see the geniculate fossa widened, intratumoral bony spicules, and "honeycomb" appearance of adjacent bone. A stippled pattern of calcification at the geniculate ganglion and along the course of facial nerve may be apparent. The mid-cranial fossa is almost always dehiscent over large hemangiomas of the geniculate ganglion.[231] However, because these lesions become symptomatic early, and while very small, there may be no bony changes, and the tumor may not be visible. On MR images, the vascular tumors have features which are identical to those of schwannomas. Small lesions are hypo, iso, or hyperintense on T1, hyperintense on T2-weighted images, and enhance intensely with contrast.[232] Larger lesions may appear more heterogeneous secondary to the presence of bony spicules. It is more common for hemangiomas to have areas of calcification than schwannomas. Other lesions in this area which may appear similar include metastases, meningioma, and cholesteatoma.[232] Cholesteatomas do not enhance, differentiating them from hemangiomas and schwannomas. Meningiomas can have flecks of calcium and can originate in the dura present in the labyrinthine segment of the facial canal up to the geniculate ganglion.[225] In general, hemangiomas should be considered in any lesion with intratumoral calcium, which is enlarging the facial canal.

Treatment is surgical, with a transmastoid, translabyrinthine approach if there is no need to preserve hearing, or an extradural middle cranial fossa approach to preserve function. There have not been reports of recurrence after surgical removal. The timing of surgery versus watchful waiting is a controversial issue, as these tumors are slow growing, and there is considerable risk to the facial nerve from the surgical procedure.[231] Management decisions are aimed at optimizing facial nerve function.

External Auditory Canal Masses

Squamous cell carcinoma

The most common neoplasms of the EAC and pinna are squamous cell carcinoma (SCCa) and basal cell carcinoma (BCCa) of the skin. Carcinomas in this region spread by direct extension into the pinna, posterior auricular sulcus, or parotid gland. Extension into the middle ear cavity is a common route of spread, as the dense bone of the external auditory canal can block tumor spread.

SCCa is the most common malignant tumor of the temporal bone. The peak incidence of SCCa occurs in the seventh decade and both genders are equally affected.[233] Ultraviolet radiation is the predominant etiologic agent responsible for SCCa of the exposed skin. There is also an association with past radiotherapy in the region. SCCa of the middle ear and temporal bone, areas not exposed to sunlight, is believed to occur in with genetic predisposition.[234] A high incidence of human papillomavirus types 16 and 18 has been found in middle ear SCCa,[235] leading some to believe infectious spread from the upper respiratory tract to the middle ear is a cause.

Presenting symptoms can include an ulcerated exophytic mass that bleeds upon manipulation, a preauricular mass, or more specific for SCCa, offensive otorrhea, otorrhagia, otalgia, and facial palsy.[233] While the majority of cancers in this region will be SCCa, the gold standard of diagnosis, histological confirmation from biopsy, is necessary to rule out basal cell carcinoma, adenocarcinoma, chondrosarcoma, melanoma, Ewing's tumor, fibroxanthoma, verrucous carcinoma, and metastatic disease.[233]

Spread is primarily via local invasion. The lymphatics of the ear canal are not well developed, so lymphatic spread is uncommon until late in the disease process. SCCa does spread perineurally, and often involves the facial nerve. Tumors arising in the EAC can erode directly through bone or along vascular and neural pathways. Medial spread through the tympanic membrane or posteriorly into the mastoid allows access to the air cells to expose the otic capsule, posterior fossa dura, sigmoid sinus, eustachian tube, and carotid artery. Anterior spread to the temporomandibular joint, parotid gland, or infratemporal fossa occurs directly through the thin bone of the external auditory canal or the petrosquamous suture. Inferior extension can involve the jugular foramen and upper neck. Superior extension through the tegmen tympani can involve the dura and temporal lobe.[234] Prognosis is poor when the tumor extends medial to the tympanic membrane, when there is nodal disease at presentation, with undifferentiated tumor types, with dural involvement, and with carotid artery invasion.[233,236] Treatment is a combination of surgery and radiotherapy. Complications include osteoradionecrosis and facial weakness.[233]

SCCa is characterized by aggressive destruction of underlying bone (**Figs. 11-41** and **11-42**). The tumor has low to intermediate signal on T1-weighted images, and heterogeneous enhancement on T2-weighted images. Contrast enhancement is mild, and may be homo- or heterogeneous. Soft tissue thickening in the EAC, and obliteration of normal fat planes of the skin and pinna are seen. MR images are vital for detecting perineural spread, which can extend the tumor distally to the parotid gland or proximally to the geniculate ganglion and intralabyrinthine portion of the nerve and to the posterior cranial fossa through the IAC. MR and CT imaging are essential for staging and treatment planning.[234] Arriaga et al. devised a useful staging system based upon clinical and preoperative CT findings[237] (**Table 11-6**).

OTOSCLEROSIS AND DYSPLASIAS

Many diseases and dysplasias can affect the osseous components of the temporal bone. Some diseases such as otosclerosis are limited to the temporal bone and do not occur anywhere else in the body. Other diseases such as the various osteochondrodysplasias involve much of the skeleton with the temporal bone being but one component, and diseases such as fibrous dysplasia can involve many bones or can be localized to the temporal bone. There are also some entities that cause demineralization of the otic capsule.

Patients with these lesions frequently present with hearing loss, which may be sensorineural, conductive, or mixed, depending on the location and extent of the abnormal bone. Dysplastic bone can compress a nerve, resulting in various cranioneuropathies, or it can limit ossicular chain movement. On plain films

Chapter 11: The Temporal Bone 509

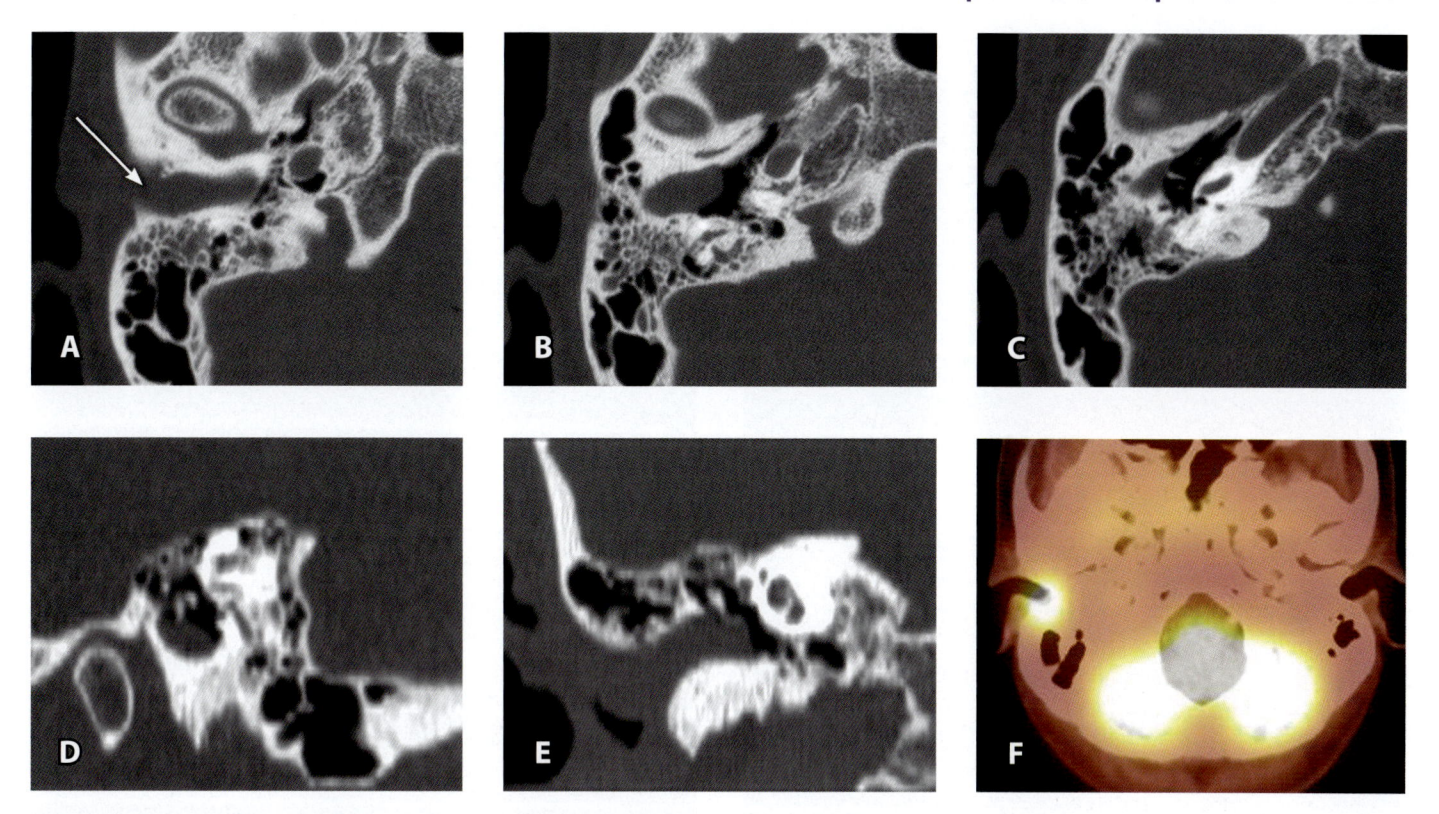

Figure 11-41 CT of a Small EAC Squamous Cell Carcinoma
Axial (**A–C**), reformatted sagittal (**D**), and coronal (**E**) CT scans show a soft tissue mass filling the right external auditory canal (EAC) (*arrow*) with minimal, if any adjacent osseous destruction. The mass invades the middle ear and abuts the ossicles. Fused PET/CT (**F**) demonstrates a focus of increase activity in the same region of the EAC and middle ear, uptake in the area consistent with a squamous cell calcinoma.

these diseases show either bone loss or sclerosis; however, due to superimposition of other osseous structures, some diagnostic findings may not be evident.

Otosclerosis

The temporal bone is unique in that there normally is persistence of primary endochondral bone as the middle layer of the otic capsule. This middle layer is between the outer periosteal layer of bone and the thin inner periosteal (endosteum) layer that lines the lumen of the labyrinth.[238,239] Resorption of the middle endochondral layer, with deposition of spongy vascular new bone, is referred to as otosclerosis (otospongiosis). This is a slowly progressive disorder with a 65% female predominance, an 80% incidence of bilaterality (which is often asynchronous), and a peak incidence in the second or third decade of life.[240–242] Although tinnitus may be the presenting symptom, hearing loss

Table 11-6 EAC Squamous Cell Carcinoma Staging

Stage	Criteria
T1	Tumor limited to EAC without bony erosion or evidence of soft tissue extension
T2	Tumor with limited EAC erosion (not full thickness) or radiological findings consistent with limited (<0.5 cm) soft tissue involvement
T3	Tumor eroding the osseous EAC (full thickness) with limited (<0.5 cm) soft tissue involvement, or involvement of middle ear/mastoid or causing facial palsy at presentation
T4	Tumor eroding the cochlea, petrous apex, medial wall of the middle ear, carotid canal, jugular foramen, or dura, or with extensive (>0.5 cm) soft tissue involvement

EAC = external auditory canal.

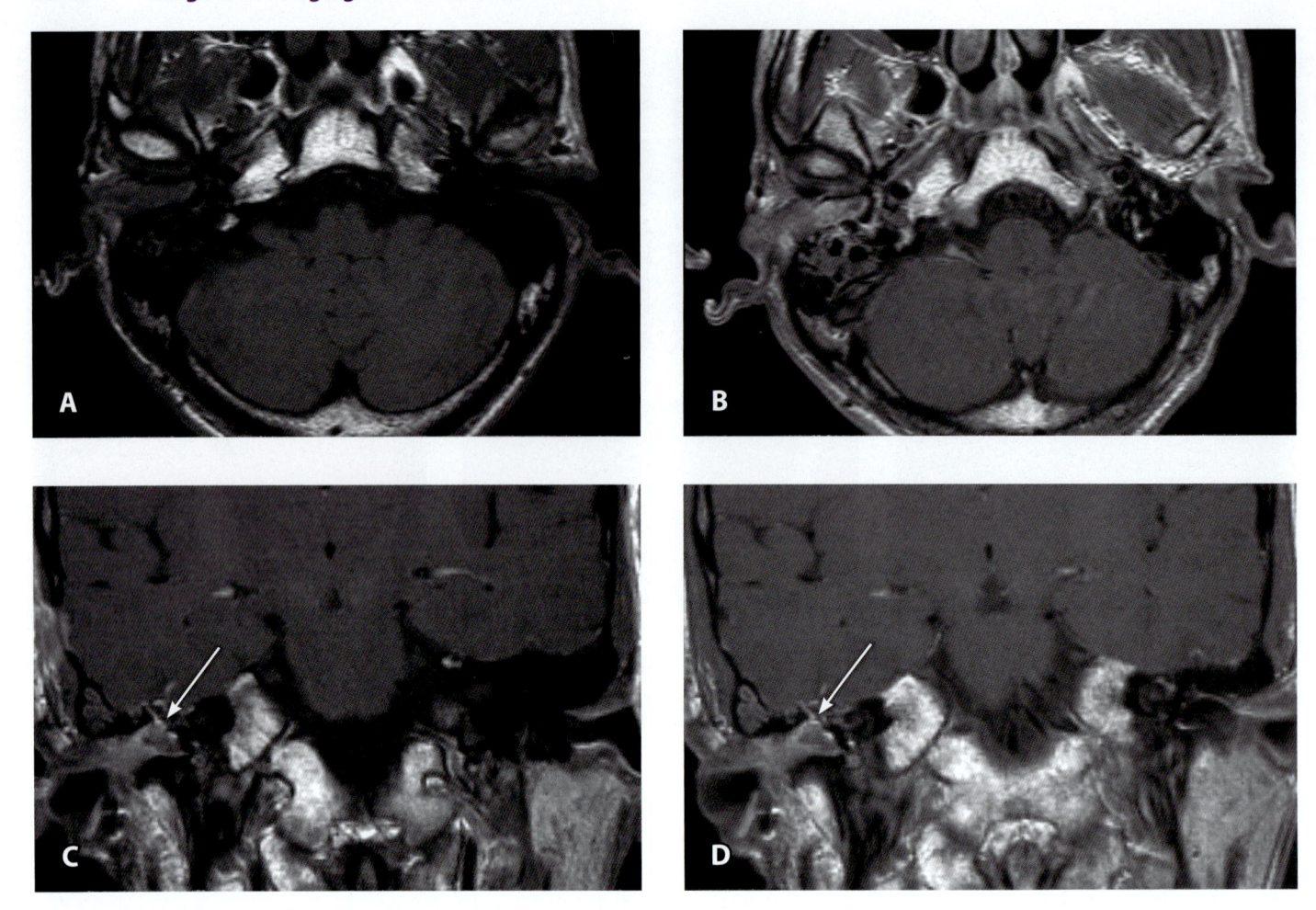

Figure 11-42 MRI of a Large EAC Squamous Cell Carcinoma
Axial (**A, B**) and (**C, D**) coronal MR scans demonstrates an aggressive destructive lesion centered on the right external auditory canal (EAC) extending anteriorly into the adjacent temporomandibular joint and posteriorly into the mastoid air cells. The contrast-enhanced images (**B–D**) demonstrate the mass to enhance heterogeneously. Coronal MR scans show that the tumor has minimally eroded through the tegmen tympani (*arrows*, **C, D**).

will always develop, and the deficit may be conductive, sensorineural, or mixed.[243]

A conductive deficit is usually present and virtually always secondary to stapediovestibular compromise. This oval window involvement is called fenestral otosclerosis. The most common lesion of otosclerosis occurs just anterior to the oval window, at the approximate location of the embryologic fissula ante fenestram.[239,243,244] The fissula is a thin crease of connective tissue stretching through the endochondral layer, roughly between the oval window and cochleariform process (point where the tensor tympani tendon turns laterally toward the malleus). Careful study of the oval window in the axial projection, using overlapping CT sections, is necessary to make the diagnosis of fenestral otosclerosis. Early disease is visualized as a small, lucent focus anterior to the oval window. This represents the abnormal "spongiotic" bone replacing the very dense bone of the otic capsule. With more pronounced disease, the "lucent" bone enlarges, protrudes slightly into the middle ear, and impinges on the anterior margin of the oval window. On CT in the axial plane, the oval window is narrowed.

Rarely, rather than being relatively lucent the abnormal focus of bone is the same density as the otic capsule. In these cases, the disease is detected by demonstrating slight enlargement of the normal density bone at the anterior oval window margin. Some researchers have postulated that this reflects the later inactive phase of otosclerosis. Complete obliteration of the oval window (obliterative fenestral otosclerosis) occurs in approximately 2% of cases, and such severe disease may also be appreciated in the coronal plane.

For a number of years, fenestral otosclerosis has been treated surgically, and many different procedures, including stapes mobilization and fenestration of the lateral semicircular canal, have been used. Currently, most surgeons perform a stapedectomy followed by a prosthesis insertion.[245]

The preoperative evaluation of individuals with a non-inflammatory conductive deficit must always include careful evaluation of the oval window for subtle otosclerotic plaque formation (**Fig. 11-43**).[246,247] Patients may have a focus of bone in the typical anterior location, a posterior focus, or both, and the contralateral ear must always be studied. The incidence of

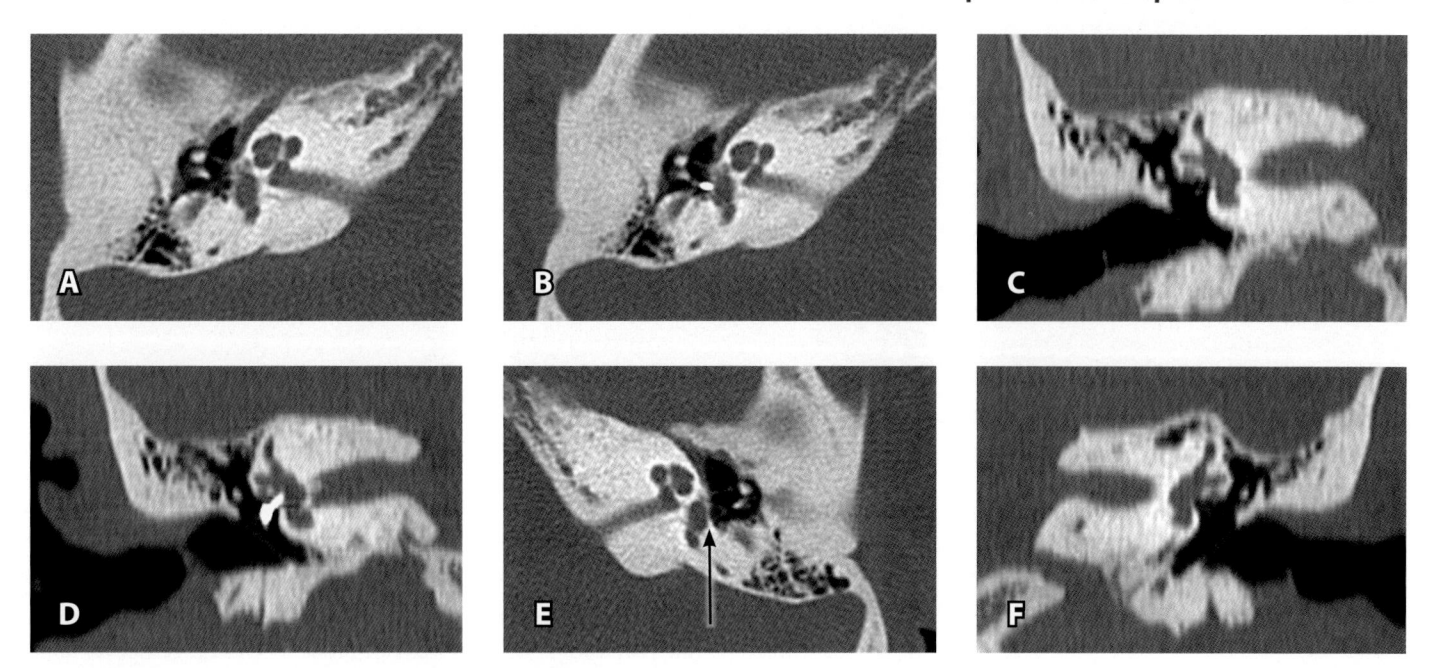

Figure 11-43 Otosclerosis with Failed Stapedial Prosthesis
Axial (**A, B**) and reformatted coronal (**C, D**) CT scans of the right temporal bone shows a piston prosthetic device that extends beyond the oval window for about 2–3 mm, that represents abnormal penetration into the vestibule, Axial (**E**) and reformatted coronal (**F**) CT scans of the left temporal bone show minute otosclerotic foci adjacent to the left oval window (*arrow*, **E**).

bilaterality is high even when no measurable air bone gap is present audiometrically. On occasion, patients will have only a subtle thickening of the stapes footplate annular ligament complex. The latter situation may also occur as a postinflammatory phenomenon (tympanosclerosis).[248] When oval window disease is not appreciated, the ossicular chain must be carefully studied for evidence of congenital anomaly. On occasion, no abnormality will be evident despite intensive careful study, and congenital stapes fixation may be the ultimate surgical diagnosis. This entity may or may not have CT manifestations.[249]

CT evaluation of the round window, facial nerve canal, jugular foramen, and cochlear aqueduct are necessary for satisfactory preoperative examination.[247] Round window obliteration secondary to otosclerosis may occur, but fortunately it is unusual. Many surgeons will not operate in this circumstance because surgical results may be compromised. A small percentage of patients with fenestral otosclerosis also have lateral ossicular fixation, usually manifested by a bony web interposed between the malleus or incus and the lateral attic wall. Facial nerve dehiscence may also be appreciated on CT, and the preoperative demonstration of this anomaly can help the surgeon avoid operative facial nerve injury.[250] In both of these cases the CT findings are best appreciated in the coronal plane.

Profuse flow of CSF following oval window manipulation (the "stapes gusher") is said to occur in individuals with a communication between the CSF and the perilymph. Although some authors have suggested a pathway through an enlarged cochlear aqueduct, there is considerable dispute in the otolaryngologic literature regarding this phenomenon. Certainly, enlargement or flaring limited to the medial aperture of the duct is of very doubtful significance.[251] The surgical hazard of a dehiscent jugular vein is obvious, but the otologist usually recognizes this anomaly.

Sensorineural hearing loss from otosclerosis is less common than conductive hearing loss, and indeed a pure sensorineural loss is rare. Areas of demineralization at various locations within the otic capsule can be appreciated on CT (**Fig. 11-44**) and when present in the cochlea, these abnormalities represent a relative contraindication to cochlear implant surgery.[12,246,249,252–257] CT scans obtained in both the axial and coronal planes should be carefully evaluated for otospongiotic foci, and there is a strong tendency for these changes to be symmetrical. Concerning MRI, there is now anecdotal evidence that pericochlear enhancement occurs on T1-weighted (T1W) images acquired after gadolinium administration.

The cause of the SNHL in otosclerosis is controversial, and cytotoxic enzymes have been implicated.[258,259] Diffusion of these enzymes into the cochlear fluid is theorized to be responsible for hyalinization of the spiral ligament and subsequent hearing loss.

The basilar membrane forms the boundary between the cochlear duct and the scala tympani, and this membrane thickens as it approaches the apical turn. High-frequency tones have maximum effective amplitude at the basilar turn, where the basilar membrane is relatively thin, and low-frequency tones have maximum effective amplitude toward the apex. The type of sensorineural hearing loss can therefore be predicted from the CT location of these foci.[247]

As with the fenestral ostosclerosis, it has been suggested that areas of demineralization (otospongiosis) in the cochlea are associated with only the active phase of this disease. Cochlear otosclerosis in the chronic phase may have no CT manifestations, other than subtle periosteal thickening. This may explain

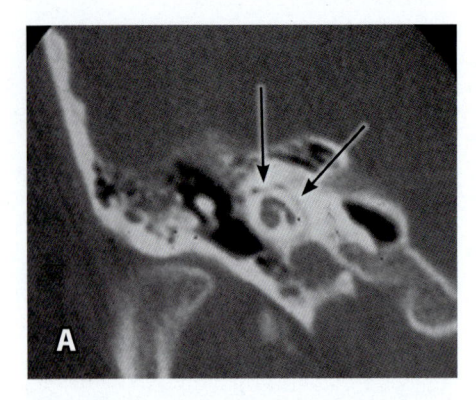

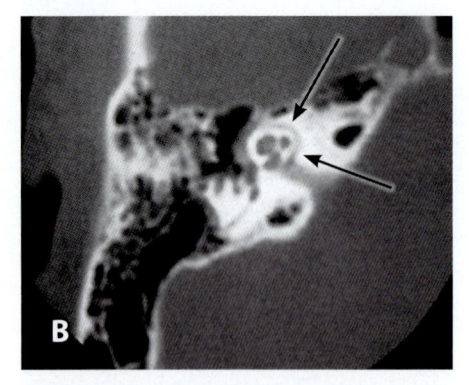

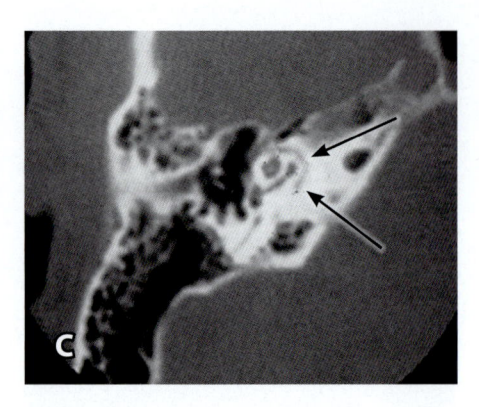

Figure 11-44 Cochlear Otosclerosis
Coronal (**A**) and axial (**B, C**) CT scans of the right temporal bone. There is halo of low density surrounding the cochlear apparatus (*arrows*), giving the appearance of a "mega-cochlea," a characteristic finding in cochlear otosclerosis.

the relatively high incidence of otherwise asymptomatic sensorineural hearing loss occurring in young individuals with normal CT scans.

The observer should be aware that diffuse labyrinthine ossification is not a consequence of otosclerosis.[260] In this situation, a history of previous labyrinthectomy should be sought. Otherwise this finding will likely represent a long standing residuum of labyrinthitis (labyrinthitis ossificans).

CT with densitometric measurements has been proposed as an objective approach to the study of otospongiosis, and comparison of densitometry readings performed before and after medical treatment may provide an opportunity to monitor the effectiveness of therapy.[261,262]

The differential diagnosis of otic capsule demineralization includes otosclerosis, osteogenesis imperfecta, and Paget's disease. Syphilitic involvement of the temporal bone (virtually always associated with systemic disease) also may result in demineralization.

Fibrous Dysplasia

Fibrous dysplasia is a common disorder characterized by proliferating fibroosseous tissues within bone. The histopathology of fibrous dysplasia shows replacement of normal bone by abnormal, slow growing fibrous tissue with abundant spindle cells in a loose, whorled arrangement. In some cases, the replaced tissue is acellular with a predominance of collagenous ground substance. The bony trabeculae of fibrous dysplasia are poorly formed with variable shapes that are likened to Chinese characters. These unusual trabeculae are composed of woven bone rather than lamellar bone, and they are sporadically dispersed within the fibrous tissue. The proliferative process may give rise to expansion, distortion, and structural weakness. Because fibrous dysplasia primarily involves the cancellous bone, and rarely involves the cortical bone, this lesion usually widens the bone by replacing the normal medullary space. In many instances the abnormal dysplastic bone is covered by a thin shell of normal cortical bone.[263–265]

There are two patterns of fibrous dysplasia. Both patterns may involve the temporal bone. The monostotic form is seen most often, accounting for about 70% of skeletal lesions. Of these lesions, 20% are located in the temporal bone. The polyostotic form is not symmetric, is mildly aggressive, and represents the remaining 30% of cases of fibrous dysplasia. Temporal bone involvement is quite common and may be seen in up to 50% of the polyostotic cases. With severe skeletal involvement, the temporal bone is affected in nearly 100% of cases. The McCune Albright syndrome is present in 3% of polyostotic cases and is associated with endocrine disturbances.[263]

Most cases of fibrous dysplasia present when the patient is between 10 and 20 years of age, and females are affected twice as often as males. The most common clinical presentations relating to the temporal bone are hearing loss (characteristically conductive), a postauricular deformity, and obstruction of the EAC.[266] Constriction of the lateral part of the EAC may lead to an external canal cholesteatoma (keratosis obturans) medial to the narrowing.[264] Malignant degeneration of fibrous dysplasia is rare, and although several forms of sarcoma may develop, osteosarcoma is the most common.[263]

The radiographic findings in fibrous dysplasia fall into three distinct patterns: pagetoid, sclerotic, and cystlike. Taken over the entire skeleton, the pagetoid form of fibrous dysplasia is most common, occurring in about 53% of cases; the patient is usually over 30 years of age. The pagetoid form has regions of bony expansion and alternating areas of radiodensity and radiolucency (**Fig. 11-45**). The sclerotic form, which occurs in 23% of cases, is usually seen in younger patients and radiographically consists of homogeneous "ground glass" radiodensities and bone expansion (**Fig. 11-46**). The cystlike form, which occurs in 21% of cases, also occurs in younger patients and is characterized by round or oval "cystic" lesions with sclerotic borders. In some cases the sclerotic and cystlike forms are precursors to the pagetoid form. In the temporal bone, fibrous dysplasia is almost always of the sclerotic form, with the cystlike form being uncommon[264,267] (**Fig. 11-47**).

High-resolution CT provides the maximum detail available for imaging fibrous dysplasia of the temporal bone. The most common CT findings include an increase in bone thickness, a homogeneous radiodensity, and a loss of trabecular pattern.[263] The CT attenuation numbers range from 70 to 130 HU.[267] The IAC may be narrowed, but the otic capsule is characteristically

Chapter 11: The Temporal Bone   513

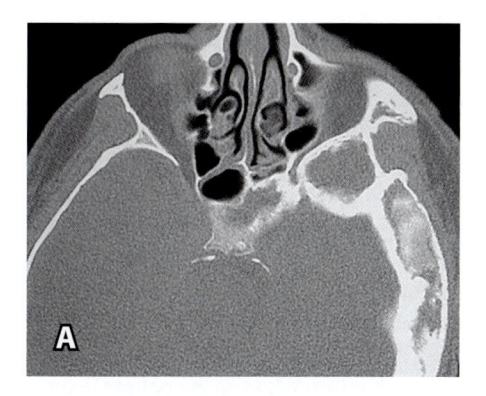

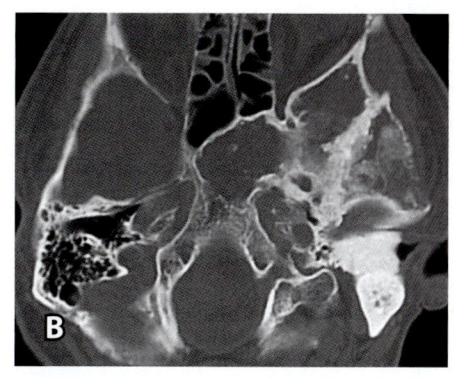

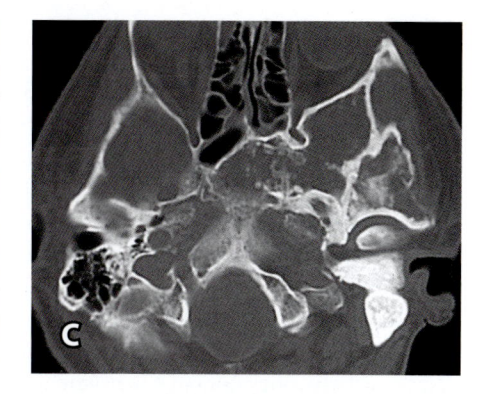

Figure 11-45 Fibrous Dysplasia Pagetoid Type
Serial axial CT scans (**A–C**) of the skull base. There is thick dense cortical bone with expansion of the diploic spaces of the left sphenoid and temporal bones. The mastoid process is completely sclerotic with loss of the air cells, characteristic of fibrous dysplasia. There are intermixed foci of both increased and decreased densities within the diploic spaces that simulate Paget disease of the skull.

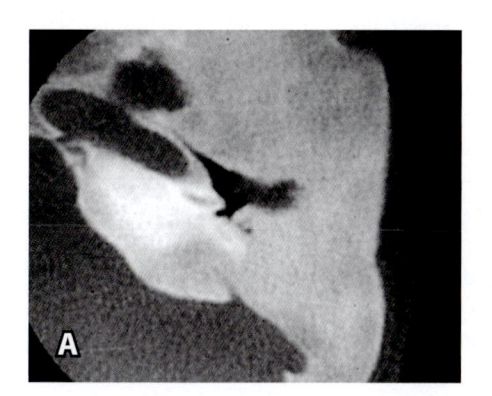

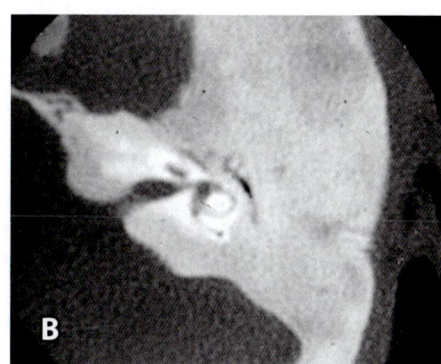

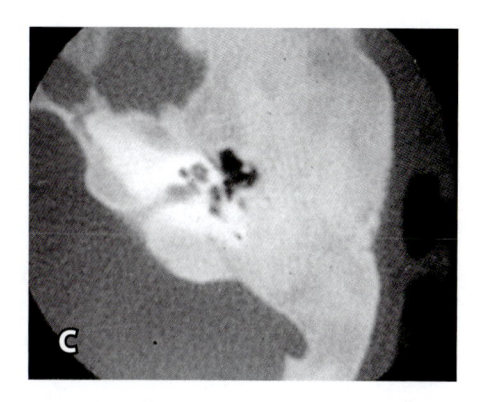

Figure 11-46 Fibrous Dysplasia Sclerotic Type
Serial axial CT scans (**A–C**) of the left temporal bone. There is dense bone that completely obliterates the mastoid air cells and the lateral portion of the external auditory canal (EAC) and portions of the middle ear cavity. There is a small amount of residual lumen of the EAC that is filled with soft tissue that represents an acquired cholesteatoma (aka keratosis obturans) (*arrow*, **A**). The dense osseous labyrinth is not destroyed, a characteristic feature of fibrous dysplasia, unlike Paget disease that may destroy the osseous labyrinth (**Fig. 11-49**).

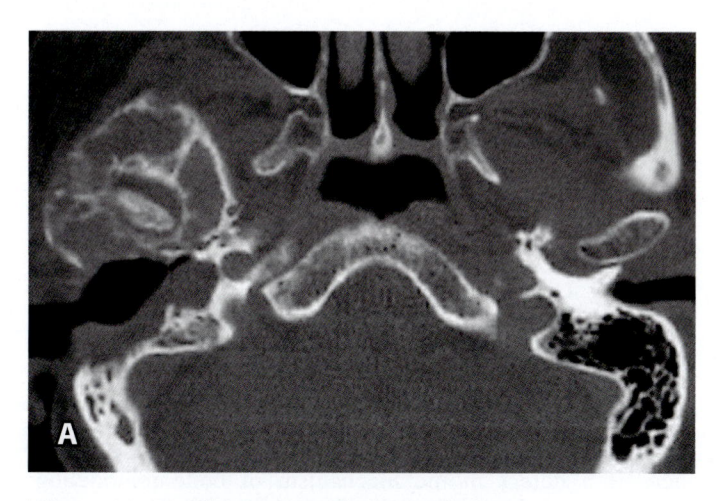

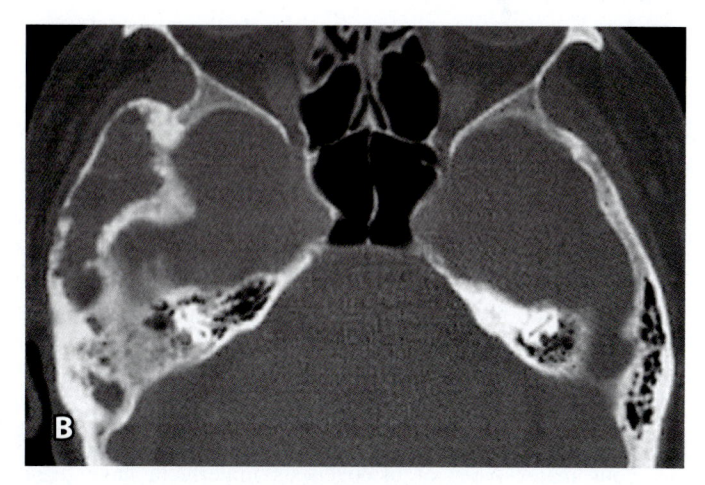

Figure 11-47 Fibrous Dysplasia Cystic Type
Axial CT scans (**A, B**) of the temporal bones. There is expansion with cortical thickening and deformity of the right squamous temporal bone and temporomandibular joint (TMJ). There is a surgical defect of the TMJ and EAC. The expanded diploic spaces show primarily cystic changes consistent with the cystic type of fibrous dysplasia.

spared, and there may be varying degrees of obliteration of the mastoid air cells, the middle ear, and the external auditory canal.

Although CT best demonstrates fibrous dysplasia, this lesion can also be seen on MRI. On both T1W and T2W images, the bone is thickened, and there is low, often homogeneous, signal intensity. Following gadolinium contrast administration, the dysplastic bone has moderate enhancement.[268]

Fibrous dysplasia of the temporal bone may simulate several other diseases. Paget's disease is usually bilateral and exhibits osteopenia with occasional areas of sclerosis. The patients are typically older than those with fibrous dysplasia, and Paget's disease usually does not have the same degree of osseous thickening seen with fibrous dysplasia.

Changes of hyperparathyroidism may be evident throughout the skeleton. These patients have cortical bone cysts, with local tenderness, and systemic hypercalcemia. Hyperparathyroidism may also cause sclerotic bone changes, particularly with the secondary form. However, there is no thickening of the involved bone.

Neurofibromatosis may on occasion simulate fibrous dysplasia whenever a neurofibroma erodes into or originates within the temporal bone. However, the additional clinical features associated with neurofibromatosis usually allow this diagnosis to be made.

Ossifying fibroma is a proliferative lesion that may involve the medullary and the cortical bone. The tumor is very similar to fibrous dysplasia but is more localized, appearing more like a tumor than an area of dysplastic bone. The lesion is typically well demarcated and has a sclerotic margin. The histopathology is quite similar to that of fibrous dysplasia, but there are differences because ossifying fibromas have lamellar bone rather than woven bone.

Sclerosteosis (endosteal hyperostosis) is an autosomal recessive disease first appearing in infancy or early childhood. There is overgrowth of the skull, vertebrae, and mandible with giantism and syndactyly. Cranial nerve palsies are common in this condition. The long bones have a sclerotic pattern dissimilar to that of fibrous dysplasia.

An aneurysmal bone cyst may occur in the temporal bone. Although this cyst is expansile, it is usually accompanied by pain and tenderness, symptoms uncommonly associated with fibrous dysplasia.[164,263,269–271]

Osteogenesis Imperfecta

Osteogenesis imperfecta represents a group of heritable disorders that result in osteoporosis and increased bone fragility. Several additional clinical manifestations are seen in osteogenesis imperfecta; blue sclera, abnormal dentinogenesis, hearing loss, hyperextensible joints, and wormian bones are present. The genetic defects leave the patients with decreased amounts of type I collagen. This form of collagen is predominant in bones and is also present in skin, connective tissues, and dentin.[269,272]

Four major types of osteogenesis imperfecta have been described with several subtypes. Type I, previously called osteogenesis imperfecta tarda, is the most common form and reflects a decreased production of type I collagen. The usual clinical presentation is a bone fracture following minimal or no trauma. Blue or grayish sclera are invariably present, and deafness is common after childhood. These patients can have joint dislocations and hyperextensibility, as well as easy bruisability. Dentine production may be normal or abnormal. Type II, previously known as osteogenesis imperfecta congenita, is the most severe form of this disease. The genetic defect is variable. Death in utero or shortly after birth is common due to multiple fractures of the skull, vertebrae, or chest wall. Type III osteogenesis imperfecta presents with marked bony deformity and frequent early fractures of the long bones. Short stature is common, as is abnormal production of dentine (dentinogenesis imperfecta). The sclera originally are blue but turn white as the patient grows. The genetic defect is not well understood. Type IV osteogenesis imperfecta has variable severity with a defect in one subunit of collagen. Some patients exhibit normal sclera and dentine with minimal bone fragility.[269,272]

Radiographs show generalized osteopenia with diminished trabeculae and a thin cortex. Wormian bones are often seen on plain films, and occasionally there is basilar invagination. The extremities show marked bowing and deformity as a result of multiple fractures. The ribs are thin, notched, and may also show evidence of fractures. The vertebrae are usually biconvex because the soft endplates mold around the intervertebral disk, and sclerosis of the vertebral bodies may occur.[273]

With temporal bone involvement, CT may show proliferation of undermineralized, thickened bone around the otic capsule. As this thickened bone extends from the labyrinth, the middle ear cavity may be narrowed, the oval window may become obstructed with the stapedial crura embedded in the dysplastic osseous mass, and the facial canal may be narrowed with corresponding damage to the facial nerve.[273–275]

The differential diagnosis of osteogenesis imperfecta includes Paget's disease, otosclerosis, or hyperparathyroidism. In Paget's disease, the patients typically will be older and do not have such prominent hypertrophic bone formation around the stapes and oval window. Otosclerosis may cause a thin zone of low density about the otic capsule, creating a similar appearance to that of osteogenesis imperfecta. Otosclerosis also may have focal areas of sclerosis, and the abnormal bone may involve the stapedial foot plate and oval window. In some cases it is virtually impossible to differentiate otosclerosis from osteogenesis imperfecta. Indeed, histologically, the two diseases are quite similar; however, the changes in osteogenesis imperfecta are usually more extensive. The abnormal bone can reach the level of the semicircular canals. The manifestations of hyperparathyroidism are seen throughout the skeleton. These patients have cortical cysts, localized tenderness, and hypercalcemia. These more general changes help differentiate this disease from osteogenesis imperfecta.[273]

Osteopetrosis

Osteopetrosis is a rare group of heritable disorders in which there is a defect in the mechanism of bone remodeling. Defective resorption of the primary spongiosa with persistence of calcified cartilage results in thick, dense, yet fragile bones.[238,276] Overproduction of immature bone causes thickening of the cortex and narrowing or obliteration of the

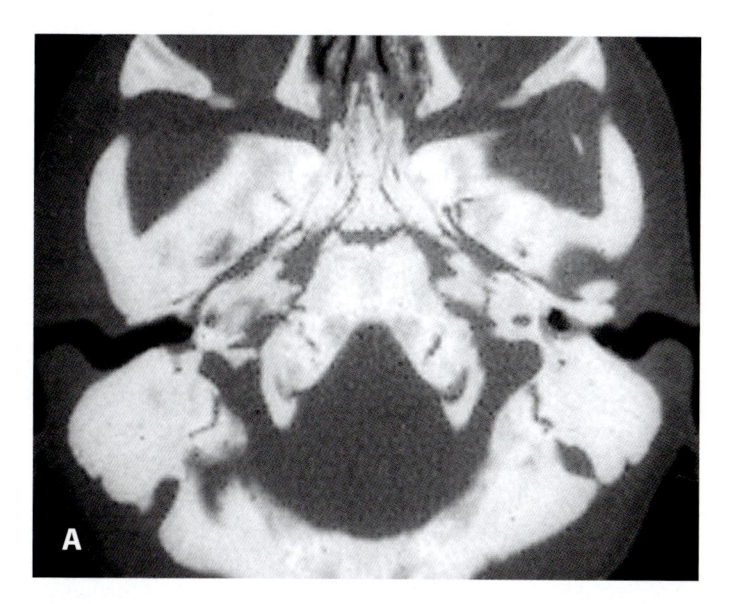

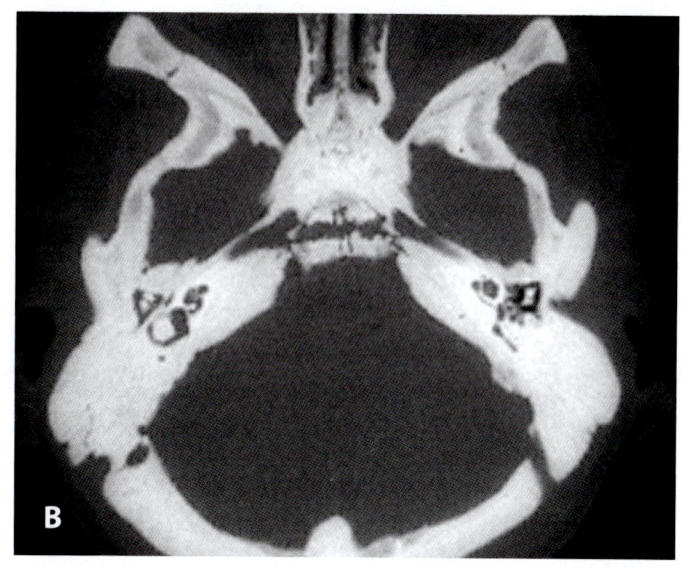

Figure 11-48 Osteopetrosis–Autosomal Dominant
Axial CT scans (**A, B**) of the skull base. There is thick, markedly dense cortical and diploic bone throughout with obliteration of nearly all the air containing cavities and narrowing of the fissures and foramina of the skull base. The fatal nature of the disease relates to the lack of marrow within the skull and axial skeleton.

medullary cavity. These osteosclerotic bones have been aptly termed chalk bones.[277,278]

Two modes of inheritance have been determined: an autosomal recessive (malignant) form and an autosomal dominant (benign) form. There may be severe and mild forms of the autosomal recessive type, which is the less common form of this disease.[279] There are frequent stillbirths, and those surviving birth rarely survive childhood. Clinical features may be severe. Compromise of the marrow cavity, obliterated by the immature bone, can lead to pancytopenia. Extramedullary hematopoiesis may be present. There may be multiple CN palsies due to foraminal stenosis. Hydrocephalus, hepatosplenomegaly, improper dental development, and deafness may also be present.[277]

The autosomal dominant pattern of osteopetrosis is separated into type I and type II, both of which may be asymptomatic. Type I patients may experience bone pain or have symptoms of foraminal stenosis. These patients may also show normal fracture rates. Type II patients often have long bone fractures with minimal trauma and may show delayed healing.

There is an intermediate recessive type that is less severe than the typical autosomal recessive type in its manifestations of anemia, hepatosplenomegaly, and frequent fractures. An autosomal recessive type with renal tubular acidosis has also been described. Affected patients have renal tubular acidosis, cerebral calcifications, hypotonia, mental retardation, and easy fracturing that improves with increasing age.[269]

The radiographic findings differ among the various types of osteopetrosis. The autosomal recessive (malignant) type shows generalized dense bone and flaring of the metaphyses from defective tubular modeling. Transverse striations are often seen as a result of alternating areas of mature and sclerotic bone.[269] In the autosomal dominant (benign) type I disease, sclerosis of the skull is pronounced and thickening of the cranial vault is evident, without involvement of the spine (**Fig. 11-48**). The long bones may have an "Erlenmeyer flask" deformity of the metaphyseal region from overproduction and faulty resorption of bone.[280] Type II disease shows end plate thickening of the vertebrae, which results in a "rugger jersey" appearance of the spine. The base of the skull shows sclerosis, but the calvarium has little involvement.[281–283] The intermediate recessive type gives rise to marked thickening and sclerosis of the base of the skull. The autosomal recessive type with renal tubular acidosis demonstrates intracranial calcifications, most commonly centered in the basal ganglia. Metaphyseal expansion and endobones (bone within bone) may also be present.[269]

In patients with the autosomal recessive (malignant) form of the disease, temporal bone CT shows increased mastoid density and a lack of pneumatization of the mastoid air cells, which may be filled with osteoporotic bone. MR shows obliteration of the mastoid and a generalized thickening of the bone. The internal auditory canals are shortened and trumpet shaped, with the largest opening medially. The subarcuate fossae are enlarged, resulting in a fetal appearance to the bone that persists past infancy, and the ossicles may be thickened and enlarged.[279,284]

In establishing the diagnosis of osteopetrosis, it is important to consider inheritance, age of manifestation, and changes in the skeleton. Paget's disease is characterized by recurrent bone resorption and formation. The temporal bone characteristically shows bony resorption with occasional sclerosis of specific portions. The age and systemic manifestations of Paget's disease will differ from osteopetrosis. Fibrous dysplasia is a disorder of proliferating fibroosseous tissues that results in widening of the diploic spaces. The medullary spaces may be filled with fibrous material. Patients with fibrous dysplasia have greater marrow involvement than patients affected by osteopetrosis. The changes of hyperparathyroidism are seen throughout the skeleton and may accompany other clinical manifestations. Although secondary hyperparathyroidism may show areas of localized sclerosis, it can be differentiated from osteopetrosis by clinical information and laboratory tests. Pycnodysostosis is an autosomal recessive disease first evident in infancy and early childhood and characterized by short stature, frequent fractures, and a large cranium with frontal and occipital bossing. Thickening of the skull base with sclerosis is often present. The osteosclerosis of pycnodysostosis is uniform, and the long bones retain their normal external shape, unlike the findings in the autosomal recessive type of osteopetrosis.[285] Sclerosteosis (endosteal hyperostosis) is an autosomal recessive disease beginning in infancy or early childhood and causing overgrowth of the skull, vertebrae, and mandible with giantism and syndactyly. There is sclerotic thickening of the cortex of long bones with an obvious endosteal component. Cranial nerve palsies are common in this condition, but the cortical thickening in the long bones does not resemble the abnormality in osteopetrosis.[269] Progressive diaphyseal dysplasia is an autosomal dominant disease usually diagnosed in childhood. It is characterized by muscle weakness, bone pain, and difficulty walking. The unusual hyperostosis of the long bones in progressive diaphyseal dysplasia gives a thick and irregular cortex rather than the more uniformly dense bone seen with osteopetrosis.[270,286]

Increased bone density of the skull base also occurs in craniometaphyseal dysplasia. Osteopathic striata (Voorhoeve syndrome) is an autosomal dominant condition, which may also result in generalized temporal bone sclerosis, and conductive hearing loss is an important symptom.[287]

Paget's Disease

In 1876, a well-known English surgeon, Sir James Paget, was the first to describe what is now known as Paget's disease of bone (osteitis deformans). The disease is fairly common, affecting 3% of the population over 40 years of age and up to 10% of patients over 80 years of age. There is an ill-defined genetic factor suggested by familial and geographic clustering. The disease is a chronic, sometimes progressive, condition that may present as a solitary monostotic form, which remains asymptomatic only to be discovered as an incidental finding, or the disease may evolve into a clinically obvious entity. In its disseminated polyostotic form, many bones in different regions of the skeleton may be affected. The pelvis is most often involved, followed in descending order of frequency by the femur, skull, tibia, and spine. Progressive involvement of the temporal bone results in an increase in size and changes in the architecture and position of the petrous pyramid, external canal, middle ear, and otic capsule.[272,288,289]

The histopathology of Paget's disease shows osteoclastic resorption of trabeculae of the spongiosa or walls of the Haversian canals of the compacta. This gives rise to the osteolytic phase of this disease, which characterizes early bone involvement. Heightened bone formation leads to an increase in vascularity. The attacked bone is replaced by densely packed, narrow trabeculae of lamellar, coarse fibered bone. This new bone is hard, dense, and less vascular than normal bone, giving rise to the sclerotic phase of Paget's disease. The sclerotic bone may undergo resorption, leading to variable densities in adjacent areas of bone and resulting in a "mosaic" pattern. The medullary cavity may be filled by a vascular, fibrous connective tissue. Skull base involvement begins in the petrous pyramids. Eventually, there is invagination of the skull base, and the petrous pyramids tilt upward as the softening bone responds to the various forces placed on the skull base. Hearing loss, which may be conductive, sensorineural, or mixed, is the most common manifestation in patients with skull base involvement. Less common symptoms include tinnitus, vertigo, and unsteadiness. Malignant degeneration is seen in about 1% of cases.[272,288,290]

The osteolytic phase of the disease is characterized by sharply demarcated areas of "washed out" radiolucency, typically seen in the skull base or calvarium. The term osteoporosis circumscripta has been applied to the appearance of the skull during the lytic phase. Progression of the disease varies in different areas of the skull and temporal bone. The lytic areas may be replaced by bone, with an increase in density and thickness. The sclerotic form of the disease is much less common in the temporal bone, and a lesion in the sclerotic phase has an "ivory" appearance, distinguishing it from the adjacent bone. Bone expansion continues until resorption occurs. A mixture of phases results in a "cotton wool" appearance caused by simultaneous osteolysis and sclerosis.[272,288]

Examination of the temporal bone by CT shows the decreased density typically seen when demineralization is ongoing. These areas may be intermixed with sites of bone thickening and sclerosis.[273,275,291] The disease begins at the petrous apex (site of greatest marrow deposition) and progresses inferolaterally, with demineralization of the otic capsule being a later manifestation. Frequently, the central skull base is also involved (**Figs. 11-49** and **11-50**). Basilar invagination occurs as the distorted skull base "sags" downward, and the cervical spine can protrude into the foramen magnum. Hearing loss, from the direct involvement of the temporal bone, may be further accentuated by stretching of the acoustic nerves that results from the basilar invagination.

In the calvarium, the outer cortical table becomes thin and may even disappear. The spongiosa may have a delicate, homogeneous, washed out appearance or may show alternating areas of translucency and opacity.

Involvement of the otic capsule is less common. When present, there are areas of resorption that tend to advance from the periphery toward the central regions, and in severe cases resorption may be seen throughout the otic capsule. The stapedial foot plate may be thickened, contributing to hearing loss. The mastoid process may show thickening, demineralization, or a mosaic pattern.[12,289]

The MRI findings are variable. Marrow replacement by fibrous tissue results in diminished T1W signal intensity; however, patchy hyperintensity may occur secondary to hemorrhage or slow flow in vascular channels. Contrast enhancement, when present, reflects the highly vascular nature of this process.[292]

The variability of findings in Paget's disease leads to an extensive differential diagnosis. Fibrous dysplasia results in widening of the diploic spaces, and the medullary spaces become filled with fibrous material with a ground glass appearance.

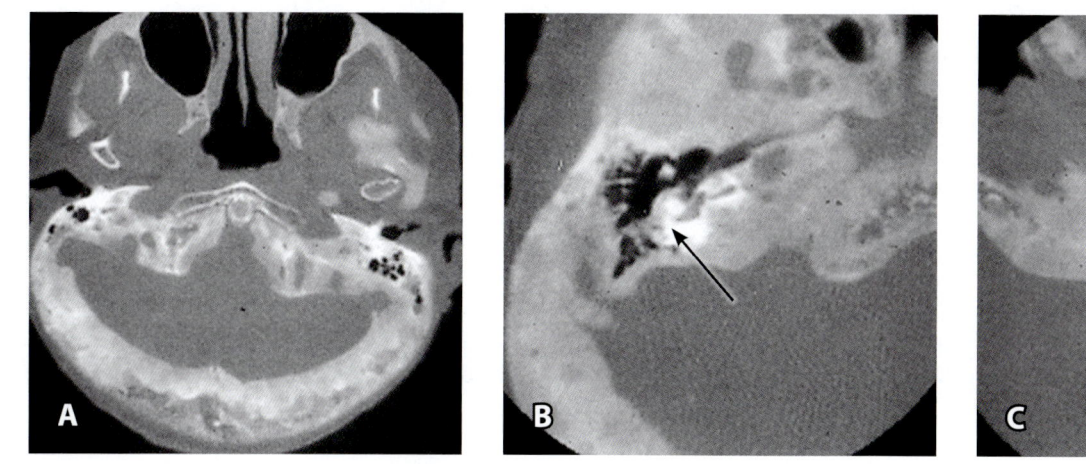

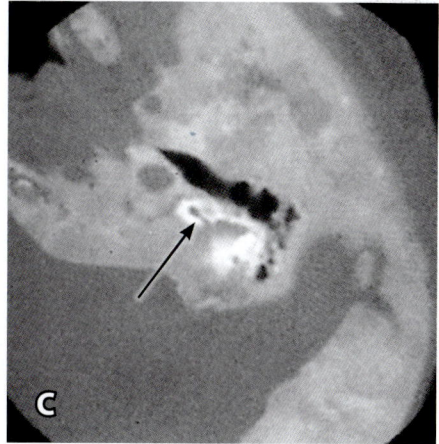

Figure 11-49 Paget Disease Bilateral
Axial CT scan of the skull base (**A**) and of both temporal bones (**B, C**). There is marked expansion of the visualized skull base. Most of the expansion involves the diploic spaces that show a heterogenous mixture of densities. There is destruction of portions of the osseous labyrinth (*arrows*, **B, C**), a characteristic finding with Paget disease unlike fibrous dysplasia that does not erode the labyrinth (**Fig. 11-46**).

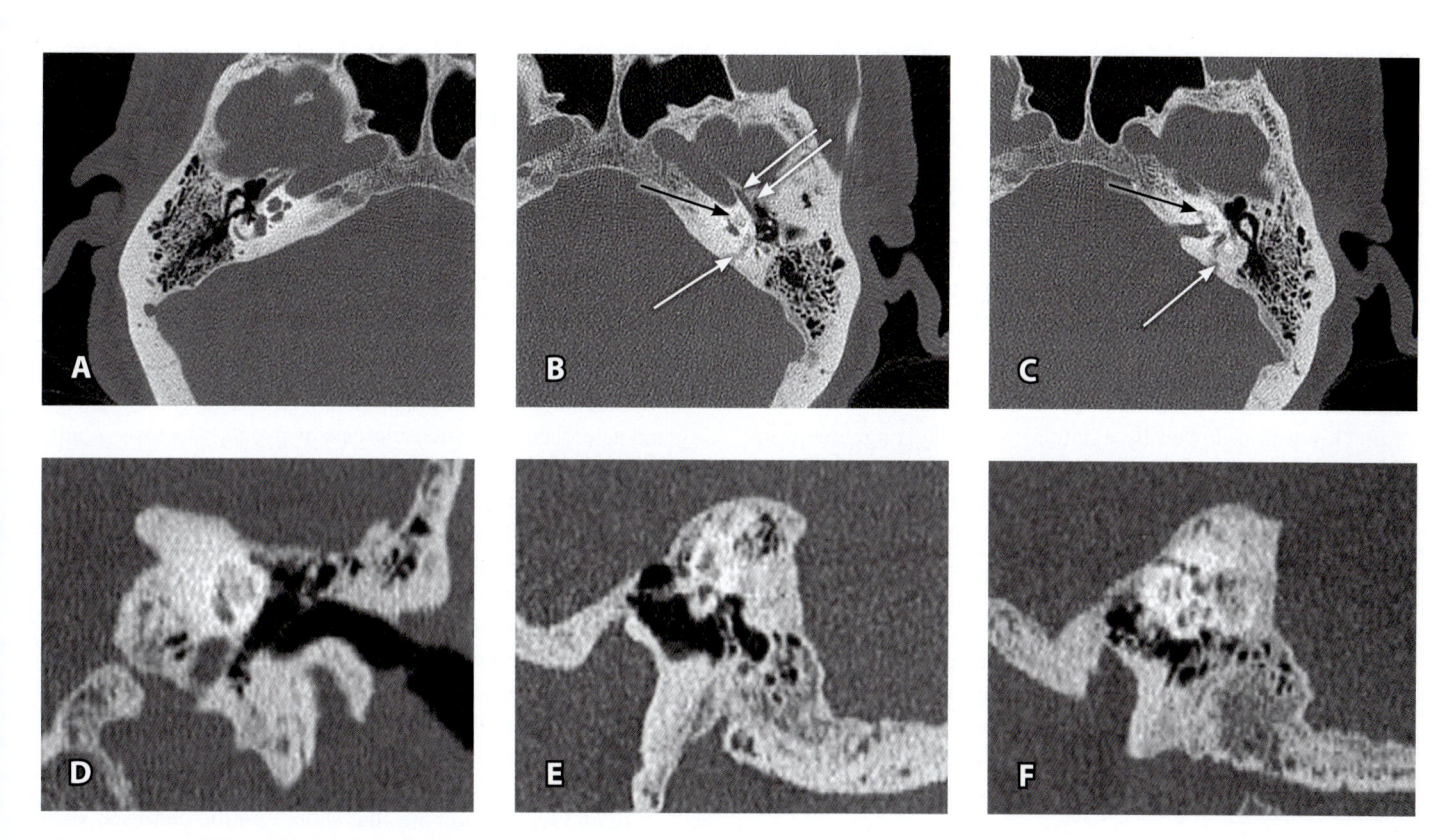

Figure 11-50 Paget Disease Unilateral
Axial (**A–C**), coronal (**D**) and sagittal reformatted (**E–F**) bone CT scans show Paget disease involving the calvarium and left temporal bone. Axial images show encroachment of the inner ear spaces with loss of the integrity of both the cochlea (black *arrows*, **B, C**) and the vestibular apparatus (*single white arrows*, **B, C**) on the left. There is irregular narrowing of the internal auditory canal and the facial canal (*double white arrows*, **B**). There is thickening of the calvarium and smudginess of the diploic spaces best seen in the sagittal view (**E, F**). Note that the middle ear and external auditory canal are normal, as are the cochlea and vestibular apparatus on the right side (**A**).

Patients affected by fibrous dysplasia are characteristically younger and have greater marrow involvement than patients with Paget's disease.[275] The lesions of hyperparathyroidism may be seen throughout the skeleton and are accompanied by other clinical and laboratory manifestations of this disease. Even though some hyperparathyroid lesions are sclerotic, particularly in patients with secondary hyperparathyroidism, such lesions do not actually thicken the bony structures. Temporal bone involvement by osteogenesis imperfecta may have some similarities to the findings in Paget's disease, but the clinical findings and radiologic survey are vastly different. Hereditary hyperphosphatasia, or juvenile Paget's disease, is an autosomal recessive disorder seen in infants who have thickening and deossification of the skull base with bowing of the extremities. Their urinary levels of hydroxyprolamine and alkaline phosphatase are elevated.[269,270] Progressive diaphyseal dysplasia (Camurati Engelmann disease) is an autosomal dominant disease usually diagnosed in childhood. It has a typical hyperostosis of the long bones that can be easily differentiated from Paget's disease.[270,286] The skull base thickening and sclerosis seen in pycnodysostosis is also uniformly present throughout the skeleton, unlike the patchy lesions of Paget's disease.[285]

Metastatic osseous lesions may mimic Paget's disease, particularly when originating from prostate or breast neoplasms. Clinical information is vital to help differentiate these entities. Meningiomas are usually sharply demarcated, and they tend to show inward growth from the inner table of the skull, which may differentiate them from Paget's disease.[164,271]

Progressive Diaphyseal Dysplasia and Other Dense Bone Dysplasias

Progressive diaphyseal dysplasia (Camurati Engelmann disease) is a rare osteosclerotic dysplasia of bone. It was initially described in 1922 by Camurati as an autosomal dominant disease. This was followed by a similar report by Engelmann in 1929. Neuhauser and his associates named this condition progressive diaphyseal dysplasia in 1948. This disease represents a slowly progressive and unpredictable hyperostotic process that is characterized by new bone formation along both the periosteal and endosteal surfaces of long bones. The calvarium and other membranous bones are commonly affected in severe cases. Patients with this disorder are typically diagnosed in childhood and experience a variety of symptoms such as bone pain, easy fatigability, headache, poor appetite, and difficulty ambulating. Clinical signs frequently observed include muscle weakness, decreased muscle mass, a waddling gait, and exophthalmos.[270,278,286,292]

The radiographic findings in progressive diaphyseal dysplasia are usually symmetric, with the upper extremities less often affected than the lower extremities. In mild cases, there is only minimal middiaphyseal thickening of the cortex. Patients with more advanced conditions exhibit more pronounced sclerosis that has spread to the metaphyseal regions, with narrowing of the medullary cavities. In some severe cases, both the skull base and calvarium show the characteristic sclerosis, and the vertebral column, shoulder girdles, metacarpal and metatarsal bones can also be affected in the more severe cases[270] (**Fig. 11-51**).

The CT examination documents the mild to moderate thickening of the skull base with hyperostosis and sclerosis. The middle ear may be completely encased by sclerotic bone along with widespread foraminal narrowing. MRI of the skull base shows a mantle of signal void around the base of the skull and calvaria on both the T1W and T2W images. Hyperostotic bone may be seen encasing the otic capsule, middle, and external ears.[270,293,294]

The diagnosis of progressive diaphyseal dysplasia should be established as early as possible, since treatment determines the severity and progression of the disease. Treatment options include alternate day administration of corticosteroids, which may yield significant relief of pain and symptoms. Calcitonin injections have also been shown to relieve symptoms. Surgery may be indicated to relieve pain and decompress the affected CNs.[285,294]

Several diseases must be considered in the differential diagnosis of progressive diaphyseal dysplasia. Generalized cortical hyperostosis, or van Buchem's disease, is one of the diseases now grouped as the endosteal hyperostoses. This autosomal recessive disorder is characterized by osteosclerosis of the skull base and calvarium, mandible, and long and short bones. An elevated level of alkaline phosphatase is typically present. Sclerosteosis, another of the endosteal hyperostoses, is an autosomal recessive disease that portrays overgrowth of the skull, vertebrae, and mandible with gigantism. Cranial nerve palsies are common in this condition, but the long bone findings can usually be differentiated from progressive diaphyseal dysplasia. The cortex is not as thick and irregular in sclerosteosis, and the skeletal distribution is also different. Craniodiaphyseal dysplasia is an autosomal recessive disease that results in facial deformity from the early sclerosis of the skull and facial bones. The CNs may be affected due to stenosis and narrowing of their foramina. Pycnodysostosis is an autosomal recessive disease of infancy and early childhood characterized by skull base thickening and sclerosis. The osteosclerosis of pycnodysostosis is uniform, and the long bones do not show the unusual hyperostosis of progressive diaphyseal dysplasia.[285] The autosomal recessive (malignant) form of osteopetrosis occurs in infants and has some features similar to those of progressive diaphyseal dysplasia. There may also be fractures of the long bones, but radiographs of the long bones will not show the hyperostosis characteristic of progressive diaphyseal dysplasia. The autosomal dominant (benign) form of osteopetrosis will have sclerosis of the base of the skull and show diaphyseal thickening, but the skeletal pattern will show sparing of the hands, feet, ribs, and shoulders.[269] Paget's disease occurs in older patients and has a different pattern of diaphyseal thickening that should not be confused with progressive diaphyseal dysplasia. The osteolytic regions seen in Paget's are not present, and the sclerosis is more uniform without the "cotton wool" pattern in the skull.

TRAUMA OF THE TEMPORAL BONE

In most traumatic lesions of the temporal bone, such as fractures and ossicular dislocations, CT is much more sensitive and specific than MRI. High-resolution CT is advised in all cases where

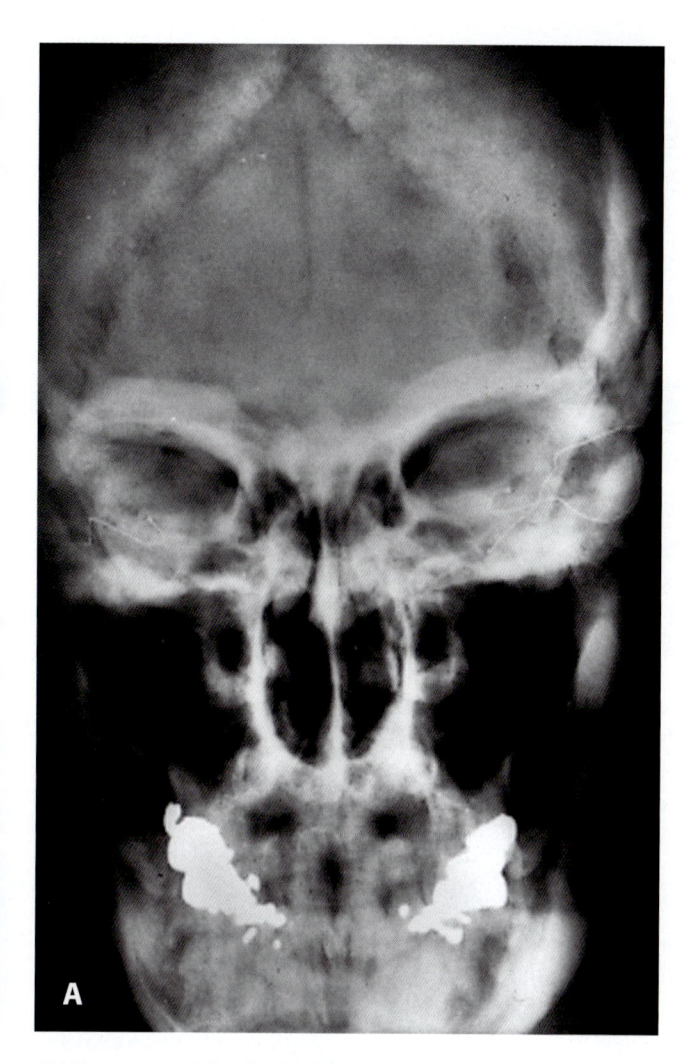

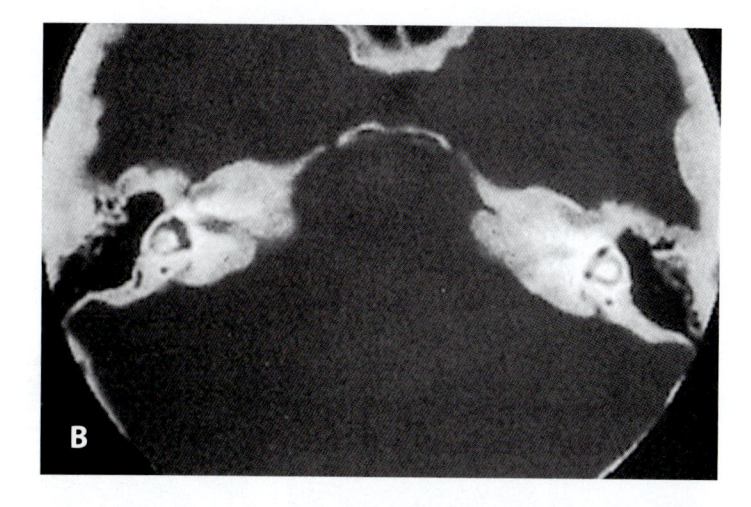

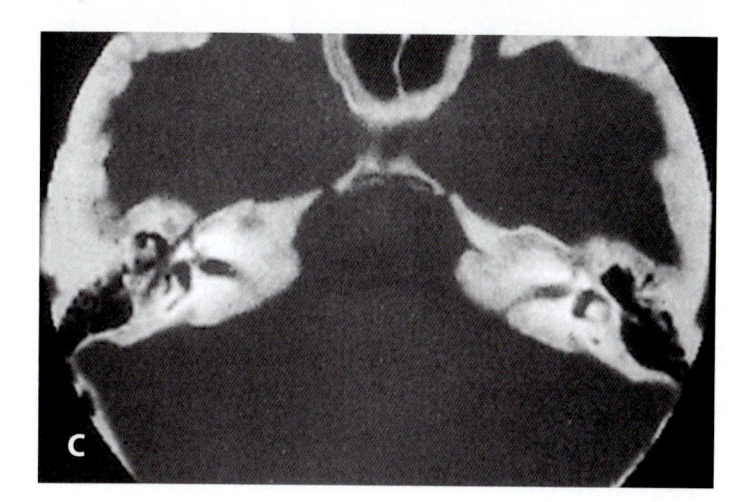

Figure 11-51 Diaphyseal Dysplasia
Caldwell view of the skull (**A**) and axial CT scans (**B, C**) of the temporal bones. There is moderate dense cortical bone throughout the skull and skull base with obliteration of the diploic spaces, but not the air-containing cavities. Deafness results from overgrowth of bone with narrowing of the internal auditory canal. The electrodes of a cochlear implant are visible on the left side.

persistent conductive hearing loss and/or facial nerve palsy is evident following injury. Neurosensory hearing loss and some cases of CSF leaks may benefit from MR studies. What follows is a brief discussion of the role of both CT and MRI in temporal bone injuries.

Traumatic hemorrhages into the air containing cavities of the temporal bone and mastoid air cells results in opacifications with or without air-fluid levels. Hemotympanum appears as nonspecific fluid density within the tympanic cavity and mastoid antrum on both CT and MRI scans.

Fracturing of the osseous components of the temporal bone is effectively diagnosed with high-resolution axial CT scans and multi-planar reformatting. These scans can detect various types of traumatic injuries to the ossicles, facial nerve canal, or internal auditory canal with a high level of confidence. Surgical relief of compressive traumatic injuries to the facial nerve canal can best be accomplished through CT imaging.[136,291]

Injuries to the contents of the IAC may be directly detected with MRI as foci of hemorrhage or edema surrounding the facial, vestibular, or acoustic nerves. Furthermore, neurosensory hearing loss following head trauma may be caused by an injury to the central auditory nuclei in the brain stem, detected as foci of hemorrhagic contusion on blood-sensitive MR sequences such as GRE and SWI.[115]

Longitudinal and Transverse Fractures

Longitudinal fractures are the most common type of temporal bone fractures. They run along the long axis of the petrous pyramid in the horizontal plane. Reformatted coronal and sagittal CT images are particularly useful in the search for longitudinal fractures. Such fractures typically extend from the temporal squamosal and posterior portion of the external auditory canal and across the tegmen tympani and tegmen antri.

Rupture of the tympanic membrane, hemotympanum, or ossicular disruption usually results in conductive hearing loss. Neurosensory loss may result from labyrinthine injury. Such an injury may be caused by a fracture through the osseous labyrinth, resulting in a "dead ear" with complete loss of both

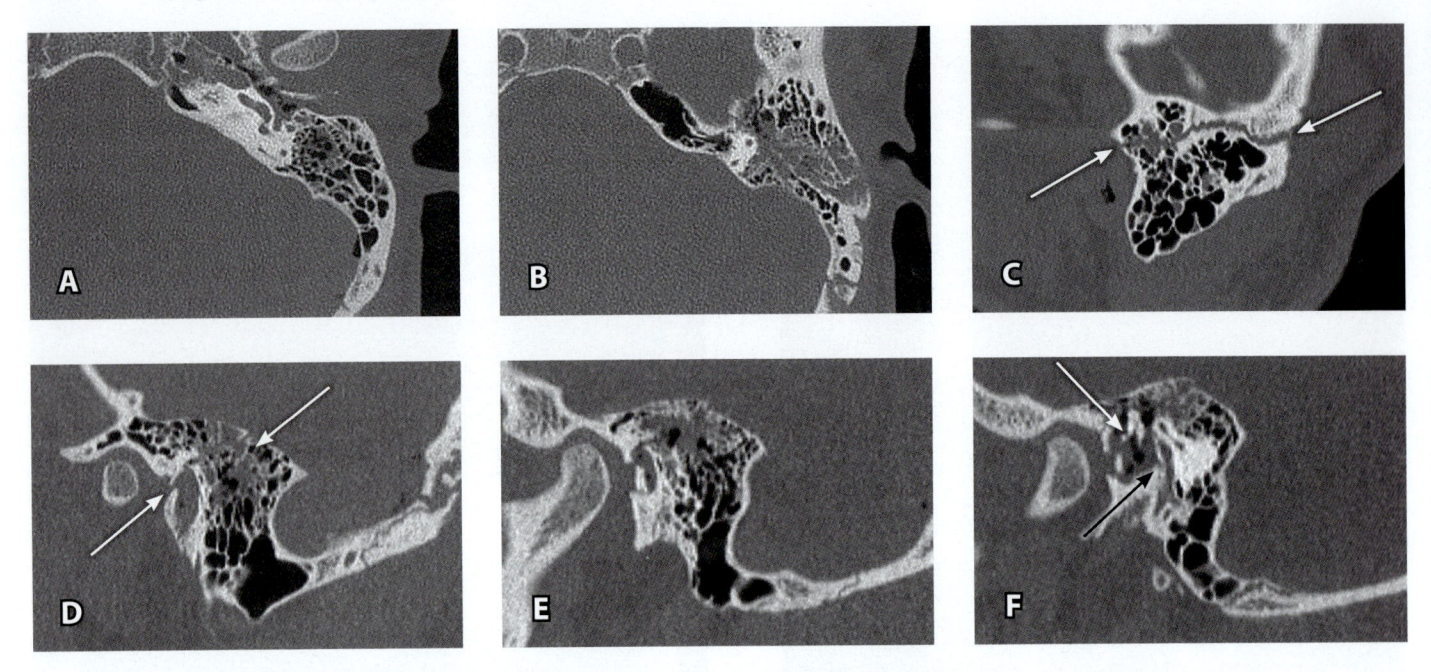

Figure 11-52 Temporal Bone Fracture with Facial Nerve Canal and Malleal Injuries
(**A, B**) Axial and (**C–F**) serial reformatted sagittal CT images of the left temporal bone. There is minimally diastatic fracturing of the mastoid process and external canal walls (*arrows*, **C** and **D**) extending into the mastoid antrum and tympanic cavity. There is a fracture into the mastoid portion of the facial nerve canal (*black arrow*, **F**) and a fracture of the long process of the malleus (*white arrow*, **F**).

auditory and vestibular functions. Facial nerve dysfunction may be caused by transection of the facial nerve in the canal or by edematous compression of the nerve in the canal (**Fig. 11-52** and **11-53**).

Transverse fractures run perpendicular to the long axis of the petrous pyramid. Axial CT scans are ideal for evaluating these fractures. Associated traumatic lesions involving the TMJ, mandibular condyle, or skull base can also be evaluated on axial images.[291]

Complex and Comminuted Fractures

In cases of severe injury following high-speed vehicular accidents, complex and comminuted fractures are being increasingly diagnosed. Such multiple fractures may show major distractions of the fracture fragments resulting in communications between the cranial cavity and temporal bone cavities. CSF otorrhea or rhinorrhea may be seen, and in some cases, there may be evidence of herniation of the temporal lobe into the middle ear or EAC (enaural encephalocele).

Injuries to the Ossicles

Conductive hearing loss, persisting sometime after the resolution of hemotympanum, with or without rupture of the tympanic membrane, requires high-resolution CT evaluation for suspected injuries to the ossicles. Axial or reformatted sagittal images are usually preferred for diagnosis of an incudomalleal dislocation. The malleus is the most firmly attached ossicle, making incudomalleal dislocation less likely than incudostapedial dislocation.

Incudomalleal separation is evident by an increased space between the head of the malleus and the body and short process of the incus (**Fig. 11-54**). The normal parallel configuration between the long process of the malleus and the long and lentiform processes of the incus may be disturbed. Fractures of the long processes should also be considered when fragments of bone are seen separately within the tympanic cavity.

Reformatted coronal or sagittal images are preferred for diagnosis of an incudostapedial dislocation. In such cases, the lentiform process of the incus points away from the oval window, with loss of the normal "V" shape between this structure and the stapes superstructure. The stapes footplate is well anchored and is rarely displaced from the oval window. However, severe injuries resulting in petrous bone diastasis may show general malposition of all ossicular components.

Traumatic damage to the ossicles may be surgically reconstructed at the time of tympanoplasty. Replacement ossicles may be implanted or removed with interposition of various types of prosthesis. Post-operative CT scanning may be used to document correct placement or displacement of the prosthesis in cases of persistent conductive deafness.[291]

Brain Herniation (Enaural Encephalocele)

Herniation of the temporal lobe into the ear cavities may occur in cases of complex or diastatic fracturing. The dehiscence may

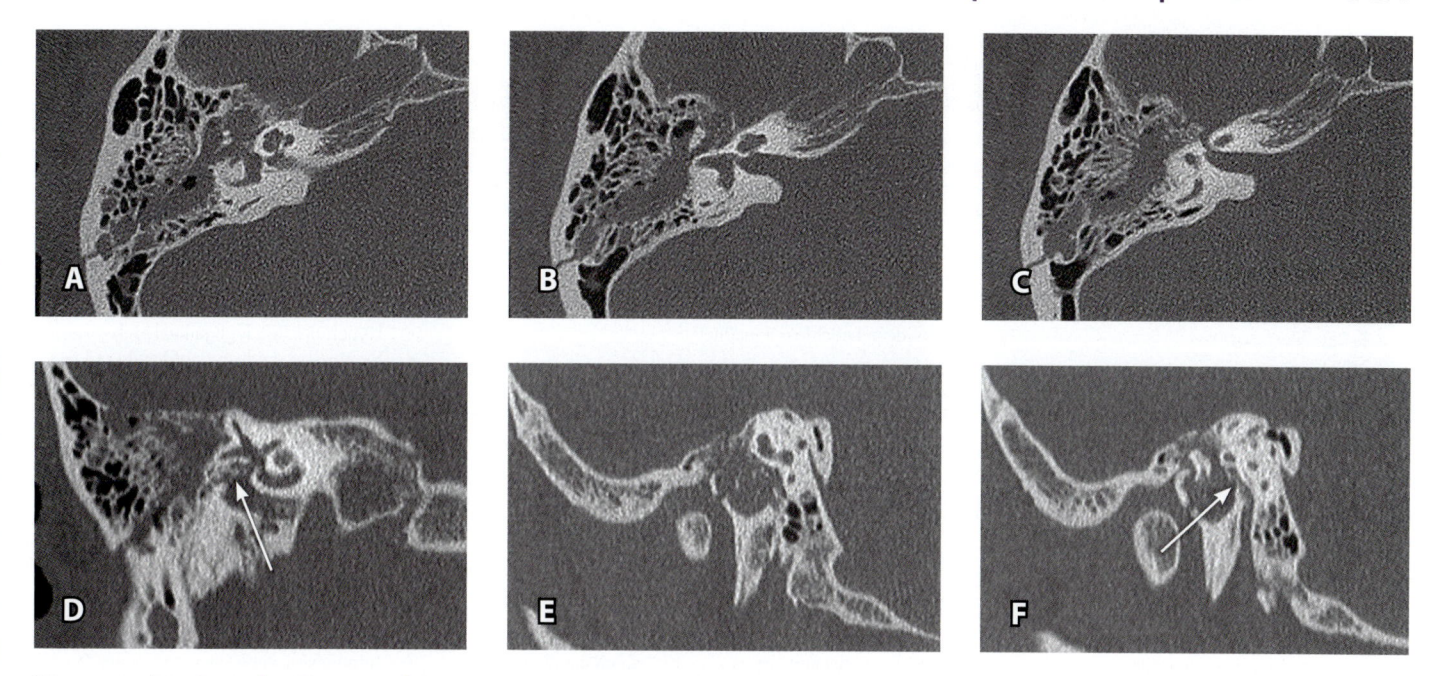

Figure 11-53 Complex Temporal Bone Fracture with Facial Canal Injury
(**A–C**) Axial, (**D**) reformatted coronal, and (**E, F**) reformatted sagittal CT scans. There are complex diastatic fractures of the mastoid and petrous portions of the right temporal bone. The tympanic portion of the facial nerve canal shows tiny fragments of bone in the course of the facial nerve (*arrows*, **D, E**) and at the junction between the tympanic and mastoid portions of the facial nerve canal (*arrow*, **F**).

be seen into the tegmen antri, tegmen tympani, or the external auditory canal. Combined dehiscences are common with both middle ear and external ear involvement. Clinically, such patients may present with hearing loss and otorrhea or rhinorrhea. Showering or bathing may initiate an acute vertiginous episode or may induce pain when water enters the external auditory canal. A mass may be seen extending inferiorly from the roof of the external auditory canal.

On CT, a soft tissue mass extending downwards into the external or middle ears may be seen. T2-W MR scans are particularly useful with detection of both meningeal structures surrounded by CSF and/or individual gyri of the temporal lobe[115,291] (**Fig. 11-55**).

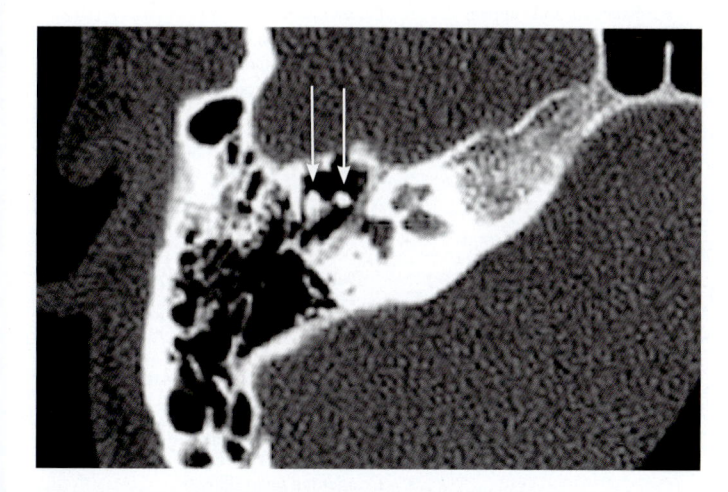

Figure 11-54 Malleoincudal Joint Dislocation
Temporal bone fracture with malleoincudal joint dislocation. Axial CT shows pathological widening (*arrows*) of the malleoincudal joint reflecting a partial subluxation in this patient with conductive hearing loss.

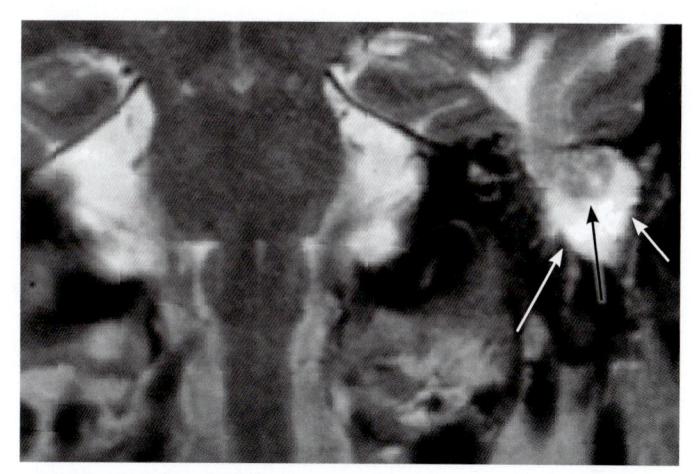

Figure 11-55 Enaural Encephalocele
Coronal T2 MRI of the skull base. On the left side there is combined herniation of the inferior temporal gyrus (*black arrow*) surrounded by a CSF-filled meningocele (*white arrows*) extending through the roof of the left middle and external ear. (Courtesy of Joel Swartz, MD.)

Appendix 11-1 Congenital Syndromes Involving the Ear

Syndrome	Ear Abnormalities External	Ear Abnormalities Middle	Ear Abnormalities Inner	Associated Anomalies
Apert Syndrome (acrocephalosyndactyly)	• Low-set ears • Stapedial footplate fixation • Incus fixation • CHL	• Enlarged IAC • Large subarcuate fossa that connects to middle fossa dura • Perilymph gushers due to widened cochlear aqueduct	• Craniosynostosis • Acrobrachycephaly • Midface hypoplasia	• Flattened facies • Saddle nose deformity • Shallow orbits with proptosis • Exotropia • Down-slanting palpebral fissures • Hypertelorism; high palatal arch • Symmetric syndactyly of hands and feet minimally involving digits 2,3, and 4
Achondroplasia	• None	• Ossicular fusion • Dense, thick trabeculae without islands of cartilage in the enchondral bone and periosteal bone	• Deformed cochlea • Thickened intracochlear partitions	• Dwarfism • Macrocephaly with prominent forehead and occiput • Midface hypoplasia • Nasal retrusion • Lordosis • Spinal stenosis • Tripod hands • Lumbar
Alagille Syndrome	• Large ears • Helices incompletely folded	• Bulky incus and stapes with immature interossicular joint	• Cochlear dysplasia • Hypoplasia or complete agenesis of posterior and anterior SCCs • Absence or stenosis of cochlear aqueduct	• Intrahepatic cholestasis secondary to decreased intrahepatic bile ducts • Peripheral pulmonary artery stenosis • Facial anomalies include prominent forehead, hypertelorism, deep-set eyes, small chin, and saddle-nose
Albers-Schonberg Disease (Marble bone disease or osteopetrosis)	• EAC sclerosis and stenosis	• Tympanic cavity narrowing with bony encroachment and/or chronic otitis media may lead to CHL • Ossicular abnormalities • Fetal form of stapes • Stenotic facial canal with secondary facial palsy • Poor mastoidal pneumatization	• IAC sclerosis and stenosis, with bony encroachment on nerves VII /VIII may lead to SNHL	• Thick, dense, and fragile bones • Stenotic cranial foramina leading to secondary blindness, strabismus, facial palsy and/or deafness • Macrocephaly with frontal and parietal bossing • Exophthalmos • Obliteration of paranasal sinuses • Anemia • Frequent fractures
Branchio-Oto-Renal Syndrome (Melnick-Fraser Syndrome)	• Small, low-set ears • Cup-shaped anteverted pinnae • Preauricular fistula or sinus	• Fixed stapedial footplate • Shortened manubrium of malleus or long process of incus • Bulky malleus and incus; absent stapes • Fixation of malleus and incus within the attic • Small middle-ear cavity • Absent OW or stapedial muscle tendon • Large and deep OW niche • Hypoplastic facial nerve • Dehiscence of bony facial canal • CHL	• Dilated vestibule • Small SCCs • Saccular wide appearance of lateral SCC • Hypoplastic cochlea • Dilated endolymphatic duct • Absent ampulla and crista in lateral SCC • SNHL	• Branchial sinuses, kidney and/or ureteric hypoplasia or agenesis • Facial nerve palsy • Cervical fistula or cysts • Long narrow facies • Lacrimal duct stenosis or atresia • Retrognathia
Carpenter Syndrome	• Low-set ears • Preauricular fistulas	• Idiopathic CHL	• Idiopathic SNHL	• Craniosynostosis • Cloverleaf skull • Preaxial polysyndactyly of feet • Short fingers with clinodactyly • Congenital heart defects • Down-slanting palpebral fissures • Epicanthic folds • Microcornea • Corneal opacity • Optic atrophy • Short neck • Small mandible • Highly-arched palate

Appendix 11-1 Congenital Syndromes Involving the Ear (Continued)

Syndrome	Ear Abnormalities External	Ear Abnormalities Middle	Ear Abnormalities Inner	Associated Anomalies
CHARGE Syndrome	• Small, low-set, short, and wide cup-shaped ears with a triangular concha; "lop ears" and "snipped-off" helical folds • Discontinuity between antihelix and antitragus • Small or absent earlobes	• Absent stapes superstructure • Foreshortened incus with absent long process • Misshapen stapes footplate • Absent stapedius tendon and pyramidal process • Absent OW and round window	• Mondini dysplasia of pars inferior • Absent pars superior • Short cochlea • Hypoplasia of vestibular sense organs and nerves	• Coloboma; heart anomalies (VSD, ASD, PDA, tetralogy of Fallot) • Choanal atresia • Growth retardation and developmental delay • Mental retardation • Genital anomaly
Crouzon Syndrome	• EAC atresia and stenosis • Microtia	• Absent TM • Ankylosis of malleus to epitympanum • Deformed stapes with bony fusion to promontory • Distortion and narrowing of middle ear space • Narrow round window niche • Eustachian tube dysfunction • Hypoplastic periosteal labyrinth • Decreased periosteal layer of petrous bone	• None	• Cranial synostosis • Midface (maxillary) hypoplasia, mandibular prognathism • High-arched or CP • Orbital hypoplasia with proptosis and exophthalmos, hypertelorism, protuberant and arched "parrot-beaked" nose due to maxillary recession; choanal atresia
Down's Syndrome Trisomy 21	• Small, low-set ears; EAC stenosis	• Bulky malleus and incus • Deformed stapes with distortion of stapedial crura • Narrowed or collapsed eustachian tube • Hypoplastic pyramidal eminence • Underdeveloped mastoid air cells • Chronic otitis media with effusion CHL	• Shortened cochlea • Utriculo-endolymphatic valve agenesis • Wide utricular space and SCC • Wide cochlear aqueduct • Hypogenesis of posterior SCC • Enlarged bony posterior SCC ampulla • SNHL	• Hypertelorism • Epicanthic fold • Slanting eyes • Strabismus • Narrowed nasal cavity • Hypoplastic paranasal sinuses • Protruding tongue • High palate • Flattened skull • VSD, ASD, PDA (cardiovascular defects)
Duane Syndrome	• Preauricular skin tags • Pinna malformation • Microtia • Hypoplasia or atresia of EAC	• Ossicular deformities • Fused ossicles • Lack of contact between fused-ossicles and OW • Closure of OW by thin membrane • Ossicular mass without connection to stapes	• None	• Abducens nerve paralysis • Limited ocular abduction, restriction of adduction and retraction (usually unilateral) • Nystagmus, epibulbar dermoid, ptosis, anisocoria • Hemifacial microsomia • Hypoplastic extremities • Thoracic scoliosis • Hemangiomas • CNS hypotonia and convulsions
Edwards Syndrome Trisomy 18	• Low-set ears • EAC atresia	• Deformed malleus, incus, and stapes • Split tensor tympani muscle in separate bony canals • Exposed stapedial muscle in tympanic cavity • Absent stapedial tendon • Anomalous course of the facial and chorda tympani nerves • Absent pyramidal eminence • CHL	• Absent utriculo-endolymphatic valve • Absent lateral limbs of superior and lateral SCCs • Enlarged endolymphatic duct • Double singular nerve • SNHL	• Ptosis • High-arched palate • Micrognathia • Flexion deformity • Hypertrophic pancreatic tissue • Failure to thrive • Mental retardation • Poor prognosis
Fanconi Syndrome	• Microtia	• Fixation of stapedial footplate	• Hypoplastic hook of cochlea and reduced length of cochlear duct	• Aplastic anemia • Skeletal deformities • Hyperpigmentation • Renal anomalies • Mental retardation

(Continued)

Appendix 11-1 Congenital Syndromes Involving the Ear (Continued)

Syndrome	Ear Abnormalities External	Ear Abnormalities Middle	Ear Abnormalities Inner	Associated Anomalies
Goldenhar Syndrome (hemifacial microsomia)	• Preauricular skin tags • Microtia/anotia	• Malformation or absence of ossicles • Absent chorda tympani nerve • Straightened tensor tympani tendon • Hypoplastic stapedius muscle • Small tympanic cavity, encroached upon by a low tegmen and thick atretic plate • Hypoplastic and under pneumatized mastoid • CHL	• Hypoplastic cochlea and petrous bone • Dysplastic and shortened lateral and superior semicircular canals • Narrow and short IAC	• Facial asymmetry with unilateral mandibular hypoplasia • Cervical vertebral dysplasia • Scoliosis • Spina bifida • Coloboma • Blepharoptosis • Narrowed palpebral fissures • Epibulbar dermoid • CP • Congenital heart defects (tetralogy of Fallot, VSD
Gorlin-Holt Syndrome (frontometaphyseal dysplasia)	• None	• Fixation of malleus • Malformation of ossicles	• Osseous infiltration around cochlea	• Decreased pneumatization of frontal sinuses • Micrognathia • Metaphyseal splaying of tubular bones • Large supraorbital ridge • Wide nasal bridge • Flaring of iliac wings
Hemifacial Microsomia (craniofacial microsomia)	• Microtia • Preauricular tags and/or pits	• Ossicular deformities • Facial nerve defect with hypoplastic facial muscles • CHL	• None	• Defects are unilateral • Orbital distortion • Mandibular hypoplasia • Hypoplasia or absence of parotid gland and muscles of mastication
Heusinger Syndrome	• Preauricular pits	• Malformation and fusion of ossicles • Bilateral abnormality in form and relationship of middle ear spaces, middle cranial fossa, and inner ears • CHL	• Hypoplastic cochlea and its neural components • Degeneration of vascular stria and organ of Corti • SNHL	• Branchial fistulae and renal anomalies
Jervell and Lange-Nielsen Syndrome	• None	• None	• Degeneration of organ of Corti; collapsed Reissner's membrane • Atrophic stria vascularis • Reduced number of spiral ganglion cells • SNHL	• Cardiac EKG abnormalities such as prolonged QT interval and large T waves, which result in arrhythmias; mild hyperchromic anemia
Klippel-Feil Syndrome (Brevicollis)	• Low-set ears; microtia • Preauricular appendage • EAC atresia or stenosis	• Ossicular agenesis • Slit-like malleoincudal joint • Short process of incus fused to attic floor • Absent lenticular process of stapes with fibrous joint between long process of incus and stapes • Fixed stapes to OW • Fistula of stapes footplate • Anomalous course of facial nerve • CHL	• Rudimentary cochlea and/or modiolus • Dilated SCCs • Wide communication between saccule and utricle • Shallow, superiorly positioned IAC • SNHL	• Fusion of cervical vertebrae, spina bifida, and Sprengel scapular deformity • Short, immobile neck with prominent soft tissue • Hairline extending down to the back • Mental retardation

Appendix 11-1 Congenital Syndromes Involving the Ear (*Continued*)

Syndrome	Ear Abnormalities External	Ear Abnormalities Middle	Ear Abnormalities Inner	Associated Anomalies
Larsen Syndrome	• None	• Bulbous lenticular process of incus • Incudostapedial joint laxity • Fixation of stapes footplate • CHL	• None	• Multiple joint dislocations and skeletal abnormalities • Anterior dislocation of knees • Dislocation of hips and elbows • Equinovarus or equinovalgus deformity of feet • None tapered cylindrical fingers with spatulate thumbs • Hypertelorism; frontal bossing • Depressed nasal bridge
Levy-Hollister Syndrome (lacrimo-auriculo-dento-digital syndrome)	• Cup-shaped ears; short helix; hypoplastic antihelix	• Idiopathic CHL	• Idiopathic SNHL	• Nasolacrimal duct obstruction • Hypoplastic or absent lacrimal glands • Epiphora • Dental anomalies such as hypodontia, peg-shaped incisors and enamel hypoplasia • Premature tooth decay • Upper limb anomalies • Hypoplastic or absent salivary glands • Renal anomalies
Melnick-Needles Syndrome (osteodysplasty)	• Small, distorted pinnae • Narrow EAC	• Absent round window • Mastoid sclerosis	• None	• Late closure of fontanelles • Dense base of skull • Small facial bones • Prominent eyes • Delayed paranasal sinus development • Small mandible • Short upper extremities • Short distal phalanges • Bowing radius and tibia • Flaring of distal humerus • Tibia and fibula
Mobius Syndrome (facial diplegia)	• Microtia; EAC atresia • Auricular deformity	• Ossicular mass without identifiable stapes/OW/round window • Absent facial nerve	• Dilated vestibule and SCC system	• CN VII and VI palsies due to intracerebral nuclear defects • Motionless facial expression; nasolabial grin • Strabismus • Hypoglossia • Microstomia • Speech disorders secondary to facial muscle paralysis
Mohr Syndrome (oral-facial-digital syndrome 2)	• None	• Malformation of ossicles • Absent lenticular process of incus • Otitis media and serous otitis secondary to muscular dysfunction of CP	• None	• Lobed tongue • High-arched or CP • Broad bifid nasal tip • Supernumerary digits with ulnar Hexadactyly • Polysyndactyly of hallucus • Mental retardation • Poor coordination • Muscular hypotonia • Microcephaly
Nager Syndrome (acrofacial dysostosis)	• Malformation of pinna • Low-set ears • Stenotic EAC	• Ossicular deformities • Fixation of malleus and incus • Ankylosis or absence of stapes • CHL	• Abnormalities of the labyrinth • SNHL	• Similar to Treacher Collins syndrome, except without coloboma • Severe CP • Hypoplasia or agenesis of radius and thumb • Short stature • Infants have respiratory and feeding difficulty

(*Continued*)

Appendix 11-1 Congenital Syndromes Involving the Ear (Continued)

Syndrome	Ear Abnormalities External	Ear Abnormalities Middle	Ear Abnormalities Inner	Associated Anomalies
Neurofibromatosis 2 Vestibular Schwannoma	• None	• None	• Tinnitus; vertigo • SNHL, usually bilateral	• Acoustic tumors are benign and asymptomatic until pressure exerted on surrounding structures gives rise to: meningiomas • Gliomas • Neurofibromas • Schwannomas • Café au lait macules • Facial nerve neuromas • Juvenile posterior subcapsular lenticular opacity; cranial nerve deficits
Noonan Syndrome (pseudo-Turner Syndrome)	• Anteverted ear lobes secondary to fetal cystic hygroma	• Ossicular deformities • Absent long process of incus • Chronic otitis media • CHL	• Idiopathic SNHL	• Short stature • Hypertelorism • Webbed neck • Cubitus valgus • Pectus • Hypogonadism • Ptosis; strabismus • Amblyopia • Cherubism • Cardiac anomalies including pulmonary valve defects with pulmonary hypertension • Partial factor XI deficiency with bleeding diathesis; autoimmune thyroiditis; idiopathic hepatosplenomegaly
Oculo-Auriculo-Vertebral Syndrome	• Microtia	• Fusion of incus and malleus; hypoplastic or absent ossicles • CHL	• None	• Hemifacial microsomia • Hypoplastic maxilla and mandible • Microstomia • CNS abnormalities • Epibulbar dermoids • Vertebral defects
Patau Syndrome Trisomy 13	• Low-set ears • EAC stenosis • Small TM	• Thick manubrium of malleus • Distorted incudostapedial joint • Deformed stapes • Small facial nerve • Wide angle of facial genu • Absent stapedial muscle and tendon • Persistent stapedial artery • Dehiscence of facial canal • Absent pyramidal eminence • Small antrum • Small mastoid	• Shortened cochlea • Absent hook of cochlea • Absent or hypoplastic modiolus; malformed scala vestibule with small space in the basal turns • Large and patent cochlear aqueduct • Shortened utriculoendolymphatic valve • Direct communication between utricle and saccule • SCC deformities • Shallow and wide IAC	• Microcephaly • Arrhinencephaly; multiple eye anomalies • Hypertelorism • Cleft lip and CP • VSD • Simian creases • Hyperconvexity of nails
Pendred Syndrome	• None	• None	• Hypoplastic cochlea • Flattened promontory • Atrophy of organ of Corti and tectorial membrane • Absent inner/outer hair cells • Few spiral ganglion cells • Mondini defect • SNHL	• Euthyroid goiter

Chapter 11: The Temporal Bone   527

Appendix 11-1 Congenital Syndromes Involving the Ear (*Continued*)

Syndrome	Ear Abnormalities External	Ear Abnormalities Middle	Ear Abnormalities Inner	Associated Anomalies
Pfeiffer Syndrome (Types 1, 2, and 3)	• Preauricular tag • Absent EAM	• Ankylosis of stapedial footplate • Fusion of incus to epitympanum • Fixation of incudomalleal joint • Stapes crural malformation hypoplastic mastoid • CHL	• None	• Craniosynostosis-bilateral coronal suture fusion • Midface hypoplasia • Ocular proptosis • Broad great toes and thumbs • Brachydactyly • Syndactyly of hands • Cloverleaf skull with hydrocephalus and severe ocular proptosis in type 2
Pierre Robin Syndrome	• Cup-shaped, low-set ears	• Thickened stapes crura and footplate • Small facial nerve • Dehiscence of facial canal • Absent middle ear cavity	• Scala communis between apical and middle cochlear turns • Hypoplastic modiolus • Narrowed communication between crus commune and utricle • Small and narrow IAC	• Mandibular hypoplasia and retromandibulism; glossoptosis • CP • Micrognathia; posteriorly prolapsed tongue may lead to airway obstruction in infants • Feeding problems • Hydrocephalus • Microcephaly • Microphthalmia • Myopia • Cataracts • Retinal detachment • Congenital heart anomalies
Pyle Disease (craniometaphyseal dysplasia)	• None	• Malleal encasement by bony promontory • Deformed incus fixed to promontory • Stapes head in OW filled with bone • Enlarged chorda tympani nerve • CHL	• IAC stenosis • SNHL	• Hypertelorism • Nasal dorsum deformity • Saddle nose • Prognathism • Posterior choanal atresia • Defective dentition; metaphyseal widening of long bones • Nystagmus • Optic atrophy • CN VII palsy • Narrowing of nasal passage • Obliterated paranasal sinus • Nasolacrimal duct obstruction
Saethre-Chotzen Syndrome (acrocephalosyndactyly type III)	• Small, low-set ears • Prominent crus and antihelix; stenotic EAC	• None	• None	• Craniosynostosis • Ptosis of upper eyelids • Low-set frontal hairline • Facial asymmetry • Deviated nasal septum • Strabismus • Lacrimal duct stenosis • High-arched palate • Brachydactyly • Partial cutaneous syndactyly • Other skeletal anomalies
Stickler Syndrome	• None	• None	• Idiopathic SNHL	• Orofacial and ophthalmologic abnormalities • Deafness • Arthritis • Flat and hypoplastic midface • Depressed nasal bridge • Short nose • Anteverted nares • Micrognathia • Cleft palate • Abnormal architecture of vitreous gel with severe myopia • Cataracts • Retinal detachment • Joint hypermobility in infancy • Juvenile-onset arthritis • Mitral valve prolapse

(*Continued*)

Appendix 11-1 Congenital Syndromes Involving the Ear (*Continued*)

Syndrome	Ear Abnormalities External	Ear Abnormalities Middle	Ear Abnormalities Inner	Associated Anomalies
Thalidomide Embryopathy	• Malformation or absence of pinna • EAC atresia • Deformed TM	• Fixation of malleus • Displaced long process of incus; absent stapes • Absent facial and chorda tympani nerves • Persistent stapedial artery • Slit-shaped tympanic cavity • Absent OW	• Aplastic inner ear • Absent facial nerve and statoacoustic nerve in IAC	• Deformity, shortening, or absence of long bones • Capillary hemangiomas of forehead, nose, lips • Colobomas • Microphthalmia • Congenital heart defects • Intestinal atresia • Renal hypoplasia or agenesis • CN palsies
Townes-Brocks Syndrome	• Overturned helices "lop ears" • Microtia • Preauricular tags	• None	• Idiopathic SNHL	• Triphalangeal or hypoplastic thumbs • Abnormal wrist bones • Hypoplastic third toes • Cone-shaped epiphyses • Imperforate anus or anal stenosis • Cardiac anomalies • Urogenital anomalies such as hypospadias and cryptorchidism
Treacher Collins Syndrome (mandibulofacial dysostosis)	• Mild to severe microtia • EAC atresia or stenosis	• TM replaced by bony plate • Ossicular deformities and dysjunction • Fusion of malleoincudal joint • Absent tensor tympani muscle, stapedial muscle, and tendon of stapedius muscle • Absent pyramidal eminence, cochleariform process and mastoid antrum • Absent chorda tympani and superficial petrosal nerves • Small middle ear cavity • CHL	• Large cochlear aqueduct and a blind-pouch horizontal canal • SNHL	• Fish-like facial appearance • Micrognathia • Microgenia • Macrostomia • Cleft palate • Antimongoid palpebral fissures and colobomas of lower eyelids and iris • Absent lashes from medial two-thirds of lower lid • Malar hypoplasia • Choanal atresia • Orbital dysplasia • Pharyngeal hypoplasia • Parotid salivary gland absence or hypoplasia
Usher's Syndrome	• None	• None	• Vestibular hypofunction • Atrophic changes in organ of Corti and spiral ganglia in basal turn • Atrophy of stria vascularis, limbus, tectorial membrane, and Reissner's membrane • No known radiographic abnormality • SNHL	• Retinitis pigmentosa • Posterior subcapsular cataracts • Mental retardation
VATER Syndrome	• None	• Hypoplasia of facial, chorda tympani, and greater superficial petrosal nerves • Decreased cells in geniculate ganglion • Anteriorly curved superstructure of stapes • Hypertrophic anterior annular ligament	• Irregular course of lateral SCC and duct • Superiorly-positioned utricle and saccule • Large endolymphatic sinus, duct, and sac • Decreased spiral ganglion cells	• Vertebral defects • Anal atresia • Tracheoesophageal fistula with esophageal atresia • Renal defects • Radial limb dysplasia • Large fontanelles • Cardiac defects • Single umbilical artery • Genital anomalies
Van Buchem Syndrome (generalized cortical hyperostosis)	• None	• Impingement of hyperostotic bone on ossicle and facial nerve • CHL	• Impingement of hyperostotic bone in IAC • SNHL	• All bones markedly hyperostotic with increased density and thickness • Significantly elevated serum alkaline phosphatase • Mandibular enlargement • Calvarium thickened • Papilledema progressing to optic atrophy and blindness

Appendix 11-1 Congenital Syndromes Involving the Ear (Continued)

Syndrome	Ear Abnormalities External	Ear Abnormalities Middle	Ear Abnormalities Inner	Associated Anomalies
Velocardiofacial Syndrome-VCFS (Shprintzen Syndrome)	• None	• Chronic otitis media; CHL	• None	• Retrognathia • Long face • Prominent nose • Microcephaly • Speech abnormalities due to incompetent pharyngeal musculature • Congenital heart defects (VSD, right-sided aortic arch, and tetralogy of Fallot) • Carotid arteries with anomalous course
Waardenburg's Syndrome	• None	• None	• Atrophic changes in spiral ganglion and nerve • Degeneration of organ of Corti • Thickening of basal membrane • Diminished vestibular function • SNHL	• Dystopia canthorum • Flat nasal root • Confluent eyebrows • Heterochromic irides • White forelock • Pigmentary abnormalities • Cleft lip and CP • Hirschsprung aganglionosis of bowel • VSD • Premature graying of hair
Wildervanck Syndrome (cervico-oculoacoustic syndrome)	• Preauricular tags • Posteriorly displaced pinnae • Small ears • Hypoplastic EAC	• Rudimentary ossicles • Fusion of malleus and incus • Absent stapes and OW • Fixation of stapes • Ossified stapedius tendon • CHL	• Abnormal SCC • Hypoplastic bony labyrinth • Stenosis or bony septum within IAC • SNHL	• Duane retraction syndrome abducens nerve palsy with limited abduction and retraction of globe • Narrowed palpebral fissures during eye adduction • Epibulbar dermoid cysts • Lens subluxation • CP • Cardiac anomalies • Klippel-Feil anomaly • Cervical vertebral fusion • Torticollis • Rib anomalies

EAC = external auditory canal, EAM = external auditory meatus, IAC = internal auditory canal, SCC = semicircular canal, TM = tympanic membrane, CHL = conductive hearing loss, SNHL = sensorineural hearing loss, CN = cranial nerve, CP = cleft palate, OW = oval window, CNS = central nervous system.

Adapted From:
1. Bluestone CD, Stool SE, and Kenna MA: Pediatric otolaryngology. 3rd ed. Philadelphia: WB Saunders, 1996.
2. Fritsch MH and Sommer A: Handbook of congenital and early onset hearing loss. New York: Igaku-Shoin Medical Publishers, 1991.
3. Kerr AG, Adams DA, and Cinnamond MJ: Scott-Brown's otolaryngology: paediatric otolaryngology. 6th ed. Oxford: Butterwoth-Heinemann, 1997.
4. Friedmann I and Arnold W: Pathology of the ear. Edinburgh: Churchill Livingstone, 1993.
5. Phelps PD and Stansbie JM: Clinical ENT radiology. Oxford: Butterworth-Heinemann, 1993.
6. Stricker M, Van der Meulen JC, Raphael B, Mazzola R, and Tolhurst DE: Craniofacial malformations. Edinburgh: Churchill Livingstone, 1990.
7. Canalis RF and Lambert PR: The ear: comprehensive otology. Philadelphia: Lippincott Williams & Wilkins, 2000.
8. Cohen MM and MacLean, RE: Craniosynostosis: diagnosis, evaluation, and management. 2nd ed. New York: Oxford University Press, 2000.
9. Goodrich JT and Hall CD: Craniofacial anomalies: growth and development from a surgical perspective. New York: Thieme Medical Publishers, 1995.
10. Dufresne CR, Carson BS, and Zinreich SJ: Complex craniofacial problems. New York: Churchill Livingstone, 1992.
11. Swartz JD and Harnsberger HR: Imaging of the temporal bone. 3rd ed. New York: Thieme, 1998.
12. Valvassori GE, Mafee MF, and Carter, BL: Imaging of the head and neck. New York: Thieme, 1995.
13. Som PM and Curtin HD: Head and neck imaging. 4th ed. St. Louis: Mosby, 2003.
14. Stevenson RE, Hall JG, and Goodman RM: Human malformations and related anomalies. New York: Oxford University Press, 1993.
15. Wilson GN and Cooley WC: Preventive management of children with congenital anomalies and syndromes. Cambridge: Cambridge University Press, 2000.

REFERENCES

1. Som PM and Bergeron RT: Head and neck imaging. 2nd ed. St. Louis: Mosby-Year Books; 1991:1152.
2. Gray H, Williams PL, and Bannister LH: Gray's anatomy : the anatomical basis of medicine and surgery. 38th ed. New York: Churchill Livingstone; 1995:2092.
3. Gulya AJ and Schuknecht HF: Anatomy of the temporal bone with surgical implications. 2nd ed. New York: Parthenon Pub. Group; 1995:350.
4. Leonard RJ and Ebrary Inc: Human gross anatomy: an outline text. New York: Oxford University Press; 1995:437.
5. Colman BH and Hall IS: Hall & Colman's diseases of the nose, throat and ear, and head and neck: a handbook for students and practitioners. 14th ed. New York: Churchill Livingstone; 1992:293.
6. O'Donoghue GM, Narula AA, and Bates GJ: Clinical ENT: a primer. 2nd ed. San Diego: Singular Pub. Group; 2000:257.
7. Phelps PD and Lloyd GAS: Diagnostic imaging of the ear. 2nd ed. New York: Springer-Verlag; 1990:218.
8. Newton TH, Hasso A, and Dillon W: Modern neuroradiology: CT of the head and neck. San Anselmo, CA: Clavadel Press; 1988.
9. Bergeron RT and Osborn AG: Head and Neck imaging excluding the brain. St. Louis: C.V. Mosby Co.; 1984:896.
10. Jensen J: Congenital anomalies of the inner ear. Radiol Clin North Am 1974;12(3):473–482.
11. Anson BJ and Donaldson JD: Surgical anatomy of the temporal bone. 3rd ed. Philadelphia: Saunders; 1981:734.
12. Vignaud J, Rosen L, and Jardin C: The ear, diagnostic imaging: CT scanner, tomography, and magnetic resonance. New York: Masson Pub. U.S.A.; 1986:365.
13. Wright JW Jr.: Polytomography and congenital external and middle ear anomalies. Laryngoscope 1981;91(11):1806–1811.
14. Jahrsdoerfer R: Congenital malformations of the ear. Analysis of 94 operations. Ann Otol Rhinol Laryngol 1980;89(4Pt1):348–352.
15. Swartz JD and Faerber EN: Congenital malformations of the external and middle ear: high-resolution CT findings of surgical import. Am J Roentgenol 1985;144(3):501–506.
16. Tasar M, et al.: Preoperative evaluation of the congenital aural atresia on computed tomography: an analysis of the severity of the deformity of the middle ear and mastoid. Eur J Radiol 2007;62(1):97–105.
17. De la Cruz A and Hansen M: Reconstruction of the ear: auditory canal and tympanum, in head & neck surgery—otolaryngology. In: Bailey BJ, Johnson JT, and Newlands SD, eds. Philadelphia, PA: Lippincott Williams & Wilkins; 2006.
18. Mayer TE, et al.: High-resolution CT of the temporal bone in dysplasia of the auricle and external auditory canal. Am J Neuroradiol 1997;18(1):53–65.
19. Lambert PR: Congenital aural atresia, in head & neck surgery—otolaryngology. In: Bailey BJ, Johnson JT, and Newlands SD, eds. Philadelphia, PA: Lippincott Williams & Wilkins; 2006:2027–2040.
20. Jahrsdoerfer RA, et al.: Grading system for the selection of patients with congenital aural atresia. Am J Otol 1992;13(1):6–12.
21. Shonka DC Jr., Livingston WJ, 3rd, and Kesser BW: The Jahrsdoerfer grading scale in surgery to repair congenital aural atresia. Arch Otolaryngol Head Neck Surg 2008;134(8):873–877.
22. Robson CD, Robertson RL, and Barnes PD: Imaging of pediatric temporal bone abnormalities. Neuroimaging Clin N Am 1999;9(1):133–155.
23. Kosling S, Omenzetter M, and Bartel-Friedrich S: Congenital malformations of the external and middle ear. Eur J Radiol 2009;69(2):269–279.
24. Sone M, et al.: Imaging findings in a case with cholesteatoma in complete aural atresia. Am J Otolaryngol 2009:297–299.
25. Lapayowker MS: Congenital anomalies of the middle ear. Radiol Clin North Am 1974;12(3):463–471.
26. Petasnick JP: Congenital malformations of the ear. Otolaryngol Clin North Am 1973;6(2):413–428.
27. Moore KL: The developing human: clinically oriented embryology. 4th ed. Philadelphia, PA: Saunders; 1988:462.
28. Rodriguez K, Shah RK, and Kenna M: Anomalies of the middle and inner ear. Otolaryngol Clin North Am 2007;40(1):81–96.
29. Nandapalan V and Tos M: Isolated congenital stapes ankylosis: an embryologic survey and literature review. Am J Otol 2000;21(1):71–80.
30. Park K and YH Choung: Isolated congenital ossicular anomalies. Acta Otolaryngol 2009;129(4):419–422.
31. Casqueiro JC, et al.: Imaging case of the month. Congenital absence of the stapes superstructure. Otol Neurotol 2009;30(8):1230–1231.
32. Harada T, et al.: Temporal bone histopathologic findings in congenital anomalies of the oval window. Otolaryngol Head Neck Surg 1980;88(3):275–287.
33. Zeifer B, Sabini P, and Sonne J: Congenital absence of the oval window: radiologic diagnosis and associated anomalies. Am J Neuroradiol 2000;21(2):322–327.
34. de Alarcon A, Jahrsdoerfer RA, and Kesser BW: Congenital absence of the oval window: diagnosis, surgery, and audiometric outcomes. Otol Neurotol 2008;29(1):23–28.
35. Jackler RK, Luxford WM, and House WF: Congenital malformations of the inner ear: a classification based on embryogenesis. Laryngoscope 1987;97(3 Pt 2 Suppl 40):2–14.
36. Jackler RK: Congenital malformations of the inner ear, in cummings otolaryngology head & neck surgery. In: Cummings CW, ed. Philadelphia, PA: Elsevier Mosby; 2005:4523.
37. Bluestone CD, Stool SE, and Kenna MA: Pediatric otolaryngology. 3rd ed. Philadelphia, PA: Saunders; 1996.
38. Kwee HL: The occurrence of the Tullio phenomenon in congenitally deaf children. J Laryngol Otol 1976;90(6):501–507.
39. Sando I, Takahara T, and Ogawa A: Congenital anomalies of the inner ear. Ann Otol Rhinol Laryngol Suppl 1984;112:110–118.
40. Parnes LS and Chernoff WG: Bilateral semicircular canal aplasia with near-normal cochlear development. Two case reports. Ann Otol Rhinol Laryngol 1990;99(12):957–959.
41. Swartz JD and Mukherji SK: The inner ear and otodystrophies, in imaging of the temporal bone. In: Swartz JD, and Harnsberger HR, eds. New York: Thieme; 2009:298–411.
42. Belden CJ, et al.: CT evaluation of bone dehiscence of the superior semicircular canal as a cause of sound- and/or pressure induced vertigo. Radiology 2003;226(2):337–343.
43. Minor LB: Clinical manifestations of superior semicircular canal dehiscence. Laryngoscope 2005;115(10):1717–1727.
44. Krombach GA, et al.: Semicircular canal dehiscence: comparison of T2-weighted turbo spin-echo MRI and CT. Neuroradiology 2004;46(4):326–331.
45. Lagundoye SB, Martinson FD, and Fajemisin AA: The syndrome of enlarged vestibule and dysplasia of the lateral semicircular canal in congenital deafness. Radiology 1975;115(2):377–378.
46. Marsot-Dupuch K, et al.: CT and MR findings of Michel anomaly: inner ear aplasia. Am J Neuroradiol 1999;20(2):281–284.
47. Ozgen B, et al.: Complete labyrinthine aplasia: clinical and radiologic findings with review of the literature. Am J Neuroradiol 2009;30(4):774–780.
48. Philippon D, et al.: Cochlear implantation in postmeningitic deafness. Otol Neurotol 2010;31(1):83–87.
49. Parry DA, Booth T, and Roland PS: Advantages of magnetic resonance imaging over computed tomography in preoperative evaluation of pediatric cochlear implant candidates. Otol Neurotol 2005;26(5):976–982.
50. Reilly G, Lalwani AK, and Jackler RK: Congenital anomalies of the inner ear, in pediatric otology and neurotology. In: Lalwani AK, and Grundfast K, eds. Philadelphia, PA: Lippincott-Raven; 1998:728.
51. Mylanus EA, Rotteveel LJ, and Leeuw RJ: Congenital malformation of the inner ear and pediatric cochlear implantation. Otol Neurotol 2004;25(3):308–317.
52. Schuknecht HF: Mondini dysplasia; a clinical and pathological study. Ann Otol Rhinol Laryngol Suppl 1980;89(1 Pt 2):1–23.
53. Casselman JW, et al.: CT and MR imaging of congenital abnormalities of the inner ear and internal auditory canal. Eur J Radiol 2001;40(2):94–104.
54. Paparella MM: Mondini's deafness. A review of histopathology. Ann Otol Rhinol Laryngol Suppl 1980;89(2 Pt 3):1–10.
55. Miyasaka M, et al.: CT and MR imaging for pediatric cochlear implantation: emphasis on the relationship between the cochlear nerve canal and the cochlear nerve. Pediatr Radiol 2010:1509–1516.

56. Robson CD: Congenital hearing impairment. Pediatr Radiol 2006;36(4): 309–324.
57. Shu MT, et al.: Hypoplasia of the cochlear nerve in the internal auditory canal. Otol Neurotol 2007;28(7):990–991.
58. Carner M, et al.: Imaging in 28 children with cochlear nerve aplasia. Acta Otolaryngol 2009;129(4):458–461.
59. Adunka OF, et al.: Internal auditory canal morphology in children with cochlear nerve deficiency. Otol Neurotol 2006;27(6):793–801.
60. Casselman JW, et al.: Aplasia and hypoplasia of the vestibulocochlear nerve: diagnosis with MR imaging. Radiology 1997;202(3):773–781.
61. Butman JA, Patronas NJ, and Kim HJ: Imaging studies of the temporal bone, in head & neck surgery—otolaryngology. In: Bailey BJ, Johnson JT, and Newlands SD, eds. Philadelphia, PA: Lippincott Williams & Wilkins; 2006:1961–1985.
62. Casselman JW, et al.: Magnetic resonance examination of the inner ear and cerebellopontine angle in patients with vertigo and/or abnormal findings at vestibular testing. Acta Otolaryngol Suppl 1994;513:15–27.
63. Casselman JW, et al.: Inner ear malformations in patients with sensorineural hearing loss: detection with gradient-echo (3DFT-CISS) MRI. Neuroradiology 1996;38(3):278–286.
64. Casselman JW, et al.: Constructive interference in steady state-3DFT MR imaging of the inner ear and cerebellopontine angle. Am J Neuroradiol 1993;14(1):47–57.
65. Tien RD, Felsberg GJ, and Macfall J: Fast spin-echo high-resolution MR imaging of the inner ear. Am J Roentgenol 1992;159(2):395–398.
66. Krombach GA, et al.: MRI of the inner ear: comparison of axial T2-weighted, three-dimensional turbo spin-echo images, maximum-intensity projections, and volume rendering. Invest Radiol 2000;35(6): 337–342.
67. Kim HJ, et al.: Common crus aplasia: diagnosis by 3D volume rendering imaging using 3DFT-CISS sequence. Clin Radiol 2004;59(9): 830–834.
68. Hans P, et al.: Comparison of three-dimensional visualization techniques for depicting the scala vestibuli and scala tympani of the cochlea by using high-resolution MR imaging. Am J Neuroradiol 1999;20(7): 1197–1206.
69. Klingebiel R, et al.: A post-processing protocol for three-dimensional visualization of the inner ear using the volume-rendering technique based on a standard magnetic resonance imaging protocol. Acta Otolaryngol 2001;121(3):384–386.
70. Clark JL, DeSanto LW, and Facer GW: Congenital deafness and spontaneous CSF otorrhea. Arch Otolaryngol 1978;104(3):163–166.
71. Pimontel-Appel B and Vignaud J: Liquorrhea in congenital malformation of the petrosal bone. J Belge Radiol 1980;63(2–3):283–289.
72. Sykora GF, Kaufman B, and Katz RL: Congenital defects of the inner ear in association with meningitis. Radiology 1980;135(2):379–382.
73. Curtin HD, Vignaud J, and Bar D: Anomaly of the facial canal in a Mondini malformation with recurrent meningitis. Radiology 1982;144(2): 335–341.
74. Tyagi I, Syal R, and Goyal A: Cerebrospinal fluid otorhinorrhoea due to inner-ear malformations: clinical presentation and new perspectives in management. J Laryngol Otol 2005;119(9):714–718.
75. Carter BL, Wolpert SM, and Karmody C: Recurrent meningitis associated with an anomaly of the inner ear. Neuroradiology 1975;9:55.
76. Levy LM, et al.: Flow-sensitive magnetic resonance imaging in the evaluation of cerebrospinal fluid leaks. Am J Otol 1995;16(5):591–596.
77. Jegoux F, et al.: Hyrtl's fissure: a case of spontaneous cerebrospinal fluid-otorrhea. Am J Neuroradiol 2005;26(4):963–966.
78. Mukherji SK, et al.: Enlarged cochlear aqueduct. Am J Neuroradiol 1998;19(2):330–332.
79. Weissman JL, Weber PC, and Bluestone CD: Congenital perilymphatic fistula: computed tomography appearance of middle ear and inner ear anomalies. Otolaryngol Head Neck Surg 1994;111(3 Pt 1):243–249.
80. Yanagihara N and Nishioka I: Pneumolabyrinth in perilymphatic fistula: report of three cases. Am J Otol 1987;8(4):313–318.
81. McGhee MA and Dornhoffer JL: A case of barotrauma-induced pneumolabyrinth secondary to perilymphatic fistula. Ear Nose Throat J 2000;79(6):456–459.
82. Lovblad KO, et al.: CT cisternography in congenital perilymphatic fistula of the inner ear. J Comput Assist Tomogr 1995;19(5):797–799.
83. Kim S, Park CH, and Park K: Cerebrospinal fluid rhinorrhea caused by a congenital defect of stapes mimicking otorrhea: radionuclide cisternographic findings. Clin Nucl Med 2000;25(8):634–635.
84. Nakashima T, et al.: Imaging of a congenital perilymphatic fistula. Int J Pediatr Otorhinolaryngol 2003;67(4):421–425.
85. Talbot JM and Wilson DF: Computed tomographic diagnosis of X-linked congenital mixed deafness, fixation of the stapedial footplate, and perilymphatic gusher. Am J Otol 1994;15(2):177–182.
86. Swartz JD, et al.: Aberrant internal carotid artery lying within the middle ear. High resolution CT diagnosis and differential diagnosis. Neuroradiology 1985;27(4):322–326.
87. Sinnreich AI, et al.: Arterial malformations of the middle ear. Otolaryngol Head Neck Surg 1984;92(2):194–206.
88. Glasscock ME, 3rd, et al.: Vascular anomalies of the middle ear. Laryngoscope 1980;90(1):77–88.
89. Saito H, Chikamori Y, and Yanagihara N: Aberrant carotid artery in the middle ear. Arch Otorhinolaryngol 1975;209(2):83–87.
90. Lapayowker MS, et al.: Presentation of the internal carotid artery as a tumor of the middle ear. Radiology 1971;98(2):293–297.
91. Keen J: Absence of both internal carotid arteries. Clin Proc 1946;4: 588–594.
92. Overton SB and Ritter FN: A high placed jugular bulb in the middle ear: a clinical and temporal bone study. Laryngoscope 1973;83(12):1986–1991.
93. Jahrsdoerfer RA, Cail WS, and Cantrell RW: Endolymphatic duct obstruction from a jugular bulb diverticulum. Ann Otol Rhinol Laryngol, 1981;90(6 Pt 1):619–623.
94. Lo WW and Solti-Bohman LG: High-resolution CT of the jugular foramen: anatomy and vascular variants and anomalies. Radiology 1984;150(3):743–747.
95. Lloyd TV, Van Aman M, and Johnson JC: Aberrant jugular bulb presenting as a middle ear mass. Radiology 1979;131(1):139–141.
96. Swartz JD: The middle ear and mastoid, in imaging of the temporal bone. In: Swartz JD, and Harnsberger HR, eds. New York: Thieme; 2009:58–246.
97. Maroldi R, et al.: Computed tomography and magnetic resonance imaging of pathologic conditions of the middle ear. Eur J Radiol 2001;40(2): 78–93.
98. Nemzek WR and Swartz JD: Temporal bone: inflammatory disease, in head and neck imaging In: Som PM, and Curtin HD, eds. St. Louis: Mosby; 2003:1173–1229.
99. Mafee MF, et al.: Acute otomastoiditis and its complications: role of CT. Radiology 1985;155(2):391–397.
100. Antonelli PJ, et al.: Computed tomography and the diagnosis of coalescent mastoiditis. Otolaryngol Head Neck Surg 1999;120(3):350–354.
101. Wetmore RF: Complications of otitis media. Pediatr Ann 2000;29(10): 637–646.
102. Chole RA and Sudhoff H: Chronic otitis media, mastoiditis, and petrositis, in cummings otolaryngology head & neck surgery. In: Cummings CW, ed. Philadelphia, PA: Elsevier Mosby; 2005:4523.
103. Harker L and Clough S: Complications of temporal bone infections, in cummings otolaryngology head & neck surgery. In: Cummings CW, ed. Philadelphia, PA: Elsevier Mosby; 2005:4523.
104. Bousser MG, and Ferro JM: Cerebral venous thrombosis: an update. Lancet Neurol 2007;6(2):162–170.
105. Davison SP, et al.: Use of magnetic resonance imaging and magnetic resonance angiography in diagnosis of sigmoid sinus thrombosis. Ear Nose Throat J 1997;76(7):436–441.
106. Rollins N, et al.: Cerebral MR venography in children: comparison of 2D time-of-flight and gadolinium-enhanced 3D gradient-echo techniques. Radiology 2005;235(3):1011–1017.
107. Roche J and Warner D: Arachnoid granulations in the transverse and sigmoid sinuses: CT, MR, and MR angiographic appearance of a normal anatomic variation. Am J Neuroradiol 1996;17(4): 677–683.
108. Seven H, Ozbal AE, and Turgut S: Management of otogenic lateral sinus thrombosis. Am J Otolaryngol 2004;25(5):329–333.
109. Stam J: Thrombosis of the cerebral veins and sinuses. N Engl J Med 2005;352(17):1791–1798.
110. Neely JG and Arts HA: Intratemporal and intracranial complications of otitis media, in head & neck surgery—otolaryngology. In: Bailey BJ,

110. Johnson JT, and Newlands SD, eds. Philadelphia, PA: Lippincott Williams & Wilkins; 2006:2041–2056.
111. Mishra AM, et al.: Biological correlates of diffusivity in brain abscess. Magn Reson Med 2005;54(4):878–885.
112. Dorenbeck U, et al.: Diffusion-weighted echo-planar MRI of the brain with calculated ADCs: a useful tool in the differential diagnosis of tumor necrosis from abscess? J Neuroimaging 2003;13(4):330–338.
113. Walsh RM, et al.: Management of retraction pockets of the pars tensa in children by excision and ventilation tube insertion. J Laryngol Otol 1995;109(9):817–820.
114. Yates PD, et al.: CT scanning of middle ear cholesteatoma: what does the surgeon want to know? Br J Radiol 2002;75(898):847–852.
115. Harnsberger HR: Diagnostic imaging. head and neck. 1st ed. Salt Lake City: UT: Amirsys; 2005:1 v. (various pagings).
116. Martin N, Sterkers O, and Nahum H: Chronic inflammatory disease of the middle ear cavities: Gd-DTPA-enhanced MR imaging. Radiology 1990;176(2):399–405.
117. Mafee MF: MRI and CT in the evaluation of acquired and congenital cholesteatomas of the temporal bone. J Otolaryngol 1993;22(4):239–248.
118. Fitzek C, et al.: Diffusion-weighted MRI of cholesteatomas of the petrous bone. J Magn Reson Imaging 2002;15(6):636–641.
119. Aikele P, et al.: Diffusion-weighted MR imaging of cholesteatoma in pediatric and adult patients who have undergone middle ear surgery. AJR Am J Roentgenol 2003;181(1):261–265.
120. Lemmerling MM, et al.: Imaging of the opacified middle ear. Eur J Radiol 2008;66(3):363–371.
121. Bowes AK, et al.: Brain herniation and space-occupying lesions eroding the tegmen tympani. Laryngoscope 1987;97(10):1172–1175.
122. Isaacson B, Kutz JW, and Roland PS: Lesions of the petrous apex: diagnosis and management. Otolaryngol Clin North Am 2007;40(3):479–519.
123. Le BT and Roehm PC: Petrous apex mucocele. Otol Neurotol 2008;29(1):102–103.
124. Browning GG, et al.: Chronic otitis media, in Scott-Brown's otorhinolaryngology, head and neck surgery. In: Gleeson M, ed. London: Hoddler Arnold; 2006:3395–3445.
125. Stangerup SE, et al.: Recurrence of attic cholesteatoma: different methods of estimating recurrence rates. Otolaryngol Head Neck Surg 2000;123(3):283–287.
126. Darrouzet V, et al.: Preference for the closed technique in the management of cholesteatoma of the middle ear in children: a retrospective study of 215 consecutive patients treated over 10 years. Am J Otol 2000;21(4):474–481.
127. Vartiainen E: Ten-year results of canal wall down mastoidectomy for acquired cholesteatoma. Auris Nasus Larynx 2000;27(3):227–229.
128. Thomassin JM and Braccini F: Role of imaging and endoscopy in the follow up and management of cholesteatomas operated by closed technique. Rev Laryngol Otol Rhinol (Bord) 1999;120(2):75–81.
129. Williams MT and Ayache D: Imaging of the postoperative middle ear. Eur Radiol 2004;14(3):482–495.
130. Blaney SP, et al.: CT scanning in "second look" combined approach tympanoplasty. Rev Laryngol Otol Rhinol (Bord) 2000;121(2):79–81.
131. Williams MT, et al.: Detection of postoperative residual cholesteatoma with delayed contrast-enhanced MR imaging: initial findings. Eur Radiol 2003;13(1):169–174.
132. Venail F, et al.: Comparison of echo-planar diffusion-weighted imaging and delayed postcontrast T1-weighted MR imaging for the detection of residual cholesteatoma. Am J Neuroradiol 2008;29(7):1363–1368.
133. Vercruysse JP, et al.: The value of diffusion-weighted MR imaging in the diagnosis of primary acquired and residual cholesteatoma: a surgical verified study of 100 patients. Eur Radiol 2006;16(7):1461–1467.
134. De Foer B, et al.: Detection of postoperative residual cholesteatoma with non-echo-planar diffusion-weighted magnetic resonance imaging. Otol Neurotol 2008;29(4):513–517.
135. Dhepnorrarat RC, Wood B, and Rajan GP: Postoperative non-echo-planar diffusion-weighted magnetic resonance imaging changes after cholesteatoma surgery: implications for cholesteatoma screening. Otol Neurotol 2009;30(1):54–58.
136. Valvassori GE: Imaging of the temporal bone, in Valvassori's imaging of the head and neck In: Mafee MF, Valvassori GE, and Becker M, eds. New York: Thieme; 2005:3–132.
137. Hussam K and Lee A: Tympanoplasty and ossiculoplasty, in cummings otolaryngology head & neck surgery. In: Cummings CW, eds. Philadelphia, PA: Elsevier Mosby; 2005:2989–3012.
138. Stone JA, et al.: CT evaluation of prosthetic ossicular reconstruction procedures: what the otologist needs to know. Radiographics 2000;20(3):593–605.
139. Syms AJ and Petermann GW: Magnetic resonance imaging of stapes prostheses. Am J Otol 2000;21(4):494–498.
140. White DW: A method to intraoperatively assess stapes prostheses for magnetic attraction. Laryngoscope 2003;113(12):2067–2068.
141. Martin AD, et al.: Safety evaluation of titanium middle ear prostheses at 3.0 tesla. Otolaryngol Head Neck Surg 2005;132(4):537–542.
142. Wild DC, Head K, and Hall DA: Safe magnetic resonance scanning of patients with metallic middle ear implants. Clin Otolaryngol 2006;31(6):508–510.
143. Williams MD, et al.: Middle ear prosthesis displacement in high-strength magnetic fields. Otol Neurotol 2001;22(2):158–161.
144. Grandis JR, Curtin HD, and Yu VL: Necrotizing (malignant) external otitis: prospective comparison of CT and MR imaging in diagnosis and follow-up. Radiology 1995;196(2):499–504.
145. Linstrom CJ and Lucente FE: Infections of the external ear, in head & neck surgery—otolaryngology. In: Bailey BJ, Johnson JT, and Newlands SD, eds. Philadelphia, PA: Lippincott Williams & Wilkins; 2006:1987–2001.
146. Rubin Grandis J, Branstetter BFT, and Yu VL: The changing face of malignant (necrotising) external otitis: clinical, radiological, and anatomic correlations. Lancet Infect Dis 2004;4(1):34–39.
147. Levin WJ, et al.: Bone scanning in severe external otitis. Laryngoscope 1986;96(11):1193–1195.
148. Karantanas AH, et al.: CT and MRI in malignant external otitis: a report of four cases. Comput Med Imaging Graph 2003;27(1):27–34.
149. Stokkel MP, Boot CN, and van Eck-Smit BL: SPECT gallium scintigraphy in malignant external otitis: initial staging and follow-up. Case reports. Laryngoscope 1996;106(3 Pt 1):338–340.
150. Isaacson B, et al.: Labyrinthitis ossificans: how accurate is MRI in predicting cochlear obstruction? Otolaryngol Head Neck Surg 2009;140(5):692–696.
151. Lemmerling M, et al.: CT and MRI of the semicircular canals in the normal and diseased temporal bone. Eur Radiol 2001;11(7):1210–1219.
152. Lemmerling MM, et al.: Imaging of inflammatory and infectious diseases in the temporal bone. Neuroimaging Clin N Am 2009;19(3):321–337.
153. DeSautel MG and Brodie HA: Effects of depletion of complement in the development of labyrinthitis ossificans. Laryngoscope 1999;109(10):1674–1678.
154. Rodriguez D and Young Poussaint T: Neuroimaging findings in neurofi-bromatosis type 1 and 2. Neuroimaging Clin N Am 2004;14(2):149–170.
155. Grant G, Mayber MR: Vestibular schwannomas, in neuro-oncology: the essentials. In: Bernstein M, et al., eds. New York: Thieme Medical Publishers; 2000:508.
156. Ellison D: Neuropathology: a reference text of CNS pathology. London;Chicago: Mosby; 1998:1 v. (various paging).
157. Yoshimoto Y: Systematic review of the natural history of vestibular schwannoma. J Neurosurg 2005;103(1):59–63.
158. Rutherford SA and King AT: Vestibular schwannoma management: what is the 'best' option? Br J Neurosurg 2005;19(4):309–316.
159. Kondziolka D, Lunsford LD, and Flickinger JC: Comparison of management options for patients with acoustic neuromas. Neurosurg Focus 2003;14(5):e1.
160. Driscoll C: Vestibular schwannoma in tumors of the ear and temporal bone. In: Jackler RK, and Driscoll CLW, eds. Philadelphia, PA: Lippincott Williams & Wilkins; 2000:494.
161. Irving R: Meningiomas of the internal auditory canal and cerebellopontine angle, in tumors of the ear and temporal bone. In: Jackler RK and Driscoll CLW, eds. Philadelphia, PA: Lippincott Williams & Wilkins; 2000:494.
162. Kleihues P and Cavenee WK: World Health Organisation classification of tumours: pathology and genetics of tumours of the nervous system. Lyon: IARC Press; 2000.
163. Jackler RK and Driscoll CLW: Tumors of the ear and temporal bone. Philadelphia, PA: Lippincott Williams & Wilkins; 2000:494.

164. Som PM and Curtin HD: Head and neck imaging. 3rd ed. St. Louis: Mosby; 1996:2 v. (xii, 1549, I-59 p.), [16] p. of plates.
165. Whittle IR, et al.: Meningiomas. Lancet 2004;363(9420):1535–1543.
166. Black P: Meningiomas in neuro-oncology: the essentials. In: Bernstein M and Berger MS, eds. New York: Thieme; 2008:477.
167. Goldsher D, et al.: Dural "tail" associated with meningiomas on Gd-DTPA-enhanced MR images: characteristics, differential diagnostic value, and possible implications for treatment. Radiology 1990;176(2): 447–450.
168. Kalkanis SN, et al.: Correlation of vascular endothelial growth factor messenger RNA expression with peritumoral vasogenic cerebral edema in meningiomas. J Neurosurg 1996;85(6):1095–1101.
169. Davidson HC: Imaging of the temporal bone. Magn Reson Imaging Clin N Am 2002;10(4):573–613.
170. Nakamura M, et al.: Meningiomas of the internal auditory canal. Neurosurgery 2004;55(1):119–127.
171. Bacciu A, et al.: Intracanalicular meningioma: clinical features, radiologic findings, and surgical management. Otol Neurotol 2007;28(3): 391–399.
172. Asaoka K, et al.: Intracanalicular meningioma mimicking vestibular schwannoma. Am J Neuroradiol 2002;23(9):1493–1496.
173. Goldsmith B and McDermott MW: Meningioma. Neurosurg Clin N Am 2006;17(2):111–120.
174. Zachenhofer I, et al.: Gamma-knife radiosurgery for cranial base meningiomas: experience of tumor control, clinical course, and morbidity in a follow-up of more than 8 years. Neurosurgery 2006;58(1):28–36.
175. Smirniotopoulos JG, Yue NC, and Rushing EJ: Cerebellopontine angle masses: radiologic-pathologic correlation. Radiographics 1993;13(5): 1131–1147.
176. Ikushima I, et al.: MR of epidermoids with a variety of pulse sequences. Am J Neuroradiol 1997;18(7):1359–1363.
177. Eisenman D, Voigt E, and Selesnick S: Unusual tumors of the internal auditory canal and the cerebellopontine angle, in tumors of the ear and temporal bone. In: Jackler RK and Driscoll CLW, eds. Philadelphia, PA: Lippincott Williams & Wilkins; 2000:236–275.
178. Truwit CL and Barkovich AJ: Pathogenesis of intracranial lipoma: an MR study in 42 patients. Am J Roentgenol 1990;155(4):855–864.
179. Brodsky JR, et al.: Lipoma of the cerebellopontine angle. Am J Otolaryngol 2006;27(4):271–274.
180. Cohen TI, Powers SK, and Williams DW, 3rd: MR appearance of intracanalicular eighth nerve lipoma. Am J Neuroradiol 1992;13(4): 1188–1190.
181. Dahlen RT, et al.: CT and MR imaging characteristics of intravestibular lipoma. Am J Neuroradiol 2002;23(8):1413–1417.
182. Tankere F, et al.: Cerebellopontine angle lipomas: report of four cases and review of the literature. Neurosurgery 2002;50(3):626–631.
183. Pradilla G and Jallo G: Arachnoid cysts: case series and review of the literature. Neurosurg Focus 2007;22(2):E7.
184. Jallo GI, et al.: Arachnoid cysts of the cerebellopontine angle: diagnosis and surgery. Neurosurgery 1997;40(1):31–37.
185. Becker T, et al.: Do arachnoid cysts grow? A retrospective CT volumetric study. Neuroradiology 1991;33(4):341–345.
186. Romo LV, Casselman J, and Robson CD: Temporal bone: congenital anomalies, in head and neck imaging. In: Som PM, and Curtin HD, eds. St. Louis: Mosby; 2003:1109–1172.
187. Myssiorek D: Head and neck paragangliomas: an overview. Otolaryngol Clin North Am 2001;34(5):829–836.
188. Kahn LB: Vagal body tumor (nonchromaffin paraganglioma, chemodectoma, and carotid body-like tumor) with cervical node metastasis and familial association: ultrastructural study and review. Cancer 1976;38(6): 2367–2377.
189. Manolidis S, et al.: Malignant glomus tumors. Laryngoscope 1999;109(1): 30–34.
190. Hiraide F, Inouye T, and Miyakogawa N: Experimental cholesterol granuloma. Histopathological and histochemical studies. J Laryngol Otol 1982;96(6):491–501.
191. Jackler RK and Cho M: A new theory to explain the genesis of petrous apex cholesterol granuloma. Otol Neurotol 2003;24(1):96–106.
192. Pfister MH, Jackler RK, and Kunda L: Aggressiveness in cholesterol granuloma of the temporal bone may be determined by the vigor of its blood source. Otol Neurotol 2007;28(2):232–235.
193. Brodkey JA, et al.: Cholesterol granulomas of the petrous apex: combined neurosurgical and otological management. J Neurosurg 1996;85(4): 625–633.
194. Eisenberg MB, Haddad G, and Al-Mefty O: Petrous apex cholesterol granulomas: evolution and management. J Neurosurg 1997;86(5):822–829.
195. Colli BO and Al-Mefty O: Chordomas of the skull base: follow-up review and prognostic factors. Neurosurg Focus 2001;10(3):E1.
196. Forsyth PA, et al.: Intracranial chordomas: a clinicopathological and prognostic study of 51 cases. J Neurosurg 1993;78(5):741–747.
197. Pickett BP and Kelly JP: Neoplasms of the ear and lateral skull base, in head & neck surgery–otolaryngology. In: Bailey BJ, Johnson JT, and Newlands SD, eds. Philadelphia, PA: Lippincott Williams & Wilkins; 2006:1961–1985.
198. Wenig BM: Atlas of head and neck pathology. 2nd ed. Philadelphia, PA: Saunders Elsevier; 2008:1139.
199. McDermott AL, et al.: Maffucci's syndrome: clinical and radiological features of a rare condition. J Laryngol Otol 2001;115(10):845–847.
200. Perry BE, McQueen DA, and Lin JJ: Synovial chondromatosis with malignant degeneration to chondrosarcoma. Report of a case. J Bone Joint Surg Am 1988;70(8):1259–1261.
201. Meyers SP, et al.: Chondrosarcomas of the skull base: MR imaging features. Radiology 1992;184(1):103–108.
202. Brackmann DE and Teufert KB: Chondrosarcoma of the skull base: long-term follow-up. Otol Neurotol 2006;27(7):981–991.
203. Tzortzidis F, et al.: Patient outcome at long-term follow-up after aggressive microsurgical resection of cranial base chondrosarcomas. Neurosurgery 2006;58(6):1090–1098.
204. Liu JK, et al.: Aneurysms of the petrous internal carotid artery: anatomy, origins, and treatment. Neurosurg Focus 2004;17(5):E13.
205. Moonis G, et al.: Otologic manifestations of petrous carotid aneurysms. Am J Neuroradiol 2005;26(6):1324–1327.
206. Depauw P, et al.: Endovascular treatment of a giant petrous internal carotid artery aneurysm. Case report and review of the literature. Minim Invasive Neurosurg 2003;46(4):250–253.
207. Branstetter BFT and Weissman JL: The radiologic evaluation of tinnitus. Eur Radiol 2006;16(12):2792–2802.
208. Koesling S, Kunkel P, and Schul T: Vascular anomalies, sutures and small canals of the temporal bone on axial CT. Eur J Radiol 2005;54(3): 335–343.
209. Silbergleit R, et al.: The persistent stapedial artery. Am J Neuroradiol 2000;21(3):572–577.
210. Mukherji SK, et al.: Papillary endolymphatic sac tumors: CT, MR imaging, and angiographic findings in 20 patients. Radiology 1997;202(3): 801–808.
211. Manski TJ, et al.: Endolymphatic sac tumors. A source of morbid hearing loss in von Hippel-Lindau disease. JAMA 1997;277(18):1461–1466.
212. Stanley J and Pickett B: Endolymphatic sac tumors, in tumors of the ear and temporal bone. In: Jackler RK and Driscoll CLW, eds. Philadelphia, PA: Lippincott Williams & Wilkins; 2000:494.
213. Patel NP, Wiggins RH, 3rd, and Shelton C: The radiologic diagnosis of endolymphatic sac tumors. Laryngoscope 2006;116(1):40–46.
214. Neff BA, Willcox TO Jr, and Sataloff RT: Intralabyrinthine schwannomas. Otol Neurotol 2003;24(2):299–307.
215. Green JD, Jr. and McKenzie JD: Diagnosis and management of intralabyrinthine schwannomas. Laryngoscope 1999;109(10):1626–1631.
216. Montague ML, et al.: MR findings in intralabyrinthine schwannomas. Clin Radiol 2002;57(5):355–358.
217. Green JD, Jr.: Intralabyrinthine schwannoma, in tumors of the ear and temporal bone. In: Jackler RK and Driscoll CLW, eds. Philadelphia, PA: Lippincott Williams & Wilkins; 2000:494.
218. Kennedy RJ, et al.: Intralabyrinthine schwannomas: diagnosis, management, and a new classification system. Otol Neurotol 2004;25(2):160–167.
219. Phillips CD and Bubash LA: The facial nerve: anatomy and common pathology. Semin Ultrasound CT MR 2002;23(3):202–217.
220. Schaitkin BM: Facial nerve schwannoma, in tumors of the ear and temporal bone. In: Jackler RK, and Driscoll CLW, eds. Philadelphia, PA: Lippincott Williams & Wilkins; 2000:494.
221. Wiggins RH 3rd, et al.: The many faces of facial nerve schwannoma. Am J Neuroradiol 2006;27(3):694–699.
222. Kertesz TR, et al.: Intratemporal facial nerve neuroma: anatomical location and radiological features. Laryngoscope 2001;111(7):1250–1256.

223. Shelton C, et al.: Intratemporal facial nerve hemangiomas. Otolaryngol Head Neck Surg 1991;104(1):116–121.
224. Batsakis JG: Tumors of the head and neck: clinical and pathological considerations. 2nd ed. Baltimore: Williams & Wilkins; 1979:573.
225. Curtin HD, et al.: "Ossifying" hemangiomas of the temporal bone: evaluation with CT. Radiology 1987;164(3):831–835.
226. Lenarz M, et al.: Cavernous hemangioma of the internal auditory canal. Eur Arch Otorhinolaryngol 2007;264(5):569–571.
227. Friedman O, et al.: Temporal bone hemangiomas involving the facial nerve. Otol Neurotol 2002;23(5):760–766.
228. Piccirillo E, et al.: Management of temporal bone hemangiomas. Ann Otol Rhinol Laryngol 2004;113(6):431–437.
229. O'Donoghue G: Tumors of the facial nerve, in neurotology. In: Jackler RK and Brackmann DE, eds. Philadelphia: Elsevier Mosby; 2005:1411.
230. Brackmann DE, Weisskopf PA, and Lo WW: Ossifying hemangioma of the internal auditory canal. Otol Neurotol 2005;26(6):1239–1240.
231. Isaacson B, et al.: Hemangiomas of the geniculate ganglion. Otol Neurotol 2005;26(4):796–802.
232. Pappas DG, et al.: Cavernous hemangiomas of the internal auditory canal. Otolaryngol Head Neck Surg 1989;101(1):27–32.
233. Moffat DA and Wagstaff SA: Squamous cell carcinoma of the temporal bone. Curr Opin Otolaryngol Head Neck Surg 2003;11(2):107–111.
234. Barrs DM: Temporal bone carcinoma. Otolaryngol Clin North Am 2001;34(6):1197–1218.
235. Jin YT, et al.: Prevalence of human papillomavirus in middle ear carcinoma associated with chronic otitis media. Am J Pathol 1997;150(4):1327–1333.
236. Gillespie MB, et al.: Squamous cell carcinoma of the temporal bone: aradiographic-pathologic correlation. Arch Otolaryngol Head Neck Surg 2001;127(7):803–807.
237. Arriaga M, et al.: The role of preoperative CT scans in staging external auditory meatus carcinoma: radiologic-pathologic correlation study. Otolaryngol Head Neck Surg 1991;105(1):6–11.
238. Valvassori GE: Otodystrophies, in modern thin-section tomography. In: Berrett A, Brünner S, Valvassori GE, Berrett A, Brünner S, and Valvassori GE, eds. Springfield: Thomas; 1973:337.
239. Valvassori GE: Otosclerosis. Otolaryngol Clin North Am 1973;6(2):379–389.
240. Goodhill V: Ear diseases, deafness, and dizziness. Hagerstown: MD: Medical Dept. Harper and Row; 1979:781.
241. Lindsay J: Otosclerosis, in otolaryngology. In: Paparella MM, and Shumrick SA, eds. Philadelphia, PA: Saunders; 1980:3020.
242. Ruedi L: Pathogenesis of Otosclerosis. Arch Otolaryngol 1963;78:469–477.
243. Rovsing H: Otosclerosis: fenestral and cochlear. Radiol Clin North Am 1974;12(3):505–515.
244. Bretlau P: Relation of the otosclerotic focus to the fissula ante-fenestram. J Laryngol Otol 1969;83(12):1185–1193.
245. Swartz JD, et al.: Stapes prosthesis: evaluation with CT. Radiology 1986;158(1):179–182.
246. Mafee MF, et al.: Use of CT in stapedial otosclerosis. Radiology 1985;156(3):709–714.
247. Swartz JD, et al.: Fenestral otosclerosis: significance of preoperative CT evaluation. Radiology 1984;151(3):703–707.
248. Gussen R: Early Paget's disease of the labyrinthine capsule. Case report and bone study. Arch Otolaryngol 1970;91(4):341–345.
249. Swartz JD and Harnsberger HR: Imaging of the temporal bone. 3rd ed. New York: Thieme; 1998:497.
250. Swartz JD: The facial nerve canal: CT analysis of the protruding tympanic segment. Radiology 1984;153(2):443–447.
251. Jackler RK and Hwang P: Enlargement of the cochlear aqueduct: factor fiction? Otolaryngol Head Neck Surg 1993;109(1):14–25.
252. Ball JB Jr., Miller GW, and Hepfner ST: Computed tomography of single-channel cochlear implants. Am J Neuroradiol 1986;7(1):41–47.
253. Swartz JD, et al.: Fenestral and cochlear otosclerosis: computed tomographic evaluation. Am J Otol 1985;6(6):476–481.
254. Swartz JD, et al.: Cochlear otosclerosis (otospongiosis): CT analysis with audiometric correlation. Radiology 1985;155(1):147–150.
255. Balkany TJ, Dreisbach JN, and Seibert CE: Radiographic imaging of the cochlear implant candidate: preliminary results. Otolaryngol Head Neck Surg 1986;95(5):592–597.
256. Harnsberger HR, et al.: Cochlear implant candidates: assessment with CT and MR imaging. Radiology 1987;164(1):53–57.
257. O'Donoghue GM, et al.: Cochlear implantation in children: the problem of head growth. Otolaryngol Head Neck Surg 1986;94(1):78–81.
258. Antoli-Candela F, Jr., McGill T, and Peron D: Histopathological observations on the cochlear changes in otosclerosis. Ann Otol Rhinol Laryngol 1977;86(6 Pt 1):813–820.
259. Parahy C and Linthicum FH, Jr.: Otosclerosis: relationship of spiral ligament hyalinization to sensorineural hearing loss. Laryngoscope 1983;93(6):717–720.
260. Swartz JD, et al.: Labyrinthine ossification: etiologies and CT findings. Radiology 1985;157(2):395–398.
261. Valvassori GE: CT densitometry in otosclerosis. Adv Otorhinolaryngol 1987;37:47–49.
262. Valvassori GE and Dobben GD: CT densitometry of the cochlear capsule in otosclerosis. AJNR Am J Neuroradiol 1985;6(5):661–667.
263. Nager GT, Kennedy DW, and Kopstein E: Fibrous dysplasia: a review of the disease and its manifestations in the temporal bone. Ann Otol Rhinol Laryngol Suppl 1982;92:1–52.
264. Lambert PR and Brackmann DE: Fibrous dysplasia of the temporal bone: the use of computerized tomography. Otolaryngol Head Neck Surg 1984;92(4):461–467.
265. Kransdorf MJ, Moser RP, Jr., and Gilkey FW: Fibrous dysplasia. Radiographics 1990;10(3):519–537.
266. Barrionuevo CE, et al.: Fibrous dysplasia and the temporal bone. Arch Otolaryngol 1980;106(5):298–301.
267. Daffner RH, et al.: Computed tomography of fibrous dysplasia. Am J Roentgenol 1982;139(5):943–948.
268. Casselman JW, et al.: MRI in craniofacial fibrous dysplasia. Neuroradiology 1993;35(3):234–237.
269. Herman TE and McAlister WH: Inherited diseases of bone density in children. Radiol Clin North Am 1991;29(1):149–164.
270. Kaftori JK, Kleinhaus U, and Naveh Y: Progressive diaphyseal dysplasia (Camurati-Engelmann): radiographic follow-up and CT findings. Radiology 1987;164(3):777–782.
271. Leeds N and Seaman WB: Fibrous dysplasia of the skull and its differential diagnosis. A clinical and roentgenographic study of 46 cases. Radiology 1962;78:570–582.
272. Harrison TR and Isselbacher KJ: Harrison's principles of internal medicine. New York: McGraw-Hill; 1994:xxxii, 2496, 154.
273. Jardin C, Ghenassia M, and Vignaud J: Tomographic and CT features of the petrous bone in Lobstein's disease. One case and a review of the literature. J Neuroradiol 1985;12(4):317–326.
274. Tabor EK, et al.: Osteogenesis imperfecta tarda: appearance of the temporal bones at CT. Radiology 1990;175(1):181–183.
275. d'Archambeau O, et al.: CT diagnosis and differential diagnosis of otodystrophic lesions of the temporal bone. Eur J Radiol 1990;11(1):22–30.
276. Schuknecht HF: Pathology of the Ear. 2nd ed. Philadelphia, PA: Lea & Febiger; 1993:672.
277. Hawke M, Jahn AF, and Bailey D: Osteopetrosis of the temporal bone. Arch Otolaryngol 1981;107(5):278–282.
278. Greenspan A: Sclerosing bone dysplasias–a target-site approach. Skeletal Radiol 1991;20(8):561–583.
279. Bartynski WS, Barnes PD, and Wallman JK: Cranial CT of autosomal recessive osteopetrosis. Am J Neuroradiol 1989;10(3):543–550.
280. Jackson WP, et al.: Metaphyseal dysplasia, epiphyseal dysplasia, diaphyseal dysplasia, and related conditions. I. Familial metaphyseal dysplasia and craniometaphyseal dysplasia; their relation to leontiasis ossea and osteopetrosis; disorders of bone remodeling. AMA Arch Intern Med 1954;94(6):871–885.
281. Andersen PE, Jr. and Bollerslev J: Heterogeneity of autosomal dominant osteopetrosis. Radiology 1987;164(1):223–225.
282. Bollerslev J and Andersen PE, Jr.: Radiological, biochemical and hereditary evidence of two types of autosomal dominant osteopetrosis. Bone 1988;9(1):7–13.
283. Bollerslev J and Mosekilde L: Autosomal dominant osteopetrosis. Clin Orthop Relat Res 1993;(294):45–51.
284. Elster AD, et al.: Cranial imaging in autosomal recessive osteopetrosis. Part II. Skull base and brain. Radiology 1992;183(1):137–144.

285. Whyte MP: Heritable metabolic and dysplastic bone diseases. Endocrinol Metab Clin North Am 1990;19(1):133–173.
286. NavehY, et al.: Progressive diaphyseal dysplasia: genetics and clinical and radiologic manifestations. Pediatrics 1984;74(3):399–405.
287. Odrezin GT and Krasikov N: CT of the temporal bone in a patient with osteopathia striata and cranial sclerosis. Am J Neuroradiol 1993;14(1):72–75.
288. Nager GT: Paget's disease of the temporal bone. Ann Otol Rhinol Laryngol 1975;84(4 Pt 3 Suppl 22):1–32.
289. Kelly JK, et al.: MR imaging of lytic changes in Paget disease of the calvarium. J Comput Assist Tomogr 1989;13(1):27–29.
290. Swartz JD, et al.: High resolution computed tomography: Part 6. Craniofacial Paget's disease and fibrous dysplasia. Head Neck Surg 1985;8(1):40–47.
291. Newton TH, Hasso AN, and Dillon WP: Computed tomography of the head and neck. modern neuroradiology. vol. 3. New York: Raven Press; 1988:451.
292. Ginsberg LE, Elster AD, and Moody DM: MRI of Paget disease with temporal bone involvement presenting with sensorineural hearing loss. J Comput Assist Tomogr 1992;16(2):314–316.
293. Applegate LJ, Applegate GR, and Kemp SS: MR of multiple cranial neuropathies in a patient with camurati-engelmann disease: case report. Am J Neuroradiol 1991;12(3):557–559.
294. Dannenmaier B and Weber B: Observations on the Camurati-Engelmann syndrome. Demonstration of changes of the petrous bone using high-resolution computed tomography. Rofo 1989;151(2):175–178.

Index

Note: Page numbers followed by "f" denote figures; those followed by "t" denote tables.

A

Aberrant internal carotid artery, 502–503
Abscess, 218
Accessory parotid tissue, 261
Achondroplasia, 427, 427f, 428f
Acinic cell carcinoma
   of parotid space, 280, 282–283
Ackerman tumor. *See* Verrucous carcinoma
Acquired immunodeficiency syndrome (AIDS), 68, 263
Acrocephalosyndactyly type 1. *See* Apert syndrome
Acrocephalosyndactyly type II. *See* Crouzon syndrome
Acute bulbar hemorrhages, 81f
Acute disseminated encephalomyelitis (ADEM), 367
   of optic tract, 373f
Acute disseminated encephalomyelopathy, 371t
Acute infectious thyroiditis, 318
Acute labyrinthitis, 492
Acute otitis media (AOM), 481–483, 483f
Acute retroviral syndrome (HIV), 370
Acute sialadenitis. *See* Sialadenitis, acute
Acute sinusitis, 152–153
Acute subperiosteal hematoma, 78
Acute suppurative sialadenitis. *See* Suppurative sialadenitis, acute
Acute viral sialadenitis. *See* Viral sialadenitis, acute
Acyclovir, 370
"Adam's apple", 193
Adenocarcinoma, 178–180, 214–215
Adenoid cystic carcinoma (ACC), 72, 161, 214, 256, 257f
   acinic cell carcinoma, 280, 282–283
   of left lacrimal gland, 73f
   lymphoma, 283
   of parotid space, 280–284
   of submandibular and sublingual spaces, 291
   squamous cell carcinoma, 283–284
Adenoidal hypertrophies, 263
Adenomatous polyposis coli (APC), 170
Adenosquamous carcinoma, 214
Adnexal structures, 17
Agger nasi, 91
Agger nasi cell, 91
Aggressive fibromatosis (AF), 170, 258
   of masticator space, 297–299
Aggressive mandibular fibromatosis, 171f
Aglossia-adactylia syndrome, 117–118
Agnathia, 118–119, 119f
Agnathia-holoprosencephaly, 118
Agnathia-synotia-microstomia syndrome, 118
Allergic fungal sinusitis (AFS), 157, 158f
Alobar holoprosencephaly, 119
Alveolar ridge carcinoma, 250, 252f, 253f
Amblyopia, 13
Ameloblastomas, 172–173
American Joint Committee on Cancer (AJCC)
   nodal anatomic subsites, 314t–315t
American Society of Clinical Oncology (ASCO), 212
Ampulla, 463
Amyloidosis, 159, 217
Anaplastic carcinoma, 322
Andersen-Warburg syndrome. *See* Norrie disease
Aneurysm, 382–383, 384f
   and pseudoaneurysm, of parapharyngeal space, 310
Aneurysmal bone cysts (ABC), 441
Angiofibroma, 165
Anisometropia, 13
Ankyloglossia, 120–121
Anomalous internal carotid artery
   of retropharyngeal space, 306–307
Anophthalmia, 22
Anterior chamber hemorrhage, 79
Anterior ethmoid artery variants, 95–96
Anterior midbrain lesion. *See* Weber syndrome
Anterior sclera, 69
Anterior spread, of NPC, 234
Anterior staphylomas, 59
Anterior tonsillar pillar carcinoma, 238
Anterior tympanic artery, 460
Antrochoanal polyp, 154f
Apert syndrome, 122, 122f
Aplasia, 43
Apparent diffusion coefficient (ADC), 8
Arachnoid cyst
   and vestibular schwannoma, 401f
Arachnoid cyst, 49, 498
Arhinia, 112
Arm, dermatomes of, 332f
Arteriovenous malformation (AVM), 446, 447
Arteriovenous malformations (AVM), 350–353, 352f
Arytenoid swellings, 193,
Aspergillosis, 31158–159
Atlanto-occipital assimilation, 423–424, 423f
Atlanto-occipital joint axis angle, 421f
Atlantoaxial subluxation, 431
Atrophia bulborum hereditaria Fetal Iritis Syndrome. *See* Norrie disease
AV fistula, of maxillary artery, 352f
Axillary artery, 328f

B

Bacterial sialadenitis, chronic, 274
Bacteroides, 274, 299
Basal cell carcinoma (BCCa), 508
Basal cephaloceles, 97f, 99, 101
Basaloid cell carcinoma, 214
Basaloid squamous cell carcinoma, 252–254
Basilar artery, 360t
Basilar invagination, 422–424, 423f, 423t, 424f
Basiocciput hypoplasia, 423
Basion, 421
Beckwith-Wiedemann syndrome, 120
Bell's palsy, 370, 393–395, 397
   differential diagnosis of, 398t
Benedikt syndrome, 382t
Benign fibro-osseous lesion, 167–168
Benign fibrous histiocytoma, 170
Benign intracranial hypertension, 44
Benign lesions, 163–165
   of thyroid gland, 319–320
Benign masseteric hypertrophy, 263–264
Benign mixed tumor, 291. *See also* Pleomorphic adenomas
Benign neoplasms, 216–217, 257–259, 437–443, 438f, 439f, 440f, 443f
   aggressive fibromatosis, 258
   exostoses, 259
   lipomas, 259
   pleomorphic adenomas, 258
Benign thyroid cysts, 319–320
Benign tumors
   of submandibular and sublingual spaces, 290–291

537

Benign tumors
    of carotid space, 302–303
    of masticator space, 294–295
    of parapharyngeal space, 311–312
    of parotid space, 276–280
    of retropharyngeal space, 308
Bifid mandibular condyle, 121
Bifid nose, 109
Bilateral Bell's palsy, 397f
Bilateral cleft nose, 108
Bilateral CN VII palsy
    causes of, 395t
Bilateral nodal metastasis
    hypopharynx squamous cell carcinoma with, 246f
Bilateral staphylomas
    in elderly female, 61f
    in young adult, 61f
Bilateral tumors, 66
Binocular diplopia, 13
Bleomycin, 347
Blow down fracture, 76f
Blow-in fractures, 76
Blow-out fractures, 76, 149
Bone erosion, 486
Bony labyrinth, 460–461, 469
Bony lesions, of brachial plexus, 332
Bony orbit and fibrous septae, 18–19, 18f
Borrelia burgdorferi, 367
Bound protons, 4
Bourneville diseas, 65
Brachial plexus, 327, 329t
    anatomy, 327–328
    arteries of, 328t
    axillary segment of, 328f
    C7 Ramus, schwannoma of, 334f
    cervical rib, 334f
    clinical application, 330–335
    imaging, 328–330
    MR Protocols for plexopathies, 329t
    neck metastasis, melanoma with, 333f
    neurofibroma, 333f
    schematic, 327f
    schwannoma, of superior trunk, 334f
Brain abscess, 485
Brain herniation, 520–521
Brain herniation post-trauma, 75f
Branchial apparatus, 267–268
Branchial arches, derivatives of, 268f
Branchio oto-renal syndrome, 126
Branchio-oculo-facial (BOF) syndrome, 126
Branchio-oto-renal (BOR) syndrome, 125–126
Buccal space spindle cell liposarcoma, 259f
Buccomasseteric region, 230
Buccopharyngeal fascia, 227
Bulbar fascia, 19
Bulla frontalis, 94
Buphthalmos, 24
Burkitt lymphoma, 255
Burkitt lymphoma, of carotid space, 305f

C

Calcified nodal metastasis
    thyroid papillary carcinoma with, 321f
Calcifying epithelial odontogenic tumor, 173
Calcium phosphate, 15
Calcium pyrophosphate dihydrate deposition (CPPD), 433
Campylobacter jejuni, 365
Camurati Engelmann disease, 518
Capillary hemangiomas, 347
Capillary malformations, 347, 348f
Caroticotympanic nerves, 460
Carotid artery dissection and pseudoaneurysm
    of carotid space, 299–300
Carotid cavernous fistula, 43
Carotid paragangliomas
    of carotid space, 302
Carotid space (CS), 299
    anatomy of, 299
    benign tumors of, 302–303
    malignant tumors of, 303–306
    vascular lesions of, 299–301
Cartilaginous nasal capsule, 87
Cavernomas. *See* Cavernous malformation
Cavernous angiomas. *See* Cavernous malformation
Cavernous carotid aneurysm, with CN VI palsy, 384f
Cavernous hemangiomas, 58, 59f. *See also* Cavernous malformation
Cavernous internal carotid artery
    multilobular aneurysm involving, 384f
Cavernous malformation, 364–365
Cavernous sinus syndrome, 381f, 382t
Cellulites, 26–29, 27t, 28f, 30f
    and abscess
    of masticator space, 294
    of submandibular and sublingual spaces, 287–288
    of retropharyngeal space, 307
Cementing ossifying fibroma, 169f
Central and peripheral CN VII palsy, 396f
Cephaloceles, 26, 96–99, 98t, 99f, 106t
Cerebellopontine angle
    melanoma metastasis to, 404f
Cerebellopontine angle (CPA), 365, 387f, 494–498, 494f, 495f
    epidermoid cyst of, 401–403
    meningioma at, 401
    metastases to, 403–404
Cerebellopontine angle meningioma, 403f
Cerebellopontine angle nerves, 358, 359t, 390–404
Cerebrospinal fluid (CSF), 76, 135, 473, 474
Cervical fascia
    layers of, 271
Cervical rib, 334f
Cervical subluxations, 431
Cervicofacial AVMs, 350
Cervicomedullary arteriovenous malformation, 446

Chamberlain line, 420f, 421
Charcot-Marie-Tooth disease, 365
CHARGE syndrome, 23, 377
Cheek neurofibroma, 360f
Chemical shift, 8
Chemically selective saturation, 4–5
Chiari I and II malformations, 425–427, 426f
Choanal atresia, 109
Choanal stenosis, 112
"Chocolate" cysts, 485
Cholesteatoma, 465
Cholesterol granuloma (CG), 7879, 485, 500
Chondromas, 216
Chondrosarcoma, 182, 214, 297, 444, 445, 502
    of petrous apex, 386f
Chordal eminence, 458
Chordomas, 256, 500–502
Choroidal detachment, 79, 80
Choroidal hemangioma, 63
Choroidal nevus, 64
Choroidal osteoma, 63–64, 63f, 64f
Chronic atlantoaxial subluxation, 449
Chronic bacterial sialadenitis. *See* Bacterial sialadenitis, chronic
Chronic hematic cysts, 78
Chronic inflammatory demyelinating polyradiculopathy, 365
Chronic low-grade compression, 430
Chronic otitis media, 482
Chronic otomastoiditis, 485–486, 487f, 488f, 489f
Chronic sclerosing sialadenitis (CSS), 290
Chronic sialadenitis. *See* Sialadenitis, chronic
Chronic sinusitis, 153
Chronic subperiosteal hematoma, 78
Chronically inspissated secretions, 156
Ciliary staphylomas, 59
Classic Mondini's malformation, 471
Clivus invasion, 442
Clivus meningioma, 438
Cluster headache, 392–393
CMV retinitis, 68
Coats' disease
    imaging of, 62
Coats' disease, 62
Cobb syndrome, 347
Cochlear aplasia, 470
Cochlear branch, of CN VIII, 390
Cochlear hypoplasia, 471
Cochlear nerve aplasia, 471
Coherent (unspoiled) gradient echo, 7–8
Collet-Sicard syndrome, 408t
Coloboma, 24, 24f, 25t
Colobomatous cyst, 24–26, 25f, 25t
Colobomatous *versus* congenital cysts
Combined cleft lip, 108
Combined malformations, 353, 353f, 354f
Complete labyrinthine aplasia, 469–470
Completesyndrome, 466
Complex anterior syngnathia, 117
Complex microphthalmos, 23

Complex zygomatico-mandibular syngnathia, 117
Concha bullosa, 94
Condylar foramen, 421
Condylar hypoplasia, 423f
Condyloid canal, 421
Condylus tertius, 425
　with pseudogout, 425f
Condylus tertius, 425, 425f
Congenital anomalies
　of brachial plexus, 330
　of parapharyngeal space, 310
　of parotid space, 272
　of pediatric neck, 323–327
　of submandibular and sublingual spaces, 285–287
Congenital cholesteatomas, 496, 505
Congenital cysts *versus* colobomatous
Congenital lesions, 217
Congenital mandibular hypoplasia, 114
Congenital midline nasofrontal masses, 96
Congenital optic atrophy, 44
Congenital subglottic hemangioma, 217
Congenital tubular nose, 112–113
Contrast-enhanced Fourier acquired steady-state technique (CE-FAST)
Contrast-enhanced MRA, 9
Conventional spin echo (CSE). *See* Spin echo (SE)
Corniculate cartilages, 194
Cranial nerves, 20, 21t, 356
　cerebellopontine angle nerves (CN V, VII, and VIII), 385–404
　embryology, 356–357
　　pharyngeal arch abnormalities, 356–357
　　pharyngeal arches, 356, 357t
　　pharyngeal grooves, 356
　　pharyngeal membranes, 356
　　pharyngeal pouches, 356, 357t
　extraocular muscle nerves (CN III, IV, and VI), 378–385
　function and pathology, 357, 365t
　　anatomy of, 358f
　　cranial nerve pathologies, 358–372
　　overview of, 359t
　　vascularization, of cranial nerves, 357
　hypoglossal nerve (CN XII), 414–415
　jugular foramen nerves (CN IX, X and XI), 404–414
　olfactory nerve (CN I), 372–377
　optic nerve (CN II), 377–378
Cranial neuritis, 365, 365t, 371t
Craniocervical junction (CCJ), 419
　anatomy, 419–421, 419f, 420f, 421f
　clinical findings, 421–422
　congenital and developmental lesions, 422
　　achondroplasia, 427, 427f, 428f
　　basilar invagination, 422–424, 423f, 423t, 424f
　　chiari I and II malformations, 425–427, 426f
　　condylus tertius, 425, 425f

Down's syndrome, 427
　fibrous dysplasia, 430
　Klippel-Feil syndrome, 427–428, 429f
　mucopolysaccharidosis type II, 428, 430
　mucopolysaccharidosis type IV, 430
　Os odontoideum, 424–425, 425f
　platybasia, 422
degenerative lesions
　fibrous pseudotumor, 449–451
embryology, 421, 422f
inflammatory/infectious lesions, 431
　gout, 433–434
　multicentric reticulohistiocytosis, 434, 435f
　nonpyogenic infections, 436, 438f
　pseudogout, 433, 434f
　psoriatic arthritis, 431, 433f
　pyogenic infections, 434, 436, 436f, 437
　rheumatoid arthritis (RA), 431, 432f
neoplastic lesions, 437
　benign neoplasms, 437–443, 438f, 439f, 440f, 443f
　malignant neoplasms, 443–446
traumatic lesions, 448–449, 449f, 450f
vascular lesions, 446–447, 446f, 447f
Craniocervical junction, 430
Craniofacial chondrosarcomas, 444
Craniofacial osteosarcoma, 186, 445
Craniosynostosis, 123
Cricoid cartilage fractures, 193, 218
Cricovocal membrane, 194
Crouzon syndrome, 122–123, 124f
　with cloverleaf skull, 124f
　without cloverleaf skull, 125f
Crumple zone buttress system, 136, 137, 139t
Cryptophthalmos, 22
CT Protocol
　of nasopharynx, 232t
　of oropharynx, 232t
　of tongue, 232t
Cutaneous capillary malformations, 353
Cutaneous neurofibromas, 166
Cystic hygromas. *See* Lymphatic malformation
Cysticercosis, 27
Cytomegalovirus (CMV) retinitis, 68, 365
Cytomegalovirus, 371t

D

Dacryocystitis, 71
Dacryocystocele, 113–114
Dacryocystography, 69, 70f
Dacryostenosis, 114
De Morsier syndrome, 44
De Quervain's thyroiditis. *See* Granulomatous subacute thyroiditis (GST)
Deep auricular artery, 460
Deep cervical fascia (DCF), 269
Dejerine-Sottas disease, 365
Denervation muscle atrophy, 263

Dentigerous cyst, 170, 172f
Dermoid, 40f, 102–104, 106t
　of submandibular and sublingual spaces, 290–291
Dermoid cysts, 261
Desmoid tumor, 298f. *See also* Aggressive fibromatosis (AF)
Developmental lesions, 259–261
　accessory parotid tissue, 261
　dermoid cysts, 261
　digastric muscle anomalies, 261
　extracranial craniopharyngioma, 260
　lingual thyroid, 261
　nasopharyngeal teratoma, 260–261
　thyroglossal duct cysts, 261
　Tornwaldt's cyst, 259–260
Diabetes insipidus, 32
Diffuse large b-cell lymphoma (DLBCL), 182
Diffusion weighted imaging (DWI), 8, 485, 490
Digastric muscle, 229
Digastric muscle anomalies, 261
DiGeorge anomaly, 356
Diplopia, 13, 78
Direct subarachnoid space, 475
"Dirty CSF", 497
Double vision. *See* Diplopia
Down syndrome, 120, 427
Dural arteriovenous fistula (DAVF), 447
Dural ectasia, 49
Dural sinus occlusive disease, 484
Dural sinus thrombosis, 484, 484f
Dysphonia, 219
Dysplasias, 466, 508
　fibrous dysplasia, 512–514, 513f
Dystrophic calcification, 15, 16t

E

Eardrum, 456
Eccrine tumor metastasis to parotid, 281f
Echinococcus, 27
Echinococcus granulosus, 31
Echo planar imaging (EPI), 1, 8
Echo spacing, 5
Echo train length (ETL), 5
Edwards syndrome. *See* Trisomy 18
Enaural encephalocele, 520–521, 521f
Encapsulated venous malformation, 58
Encephalocele. *See* Cephalocele
Endocrine orbitopathy, 41
Endolymphatic hydrops, 503
Endolymphatic sac tumor (ELST), 503
Endophthalmitis, 67–68
Enophthalmos, 15
Epidermoid, 37–39, 39f, 39t, 40f
Epidermoid cyst, 39f, 40f, 102–104, 106t, 107f
　of CPA, 401–403
　of submandibular and sublingual spaces, 290–291
Epidermoid inclusion cysts, 496
Epidermoids, 494, 496–498

Epidural abscesses, 485
Epiphora, 15
Episcleritis, 69
Episkopi Blindness. *See* Norrie disease
Epithelial tumors, 72
Epitympanic recess, 456
Epstein-Barr virus (EBV), 182, 234, 261, 365
Erdheim Chester disease, 32, 371t
Escherichia coli, 274, 289
Esthesioneuroblastoma, 175–177, 376, 377t
Ethanol, 350
Ethibloc®, 347
Ethmoid bulla, 93
　variations, 93
Ethmoid mucocele, 155f
Ethmoid osteoma, 167
Ethmoid roof, 95
Ethmoid sinus, 26, 89–91
Ethmoid sinus fractures, 147, 155f
Ethmoidal infundibulum, 93
Ethmoidal sulcus, 95
Ethmomaxillary sinus, 95
Ethmoturbinals, 89
Ethyl alcohol, 347
Evisceration, 83
Ewing's sarcoma, 187–188, 445
Exophthalmometer, 15
Exophthalmos, 15
Exorbitism, 15
Exostoses, 167
Exostoses, 259
External auditory canal (EAC), 285f, 454, 455, 464
External auditory canal masses, 508
External carotid artery, 360t
Extraconal varix, 57f
Extracranial craniopharyngioma, 260
Extracranial meningiomas, 166
Extracranial schwannoma
　of CN X, 412f
Extradural neoplasms, 443
Extraocular muscle nerves (CN III, IV, and VI), 358, 359t, 378
　function of, 378–381, 380t
　pathology of, 381–385, 382t
　　aneurysm, 382–383, 384f
　　microvascular disease, 383
　　ophthalmoplegic migraine, 385
　　petrous apex pathology, 385
　　syndromes, 381, 382t
　　Tolosa-Hunt syndrome, 385
　　trauma, 383
Extraocular muscles, 19, 19f
Extraocular orbital hemorrhage, 78
Extrinsic muscles, of tongue, 228
EYA1 gene, 125

F

Facial angiomas, 62–63
Facial fractures
　classification, 139–152, 140t, 141t, 142t, 143f, 144f, 145f, 146f
　crumple zone buttress system, 136, 137, 139t
　diagnosis, 136, 137t, 138t, 139t
　imaging techniques, 136
Facial nerve canal, 465, 466
Facial nerve hemangioma, 507–508
Facial nerve masses, 505–508
Facial nerve schwannoma, 399, 402, 402f, 505–507
Facial recess, 458
Farsightedness, 13
Fascial layers and spaces, 226–227
Fast field echo (FFE), 8
Fast imaging with steady-state precession (FISP), 7–8
Fast low-angle shot (FLASH), 8
Fast spin echo (FSE), 5
Fat-sat technique, 4
Fenestral otosclerosis, 510
Ferumoxtran-10, 3
Fetal alcohol syndrome, 345
FGFR2 gene, 122
FGFR3 gene, 122
Fibroblast growth factor receptor-1 (FGFR1), 375
Fibromatosis, 170
Fibromyxoma, 174
Fibrosarcoma, 183–184, 295–296, 340
Fibrous dysplasia, 167–168, 168f, 430, 512–514, 513f
Fibrous pseudotumor, 449–451
Fibrous thyroiditis. *See* Reidel thyroiditis (RT)
First arch syndrome, 466
First branchial arch dysplasia, 466
First branchial cleft cyst,
　of parotid space, 272, 273f
　of pediatric neck, 323–325
Fistulas, 102–104
"Flat tire" sign, 79
Floor of mouth adenoid cystic carcinoma, 257f
Floor of mouth carcinoma, 248–249, 248f, 249f
Floor of the mouth, 229
Fluid attenuated inversion recovery (FLAIR), 7
Follicular carcinoma, 321
Fonticulus frontalis, 90
Foramen cecum thyroglossal duct cyst, 325f
Foreign bodies and penetrating injury, of retropharyngeal space, 307
Fourier acquired steady-state technique (FAST), 8
Frankfurt Horizontal (FH) plane, 136
Frequency-encoding gradient, 1
Frontal cells, 94
Frontal cephaloceles, 99, 100f
Frontal mucocele, 156
Frontal recess, 94
Frontal sinus, 90, 94
Frontal sinusotomy, 134
Frontonasal cephaloceles, 99, 100f
Frontonasal dysplasia, 109
FSE image, 5
Functional endoscopic sinus surgery (FESS), 93, 131, 133, 134
　complications, 134–135, 135t
　for chronic rhinosinusitis, 132–133
　facial fractures
　　classification, 139–152, 140t, 141t, 142t, 143f, 144f, 145f, 146f, , 147t, 148f, 149f, 150t, 151f, 152f
　　crumple zone buttress system, 136, 137, 139t
　　diagnosis, 136, 137t, 138t, 139t
　　imaging techniques, 136
　indications for, 134, 135t
　infections and inflammation
　　acute sinusitis, 152–153
　　allergic fungal sinusitis (AFS), 157, 158f
　　amyloidosis, 159
　　aspergillosis, 158–159
　　chronic sinusitis, 153
　　chronically inspissated secretions, 156
　　granulomatous lesions, 159
　　mucoceles, 153, 155f–156f
　　nasal cycle, 153
　　noninvasive fungal sinusitis, 156, 157f
　　retention cysts and polyps, 153, 154f
　　rhinocerebral mucormycosis, 157–158
　　sinonasal infections, 159
　postoperative sinus CT, 135–136
　prinvciples, 131, 132t
　sinonasal neoplasms
　　benign lesions, 163–165
　　clinical features, 159–160
　　imaging characteristics, 160–163, 161t, 161t
　　lymphomas, 182
　　malignancies, 174–181
　　neurogenic tumors, 166–167
　　odontogenic cysts and tumors, 170–174
　　odontogenic malignancies, 188
　　osseous malignancies, 185–188
　　osseous tumors, 167–170,
　　sarcomas, 182–185
　types
　　frontal sinusotomy, 134
　　functional endoscopic sinus surgery, for chronic rhinosinusitis, 132–133
　　minimally invasive sinus technique, 133–134
　　sphenoethmoid recess, 134

G

Gadolinium, 349
Gadolinium contrast agents, 2–3, 3t
Gamma knife radiosurgery (GKR), 494–495
Ganglion cysts, 442
Gardner's syndrome, 167
Geniculate ganglion, 402f

Geniohyoid muscle, 229
Giant cell tumor, 185–186, 441
Giant cholesterol cysts, 485
Gingival/buccal mucosa carcinoma, 249, 251f
Glomus jugulare paraganglioma, 410f
Glomus paragangliomas, 408–409
Glomus tumor, 407t
Glomus tympanicum paraganglioma (GTP), 498–500
Glomus vagale tumor
Glossopharyngeal nerve, 460
Glossopharyngeal nerve. See CN IX
Glottic, 214
Glottic carcinoma, 210, 205, 206f, 207
"Glue ear", 482
Glycosarninoglycans (GAG), 41, 428, 430
Goldenhar syndrome, 115, 123
Gout, 433–434
Gradient echo sequences, 7
Gradient moment nulling, 4
Gradient recalled and spin echo (GRASE), 8
Gradient recalled acquisition in the steady state (GRASS), 7
Gradient recalled echo (GRE), 7
Granular cell tumors, 216
Granulation tissue (GT), 485
Granulomatous disease, of parotid space, 275–276
    postirradiation sialadenitis, 276
    sarcoidosis, 275
    Sjogren's syndrome (SS), 275–276
Granulomatous lesions, 159
Granulomatous subacute thyroiditis (GST), 317–318
Graves' disease, 41, 42f, 318
Guillain-Barré syndrome, 371t
    with polyneuritis cranialis, 372f
Guillain-Barré syndrome, 365–366

H

Haemophilus influenzae, 274, 289, 482
Haller cell mucocele, 156f
Haller's cells, 94
Hard palate and retromolar trigone, 230
Hard palate carcinoma, 250
Hard palate mucoepidermoid, 258f
Hashimoto thyroiditis, 316–317
    with lymphoma, 317f
Hashimoto thyroiditis, 41
HASTE (halfacquisition single-shot turbo echo), 5
Heerfordt syndrome, 68
Heerfordt's syndrome, 363
Hemangioma
    of submandibular and sublingual spaces, 285, 287
    differential diagnosis, 341t
    MR imaging of, 340, 342t
    noninvoluting congenital hemangioma, 341f, 342f, 343f, 344f, 345f
    Hemangiomas, 58

Hemangiopericytoma, 442–443
Hematic cyst, 78–79
Hemifacial microsomia, 115–116, 117f, 356
Hemorrhage, 79
Hemorrhagic choroidal detachments, 79
Hemorrhagic venolymphatic malformation, 354f
Hepatitis A, 365
Hepatitis C, 365
"Herald spot", 58
Herpes simplex virus, 370, 371t
Hiatus semilunaris, 93
"Hidden eye", 22
High jugular bulb, 479
High spinal cord compression, 430
Hindbrain hernia, 425
Hodgkin's lymphoma
    of carotid space, 304–306
Hodgkin's lymphoma (HL), 254–255
Hunter's syndrome, 428, 430
Hyaloid artery, 16
Hyaloid artery, 62
Hydatid infections, 31–32
Hyperopia, 13
Hypertelorism, 15
Hyphema, 79
Hypoglossal nerve (CN XII), 358, 359t, 414–415
Hypomandibular craniofacial dysostosis, 118
Hypopharyngeal carcinoma, 241–242, 245f
Hypopharyngeal carcinoma tumor staging, 247t
Hypopharyngeal retrocricoid carcinoma with retrotracheal extension, 247f
Hypopharynx, 230–231
    blood supply, 230–231
    innervation, 231
    lymphatic drainage, 231
Hypoplasia, 472
Hypotelorism, 15
Hyrtl's fissure, 475

I

"Ice cream cone", 459, 494
Idiopathic optic neuropathy, 44
Idiopathic orbital pseudotumor (IOP), 32–36, 33t, 34f, 34t, 35f
IJV thrombosis, 301f
Immune/diopathic demyelinating cranial neuropathies, 371t
Incoherent (spoiled) gradient echo, 8
Incomplete cleft lip, 108
Incudomalleal separation, 520
Infectious cranial neuritis, 371t
Infectious mononucleosis, 261–262
Inferior orbital fissure, 19
Inferior spread, of NPC, 234
Inferior thyroid artery, 269
Inferior thyroid vein, 269
Inferior turbinate, 94–95
Infraorbital ethmoidal cells. See Haller's cells
Inner ear masses, 503–505, 504f, 505f

Interarytenoid muscle, 195
Interferon-alpha-2, 343
Internal auditory canal (IAC), 387f, 463, 471, 474
Internal auditory canal and cerebellopontine angle (IAC-CPA) schwannoma, 399
Internal auditory canal, vascular conflict at, 393f
Internal carotid artery (ICA), 299, 360t, 502
    anomalies, 477–479, 479f
Internal carotid artery pseudoaneurysm, 300f
Intersinus septum, 95
Interstitial neodymium:yttrium-aluminum-garnet laser therapy, 349
Intestinal-type adenocarcinoma (ITAC), 179
Intraconal varix, with thrombosis, 57f
Intracranial chordoma, 443
Intralabyrinthine schwannoma (ILS), 503–505, 504f, 505f
Intranasal gliomas, 101
Intraocular air, 79
Intraocular metallic foreign body, 82f
Intrinsic muscles, of tongue, 228
Invasive nasopharyngeal carcinoma, 237f
Invasive nasopharyngeal carcinoma, 363
Inversion recovery (IR), 7
Inversion time (TI), 7
Inverted papilloma, 163, 164f
Involuting congenital hemangioma, 343f, 344f, 345f
Ischemia, 371t
Isotropic, 8

J

Jackson syndrome, 408t
Jacobson's nerve, 405
Jadassohn disease, 64
Jugular agenesis, 480
Jugular diverticulum, 480
Jugular foramen cranial nerve, 404–414
    developmental abnormalities of, 414
    function, 406t
    glomus paragangliomas, 408–409
    imaging patterns, 407t
    jugular foramen meningioma, 410, 413
    jugular foramen schwannomas, 409–410
    lower cranial nerve syndromes, 407–408
    metastases to, 413–414
    uncommon pathology of, 407t
Jugular foramen meningioma, 410, 413
Jugular foramen nerves (CN IX, X and XI), 358, 359t
Jugular foramen schwannomas, 409–410
Jugular foramen syndrome, 408t
Jugular foramen tumors, 498–500
Jugular vein anomalies, 479–481
Jugular vein thrombosis, 300–301
Jugulotympanic paraganglioma, 302
Juvenile active ossifying fibroma, 168, 170
Juvenile angiofibroma, 165f
Juvenile nasopharyngeal angiofibroma (JNA), 165

K

K space, 2
Kadish staging system, 176
Kallmann syndrome, 374–376, 376f
Kaposi's sarcoma, 215–216
Kasabach-Merritt syndrome, 340
Kerckning's process, 421
Kimura disease, 37, 38f
"Kissing choroids", 80
Klippel-Feil syndrome, 427–428, 429f
Kupffer cells, 3
Kuttner tumor. *See* Chronic sclerosing sialadenitis (CSS)

L

Labyrinthine fistula, 486
Labyrinthitis, 492–493, 493f
Lacrimal apparatus and eyelids, 21
Lacrimal dysfunction, 15
Lacrimal gland, 71–73, 73f
Lacrimal glands, 68
Lacrimal sac abscess, 72
Lactate, 9
Lamina papyracea, 95
Langerhans cell histiocytosis (LCH), 32, 442, 371t
Larmor frequency, 1
Laryngeal trauma, 217
Laryngoceles, 217
Laryngotracheal groove, 193
Larynx, 193
 blood supply, 196
 computed tomography (CT), 198, 199f
 divisions, 197
 embryology and development, 193
 innervation, 196
 laryngeal skeleton, 193–194
 laryngoscopy *versus* CT/MRI, 197–198
 ligaments and membranes, 194, 194f, 194t
 lymphatic drainage, 197
 magnetic resonance imaging (MRI), 198, 201f
 muscles of, 195–196, 196f
 neoplastic invasion of cartilage, 198, 200, 204
 pathology
  benign neoplasms, 216–217
  congenital lesions, 217
  inflammation/infection, 218–219
  malignant neoplasms, 205–216
  postsurgical changes, 221–223
  radiation changes, 219, 221
  trauma, 217–218
  vocal cord paralysis, 219, 220f
 physiology and function
  airway provision and protection, 197
  phonation, 197
  subglottic pressure gradient, 197
 positron emission tomography, 204–205
 spaces and sinuses, 195, 195f, 195t
Lateral spread, of NPC, 234
"Lazy eye", 13

Le Fort, Rene, 139, 140
Leber's disease, 44
Leber's Hereditary Optic Neuropathy (LHON), 44
Legal blindness, 13
Leiomyosarcoma, 215, 215f
Leprosy, 371t
Leukocoria, 66
Linear nevus sebaceous syndrome, 64
Lingual and sublingual thyroid of pediatric neck, 326–327
Lingual septum, 228
Lingual thyroid, 261
Lip, tumor staging, 254t
Lip carcinoma, 248
Lipoid dermato-arthritis, 434
Lipoma, 216, 259, 498
 of parapharyngeal space, 311–312, 312f
 of parotid space, 280
 of retropharyngeal space, 308
 of submandibular and sublingual spaces, 291
Liposarcoma, 42–43, 215, 256–257
 of neck, 312f
Lips and gingivobuccal region, 229–230
Lobar holoprosencephaly, 119
Lofgren's syndrome, 68
Lower cranial nerve syndromes, 407–408
Lower cranial nerve syndromes, 408t
Ludwig's angina, 263. *See also* Cellulitis
Lupus pernio, 68
Luteinizing hormone-releasing hormone (LHRH), 375
Lyme disease, 367, 371t
Lymph nodes, 162, 269
Lymphangiomas, 58–59, 60f. *See also* Lymphatic malformations
Lymphatic drainage, 197, 207
Lymphatic malformations, 344–347, 346f, 353
 differential diagnosis, 346t
 MR imaging of, 347t
 of submandibular and sublingual spaces, 287
Lymphatic spread, 207, 209f
 of NPC, 235–236
 of oropharyngeal and hypopharyngeal carcinoma, 242
Lymphoepithelial cysts, of parotid space, 276
Lymphoma, 41, 182, 254256, 322–323
 hashimoto thyroiditis with, 317f
 of carotid space, 303–304
 of parotid space, 283
 of retropharyngeal space, 309
 of submandibular and sublingual spaces, 292
Lymphoproliferative disease, 37t
Lymphoproliferative disease, 36–37, 36f, 37t

M

Macroglossia, 119–120, 120t, 264
Macrostomia, 108

Magnetic resonance angiography (MRA), 1, 9, 447
Magnetic resonance spectroscopy (MRS), 8
Magnetization transfer (MT) contrast, 4
Malformational mandibular hypoplasia, 114–115
Malignancies, 174–181
Malignant external otitis (MEO), 492
Malignant fibrous histiocytoma (MFH), 184–185, 257
Malignant lesions, of thyroid gland, 320–323
Malignant melanoma, 64, 177
Malignant neoplasms, 205–216, 443–446
Malignant odontogenic tumors, 188
Malignant tumors, of carotid space, 303–306
 of masticator space, 295–299
 of parapharyngeal space, 312
 of parotid space, 280–284
 of retropharyngeal space, 308–309
Mandible lateral view, 149f
Mandibular aplasia, 118
Mandibular deformity, 116
Mandibular hypoplasia, 114–115, 114t
Masticator space (MS), 292
 anatomy of, 293
 benign tumors of, 294–295
 inflammatory lesions of, 294
 malignant tumors of, 295–299
 vasoformative anomalies of, 293–294
Masticator space rhabdomyosarcoma, 296f
Masticator space, venolymphatic malformation of, 353f
Mastoid part, 454
Mastoid process, 454
Mastoidectomy, 490
Mastoiditis, 482
Maxillary ameloblastoma, 173f
Maxillary artery, AV fistula of, 352f
Maxillary sinus, 89, 94
Maxillary sinus hypoplasia (MSH), 94
Maxillary sinusitis, 152
Maxillo-alveolar buttress fractures, 144
Maxillomandibular anomalies, 114–121
Maxillomandibular fusion, 116–118, 118f
Maximum intensity projection (MIP), 9, 473
Meckel's cave, CSF cephalocele in, 391f
Median cleft face syndrome, 109
 in adult, 110f
 in infant, 110f
Medullary carcinoma, 321–322
Melanoma, 177–178
Melanoma metastasis, 404f
Melnick-Fraser syndrome, 125
Membranous choanal atresia, 111f
Membranous labyrinth, 461–462, 469
Meningioma, 166167, 361–362, 365t, 400t, 403f, 401, 407t, 437–438, 438f, 496
Meningogenic labyrinthitis, 492
Meninx primitive, 498
Mesotympanum, 456
Metachromatic leukodystrophy, 371t

Metastasis, 40
  to CPA, 403–404
  to jugular foramen, 407t, 413–414
  to thyroid and neck, 320f
Metastatic calcification, 15, 17t
Metastatic disease, 41, 64, 216, 445
Metastatic neuroblastoma, 58
Metastatic parotid spindle cell tumor, 282f
Metastatic spread, to cranial nerves, 362
Metastatic tumors, 162–163
Michel's deformity, 469
Microform clefts, 108
Microglossia, 120
Micrognathia, 119, 120t
Microphthalmia, 60
Microphthalmos, 22, 23
Microvascular disease, 383
Mid-cranial fossa, 508
Middle ear fistulas, 475
Middle ear masses, 505
Middle thyroid vein, 269
Middle turbinate, 94
Midface, 87, 88
Midface anomalies, 97
Midface clefts, 104, 106
Midface fractures, 145f
Miller Fisher syndrome, 365, 371t
Minimally invasive sinus technique (MIST), 133134
Minor salivary glands, 271
Missed ostium sequence, 133
Mobile protons, 4
Mobius syndrome, 120
Monocrystalline iron oxide nanoparticles (MION), 3
Monocular blindness, 13
Monocular diplopia, 13
Monostotic fibrous dysplasia, 167
Monostotic lesion, 442
"Morning glory" lesion, 25
Morquio's disease, 430
Motion artifact suppression technique (MAST), 4
Motor trigeminal division, of CN V, 386–387
  dysfunction, 389t
  function, 389t
MOTSA (multiple overlapping thin slab acquisition), 9
MR contrast agents, 2
  gadolinium contrast agents, 2–3, 3t
  superparamagnetic iron oxide particles, 3–4
MR imaging
  of brachial plexus, 328–330
  of hemangiomas, 342t
  of lymphatic malformations, 374t
  of neck lymph nodes, 312
  of thyroid gland, 316
MR prepulse sequences
  chemically selective saturation, 4–5
  gradient moment nulling, 4

  magnetization transfer (MT) contrast, 4
  spatially selective saturation, 4
Mucoceles, 153, 155f–156f
  of petrous apex, 487, 490
Mucoceles. See Ranulas
Mucoepidermoid carcinoma, 74f, 214, 256, 280, 291–292
Mucopolysaccharidosis type II, 428, 430
Mucopolysaccharidosis type IV, 430
Mucormycosis, imaging of, 30
Mucous retention cysts, 153
"Mulberry lesions", 66
Multicentric reticulohistiocytosis, 434, 435f
Multicentric reticulohistiocytosis, 435f
Multidetector CT (MDCT), 231
Multiple periapical cysts, 171f
Multiple sclerosis (MS), 366
Multiple sclerosis (MS), 44
Multiple sclerosis, 371t
Musculotubal canal, 457
Mycobacterium pneumoniae, 365
Mycotic infections, 30, 30t
Mycotic orbital infection, 27
Myelomalacia, 449
Mylohyoid muscle, 229
Myopia, 13
Myringoplasty, 490
Myxoma, 174

N

Nanophthalmos, 23
Nasal bone fractures, 146–147
  classification, 147t
Nasal capsule, 88
Nasal cavities, 88, 96
Nasal cerebral heterotopias, 101, 102
Nasal cycle, 153
Nasal dermoid, 107f
Nasal gliomas, 101, 105f, 106t
Nasal septal deviation, 96
Nasal septum, 88
  olfactory nerve and, 374f
Naso-orbital cephaloceles, 99, 102f, 103f
Naso-orbital-ethmoidal fracture, 77f
Nasoethmoidal cephaloceles, 99, 101f
Nasoethmoidal fractures, 144
Nasofrontal region, 90
Nasofrontoethmoidal fractures, 142, 144
Nasolacrimal apparatus, 90
Nasolacrimal duct papilloma, 70
Nasolacrimal duct stenosis, 114
Nasolacrimal mucocele, 70
Nasolacrimal sac and duct, 69–71, 70f, 71f
Nasolacrimal sac mucocele, 70, 71, 113–114
Nasomaxillary buttress fractures, 144
Nasoorbital fractures, 142
Nasopharyngeal carcinoma (NPC), 234, 235f, 236f, 363, 370f
  tumor classification and staging, 236–237, 238t

  tumor origin and spread
    anterior spread, 234
    inferior spread, 234
    lateral spread, 234
    lymphatic spread, 235–236
    posterior spread, 234
    superior spread, 234–235
Nasopharyngeal teratoma, 260–261
Nasopharynx, 225–227, 226f
  blood supply, 226t, 227
  CT Protocol, 232t
  from posterior side, 227f
  fascial layers and spaces, 226–227
  innervation, 226t, 227
  lymphatic drainage, 227
  MRI Protocol, 233t
  pharyngeal tonsil and pharyngeal bursa, 226
  structures, 226t
Nd:YAG laser, 342
Neck
  anatomy of, 269–272
  embryology of, 267–269
Neck lymph nodes, 312
  evaluation of, 315
  imaging of, 313, 315
  staging of, 316
Neodymium:yttrium-aluminum-garnet laser therapy, 349
Neopharynx, 221
Neoplasia
  affecting CN I, 376
Nerve injuries, 78
Nerve syndromes, of extraocular muscles, 381, 382t
Neural crest cell abnormalities, 356
Neuroblastoma, 40
Neuroborreliosis. See Lyme disease
Neurocutaneous syndromes, 50t, 358
Neurofibromatosis 1 (NF-1), 358
Neurofibroma, 51, 53, 340, 166
  brachial plexus, 333f
  imaging, 55t
  of masticator space, 295
  of parapharyngeal space, 311
Neurofibromatoses, 358–361, 362f, 514
  type 1, 48, 53, 166, 399
  type 2, 359, 399
Neurogenic paralysis, of vocal cords, 219
Neurogenic tumors, 166–167
Neuroma, 216
Neuromyelitis optica, 366, 371t
Neurosarcoidosis, 363–364, 373, 375f
Neurovascular injuries, 77–78
Neurovascular structures, 19–20, 20f, 21f, 21t, 22f
"Nevus flammeus", 62–63
Non-Hodgkins lymphoma (NHL), 182, 255
  of carotid space, 304
Noninvasive fungal sinusitis, 156, 157f
Noninvoluting congenital hemangioma, 341f, 342f

Nonpyogenic infections, 436, 438f
Nonsyndromic malformational mandibular hypoplasia, 115
Noonan's syndrome, 345
Norrie disease, 26
Norrie syndrome. See Norrie disease
Norrie-Warburg disease. See Norrie disease
Nuerofibromas, 216

O

Obstructed frontal mucocele, 157f
Occipital cephalocele, 99f
Occipital condyle fractures, 448
Occipital condyle hypoplasia, 423
Ocular hypotony, 80
Ocular injuries, 79–81, 81f
Ocular structures, 20–21
Oculo-auriculovertebral (OAV) complex, 115, 123
Oculomotor muscle nerves. See Extraocular muscle nerves
Odontogenic abscesses, 263, 294
Odontogenic cysts
   dentigerous cyst, 170, 172f
   odontogenic keratocysts, 171, 172
   periapical cysts, 170, 171f
Odontogenic cysts and tumors, 170–174
Odontogenic keratocysts, 171, 172
Odontogenic malignancies, 188
Odontogenic myxoma, 174
Odontogenic submandibular cellulitis, 288f
Odontoid process dysplasia, 424
Ohngren's line, 174
Olfactory groove meningioma, 376f
Olfactory nerve, 357, 359t, 372
   and nasal septum, 374f
   pathology, 373–377
Olfactory neural tissue, 375
Olfactory neuroblastoma. See Esthesioneuroblastoma
Olfactory neurosarcoidosis, 375f
OMENS, 115
OMENS-Plus classification system, 115–116, 116t
Oncocytoma
   of parotid space, 278–279
Onodi cell, 95
Ophthalmic artery, 20
Ophthalmoplegia, 13, 14t, 42
Ophthalmoplegic migraine, 371t, 385
Opisthion, 421
Optic atrophy, 44
Optic disc swelling, 44
Optic drusen, 46f, 47f
Optic hydrops, 49
Optic nerve, 19–20, 20f, 357, 359t, 377
   atrophy of, 44
   characteristic portions of, 21f
   drusen deposits, 44
   enlargement, 43t
   pathology, 377–378
   visual pathway of, 378f

Optic nerve and orbit, 16–17
Optic nerve aplasia and hypoplasia, 43–44
Optic nerve glioma, 48–50, 50f, 51t
   imaging, 51t
Optic nerve sheath cyst, 49
Optic neuritis, 44, 47t, 48, 48f, 49f
   arthropathies associated with, 47t
   differential diagnosis, 47t
   in young woman, 49f
Optic Neuritis Treatment Trial, 44
Optic pits, 15
Optic sheath meningioma, 50, 52f
Optic sheath sarcoid, 52f
Optic tract, ADEM of, 373f
Oral carcinoma, 246–250
   tumor origin and spread
      floor of mouth, 248–249, 248f, 249f
      gingival/buccal mucosa, 249, 251f
      hard palate, 250
      lip, 248
      oral tongue, 249, 250f, 251f
      retromolar trigone, 249–250, 252f
Oral cavity, 228–230, 228f
   buccomasseteric region, 230
   CT Protocol, 232t
   floor of the mouth, 229
   hard palate and retromolar trigone, 230
   lips and gingivobuccal region, 229–230
   MRI Protocol, 233t
   oral tongue, 228–229
   tumor staging, 254t
Oral nerves, 229f
Oral tongue, 228–229
Oral tongue carcinoma, 249, 250f, 251f
Orbit and globe
   anatomy, 17
      bony orbit and fibrous septae, 18–19, 18f
      extraocular muscles, 19, 19f
      lacrimal apparatus and eyelids, 21
      neurovascular structures, 19–20, 20f, 21f, 21t, 22f
      ocular structures, 20–21
   clinical signs and symptoms, 13, 14t
      enophthalmos, 15
      hypertelorism, 15
      hypotelorism, 15
      lacrimal dysfunction, 15
      orbital calcification, 15, 16t, 17t
      proptosis, 13, 14f, 15
   congenital and developmental disorders
      cephalocele, 26
      coloboma, 24, 24f, 25t
      colobomatous cyst, 24–26, 25f, 25t
      disorders of globe, 22–24, 23f, 24f
      Norrie disease, 26
      proteus syndrome, 26
   embryologic development of, 15
      adnexal structures, 17
      optic nerve and orbit, 16–17
      vessels, 15–16, 17f

extraconal lesions, 26
   cellulites, 26–29, 27t, 28f, 30f
   dermoid, 37–39, 39t, 40f
   epidermoid, 37–39, 39f, 39t, 40f
   Erdheim-Chester disease, 32
   hydatid infections, 31–32
   idiopathic orbital pseudotumor (IOP), 32–36, 33t, 34f, 34t, 35f
   Kimura disease, 37, 38f
   Langerhans cell histiocytosis, 32
   lymphoproliferative disease, 36–37, 36f, 37t
   metastasis, 40
   mycotic infections, 30, 30t
   orbital infections, 26, 29t
   teratoma, 37–39, 39t
extraocular muscle lesions, 40, 43t
   carotid cavernous fistula, 43
   endocrine orbitopathy, 41
   Graves' disease, 41, 42f
   liposarcoma, 42–43
   rhabdomyosarcoma, 42–43
   Tolosa-Hunt syndrome, 41–42
intraconal lesions
   optic atrophy, 44
   optic nerve aplasia and hypoplasia, 43–44
   optic nerve gliomas, 48–50, 50f, 51t
   optic neuritis, 44, 47t, 48, 48f, 49f
   perioptic (optic sheath) meningioma, 50–51, 51t, 52f
   peripheral nerve sheath tumors, 51, 53–54, 53f, 54f, 55t
   pseudotumor cerebri, 44, 46f, 47f
   radiation-induced optic neuropathy (RION), 48
   septo-optic dysplasia, 44, 45f
lacrimal gland and nasolacrimal apparatus, 69, 69t
   dacryocystography, 69, 70f
   lacrimal gland, 71–73, 73f
   nasolacrimal sac and duct, 69–71, 70f, 71f
lesions of globe
   choroidal osteoma, 63–64, 63f, 64f
   Coats' disease, 62
   persistent hyperplastic primary vitreous (PHPV), 62, 63f
   retinal angiomatosis, 64–65
   retinal astrocytomas, 65–66
   retinoblastoma, 66–67, 66f, 67f
   retinopathy of prematurity (ROP), 60, 62f
   retinoschisis, 59–60
   staphyloma, 59, 61f
   uveal melanoma, 64, 65f
ocular infections and inflammations, 67
   CMV retinitis, 68
   endophthalmitis, 67–68
   episcleritis, 69
   sarcoidosis, 68
   scleritis, 69
   toxocariasis, 68

surgical materials, 83, 83f
surgical procedures, 83
trauma, 73, 75f
   cholesterol granuloma, 78–79
   foreign body, 81–83
   fractures, 74, 76, 76f, 77f
   hematic cyst, 78–79
   neurovascular injuries, 77–78
   ocular injuries, 79–81, 81f
   soft tissue injury, 74
   subperiosteal hematoma, 78–79
vasoformative anomalies
   cavernous hemangioma, 58, 59f
   lymphangiomas, 58–59, 60f
   proliferating hemangioma, 58
   venous varices, 54–55, 55t, 56f, 57f
Orbital apex syndrome, 26, 382t
Orbital calcification, 15, 16t, 17t
Orbital cellulites, 26, 66
  classification, 27t
Orbital decompression surgery, 41
Orbital emphysema, 76
Orbital hemangioma, 58
Orbital lymphoma, 36f
Orbital plexiform neurofibroma, of oculomotor nerve, 53f
Orbital roof, 18
Orbital trauma, 73
Orbital varix, 54, 55, 56f
Orofacial, 104, 106
Orofacial clefts, 104, 106
Oronasal membrane, 88
Oropharyngeal and hypopharyngeal carcinoma, 237
  tumor origin and spread
    anterior tonsillar pillar, 238
    hypopharyngeal carcinoma, 241–242
    lymphatic spread, 242
    posterior oropharyngeal wall, 241
    posterior tonsillar pillar, 238
    soft palate, 240
    tongue base, 240–241
    tonsillar fossa, 238–240
    treatment based on staging, 243–246
    tumor classification and staging, 242–243
Oropharyngeal abscess, 311f
Oropharyngeal carcinoma tumor staging, 247t
Oropharynx, 227–228
  blood supply, 228
  CT Protocol, 232t
  innervation, 228
  lymphatic drainage, 228
  MRI Protocol, 233t
Os odontoideum, 424–425, 425f
Osseomembranous choanal atresia, 111f
Osseos choanal atreseia, 111f
Osseous malignancies, 185–188
Osseous tumors, 167–170
Ossiculoplasty, 490–491
Ossified cartilage, 207

Ossifying fibroma, 168, 169f, 514
  of maxillary sinus, 169f
Ossifying labyrinthitis, 493f
Osteochondromas, 440
Osteogenesis imperfecta, 514
Osteoid osteoma, 440
Osteomas, 167
Osteomyelitis, 436
  of masticator space, 294
Osteopetrosis, 514–516
Osteoradionecrosis, 294
Osteosarcoma, 182, 186–187, 186f, 445
  of masticator space, 296–297
Ostiomeatal complex (OMC), 96
Ostiomeatal unit/complex, 93
"Otitic hydrocephalus", 484
Otitis media with effusion (OME), 482
Otocephaly, 118–119, 119f
Otocephaly agnathia syndrome, 119f
Otocephaly. See Agnathia
Otocervical syndromes, 477
Otocraniofacial syndromes, 476–477
Otosclerosis, 508–512
Otoskeletal syndromes, 477

P

Paget's disease, 514, 515, 516–518
Palate, 87–88
Papillary carcinoma, 321
Papillary cystadenoma lymphomatosum. See Warthin's tumor
Papilledema, 46f
Papillomas, 163, 216
Paradoxical middle turbinate, 94
Paraganglioma, 217, 408, 498–499
  of carotid space, 302
  classification of, 409t
Paranasal sinuses, 88–89
Parapharyngeal branchial cleft cyst, 310f
Parapharyngeal space, 227, 309
  anatomy of, 309
  aneurysm and pseudoaneurysm of, 310
  benign tumors of, 311–312
  congenital anomalies of, 310
  inflammatory lesions of, 310–311
  malignant tumors of, 312
Parathyroid glands, 268–269, 270
Parenchymal atrophy, 450
Parkes-Weber syndrome, 353
Parotid adenoid cystic carcinoma, 284f
  with perineural and meningeal spread, 283f
Parotid facial nerve schwannoma, 402f
Parotid gland, 270
Parotid lymphangioma, with hemorrhage, 273f
Parotid metastatic melanoma, 280f
Parotid mucoepidermoid with nodal metastasis, 282f
Parotid space, 272
  anatomy of, 272
  benign tumors of, 276–280

  congenital anomalies of, 272
  inflammatory lesions of, 272, 274–276
  lymphoepithelial cysts of, 276
  malignant tumors of, 280–284
Pars flaccida cholesteatomas, 486
Pars tensa cholesteatoma, 486
Partial ossicular reconstructive prosthesis (PORP), 490
Patau syndrome. See Trisomy 13
Pediatric neck
  congenital anomalies of, 323–327
Peptostreptococcus, 274
Percutaneous sclerotherapy, 347
Periapical cysts, 170, 171f
Perilymphatic fistula, 476
Perineural spread, 362–363, 365t
  along CN V and CN VII, 367f
  of cranial nerve V1, 368f, 369f
  of head and neck cancers, 366f
  parotid adenoid cystic carcinoma with, 283f
Perioptic cysts, 51
Perioptic hygroma, 49
Perioptic meningiomas, 50–51, 51t, 52f
  imaging, 51, 51t
Periorbita, 19
Peripheral nerve sheath tumors, 51, 53–54, 53f, 54f, 55t, 358
  neurofibromatoses, 358–361, 362f
  schwannoma, 361
Peripheral primitive neuroectodermal tumors (PNET), 187
Persistent hyperplastic primary vitreous (PHPV), 62, 63f
Petrous apex infections, 486–487, 489f
Petrous apex masses, 500–503, 501f
Petrous apex pathology, 385
  causes of, 385t
Petrous apicitis, 483–484, 486
Petrous bone, 473–474
Petrous part, 454–455
PHACES, 340
Phakomatoses, 50t
Pharyngeal arch abnormalities, 356–357
Pharyngeal arches, 356, 357t
Pharyngeal bursa, 226
Pharyngeal grooves, 356
Pharyngeal membranes, 356
Pharyngeal pouches, 356, 357t
Pharyngeal tonsil, 226
Pharyngobasilar fascia, 226
Pharynx
  anatomy, 225–231
  embryology and development, 225
  imaging, 231–233
  musculature, 230f
  and oral cavity, 225
  pathology, 234–264
  physiology and function, 231
    deglutition, 231
    respiration, 231
Phase contrast, 9

Phase encoding, 1–2
Phleboliths, 55, 349
Phthisis bulbi, 79, 81f
Picibanil (OK-432), 347
Pierre-Robin sequence, 123, 125, 126f
Pindborg tumor, 172–173
Platybasia, 422
Pleomorphic adenoma, 163–165, 258
  of parapharyngeal space, 311
Pleomorphic adenoma. *See* Benign mixed tumors (BMT)
Plexiform neurofibroma, 53, 166, 361f
  in child, 54f
Plummer-Vinson syndrome, 242
Pneumocephalus, 76
Polidocanol, 350
Polyneuritis cranialis, 365, 371t
  Guillain-Barré syndrome with, 372f
Polyostotic fibrous dysplasia, 167
Polyrhinia, 113
Popliteal pterygium syndrome, 117, 118
Port-wine stain, 348f
Positron emission tomography (PET), 233
Postassium titanyl phosphate, 349
Postassium-titanyl-phosphate laser therapy, 349
Postcricoid tumors, 242
Posterior communicating artery (PCA), 382
Posterior condylar canal, 421
Posterior ethmoid sinus, 95
Posterior oropharyngeal wall carcinoma, 241
Posterior sclera, 69
Posterior scleritis, 33
Posterior spread, of NPC, 234
Posterior tonsillar pillar carcinoma, 238
Postirradiation sialadenitis
  of parotid space, 276
Postoperative middle ear and mastoid, 490–491
Postradiation optic tract degeneration, 374f
Postsphenoid, 90
Postsurgical changes, 221–223
Potassium titanyl phosphate laser (KTP), 342–343
Preseptal cellulites, 26, 28f
Presphenoid, 90
Primary cavernous malformations, 365
Primary malignancies, extension of, 299
Primary osteosarcoma, 186
Primary retinal telangiectasia. *See* Coats' disease
Primitive optic stocks, 15
Proboscis lateralis, 112–113
Progressive diaphyseal dysplasia, 518, 519f
Proliferating hemangioma, 58
Proptosis, 13, 14f, 15
Proteus syndrome, 26
Protruding jugular bulb, 479, 480f
Pseudogout, 433, 434f
  of CCJ, 434f
Pseudomonas, 263
Pseudotumor cerebri, 44, 46f, 47f

Psoriatic arthritis, 431, 433f
Pterygopalatine fossa (PPF), 161, 234
Pulsed dye, 349
Pycnodysostosis, 516, 518
Pyogenic empyema, 437f
Pyogenic infections, 434, 436, 436f, 437
Pyogenic osteomyelitis, 434
Pyramidal eminence, 458
Pyriform aperture stenosis, 112, 113f

R

Radiation changes, 219, 221
Radiation-induced neuritis, 371t
Radiation-induced optic neuropathy (RION), 48
Radiation-induced sarcoma (RIS)
  of masticator space, 297
Radiation neuritis, 372
Ramsay Hunt syndrome, 370, 395–396, 398f
  differential diagnosis of, 398t
Ranula, 288–289
Reactive lymphadenopathy, of retropharyngeal space, 307–308, 308f
Receiver coils, 1
Recessus terminalis, 93
Red nucleus lesion. *See* Benedikt syndrome
Refsum's disease, 365
Regional malignancies extension
  of carotid space, 303
  of parapharyngeal space, 312
Relative cerebral blood volume (rCBV), 362
Renal cell carcinoma, 163
Renal dysplasia, 125
Retention cysts and polyps, 153, 154f
Reticuloendothelial system (RES), 3
Retinal angiomatosis, 64–65
Retinal astrocytomas, 65–66
Retinal capillary angioma, 64–65
  fundoscopic examination, 65
Retinal colobomas, 24f
Retinal colobomatous cyst, 25f
Retinal detachment, 79
Retinoblastoma, 66–67, 66f, 67f
Retinopathy of prematurity (ROP), 60, 62f
Retinoschisis, 59–60
  children with, 60
  infants with, 60
Retrolental fibroplasias. *See* Retinopathy of prematurity (ROP)
Retromolar trigone carcinoma, 249–250, 252f
Retropharyngeal infections, 262
Retropharyngeal space (RPS), 227, 271, 306
  anatomy of, 306
  benign tumors of, 308
  foreign bodies and penetrating injury of, 307
  inflammatory lesions of, 307
  malignant tumors of, 308–309
  reactive lymphadenopathy of, 307–308, 308f
  vascular anomalies of, 306–307
  vasoformative anomalies of, 306

Retropharyngeal squamous cell carcinoma, 244f
RF pulse, 1
RF-spoiled Fourier acquired steady-state technique (FAST), 8
Rhabdomyoma, 217
Rhabdomyosarcoma, 42–43, 58, 182–183, 256, 340
  of masticator space, 296
Rheumatoid arthritis (RA), 219, 431, 432f
Rhinocerebral mucormycosis, 30, 157–158
Riedel thyroiditis (RT), 317
Robin sequence, 356

S

Saccule, 195
Salivary glands, 268, 270
Sarcoidosis, 68, 159, 363, 365t, 373–374
  of parotid space, 275
Sarcoma, 182–185
  of masticator space, 295
Scala vestibule, 461
Scheibe's dysplasia, 469
Schmidt's syndrome, 408t
Schwannoma, 51, 53, 166, 216, 361, 363t, 365t, 399–401, 407t, 438–443, 439f, 440f, 443f, 494
  of C7 Ramus, of brachial plexus, 334f
  of carotid space, 303
  of CN V2, 403f
  of CN V3 and X, 364f
  of CN IX, 413f
  of CN X, 411f
  imaging, 55t
  of masticator space, 294–295
  of parotid space, 279–280
  of parapharyngeal space, 311
  of superior trunk, of brachial plexus, 334f
  treatment of, 54
  vagus nerve, 439f
  of Xth nerve, 304f
Scleritis, 69
Sclerosteosis, 514, 518
Sclerotherapy, 349
Second branchial arch dysplasias, 466
Second branchial cleft cyst, 286f, 287
  of parapharyngeal space, 310
  of pediatric neck, 325
  of submandibular and sublingual spaces, 285
Second branchial cleft fistula, remnant of, 324f
Secondary anophthalmia, 22
Secondary osteosarcoma, 186
Section (slice) selection, 1
Section-select gradient, 1
Semilobar holoprosencephaly, 119
Sensorineural hearing loss (SNHL), 466, 467t–468t, 511
Sensory ganglia, 356

Sensory trigeminal division, of CN V, 385
  dysfunction, 389t
  function, 389t
Septo-optic dysplasia, 44, 45f
  with pachygyria, 45f
Serous choroidal detachments, 79–80
Short inversion time inversion recovery (STIR), 7
Simple and multinodular goiter, 318–319
Simple anterior syngnathia, 117
Simple microphthalmos, 23
Simple zygomatico-mandibular syngnathia, 117
Simultaneous acquisition of spatial harmonics (SMASH), 1
Simultaneous detection of spatial harmonics (SENSE), 1
Sincipital cephaloceles, 97f, 99
Single photon emission computed tomography (SPECT), 40
Single-shot FSE (SS-FSE), 5
Sinonasal anomalies, 109–121
Sinonasal infections, 159
Sinonasal lymphomas, 182
Sinonasal mucosal malignant melanomas, 177, 178
Sinonasal polyposis, 154f, 373
Sinonasal schwannomas, 166
Sinonasal undifferentiated carcinoma (SNUC), 180–181
Sinus lateralis, 93
Sinus tympani, 458
Sjogren's syndrome (SS)
  of parotid space, 275–276, 275f
Skull base chondrosarcomas, 445
Sluder's neuralgia. See Sphenopalatine neuralgia
Sodium tetradecyl sulfate. See Sotradecol
Soft palate carcinoma, 240, 241f
Soft palate pleomorphic adenoma, 260f
Soft tissue injury, 74
Solitary neurofibromas, 53
  treatment of, 54
Sotradecol, 350
Spaces, of neck, 271–272
Spasmus mutans, 49
Spatially selective saturation, 4
Sphenoethmoid recess, 134
Sphenoethmoidal cell, 95. See also Onodi cell
Sphenoethmoidal cephaloceles, 99, 101, 103f
Sphenoethmoidal recess, 95
Sphenoid mucocele, 155f, 395f
Sphenoid sinus, 90, 95
Spheno-orbital cephaloceles, 101
Sphenomaxillary cephaloceles, 101
Sphenopalatine ganglion, 395f
Sphenopalatine neuralgia, 392–393
Sphenotemporal buttress fractures, 146
Spin echo (SE), 5
Spinal osteosarcoma, 445
Spindle cell carcinoma, 214
Spoiled gradient recalled echo (SPGR), 8

Squamous cell carcinoma, (SCCa), 174–175, 205, 228, 508
  from external auditory canal, 285f
  of parotid space, 283–284
  of submandibular and sublingual spaces, 292
Squamous cell carcinoma variants, 252–254
Squamous part, 454
Stapedial artery, 477
Stapedius muscles, 460
Staphylococcus aureus, 274, 434
Staphyloma, 59, 61f
Steady-state free precession (SSFP), 7, 8
"Strawberry nevi", 58
"Strawberry" hemangiomas. See Superficial hemangiomas
Streptococcus pneumonia, 274, 482
Streptococcus pyogenes, 274, 289
Streptococcus viridans, 274, 289
Sturge-Weber syndrome, 62, 63, 347, 353
Styloid process, 455
Subacute endophthalmitis, 68
Subaxial subluxation, 431
Subclavian artery, 328f
Subglottic carcinoma, 207, 208f, 210
Subglottic pressure gradient, 197
Sublingual glands, 271
Sublingual space (SLS), 284–292
Submandibular and sublingual spaces, 284
  anatomy, 284–285
  benign tumors of, 290–291
  congenital anomalies of, 285–287
  inflammatory lesions of, 287–290
  malignant tumors of, 291–292
Submandibular adenoid cystic carcinoma, 292f
Submandibular gland, 271
Submandibular gland tumor, 291
Subperiosteal abscess, 28, 31f, 482
Subperiosteal hematoma, 78–79
Superficial cervical fascia (SCF), 271
Superficial hemangiomas, 339, 340
Superior orbital fissure syndrome, 382t
Superior spread, of NPC, 234–235
Superior thyroid artery, 269
Superior thyroid vein, 269
Supernumerary nostril, 113
Superparamagnetic iron oxide particles (SPIO), 2, 3–4
Suppurative sialadenitis, acute, 274
Suppurative thyroiditis. See Acute infectious thyroiditis
Suprabullar and retrobullar recesses, 93
Supraglottic abscess, 218f
Supraglottic carcinoma, 205, 210
Supraglottic laryngectomy, 221
Suprahyoid epiglottic tumors, 205
Surgical banding, 83–84, 83f
Surgical excision, 349
Syngnathia, 116–118
Synkinesia, 375
Synovial cysts, 442

Synovial sarcoma, 309
Syphilis, 367, 371t
Syringobulbia, 426
Syringohydromyelia, 426

T

T1 fast field echo (T1-FFE), 8
T1-weighted imaging
  coherent (unspoiled) gradient echo, 7–8
  diffusion-weighted imaging (DWI), 8
  echo planar imaging (EPI), 8
  fast spin echo (FSE), 5
  FSE image, 5
  gradient echo sequences, 7
  gradient recalled and spin echo (GRASE), 8
  incoherent (spoiled) gradient echo, 8
  inversion recovery (IR), 7
  spin echo (SE), 5
    differences from, 5
  steady-state free precession (SSFP), 8
  turbo spin echo, 5
T3 supraglottic carcinoma, 209f
Tapia syndrome, 408t
Teflon vocal cord injection, 221f
Temporal bone
  dysplasias, 508
    fibrous dysplasia, 512–514, 513f
  embryology and congenital anomalies, 462
    congenital syndromes, 476–477
    direct subarachnoid space, 475
    normal variations, 463
    outer ear, anomalies of, 463–465
    perilymphatic fistulas, 476
    petrous bone, 473–474
    translabyrinthine fistulas, 474–475, 475f
    wide cochlear aqueduct, 475–476
  external ear
    external auditory canal and pinna, 455
    sensory innervation, 456
    vessels, 456
  infections
    acute otitis media, 481–482
    acute otomastoiditis, 482–483, 483f
    brain abscess, 485
    chronic otitis media, 482
    chronic otomastoiditis, 485–486, 487f, 488f, 489f
    dural sinus thrombosis, 484, 484f
    labyrinthitis, 492–493, 493f
    malignant external otitis (MEO), 492
    petrous apex infections, 486–487, 489f
    petrous apicitis, 483–484
    postoperative middle ear and mastoid, 490–491
  inner ear
    anomalies of, 466–473, 467t–468t, 470f, 472f, 473f, 474t
    bony labyrinth, 460–461
    membranous labyrinth, 461–462
  mastoid part, 454

Temporal bone (*Continued*)
  middle ear
    anomalies of, 465–466
      tympanic cavity, 456–460, 457f
      tympanic membrane, 456
  osteogenesis imperfecta, 514
  osteopetrosis, 514–516
  otosclerosis, 508–512
  Paget's disease, 516–518
  petrous part, 454–455
  progressive diaphyseal dysplasia, 518, 519f
  squamous part, 454
  styloid process, 455
  trauma, 518
    brain herniation , 520–521
    complex and comminuted fractures injuries to ossicles, 520
    longitudinal and transverse fractures, 519–520
  tumors and mimics
    cerebellopontine angle masses, 494–498, 494f, 495f
    external auditory canal masses, 508
    facial nerve masses, 505–508
    glomus tympanicum paraganglioma (GTP), 498–500
    inner ear masses, 503–505, 504f, 505f
    jugular foramen tumors, 498–500
    middle ear masses, 505
    petrous apex masses, 500–503, 501f
  tympanic part, 455
  vascular anomalies
    internal carotid artery anomalies, 477–479, 479f
    jugular vein anomalies, 479–481
    magnetic resonance imaging of, 481
Temporomandibular joint (TMJ), 116, 150, 465
Tenon's capsule, 19
Tensor tympani, 460
Teratoid cysts, 290–291
Teratoma, 37–39, 39t
Tertiary anophthalmia, 22
"Third occipital condyle", 425
3D imaging, 2
3D-TOF techniques, 9
Thymus and inferior parathyroid glands, 268–269, 270
Thyroglossal duct cyst, 261, 286f, 326, 326f
  of pediatric neck, 325–236
  of submandibular and sublingual spaces, 285
Thyroid adenoma, 319
Thyroid gland, 268, 269–270
  anatomy of, 316
  benign lesions of, 319–320
  inflammatory and metabolic lesions of, 316–319
  malignant lesions of, 320–323
  MR imaging of, 316
Thyroid gland, 269

Thyroid gland colloid cysts, 319f
Thyroid medullary carcinoma, 324f
Thyroid ophthalmopathy, 14f
Thyroid papillary carcinoma, 321f
Thyroiditis, 316
Tic douloureux. *See* Trigeminal neuralgia
Time of flight (TOF), 9
Tolosa-Hunt syndrome, 41–42, 385
Tongue
  CT Protocol, 232t
  MRI Protocol, 233t
Tongue base carcinoma, 240–241, 242f, 243f
Tongue swelling, 264
Tongue-tie. *See* Ankyloglossia
Tonsil carcinoma, 239f, 240f
Tonsillar fossa, 227
Tonsillar fossa carcinoma, 238–240
Tonsillar herniation, 425
Tonsillitis, 311f
  and peritonsillar abscess, 262, 262f
Tophaceous gout, 434
Tornwaldt's cyst, 259–260
Total and partial ossicular reconstructive prosthesis (TORP), 490–491
Total laryngectomy, 221
Toxocariasis, 68
"Tram-track" sign.
Transalar cephalocele, 105f
Transethmoidal cephaloceles, 99
Transglottic carcinoma, 207
Translabyrinthine fistulas, 474–475, 475f
Transoral laser microsurgery, 212
Trans-sphenoidal cephaloceles, 101
  in adult, 104f
  in infant, 104f
Transverse facial cleft, 108
Trauma, 217–218, 383
  of brachial plexus, 330
Traumatic carotid artery dissection, 301f
Traumatic carotid artery pseudoaneurysm, 300f
Traumatic hemorrhages, 519
Traumatic optic neuropathy (TON), 78
Treacher Collins syndrome, 115, 356
Treponema pallidum, 367
Trigeminal nerve branches, 388f
Trigeminal neuralgia, 390, 392t
Trigeminal root anatomy, 392f
Trigeminal vascular conflict, 392f
Trilateral retinoblastoma, 66
Triple combination chemotherapy, 42
Trisomy 13, 121
Trisomy 18, 121–122
Trisomy 21, 427
Tuberculosis, 21–219
Tuberculous abscess, 438
Tuberous sclerosis, 65
Tullio's phenomenon, 469
Tumor staging
  of lip, 254t
  oral cavity, 254t

Tumors and mass lesions, of brachial plexus, 330–332
Turbo spin echo, 5
Turner's syndrome, 345
Tympanic cavity, 456–460, 457f
Tympanic membrane, 456
Tympanic part, 455
Tympanic ring aplasia, 465–466
Tympanic ring dysplasia, 465
Tympanogenic labyrinthitis, 492
Tympanoplasty, 490

U

Ultrasmall superparamagnetic iron oxide particles (USPIO), 2, 3, 4
Ultrasonography, 233
Uncinate process, 91
Uncinate process variants, 91–93, 92t
Undifferentiated nasopharyngeal carcinoma, 236f
Unilateral cleft nose, 108
Uveal melanoma, 64
Uveal melanoma, 64, 65f
Uveoparotid fever, 68

V

Vagal paraganglioma, 302–303
van Buchem's disease, 518
van der Woude syndrome, 117, 118, 121
Varicella zoster, 371t
Varicella zoster virus (VZV), 367, 370
Vascular anomalies and vascular tumors, 339, 340f
  hemangiomas, 339–343, 341f, 341t, 342f, 342t, 343f, 344f, 345f
  vascular malformations, 339, 343–354
    arteriovenous malformations (AVM), 350–353
    capillary malformations, 347
    combined malformations, 353–354
    lymphatic malformations, 344–347
    venous malformations, 347–350
Vascular anomalies, of retropharyngeal space, 306–307
Vascular conflict, 394f
  at internal auditory canal, 393f
Vascular conflict syndromes, 390, 392
Vascular lesions, of carotid space, 299–301
Vascular loop syndromes. *See* Vascular conflict syndromes
Vascular malformations, 339, 343–354
  arteriovenous malformations (AVM), 350–353
  capillary malformations, 347
  combined malformations, 353–354
  lymphatic malformations, 344–347, 346f
  venous malformations, 347–350
Vascularization, of cranial nerves, 357, 360t
Vasculitis, 371t
Vasoformative anomalies
  of masticator space, 293–294

of parotid space, 272
of retropharyngeal space, 306
Vasoformative malformations
   of submandibular and sublingual spaces, 285, 287
      hemangioma, 285, 287
      lymphatic malformation, 287
Vasoformative malformations. *See* Vascular anomalies and vascular tumors
Vasoformative tumors, 217
Veno-lymphatic malformation, 59
Venolymphatic malformation, of masticator space, 353f
Venous engorgement, 426
Venous malformations, 347–350, 348f, 349f, 350f, 351f, 353
Vernet syndrome, 408t
Verrucous carcinoma, 252
Vertebral artery, 328f
Vertebrobasilar dolichoectasia, 447
Vertical hemilaryngectomy, 221, 223
Vestibular branch, of CN VIII, 390
Vestibular schwannoma, 399, 400f, 401f, 494
   differential diagnosis of, 400t
Vestibulocochlear nerve aplasia, 472
Villaret's syndrome, 408t
Viral sialadenitis, acute, 274
Visual disturbances, 13, 14t
Visual pathway, of optic nerve, 378f
Vitreoretinal traction, 62
Vocal cord paralysis, 219, 220f
von Hippel-Lindau disease (VHLD), 65, 503

W

Wackenheim clivus baseline, 420f, 421
Waldeyer's Ring Lymphoma, 255f
Warthin's tumor, 277–278, 278f, 279f
Weber syndrome, 382t
Wegener granulomatosis, 159, 373–374
Welcher basal angle, 420f
Whitnall-Norman syndrome. *See* Norrie disease
Wide cochlear aqueduct, 475–476
Wyburn-Mason syndrome, 347

X

Xanthoma, 170

Z

Zonular fibers, 81
Zygomaticomaxillary complex fractures, 144–146
Zygomaticomaxillary complex tripod fracture, 146f
Zygomycetes, 157